Managing Health Services Organizations and Systems

Fourth Edition

Managing Health Services Organizations and Systems

Fourth Edition

Beaufort B. Longest, Jr., Ph.D., FACHE
University of Pittsburgh

Jonathon S. Rakich, Ph.D.
Indiana University Southeast

Kurt Darr, J.D., Sc.D., FACHE
The George Washington University

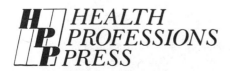
HEALTH
PROFESSIONS
PRESS

Baltimore • London • Winnipeg • Sydney

Health Professions Press, Inc.
Post Office Box 10624
Baltimore, Maryland 21285-0624

www.healthpropress.com

Typesetting by Barton Matheson Willse & Worthington, Baltimore, Maryland.
Printed in the United States of America by Hamilton Printing Company, Rensselaer, New York.

Because website addresses change frequently, some of the addresses provided in this volume may not be valid. If you get a 404 message, try an Internet search engine or directory to search for the organization by name.

Second printing, December 2001.
Third printing, May 2003.
Fourth printing, September 2004.

Library of Congress Cataloging-in-Publication Data
Longest, Beaufort B.
    Managing health services organizations and systems / Beaufort B. Longest, Jr., Jonathon S. Rakich, Kurt Darr—4th ed.
        p. cm.
    Includes bibliographical references and indexes.
    ISBN 1-878812-57-2
    1. Health facilities—Administration. I. Rakich, Jonathon S. II. Darr, Kurt. III. Title.

RA971.R26 2000
362.1′068—dc21   00-021493

British Cataloguing in Publication Data are available from the British Library.

Contents

About the Authors

Beaufort B. Longest, Jr., Ph.D., FACHE, M. Allen Pond Professor of Health Policy & Management, Professor and Director, Health Policy Institute, Graduate School of Public Health, University of Pittsburgh, Pittsburgh, Pennsylvania 15261

Beaufort B. Longest, Jr., is the M. Allen Pond Professor of Health Policy & Management, as well as Professor of Health Policy and Management in the Department of Health Services Administration, Graduate School of Public Health, at the University of Pittsburgh. He holds a secondary appointment as Professor of Business Administration in the University of Pittsburgh's Katz Graduate School of Business. He also is Director of the University of Pittsburgh's Health Policy Institute.

Professor Longest received his undergraduate education at Davidson College and the Master of Health Administration and Doctor of Philosophy degrees from Georgia State University. He is a Fellow of the American College of Healthcare Executives and a member of the Academy of Management, Beta Gamma Sigma Honor Society in Business, and Delta Omega Honor Society in Public Health.

His research on issues of health policy and management has generated substantial grant support and has led to the publication of numerous peer-reviewed articles. In addition, he has authored or coauthored 8 books and 16 chapters. His book *Health Policymaking in the United States, Second Edition*, is one of the most widely used textbooks in health policy programs.

Longest consults with health care organizations and systems, universities, associations, and government agencies on health policy and management.

Jonathon S. Rakich, Ph.D., Professor of Management, School of Business, Indiana University Southeast, New Albany, Indiana 47150

Jonathon S. Rakich received his Master of Business Administration from the University of Michigan–Ann Arbor and his Ph.D. from Saint Louis University. His university instructional areas are strategic management and health services administration. During his 33-year teaching career, Rakich has written or coauthored 3 books in 11 editions, 40 journal articles (including those in *Health Care Financing Review, Health Care Management Review, Hospital & Health Services Administration, Journal of Health and Social Policy*, and *Hospital Topics*), and more than 35 conference proceedings and professional papers.

Professor Rakich has been awarded a postdoctoral Federal Faculty Fellowship with the U.S. Department of Health and Human Services and has served on the board of trustees of a home health agency and health systems agency. While on sabbatical in 1979, he served an administrative residency at Summa Health System. During a 1989 sabbatical, he conducted onsite research of the Canadian health care system.

Rakich is a member of the Academy of Management, the Association for Health Services Research, and the Decision Sciences Institute. He holds personal membership in the Association of University Programs in Health Administration and is a faculty affiliate of the American College of Healthcare Executives.

Professor Rakich is Distinguished Professor Emeritus of Management and Health Services Administration at the University of Akron, where he taught from 1972 to 1999. During that period he held administrative positions as Director of Graduate Programs in Business, Director of Executive Development Programs, and coordinator of the MBA-Health Services Administration option program.

Kurt Darr, J.D., Sc.D., FACHE, Professor, Department of Health Services Management and Policy, School of Public Health and Health Services, The George Washington University Medical Center, Washington, DC 20037

Kurt Darr is Professor of Hospital Administration in the Department of Health Services Management and Policy and Professor of Health Care Sciences at The George Washington University. He holds a Doctor of Science from The Johns Hopkins University and a Master of Hospital Administration and a Juris Doctor from the University of Minnesota.

Professor Darr completed his administrative residency at Rochester (Minnesota) Methodist Hospital and subsequently worked as an administrative associate at the Mayo Clinic. After being commissioned in the U.S. Navy, he served in administrative and educational assignments at St. Albans Naval Hospital and Bethesda Naval Hospital. He completed postdoctoral fellowships with the Department of Health and Human Services, the World Health Organization, and the Accrediting Commission on Education for Health Services Administration.

Professor Darr is a Fellow of the American College of Healthcare Executives, is a member of the District of Columbia and Minnesota Bars, serves as an arbitrator and mediator for the National Health Lawyers Association, and is a mediator for the Superior Court of the District of Columbia.

He regularly presents seminars on health services ethics, hospital organization and management, quality improvement, and the application of the Deming method in health services. Darr is the author and editor of numerous books used in graduate health services administration programs and numerous articles on health services topics.

Preface

Leading the way, some health services organizations and systems are setting the benchmarks and establishing the best practice standards for the 21st century. They are simultaneously satisfying their customers, improving the quality of care they provide, and meeting cost objectives. The benchmarks of excellence in health services delivery are being established in organizations and systems that share one common characteristic: They have excellent managers as well as excellent clinicians.

Our purpose in this fourth edition, as in the previous editions, is to present information and insight that can help set the benchmarks of excellence in the management of health services. We want the book to be useful to two groups. Primarily, we want it to assist students as they prepare for health services management careers through programs of formal study. Also, we continue to hope that current health services managers, as part of their ongoing programs of professional development, will find the book a useful supplement to their experience and a new source of knowledge of applied management theory. We hope that both students and current managers will find the book a useful addition to their reference libraries.

Readers who are familiar with previous editions will note a change in the title, which reflects an important shift in the health services industry by adding "systems." This change reflects the extensive attention given in this edition to managing health systems (HSs), as well as the continuation of attention to managing health services organizations (HSOs). Hospitals and long-term care organizations continue to be prominent HSOs; as such, they receive a great deal of attention. Managed care organizations, ambulatory care organizations, home health agencies, and hospice, among other HSOs, also are covered. Whether HSOs operate as independent entities or align themselves into a variety of forms of HSs, all face dynamic environments—a mosaic of external forces that includes new rules, regulations, and technologies; changing demographic patterns; increased competition; public scrutiny; heightened consumer expectations; greater demands for accountability; and more constraints on resources. In this context, managerial excellence helps establish the benchmarks.

Pedagogically, our objective is to present management theory in a way that demonstrates its widespread applicability to all types of HSOs/HSs. This objective is accomplished by using a process orientation that focuses on how managers manage. We examine management functions, concepts, and principles as well as managerial roles, skills, and competencies within the context of HSOs/HSs and their external environment. For nascent managers, we introduce new terminology and concepts to provide a foundation for lifelong learning and professional development. For experienced managers, we seek to reinforce existing skills and experience while providing and applying new theory, as well as traditional theory and concepts in new ways.

The book's structure and content are described more fully at the end of Chapter 1. Briefly, it is divided into three parts covering management and how it occurs in the health services environment, managerial tools and techniques useful in this environment, and managing relationships. Each chapter includes discussion questions and a number of cases to stimulate discussion about the chapter's content.

In *Part I, Managing in the Health Services Environment*, the six chapters cover a comprehensive model of managing in HSOs/HSs, an extensive description of the health care system, the organizational designs of HSOs and HSs, and the increasingly important role that technology plays in contemporary health services.

Part II, Managerial Tools and Techniques, contains six chapters devoted to methods for managing effectively in the HSO/HS environment. These chapters address how managers solve problems and make decisions; their conduct of strategic planning and marketing; the roles played by quality and productivity in establishing and maintaining competitive position and how managers can effectively nurture a continuous quality improvement (CQI) philosophy; controlling and allo-cating resources; human resources and labor relations; and managing change.

Part III, Managing Relationships, is composed of five chapters that address how managers seek to manage the complex human relationships that exist within HSOs/HSs and among HSOs/HSs and external stakeholders. These chapters provide background in ethics and law for managers, as well as the roles played by leadership, motivation, and communication in managing the myriad relationships in which effective HSO/HS managers must engage.

In sum, these seventeen chapters form an integrated whole about how managers manage in HSOs/HSs. We hope the book will be useful to readers who aspire to establish the new benchmarks of excellence in this extraordinarily complex and important process.

Acknowledgments

Professor Longest thanks Carolyn, whose presence in his life continues to make many things possible and doing them seem worthwhile. He extends appreciation to Herbert S. Rosenkranz, Ph.D., Interim Dean of the Graduate School of Public Health, and to Arthur S. Levine, M.D., Senior Vice Chancellor for Health Sciences at the University of Pittsburgh, for encouraging and facilitating a work environment that is conducive to creative and scholarly endeavors by faculty members. He thanks Denise Thrower for help with many details. Special appreciation is extended to Linda Kalcevic for her tireless and professional efforts in editing the manuscript.

Professor Rakich especially thanks his wife, Tana, for her encouragement, support, and patience during the multiple years it took to revise this book; it would not have been possible without her understanding. Special appreciation is given to his employers for their assistance in numerous ways: Stephen Hallam, Dean of the College of Business Administration at The University of Akron, and since July 1999, Uric Dufrene, Dean of the School of Business at Indiana University Southeast. Special recognition is given to his graduate assistants, Yin Chan and Ryan Ledbetter, both of whom provided immeasurable research support.

Professor Darr is grateful to Anne for her unstinting support and for never once asking, "Isn't it done yet?" A book of this magnitude—even a revision—cannot be researched and written without the help of others. Special thanks are owed the long-suffering assistants who worked diligently, usually without complaint and often under severe time constraints, to bring this fourth edition to fruition. Dina Awad, Melissa Gozdieski, Tracy Hernandez, and Cynthia Mahood were indispensable helpmates. It was delightful to work with them and he wishes them every success in the world of health services management.

The authors wish to thank several people at Health Professions Press for their assistance with this book. Mary Magnus, Director of Publications; Meghan Moore, Marketing Manager; and Megan Westerfeld, copyeditor, each in her own way made important contributions. We are especially grateful to Anita McCabe, Editorial & Production Director, for her untiring efforts to make the book as good as it could be. She saw us through the project with good cheer and much assistance.

We also thank the publishers and authors who granted permission to reprint material to which they hold the copyright. Last, but certainly not least, we are grateful to the many users of previous editions of this book, whose comments and critiques aided us in improving the fourth edition.

Managing
in the
Health Services Environment

1 Management and Managers

The leading health care organizations are demonstrating how to satisfy customers, improve quality of care, and meet cost goals simultaneously. These organizations are setting the benchmarks and best practices for the 21st century[1]

The work of managers is one of three distinct but interrelated types of work performed in organizations and systems,[2] including in health services organizations (HSOs) and health systems (HSs). Direct work in these settings entails performance of some combination of patient care, research, education, and the production of products or services. A second type of work done in HSOs/HSs, support work, is a necessary and facilitative adjunct to the direct work. In these settings, people doing support work are involved in such activities as fund-raising and development, provision of legal counsel, marketing, public relations, finance, or human resources, for example. The third type of work done in HSOs/HSs is management work. Management work involves establishing organizational objectives and creating an organizational environment in which the direct work, aided by support work, can lead to the accomplishment of the objectives.

The people who perform management work in HSOs/HSs—those who occupy positions of managerial authority—face unprecedented challenges. These challenges result from many forces: remarkable scientific and technological advances in medicine, new organizational forms and relationships through which to provide health services, and new policies and programs for financing the provision of these services, to name some of the most important. It is fair to say that managers in HSOs/HSs are accustomed to challenges. They have routinely faced high expectations by consumers and patients, by clinicians, and by those who pay for health care. They have long been scrutinized for the costs and quality of the services they provide. Demands for greater efficiency in the delivery of services and for effectiveness in service delivery are familiar to these managers.

As can be seen in this introductory chapter, there are several ways in which management work can be assessed and studied. The work of managers can be approached in terms of the functions managers perform, the skills they use in doing their work, the roles that managers play in performing

3

their work, and the competencies they need to do the work well. Each of these approaches is considered in this chapter and used to illustrate important aspects of management work throughout the book. Overall, however, the book focuses on the process of management, that is, on what managers actually do as they manage. Before discussing the approaches to the work of managers, some key definitions are necessary. Following these definitions, consideration is given to the vital relationships between management and the culture and philosophies of HSOs/HSs, and between management and the overall performance of HSOs/HSs. Using the content of these sections as background, the chapter concludes with the description of a comprehensive model of management in HSOs/HSs; this model forms the framework for the entire book.

KEY DEFINITIONS

The terms *health, health care, health services, health services organizations,* and *health systems* must be defined because they provide the book's context. *Managers* and *management* require definition because managers and their work are the focus of the book.

Health

There are many ways to think about the health of human beings. Health is conceptualized by different people in both negative and positive terms and both narrowly and broadly.[3] Negatively, health is viewed as the minimization, if not the absence, of some variable, as in the absence of infection or the shrinking of a tumor; at the extreme it is the absence of disease. Positively, health is viewed as a state in which some variable is maximized. For example, viewing health positively and broadly, the World Health Organization defines it as a state or condition of complete physical, mental, and social well-being, not merely the absence of disease.

The definition of health is important in managing in the health sector because the way that a society conceptualizes and defines health reflects its values and how far it will to go to maximize health. A society that defines health in negative terms and narrowly, for example, might intervene only in life-threatening traumas and illnesses. Conversely, if health is defined in positive terms and broadly, a society will pursue a variety of significant interventions to enhance the health of its members. Western societies have increasingly defined health in more positive and broader terms. A useful contemporary definition holds that health is *the maximization of the biological and clinical indicators of organ function and the maximization of physical, mental, and role functioning in everyday life.*[4]

The consequences of a society's defining health positively and broadly are substantial. In contrast to focusing on treatment of illness or injury to minimize an undesired variable, such a definition encourages society to seek proactive interventions aimed at many variables in the quest for health. The enormous range of targets for intervention in health care is made possible by the fact that health is determined by several synergistically related factors. Among these health determinants, none are more important than the physical, social, and economic environments in which people live.[5] In addition, health is strongly influenced by lifestyles and by heredity, as well as by the type, quality, and timing of health services that people receive.

Health Care and Health Services

Health care is *the total societal effort, undertaken in the private and public sectors, focused on pursuing health.* Within the larger domain of health care, health services are *specific activities undertaken to maintain or improve health or to prevent decrements of health.* These services can be preventive (e.g., blood pressure screening, mammography), acute (e.g., surgical procedures, antibiotics to fight an infection), chronic (e.g., control of diabetes or hypertension), restorative (e.g., physical rehabilitation of a stroke or trauma patient), or palliative (e.g., pain relief or comfort in terminal stages of disease) in nature.

In general, health services can be divided into two basic types. Public health services are activities that are conducted on a communitywide or populationwide basis, such as communicable disease control, the collection and analysis of health statistics, and air pollution control. Personal health services, in contrast, are activities directed at individuals and include promotion of health, prevention of illness, diagnosis, treatment (sometimes leading to a cure), and rehabilitation. Thus activities as diverse as the emergency room treatment of a child with acute asthma or the conduct of education programs about the practice of safe sex to prevent the spread of human immunodeficiency virus (HIV) are examples of health services.

Health Services Organizations

Health services are provided through a variety of organizational arrangements. HSOs are *entities that provide the organizational structure within which the delivery of health services is made directly to consumers, whether the purpose of the services is preventive, acute, chronic, restorative, or palliative.* Historically, HSOs were predominantly independent, freestanding organizations. In a movement beginning in the 1970s and gaining momentum through the 1980s and 1990s, however, many HSOs have joined together to form systems of organizations.

One way to envision the diversity of HSOs is to consider a continuum of clinical health services that people might use during the course of their lives and to think of the organizational settings that provide them. Prebirth, the continuum could begin with HSOs that minimize negative environmental impact on human fetuses or that provide genetic counseling, family planning services, prenatal counseling, prenatal ambulatory care services, and birthing services. This would be followed early in life by pediatric ambulatory services; pediatric inpatient hospital services, including neonatal intensive care units (NICUs) and pediatric intensive care units (PICUs); and both ambulatory and inpatient psychiatric services for children.

For adults, the most relevant HSOs are those providing adult ambulatory services, including ambulatory surgery centers and emergency and trauma services; adult inpatient hospital services, including routine medical, surgical, and obstetrical services, as well as specialized cardiac care units (CCUs), medical intensive care units (MICUs), surgical intensive care units (SICUs), and monitored units; stand-alone cancer units, with radiotherapy capability and short-stay recovery beds; ambulatory and inpatient rehabilitation services, including specific subprograms for orthopedic, neurological, cardiac, arthritis, speech, otological, and other services; ambulatory and inpatient psychiatric services, including specific subprograms for people with psychosis, day programs, counseling services, and detoxification; and home health care services.

In their later years, people might add to the list of relevant HSOs those providing skilled and intermediate nursing services; adult day services; respite services for caregivers of homebound patients, including services such as meal provision, visiting nurses and home health aides, electronic emergency call capability, cleaning, and simple home maintenance; and hospice care and associated family services, including bereavement, legal, and financial counseling.

Health Systems

The continuum of health services outlined previously has been provided traditionally by autonomous or independent HSOs, often in an uncoordinated and disjointed manner. However, many HSOs have significantly changed how they relate to one another. Mergers, consolidations, acquisitions, and affiliations between and among previously independent HSOs are pervasive. At the extreme end of this activity is vertical integration, in which HSOs join into unified organizational arrangements or systems of organizations.[6] This phenomenon of integration is likely to continue into the foreseeable future.[7] In fact, among the most important contemporary developments in the infrastructure of health care is the integration of HSOs into HSs. HSs are *formally linked HSOs, possibly including financing arrangements, joined together to provide more coordinated and comprehensive health services.*

The development of vertically integrated HSs capable of providing a largely "seamless" continuum of health services, including primary, acute, rehabilitation, long-term, and hospice care, increasingly characterizes the organizational context of health care. Many HSOs participate in a variety of forms of organizational integration, a phenomenon that began in the 1970s and is intensifying (see Figure 1.1).

The most extensively integrated situations arise in the formation of integrated delivery systems, or IDSs (synonymous with organized delivery systems or integrated delivery networks). Whatever the name, these highly integrated systems or networks of HSOs are distinguished by the fact that each "provides or arranges to provide a coordinated continuum of services to a defined population and is willing to be held clinically and fiscally accountable for the outcomes and the health status of the population served."[8]

Of course, not all HSOs are part of HSs. Furthermore, a number of people question the rationale for vertical integration among HSOs and its potential growth.[9] As has been pointed out, if integration among HSOs is to achieve its promise,

> there would first have to be a major restructuring of both markets and systems (which, admittedly, is already under way), a removal of barriers that have historically separated providers at the local level, and a significant investment in the components of system building (e.g., integrated information systems) that are essential for ensuring the coordination of care across the full spectrum of healthcare providers and services. And if integrated systems are to achieve the mythical end stage in system evolution—reaching out to communities to serve the needs of defined populations—they will need to evolve competencies heretofore untested and undemonstrated in establishing delivery system modalities. All of this is a very tall order, indeed.[10]

Although the question of how far HSOs will integrate remains unanswered, it is a reality that more integration will characterize health services in the future. The implications of HSOs integrating into HSs are considered throughout this book. Whether autonomous or integrated, however, all HSOs and HSs must be managed. Thus definitions of managers and of management are important; they form the substance and focus of this book.

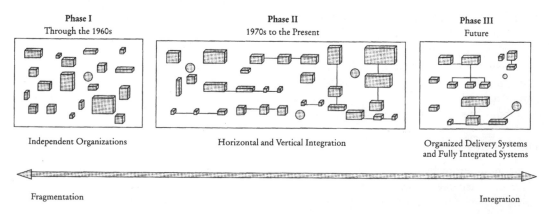

Figure 1.1.   The changing structure of health services organizations and systems. (Adapted from Longest, Beaufort B., Jr. *Health Policymaking in the United States,* 2nd ed., 22. Chicago: Health Administration Press, 1998; reprinted by permission.)

Managers

HSO/HS managers are *people formally appointed to positions of authority in organizations or systems who enable others to do their direct or support work effectively, who have responsibility for resource utilization, and who are accountable for work results.* In HSOs/HSs this broad definition includes people with titles such as nurse team manager; maintenance director; dietary, surgery, or medical records director or supervisor; director of pharmacy, laboratory, outpatient clinic, social services, or business office; medical director; or president or vice president. The variety of managers in HSOs/HSs can be identified, in part, by the level of the organization at which they work.

Classification schemes typically identify managers as top or senior management, middle-level management, and supervisory or first-level management. Sometimes the classifications are policy level, administrative or coordinative level, and operations level.[11] Griffith distinguishes between decision-oriented and implementation-oriented managers. The former typically are positioned higher in the HSO/HS and help it establish its objectives and address its most sensitive and difficult decisions: "weighing the importance and permanence of environmental changes, recommending budget guidelines, and resolving serious disputes."[12] Implementation-oriented managers focus more on getting things done, often through direct supervision of others or through leading teams. Regardless of title, level, or orientation, managers have several common attributes: 1) they are formally appointed to positions of authority, 2) they are charged with directing and enabling others to do their work effectively, 3) they are responsible for utilizing resources, and 4) they are accountable to superiors for results.

The primary differences between levels of managers are the degree of authority and the scope of responsibility at each level. For example, senior managers, presidents, or chief executive officers (CEOs) and vice presidents in HSOs have authority over and are responsible for entire organizations—all staff, resources, and individual and organizational results. CEOs are accountable to the governing body. Increasingly, with the rapid movement to more integration, some senior managers are responsible for systems (HSs) with many organizations (HSOs).

Reporting to senior managers are numerous middle-level managers, each of whom is responsible for smaller segments of the organization. Middle-level managers, such as department heads and heads of services, have authority over and are responsible for a specific segment, in contrast to the organization or system as a whole. Finally, first-level managers, who generally report to middle-level managers, have authority over and are responsible for overseeing specific work and a particular group of workers.

> *Senior-, middle-, and first-level managers are responsible for very different types of activities. But all of these activities are important and no organization can be successful unless the management work at each level is done well and unless the work at each level is carefully integrated with that done at the other levels.*[13]

Management

No matter what their level, all managers in HSOs/HSs perform management work. That is, they engage in the process of management. Management is defined as *the process, composed of interrelated social and technical functions and activities, occurring in a formal organizational setting for the purpose of accomplishing predetermined objectives through the use of human and other resources.* Management at all levels has four main elements:

- It is a process—a set of interactive and interrelated ongoing functions and activities.
- It involves accomplishing organizational objectives.
- It involves achieving these objectives through people and the use of other resources.

- It occurs in a formal organizational setting, whether a single, independent organization or a system of organizations; organizations invariably exist in the context of larger external environments.

By definition, managers in HSOs/HSs focus on establishing and achieving organizational objectives. The scope of managerial work includes providing the organizational context within which direct and support work can be performed effectively. Managerial work also includes preparing an organization or system to deal with both the threats and opportunities in its external environment. Managers influence all work in HSOs/HSs because they influence premises of decisions about work and conditions under which it is done. In effect, managers help shape the culture and philosophy of the organizations or systems that they manage in important ways; more than anyone, they determine the overall performance that is achieved by their organizations or systems.

MANAGEMENT AND ORGANIZATIONAL CULTURE, PHILOSOPHY, AND PERFORMANCE

This section discusses the vital relationships between management and the development and maintenance of appropriate organizational cultures and philosophies in HSOs/HSs and between management and organizational performance. Managers make unique contributions to the cultures, philosophies, and performance of HSOs/HSs, and these contributions justify their presence.

Management and Organizational Culture and Philosophy

All organizations have identifiable cultures; HSOs/HSs are no exception.[14] HSOs/HSs typically have cultures that are very different from business enterprises because they provide services that are unique in society and because they are humanitarian in nature. HSO/HS managers manage in the special context of the HSO's/HS's culture. This culture is the pattern of shared values and beliefs—along with associated behaviors, symbols, and rituals—that is acquired over time by members of the HSO/HS.[15] It is the historically developed sense of the institution's "legacy"—what it is and what it stands for—that permeates the entire organization or system and is known to all who work in it.[16] Examples of important values are duty, respect, trust, integrity, honesty, equity, and fairness.[17] Examples of shared beliefs are the commitment to patients and to meeting their needs and respecting them as individuals, with the unshakable belief that they are the primary reason for the HSO's/HS's existence. These values and beliefs shape organizational objectives and prescribe acceptable behavior for members—managers and employees—as well as acceptable relationships between the HSO/HS and its external stakeholders. By adhering to these values and beliefs, HSOs/HSs retain their unique character and the privileges that society has accorded them.[18]

An organization's philosophy is its explicit and implied view of itself and what it is. Generally expressed in its mission statement, the philosophy is directly linked to and rooted in the organization's cultural values and beliefs.[19] An organization's philosophy and culture must be compatible, and each must reflect the other. One important aspect of a HSO's/HS's philosophy is that it depicts the desired nature of relationships between it and its stakeholders.

Managers, especially senior managers, are important in establishing and maintaining the HSO's/HS's culture. They "have a critical role as the conscience of the enterprise like it or not, for good or ill."[20] As Zuckerman observed,

> the CEO must lead the organization in adapting to the external environment and in managing the internal organization. The CEO also plays an overarching role, however, in providing strategic direction and vision to the organization, serving as the keeper of the corporate values, and assuring that the organization achieves its mission.[21]

The conduct of managers conveys to internal and external stakeholders the HSO's/HS's values and beliefs (its culture) and its philosophy about itself. Culture and philosophy are expressed through approaches to customer service, attitudes about staff, and attitudes about stakeholder relations in general.[22] A philosophy that reflects commitment to customer service and quality patient care—a philosophy prevalent in HSOs/HSs and rooted in their values—is continuous quality improvement (CQI). Based on the tenets of Philip B. Crosby, W. Edwards Deming, and Joseph M. Juran,[23] CQI focuses on improving processes in the organization. Improved processes lead to higher levels of quality in outcomes and to more patient satisfaction.[24]

An organization's philosophy about staff is also rooted in its values. A HSO's/HS's philosophy about its staff may include concepts such as respect for them as individuals, whether they are viewed as the principal component in accomplishing organizational objectives, the extent of their involvement and participation in decision making about work and work systems design, and the way in which management oversees their work.[25]

Stakeholders are individuals, groups, or organizations who are affected by the HSO/HS and who may seek to influence it.[26] A well-thought-out and implemented philosophy about stakeholders is prerequisite to strategic planning, resource allocation and utilization, customer service, and ability to cope with the external environment. A HSO's/HS's stakeholders can be classified into three groups.[27] Internal stakeholders operate entirely within the HSO/HS and typically include management and professional and nonprofessional staff members. Interface stakeholders function both internally and externally to the HSO/HS and include members of the professional staff organization (PSO), the governing body, and stockholders in the case of for-profit HSOs/HSs. External stakeholders include suppliers, patients, third-party payers, competitors, interest groups, local communities, labor organizations, and regulatory and accrediting agencies.

HSO/HS managers must determine which stakeholders are relevant, which represent potential threats, and which have the potential to cooperate.[28] Appropriate HSO/HS behavior toward stakeholders is based on these assessments, and ranges from ignoring to negotiating to co-opting and cooperating. Careful assessments also can indicate which of the conflicting priorities, needs, demands, and pressures presented by stakeholders should be addressed by the HSO/HS. Balancing the demands of multiple stakeholders with different interests is a major challenge, requiring managers to apply the HSO's/HS's philosophy. Balancing maintains ethical values and social responsibility and prevents inappropriate demands made by single-interest stakeholders from predominating.[29]

Management and Organizational Performance

HSOs/HSs are formed by conscious and formal efforts for the purpose of accomplishing certain objectives that participants in organizations or systems could not achieve as well acting as individuals. From this fact arises the central purpose of management work and of all managers: to help achieve high performance in relation to organizational objectives. The term *organizational effectiveness* means the degree to which organizational objectives are successfully met.[30] A higher-performing organization meets more of its objectives than a lower-performing organization. Managers, because they occupy positions that permit them to make unique contributions to organizational effectiveness, are judged by these contributions.

There is no universally accepted formula by which managers maximize their contributions to their organizations. However, the evidence of the contributions managers make to organizational performance is substantial. For example, studies conducted in a variety of HSOs/HSs have demonstrated that the way managers set standards,[31] coordinate and integrate various workgroups,[32] make decisions,[33] and design their organizations[34] affects organizational performance. Effective managers create work environments and conditions that are conducive to superior performance. The next section describes how the functions, skills, roles, and competencies that managers fulfill, use, play, and possess permit them to do this.

MANAGEMENT FUNCTIONS, SKILLS, ROLES, AND COMPETENCIES

As noted earlier, there are several different possible approaches to considering management work. In this section, the most important ones—functions, skills, roles, and competencies—are considered. Table 1.1 summarizes them. No one approach provides a comprehensive framework for considering management or the management work performed in HSOs/HSs. Each contributes something to understanding management; together, they provide a comprehensive framework. The functions that are fulfilled in the management process are considered first.

Management Functions

The set of social and technical functions inherent in the management process (see the definition of management presented earlier) includes planning, organizing, staffing, directing (motivating, leading, and communicating), and controlling. Decision making pervades each of these functions, and, although some authorities list it as a separate function, it is best viewed as integral to each of the management functions.

These management functions are the logical grouping of generic management activities. All HSO/HS managers perform these functions to some degree regardless of hierarchical level. Figure 1.2 illustrates the interdependence among the management functions. In considering management in terms of its functions, it is convenient to separate them so that each can be discussed independently. The danger is that the management process may be seen as a series of separate functions. This is not the case, nor are the functions performed sequentially. In practice, a manager performs these functions simultaneously and as part of an interdependent mosaic of functions, as shown in Figure 1.2. The separation of management functions is necessary for purposes of discussion, but it is an artificial treatment of the reality of managing.

The Planning Function

In essence, planning in HSOs/HSs means deciding prospectively what to do—charting a course of action for the future. Planning establishes and devises the means to achieve organizational objectives. Without planning, disjointed, even random activities will prevail. Planning is a necessary precursor to the other management functions. It lays the foundation for organizing; an organizational structure is designed to carry out plans. It dictates the objectives and activities toward which managers lead other members of the organization. Part of the planning function is establishing desired objectives and standards against which actual performance can be measured when managers carry out their controlling function.

There are a number of reasons that planning is crucial to the successful operation of HSOs/HSs. None is more important than that planning focuses attention on objectives. Good planning yields appropriate organizational objectives and develops the means through which they can be met. In this way planning contributes to integrating the actions of organizational participants toward common ends.

TABLE 1.1. APPROACHES TO CONSIDERING MANAGEMENT WORK

Functions	Skills	Roles	Competencies
Planning	Technical	Interpersonal	Conceptual
Organizing	Human	Informational	Technical managerial/clinical
Staffing	Conceptual	Decisional	Interpersonal/collaborative
Directing		—	Political
(motivating, leading, and communicating)		Designer	Commercial
Controlling		Strategist	Governance
Decision making		Leader	

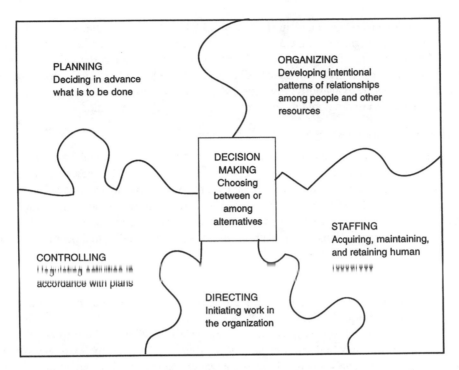

Figure 1.2.   The management functions are interrelated like the pieces of a puzzle.

Another reason that planning is important is because it helps offset the pervasive uncertainty that HSOs/HSs face. For the typical HSO or HS, the only certainty about the future is uncertainty. However, when managers think systematically about the future and plan for contingencies, they greatly reduce the chances of being unprepared. The profound changes occurring in delivering and financing health services require that HSOs/HSs be adaptable and flexible; planning is critical for both.

A third reason that planning is important to contemporary HSOs/HSs is because it enhances efficiency and effectiveness. Health services are expensive, and, whereas many aspects of their cost are beyond the manager's control, others can be minimized through planning for efficient operation. Planning substitutes integrated effort for random activity, controlled flow of work for uneven flow, and thoughtful decisions for snap judgments. As the delivery of health services becomes more dependent on costly technologies and more and more centered in complex organizations and systems, the managerial function of planning in these settings becomes increasingly important to contain service costs.

Finally, planning in HSOs/HSs is important because it facilitates fulfillment of the management function of controlling. Controlling implies comparing actual results with predetermined desired results and correcting deviations when they occur. The planning function yields information that can be used to set standards against which actual results can be compared. As third parties, principally government and private employers, have assumed a greater share of the financial burden of health services, they have required significantly more accountability from service providers. This accountability goes beyond costs to include both the quality of care and the manner in which it is delivered. The trend toward more accountability and the concurrent necessity for control that it implies will become increasingly important in HSOs/HSs in the years ahead. The effect of planning on managers' efforts to control the activities for which they are responsible is one of the most important values in effective planning.

Planning is done by all managers in HSOs/HSs, although the work varies by level. Senior managers typically are concerned with the planning function activities of external environment assessment and of objective and strategy formulation for the organization or system. Objectives that are consistent with and support organizationwide objectives are set by middle-level and first-level managers for their areas of responsibility. Planning by these managers focuses on program and operations design, as well as on implementation procedures and work scheduling.

The Organizing Function

Objectives are established by planning, but managers must design an organization that is capable of achieving them if they are to become reality. If the objectives of HSOs/HSs are to be effectively pursued, their managers must develop intentional patterns of relationships among staff and other resources in the HSOs/HSs. The resulting structure is called the organization design, and the developmental efforts and activities are the organizing function of management.

The design of organizations begins with the establishment of individual positions, which typically are determined by how an organization's work has been divided and specialized. Conceptually, organization design proceeds from individual positions to clustering positions into workgroups such as departments and units, then further clustering of workgroups into larger subdivisions of the organization, and, eventually, clustering these into an entire organization and, in some cases, into systems or networks of organizations.

Successful designs in HSOs/HSs depend on appropriate distributions of responsibility and authority as the organization is built through successive rounds of clustering. Authority is the power that is derived from a person's position in an organization. Responsibility can be thought of as the obligation to execute work, whether it is direct, support, or management work. All staff in organizations have responsibilities as a result of their organizational positions. The source of responsibility is one's superior in the organization. By delegating responsibility to a subordinate, the superior creates a relationship based on obligation between superior and subordinate. When responsibility is delegated to staff in organizations, they also must be given the authority to make commitments, use resources, and take the actions necessary to fulfill their responsibilities.

In HSOs, which typically are departmentalized functionally and in which effective interactions among the departments are essential, integration and coordination among departments are important. In HSs integration and coordination among the components are essential to success. One must recognize the relationship between the degree to which an organization's work is divided and specialized and subsequent requirements for integration and coordination of the work. The more differentiation of work and specialization of workers, the more difficult the integration task. HSOs/HSs, especially large hospitals or multiunit systems, are among the most complex organizations in terms of differentiation of work and worker specialization. These organizations are characterized by detailed division of work into a number of different jobs. The work done in these organizations is so specialized and performed by such a variety of workers that very significant problems involving integration of work often arise. Furthermore, in HSOs/HSs the direct, support, and management work is highly interdependent. This condition of functional interdependence makes integration and coordination of work done in HSOs/HSs an important aspect of successfully carrying out the organizing function.

Successful HSO/HS organization designs include features that ensure a high level of integration of work. The essential challenge of effectively integrating the work in these organizations stems from the fact that individuals often perceive objectives differently and may also favor various methods of accomplishing them. Effectively integrating and coordinating work often means managing conflicts that may arise between and among the subparts of an organization, such as between the PSO and senior-level management or between the nursing service and the pharmacy or laboratory. There also may be conflicts involving pairs of individuals or conflicts between individuals and the organization. In situations involving multiple organizations in a system, conflicts can arise between and among organizations. Any one of these and other relationships has the potential for conflict. Not all conflict is bad, but even low levels of conflict, such as "disliking" and "difficulty in getting along with," reduce organizational effectiveness. Integration and coordination are managerial activities concerned with preventing conflicts and misunderstandings in the organization. Organization designs that facilitate integration are very important to the success that managers achieve in carrying out the organizing function.

The Staffing Function

Staffing, which involves acquiring, maintaining, and retaining human resources, is an important management function in itself. In addition, it is an important complement to the organizing function. Staffing is both technical and social. Technical aspects include human resources planning, job analysis, recruitment, testing, selection, performance evaluation, compensation and benefits administration, employee assistance, and safety and health. Social aspects are activities that influence the behavior and performance of organization members and include training and development, promotion, counseling, and discipline.

All managers engage in the staffing function, although many of its aspects are centralized in a human resources department that is responsible for human resources acquisition and retention, as well as labor relations and collective bargaining (see Chapter 11).

The Directing Function

Directing is social-behavioral in nature and focuses on initiating action in the organization or system. Effectively directing others in organizations depends on managers being able to lead, motivate, and communicate with those they direct. Leading others is important to successful directing at all levels of HSOs/HSs. First- and middle-level managers rely on their ability to lead those whom they directly manage.[35] HSOs/HSs also require leadership at the organization level. Leadership at this level reflects the ability to develop and instill in members of the HSO/HS a common vision and to direct adherence to that vision.

Leading effectively means managers must inspire and influence others to contribute to the attainment of organizational objectives. Leading requires interactions between managers and those they manage in a wide variety of organizational situations. A single pattern of leadership behavior will not fit the diversity of these situations. Thus the successful manager is not locked into a particular leadership style but chooses the method that is most appropriate in a given situation.

Success in the directing function is influenced by how effectively managers motivate others and by how well they communicate with them. Inducing people to follow directions is *caused* behavior. Thus skill at motivating people is crucial to effective directing. Similarly, managers who can effectively articulate and communicate their visions and preferences have a distinct advantage in having them followed and in providing guidance for the behaviors of their followers.

The Controlling Function

The controlling function of management involves gathering information about and monitoring activities and performance, comparing actual results with expected results, and, when appropriate, intervening to take corrective action. That is, controlling is the regulation of activities and performance in the HSO/HS in accordance with the requirements of plans. By definition, the controlling function is directly linked to the planning function because it involves measuring and correcting activities of people and things in an organization to ensure that objectives developed in the planning function are accomplished. Controlling is a function of managers at all levels, and its basic purpose is to ensure that what is intended is what is done. Senior managers focus on controlling overall results in their organization or system, such as quality of care, expenditures compared with revenues, and resource utilization. First-level managers focus on control in their areas of responsibility—for example, number of laboratory tests performed per employee per day, number of meals served, or time between dictation and transcription of medical records. The control function monitors outputs and inputs, but it also must monitor processes, or *how* work is done. CQI requires that all processes be systematically monitored, evaluated, and changed to improve quality and ensure that the needs of customers are met.

Control techniques are based on the same basic elements regardless of whether people, quality of services, money, or morale is being controlled. Control, wherever it is applied, involves four steps: establishing standards, measuring performance, comparing actual results with standards, and correcting deviations from standards.

The Pervasiveness of Decision Making

As noted earlier and as shown in Figure 1.2, decision making is intertwined with each of the functions of management. All managers are decision makers. HSO/HS managers make decisions when they monitor and control work; when they plan, establish, or change organizational arrangements and work process and content; when they acquire and assign personnel; and when they direct work activity. All managers make decisions, but their decisions vary in scope and nature, as well as in techniques used, depending on the manager's level in the organization or system. Senior managers make policy decisions that affect entire organizations or systems, and resource allocation decisions that affect the various parts of the organization; middle- and first-level managers make decisions about allocating and utilizing resources provided by senior management within their areas of authority and responsibility.

Management Skills

Consideration of the management functions of planning, organizing, staffing, directing, controlling, and decision making helps one understand what is done in management work. There is strong evidence from empirical studies that much of what managers do can be categorized into one or more of these functions.[36] However, identifying the management functions says very little about the skills needed to execute the functions properly. It has been suggested that consideration of the functions of management "is more a representation of the objectives of managerial work than it is a description of the work itself."[37] Thus another way to consider management work is to examine the set of skills that people must possess and use in doing this work well.

As shown in Table 1.1, effective managers utilize three distinct types of skills.[38] The technical skills of managers are their abilities to use the methods, processes, and techniques of managing. It is easy to visualize the technical skills of a surgeon or a physical therapist, but counseling a subordinate or developing a departmental budget also requires specific technical skills. Human or interpersonal skills are the abilities of managers to get along well with other people, to understand them, and to motivate and lead them in the workplace. Conceptual skills reflect the mental abilities of managers to visualize the complex interrelationships in a workplace—relationships among people, among departments or units of a HSO, among various organizations in a HS, and even between a HSO/HS and its external environment. Conceptual skills permit managers to understand how the various factors in particular situations fit together and interact with one another.

Not all managers use these skills to the same degree or in the same mix, although every manager must rely on all three types of skills in performing management work. For example, the management work that takes place in a hospital nursing service reflects different levels of management and requires different mixes of these technical, human, and conceptual skills. The vice president for nursing (a senior-level manager) is vitally concerned with how the nursing service fits into the hospital's operation. However, the vice president can rely on nursing service staff to accomplish the technical work. In contrast, a director of nursing (a middle-level manager), whose primary responsibility is to "troubleshoot" an entire nursing staff on one shift, may be constantly required to make decisions on the basis of technical knowledge of nursing while rarely having time to think about the relationship of the nursing service to other hospital departments. A nurse in charge of a nursing unit may use a considerable amount of technical skill because, in addition to being a manager, this individual also must practice nursing. This manager also may be required to use human relations skills on the job more than either the vice president or director of nursing because almost all of this person's work involves direct contact with other people.

The extent to which each management skill is used varies with the manager's position in the organizational hierarchy; degree of authority; scope of responsibility; and number, types, and skills of subordinates. Senior-level managers typically use disproportionately more conceptual skills in their jobs than do middle- or first-level managers. Conceptual demands include recognizing and evaluating multiple, complex issues and understanding their relationships; engaging in planning and problem solving that profoundly affect the HSO/HS; and thinking globally about the organization or system and its environment. In contrast, first-level managers tend to use job-related technical skills, or skills that involve specialized knowledge, more than do either middle-level or senior-level managers. Figure 1.3 shows the relationship of these skills, degree of authority, and scope of responsibility and activities for each management level.

Management Roles

All HSO/HS managers engage in the management functions of planning, organizing, staffing, directing, and controlling; all managers utilize some mix of technical, conceptual, and human relations skills; and all constantly engage in decision making. Yet these ways of thinking about management work do not capture all that managers do. For example, a hospital CEO or other senior-level manager may serve on an areawide mental health task force, a health maintenance organization (HMO) president may testify before a legislative body, the administrator of a nursing facility may serve on a state licensing board, the vice president of nursing at an academic medical

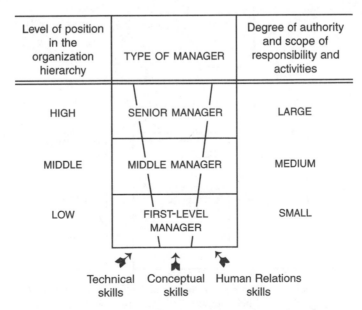

Figure 1.3. Skills used by different types of HSO/HS managers.

center may present a guest lecture in a nursing baccalaureate program, and a Department of Veterans Affairs official may provide testimony about the Veterans Administration (VA) Health System before Congress to justify budget increases. Such activities are not fully encompassed in traditional views of management functions or skills.

Interpersonal, Informational, and Decisional Roles

One of the most exhaustive studies of management work was conducted by Henry Mintzberg. He observed a sample of managers over a period of time, recording what they did. He concluded that management work can be described meaningfully in terms of roles that all managers play. Roles in HSOs/HSs are the typical or customary sets of behaviors that accompany particular organizational positions. Mintzberg compared the roles of managers to those of actors on a stage, and concluded that, just as actors play roles, managers, because they are managers, must adopt certain patterns of behavior when filling managerial positions. He viewed the work of managers as a series of three broad categories of roles—interpersonal, informational, and decisional—with each category comprising several distinct but interrelated roles.[39] Figure 1.4 summarizes them. Thus a third way to examine the work of managers is to consider the different roles that they play (see Table 1.1).

Interpersonal Roles

In Mintzberg's view, all managers are granted formal authority over the organizational units they manage, and this authority leads to their interpersonal roles as figurehead, leader, and liaison. The figurehead role is played by managers, especially by senior-level managers, when engaging in ceremonial and symbolic activities such as presiding over the opening of an addition to their organization's physical plant or giving a speech about health care to a local civic club. Managers play an influencer or leader role when they seek to motivate, inspire, and set examples through their own behavior. The liaison role allows managers in formal and informal contacts, both inside their

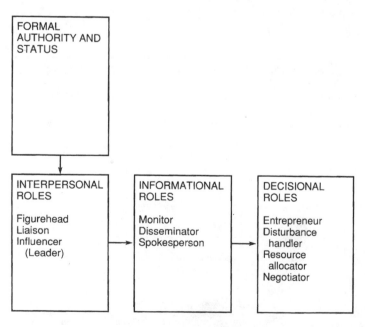

Figure 1.4.   The manager's roles. (Reprinted by permission of *Harvard Business Review* from Mintzberg, Henry. The manager's job: Folklore and fact. 53 [July–August 1975]. Copyright © 1975 by the President and Fellows of Harvard College; all rights reserved.)

HSO/HS and with external stakeholders, to establish relationships that will help them achieve organizational objectives. Playing interpersonal roles provides managers with opportunities to gather information. This fact, along with what the manager does with the information, permits a second set of roles.

Informational Roles

The informational roles of managers include monitor, disseminator, and spokesperson. As monitors, managers gather information from their networks of contacts, including those established in their liaison roles; filter the information; evaluate it; and decide whether to act as a result of the information. The disseminator role grows out of managers' access to information and ability to choose what to do with that information. In dissemination, managers have many choices about who, inside and outside their organizations or systems, should receive information. The third informational role, spokesperson, is related to their figurehead role and involves managers' communicating the positions of their HSOs/HSs to internal and external stakeholders who affect their areas of responsibility.

Decisional Roles

Managers' decisional roles include entrepreneur, disturbance handler, resource allocator, and negotiator. The authority granted by their organizations and supported by their interpersonal and informational roles permits managers to play decisional roles. As entrepreneurs, managers are initiators and designers of changes intended to improve performance in their organizational domains. When playing this role, managers act as change agents. In their disturbance handler role, managers decide how to handle a wide variety of problems or issues that arise as they carry out their daily work. Senior-level managers may face disturbances created by their professional staff, by a regulatory agency, or by the actions of a competitor. First-level managers may face a variety of disturbances ranging from a heavy snowfall that keeps key staff from their work, to conflict among subordinates, to budget cuts. The ability to make good decisions about handling disturbances is an important determinant of managerial success.

In their resource allocator role, managers must allocate human, physical, and technological resources among alternative uses. The decisions about resource allocation become more difficult, and more important, as resources are constrained. As negotiators, managers interact and bargain with employees, suppliers, regulators, customers and clients, and others. Negotiating includes deciding what objectives or outcomes to seek through negotiation and how to conduct the negotiations.

Integration of Managerial Roles

The 10 managerial roles shown in Figure 1.4 cannot be neatly separated. In practice, they are intertwined into what psychologists term a *gestalt,* or an integrated whole. Management work is much more than the algebraic sum of these 10 roles. When the interconnected roles are each played well, the result is synergistic. Being a good negotiator makes a manager a better disturbance handler. Playing the informational roles effectively improves performance in the decisional roles because managers have better information with which to make decisions.

Obviously, each manager will use different combinations of these roles. In part, the manager's level in the organization will determine the optimum mix. Senior-level managers in HSOs/HSs engage in figurehead, entrepreneur, and spokesperson roles more frequently than do other managers. Middle-level managers often are heavily involved in disturbance handler and resource allocator roles, and many of them rely on their abilities to successfully play their informational roles as a key ingredient in their work. First-level managers may play leader, disturbance handler, and negotiator roles extensively in their daily work. The point is that all managers engage in these roles, but specific circumstances, work conditions, and their responsibilities will dictate the most appropriate mix of roles.

Designer, Strategist, and Leader Roles

Another conceptualization of the roles of managers views them as playing a "trinity" of roles: designer, strategist, and leader.[40] Figure 1.5 illustrates this model of management roles. Like Mintzberg's model, this depiction of the roles of managers can apply to managers in all types of organizational settings and to the management work that occurs at the various levels of organizations and systems. In this model as well, managers in differing circumstances must use varying mixes of the roles if they are to achieve optimal performance.

The Designer Role

The designer role is fulfilled when managers establish intentional patterns of relationships among staff and other resources in their organizations. Managers at all levels of HSOs/HSs play the designer role, although in different ways. First-level managers are more concerned with designating individual positions and aggregating them into the workgroups (teams, departments, units, and so forth) that they manage. Middle-level managers cluster workgroups into the major divisions of their organizations and determine how various workgroups and clusters of workgroups are integrated and coordinated. In their designer roles senior-level managers are likely to focus on arranging the workgroups and clusters of workgroups into entire organizations, perhaps even into integrated delivery systems or networks of organizations.

The Strategist Role

The strategist role is played when managers establish suitable organizational objectives and develop and implement plans or strategies that are capable of accomplishing them. When managers think strategically, they are thinking about how to adapt their organizational domains to the external challenges and opportunities presented by the environment.[41] HSOs/HSs are dynamic, open systems that exist within complex external environments where they engage in ongoing exchanges and are influenced, sometimes dramatically, by events. Also, each part within an organization or system has similar relationships with other parts or components. When managers think strategically, they acknowledge this reality and their decisions and actions reflect it.

Important in the strategist role is that managers discern essential information in their environments. They engage in situational analysis through which they see and assess pertinent information in their environments. At the macro level, HSO/HS managers must scan an enormous amount of biological, cultural, demographic, ecological, economic, ethical, legal, political, psychological, social, and technological information to assess its potential effect on their organizations. In addition, managers must analyze internal organizational conditions, decisions, and actions to ascertain their effects.

Good situational analysis, however, includes more than merely discerning important information. It also includes organizing information and evaluating it in order to chart the issues that are

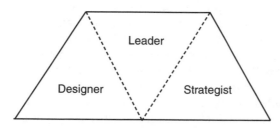

Figure 1.5.   The trinity of managerial roles. (From Zuckerman, Howard S., and William L. Dowling. The managerial role. In *Essentials of Health Care Management,* edited by Stephen M. Shortell and Arnold D. Kaluzny, 47. Albany, NY: Delmar Publishers, 1997; reprinted by permission.)

likely to have significant impact. In addition, it includes assessing the internal strengths and weaknesses of the organization or system and its mission and objectives, as well as the values held by those in the HSO/HS. Only after all of this information is considered can managers most effectively make strategic decisions about the objectives they wish to pursue and the means they wish to use in doing so.

Managers' strategist roles also involve them in acting on information garnered through situational analysis. They formulate objectives—the ends to be achieved—and decide on strategies— broad patterns of actions—that are necessary to achieve the objectives. Senior-level managers, who are sometimes called strategic managers, are responsible, along with their governing bodies, for establishing the overall strategic directions of their organizations or systems. Middle- and first-level managers who implement organization-level strategies frequently are in a position to provide valuable inputs to the formulation of these strategies. In addition, they must develop and implement objectives and the means to their accomplishment for the parts of their organizations that they directly manage. Thus all managers play strategist roles, although differently.

The Leader Role

As discussed earlier, HSOs/HSs are dependent on the quality of leadership that is exercised by their managers. Only effective leadership will encourage and motivate staff in these organizations and systems to meet organizational objectives. The leader role is not isolated from the other roles that managers play. Leadership is affected directly by the context in which it takes place. How well managers play their design and strategist roles will affect their leader roles. For example, leadership is facilitated in HSOs/HSs where

- The existence of long-standing shared values and a commonly accepted philosophy helps shape the HSO's/HS's mission and objectives and resolves conflicts among competing views about them.
- A history of service helps legitimize the HSO's/HS's claims for support from internal and external stakeholders.
- The technical ability to do good strategic planning helps provide a sense of organizational purpose, stability, and self-control.

Successfully playing the leader roles in all organizations is a challenge, but this is especially true in HSOs/HSs for several reasons. Most important is that these organizations operate in such dynamic environments. As Vladeck noted, "The most difficult leadership challenges arise when changes in the environment require transformation of organizational cultures, or reexamination of organizational goals."[42] HSOs/HSs continuously face this challenge.

A second reason that the leader role is difficult in HSOs/HSs is because their managers must satisfy diverse constituencies. The communities that are served by these organizations and systems must be considered, as must the wishes of the people who work, govern, or practice in the organizations and systems. Only rarely are the preferences of these various groups in harmony.

A third reason for the difficulty of leading in HSOs/HSs is that, unlike many other organizations, they often require extensive sharing of the leadership role. The managers of HSOs/HSs certainly play leadership roles, but so do the members of the governing body and of the professional staff. The president of a HSO/HS plays a key organizational leadership role, but it would be very difficult to play this leadership role properly without support and validation provided by the governing body. Furthermore, clinical leadership primarily resides with clinicians in HSOs/HSs—including physicians and, increasingly, others with clinical responsibilities.[43] So the issue of who provides organizational leadership in many HSOs/HSs can be cloudy. What is clear, however, is that the challenge of leadership is made more complex by the ambiguities about who is responsible for it.

Management Competencies[44]

The work of managers in HSOs/HSs has been viewed from three perspectives: the functions that they perform, the skills that they use in doing management work, and the roles that they play as managers. Each perspective contributes to understanding management work, yet none explains the competencies or underlying clusters of knowledge and skill in using them that permit managers to do their work. A person's capacity to work well depends on possession of the relevant competencies, whether the work is direct, support, or management. Thus another important approach to considering management work includes an analysis of the underlying competencies that are needed to do the work well (see Table 1.1).

Although there may be some overlap, six rather distinct competencies are required for successful management work in HSOs/HSs, especially at senior levels. The clusters of knowledge and skills that make up these competencies are 1) conceptual, 2) technical managerial/clinical, 3) interpersonal/collaborative, 4) political, 5) commercial, and 6) governance. In part, this categorization of managerial competencies builds on Katz's model of the conceptual, technical, and interpersonal skills that are used by managers.[45] The set of competencies described here includes conceptual competence, albeit of a more expansive nature than that envisioned by Katz. The set also includes a technical managerial/clinical cluster as well as an interpersonal/collaborative cluster, each of which is an extension of elements in Katz's model. The political, commercial, and governance clusters represent important additional competencies that are increasingly required, especially of senior managers. These competencies, as they apply to situations in which HSOs integrate into HSs, are discussed further in Chapter 5.

Conceptual Competence

In all organizational settings possession of an adequate cluster of conceptual knowledge and skills is a competency that permits managers to envision the places and roles of their organizations or systems in the larger society. For middle- and first-level managers, conceptual competency enables them to understand their part in the larger organization. This competency also allows managers to visualize the complex interrelationships within their workplaces—relationships among staff and other resources, among units of a HSO, and among the various organizations in a HS. In short, adequate conceptual competence allows managers to identify, understand, and interact with their organization's or system's myriad external and internal stakeholders, that is, with "those individuals, groups, or organizations who have a contractual, ethical, financial, and/or political interest (stake) in the decisions and actions of a particular organization."[46] Conceptual competence also enhances managers' abilities to comprehend organizational cultures and historically developed values, beliefs, and norms and to visualize the futures of their organizations.

Technical Managerial/Clinical Competence

The cluster of knowledge and associated skills that compose technical competence pertains to management work as well as to direct work performed in a manager's domain. In HSOs/HSs direct work includes clinical activities such as performing a surgical procedure, administering a chemotherapeutic agent, conducting a physical therapy session, or counseling a dying patient in a hospice. However, the technical aspects of management work, such as planning for a new service or facility, devising and operating an incentive-based compensation program, or arranging the financing of long-term debt, are also crucial to the HSO's/HS's success.

Traditionally, managers in HSOs/HSs had to know something of the clinical work to properly support it with the necessary resources and with the help of experts to ensure that it was done at an acceptable level of quality. They also have needed to know a great deal about management work. Knowledge and relevant skills in using or applying the knowledge in both clinical and management areas compose technical competence for HSO/HS managers. Most important, HSO/HS managers increasingly must rely on technical knowledge that is both clinically and managerially based, and some that is both simultaneously.

Interpersonal/Collaborative Competence

An important ingredient in managerial success has always been the cluster of knowledge and related skills about human interactions and relations by which managers direct or lead others in the pursuit of organizational objectives. A survey of executives to determine the management competencies that are the most important to success in management performance in ambulatory health services settings found interpersonal skills rated most highly.[47]

Interpersonal competence incorporates knowledge and skills that are useful in effectively interacting with others, including the knowledge and related skills that permit managers to develop and instill a common vision and stimulate a determination to pursue the vision and fulfill objectives related to it. The essence of the interpersonal competence of managers is knowing how to motivate people, how to communicate their visions and preferences, how to handle negotiations, and how to manage conflicts.

The core elements of traditional interpersonal competence expand considerably when HSOs are involved in greater integration, particularly in the formation and operation of HSs. This expansion results from the differences in interpersonal relationships that occur within organizations compared with those that occur among organizations in a system. Achieving and managing integration relies on knowledge and skills that facilitate synergistic interaction among the staff and organizations involved. As is discussed further in Chapter 5, this is collaborative competence.

Political Competence

Political competence, defined as the dual capability to accurately assess the impact of public policies on the performance of the manager's domains of responsibility and to influence public policy making at state and federal levels, is extraordinarily important, especially for senior-level managers.[48] Managers possess position-, reward-, and expertise-based opportunities to influence public policy making. Key is understanding the complex policy-making process at all levels of government. This process includes policy formulation, which incorporates legislative agenda setting and the development of laws, and policy implementation, which incorporates rule making and policy operation.[49]

Senior-level managers can influence their HSO's/HS's public policy environments at many points. For example, they can help define problems that policies address, they can design solutions, or they can create the political circumstances that are necessary to advance solutions through the policy-making process.[50] Their central roles in the health industry enable senior managers of HSOs/HSs to know, often intimately, about health problems that should be addressed through public policies. By permitting their organizations to serve as demonstration sites for assessing possible solutions, they can play important roles in identifying feasible solutions to problems. Effective mechanisms through which they can help shape the political circumstances surrounding a policy issue include interest groups, lobbying, and the courts.

Furthermore, individually and through interest groups, senior managers can participate in drafting legislative proposals, and they can testify at legislative hearings. They can also influence the public policymaking process in the implementation phase by focusing on rule making. Procedurally, rule making typically precedes and guides the implementation of public policies and is designed to include input from those who will be affected by the regulations in the form of formal comments on proposed rules.

Commercial Competence

In any setting, commercial competence is the ability of managers to establish and operate value-creating situations in which economic exchanges between buyers and sellers occur. Value in health services has a specific meaning. It requires that buyers and sellers think about both quality and price. Value is quality divided by price.[51] Value in health services is created when services have more of the quality attributes desired by buyers than competitors offer. Value is also created when a HSO/HS sells a set of quality attributes desired by buyers at a lower price than its competitors. Of course, determining value in health services is not quite so straightforward as these relationships might suggest.

The quality of a single health service, such as the repair of a hernia, is difficult to assess. Creating value in health services more typically involves the quality of a large and diverse package of services—up to and including all services provided by a health plan. Assessing the quality of packages of services is even more difficult than assessing that of a single service. Similarly, comparing price is difficult because packages of services are being purchased. True price comparisons require that all of the benefits or services in the various packages be the same, including any associated co-payments or deductibles. Despite these difficulties, however, the commercial success of HSOs/HSs increasingly requires that they compete on value.

Governance Competence

Each HSO/HS relies on senior managers and those who govern the organization or system, working in concert at its "strategic apex,"[52] to establish a clear vision for the organization, to foster a culture that supports the realization of the vision, to assemble and effectively allocate the resources to realize the vision, to lead the organization through various challenges, and to ensure proper accountability to multiple stakeholders.[53] Accountability, in the context of governance of HSOs/HSs, means "taking into account and responding to political, commercial, community, and clinical/patient interests and expectations."[54] Although the boundaries between management and governance are not always clear cut, governance is perceived as the unique function in the organization that "holds management and the organization accountable for its actions."[55]

The knowledge and associated skills of governance competence are important for managers—especially senior managers—for three reasons. First, most senior managers participate directly in the governance function as members of their organization's or system's governing body. Many HSOs include their CEOs on their governing bodies.[56] Chief executives of HSs are almost universally included. Other senior managers, such as chief financial and medical officers with specific expertise, also are typically added to governing bodies.

A second reason for senior managers to possess governance competence is that, at the strategic apex, it is difficult to separate what occurs under the rubric of governance from what occurs in the context of strategic management. Consequently, effective senior managers must be knowledgeable about management and governance.

A third reason that HSO/HS managers must possess governance competence is that such competence enables them to assist those with direct governance responsibilities to do a better job. This includes providing development programs for members of their organization's or system's governing body.

Governance competence enables managers to fulfill five interrelated responsibilities.[57] First, those who govern HSOs/HSs are responsible for establishing a vision for the organization or system from which a mission and associated objectives grow. Second, governing bodies ensure suitable performance from senior managers. Steps in fulfilling this responsibility typically include selecting the CEO, specifying performance expectations, and periodically appraising the chief executive's actual performance. The third area of governance responsibility is the quality of health services. The legal responsibility of governance in this area is well established and includes credentialing licensed independent practitioners on professional staffs; seeing that procedures for quality management, utilization management, and risk management issues are in place; and assessing both the processes and outcomes of care, increasingly at the level of populations.[58] HSOs/HSs face unprecedented opportunities for the application of algorithms, guidelines, or pathways to improve clinical outcomes, as well as new opportunities for improved service quality and improved levels of customer satisfaction among the populations served.

Governing bodies in HSOs/HSs also bear responsibility in a fourth area, the finances and financial performance of their organizations or systems. This responsibility entails establishing appropriate financial objectives, maintaining adequate controls over financial matters, and ensuring that the organization's or system's financial obligations, including investments, are met. The fifth area of governance responsibility is for self. That is, those who govern must do so effectively and efficiently. Fulfilling this responsibility includes establishing and maintaining appropriate bylaws to guide the governance process, selecting governing body members who can and do serve the HSO/HS well, and ensuring that processes function to evaluate board performance and develop members.

Summary

The work of managers in HSOs/HSs has been considered from four perspectives: the functions that managers perform, the skills that they use in carrying out these functions, the roles that managers fulfill in managing, and the set of management competencies that is needed to do the work well. These perspectives form a mosaic—a more complete picture than any one perspective—of management work in HSOs/HSs. Building on and integrating these perspectives on management, a comprehensive model of management in HSOs/HSs is described in the next section.

A MANAGEMENT MODEL FOR HSOs/HSs

Earlier in this chapter, management was defined as the process, composed of interrelated social and technical functions and activities, occurring within a formal organizational setting for the purpose of accomplishing predetermined objectives through the use of human and other resources. It was noted and shown in Table 1.1 that all HSO/HS managers perform the management functions of planning, organizing, staffing, directing, and controlling, and that all managers engage in decision making as they perform each of these functions. These interrelated functions enable managers to accomplish objectives through people and by using other resources in a formal organizational setting. In undertaking these functions managers use conceptual, technical, and human relations skills; fulfill interrelated interpersonal, informational, and decisional roles, as well as managerial roles as strategists, organization designers, and leaders; and rely on extensive sets of management competencies, including conceptual, technical managerial/clinical, interpersonal/collaborative, political, commercial, and governance competencies.

A schematic model of the management process in HSOs/HSs, which serves as the framework and structure for the discussion of management throughout the book, is presented and described in this section. The model shows management as an input–conversion–output process that takes place within HSOs/HSs, which are set within their larger environments. Whether independent or joined into systems or networks of organizations, HSOs are open systems that are constantly interacting with their external environment. Within HSOs/HSs, inputs (human and physical resources and technology) are converted, under the catalytic influence of management, into desired outputs (accomplishment of organizational objectives regarding services, products, and other parameters of organizational performance). Figure 1.6 depicts this conversion in the context of an organization or system, within the larger external environment. Several important relationships are illustrated.

- A HSO/HS is a formal setting where outputs are produced (objectives accomplished) through use (conversion) of inputs (resources).
- Managers and the management work that they perform are the catalyst that converts inputs to outputs.

- A HSO/HS (and its managers) interact with—are affected by and affect—the HSO's/HS's external environment; this makes HSOs/HSs open systems because inputs are obtained from the external environment and outputs go into it.

The input–conversion–output model is expanded into the more comprehensive HSO/HS management model in Figure 1.7. The expanded model incorporates the input–conversion–output perspective but is significantly more detailed. (*Note:* The discussion of this model that follows references the major components of the model by numbers in brackets.)

Inputs (Resources)

The "inputs" component [1] in Figure 1.7 shows that resources are acquired and used to generate "outputs" [3]. Inputs include human resources, material/supplies, technology/equipment, information, capital resources, and patients/customers. Examples of human resources in HSOs/HSs include managers, physicians, dentists, nurses, technologists, pharmacists, dietitians, social workers, and clerical and housekeeping staff. Material inputs (resources) are supplies of all types, such as medical forms, food, linens, drugs, and instruments. Technological resources include equipment, such as magnetic resonance imagers, heart catheterization equipment, and fetal monitors, as well as knowledge possessed by the HSO/HS staff. Internal information sources include diverse areas such as patient data, reports, schedules, and budgets. External information includes public policy, stakeholder views and opinions, economic data and forecasts, and the HSO's/HS's more immediate environment—the health care system, which includes regulation, accreditation, competition, and third-party payers. Capital resources are physical plant and funds. Finally, patients or customers are an input resource in HSOs/HSs.

A great variety of inputs are necessary for any HSO/HS to function. Eliminating or restricting them may compromise the effectiveness of the whole organization or system. For example, a rapid rise in supply costs could affect an output such as the cost of care or provision of a service, or high interest rates may prevent capital expansion. Obsolete equipment may detract from providing better care, or an inadequate supply of human resources may mean that some services are unavailable.

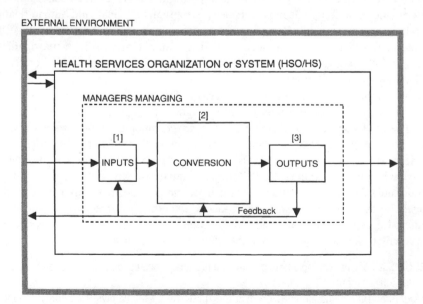

Figure 1.6. Management as an input–conversion–output process.

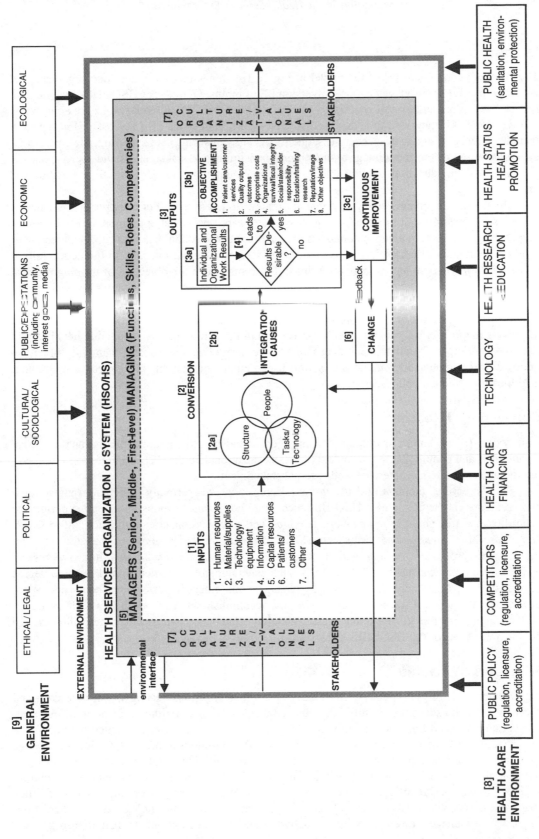

Figure 1.7. Management model for HSOs/HSs.

25

Outputs (Objectives)

The "output" component [3] of the model in Figure 1.7 shows that individual and organizational work results [3a] are produced by the conversion [2] of inputs. Outputs for HSOs/HSs include both specific individual and overall organizational work results [3a]. When work results are appropriate and desirable [4], they lead to achieving objectives [3b]. Objectives [3b] of HSOs/HSs typically include patient care and customer services; quality of care; delivering care at appropriate costs; organizational survival and fiscal integrity; meeting responsibilities to stakeholders and society; participating in medical education, training, and research; and maintaining the HSO's/HS's reputation and image.

Organizational objectives vary by type of organization or system. For example, a home health agency seeks primarily to provide high-quality patient care services at appropriate costs to clients in their homes. By comparison, a nongovernmental acute care hospital has the primary objective of providing a range of diagnostic and restorative services of different intensity to the community it serves in both inpatient and outpatient settings; it also may have the objective of training medical residents. A VA hospital may have the primary objective of caring for veterans. A community health center provides care to an indigent population. A genetics counseling center has the objective of providing counseling and appropriate referral services. A public health department seeks to improve general health through preventive measures in its community. An academic health center may have multiple objectives, including patient care; providing specialized treatment, which requires different inputs, combinations of sophisticated equipment, and medical specialists; training health care personnel; and research.

Conversion (Integration)

Conversion [2] of inputs to outputs occurs when managers [5] integrate [2b] structure, tasks/ technology, and people [2a] in the context of the organizational culture [7] and in response to meeting the needs of internal, interface, and external stakeholders.

The "structure" element [2a] in Figure 1.7 conceptualizes formally designed organizational arrangements characteristic of a HSO/HS, such as authority and responsibility and superior and subordinate relationships; grouping work activities; and coordination, communication, information, and control mechanisms. The "tasks/technology" element [2a] represents work specialization: job design; work processes, methods, and procedures; and logistical and work flows. It also represents technological characteristics of the HSO/HS, such as equipment, cybernetics, and to some degree information and knowledge that are used by managers and others in performing their work. Work occurs only through the "people" element [2a]; the accomplishment of work in HSOs/HSs requires that managers integrate [2b] structure, tasks/technology, and people within the context of the shared beliefs and values of the HSO's/HS's culture [7].

Managers Managing

As managers in HSOs/HSs manage [5] by carrying out their functions—using appropriate skills and competencies and successfully fulfilling managerial roles—they determine the nature of the model's components and link and integrate them. Figure 1.7 shows this with the dotted boundary line that surrounds the inputs [1], conversion [2], outputs [3], continuous improvement [3c], and change [6] components. When managers plan, they determine the individual and organizational work that will lead to accomplishing the HSO's/HS's objectives. Once determined, human and other input resources [1] can be identified, acquired, and allocated. When managers organize and staff, they shape the setting where conversion [2] occurs—the structure, tasks/technology, and staff relationships. When managers direct, they initiate activity that is intended to accomplish appropriate and desirable individual and organizational work results [3a]. When managers control, they monitor individual and organizational work results [3a] and compare them with standards and expectations to determine whether objectives [3b] are being achieved. If results are inconsistent with standards, expectations, or both [4], then managers make changes [6] through a feedback loop. For example, if utilization review or comparison with best clinical practices determines that care in a HSO/HS should be improved, then managers change the structure, tasks/technology, and people components, change input resources, or both. Even if objectives are being met [3b], the philosophy of CQI requires that assessment and improvement of HSO/HS activity be continuous [3c]. The essential implication of the CQI philosophy is that HSOs/HSs can improve outcomes in all organizational performance dimensions by continuously evaluating, changing [6], and improving [3c] processes that are used in conversion [2] or the inputs used [1], or both.

External Environment (An Open Systems Perspective)

HSOs/HSs are not isolated from their external environments. The gray boundary in Figure 1.7 denotes the environment that is external to the HSO/HS, which has two major components; the general environment [9] and the more proximate to able to the environment [8]. HSOs/HSs are affected by the external environment—their inputs come from it. HSOs/HSs affect the external environment—their outputs go into it. Managers seek to influence, modify, and change the external environment of their organization or system. This is denoted by the change loop arrow [6] in Figure 1.7 that extends to the environment. Advocacy and lobbying with external stakeholders are responsibilities of senior management.[59] As noted by Zuckerman,

> *the linkage between environment and organization should be a two-way interaction. . . . In essence, the CEO has a role as an advocate for the organization, for the constituents that it represents, and for the population that it serves. CEOs should and do seek to influence the formulation and implementation of public policy.*[60]

Systems theory provides a framework within which to conceptualize the relationships between a HSO/HS and its external environment. A system is a set of interrelated and interdependent parts. A subsystem is part of a system; a suprasystem is a set of systems. The HSO/HS may be viewed as a system that is composed of many subsystems, such as those for patient care, ancillary services, professional staff, financial services, and information, among others. The HSO/HS also may be viewed as a subsystem of the larger system of HSOs/HSs found in the health care environment [8], which is, in turn, part of the suprasystem called the general environment [9].

A suprasystem, its systems, and their subsystems are interrelated and interdependent, and simultaneously affect one another at all levels. The general environment [9] is a suprasystem (see Figure 1.7) composed of many systems that include ethical/legal, political, cultural/sociological, public (i.e., external stakeholders such as the community at large, interest groups, and media), economic, and ecological systems and the systems that compose the health care environment [8].

More proximate to and having a more direct effect on the HSO is the health care environment. The forces and influences in the health care environment affecting the HSO, its managers, and how they manage are presented in Figure 1.7 [8]. A variety of external stakeholders—including patients, third-party payers, and government, as well as special interests, local communities, and licensure, regulatory, and accrediting agencies—are important to HSOs/HSs. Other forces in the health care system include competition by other HSOs/HSs; numbers and skills of practitioners; public and private financing of health care; and resource entities for technology, equipment, and materials. A final, more remote group of health care environmental forces that affect HSOs/HSs includes health research and education; health status, wellness, prevalence of disease, and health promotion and awareness; and the status of public health, general sanitation, and protection from hazardous substances and injurious working conditions.

The Challenges of Management

The management model presented in Figure 1.7 is a unifying framework for the book. Managers doing management work throughout the process detailed in this model permit HSOs/HSs to reach their potential for contributing to the health of society. The challenges facing HSOs/HSs and their managers—which must be met daily—are considerable. They must be

> *concerned with the overall health status of their communities while continuing to provide direct patient services. They should take a leadership role in enhancing public health and continuity of care in the community by communicating and working with other health care and social agencies to improve the availability and provision of health promotion, education, and patient care services.*
>
> *[They] are responsible for fair and effective use of available health care delivery resources to promote access to comprehensive and affordable health care services of high quality. This responsibility extends beyond the resources of the given [HSO/HS] to include efforts to coordinate with other health care organizations and professionals and to share in community solutions for providing care for the medically indigent and others in need of specific health services.*
>
> *All [HSOs/HSs] are responsible for meeting community service obligations which may include special initiatives for care for the poor and uninsured, provision of needed medical or social services, education, [and] various programs designed to meet the specific needs of their communities.*[61]

STRUCTURE OF THE BOOK

This chapter and the next five form Part I, *Managing in the Health Services Environment.* Chapter 2, "The Health Care System," is an overview of the system for financing and delivering health services in the United States, including the remarkable impact of managed care and integration on this system. Chapter 3, "Concepts of Organization Design," provides conceptual background for understanding HSO/HS organizational structures. It contains information on general organization theory, including classical principles as well as contemporary concepts as they relate to organizations and to systems and networks of organizations. Chapter 4, "How Health Services Organizations Are Organized," details the backgrounds, structures, and functions of various HSOs, including acute care hospitals, nursing facilities, managed care organizations, ambulatory care organizations, hospice, birth centers, and home health agencies. Chapter 5, "How Health Systems Are Organized," details HS organizational forms and relationships arising as HSOs increasingly join integrated delivery systems and networks. Chapter 6, "Health Care Technology," provides an understanding of technology in the provision of health services, including its effects, assessment, and management. Together, the first six chapters provide a comprehensive perspective on managing in HSOs/HSs.

Part II, *Managerial Tools and Techniques,* contains six chapters that detail methods for effectively managing in the HSO/HS environment. In Chapter 7, "Managerial Problem Solving and Decision Making," the pervasive decision-making function is examined, particularly as it relates to the challenge of solving problems. A problem-solving model is used to structure the chapter. Chapter 8, "Strategic Planning and Marketing," details how HSO/HS managers establish appropriate organizational objectives and formulate, implement, and control strategies to accomplish them. Chapter 9, "Quality and Competitive Position," focuses on CQI and productivity improvement. The relationship of CQI to process improvement, as well as methods such as reengineering to improve productivity through better work methods, flows, job design, facilities layout, and scheduling, are discussed.

Chapter 10, "Control and Resource Allocation," presents a general model of control and focuses on controlling individual and organizational work results through techniques such as management information systems, management and operations auditing, and budgeting. Control of medical care quality through risk management and quality assessment and improvement is discussed. The chapter concludes with applications of quantitative techniques that are useful in resource allocation, such as volume analysis, capital budgeting, cost–benefit analysis, and simulation. Chapter 11, "Human Resources and Labor Relations," addresses human resource acquisition, maintenance, and retention, including recruitment, selection, training, and development. Compensation and benefits administration in HSOs/HSs, including performance appraisal, are described, and a brief discussion of labor relations is presented. Chapter 12, "Organizational Change," completes this part on managerial tools and techniques by examining the process of change in HSOs/HSs. Because they work in such dynamic organizations, managers in HSOs/HSs must possess knowledge of tools and techniques to make them effective change agents.

Part III, *Managing Relationships,* contains five chapters that address how managers seek to manage the complex human relationships that exist within HSOs/HSs and among HSOs/HSs and external stakeholders. Chapter 13, "Ethics," provides a framework that managers can use to understand, analyze, and solve ethical problems that arise. Specific administrative and biomedical ethical issues are included. An introduction to the law and the legal aspects of managing HSOs/HSs is provided in Chapter 14, "Legal Considerations." Especially useful is material on how managers can interact effectively with the legal system and legal counsel. Chapter 15, "Leadership," differentiates transactional and transformational leadership and models and defines leadership. The extensive literature on leader behavior and situational theories of leadership is reviewed. The final section integrates the theories of leadership. Chapter 16, "Motivation," presents the concept of motivation, models and defines it, and reviews the literature on content and process theories of motivation. The final section in this chapter integrates the theories of motivation. Chapter 17, "Communication," concludes this part on managing relationships by examining communication for HSO/HS managers. A communication process model is presented, and its application to communicating within HSOs/HSs and between them and their external stakeholders is discussed.

SUMMARY

This chapter on managers and their management work in HSOs/HSs establishes the book's foundation. HSO/HS managers are defined as people appointed to positions of authority who enable others to do their work effectively, who have responsibility for resource utilization, and who are accountable for work results. A classification scheme is developed for senior-, middle-, and first-level managers who must work together effectively if a HSO's/HS's organizational objectives are to be met.

The focus is on management as a process composed of interrelated social and technical functions and activities, occurring within a formal organizational setting for the purpose of accomplishing predetermined objectives through the use of human and other resources. The primary management functions of planning, organizing, staffing, directing, and controlling, with decision making intertwined throughout each, are presented. The skills and competencies needed by managers and the roles they play in carrying out their work are discussed. Organizational culture, with derivative philosophies about customers, staff, and stakeholders, is discussed as a context for managing.

A management model for HSOs/HSs, using an input–conversion–output perspective, that provides the book's conceptual framework, is presented in Figure 1.7. The input and output components of the model are described, and there is extensive discussion of the conversion component. This component of the model demonstrates that, when managers manage, they integrate the HSO's/

HS's structure–tasks/technology–people elements to achieve individual and organizational work results.

Integrating general systems theory with the management model emphasizes the importance of the external environment for HSOs/HSs. A HSO's/HS's external environment includes the health care environment and the larger general environment. Both affect HSOs/HSs, their managers, and how they are managed.

DISCUSSION QUESTIONS

1. What is the distinction among health, health care, and health services?
2. Define the term *manager*.
3. Define *management* and include the basic ingredients of the definition. Why is management a process?
4. How are managers at various levels in HSOs classified and differentiated?
5. Figure 1.4 shows various managerial roles. Relate these roles to the management functions and to management competencies.
6. What relationship do managers have to the input–conversion–output perspective of HSOs/HSs?
7. Carefully examine Figure 1.7. Describe and discuss 1) its components and how they flow and link, and 2) the way in which management functions, skills, roles, and competencies interrelate with the components.
8. Figure 1.7 shows that outputs are composed of individual and organizational work results that accomplish objectives. How do individual and organizational work results fulfill objectives? Choose a HSO/HS with which you are familiar and identify its objectives.
9. Figure 1.7 shows two external environments and the forces that affect HSOs/HSs. How do these forces affect HSOs/HSs? Are there others?
10. Identify a HSO/HS. Identify its internal, interface, and external stakeholders. For stakeholders in each group, indicate whether the stakeholder is 1) important, 2) influential, and/or 3) a positive influence or threat; and 4) whether the HSO/HS must cooperate with, co-opt, or ignore the stakeholder.
11. Identify and list values and beliefs as well as symbols and rituals that are characteristic of the culture of a HSO/HS.

CASE STUDY 1: THE CEO'S DAY

Terry Blaze, the 45-year-old president and CEO of Midvale Community Hospital, rose early on Monday morning. A busy schedule of meetings and several major issues that would require full attention and careful decisions lay ahead. While getting dressed, Blaze thought about what to say to two county commissioners at a breakfast meeting in a local restaurant at 6:30 A.M. The county coroner had called Blaze the previous Wednesday asking if Midvale Community Hospital would permit the coroner's office to use some of the hospital's facilities. As a 500-bed teaching hospital with more than 2,000 full-time employees and a medical staff of 450 physicians, Midvale was the largest of the four hospitals located in the metropolitan area, which has a population of about 400,000. Recent budget reductions to the coroner's office by the county commissioners had prompted the inquiry; consequently, the coroner was searching for ways to run his office on a reduced budget by drawing on the goodwill and resources of other community organizations.

Blaze had scheduled the meeting with the commissioners to see if they were aware of the coroner's request. Blaze was relatively open-minded about the situation, wanted to maintain the existing good relations between the commissioners and the hospital, and wanted to respond to the needs of the community provided that the hospital's basic objectives were not jeopardized or its resources inappropriately used. However, getting caught in the middle of the county's political problems could be disastrous.

At 7:30 A.M., Blaze attended a campaign fund-raiser breakfast for the state senator who represented the district in which Midvale was located. Blaze spoke to the senator about how the state's recently announced Medicaid payment reductions under their managed care program would affect Midvale and asked that the senator use his influence to try to have funding levels increased. After circulating among the other guests, Blaze went to the hospital. As soon as Blaze arrived at the office at 8:15 A.M., the executive secretary, Ms. Billings, mentioned that Dr. Smith, president of the professional staff organization (PSO), composed of physicians, dentists, podiatrists, and clinical psychologists having privileges at Midvale, insisted on speaking privately with Blaze about a problem involving a staff physician before the scheduled 9:00 A.M. meeting of the PSO executive committee. Blaze immediately called Dr. Smith, and at the end of the conversation wondered whether it had been a correct decision to tell Dr. Smith to handle the problem as he thought appropriate. Relations between administration and the PSO are always delicate, but this time it seemed best to let Dr. Smith handle the situation and keep Blaze informed.

At 8:30 A.M., the vice president for operations arrived and accompanied Blaze to the hospital's conference room. All department heads were present. Because of a recent decision by Blaze and the board to establish a satellite facility in an adjacent county, most departments would be expanded, work loads would be increased, and coordination mechanisms between the hospital and satellite facility would need to be developed. Blaze explained the reasons for the decision, described the planning that had occurred before the decision was made, indicated how Midvale would work with the state planning agency in obtaining a certificate of need, and described how it would affect Midvale and its patients, as well as other area hospitals. Blaze asked the department heads to inform their subordinates before the official announcement was made to the press on Wednesday. A question-and-answer session followed.

Blaze arrived at the 9:00 A.M. PSO executive committee meeting 10 minutes late and found that it had been postponed until the next day. Because the next meeting on the day's schedule was not until 10:00 A.M., Blaze returned to the office and asked Billings to hold all calls. Blaze had given considerable thought over several months to the governing body's directive that options be evaluated for expanding the scope of the hospital's services, particularly in light of the government's attitude favoring competition among HSOs and especially the actions of other area hospitals and area's newly formed HMO. Mindful of the hospital's resource constraints, rising costs, changing patient mix, and the continued tightening of Medicare and Medicaid reimbursement, Blaze was concerned about accomplishing the hospital's objectives during the next 5 years in this changing environment. Particularly worrisome was the restlessness of some members of the PSO, who wanted new services and an on-site medical office building.

Blaze recalled the discussions that had occurred at past governing body and management executive staff meetings. After weighing the options, Blaze realized that the hospital would need three feasibility studies to be performed by external consultants. Blaze dictated a memo to the vice president for operations and the assistant vice president for planning, instructing them to begin studies for expansion of the hospital's cardiac services and the addition of 34 psychiatric beds and a physicians' office building adjacent to the hospital. Blaze did not approve a study for a regional burn unit because this service, although desirable, would contribute less to the hospital's objectives than the others, and limited resources meant some projects could not be undertaken.

At 10:00 A.M., Blaze met with the chair of the department of psychiatry. Blaze informed him of the feasibility study, but the meeting also continued negotiations about making the psychiatry department chair a salaried position. This would be the first such position in the hospital and would set a precedent with long-term implications.

At 10:30 A.M., Blaze interviewed a finalist for the position of director of marketing. At 11:00 A.M., Dr. Loren, who had requested clinical privileges, arrived for a meeting. It was a long-standing policy for the president of the PSO and the CEO to interview all those seeking privileges.

At 11:30 A.M., Blaze returned telephone calls that required immediate attention. The first was to a governing body member whose husband was being admitted for minor surgery. The second was to a former patient with a complaint about his statement. Billings told Blaze that the former patient had already spoken to patient accounts but was still dissatisfied. Blaze spoke briefly with him and gave assurances that the matter would be rectified. The last telephone call was to the director of human resources. They decided that the human resources director should accept the mayor's invitation to serve on the health department's personnel evaluation task force. This would require approximately 8 hours per week for 6 months, but they agreed it would help the hospital and community.

As was customary, Blaze had lunch in the hospital cafeteria and circulated among the staff before and after eating. It was a simple yet effective way to stay in touch with them.

Two major meetings were scheduled in the afternoon. From 1:00 to 3:00 P.M., the budget committee reviewed next year's operations and capital expenditures budgets. The executive staff and comptroller had prepared options for review. Among those Blaze approved for presentation to the governing body were an increase in the number of nursing service employees, a reduction in the equipment budget, and the annual pay increase for nonprofessional personnel that had been discussed previously. Blaze had positive relations with the governing body and told the executive administrative staff that the recommendations would likely be approved. However, a source of displeasure was last month's adverse overtime budget variance and the cost overrun on supplies. Both were unacceptable because census and patient days were below expectations. Blaze firmly told the senior managers to monitor their areas closely and report variations weekly.

The second meeting that afternoon was with the governing body task force on diversification. Near the end of the meeting, Blaze told them about ordering the physicians' office building feasibility study and told them they should be thinking about incorporating a for-profit subsidiary to own and manage the office building. The major consideration was how reimbursement would be affected by allocating overhead to either the not-for-profit hospital or the for-profit subsidiary. The board task force asked Blaze to include these revenue–cost implications in the feasibility study.

On returning to the office at 4:00 P.M., Blaze approved the agenda for Friday's weekly senior management staff meeting, gave Billings several items for the agenda of the next governing body meeting, and returned phone calls. At 5:00 P.M., Blaze left the hospital to attend a 5:30 P.M. area hospital executives' council quarterly meeting. The meeting featured a presentation by the new dean of the medical school located in Midvale about how her plans would affect teaching hospitals and their medical education and residency programs. During the half-hour drive to and from the medical school, Blaze dictated several letters and memoranda and took a call on his cell phone. Blaze went to a restaurant at 7:00 P.M. for dinner and left at 8:00 P.M. to attend a United Way trustees board meeting. At 10:00 P.M., Blaze returned home and did paperwork for an hour before retiring.

QUESTIONS

1. Terry Blaze engaged in activities related to the functions of management and roles of managers. Identify which of Blaze's activities relate to the management functions and managerial roles presented in the chapter.

2. Use the environmental portion of the management model in Figure 1.7 to 1) identify internal, interface, and external stakeholders with whom Blaze interacted; and 2) identify other environmental forces that affected Blaze as well as Blaze's actions that affected the environment.

CASE STUDY 2: ROLE AND FUNCTIONS OF EXECUTIVE MANAGEMENT[62]

The American Hospital Association (AHA), in its statement on the "Role and Functions of Hospital Executive Management," identified the following as responsibilities of senior management:

1. *Executive management should initiate and monitor organizational mechanisms to ensure that the hospital has effective organizational structures and processes.* Executive management should develop and recommend to the governing board an effective organizational plan that takes into consideration the interdependent leadership roles of executive management, the governing board, and the medical staff, and that clearly assigns responsibilities for specific organizational programs and services to specific components and individuals. The organizational plan should clearly define relationships among the board's broad policy responsibility, the medical staff's shared responsibility for quality of care, and executive management's responsibility for overall operations.

2. *Executive management is expected to infuse the mission and philosophy of the institution into the entire organization.* This function requires an understanding by executive management of the relationships between the philosophy of the hospital as a center for community health and the goal of improving the health status of the community. It also requires a system for communicating the hospital's philosophy to the community.

3. *Executive management should assume primary responsibility for ensuring that members of the hospital organization are kept informed about public policy and environmental issues and their effects on the hospital.* Executive management is responsible for establishing mechanisms for identifying and obtaining information about public policy issues and decisions affecting the hospital and, when necessary, for developing an appropriate organizational response. Executive management should take the initiative to work with other community organizations on public policy issues and decisions affecting the health status of the community.

4. *Executive management should take the initiative in ensuring that the hospital has a broadly based strategic planning program.* Strategic planning provides the hospital with a powerful management tool to help determine its goals and objectives in relationship to changes in the environment and the needs of its community, to establish its priorities to choose the most appropriate organizational structure to achieve its goals and objectives, and to provide benchmarks for evaluating the achievements of its goals and objectives.

5. *Executive management should assume responsibility for the cost-effective management of the hospital's resources.* This responsibility requires a commitment to provide the most economical and highest quality services possible in keeping with available resources and to communicate this commitment to the entire organization and the community. This commitment implies a willingness to assume leadership, along with the governing board and the medical staff, in introducing new patient care technologies and programs that are of high quality, are medically necessary and appropriate, and are efficiently, yet compassionately, provided. It implies a responsibility to engage the medical staff in a cooperative effort to eliminate obsolete technologies and programs, and a willingness to introduce new management techniques and practices to improve the use of human and financial resources. It also implies a willingness to experiment with and make the community aware

of alternatives to traditional means of health care delivery and financing, such as health maintenance organizations, independent practice associations, consumer choice health plans, and others. Finally, it implies the existence of an effective system for financial and management reporting that enhances the monitoring and evaluation of organizational performance.

6. *Executive management should provide a work atmosphere that recognizes the vital importance of human resources to the health care organization.* The provision of a positive work atmosphere implies a moral and ethical commitment to the needs of people, a concern for their health status and quality of life, and a commitment to fostering respect and satisfaction for all.

QUESTIONS

1. For each statement (1, 2, 3, 4, 5, and 6), identify the explicit or implicit managerial functions involved.
2. For each statement (1, 2, 3, 4, 5, and 6), identify the explicit or implicit senior-level managerial skills, roles, and competencies involved.

CASE STUDY 3: THE ROLE OF THE HEALTH CARE EXECUTIVE IN A CONSOLIDATION, MERGER, ACQUISITION, OR AFFILIATION[63]

The American College of Healthcare Executives (ACHE), in a Professional Policy Statement on what senior-level managers should do when their HSO/HS is involved in a consolidation, merger, acquisition, or affiliation, as so many HSOs/HSs are, offers the following description of the issue and suggestions.

Statement of the Issue
Changes in organizational ownership or control present special challenges for health care executives. Executives must lead their organizations through the transition without self-serving motives. Perhaps most important is the challenge of community accountability—balancing the needs of the community for patient care and health improvement with the needs of the organization for adaptation.

Policy Position
ACHE believes that CEOs, their boards, and members of their senior management teams should take a systematic approach to evaluating community health status and how the stakeholders might be affected by proposed changes to organization ownership or control. To this end, ACHE offers the following as a guide.

On an ongoing basis:
• Listen to the community and identify its future health improvement requirements. This assessment should include an evaluation of current health status, available health care resources, health improvement initiatives, and anticipated future needs.
• Ensure that a plan exists for providing care to the underserved in the community and for the continuation of other essential community services.

Before considering a change in ownership or control:
• Identify your organization's values and goals.
• Understand any legal limitations of your organization's certificate of incorporation, articles of organization, charter, or other binding documents that may restrict the consideration of alternatives.

- Establish a code of conduct and specific criteria that the board, management team and other staff, and medical staff can use to evaluate proposals regarding change of ownership or control.
- Conduct a study to assess various options for change that may be available to your organization and community. The study should examine your market and understand the changes that may affect your organization's ability to fulfill its vision and mission.

When considering specific proposals related to change of ownership or control:
- Identify financial incentives that may have an undue influence on the views of board members, executives, and others involved in proposing and evaluating any change in ownership or control.
- Disclose all conflicts of interest, offers of future employment or future remuneration, and other benefits related to the transaction.
- Evaluate proposals in terms of their likely impact on community health care and health status, organization mission and values, protection of the community's assets, and financial viability. Assess the compatibility between your organization's values and philosophy and those of your potential partner.
- Gain a thorough understanding of all of the terms of the proposed transaction and of all collateral agreements.
- Develop and implement a communications plan that involves and informs all constituencies.

If the decision is made to proceed with a change of ownership or control:
- Obtain a valuation, by a party not involved in the transaction, of charitable assets being converted or restructured to ensure that reasonable value is received or used in structuring the transaction.
- Prohibit private inurement or personal financial gain by individuals involved in the transaction.
- Ensure that control and administration of any foundation or charitable trust that would be created by the transaction be distinct from the restructured health care organization and that the foundation or trust continues to serve a health care–related charitable purpose in the community.
- Require that any foundation or trust created provide regular reports to the community on its efforts to improve community health status.
- Explain to the community the issues related to the change in ownership or control, the decision-making process, and how the transaction will benefit the community.
- Provide an opportunity for public comment on the transaction before it is final.
- Publicly disclose the terms of the agreement once a letter of intent (memorandum of understanding) is signed.
- Inform the appropriate federal, state, and local officials of the terms of the transaction in accordance with their requirements.
- Develop and implement a restructuring plan that provides for fair treatment of all employees.

In addition, ACHE members have a personal responsibility to

- Abide by the standards set forth in the ACHE Code of Ethics (see discussion of this in Chapter 13).
- Place community and organizational interests above personal pride, ego, or gain.
- Carry out the fiduciary responsibilities of their positions.
- Conduct all negotiations with honesty and integrity.

As consolidation and related activities continue in the health care field, organizations and their executives will be under increased scrutiny. Executives must demonstrate, through their words and actions, that their business decisions are guided by professional ethics and a commitment to improving community health status.

QUESTIONS

1. How are these guidelines for the actions of senior-level managers in HSOs during consolidation, merger, acquisition, or affiliation decisions related to their roles as strategists, leaders, and organization designers?
2. Why is it important for senior-level managers in HSOs to have governance competence during consolidation, merger, acquisition, or affiliation activities?

CASE STUDY 4: A MANAGEMENT FUNCTION QUESTIONNAIRE

For each of the following items, circle the response that most accurately depicts the HSO/HS for which you currently work or one at which you previously worked. Support your rating with examples. If you have no experience in a HSO/HS, use any organization as a frame of reference.

		High		Low	
1.	*Culture:* how well the values and beliefs are communicated and understood by organization members.	1	2	3	4
2.	*Objectives:* how well organizational objectives are articulated by senior management and understood by members.	1	2	3	4
3.	*Planning:* how well management anticipates the future and plans for future activities.	1	2	3	4
4.	*Organizing:* whether organizational arrangements are rational and the extent of coordination and cooperation among units.	1	2	3	4
5.	*Staffing:* whether there are adequate personnel with appropriate skills.	1	2	3	4
6.	*Directing:* whether managers give guidance and clear instructions.	1	2	3	4
7.	*Motivating:* whether managers positively influence subordinates and facilitate effective behavior.	1	2	3	4
8.	*Communicating:* whether the content and flow of ommunication keeps employees informed.	1	2	3	4
9.	*Controlling:* whether control methods and systems are in place and operating properly.	1	2	3	4
10.	*Decision making:* whether major decisions by senior management are reasonable and well thought out.	1	2	3	4

NOTES

1. Griffith, John R. *Can You Teach the Management Technology of Health Administration? A View of the 21st Century.* The Andrew Pattullo Lecture, the Association of University Programs in Health Administration, Washington, DC, June 1998.
2. Charns, Martin P., and Carol Ann Lockhart. "Work Design." In *Essentials of Health Care Management,* edited by Stephen M. Shortell and Arnold D. Kaluzny, 198–219. Albany, NY: Delmar Publishers, 1997.
3. Longest, Beaufort B., Jr. *Health Policymaking in the United States,* 2nd ed., 1–2. Chicago: Health Administration Press, 1998.

4. Brook, Robert H., and Elizabeth A. McGlynn. "Maintaining Quality of Care." In *Health Services Research: Key to Health Policy,* edited by Eli Ginzberg, pp. 284–314. Cambridge, MA: Harvard University Press, 1991.

5. Blum, Henrik K. *Expanding Health Care Horizons: From a General Systems Concept of Health to a National Health Policy,* 2nd ed. Oakland, CA: Third Party Publishing, 1983.

6. Shortell, Stephen M., Robin R. Gillies, David A. Anderson, Karen Morgan Erickson, and John B. Mitchell. *Remaking Healthcare in America: Building Organized Delivery Systems.* San Francisco: Jossey-Bass, 1996.

7. Satinsky, Marjorie A. *The Foundations of Integrated Care: Facing the Challenges of Change.* Chicago: American Hospital Publishing, 1997.

8. Shortell, Gillies, Anderson, Erickson, and Mitchell, *Remaking Healthcare in America,* 7.

9. Goldsmith, Jeff. "The Illusive Logic of Integration," *Healthcare Forum Journal* 35 (August/September 1994): 26–31; Slomski, Anita J. "Maybe Bigger Isn't Better After All." *Medical Economics* 72 (February 27, 1995): 55–60.

10. Luke, Roice D., and James W. Begun. "Permeating Organizational Boundaries: The Challenge of Integration in Healthcare." *Frontiers of Health Services Management* 13 (Fall 1996): 46.

11. Bateman, Thomas S., and Carl P. Zeithaml. *Management Function and Strategy,* 25. Homewood, IL: Irwin, 1990.

12. Griffith, John R. *The Well-Managed Health Care Organization,* 4th ed., 130. Chicago: Health Administration Press/AUPHA Press, 1999.

13. Longest, Beaufort B., Jr. *Health Professionals in Management,* 43. Stamford, CT: Appleton & Lange, 1996.

14. Darr, Kurt. "Importance and Relevance of the Organizational Philosophy." *Hospital Topics* 65 (July/August 1987): 9.

15. Conner, Daryl. "Corporate Culture: Healthcare's Change Master." *Healthcare Executive* 5 (March/April 1990): 28.

16. Deal, Terrence E. "Healthcare Executives as Symbolic Leaders." *Healthcare Executive* 5 (March/April 1990): 25.

17. Brozovich, John P., and Stephen M. Shortell. "How to Create More Humane and Productive Health Care Environments." *Health Care Management Review* 9 (Fall 1984): 47.

18. Friedman, Emily. "Ethics and Corporate Culture: Finding a Fit." *Healthcare Executive* 5 (March/April 1990): 18.

19. Gibson, Kendrick C., David J. Newton, and Daniel S. Cochran. "An Empirical Investigation of Hospital Mission Statements." *Health Care Management Review* 15 (Summer 1990): 35–36.

20. Stevens, Rosemary. "The Hospital as a Social Institution, New-Fashioned for the 1990s." *Hospital & Health Services Administration* 36 (Summer 1991): 172.

21. Zuckerman, Howard S. "Redefining the Role of the CEO: Challenges and Conflicts." *Hospital & Health Services Administration* 34 (Spring 1989): 35–36.

22. Deal, "Healthcare Executives," 25.

23. Crosby, Philip B. *Quality Without Tears: The Art of Hassle-Free Management.* New York: McGraw-Hill, 1984; Deming, W. Edwards. *Out of the Crisis.* Cambridge, MA: The MIT Press, 1986; Juran, Joseph M. *Juran on Planning for Quality.* New York: The Free Press, 1988.

24. Darr, "Importance and Relevance," 9; Darr, Kurt. "Applying the Deming Method in Hospitals, Part 1." *Hospital Topics* 67 (November/December 1989): 4–5.

25. Metzger, Norman. "The Changing Health Care Workplace: A Challenge for Management Development." *Journal of Management Development* (Special Issue on Health Care) 10 (1991): 55.

26. Blair, John D., and Myron D. Fottler. "Effective Stakeholder Management: Challenges, Opportunities and Strategies." In *Handbook of Health Care Management,* edited by W. Jack Duncan, Peter M. Ginter, and Linda E. Swayne, 19–48. Malden, MA: Blackwell, 1998.

27. Fottler, Myron D., John D. Blair, Carlton J. Whitehead, Michael D. Laus, and Grant T. Savage. "Assessing Key Stakeholders: Who Matters to Hospitals and Why?" *Hospital & Health Services Administration* 34 (Winter 1989): 525–546.

28. Blair and Fottler, "Effective Stakeholder Management."

29. Levey, Samuel, and James Hill. "Between Survival and Social Responsibility: In Search of an Ethical Balance." *Journal of Health Administration Education* 4 (Spring 1986): 225–231.

30. Flood, Ann B., Stephen M. Shortell, and W. Richard Scott. "Organizational Performance: Managing for Efficiency and Effectiveness." In *Essentials of Health Care Management,* edited by Stephen M. Shortell and Arnold D. Kaluzny, 381–429. Albany, NY: Delmar Publishers, 1997.

31. Shortell, Stephen M. "High Performing Health Care Organizations: Guidelines for the Pursuit of Excellence." *Hospital & Health Services Administration* 30 (July–August 1985): 7–35.

32. Longest, Beaufort B., Jr. "Relationships Between Coordination, Efficiency, and Quality of Care in General Hospitals." *Hospital & Health Services Administration* 19 (Winter 1974): 65–86; Shortell, Stephen M., Selwyn W. Becker, and Duncan Neuhauser. "The Effects of Management Practices on Hospital Efficiency and Quality of Care." In *Organizational Research in Hospitals,* edited by Stephen M. Shortell and Montague Brown, 90–107. Chicago: Blue Cross Association, 1976.

33. Payne, Beverley C., Thomas F. Lyons, and Evelyn Neuhaus. "Relationship of Physician Characteristics to Performance Quality and Improvement." *Health Services Research* 19 (August 1984): 307–332.

34. Morlock, Laura L., Charles Nathanson, Susan Horn, and David Schumacher. "Organizational Factors Associated with the Quality of Care in Seventeen General Acute Hospitals." Paper presented at the Annual Meeting of the Association of University Programs in Health Administration, 1979, Toronto; Mark, Barbara. "Task and Structural Correlates of Organizational Effectiveness in Private Psychiatric Hospitals." *Health Services Research* 20 (June 1985): 199–224.

35. Kaluzny, Arnold D. "Revitalizing Decision-Making at the Middle Management Level." *Hospital & Health Services Administration* 34 (Spring 1989): 39–51.

36. Carroll, Stephen J., and Dennis J. Gillen. "Are the Classical Management Functions Useful in Describing Managerial Work?" *Academy of Management Review* 12 (January 1987): 38–51.

37. Zuckerman, Howard S., and William L. Dowling. "The Managerial Role." In *Health Care Management: Organization Design and Behavior,* 3rd ed., edited by Stephen M. Shortell and Arnold D. Kaluzny, 33. Albany, NY: Delmar Publishers, 1994.

38. Katz, Robert L., "Skills of an Effective Administrator." *Harvard Business Review* 52 (September–October 1974): 90–102.

39. Mintzberg, Henry. *The Nature of Managerial Work.* New York: Harper & Row, 1973; Mintzberg, Henry. "The Manager's Job: Folklore and Fact." *Harvard Business Review* 53 (July–August 1975): 49–61.

40. Zuckerman, "Redefining the Role"; Zuckerman and Dowling, "The Managerial Role."

41. Ginter, Peter M., Linda M. Swayne, and W. Jack Duncan. *Strategic Management of Health Care Organizations,* 3rd ed. Malden, MA: Blackwell, 1998.

42. Vladeck, Bruce C. "Health Care Leadership in the Public Interest." *Frontiers of Health Services Management* 8 (Spring 1992): 10.

43. Asay, Lyal D., and Joseph A. Maciariello. *Executive Leadership in Health Care.* San Francisco: Jossey-Bass, 1991.

44. This section is adapted from Longest, Beaufort B., Jr. "Managerial Competence at Senior Levels of Integrated Delivery Systems." *Journal of Healthcare Management* 43 (March/April 1998): 115–135.

45. Katz, "Skills of an Effective Administrator."

46. Savage, Grant T., Rosemary L. Taylor, Timothy M. Rotarius, and John A. Buesseler. "Governance of Integrated Delivery Systems/Networks: A Stakeholder Approach." *Healthcare Management Review* 22 (Winter 1997): 8.

47. Hudak, Ronald P., Paul P. Brooke, Jr., Kenn Finstuen, and James Trounson. "Management Competencies for Medical Practice Executives: Skills, Knowledge and Abilities Required for the Future." *Journal of Health Administration Education* 15 (Fall 1997): 219–239.

48. Longest, Beaufort B., Jr. *Seeking Strategic Advantage Through Health Policy Analysis.* Chicago: Health Administration Press, 1997.

49. Longest, *Seeking Strategic Advantage*; Longest, *Health Policymaking.*

50. Kingdon, John W. *Agendas, Alternatives, and Public Policies,* 2nd ed. New York: HarperCollins College Publishers, 1995.

51. Zelman, Walter A. *The Changing Healthcare Marketplace: Private Ventures, Public Interests.* San Francisco: Jossey-Bass, 1996.

52. Mintzberg, Henry. *Power In and Around Organizations.* Englewood Cliffs, NJ: Prentice-Hall, 1983.

53. Orlikoff, James E., and Mark K. Totten. *The Future of Health Care Governance: Redesigning Boards for a New Era.* Chicago: American Hospital Publishing, 1996.

54. Gamm, Larry D. "Dimensions of Accountability for Not-for-Profit Hospitals and Health Systems." *Healthcare Management Review* 21 (Spring 1996): 74–75.

55. Shortell, Stephen M., and Arnold D. Kaluzny. "Organization Theory and Health Services Management." In *Essentials of Healthcare Management,* edited by Stephen M. Shortell and Arnold D. Kaluzny, 19. Albany, NY: Delmar Publishers, 1997.

56. Pointer, Dennis D., and Charles M. Ewell. *Governance Trends and Practices: 1994 Panel Survey of Hospital Boards.* La Jolla, CA: The Governance Institute, 1994.

57. Pointer, Dennis D., Jeffrey A. Alexander, and Howard S. Zuckerman. "Loosening the Gordian Knot of Governance in Integrated Healthcare Delivery Systems." *Frontiers of Health Services Management* 11 (Spring 1995): 3–37.

58. Molinari, Carol, Laura L. Morlock, Jeffrey A. Alexander, and Charles A. Lyles. "Hospital Board Effectiveness: Relationships Between Governing Board Composition and Hospital Financial Viability." *Health Services Research* 28:3 (August 1993): 358–377.

59. Longest, *Seeking Strategic Advantage.*

60. Zuckerman, "Redefining the Role," 27.

61. American Hospital Association. *Ethical Conduct for Health Care Institutions: Management Advisory,* 1–2. Chicago: American Hospital Association, 1992.

62. Excerpted from American Hospital Association, Institutional Policies Committee, *Role and Functions of Hospital Executive Management: Management Advisory,* 1–4. Chicago: American Hospital Association, 1990. Reprinted by permission of the American Hospital Association, copyright 1990.

63. From *The Role of the Healthcare Executive in a Consolidation Merger, Acquisition, or Affiliation.* Chicago: American College of Healthcare Executives. Reprinted with permission of the American College of Healthcare Executives.

SELECTED BIBLIOGRAPHY

Asay, Lyal D., and Joseph A. Maciariello. *Executive Leadership in Health Care.* San Francisco: Jossey-Bass, 1991.

Bateman, Thomas S., and Carl P. Zeithaml. *Management Function and Strategy.* Homewood, IL: Irwin, 1990.

Blair, John D., and Myron D. Fottler. "Effective Stakeholder Management." In *Handbook of Health Care Management,* edited by Duncan, W. Jack, Peter M. Ginter, and Linda E. Swayne, 19–48. Malden, MA: Blackwell, 1998.

Brown, Montague. "Mergers, Networking, and Vertical Integration: Managed Care and Investor-Owned Hospitals." *Health Care Management Review* 21 (Winter 1996): 29–37.

Carroll, Stephen J., and Dennis J. Gillen. "Are the Classical Management Functions Useful in Describing Managerial Work?" *Academy of Management Review* 12 (January 1987): 38–51.

Coddington, Dean C., Keith D. Moore, and Elizabeth A. Fischer. *Making Integrated Healthcare Work.* Englewood, CO: Center for Research in Ambulatory Healthcare Administration, 1996.

Crosby, Philip B. *Quality Without Tears: The Art of Hassle-Free Management.* New York: McGraw-Hill, 1984.

Darr, Kurt. "Importance and Relevance of the Organizational Philosophy." *Hospital Topics* 65 (July/August 1987): 9.

Darr, Kurt. "Applying the Deming Method in Hospitals, Part 1." *Hospital Topics* 67 (November/December 1989): 4–5.

Darr, Kurt. "Applying the Deming Method in Hospitals, Part 2." *Hospital Topics* 68 (Winter 1990): 4–6.

Deal, Terrence E. "Healthcare Executives as Symbolic Leaders." *Healthcare Executive* 5 (March/April 1990): 25.

Deming, W. Edwards. *Out of the Crisis.* Cambridge, MA: The MIT Press, 1986.

Fottler, Myron D., John D. Blair, Carlton J. Whitehead, Michael D. Laus, and Grant T. Savage. "Assessing Key Stakeholders: Who Matters to Hospitals and Why?" *Hospital & Health Services Administration* 34 (Winter 1989): 525–546.

Gamm, Larry D. "Dimensions of Accountability for Not-for-Profit Hospitals and Health Systems." *Healthcare Management Review* 21 (Spring 1996): 74–86.

Gibson, Kendrick C., David J. Newton, and Daniel S. Cochran. "An Empirical Investigation of Hospital Mission Statements." *Health Care Management Review* 15 (Summer 1990): 35–36.

Ginter, Peter M., Linda M. Swayne, and W. Jack Duncan. *Strategic Management of Health Care Organizations,* 3rd ed. Malden, MA: Blackwell, 1998.

Goldsmith, Jeff. "The Illusive Logic of Integration." *Healthcare Forum Journal* 35 (August/September 1994): 26–31.

Griffith, John R. *The Well-Managed Health Care Organization,* 4th ed. Chicago: AUPHA Press/Health Administration Press, 1999.

Hudak, Ronald P., Paul P. Brooke, Jr., Kenn Finstuen, and James Trounson. "Management Competencies for Medical Practice Executives: Skills, Knowledge and Abilities Required for the Future." *Journal of Health Administration Education* 15 (Fall 1997): 219–239.

Juran, Joseph M. *Juran on Planning for Quality.* New York: The Free Press, 1988.

Kaluzny, Arnold D. "Revitalizing Decision-Making at the Middle Management Level." *Hospital & Health Services Administration* 34 (Spring 1989): 39–51.

Katz, Robert L., "Skills of an Effective Administrator." *Harvard Business Review* 52 (September–October 1974): 90–102.

Longest, Beaufort B., Jr. *Health Professionals in Management.* Stamford, CT: Appleton & Lange, 1996.

Longest, Beaufort B., Jr. *Seeking Strategic Advantage Through Health Policy Analysis.* Chicago: Health Administration Press, 1997.

Longest, Beaufort B., Jr. *Health Policymaking in the United States,* 2nd ed. Chicago: Health Administration Press, 1998.

Longest, Beaufort B., Jr. "Managerial Competence at Senior Levels of Integrated Delivery Systems." *Journal of Healthcare Management* 43 (March/April 1998): 115–135.

Luke, Roice D., and James W. Begun. "Permeating Organizational Boundaries: The Challenge of Integration in Healthcare." *Frontiers of Health Services Management* 13 (Fall 1996): 46–49.

Metzger, Norman. "The Changing Health Care Workplace: A Challenge for Management Development." *Journal of Management Development* (Special Issue on Health Care) 10 (1991): 55.

Mintzberg, Henry. *The Nature of Managerial Work.* New York: Harper & Row, 1973.

Mintzberg, Henry. "The Manager's Job: Folklore and Fact." *Harvard Business Review* 53 (July–August 1975): 49–61.

Mintzberg, Henry. *Power In and Around Organizations.* Englewood Cliffs, NJ: Prentice-Hall, 1983.

Molinari, Carol, Laura L. Morlock, Jeffrey A. Alexander, and Charles A. Lyles. "Hospital Board Effectiveness: Relationships Between Governing Board Composition and Hospital Financial Viability." *Health Services Research* 28 (August 1993): 358–377.

Orlikoff, James E., and Mark K. Totten. *The Future of Health Care Governance: Redesigning Boards for a New Era.* Chicago: American Hospital Publishing, 1996.

Pointer, Dennis D., Jeffrey A. Alexander, and Howard S. Zuckerman. "Loosening the Gordian Knot of Governance in Integrated Healthcare Delivery Systems." *Frontiers of Health Services Management* 11 (Spring 1995): 3–37.

Pointer, Dennis D., and Charles M. Ewell. *Governance Trends and Practices: 1994 Panel Survey of Hospital Boards.* La Jolla, CA: The Governance Institute, 1994.

Satinsky, Marjorie A. *The Foundations of Integrated Care: Facing the Challenges of Change.* Chicago: American Hospital Publishing, 1997.

Savage, Grant T., Rosemary L. Taylor, Timothy M. Rotarius, and John A. Buesseler. "Governance of Integrated Delivery Systems/Networks: A Stakeholder Approach." *Healthcare Management Review* 22 (Winter 1997): 7–20.

Shortell, Stephen M. "High Performing Health Care Organizations: Guidelines for the Pursuit of Excellence." *Hospital & Health Services Administration* 30 (July–August 1985): 7–35.

Shortell, Stephen M., Robin R. Gillies, David A. Anderson, Karen Morgan Erickson, and John B. Mitchell. *Remaking Healthcare in America: Building Organized Delivery Systems.* San Francisco: Jossey-Bass, 1996.

Shortell, Stephen M., and Arnold D. Kaluzny, Eds. *Health Care Management: Organization Design and Behavior,* 3rd ed. Albany, NY: Delmar Publishers, 1994.

Shortell, Stephen M., and Arnold D. Kaluzny, Eds. *Essentials of Health Care Management.* Albany, NY: Delmar Publishers, 1997.

Stevens, Rosemary. "The Hospital as a Social Institution, New-Fashioned for the 1990s." *Hospital & Health Services Administration* 36 (Summer 1991): 163–173.

Vladeck, Bruce C. "Health Care Leadership in the Public Interest." *Frontiers of Health Services Management* 8 (Spring 1992): 1–26.

Zelman, Walter A. *The Changing Healthcare Marketplace: Private Ventures, Public Interests.* San Francisco: Jossey-Bass, 1996.

Zuckerman, Howard S. "Redefining the Role of the CEO: Challenges and Conflicts." *Hospital & Health Services Administration* 34 (Spring 1989): 25–38.

2 The Health Care System

The health care system [functions] through complex interactions among government, health professionals, consumers, third party payers, employers, and delivery systems. These groups use competition, standards, and regulation to pursue a balance in their respective health care goals of access, finance, and quality. There is no single source of governance or health policy, nor is there a single set of shared values or goals among these groups: the health care system is an amalgamation of many different agendas.[1]

This chapter describes the U.S. health care system—the general environment in which health services organization (HSO) and health system (HS) managers work. It develops conceptual frameworks and presents information about health care resources that show historical development, nature, extent, and relationships. Resources include HSOs/HSs, programs, personnel, technology, and financing. Detailed information about several types of HSOs—including acute care hospitals, hospice, managed care organizations, nursing facilities, ambulatory care organizations, birth centers, and home health agencies—is provided in Chapter 4. In addition, Chapter 5 includes information about HSs.

Data presented here describe the manager's environment. Successful managers have a comprehensive and accurate understanding of the world beyond their organization—this includes a thorough understanding of trends and developments. The management model in Chapter 1 describes this relationship and should be referenced by readers as necessary (see Figure 1.7). Data are drawn from numerous sources. The most common source is private groups, as supplemented by the federal government. Substantial reliance is placed on figures and tables. Readers should understand the individual presentations and their interactions, and consider the effects that various system segments have on one another.

U.S. national health expenditures in 1998 were $1.1 trillion, or more than $4,000 per capita. The 13.5% of gross domestic product (GDP) spent on health care in 1998 equaled that in 1997 as the low-

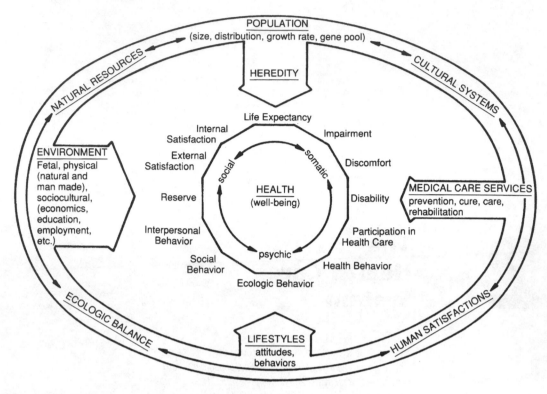

Figure 2.1.   The force-field and well-being paradigms of health. (From Blum, Henrik K. *Expanding Health Care Horizons: From a General Systems Concept of Health to a National Health Policy,* 2nd ed., 37. Oakland, CA: Third Party Publishing, 1983; reprinted by permission.)

est percentage since 1992. For 1993–1998, slow growth in health care spending combined with increases in GDP halted the steady upward trend as a percentage of GDP that had been observed since the 1960s[2] (see also Table 2.4). However, expenditures are projected to double from $1.1 trillion in 1998 to $2.2 trillion in 2008, which will be 16.2% of the GDP. Growth in health spending is projected to average 1.8 percentage points above the growth rate of the GDP for 1998–2008.[3] Such huge sums suggest the magnitude of the problems and opportunities that confront HSO/HS managers.

HEALTH AND SYSTEM GOALS

Chapter 1 distinguished the health care system from the health services system. Blum's model, shown in Figure 2.1, conceptualizes the elements affecting health. It portrays medical care services (prevention, cure, care, rehabilitation) as much less important than the environment and somewhat less important than heredity and lifestyles in affecting health (well-being). In explaining the model, Blum states that the "largest aggregate of forces resides in the person's environment. One's own behavior, in great part derived from one's experience with one's environment, is seen as the next largest force affecting health."[4] Managers must understand other influences on health status, both as factors that lead to an episode of illness and the effect that these factors have on recovery and long-term absence of illness and minimization of disability, if the individual is subjected to them again. HSO managers must have a broad view of illness and health, and this requires looking beyond the organization. They must understand that, at best, the health services system has a limited effect and can provide only stopgap measures if negative influences on health undo what has been done.

Blum suggests several goals for a health system:

- Prolonging life and preventing premature death
- Minimizing departures from physiological or functional norms by focusing attention on precursors of illness
- Minimizing discomfort (illness)
- Minimizing disability (incapacity)
- Promoting high-level "wellness" or self-fulfillment
- Promoting high-level satisfaction with the environment
- Extending resistance to ill health and creating reserve capacity
- Increasing opportunities for consumers to participate in health matters[5]

These goals are part of the conceptual framework that is applicable when using this book.

The PRECEDE-PROCEED planning model in Figure 2.2 is a more applied conceptualization of the relationships among activities that are part of health promotion planning and evaluation and that should be part of the efforts to deliver comprehensive health care.[6] Phase 1 is a social diagnosis that recognizes the relationship between health and social issues by identifying a target population's social, economic, cultural, and other nonmedical concerns and goals. The epidemiological diagnosis

PRECEDE

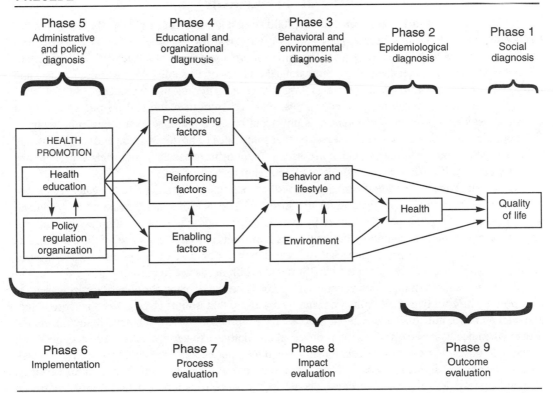

Figure 2.2. The PRECEDE-PROCEED model for health promotion planning and evaluation. (From *Health Promotion Planning: An Educational and Environmental Approach, Third Edition* by Lawrence W. Green and Marshall W. Kreuter. Copyright ©1999 by Mayfield Publishing Company. Reprinted by permission of the publisher.)

in Phase 2 appraises morbidity, disability, mortality, and demographic patterns of health problems that are linked to social concerns. The health concerns that need amelioration are listed in rank order after the objectively appraised health problems identified in Phase 2 are compared with subjectively appraised quality-of-life issues identified in Phase 1. In Phase 3 behavioral and environmental factors associated with preventing and controlling health concerns are appraised for relative importance and changeability, and intervention goals and health objectives are specified. Phase 4 compares behavioral and environmental changes needed as identified in Phase 3 with educational and organizational objectives.

The administrative and policy diagnosis in Phase 5 denotes the transition to the PROCEED portion of the model. This phase identifies available and needed resources, including staff, time, and finances. Political, bureaucratic, and organizational supports and barriers are addressed so that the strategies identified can be implemented. The result is the implementation in Phase 6. Phases 7, 8, and 9 evaluate the program in terms of process, impact, and outcome, respectively. Evaluation criteria are linked to objectives defined in the corresponding steps of the PRECEDE portion of the model. The increasing emphasis on health promotion and prevention make the PRECEDE-PROCEED model a useful tool in planning and delivering comprehensive health care, especially in integrated delivery systems.

LACK OF SYNCHRONY

The wide geographic variation in rates of hospitalization and lengths of hospital stay by diagnosis has been known for decades. Similar geographic variation was found in the 1990s in the use of nursing facilities by Medicare beneficiaries.[7] The variation in hospital use is a true difference that cannot be explained by understanding or estimating the effect of variables such as age, gender, and climate. Even more puzzling is that there are large differences in rates of hospitalization and lengths of stay by diagnosis within geographic regions, and even within individual hospitals. The most plausible explanation of these differences is physician practice patterns—variation in how physicians practice medicine. It can be hypothesized that some rates of hospitalization and lengths of stay are more appropriate than others, which means that these differences have significant implications for managers of HSOs/HSs as they strive to effectively use resources.

Other data have shown significant differences between morbidity and mortality caused by a disease and the amount of hospitalization for that disease.[8] The lack of synchrony could be explained in various ways: hospitals are constrained by available technology; hospitalization may be inappropriate to treat the medical condition that causes death or limits activity; and some medical conditions require more attention to prevention—a historical deficit for acute care hospitals. Achieving synchrony suggests that services provided by HSOs and health needs are in harmony.

There are important distinctions between the need and the demand for health services. Need is measured by morbidity and mortality data and by disability that limits activity. Need is more objective than demand, but conclusions about need are based on value judgments, nevertheless. Demand occurs when need (or perceived need) is converted into delivery of services. As suggested, need and demand do not have a one-to-one relationship. Need may not become demand because people lack knowledge about a disease or because social or cultural mores dissuade them from seeking services. Demand may be less than need because people lack financial resources or because there are no HSOs to provide health services. Furthermore, some demand is subjective; cosmetic surgery is a commonly cited example. Relationships between need and demand must be considered as health services are planned. Ethical dimensions of need and demand are addressed in Chapter 13.

A BRIEF HISTORY OF HEALTH SERVICES IN THE UNITED STATES

Technology

The importance of public health measures, such as ensuring the availability of pure food and water, was demonstrated during the "great sanitary awakening" in the mid-19th century, and this led to the establishment of state and local health departments. At about the same time, major contributions to medical knowledge resulted from the work of Pasteur, Lister, and Koch. Their efforts led to anti-sepsis and, later, asepsis, which, in addition to technology such as radiographs, inhalation anesthesia, blood typing, and improved clinical laboratories in the late 19th century, permitted efficacious surgical interventions with greatly reduced morbidity and mortality. These developments required an organization, human resources, and systems to deliver the new wonders that medicine had to offer. Acute care hospitals were an obvious choice.

It was common for acute care hospitals to be sponsored by private, not-for-profit corporations that had been formed by religious groups, concerned citizens, and wealthy benefactors; local governments sponsored others. Historically, many small "hospitals" were established as for-profit corporations, often by individual physicians who needed a place to hospitalize patients. Long-term care facilities, often called nursing homes, were rare because extended families assisted one another. People with mental illness were warehoused and isolated from society in facilities owned almost exclusively by state governments. Effective, large-scale treatment for them did not occur until after World War II with the development of psychoactive drugs. Another type of IISO sponsored by local governments was public health departments.

Mortality and Morbidity

Table 2.1 shows male and female age-adjusted death rates by causes of death since 1970, with projections to 2020. Heart disease and cancer continue to be the leading causes of death. Notably, cancer age-adjusted death rates have increased since 1970 and are projected to continue increasing well into the 21st century, before beginning to decline. Vascular disease includes stroke, which historically has been the third leading cause of death.

Except for tuberculosis, which declined rapidly by the end of the 19th century because of improved nutrition and housing, and leprosy, which never was a major medical problem in the United States, there were few chronic diseases before the 20th century. Primarily, people died of acute gastrointestinal and respiratory tract infections that usually occurred before they could develop a chronic disease. Health problems common in the mid-19th century were solved largely through the preventive measures taken by public health departments. Pure food and water and improved sanitation were major contributors.

Causes of mortality and morbidity in the 20th century were much less amenable to easy prevention or inexpensive treatment. The greater emphasis on acute services that resulted has substantially increased costs. Table 2.1 shows overall age-adjusted mortality rates steadily declining well into the 21st century. This means increased longevity and a greater likelihood of chronic diseases, which are almost certain to increase total health care costs. Figure 2.1 shows a link between lifestyle and medical problems. To be effective, many types of prevention require behavior modification, but such efforts raise questions of individual choice and liberty rights, which are more complex than purifying water and protecting food supplies. Behavior modification raises questions such as: What should be the limits of society's efforts to force people to live healthfully? What is society's obligation to aid people whose illnesses can be linked to activities known to be unhealthy?

TABLE 2.1.   FEMALE AND MALE AGE-ADJUSTED DEATH RATES BY CAUSE OF DEATH, SELECTED YEARS PER 100,000

Year	Total	Heart disease	Cancer	Vascular disease	Violence	Respiratory disease	Infancy	Digestive disease	Diabetes mellitus	Cirrhosis (liver)	AIDS	Other
Female												
1970	803.6	308.4	141.0	144.9	45.6	38.5	24.7	19.0	21.2	10.3	0.0	50.0
1975	709.1	265.2	141.4	119.8	39.6	34.3	18.2	15.8	17.4	9.5	0.0	48.0
1980	668.1	250.1	146.0	92.1	36.0	37.0	14.5	16.8	15.1	8.8	0.0	51.7
1985	638.0	227.6	150.7	73.6	31.3	45.5	11.9	16.3	14.3	7.1	0.4	59.2
1990	620.9	206.8	153.6	61.3	30.2	52.5	10.3	15.9	13.8	6.2	3.5	66.7
1991	615.0	202.5	154.2	58.5	29.6	53.1	9.9	15.8	13.5	6.1	4.5	67.4
1992	609.5	198.4	154.4	55.9	28.9	53.6	9.5	15.7	13.2	6.0	5.5	68.2
1995	594.6	186.5	156.4	48.6	27.1	55.4	8.3	15.4	12.2	5.7	8.0	70.8
2000[a]	573.5	168.4	159.3	38.9	24.5	58.7	6.8	15.1	10.9	5.4	10.1	75.5
2005[a]	553.9	153.4	161.7	32.6	22.6	61.2	5.8	14.8	9.9	5.2	7.8	78.9
2010[a]	537.0	142.6	161.5	29.2	21.7	61.7	5.3	14.5	9.4	5.1	6.5	79.4
2015[a]	521.5	134.2	159.9	26.7	21.1	61.2	4.9	14.2	9.1	5.1	6.4	78.8
2020[a]	506.7	126.5	158.0	24.5	20.5	60.5	4.5	13.9	8.8	5.0	6.4	78.0
Male												
1970	1,359.5	554.3	221.1	187.5	126.0	93.3	31.5	29.0	19.9	22.2	0.0	74.7
1975	1,237.5	491.8	229.8	156.2	113.3	87.9	22.7	23.6	17.1	21.6	0.0	73.5
1980	1,165.1	454.1	240.6	119.8	108.6	88.4	17.8	23.5	15.6	19.2	0.0	77.6
1985	1,096.4	408.5	243.2	95.1	92.2	97.7	14.8	22.5	15.2	15.7	5.5	86.0
1990	1,055.0	360.7	246.2	80.0	88.1	101.4	12.5	21.1	15.3	14.4	26.1	89.2
1991	1,047.9	353.1	247.3	76.4	86.6	101.7	11.9	20.8	15.1	14.2	31.2	89.8
1992	1,040.9	345.6	248.5	72.9	85.0	102.0	11.4	20.5	14.8	13.9	35.8	90.5
1995	1,019.3	324.4	252.1	63.5	80.6	102.9	9.9	19.6	14.1	13.1	46.4	92.6
2000[a]	981.0	292.3	258.3	50.8	73.9	105.0	8.0	18.4	13.0	12.0	52.9	96.4
2005[a]	934.0	265.8	263.2	42.5	69.0	106.8	6.8	17.5	12.1	11.3	39.7	99.3
2010[a]	900.1	246.9	263.6	38.1	66.5	106.8	6.2	17.0	11.6	11.0	32.9	99.6
2015[a]	874.0	231.9	261.1	34.8	65.1	105.9	5.7	16.6	11.2	10.9	32.0	98.7
2020[a]	850.1	218.4	258.2	32.0	63.9	104.8	5.3	16.3	10.9	10.7	31.9	97.8

Source: *Source Book of Health Insurance Data: 1997–1998*, 157–158. Washington, DC: Health Insurance Association of America, 1998.

[a]Projected.

Social Welfare

A major shift in the locus of responsibility for social welfare occurred with the Social Security Act of 1935, whose enactment resulted from the Great Depression's catastrophic economic and social problems. Before 1935, local and state governments provided social welfare. City and county governments might own a "poor farm," for example, where needy people could live and work until they could regain their independence. Since 1935 there has been a massive shift of perceived and actual responsibility for social welfare from state and local governments to the federal government. This accretion continued virtually uninterrupted until revenue sharing and other federal programs were developed in the 1970s and 1980s.

Federally sponsored national health insurance programs were proposed and seriously considered at various times during the 20th century, notably in the late 1940s and late 1960s. Such national programs were considered again in the early 1990s. At all three times these proposals covered the gamut from all-encompassing to modest interventions. They were, nevertheless, potentially costly programs. Before the 1990s, numerous factors caused the defeat of these proposals. Organized medicine's opposition is often mentioned, but its role is overstated. As important has been a lack of voter interest—many people had employer-provided private hospitalization insurance. The momentum for a universal scheme dwindled after enactment of Medicare and Medicaid in the mid-

1960s provided significant coverage for millions who had inadequate access, and as it became clear how expensive such programs could be. Distrust of government-controlled health care and the growth of managed care in the 1990s blunted the public's interest in national health insurance, developments that are likely to continue well into the 21st century.

In 1998, 12.7% of the population was age 65 or older; by 2050 it is projected that this proportion will grow to 20.0%.[9] These data suggest that there will be greatly increased demand for health services in geriatrics, chronic diseases, rehabilitation, and institutional long-term care. Unanswered is how these needs will be financed.

Federal Initiatives

The beneficiaries of early federal programs were primarily not-for-profit acute care hospitals, including those operated by state and local governments. From 1946 to 1981, the Hill-Burton Act (Hospital Survey and Construction Act of 1946, PL 79-725)[10] provided more than $4 billion in grants, loans, and guaranteed loans in a federal–state matching program. Hill-Burton aided nearly 6,000 hospitals and other health services facilities in more than 4,000 communities. Initially, the funds were used to construct new inpatient (acute care hospital) facilities; later they were used to remodel and construct outpatient facilities. The number of hospitals increased by more than 800 in this period. In return for Hill-Burton assistance, organizations agreed to provide a reasonable volume of services to people unable to pay (uncompensated services) for lengths of time that varied by the type of assistance. The annual dollar volume of uncompensated services to be provided was equal to the lesser of 3% of operating costs or 10% of the amount of federal assistance received, adjusted for inflation.[11] These repayment obligations have been met.

Figure 2.3 shows trends in the U.S. health services system since 1945. "Escalation in health care costs" and the "emphasis on secondary and tertiary care and inadequate attention to other levels of care" effects are important in the "reactions" and "results" sections of the figure. Figure 2.3 provides an important contextual framework for understanding health care and health services in the United States.

Other federal government programs provided additional resources, including generous funding for research activities that became the National Institutes of Health (NIH), which began experimentation on cancer in the 1930s. In 1999 there were 18 institutes and 7 centers and related activities, such as the National Library of Medicine and the Clinical Center.[12] In 1999 the NIH budget was $15.6 billion, more than double the $7.6 billion in 1990 and nearly quintuple the $3.4 billion in 1980 (for nine institutes and related activities). NIH provides grants to more than 25,000 research projects in universities, medical schools, and independent research institutions.[13]

Federal programs to educate more physicians, nurses, technicians, and managers were established and funded in the 1960s. It was clear to Congress that the knowledge produced by NIH and the hospitals built by Hill-Burton could improve health status only if members of the health professions were available in sufficient numbers.

During the same postwar period, the federal government built large numbers of Veterans Administration (now Department of Veterans Affairs [DVA]) hospitals to provide services to former military personnel. The DVA system is separate from services that are provided to groups in special categories, including inmates in federal prisons, Native Americans, and active-duty and retired military personnel and their dependents in Army, Navy, and Air Force hospitals.

In 1965 amendments to the Social Security Act of 1935 directed the federal government to pay for health services to two large groups, under the Medicare and Medicaid programs. (The appendix at the end of this chapter provides a brief but concise overview of the Medicare and Medicaid programs.) An exclusively federal program, Medicare pays for services rendered to people ages 65 and older and to people with severe and permanent disabilities. Originally, Medicare comprised only

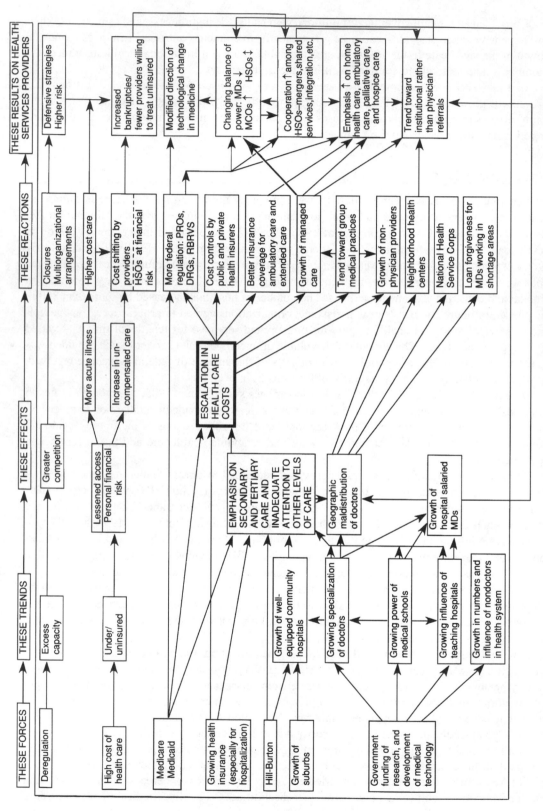

Figure 2.3. Trends in the U.S. health care system since 1945. (From Cambridge Research Institute. *Trends Affecting the U.S. Health Care System* [Health Planning In-formation Series], 409. Washington, DC: Human Resources Administration, 1976. Revised and updated by the authors, 2000.)

Parts A and B, benefits for both of which have been substantially enhanced in the interim. Part A paid for inpatient hospital services; Part B paid for physicians' services. The Balanced Budget Act of 1997 (PL 105-33)[14] added Part C, which expands the types of health plans from which Medicare beneficiaries may choose to receive their Medicare benefits. Choices include fee-for-service, coordinated care plans, provider service organizations, and medical savings accounts.[15] Medicaid is a state–federal cost-sharing program that pays for certain health services of people who meet eligibility criteria based on income levels set by each state. Both Medicare and Medicaid have become major programs as measured in numbers of beneficiaries and expenditures.

Meanwhile, there were federal efforts to rationalize the health services system.[16] The Comprehensive Health Planning and Public Health Service Amendments Act of 1966 (PL 89-749) was the first effort. It built on existing voluntary planning and the modest planning requirements in the Hill-Burton Act and was designed to enhance the use of planning processes and techniques in the health services system. This legislation was amplified and expanded with passage of the National Health Planning and Resources Development Act of 1974 (PL 93-641). This law was a major change that increased the control that planning agencies had over the expansion of hospitals and services— in an attempt to regulate the number of services. An effort to monitor the use and quality of services provided under Medicare and Medicaid programs was enacted when the Social Security Amendments of 1972 (PL 92-603) established professional standards review organizations (PSROs). Political changes caused a reassessment of the usefulness of the planning and PSRO programs. Federal support of planning ended. PSROs were replaced by peer review organizations (PROs), which are discussed later in this chapter.

Such regulatory controls were thought to be essential to slow rapid increases in health care costs. In general, however, they proved ineffective. Except for four years between 1969 and 1996, medical care items measured in the consumer price index (CPI) had the highest rates of increase, usually by wide margins. In several years, the average annual percentage changes for hospital services were two or three times the annual percentage changes for all items measured by the CPI.[17] Health care costs are discussed in more detail later in this chapter.

The Tax Equity and Fiscal Responsibility Act of 1982 (PL 97-248) and the Social Security Amendments of 1983 (PL 98-21) established a prospective payment system to address the problem of cost increases in hospitals.[18] Medicare reimbursement is determined prospectively and is based on diagnosis-related groups (DRGs), which tie the payment from the federal government for Medicare patients to a hospital's case mix. Since the mid-1970s, state governments also have been concerned about rising health services costs. They focused on certificate of need (CON) and rate review. States control Medicaid expenditures by setting arbitrary limits on what they will pay, typically causing providers to incur losses for Medicaid patients.

These federal legislative initiatives forced hospitals to become more efficient. Hospitals cannot control their environments, however. In addition, they may have to provide large amounts of uncompensated care. Under such circumstances, hospitals can survive only if they find other revenue sources. Previously, unpaid costs were shifted to Blue Cross, commercial insurance companies, and private-pay patients. Third-party payers have become unwilling to bear this cost shifting. This leaves only private-pay patients—a group that is too small to make up the difference. Beyond the issue of fairness, cost shifting is a major political issue, especially with regard to the uninsured and the costs of medical education. To protect themselves financially, hospitals and other HSOs are developing new organizational entities and relationships through corporate restructuring, joint ventures, and participation in HSs. The result is a mix of not-for-profit and for-profit organizations that may produce an enhanced revenue stream to offset deficits. These developments are discussed in Chapter 5.

Managed care, largely delivered through health maintenance organizations (HMOs), has been important in moderating the rate of increase in health care costs. Managed care may have achieved its maximum economic effect, however. Evidence for this includes a need for managed care organizations to recoup losses, higher prescription drug costs, the difficulty of wresting additional price concessions from physicians and hospitals, and the fact that the one-time savings that resulted when employees changed to managed care has been realized. HMO costs are estimated to be growing as fast as or faster than the costs of traditional health insurance.[19] In addition, anecdotes that assert that economics drive certain physician decision making may be overstated, as in the case in which equalizing payments to physicians for caesarean sections and vaginal deliveries did not decrease the number of caesarean sections. The opportunity costs of waiting out a difficult labor, the fear of malpractice suits, and the impact of a bad outcome on self-respect, reputation, and long-term profits may be more important to caesarean decisions than current fees.[20]

OTHER WESTERN SYSTEMS

By comparison, Western Europe, notably Germany and England, had government involvement in financing health services much earlier than did the United States. In 1883 Chancellor Otto von Bismarck achieved passage of a social insurance scheme, including a health services component, for certain working-class Germans. In 1911 England adopted a national health insurance program, and in 1948 the United Kingdom established the National Health Service, which included government ownership of the health services system. Western European and Canadian health services systems have, in general, much more governmental control and proportion of financing than do those in the United States.

It is noteworthy that, despite greater government involvement in planning and financing, in the past many of these countries experienced inflation in health services costs that was similar to that in the United States. However, since about 1985, U.S. increases have been well ahead of those in all other countries.[21] Countries where budgetary allocations to health services are determined prospectively spend substantially less than the United States. For example, in 1996 Canada spent 9.2% ($2,002 per capita) of its GDP on health services, Germany spent 10.5% ($2,222 per capita), the United Kingdom spent 6.9% ($1,304 per capita), and the United States consumed 14.2% ($3,708 per capita) of GDP.[22] One reason for the difference is that the United Kingdom and Canada spend far less on high technology. Furthermore, elective and nonemergent procedures may be available only after long waiting periods, called queues.

One gains a unique perspective of international health expenditures by comparing governmental and discretionary expenditures. In 1997 the percentage of GDP spent on health by the governments of Australia (5.7%), Canada (6.4%), New Zealand (5.9%), the United Kingdom (5.7%), and the United States (6.4%) were remarkably alike. It is private (discretionary) spending—only 1.0% in the United Kingdom (New Zealand, 1.7%; Australia, 2.6%; and Canada, 2.9%) but 7.2% in the United States—that puts total U.S. health expenditures at such a high level.[185]

PRESENT STRUCTURE OF THE HEALTH SERVICES SYSTEM

Various types of HSOs/HSs are found in the private (owned by individuals or groups) and public (owned by government) sectors. HSOs may be institutions, the most prominent of which are hospitals and nursing facilities, or they may be agencies and programs such as public health departments and visiting nurse associations (VNAs). Information about selected HSOs is found in Chapter 4. Various HSOs are aggregated into HSs for greater efficiency and a seamless web of services, and in this regard they are orienting their activities toward the health of populations and communities. HSOs and HSs depend on their environments (see Figure 1.7). The range of health services delivery and various providers is shown in Figure 2.4.

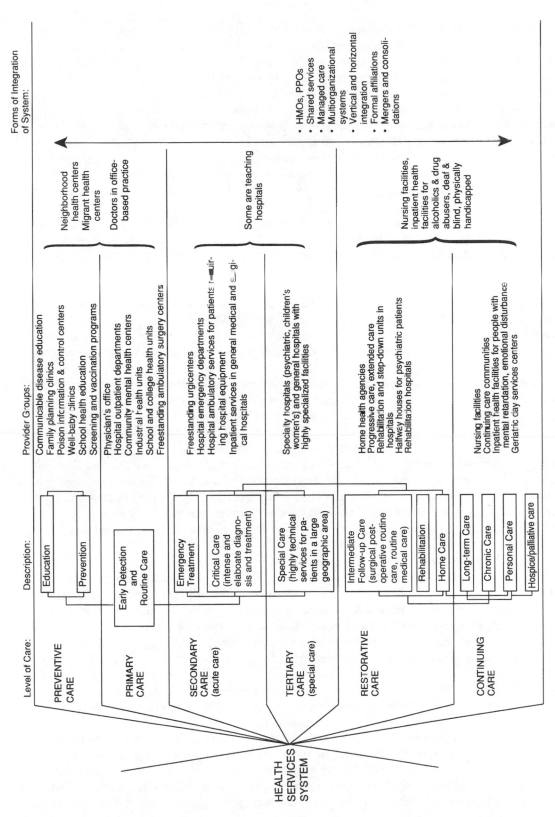

Figure 2.4. Spectrum of health services delivery. (From Cambridge Research Institute. *Trends Affecting the U.S. Health Care System* [Health Planning Information Series], 262. Washington, DC: Human Resources Administration, 1976. Revised and updated by the authors, 2000.)

One way in which HSOs/HSs can improve their focus on populations and communities is to develop community care networks, which have the following objectives: increasing access and coverage, enhancing accountability to the community, imbuing the health care system with a community health focus, improving coordination among the many parts of the health care system, and using health care resources more efficiently. Participants include insurers, business alliances, schools, churches, social services agencies, public health departments, local governments, and community-based organizations, in addition to health systems, hospitals, clinics, and physician groups. An estimated 26% of hospitals participated in community care networks in 1996.[23] Health departments can take a leading role in coordinating disparate providers and minimizing political and competitive issues to deliver integrated and comprehensive community health services.[24] Delivery of integrated services is discussed in Chapter 5, and community health information networks are discussed in Chapter 6.

Preventive care is an essential part of meeting the needs of a population. It comprises two parts, education and prevention. Health education is a long-standing part of general education in grammar and high schools, and occurs when health services are delivered. Prevention can be divided into three parts—primary, secondary, and tertiary. Primary prevention involves prevention of the disease or injury itself. Examples of primary prevention include improved design of highways, school education programs concerning use of tobacco and substance abuse, and immunization against poliomyelitis or measles. Secondary prevention blocks progression of an injury or disease from an impairment to a disability. Use of the Papanicolaou smear (Pap test) to identify early cellular changes that are precursors of cervical cancer is a type of secondary prevention. Impairment has already occurred, but disability (or death) may be prevented through early intervention. Treatment of certain streptococcal infections with penicillin can prevent the occasional development of rheumatic fever and serious heart disease. Early detection and treatment of high blood pressure can reduce the probability of a heart attack or stroke. Tertiary prevention blocks or retards the progression of a disability to a state of dependence. The early detection and effective management of diabetes can prevent some of the dependencies associated with the disease, or at least slow the rate of progression. Prompt medical care followed by rehabilitation can limit the damage caused by a cerebrovascular accident (stroke); the same is true for heart attacks. Good vehicular design can reduce the dependency that might otherwise occur as a result of an accident.[25] HSOs such as state and local public health departments have programs at all three levels of prevention. Traditionally, hospitals and nursing facilities, for example, were more likely to engage in secondary and tertiary prevention than in primary prevention.

As indicated in Figure 2.4, primary care is delivered in a number of settings, the most common of which are physicians' offices, clinics, and outpatient units of acute care hospitals. Primary care is a source not only of routine care but also of early detection, which overlaps with secondary and perhaps tertiary prevention. In addition, acute care hospitals provide secondary and tertiary services through emergency treatment and inpatient services. Restorative care may be provided in acute care hospitals but is also available in specialized hospitals, in nursing facilities, and in the home. Continuing care is available in a variety of settings, including the home, nursing facilities, and hospice.

Holistic, alternative, and complementary medicine are similar concepts that greatly broaden the theories about disease prevention, causation, and treatment. They focus on nontraditional medicine, with special emphasis placed on interventions that are less dramatic than chemicals and surgery, are more focused on self-help, and stress health promotion and prevention. Such measures are increasingly considered an adjunct to allopathy. Allopathic medicine is traditional Western medicine, which emphasizes dramatic interventions such as use of chemicals and surgery to return the body to normal functioning.[26] Increased use of nontraditional medicine will significantly affect HSOs/HSs, physician (allopathic) practice, and health care financing. It is likely that using alternative sources will only shift where payment is made, not reduce total costs to the system. In fact, total costs are likely to increase at least in proportion to the increases in the number of alternate sources of care. The issues of third-party coverage and payment and the effects on total costs and the delivery of care are only beginning to be addressed.

The majority of physician–patient interactions occur in physicians' offices. In 1995, 56.6% of interactions occurred in physicians' offices; only 12.6% occurred in hospital outpatient clinics, emergency departments, and other hospital contacts.[27] Despite a trend for physicians to be employed by HSOs/HSs, most remain self-employed entrepreneurs who may share a receptionist, billing, patient coverage, and perhaps diagnostic equipment with another physician, or they may be in a partnership or may be "employees" of a physician (professional) corporation such as a multi-specialty group practice.

CLASSIFICATION AND TYPES OF HSOs

Profit or Not for Profit

HSOs/HSs may be classified by whether they seek to make a profit (for profit or investor owned) that is paid to owners (investors), or whether the profit (sometimes called excess of income over expense) is not available to any person or corporation (not for profit) and is used by the HSO/HS to enhance the content or quality of health services or to reduce charges. Government-sponsored HSOs/HSs are not for profit, even though they are publicly owned, as compared with private ownership through either a for-profit or not-for-profit corporation.

During the mid-1990s a number of for-profit hospitals converted to not-for-profit status. One analysis found that the welfare of the communities where these conversions occurred did not uniformly benefit. Most conversions resulted in more uncompensated care being delivered, but the amount was insufficient to offset the decrease in property tax revenue to the local jurisdictions. The existing relationship with the community may be the most important consideration in judging the benefit that will result.[28] Similarly, a number of not-for-profit hospitals converted to for-profit status, which raised issues such as valuation of assets, charitable mission, private inurement (see Chapter 14), and the mission and activities of the charitable foundation that are usually established with the proceeds of the sale.[29] Such changes will continue as the health system evolves and realigns.

Ownership

Another way to classify HSOs/HSs is by ownership. In addition to private ownership, such as sectarian or nonsectarian and not for profit or investor owned, many HSOs are owned by a government (public) entity. Cities or counties establish and control public health departments. They also own acute care hospitals, some of which are financed by special tax districts. HSOs owned by state governments include health departments and psychiatric hospitals or institutions for people with mental disabilities. Many states own academic health (medical) centers, which are often university teaching hospitals that treat acute illness, conduct research, and educate people in various health occupations.

Historically, the federal government has been involved in financing and, to a lesser extent, delivering health services—preventive, acute, and long-term care for special groups. There are several examples. The U.S. Public Health Service (USPHS) hospitals were established in the late 18th century to care for merchant mariners. USPHS hospitals treating general acute care problems were operated until 1981, when the few remaining hospitals were closed or converted to other purposes. The Gillis W. Long Hansen's Disease Center in Carville, Louisiana, is the last USPHS hospital and provides diagnosis, treatment, and rehabilitation for people with leprosy (Hansen's disease).[30] In

1996 the Indian Health Service (part of USPHS, which is a division of the Department of Health and Human Services [DHHS]) operated 37 hospitals, 64 health centers, 50 health stations, and 5 school health centers.[31]

In 1999 DVA, through VHA, operated 173 medical centers (hospitals), 126 nursing facilities, and 32 domiciliary residences for former military personnel with service-connected medical problems.[32] DVA's role in medical education is discussed later. In addition, acute care hospitals and clinics operated by the U.S. Army, Navy, and Air Force serve active-duty and retired military personnel and their dependents.

Length of Patient Stay

A third way to classify HSOs is by the length of time a patient is in treatment. A general dichotomy divides them by whether services are delivered to inpatients, generally defined as patients whose treatment is 24 hours or longer, or to outpatients, whose treatment is less than 24 hours. In turn, inpatient HSOs are divided into short term (acute) and long term. The American Hospital Association (AHA) defines a short-term hospital as one in which the average length of stay is less than 30 days; a long-term hospital has patient stays that average 30 days or longer. Nursing facilities typically treat only inpatients, and lengths of stay are measured in months or years. HSOs such as home health agencies and physician group practices treat only outpatients. Some, such as hospice, have inpatients but also may provide services to patients in their homes.

Role in Health Services System

A fourth way to classify HSOs is by their roles in delivery of services. Health services may be provided in public health department screening programs, in family planning and substance abuse treatment centers, or through sanitation efforts that protect food and water supplies. There are thousands of privately and publicly owned and operated emergency medical units, such as rescue squads and ambulance services, often organized into emergency medical services systems. In addition, there are programs more oriented to social welfare activities; some only raise funds, others deliver specialized services. Depending on their activities, they may or may not be considered HSOs. The total number of HSOs in the United States is in the tens of thousands; Chapter 4 describes the history, numbers, functions, and organization of several types.

Unique Institutional Providers

In addition to inpatient HSOs such as hospitals and nursing facilities, there are many other types of inpatient facilities that provide health and health-related services. Data collection about them is sparse to nonexistent. They include residential facilities or schools for special groups such as people who are blind or deaf, people with emotional or physical disabilities, people with mental disabilities, dependent children, unwed mothers, alcoholics, drug abusers, and people with multiple physical and mental disorders.

In 1996, for example, more than 137,000 individuals with mental retardation, developmental disabilities, or both received training and support in 7,191 facilities, which is about half the number of individuals and facilities reported a decade earlier. Privately operated facilities accounted for 83% of all facilities and served 50% of clients. Forty-five percent of clients resided in state-owned/operated facilities. The remaining 5% were in city, county, or town-based facilities. The trend in recent years has been away from care provided in large state-run institutions to care provided in smaller, privately run facilities that have fewer than 15 beds.[33]

Community services may reduce the need for long-term inpatient care. Examples of community services include diagnostic and evaluation clinics, day care centers, early childhood education facilities, rehabilitation programs, and summer camps and recreational facilities. All offer alternatives to institutional placement. Community-sponsored educational services are provided by local school districts under the direction of state special education programs. Developmental disability programs are operated at local levels with state funding.

Mental Health Organizations

Mental health organizations are defined as HSOs that primarily provide mental health services to people with mental illness or emotional disturbances. Included are public or private psychiatric hospitals, psychiatric services in general hospitals, outpatient psychiatric clinics, and mental health day/night facilities. Since 1955 there have been significant changes as to where mental health services are delivered. In the mid-1950s state and county mental hospitals accounted for 77% of inpatient services; 23% were outpatient. By 1975 a reversal had occurred and 76% of services were outpatient.[34] Inpatient treatment continues to be a major type of care, however, and there were 3,319 inpatient and residential mental health organizations with more than 250,000 beds in 1994.[35]

Teaching Hospitals

There are approximately 1,100 hospitals involved in graduate medical education in the United States,[36] a decline of 200 since 1990.[37] They fall under the general rubric of teaching hospital and offer a wide range of secondary and tertiary medical services. These 1,100, plus an unknown but large number of other hospitals, participate in training a wide variety of people in the health care occupations. Many teaching hospitals are part of a medical center complex that includes a medical school. Those without a medical school are almost always affiliated with one. Their prominence in medical education, plus activities in research and publishing in the medical and scientific literature, make teaching hospitals a vital resource in the health services field.

Membership as a teaching hospital in the Council of Teaching Hospitals and Health Systems (COTH), a division of the Association of American Medical Colleges, is limited to organizations that have a documented affiliation agreement with a medical school that is accredited by the Liaison Committee on Medical Education (LCME). These organizations must sponsor or participate significantly in at least four approved active residency programs. At least two of the approved residency programs should be in medicine, surgery, obstetrics-gynecology, pediatrics, family practice, or psychiatry.[38] In 1999 there were 400 COTH member institutions, but because they train approximately 75% of the medical and surgical residents in the United States, their influence is far greater than this number suggests.[39]

A unique HSO that may fit into more than one of the categories described earlier merits special mention. The premier institution among all HSOs is the academic health (medical) center hospital, which is a subset of teaching hospitals. Academic health center hospitals are those in which a majority of the chiefs of service at the hospital chair the academic departments in a medical school. In 1997 there were 116 integrated academic medical (health) center hospitals in the United States as defined by COTH.[40]

HEALTH SERVICES WORKERS

Table 2.2 shows selected active health personnel in the United States in 1980, 1990, and 1995. The increase in active physicians from 1980 to 1995 of more than 50% is especially notable. A doubling of registered nurses (RNs) with baccalaureate degrees and a tripling of RNs with master's and doctoral degrees between 1980 and 1995 suggest the direction of contemporary nursing—less "the physician's handmaiden" and much more a highly qualified provider. Such enhanced credentials significantly increase salary costs in HSOs.

In 1999 almost 10 million people were employed in physicians' offices and clinics, nursing and personal care facilities, hospitals, and home health services.[41] Table 2.3 shows the number employed in a professional specialty, in service occupations, and as technicians in 1996. The "Percent Change" column shows potential significant growth in almost all of these health occupations. Health services is among the most rapidly growing industries in the United States, which suggests strong demand and significant challenges for health services managers.

Physicians

Allopathic medicine, which traces its lineage to Hippocrates (420–340 [?] B.C.), emerged as the dominant theory of treating disease at the beginning of the 20th century. As noted earlier, allopathy holds that interruptions of the body's normal functioning must be treated with significant interventions to restore normal bodily functioning (health). Development of the germ theory of disease causation and increasingly efficacious surgery in the late 19th century gave allopathy a scientific basis, which secured its place and dominance in Western medical practice. The increase in effective chemical therapies early in the 20th century enhanced its stature, as did the scientific knowledge developed throughout the 20th century.

TABLE 2.2.   ACTIVE HEALTH PERSONNEL ACCORDING TO OCCUPATION: U.S., 1980, 1990, AND 1995[a]

Year, occupation	No. of active health personnel	U.S. No./100,000 population[b]
1980		
Physicians	427,122	189.8
Federal	17,642	7.8
Doctors of medicine[c]	16,585	7.4
Doctors of osteopathy	1,057	0.5
Nonfederal	409,480	182.0
Doctors of medicine[c]	393,407	174.9
Doctors of osteopathy	16,073	7.1
Dentists[d]	121,240	53.5
Optometrists	22,330	9.8
Pharmacists	142,780	62.5
Podiatrists[e]	7,000	3.0
Registered nurses	1,272,900	560.0
Associate and diploma	908,300	399.9
Baccalaureate	297,300	130.9
Master's and doctorate	67,300	29.6
1990		
Physicians	567,611	230.2
Federal	20,784	8.4
Doctors of medicine[c]	19,166	7.7
Doctors of osteopathy	1,618	0.7
Nonfederal	546,826	221.8
Doctors of medicine[c]	520,450	211.1
Doctors of osteopathy	26,376	10.7
Dentists[d]	146,600	58.8
Optometrists	26,000	10.4
Pharmacists	161,900	64.4
Podiatrists[e]	10,600	4.2
Registered nurses	1,789,600	713.7
Associate and diploma	1,107,300	441.6
Baccalaureate	549,000	218.9
Master's and doctorate	133,300	53.2

(continued)

TABLE **2.2.** *(continued)*

Year, occupation	No. of active health personnel	U.S. No./100,000 population[b]
1995		
Physicians	672,859	255.9
Federal	21,153	8.0
Doctors of medicine[c]	19,830	7.5
Doctors of osteopathy	1,323	0.5
Nonfederal	651,706	247.9
Doctors of medicine[c]	617,362	234.8
Doctors of osteopathy	34,344	13.1
Dentists[d]	—[f]	—[f]
Optometrists	28,900	10.9
Pharmacists	182,300	68.9
Podiatrists[e]	10,300	3.9
Registered nurses	2,115,800	797.6
Associate and diploma	1,235,000	465.5
Baccalaureate	673,200	253.8
Master's and doctorate	117,500	78.7

Sources: Division of Health Professions Analysis, Bureau of Health Professions: Supply and Characteristics of Selected Health Personnel. DHHS Pub. No. (HRA) 81–20. Health Resources Administration. Hyattsville, MD, June 1981; unpublished data; American Medical Association. Physician characteristics and distribution in the U.S., 1981, 1992, and 1996/97 editions. Chicago, 1982, 1992, and 1997; American Osteopathic Association. 1980–81 Yearbook and Directory of Osteopathic Physicians. Chicago, 1980. American Association of Colleges of Osteopathic Medicine. Annual statistical report, 1990 and 1996 editions. Rockville, MD, 1990 and 1996; unpublished data.

From National Center for Health Statistics. *Health, United States, 1998,* 326. Washington, DC: U.S. Department of Health and Human Services, 1999.

[a]Data are compiled by the Bureau of Health Professions.

[b]Ratios for physicians and dentists are based on civilian population; ratios for all other health occupations are based on resident population.

[c]Excludes physicians not classified according to activity status and inactive from the number of active health personnel.

[d]Excludes dentists in military service, U.S. Public Health Service, and Department of Veterans Affairs.

[e]Patient care.

[f]Data not available.

Some numbers for 1990 have been revised and differ from previous editions of *Health, United States.* Starting in 1989, data for doctors of medicine are as of January 1; in earlier years, these data are as of December 31.

Major competing theories of disease causation and cure in the mid- to late 19th century were naturopathy, homeopathy, osteopathy, and chiropractic. After virtually disappearing, the public's interest in alternative and complementary medicine has stimulated a new look at naturopathy and homeopathy, although they remain at the fringe of medical practice. Osteopathy has largely merged with allopathy. Chiropractic is more accepted than at any time in its history; nevertheless, orthodox medicine still considers it a manipulative therapy with no clear scientific basis.

Osteopathy evolved from the practices of the bonesetters of England, a cult with the ability to reposition dislocated collar bones, cartilages, and other joints that was spurned by orthodox medicine.[42] The philosophy and science of osteopathic medicine were first described in 1874 by Andrew Taylor Still, a physician who founded the American School of Osteopathy in 1892. Osteopaths are educated in osteopathic medical schools, which emphasize the structure and functioning of the musculoskeletal system and an appreciation for the body's ability to heal itself when it is in its normal functional relationship and has a favorable environment and nutrition.[43] Osteopathic health care em-

TABLE 2.3. PEOPLE EMPLOYED IN THE HEALTH SERVICES INDUSTRY, BY OCCUPATION, 1996

	No. (000)	1996–2006 % change (proj.)
Professional specialty		
Social workers	146	46.1
Physical therapists	103	71.7
Respiratory therapists	81	45.8
Occupational therapists	41	71.5
Speech-language pathologists and audiologists	31	NA
Dietitians and nutritionists	28	15.9
Computer systems analysts	27	87.7
Service		
Nursing assistants and psychiatric aides	1,086	29.8
Home health aides	347	91.5
Medical assistants	222	74.7
Dental assistants	195	39.4
Physical therapy aides	81	80.6
Technicians		
Licensed practical nurses	569	23.4
Clinical lab technologists and technicians	251	14.4
Radiologic technologists	170	29.4
Dental hygienists	131	48.9
Health information technicians	77	55.1
Psychiatric technicians	60	2.4
Surgical technologists	49	31.7
Emergency medical technicians	37	60.5
Dispensing opticians	35	13.7

Source: Bureau of Labor Statistics, 1997.

Adapted from *Source Book of Health Insurance Data, 1997–1998,* 146. Washington, DC: Health Insurance Association of America.

phasizes manipulative methods of detecting and correcting structural problems, but it also utilizes generally accepted conventional medical and surgical treatment. Osteopathic medical training is similar to that of allopathic medicine, and in most respects osteopaths are the same as allopaths. Many osteopaths enter allopathic residency training programs; they are licensed under the same state statutes.

Chiropractic is an offshoot of osteopathy, with special emphasis on manipulation to correct anatomical faults that cause functional disturbances in the body. It is a uniquely American medical development. Daniel David Palmer established the first school of chiropractic medicine in Iowa in 1895. Palmer's theories stressed the importance of minor spinal displacements, or subluxations, as chiropractors later called them. Subluxations are less severe than dislocations, but cause nerve irritation that leads to disturbances of the nervous system and eventually to illness. Medical orthodoxy's mistake, according to Palmer, is that it treats disorders without understanding their source—the spinal column—and chiropractic could remedy that problem.[44]

Physician Numbers

Table 2.2 shows the number of active physicians from 1980 to 1995. Calculating the number of active physicians per 100,000 population permits accurate comparisons over time; this number increased by one third between 1980 and 1995.

Two major studies in the late 1970s reported that more allopathic medical schools and greater numbers of students would cause a physician surplus by the late 1980s. This led to decreased state and federal financial support. The end of federal capitation grants to medical schools (a fixed payment per student) meant that tuition or subsidies from other sources had to be increased. The extent of public support in the past is shown by the fact that in 1979 medical student tuition and fees paid only a little more than 5% of the cost; 55% was paid directly by the government. Income from hospitals and clinics, nongovernmental grants and contracts, and endowment and philanthropy covered the difference.[45] In 1996–1997 tuition and fees contributed only 2.8% of revenues in public and 5.1% in private medical schools. For both, the largest contributions came from practice plans (33.1% and 35.4%, respectively), state and local governments (16.0% and 0.9%, respectively), hospital/medical school programs (14.7% and 16.7%, respectively), and federal research grants and contracts (15.6% and 20.4%, respectively).[46] Out-of-state tuition at some public medical schools and tuition at some private (nongovernmental) medical schools is more than $30,000/year.

Concerns about a physician surplus surfaced again in the late 1990s. The Balanced Budget Act of 1997 limited federal financial support for graduate medical education with the expectation that reducing training sites and programs would reduce the number of new physicians.[47] In 1997 more than 98,000 residents were in Accreditation Council for Graduate Medical Education–accredited and combined special programs, including 67,000 U.S. medical graduates, 25,000 international medical graduates, 3,000 doctors of osteopathy, and 500 Canadian medical graduates.[48]

There are projections that physician supply per capita in the decade 2000–2010 will exceed demand. This does not address the geographic maldistribution of physicians and nonphysician clinicians, with strong evidence that the latter are as disinterested in underserved areas as are physicians.[49] Driven by lack of attention to a need for specialists in delivery settings and by consumer demand for specialist services, the almost-exclusive emphasis on primary care physicians in the mid-1990s subsided, and specialist physicians were once again in demand at the end of the 1990s.[50] Such cycles are to be expected as more efforts are made to "manage" delivery of services and availability of various types of clinical manpower. The Pew Health Professions Commission is a private group that has been influential in health professions education and development of policies regarding the nation's health care workforce needs.[51]

Nonphysician Clinicians

Of concern, too, is that the number of nonphysician caregivers has increased and will continue to increase dramatically. "Between 1992 and 1997, there has been a 2- to 4-fold increase in the number of graduates of nurse practitioner, certified nurse midwifery, and physician assistant programs and a doubling or more of graduates from chiropractic and acupuncture schools."[52] The greatest growth is projected among nonphysician clinicians who provide primary care services, and the greatest concentration will occur in states that already have the greatest abundance of physicians.[53]

This growth in nonphysician practitioners is occurring when it is generally agreed that the United States has an oversupply of physicians, and the supply of physicians is projected to increase more than 10% between 1995 and 2005.[54] A surplus suggests various potential problems while concomitantly creating opportunities for HSO/HS managers. With or without a surplus, however, a more significant problem has been and will continue to be the maldistribution of physicians, a special problem for rural areas.

Licensed Independent Practitioners

Physician and nonphysician clinicians with independent access to patients are known as licensed independent practitioners (LIPs); the regulation and education of the various types of LIPs are discussed later in this chapter. LIPs are likely to be competitors, with largely unknown implications for the cost of health services. Quality and productivity may be less of an issue, however; nurse practitioners (NPs) and physician assistants (PAs) can provide care of equivalent quality as they perform many of the tasks of primary care physicians.[55]

Chapter 11 addresses human resources management. A brief comment here provides a context for the subsequent discussion of health services workers (see "Regulation and Education of Caregivers"). Most physicians and many other types of LIPs are self-employed private entrepreneurs, even though they may receive some part of their income from an employment relationship. In contrast, non–LIPs, or dependent caregivers, are employed in the practices of LIPs or in a HSO such as a nursing facility or hospital. Physicians in residency programs are usually employed by the residency site. These relationships are part of the context for human resources issues in HSOs/HSs.

REGULATION AND EDUCATION OF MANAGERS

Regulation

In 1999 no state licensed hospital administrators, whereas all states licensed nursing facility administrators. Managers in other types of HSOs are unlikely to be licensed. State regulation of an industry occurs when problems suggest that a profession's self-regulation and self-discipline are ineffective to protect the public. This was the case in the long-term care industry prior to 1965.

Education

Hospital administration was identified as a distinct educational discipline when the University of Chicago established the first professional master's degree program in 1934, which followed the founding of the American College of Hospital Administrators, now the American College of Healthcare Executives (ACHE). These are milestones in the development of a professional identity. In 1999, 67 hospital administration graduate programs were accredited by the Accrediting Commission on Education for Health Services Administration, which is composed of representatives from health services professional associations. Five are in Canada.[56] Graduate and undergraduate programs exist or are being developed worldwide. It is estimated that there are more than 30,000 graduates of North American master's degree programs.

Consistent with changes in their environment, education programs for HSO/HS managers are eclectic, emphasizing generic education in management. Some offer specialty preparation in hospital, nursing facility, or ambulatory services management. The didactic portion for accredited programs is 2 academic years—four semesters. A field experience is typical; some programs require a 1-year, full-time residency that allows application of the academic preparation under the guidance of an on-site preceptor.

The basic curriculum of master's degree programs covers study in three principal areas: management theory, concepts, and skills, including leadership, financial management, economics, law, organizational behavior, quantitative methods, and planning; the health care industry, including epidemiology, health and human behavior, and medical care organization; and an integrative experience that applies management concepts to the health care industry in a major project, paper, or exam.[57] Professional master's degrees in health services management have a variety of titles and are found in various academic settings.

As with graduate programs, rapid growth in the number of undergraduate programs that prepare health services management personnel occurred in the late 1960s and early 1970s. There are 35 undergraduate programs affiliated with the Association of University Programs in Health Administration.[58] However, there are scores of other programs in the United States, in addition to which there are health services curricula of various types. Foci of the two levels of education are different. Master's programs prepare graduates to become senior-level line or staff managers; baccalaureate programs train middle-level supervisors or department managers. A continuing problem is articulating graduate and undergraduate programs.

REGULATION AND EDUCATION OF CAREGIVERS

Licensure, Certification, and Registration

Except for managers, licensing of the health care occupations is ubiquitous. In 1990 every state and the District of Columbia licensed 14 of 44 health care occupations studied by AHA. Five states regulated 30 or more of these 44 health care occupations. There is a trend toward greater regulation of health personnel.[59] For example, the Omnibus Budget Reconciliation Act of 1987 (PL 100-203; commonly known as OBRA '87) required states to register nursing assistants.

There are important distinctions among licensure, registration, and certification:

> *Licensure:* an approval granted by government that allows someone to engage in an occupation after a finding that the applicant has achieved a certain minimum competency. Licensing is a state function under the police powers. Physicians and dentists are always licensed, for example.

> *Registration:* a listing of qualified individuals on an official roster maintained by a government or nongovernment body. States may require registration for someone to engage in a health occupation; thus registration has the effect of licensure. Persons who are registered may use that designation. The registered nurse and registered dietitian are examples.

> *Certification:* a process by which a nongovernment agency or association grants recognition to someone who meets its qualifications. States may require certification for someone to engage in a health occupation, thus giving certification the effect of licensure. Nurse-midwives are certified, for example.

Physicians (MD [medical doctor]) or osteopaths (DO [doctor of osteopathy]) are the only LIPs who are granted unlimited licenses. It is rare that state licensing authorities limit a physician's license because disciplinary actions against physicians are uncommon. For all intents and purposes, physicians and osteopaths are equivalent and are called physicians in this discussion.

In general, nonphysician health services workers may be divided into two groups: those who are licensed to treat patients independently (also called LIPs), and those who may or may not be licensed but who are dependent on the orders of a LIP to allow them to deliver health services. Nonphysician LIPs have state licenses that limit their practice to certain parts of the body or specific medical problems; optometrists, podiatrists, dentists, and chiropractors are examples. In many states, nurse-midwives and some types of NPs are LIPs as well. Some states allow RNs without specialty training to perform specified examinations and procedures. Applying the general principle of independent-versus-dependent practice is complicated because many types of HSOs, but always acute care hospitals, limit further the scope of practice of health services workers (even of physicians) to clinical activities in which they have demonstrated competence. Similarly, HSOs may limit the license of nonphysician LIPs to activities ordered or supervised by physicians.

Dependent caregivers may or may not be licensed, registered, or certified, but they provide services only on receiving an order from a LIP. Distinctions beyond this are blurred. Dependent caregivers include medical technologists, pharmacists, radiographers, licensed practical nurses (LPNs), and nursing assistants. RNs and pharmacists use "registered" as a synonym for licensure. Dietitians are registered by a private association and are licensed or statutorily certified or registered in a number of states.[60]

Certification is a process of approval involving a professional association and often the American Medical Association (AMA). Certificates are issued after passing an examination, the eligibility for which requires specified academic preparation. A confusing aspect of the process is that sometimes the certificate is issued by a body that uses the title "registry." Often a group of specialty physicians also certifies. For example, the American Society of Clinical Pathologists certifies medical technologists through its board of registry.[61] People who are unable to meet the private certifying group's standards are likely to be unemployable in HSOs; this gives certification the effect of licensure. Concomitantly, if the person who is certified does not continue to meet the group's standards and certification is withdrawn, employment is likely to be forfeited.

Education and Regulation of Sample Health Occupations

Physicians

Medicine is one of the learned professions and, historically, physicians have been held in high regard. The most important modern effort to improve allopathic medical education occurred in 1910, when Abraham Flexner's study of medical education in the United States showed its weaknesses. The science curriculum was enhanced, the didactic portion was lengthened, and the clinical component was strengthened. Weak allopathic medical schools failed when they could not meet the more stringent standards.

In 1950 there were 79 U.S. allopathic medical schools; by 1970 there were 103, and by 1990 there were 126.[62] In 1998 there were 124 accredited allopathic medical schools with 66,748 students, and graduates numbering 14,114.[63] The number of MD graduates declined considerably from 16,781 in 1989.[64] Medical schools are accredited by LCME, whose 17 members include medical educators and administrators, practicing physicians, public members, and medical students.[65] In 1998, 88,000 faculty were involved in educating more than 160,000 medical students and residents.[66] In 1997 Canada's 16 accredited medical schools (none of them osteopathic) graduated 1,582 MDs.[67]

Doctors of osteopathy (DOs) are educated at 19 American Osteopathic Association (AOA)–accredited colleges of osteopathic medicine, with 9,628 students in 1998. DOs may be board certified in 19 general medical specialties, in addition to various subspecialties. In 1999 there were more than 43,000 DOs in the United States.[68]

Postgraduate Education

Following graduation from medical school, which is either a 4-year postbaccalaureate education or sometimes part of a 6- or 7-year combined baccalaureate–MD degree, the new allopathic physician begins a residency.[69]

Historically, "intern" designated graduates in the first year of hospital training or the first year of any residency program. The correct title, however, is resident; intern has not been used officially for allopaths in training since 1975.[70] Residents are designated by postgraduate year (PGY) or graduate year (GY). For example, a PGY-2 has had 1 year of clinical experience after medical school and is in the second. Clinical activities of residents are supervised by more senior residents, fellows (postresidency physicians in training), and teaching faculty (physicians) who are active staff at the HSO, usually a hospital. Residencies are accredited by the Accreditation Council for Graduate Medical Education, which is composed of professional associations in the medical field. Each specialty has a residency review committee that sets standards for specialty training and accredits the program.

Medical specialties determine the number of PGYs and the specific clinical content of those years so that the program may be accredited and provide the basis for eligibility to be certified in that specialty. For example, anesthesiology requires 1 year of initial specialty training (general residency) and 3 years of advanced specialty training (residency in anesthesiology); family practice requires 3 years of advanced specialty training (residency in family practice); and neurological surgery requires 1 year of initial specialty training (general residency) and 5 years of advanced specialty training (neurological surgery residency).[71]

In 1997, 75% of VHA's medical centers had major affiliations with medical schools, about 70% of VHA staff physicians had medical school faculty appointments, and about 9% of medical residents training in the United States were funded by DVA.[72] More than half of practicing physicians received some part of their professional training in a DVA medical center.[73]

Licensure

U.S. and Canadian medical graduates are licensed in most states after passing the U.S. Medical Licensing Examination and completing 1 year of residency. Several states require 2 years of residency, and a few require 3 years. In addition, 31 states require a minimum number of continuing medical education credits to remain licensed.[74] State licenses are unlimited in terms of the medical activities that physicians may undertake. Thus physicians may legally prescribe all medications (except some narcotics and experimental drugs) and perform all medical and surgical activities. It is only in HSOs that the scope of this otherwise unlimited right to practice medicine is modified, if at all.

Limiting practice activities to those consistent with demonstrated current competence is especially important in acute care hospitals because of the acuity of illnesses and the significant treatments provided there. However, protecting patients by ensuring the competence of physicians and other LIPs, such as podiatrists and dentists, is vital in all HSOs. Protection is achieved through the credentialing process, which includes a review of didactic and clinical experience, licensure, specialty certification, and health status, among other aspects. Periodic review of clinical performance in the HSO is part of the recredentialing process that is necessary for the practitioner to continue to have privileges in that HSO. Credentialing and recredentialing are detailed in Chapter 4. In the early 1990s state medical boards came under heavy criticism for being insufficiently aggressive in disciplining physicians with problems related to their professional activities.[75] This continuing problem is detailed in Chapter 14.[76]

Nonphysician Caregivers

Nowhere is there greater fragmentation and specialization of work than in HSOs. Each new technology seems to require another type of technical expertise. In the early years of modern medicine, physicians usually worked independent of other caregivers. As support became necessary, some physician activities were performed by technicians. Nursing is the earliest example, and sonographers are among the most recent.

Changes in staffing needs will continue as old technologies evolve and others are introduced. The use of roentgen rays (x-rays), which were discovered by Wilhelm Roentgen in 1895, is an instructive example. Roentgenology became radiology, which bifurcated into diagnostic radiology and therapeutic radiology. Diagnostic radiology has added computers, analysis of cellular emissions, and use of sound waves, and has become known as diagnostic imaging. Similarly, therapeutic radiology now includes linear accelerators added to x-ray equipment, and the use of radioactive sources has spawned the specialty of nuclear medicine. Organization and specialization are needed to deliver state-of-the-art medicine, but such services are available only at considerable economic and organizational cost.

Dentists

Dentists are LIPs who typically provide services in an office or a clinic. In addition, they may be employed or be on an HSO's attending staff. If they are, they should be subject to a credentialing process; it is required in hospitals.

Dentistry is the art and science of healing concerned with the oral region of the human body. Dentists are educated in 55 accredited dental schools in the United States and 10 in Canada, which graduated 3,930 and 426 dentists, respectively, in 1997. To become a doctor of dental surgery (DDS) or doctor of dental medicine (DMD) typically requires a baccalaureate degree plus 4 years of dental education. The dental school curriculum concentrates on basic sciences, applying health sciences to delivery of oral health services, and applying basic biomedical and dental sciences to the practice of dentistry.[77] In 1995 approximately 20% of dentists practiced in a specialty.[78] The American Dental Association recognizes eight specialties: dental public health, endodontics, oral and maxillofacial pathology, oral and maxillofacial surgery, orthodontics and dentofacial orthopedics, pediatric dentistry, periodontics, and prosthodontics.[79] Specialization requires a minimum of 2 years of advanced study and practice at the postdoctoral level. In 1997, 10 states issued specialty licenses and 7 issued certifications in most of these specialty areas. In addition, a number of states set standards for dentists who wish to announce specialty practice.[80] This level of state regulation distinguishes dentistry from medicine. Certification by medical specialty boards, albeit by a private organization, has a similar effect. There were approximately 153,000 dentists in the United States in 1996.[81]

Podiatrists

Podiatrists are LIPs who typically provide services in an office or a clinic. If they are employed by or part of a HSO's attending staff, they should be subject to a credentialing process; it is required in hospitals.

Podiatry is the branch of the healing arts and sciences that treats the foot and its related or governing structures by medical, surgical, or other means. Applicants to the seven colleges of podiatric medicine in the United States should hold a baccalaureate degree, but exceptions are made. The first 2 years of instruction emphasize basic medical sciences, such as anatomy, physiology, microbiology, biochemistry, pharmacology, and pathology. The second 2 years emphasize clinical sciences, including general diagnosis, therapeutics, surgery, anesthesia, and operative podiatric medicine. Graduates are awarded the degree of doctor of podiatric medicine (DPM). Most graduates take a residency of 1–4 years. Podiatrists are licensed in all states. The American Podiatric Medical Association has approved two specialty boards that certify in podiatric orthopedics, podiatric surgery, and primary podiatric medicine.[82] Table 2.2 shows 10,300 active podiatrists in 1995.

Nurses

Early recognition and increased stature of nursing were achieved largely through the efforts of Florence Nightingale, an Englishwoman who worked in the mid-19th century. Until then, secular nursing had a poor reputation. Dorothea Dix was an early nursing leader in the United States. As education and professional standards improved and licensing was introduced in the United States, RNs became second only to physicians on the patient care team. Nurse licensing began in the early 1900s and initially concentrated on state registration. In 1903 North Carolina nurses were the first to establish state registration, and only individuals found to be qualified by a board of examiners could be listed as registered nurses in a county and use the designation RN. Voluntary licensure has been superseded by mandatory licensure for RNs in all states and the District of Columbia.[83] RNs may be LIPs, depending on specialty preparation.

Of the 2.56 million licensed RNs in 1996, it was estimated that 2.12 million were employed in nursing.[84] The largest source of employment is acute care hospitals (42%), followed by community/home care (15%), nursing facilities (14%), and managed care (10%). The remainder work in various settings, including outpatient facilities, psychiatric hospitals, physicians' offices, and industry and schools.[85]

Contributing to the nursing shortage that began in the mid-1980s have been changes in hospital staffing patterns (focus on primary nursing [all-RN staff]); decreasing use of other types of nursing personnel, which are described later; demand for RNs outside the acute care hospital; and failure of beginning RN salaries to keep pace with inflation.[86] The early 1990s witnessed a renewed interest in nursing education,[87] but by the late 1990s most hospitals reported a shortage of RNs.[88]

Declining enrollments in baccalaureate degree programs suggest shortages will grow,[89] but a crisis is unlikely.[90]

RNs are educated in programs of varying length in different educational settings: baccalaureate (4-year, university based, leading to a bachelor of science in nursing [BSN]), diploma (3-year, hospital based, leading to a diploma in nursing), and associate (2-year, junior or community college–based, leading to an associate of arts [AA]). Graduates of all three programs may be licensed (registered) as RNs. Organized nursing developed a strong preference for baccalaureate-trained nurses, which led to a rapid decline in the number of diploma programs in the late 1960s and early 1970s. This caused major dislocations in the health services field and contributed directly to the RN shortage in the 1970s and indirectly to that in the 1980s.

In addition to RNs, there are LPNs, who may be known as licensed vocational nurses (LVNs). Nursing assistants, who are sometimes called nurse's aides and may be certified, are another common category of nursing personnel. Practical nurses and nursing assistants are clinically and usually administratively subordinate to the RN. Table 2.3 shows more than 500,000 employed LPNs in 1996.

In the late 1970s the American Nurses Association (ANA) began a RN certification program, which became the American Nurses Credentialing Center. In 1999 RNs could be certified in 13 generalist areas such as college health, pediatrics, cardiac rehabilitation, and nursing administration. In addition, advanced practice board certification was offered in 13 areas of advanced practice, including NPs in areas such as acute care, family, pediatric, and gerontological nursing, and clinical nurse specialists (CNSs) in areas such as community health, gerontology, medical-surgical, and administration.[91] Each has different requirements but all include clinical experience and passing an examination, as well as current licensure.[92] The 11,000 RNs certified by ANA in 1982[93] increased to 77,000 by 1991[94] and to 120,000 by 1998.[95]

Most states have categories of caregivers who were RNs first and then gained preparation in a specialty. NPs, for example, have independent practice authority in 21 states.[96] Some types of independent practice nurses are certified by private associations (e.g., certified registered nurse-anesthetists [CRNAs] and certified nurse-midwives [CNMs]). A majority of states allow CRNAs to administer anesthesia without a physician's supervision. Use of CRNAs will increase if Medicare regulations are changed so that an anesthesiologist's supervision is not required.[97] CNSs are licensed as RNs, certified by the American College of Nurse-Midwives, and licensed in almost half of the states as nurse-midwives. Advanced practice nurses generally include NPs, CNSs, CRNAs, and CNMs, who are likely to be credentialed by HSOs, either as a group or individually. Such providers are LIPs.

HSO/HS managers will be challenged to recruit and retain RNs, as well as use RN resources effectively.[98] Productivity is addressed in Chapter 9, and employee recruitment and retention are discussed in Chapter 11.

Pharmacists

A type of nonphysician caregiver commonly found in HSOs is the pharmacist. Professional pharmacists emerged later than professional nurses, and their role in the spectrum of care is narrower than that of nurses. Pharmacists are educated in 75 accredited colleges and schools of pharmacy in the United States. A baccalaureate in pharmacy is earned in a 5-year program, a doctorate in a 6-year program. Licensure requires graduating from an accredited program, completing an internship, and passing a state board examination. Pharmacists are not LIPs and dispense medications on the orders of LIPs such as physicians, podiatrists, and dentists.[99] Table 2.2 shows that there were 182,300 active pharmacists in the United States in 1995.

Dietitians

A type of nonphysician caregiver always found in hospitals and nursing facilities is the clinical or therapeutic dietitian, who plans therapeutic diets and implements preparation and service of meals for patients in hospitals, nursing facilities, and other, primarily inpatient HSOs. Nutritional counseling is done in HMOs and other, primarily outpatient HSOs by dietitians who may be called nutritionists. Like pharmacists, dietitians emerged later than nurses and their role in the spectrum of care is narrower. Historically, dietitians have been registered by a professional society, the American Dietetic Association. In the mid-1980s states began licensing or certifying them. In 1999 states licensed (27) or had statutory certification (13) or registration (1) for dietitians, nutritionists, or both. Minimum preparation to become a registered dietitian includes a bachelor's degree, a 6- to 12-month internship, and passing a national, written exam administered by the Commission on Dietetic Registration.[100] Table 2.3 shows 28,000 employed dietitians and nutritionists in 1996.

Technologists

In 1999, 220,000 registered radiologic technologists were practicing in the United States, including radiographers, cardiovascular-interventional technologists, sonographers, radiation therapists, mammographers, nuclear medicine technologists, computerized tomography technologists, and magnetic resonance imaging technologists.[101] The titles reflect job responsibilities and the extent of specialization. Radiographers are trained in 2-year academic or nonacademic programs or 4-year programs leading to a baccalaureate degree. Radiographers are registered by passing one of several national certifying examinations. Most states have specific licensing laws.[102] Table 2.3 shows 170,000 employed radiologic technologists in 1996.

About 60% of the almost 300,000 clinical laboratory or medical technologists are employed in hospitals. Typically, they hold a baccalaureate degree in medical technology or one of the life sciences. They perform various laboratory tests and may specialize in clinical chemistry, blood bank technology, cytotechnology, hematology, histology, microbiology, or immunology. Training programs are offered by colleges, universities, and hospitals. Technologists are certified by various groups, including the Board of Registry of the American Society of Clinical Pathologists and the American Medical Technologists. Many states require medical technologists to be licensed or registered.[103] Table 2.3 shows 25,000 employed clinical laboratory technologists and technicians in 1996. Both radiologic technicians and medical technologists are dependent nonphysician caregivers in that they have no independent access to patients and respond to a LIP's order.

Physician Assistants

Another type of dependent caregiver commonly found in HSOs is the PA, the concept for which originated in the 1960s and was based on the military medic or corpsman. Typically, PAs are trained in a 2-year general medical (primary care) curriculum, approximately half of which is devoted to clinical rotations in a wide range of inpatient and outpatient settings. A number of programs award baccalaureate degrees; and there is a trend to award master's degrees. In 1997, 111 accredited programs educated PAs.[104] Historically, PAs worked under the direction or supervision of a physician, who was accountable for their activities. There is a trend toward more independence, reflected in the fact that states are beginning to regulate PAs, who may be licensed, registered, or certified. The National Commission on Certification of Physician Assistants certifies PAs, and this certification is used by the states in regulating PAs.[105] In 1997 more than 34,500 PAs were in active practice in the United States.[106] Almost half are in primary care; in addition, they may specialize in areas such as orthopedics, emergency medicine, and cardiology. Almost all states allow physicians to delegate prescriptive authority to the PAs they supervise. Most PAs practice in ambulatory care settings. About 23% are employed by hospitals, many as house staff. The demand for PAs is expected to continue to increase.[107]

STATE AND FEDERAL REGULATION OF HSOs

When the states delegated certain powers to a federal government and ratified the U.S. Constitution, they retained a wide range of authority traditionally held by the sovereign. In sum, these are known as the police powers, defined as the powers to protect the health, safety, public order, and welfare of the public. Consistent with the police powers, states have enacted legislation to regulate and license a wide variety of HSOs. Licensure as it applies to specific types of HSOs is described in Chapter 4. Suffice it to say that HSOs that are required to obtain and retain a license must submit to inspections and other regulation.

Inspections

Licensure and Regulation

All types of HSOs are subject to state and local laws (ordinances), which result in inspections that are linked to licensure for that type of HSO for general public use and accommodation. Many states accept accreditation in lieu of licensure and other types of regulatory activity. For example, accreditation by the Joint Commission on Accreditation of Healthcare Organizations (Joint Commission) is recognized by 44 states.[108]

Regulation by state and local authorities concentrates on physical plant and safety. The *Life Safety Code* and *Fire Prevention Code* published by the National Fire Protection Association, a private voluntary association, are prominent sources of standards for public and private groups. Unless a patient care–related problem is being investigated, however, state and local government authorities pay scant attention to quality of care. City and county ordinances also apply to HSOs (because some state police powers have been delegated to local government), but these tend to address matters such as radiation safety, sanitation of food and water, and disposal of wastes. In some of these activities, local governments may be acting on behalf of the state.

Conditions of Participation

The 1965 Medicare law recognized that hospitals that were accredited by the Joint Commission on Accreditation of Hospitals (JCAH; now the Joint Commission) were in "deemed" status (eligible) for purposes of reimbursement. Concerns were raised about delegating governmental authority to a private group. In 1966 "conditions of participation" (COPs) and applicable procedures were distributed to hospitals by the Department of Health, Education and Welfare, now DHHS. The COPs were similar to the Joint Commission's 1965 standards and focused on minimum levels of performance. Legislation in 1972 mandated federal oversight of Joint Commission accreditation: The secretary of DHHS was authorized to develop COPs that were more stringent than Joint Commission standards and to review accredited hospitals on the basis of random sampling or complaints. The COPs emphasized physical plant and safety (e.g., *Life Safety Code*) and minimized interest in the content and processes of clinical practice and organization; Joint Commission emphases were the opposite. Revised COPs became effective in 1986. The 1998 revisions to the COPs focused on outcomes, not processes, and hospitals will be expected to monitor and improve the quality of care and document it; patient assessment, quality assessment, patient rights, and performance improvement are emphasized.[109] The two programs have evolved toward each other, with most of the change falling on the COPs. Other private accrediting groups, such as the Community Health Accreditation Program (CHAP) and AOA, have achieved "deemed" status as well.

Planning and Rate Regulation

Much of what happens in the states is stimulated by the federal government. As noted, the Hill-Burton Act of 1946 suggested statewide planning for hospital services. In 1966 the Comprehensive

Health Planning and Public Health Service Amendments Act encouraged use of planning methodologies to allocate resources and improve access to health services and contain costs. States were expected to develop health planning agencies known as "a" and "b" agencies to assist in health planning.

In the late 1960s states began enacting laws to control increasing health services costs. They were especially concerned about cost increases in Medicaid, whose funding they shared. These initiatives sought to control capital expenditures and the costs of health services through rate review. States such as New York and Maryland were among the first to enact capital expenditure review laws. Others were prompted by the Social Security Amendments of 1972 (PL 92-603). This law included two provisions important to HSOs. One established PSROs to review the quantity and quality of care provided for Medicare patients in hospitals. PSROs complemented the planning legislation by seeking to control use of health services, thus reducing costs. In addition, Section 1122 of the law required capital expenditure review, which enhanced planning agency control. Hospitals consume disproportionately more resources than other types of HSOs, and policy makers have given them a great deal of attention.

The National Health Planning and Resources Development Act of 1974 (PL 93-641) mandated that each state have a health planning and development agency and a network of health systems agencies (HSAs). HSAs superseded the scattered areawide health planning agencies ("b" agencies) established in the 1966 law and made recommendations to the state health planning and development agency or the state health coordinating council, which applied state CON laws and gave final approval. Planning laws sought to control costs by focusing on the supply of services.

CON laws required HSOs to obtain approval to add a new service or for construction or renovation projects exceeding a certain cost, usually several hundred thousand dollars. The purpose was to ration the supply of health services by controlling capital expenditures and preventing unneeded expansion. Critics of CON argued that this artificial limitation on the supply of services caused inflation. In the late 1970s criticism about the usefulness of mandated planning grew. The antiregulatory mood in health services fit with the movement toward deregulation elsewhere in the economy. In 1987 the National Health Planning and Resources Development Act was repealed.[110] In the years since, states have scaled back their involvement in planning. By 1989, 11 states had repealed CON review programs and 5 others had deregulated hospitals and other acute care services.[111] "Most states, [took] a . . . moderate approach, streamlining programs, deregulating services and providers—particularly those perceived as not contributing to long-term health cost increases—and raising expenditure threshold levels to exempt all but the most costly projects."[112] In 1999, 37 states and the District of Columbia had CON laws; Maine's were the most restrictive, with a review of 24 types of services, and Ohio's the least restrictive, with a review of 1 type of service.[113]

As of 1983 mandatory health services rate review (cost review) programs had been enacted in six states.[114] In addition, there were more than 20 voluntary programs. By regulating what HSOs—primarily hospitals—charged or were paid, the states treated them as public utilities. States with rates of increase in health services costs below the national average were exempt from the federal DRG (prospective payment) system for Medicare patients. In the mid-1980s exempt states included New York, New Jersey, Maryland, and Massachusetts.[115] By 1999 only Maryland was exempt. Since 1971 Maryland has had a highly regulated, all-payer system to pay for hospital-based inpatient and outpatient care. The system allows only limited discounts, which inhibits Maryland hospitals' ability to compete, especially in border areas. Beyond the competitive disadvantage, it is uncertain how long Maryland's costs can remain below the national average.

Utilization Review, PSROs, and PROs[116]

Utilization review was a mandated part of hospital participation in the original Medicare law. Hospitals were required to certify the necessity of admission, continued stay, and professional services that were rendered to Medicare beneficiaries. Review was delegated to hospitals.

Rapid Medicare cost increases in the late 1960s suggested that hospital-based utilization review programs were ineffective. PSROs were established by the Social Security Amendments of 1972 (PL 92-603) as federally funded physician organizations responsible to ensure the appropriateness, medical necessity, and quality of care furnished to Medicare beneficiaries. As with utilization review, emphasis in the PSRO program was on hospital review. The three related functions of PSRO were admission and continued stay review, quality assurance, and profile analysis (patterns of care).

Ten years later PSROs had neither proved cost-effective nor had they had a significant effect on quality. As a remedy, Congress established PROs as part of the Tax Equity and Fiscal Responsibility Act of 1982. PROs were outcome rather than process and structure oriented, and outcomes were measured against performance standards. The core of PRO activities is to deny Medicare payment for medically unnecessary care, care rendered in an inappropriate setting, or care of substandard quality. In addition, they educate problem providers, review 100% of problem cases, exert peer pressure, and, if correction is not achieved or if a gross and flagrant quality problem occurs, recommend excluding the provider from Medicare.

Since the inception of PROs, their work has been expanded to include all federal payments for medical services. Part of this trend is to include care in physicians' offices. A major initiative in the early 1990s was implementing a uniform clinical data set that enables PROs to consistently select cases that require review. This database will allow epidemiological studies and inter-PRO comparisons. In future, PROs will emphasize quality rather than utilization. In general, PROs are statewide; in 1998, 42 PROs had 53 contracts in the United States and territories.[117]

The critics of PROs focus on how few physicians and hospitals have been disciplined by them. Historically, PROs have issued few, if any, sanctions against providers. In addition, the inspector general of DHHS has estimated that far more hospital admissions are inappropriate than have been found by PROs.[118] It would seem that much work remains.

Government Payment Schemes

Diagnosis-Related Groups

Initially, Medicare reimbursement was based on the hospital's costs; the lack of incentives to be efficient caused runaway cost increases. By the early 1980s a more direct means of cost control was begun when the Tax Equity and Fiscal Responsibility Act of 1982 and the Social Security Amendments of 1983 (PL 98-21) mandated a prospective payment system for Medicare through DRGs. A division of DHHS, the Health Care Financing Administration (HCFA) is responsible for administering Medicare and Medicaid and establishing and reviewing the DRG rates for each Medicare inpatient admission. Discharged Medicare patients are assigned to one of almost 500 DRGs based on diagnosis, surgery, patient age, discharge destination, and gender. Each DRG's weight is based primarily on Medicare billing and cost data and reflects the relative cost, across all hospitals, of treating cases that are classified in that DRG.[119] Hospitals that can provide services at lower costs keep the difference. Those exceeding the DRG rate must recoup the difference elsewhere.

The change from cost-based reimbursement to payment according to rates prospectively determined by HCFA has had and will continue to have major effects on hospitals. One is that hospitals "unbundled" (separated) postacute services such as subacute, recuperative, and rehabilitative care from the acute-episode hospital stay. For example, hospital-based nursing facility beds were established to provide transitional care. Under prospective payment, hospitals must be certain that their average costs per DRG do not exceed HCFA rates. Managers and physicians must collaborate to eliminate unnecessary tests and procedures and reduce length of stay, and, in general, hospitals must become more efficient. Initially, the DRG payment system applied only to Medicare patients, but state Medicaid programs, Blue Cross, and other third-party payers have adopted it for inpatient services. Similar, DRG-like prospective payment system methodologies are being used for nursing facilities and outpatient clinics as well.

Resource Utilization Groups

DRGs are applied to hospitalized Medicare beneficiaries. Long-term care has developed its own classification system in which nursing facility residents with similar resource needs (utilization) are put into groups. Initially, these groups were based on the ability of nursing facility residents to engage in activities of daily living (ADLs), which are major explanatory factors in resource use. Since the mid-1980s these resource utilization groups (RUGs) have undergone significant derivation and validation and have evolved through RUG-II, which was used to determine nursing facility payment for Medicaid in New York and Texas.[120] RUG-III was mandated for Medicare residents by the Balanced Budget Act of 1997. It set 44 reimbursement levels (26 for Medicare, 18 for Medicaid) based on resident condition and use of services. RUG-III uses 300 elements of care to measure a resident's acuity based on differences in ADLs; need for specialized therapies, nursing, and ancillary services; and presence of depression. National rates will be phased in over 3 years and will be lower than the rates used during RUG-III phase-in. Rates will be adjusted for wage levels and whether the nursing facility is located in an urban or a rural area and will change as residents' conditions change.[121] As with other federally mandated schemes (e.g., DRGs), other payers are likely to adopt RUG-III in determining payments to nursing facilities.

Ambulatory Patient Groups and Ambulatory Payment Categories

Other providers of services have drawn the attention of regulators and lawmakers. Research in the late 1980s led to the development of ambulatory patient groups (APGs), a system of codes that explains the amount and type of resources used in an ambulatory visit. The variety of outpatient service settings, wide variation in why outpatient care was required, and the high percentage of costs associated with ancillary services necessitated a classification scheme that could reflect the range of services rendered. Like DRGs, patients in each APG are assumed to have similarities in clinical characteristics, resource use, and costs. Also like DRGs, a primary APG or a significant procedure is subdivided into groups by body systems. Unlike DRGs, variables for additional services are based on clinically similar classes, and multiple APGs can be applied per patient encounter. APGs will eventually encompass the full range of ambulatory settings, including same-day surgery units, hospital emergency rooms, and outpatient services. They will not address telephone contacts, home health visits, nursing facility care, or inpatient services.[122]

HCFA has adapted ambulatory payment categories (APCs) from APGs. APCs group thousands of procedure and diagnosis codes into more than 300 categories, with separate classifications for surgical, medical, and ancillary services. Each group includes clinically similar services that require comparable levels of resources. A relative weight based on median resource use is assigned to each classification. Payment for each APC is determined by multiplying the relative weight by a conversion factor, which is the average rate for all APC services. The system is expected to apply to all Medicare Part B outpatient facility costs, except those covered by a separate schedule, such as ambulance, durable medical equipment, laboratory, and implantable-device costs.[123]

Resource-Based Relative Value Scale

In 1992 HCFA began implementing a fee schedule for physicians who participate in Medicare Part B, a change mandated by the Omnibus Budget Reconciliation Act of 1989 (PL 101-239, OBRA '89).[124] Previously, physician payment under Part B was based on usual, customary, and reasonable charges. Among the most important effects of charge-based payment was that procedure-based specialties such as surgery were more highly paid than specialties that are based on cognitive skills (e.g., evaluation, management), such as internal medicine. The new schedule used a resource-based relative value scale (RBRVS) that resulted in dramatic changes in physician payment patterns. The prospectively set reimbursement is based on the resources that are used to produce physician services and is divided into three components: physician work, practice expenses, and malpractice insurance.[125] Nonphysician practitioners whose services are paid under Medicare Part B will continue to have their fees tied to those of physicians, and their fees will move in the same direction.[126]

The RBRVS system increased reimbursement for family and general practice physicians by about 15%; payments to ophthalmologists and anesthesiologists declined the most (approximately 35%), but those to other procedure-based specialists such as surgeons decreased as well.[127] Publication in mid-1991 of a proposed physician fee schedule that projected a 16% decrease in payments to all physicians by 1996 caused a storm of controversy.[128] To prevent physicians who have not signed a Medicare participation agreement (accepting Medicare as full payment for services [sometimes called assignment]) from balance-billing patients (when physicians bill patients for the difference between what Medicare pays and the physicians' charges), the statute imposed a cap on the amount that a nonparticipating physician may balance-bill a Medicare beneficiary.[129] Regulations developed pursuant to the Balanced Budget Act of 1997 allow physicians (and other health care practitioners) to opt out of Medicare and provide services through private contracts. However, physicians who wanted a private charging relationship with only one Medicare beneficiary had to remove themselves entirely from the Medicare program, on any level, whether fee-for-service or capitated, for 2 years. This extreme penalty meant that few physicians were likely to engage in private contracting.[130] A legal challenge to the private charging relationship regulations, however, resulted in a federal appeals court ruling that prohibited HCFA from interfering with private payment relationships between Medicare beneficiaries and their physicians.[131]

The federal application of RBRVS is only to Medicare. However, RBRVS is very likely to be used by other third-party payers, as they have used DRGs. The effect will be a major change in how physicians are paid. Other likely effects are that physicians employed in high-technology practices will generate less income for their employers; physicians will try to unbundle services and move more of them out of hospitals to their offices; physicians may seek to have lost income made up by hospitals; physicians may limit their willingness to care for Medicare beneficiaries; and adjustments in how physicians are paid in rural areas as compared with urban areas will make it easier for rural hospitals to attract physicians, thus increasing access to care by rural beneficiaries while potentially decreasing it for urban beneficiaries.[132]

Summary

The incentives in DRGs, RUGs, and APG/APCs may lead to underuse of services and consequently to inappropriate treatment of patients. DRGs are causing patients to be discharged from hospitals earlier. A Rand Corporation study reported in 1990 that the mortality rates of Medicare patients have been unchanged by DRGs, but also it showed that more patients are medically unstable when released from hospitals.[133] This finding has significant implications for home health agencies, nursing facilities, and hospitals. Continued surveillance is needed.

The incentives in RBRVS are to overuse services because the physician is paid for each treatment. Treatment by some specialties may be more effective, with lower total cost than the same diagnosis treated by a family practitioner, however. A more likely long-term effect of RBRVS will be to alter the ratios of physicians by specialty because of changes in incomes.

Other Regulators

In addition to DHHS, which affects reimbursement through HCFA, a multitude of federal regulators affect the management of HSOs. These activities are based on authority in the U.S. Constitution, as interpreted by the U.S. Supreme Court, to regulate interstate commerce and to provide for the general welfare. Regulators include independent agencies and various other executive branch departments and bureaus. The Department of Justice and the Federal Trade Commission enforce the Sherman Antitrust Act (1890) and the Clayton Act (1914) and their various amendments prohibiting anticompetitive practices. The National Labor Relations Board applies provisions of the National Labor Relations Act (1935) and its amendments to the process of union organizing and collective bargaining. The Occupational Safety and Health Administration enforces provisions of the Occupational Safety and Health Act (1970) to safeguard the work environment. The Food and Drug Administration enforces provisions of the Food, Drug, and Cosmetic Act of 1906 and its amendments and regulates drugs and medical devices. The Securities and Exchange Commission enforces the Securities Exchange Act of 1934, as amended, and affects how investor-owned HSOs market, sell, and trade stock. The Nuclear Regulatory Commission enforces provisions of the Atomic Energy Act (1954) and regulates and licenses the nuclear industry, thus regulating hazards arising from storage, handling, and transportation of nuclear materials. The Equal Employment Opportunity Commission enforces the Equal Pay Act of 1963, Title VII of the Civil Rights Act of 1964, and the Age Discrimination in Employment Act of 1967, among others, and investigates complaints about treatment of employees and prospective employees. The Bureau of Alcohol, Tobacco, and Firearms of the Treasury Department enforces the alcohol and tobacco tax provisions of the Internal Revenue Code and the Alcohol Administration Act of 1935 and regulates the use of tax-free alcohol. It is noteworthy that many federal regulatory, review, and control activities have applied to HSOs only since the early 1970s.

HEALTH SERVICES DELIVERY ACCREDITATION

Joint Commission

No voluntary, private organization has affected HSOs, especially hospitals, as has the Joint Commission on Accreditation of Healthcare Organizations. The Joint Commission was known as the Joint Commission on Accreditation of Hospitals until 1986, by which time a greatly broadened mission that included accreditation programs for several types of HSOs had made the word "hospitals" in its name a misnomer. The Joint Commission traces its lineage to the "Hospital Standardization" program established by the American College of Surgeons (ACS), which began surveying hospitals in 1918. Until 1951 ACS singlehandedly worked to improve hospital-based medical practice. Its director during most of this highly formative period was Malcolm T. MacEachern, a physician and early leader in the health services field, whose book, *Hospital Organization and Management,* is a classic in the field.

In 1951 the Joint Commission was formed by ACS, AMA, AHA, the American College of Physicians (ACP), and the Canadian Medical Association, which later left the Joint Commission and assisted in establishing the Canadian Council on Health Facilities Accreditation. The new Joint Commission began accrediting hospitals in 1953. As noted earlier, the importance of being accredited by the Joint Commission was greatly enhanced in 1965 with the passage of Medicare, which specified that Joint Commission–accredited hospitals were in "deemed" status (eligible) for purposes of Medicare reimbursement. By 1970 the Joint Commission's *Accreditation Manual for Hospitals* emphasized optimum achievable rather than minimal standards and had grown from 10 pages in 1965 to 152 pages.[134] This evolution continues and, just as Joint Commission standards have shifted to emphasize outcomes of clinical services, so too have HCFA's Conditions of Participation (COPs).

In 2000 the Joint Commission's governing body had 28 commissioners. In addition to representatives from ACS, AMA, AHA, ACP, and the American Dental Association, there were six public commissioners and one at-large nursing representative.[135] The Joint Commission has seven accreditation programs: ambulatory care, behavioral health, home care, hospitals, laboratories, long-term care, and networks. In 2000 it accredited nearly 20,000 health care organizations.[136] Each program has its own standards, but combined visits to survey common standards such as physical plant, licensure, and corporate bylaws minimize duplication for multiprogram HSOs/HSs. Joint Commission accreditation is expected for hospitals, and the vast majority are accredited.

Standards for various services and facilities are developed by professional and technical advisory committees composed of experts who may also represent health services professional and trade associations. In this sense the Joint Commission leads the various components of the health services system that it accredits, but it simultaneously reflects their level of development. Being too far ahead of the field makes standards overly demanding and difficult or impossible to meet, but merely reflecting the state of development limits progress.

The Joint Commission claims several benefits of accreditation:

Improves patient care

Strengthens community confidence

Provides professional consultation and enhances staff education

Provides ongoing support

Enhances internal quality improvement efforts

Enhances staff recruitment

May substitute for Medicare and Medicaid certification

Fulfills licensure requirements in many states

Is recognized by insurers and other third parties

Attracts professional referrals[137]

In 1986 the Joint Commission began its "Agenda for Change," a major philosophical shift to make accreditation standards performance focused, organize them around important patient care functions, and integrate them into the accreditation process.[138] This effort became known as ORYX. Its long-range goal is to establish a data-driven, continuous survey and accreditation process to complement the standards-based assessment. Each Joint Commission accreditation program will identify a set of standardized performance indicators to be used in accreditation. The measurement systems with which HSOs contract for comparative data will be expected to add some of the Joint Commission's standardized measures to their menu of measures, thus supporting the use of common measures by similar HSOs. The number of clinical measures will increase each year, and the proportion of the resident or patient population that is addressed by the measures will increase each year as well. Health status and patient-perception-of-care measures are likely to be added. The use of outcomes-related data will stimulate HSOs/HSs to examine their processes of care and take action to improve the results of care. ORYX will allow inter-HSO comparisons that are likely to be made available to the public.[139] However, there is concern about making valid interhospital comparisons and lack of standardized performance measures.[140]

In 1998 the Joint Commission began requiring HSOs to develop a definition of "sentinel events" and to identify and respond appropriately to them. The contextual definition that HSOs must use is that a

sentinel event is an unexpected occurrence involving death or serious physical or psychological injury, or the risk thereof. Serious injury specifically includes loss of limb or function. The phrase, "or risk thereof" includes any process variation for which a recurrence would carry a significant chance of a serious adverse outcome.[141]

Two subsets of sentinel events are reviewed by the Joint Commission: 1) those that result in an unanticipated death or major permanent loss of function, not related to the natural course of the illness or underlying condition; and 2) any of the following: suicide of a patient (in certain settings), infant abduction or discharge to the wrong family, rape, hemolytic transfusion reaction (certain types), and surgery on the wrong patient or wrong body part. Such events are called sentinel because they signal the need for immediate investigation and response. HSOs perform a root cause analysis that identifies the basic or causal factors that resulted in failure(s) in systems and processes that caused the sentinel event, not individual performance. Root cause analysis proceeds from special cause variation in clinical performance to common cause variation in organizational processes and identifies potential improvements. The result is an action plan of strategies that the organization will implement to reduce the risk of similar events in the future.[142]

The Joint Commission will continue to be a major force in developing performance expectations for HSOs/HSs. Even those that choose not to be accredited by the Joint Commission will benefit from considering its standards in developing and managing their programs. In 2000 and beyond, the Joint Commission will emphasize outcomes and continuous quality improvement, the theory and application of which are described in Chapter 10. The Joint Commission will remain viable only if its standards are state of the art, if HSOs/HSs continue to see the value of accreditation, and if the survey is worth the thousands of dollars it costs. As they evolve, the COPs developed by HCFA pose a substantial risk to a continued need for the Joint Commission. In addition, competing private specialty and programmatic accreditation efforts, several of which are described later, will almost certainly challenge the Joint Commission's preeminent position.

American Osteopathic Association

Osteopathic hospitals may be accredited by AOA as well as by the Joint Commission. Through its Bureau of Healthcare Facilities Accreditation, AOA accredits acute care hospitals, mental health centers, substance abuse centers, and physical rehabilitation centers. AOA accreditation is recognized by HCFA as granting "deemed" status for purposes of Medicare reimbursement.[143] In 1996 AOA accredited 144 health care facilities.[144]

International Organization for Standardization (ISO)

The International Organization for Standardization in Geneva is a nongovernmental organization that was established in 1947. ISO is a worldwide federation of national standards bodies from 130 countries. Its mission is "to promote the development of standardization and related activities in the world with a view to facilitating the international exchange of goods and services, and to developing cooperation in the spheres of intellectual, scientific, technological and economic activity."[145] Its work results in international agreements that are published as International Standards. The technical work of ISO is highly decentralized and is carried out in a hierarchy of 2,850 technical committees, subcommittees, and working groups that involve 30,000 experts in standards development. The benefits of international standards are obvious.

Most ISO standards are highly specific to a particular product, material, or process. Neither the ISO 9000 family nor the ISO 14000 family are product standards, however. They are families of generic management system standards that focus on processes and not directly on the results of process activities, even though what happens in the process affects the outcome. This means that they can be applied to any organization in any sector of activity, including HSOs. The ISO 9000 family is concerned primarily with quality management, which means that the features of a product or of services conform to customer requirements. The ISO 14000 family is primarily concerned with environmental management, which means what the organization does to minimize harmful effects on the environment caused by its activities.[146] Organizations or components of organizations that seek certification or registration using ISO 9000 or ISO 14000 standards are surveyed by independent, ISO–qualified auditors, not by ISO representatives.[147] The certification or registration is not officially recognized by ISO, even though its standards are used. ISO does not "accredit" organizations or components of organizations against its standards, as do groups such as the Joint Commission and the National Committee for Quality Assurance (NCQA), which is described later.

HSOs are beginning to implement standards such as the ISO 9000 series, which provides a framework for quality management and quality assurance. The application of ISO 9000 standards in HSOs is discussed in Chapter 9.

Community Health Accreditation Program

CHAP specializes in home care and community health. CHAP, a subsidiary of the National League for Nursing (NLN), began accreditation activities in 1965.[148] It accredits programs including community nursing centers, home health care aide services, home health organizations, infusion therapy services, home medical equipment, hospice, private duty nursing, public health organizations, and supplemental staffing services.[149] CHAP accreditation has conferred Medicare "deemed" status for home health care since 1992.[150] CHAP standards emphasize organizational structure and function; quality of services and products; adequacy of human, financial, and physical resources; and long-term viability. Its accreditation process is like that of the Joint Commission, including application for survey, self-study, site visit, and review by the CHAP board of review.[151]

National Committee for Quality Assurance

NCQA began accrediting health plans in 1991. More than half of the nation's HMOs (covering 75% of all HMO enrollees) participate in NCQA's accreditation program, which at the end of 1998 had granted accreditation to 236 health plans.[152] In 1992 NCQA began developing the Health Plan Employer Data and Information Set (HEDIS), which is widely used by employers and HMOs in judging and comparing quality. As part of its accreditation effort, NCQA requires health plans to submit audited results for clinical quality and consumer survey measures. Examples of clinical quality are childhood and adolescent immunization status, breast cancer and cervical cancer screening, advising smokers to quit, and postpartum check-ups. Examples of consumer survey measures are getting care quickly, doctors who communicate, courteous and helpful office staff, getting needed care, claims processing, and customer service. Most health plans offer several different types of products, such as a Medicare plan, a Medicaid plan, an HMO, and a point-of-service plan; NCQA reports on these products separately.[153]

Utilization Review Accreditation Commission

The Utilization Review Accreditation Commission (URAC) was established in 1990 to accredit utilization review organizations. In 1997 its name was changed to the American Accreditation Health-Care Commission (Commission/URAC) to reflect a broadened scope of activities to establish accreditation standards for managed health care company services, especially utilization management and health networks.[154] Member organizations of the Commission/URAC include AHA, AMA, ANA, Blue Cross Blue Shield Association, the American Association of Health Plans, the Association of Managed Health Care Organizations, and the Health Insurance Association of America. Standards are drafted by a committee composed of all interested parties and are then available for public review and comment. Changes are incorporated and standards are tested in managed care organizations and revised as necessary before final approval and use in surveys.

In 1998 utilization management, health networks, health care practitioner credentialing, workers' compensation utilization management, workers' compensation networks, and preferred provider organizations were accredited by Commission/URAC. Nineteen states and the District of Columbia have incorporated one or more of Commission/URAC's accreditation standards into their regulatory process.[155] Future accreditation standards will include credentials verification organizations, telephone health information and triage programs, and case management programs. By 1998 Commission/URAC had awarded 1,000 accreditation certificates to different accredited programs in approximately 200 organizations.[156]

ASSOCIATIONS FOR INDIVIDUALS AND ORGANIZATIONS

The health services field has numerous professional and trade associations for personal and institutional providers, both in generic groups and in an increasing number of subsets.

Professional Associations for Individuals

Managers

The premier professional association for HSO/HS managers is ACHE, formerly the American College of Hospital Administrators, which was established in 1933. It has more than 30,000 affiliates. Membership includes those in managerial positions running the gamut of HSOs. The important categories of affiliation are member, diplomate, and fellow. Each is separated by time and achievement requirements, including years in category, passing an examination, or submitting case studies. ACHE offers continuing education programs and publishes and enforces a code of ethics.

The Medical Group Management Association (MGMA) was established in 1926. It has 18,000 members who are actively engaged in the business management of medical groups that consist of three or more physicians in medical practice with centralized business functions. MGMA sponsors educational training programs, provides revenue and expense data on medical group practices, reports on current legislative activities and trends in health care, and provides placement and information services.[157]

Examples of other professional groups include specialized managerial personnel in HSOs: the Academy of Medical Group Management, the American College of Mental Health Administrators, the American College of Health Care Administrators (nursing facilities), the National Association of Healthcare Executives, and the College of Osteopathic Healthcare Executives. Some have levels of affiliation and advancement requirements. All provide a forum and educational activities to improve the content and quality of professional practice. The American Public Health Association does not focus on managers but has a broad membership of those in public health and other types of HSOs.

Physicians

Preeminent among physician groups is AMA, which was formed in 1847. In 1998 AMA had 290,917 members, including physicians, medical students, and residents.[158] This reflects only modest growth from its 288,275 members in 1991.[159] AMA is synonymous with "organized medicine," and it has been both a conservative and a progressive force in health care. Its conservatism is exemplified by historical opposition to government-sponsored health insurance and resistance to salaried physician arrangements as well as to innovations such as HMOs, which were seen as infringing on professional independence and total commitment to patients. AMA has been a progressive force by embracing programs such as Medicare once enacted, and by encouraging federal expenditures for basic and applied research and medical and paramedical education. Its involvement in establishing standards for medical education and licensure has contributed significantly to the unequalled standards of American medicine. AMA publishes and enforces a code of ethics.

There are many other associations for physicians. The National Medical Association represents more than 20,000 African American physicians and has goals similar to those of AMA.[160] In addition, there are associations, usually termed "colleges" or "academies," whose membership is based on medical specialties. Among the most prominent are ACP and ACS. "Fellow" or "diplomate" are titles used to refer to affiliates. As with ACHE, these associations represent the interests of affiliates and assist them in continuing education.

Nonphysician Affiliations

The list of other associations of individuals in health services is almost endless. Each new type of provider sees the need for a professional association to focus common interests. Some are old; ANA was established in 1896.[161] Other examples of nonphysician providers include the American Dental Association, the American Podiatry Association, the American Psychological Association, the Association of Operating Room Nurses, the National Association of Social Workers, the American Pharmaceutical Association (pharmacists), the National Federation of Licensed Practical Nurses, and the American Academy of Physician Assistants. The hundreds of professional associations for organizational and personal providers and managers in the health services field are a measure of its specialization and fragmentation.

Professional Associations for HSOs/HSs

American Hospital Association

With 4,975 institutional members, which includes 286 companies, AHA is the most prominent association for hospitals.[162] Founded in 1898, AHA educates and represents its members. Increasingly, it is the focal point for hospitals' efforts to participate in the political process. In 1991 AHA's executive offices were moved to Washington, D.C., while its other activities remained in Chicago. In many respects AHA is an umbrella organization—members are likely to belong to other institutional associations with more specialized orientations. Examples are described later. Representing hospitals with divergent goals and objectives makes AHA's role difficult.

Federation of American Health Systems

The Federation of American Health Systems is the investor-owned counterpart to AHA. It was established in 1966 and in 1998 had 1,000 members. The Federation monitors health legislation, regulatory and reimbursement matters, and developments in the health care industry at the state and national levels. In addition, it compiles statistics on the investor-owned hospital industry.[163]

American Osteopathic Healthcare Association

Formerly the American Osteopathic Hospital Association, the American Osteopathic Healthcare Association (AOHA) is the trade association for osteopathic hospitals and related organizations. In 1998 it had 160 members. AOHA promotes the common interests of osteopathic health care and provides advocacy and education to members.[164] The unique aspects of osteopathic health care were described earlier.

Other Hospital Associations

The Catholic Health Association of the United States represents a subset of hospitals with sectarian ownership and interests. In 1999 it had 1,200 members.[165] In addition to national hospital associations, there are regional and state hospital associations that link affiliation to geographical or state communities of interest. State hospital associations became much more important as the states became increasingly involved in regulating hospitals.

American Health Care Association

Founded in 1949, the American Health Care Association (AHCA) is a federation of 50 state health organizations that together represent nearly 12,000 not-for-profit and for-profit assisted-living, nursing facility, and subacute care providers.[166] AHCA promotes standards for professionals in long-term health care delivery and quality care for patients and residents in a safe environment. It focuses on issues such as availability, quality, affordability, and fair payment, and it acts as a liaison with government and is active in the federal political process as an advocate for members.[167]

American Association of Homes and Services for the Aging

The American Association of Homes and Services for the Aging (AAHSA) is the trade association for not-for-profit nursing facilities, continuing-care retirement communities, senior housing facilities, and assisted living and community services. Its 5,000 member organizations serve more than 1 million people. AAHSA represents its members' concerns with Congress and federal agencies. It enhances the professionalism of practitioners and facilities by certification, accreditation through the Continuing Care Accreditation Commission, conferences and programs, and publications. The financial strength of members is enhanced with group purchasing and insurance programs.[168]

American Association of Health Plans

The American Association of Health Plans (AAHP) was created in 1996 by the merger of the Group Health Association of America and the American Managed Care and Review Association. AAHP is the trade association for HMOs, preferred provider organizations, utilization review organizations, and other network-based plans; its 1,000 members provide care to more than 100 million Americans. In addition to representing member interests, it is committed to maintaining high standards of quality and professional ethics and the principle that patients come first.[169]

EDUCATIONAL ACCREDITORS

The quality of didactic and clinical programs that educate health services workers is ensured by monitoring groups that are organized like the Joint Commission. Various accreditors have boards (policy-making bodies) composed of representatives from professional groups in their fields. Accrediting committees, commissions, and groups have greater importance if they are recognized by the Office of Postsecondary Education of the Department of Education. Accreditation by a recognized accreditor is one of eight criteria that make a program eligible for federal support. There are, however, alternatives to accreditation that are acceptable to the Department of Education.

Managers

Programs for graduate education of health services managers are accredited by the Accrediting Commission on Education for Health Services Administration (ACEHSA). ACEHSA's corporate sponsors include ACHE, the American College of Medical Practice Executives, the American College of Physician Executives, AHA, AMA, the American Organization of Nurse Executives, the American Public Health Association, the Association of University Programs in Health Administration (the programs' trade association), the Canadian College of Health Services Executives, the Healthcare Financial Management Association, and the Healthcare Information and Management Systems Society. These sponsors appoint ACEHSA's commissioners (governing body). In 1999 ACEHSA accredited 67 graduate programs in North America.[170] The accreditation process is like that of the Joint Commission.

The Council on Education for Public Health (CEPH) accredits schools of public health and certain graduate public health programs offered in educational settings other than schools of public health. Schools of public health may emphasize management in their curricula. CEPH is composed of representatives from the American Public Health Association, the Association of Schools of Public Health, and graduate program and public representatives. In 1999 CEPH accredited 28 schools of public health, 12 graduate programs in community health education, and 21 graduate programs in community health/preventive medicine.[171]

Accreditors cooperate with one another when health services management education is sited in schools or degree programs that are accredited by more than one of them. For example, the International Association for Management Education, formerly the American Assembly of Collegiate Schools of Business, accredits graduate and undergraduate business programs. The unit that provides graduate education for both health services and business may request that accreditation activities be coordinated.[172]

Physicians

Figure 2.5 shows the relationships among various medical groups and accreditors of medical education at different levels. At the far left, the Council for Medical Affairs provides policy development and review activities. The Liaison Committee on Medical Education, the Accreditation Council for Graduate Medical Education, and the Accreditation Council for Continuing Medical Education accredit various levels of medical training and education. The importance of continuing medical education as part of a lifelong learning experience is apparent.

Nurses

In 1917 the predecessor to NLN released a standard curriculum for schools of nursing. Since then it has been a strong force in nursing education. NLN's mission is to improve education and health outcomes by linking communities and information through collaborating, connecting, creating, serving, and learning. Its members include individuals, schools of nursing, and health care agencies.[173] NLN established the National League for Nursing Accrediting Commission (NLNAC) as an independent subsidiary to assume the responsibility for accrediting all types of nursing education programs, including master's, baccalaureate and associate's degrees, diploma, and licensed practical nursing. In 1997 NLNAC accredited 1,249 of the 1,508 basic RN programs in the United States, including 513 baccalaureate degree, 627 associate's degree, and 109 diploma programs.[174]

Medical Specialty Boards for Allopaths

In 1998 there were 24 specialty boards in various branches of allopathic medicine and surgery. Recognition of specialization came relatively late in the development of medicine in the United States and undoubtedly gained impetus from the great expansion of medical technology that occurred early in the 20th century. The American Board of Ophthalmology, incorporated in 1917, was the first; the American Board of Medical Genetics was approved in 1991. Each board offers at least one general certification of specialization. In addition, most boards recognize subspecialization. In 1998 the 24 member boards of the American Board of Medical Specialties (ABMS) offered 37 areas of general specialization and subspecialty certificates in 75 areas.[175]

Boards play a vital role by certifying training and monitoring continued competence of physicians who claim special expertise and skills. Through their association, ABMS, the boards play a significant role in undergraduate, postgraduate, and continuing medical education. Figure 2.5 shows these relationships. It is notable that various specialty boards are composed of representatives of associations organized for that specialty.

PARENT ORGANIZATIONS OF THE CFMA, LCME, ACGME, AND ACCME
PARENT ORGANIZATIONS ESTABLISH POLICY

ABMS AMA AHA AAMC CMSS	AMA / AAMC	ABMS AMA AHA AAMC CMSS	ABMS AMA AHA AAMC CMSS AHME FSMB
COUNCIL FOR MEDICAL AFFAIRS	**LIAISON COMMITTEE ON MEDICAL EDUCATION**	**ACCREDITATION COUNCIL FOR GRADUATE MEDICAL EDUCATION**	**ACCREDITATION COUNCIL FOR CONTINUING MEDICAL EDUCATION**

FUNCTION:
Forum for discussion of issues relevant to medical education

REPRESENTATIVES
Two senior elected officers and the Chief Executive Officer of:
ABMS
AMA
AHA
AAMC
CMSS

CFMA Secretary
P.O. Box 10944
Chicago, IL 60610

FUNCTION:
Accrediting M.D. programs

REPRESENTATIVES
AMA (6)
AAMC (6)
CACMS (1)
Public (2)
Participants (nonvoting):
Students (2)
Federal (1)

LCME Secretary
(odd-numbered years)
515 N. State Street
Chicago, IL 60610-4377

(even-numbered years)
2450 N Street, NW
Washington, DC 20037-1126

FUNCTION:
Accrediting GME programs

REPRESENTATIVES
ABMS (4)
AMA (4)
AHA (4)
AAMC (4)
CMSS (4)
Resident Physicians Section AMA (1)
Public (1)
Federal (nonvoting) (1)
RRC Council Chairperson (1)

ACGME Secretary
515 N. State St., Suite 2000
Chicago, IL 60610-4377

FUNCTION:
Accrediting GME programs

REPRESENTATIVES
ABMS (3)
AMA (3)
AHA (3)
AAMC (3)
CMSS (3)
AHME (1)
FSMB (1)
Public (1)
Federal (nonvoting) (1)

ACCME Secretary
515 N. State St., Suite 7340
Chicago, IL 60610-4377

AAMC	Association of American Medical Colleges	AHME	Association For Hospital Medical Education	CMSS	Council of Medical Specialty Societies
ABMS	American Board of Medical Specialties	AMA	American Medical Association	FSMB	Federation of State Medical Boards
AHA	American Hospital Association	CACMS	Committee on Accreditation of Canadian Medical Schools		

Figure 2.5. Relationships among various medical groups and accreditors of medical education at different levels. (From American Board of Medical Specialties, Research & Education Foundation. *2000 Annual Report & Reference Handbook*, 69. Evanston, IL: American Board of Medical Specialties, 2000; reprinted by permission.)

Although the Accreditation Council for Graduate Medical Education accredits residencies, the content of residency education is largely determined by each medical specialty board's residency review committee. The Accreditation Council for Continuing Medical Education accredits the continuing medical education programs required by specialty boards for continued certification. In addition, by 1998 all 24 boards had proposed time-limited certificates requiring recertification at intervals of 7–10 years, which means specialists must demonstrate continuing competence to remain certified. About 85% of licensed physicians are board certified by an ABMS board.[176]

Managers and professional staff organization members must be vigilant about board certification. There are scores of self-designated medical specialty boards with no ABMS recognition; some states have sought to protect the public by regulating use of the terms "board certification" and "board certified."[177] A proliferation of "boards" dilutes a major reason for specialty certification—to allow the public to identify practitioners who have earned significant, accepted formal recognition of skills in a specialty. This problem is most significant outside HSOs/HSs, where there are few controls.

Neither licensure nor board certification entitles any physician to clinical privileges in a HSO. Licensure is more basic, and lawful medical practice is impossible without it, especially certification is only one indicator of competence. The HSO has an independent ethical and legal duty to determine competence initially and then to continually monitor the care delivered in it by LIPs, whether or not they are board certified. The credentialing process is detailed in Chapter 4.

FINANCING HEALTH SERVICES

Expenditure Trends

Since the 1960s the percentage of GDP devoted to health expenditures has increased. Table 2.4 provides a wealth of information about aggregate and per capita national health expenditures, as well as percentage distribution and average annual percentage growth by sources of fund. Expenditures are shown in 1999 dollars (unadjusted for inflation), with projections to 2007. Table 2.4 shows that in 1996 national health expenditures consumed 13.6% of GDP, or $1,035 billion. As discussed previously, the percentage of GDP that is consumed by health care declined in 1997 and was unchanged in 1998. It is projected that health care will consume $2.8 trillion by 2010 and $7.8 trillion by 2020.[178] The period of rapid inflation occurred soon after the passage of Medicare and Medicaid in 1965; this demand–push stimulation was undoubtedly instrumental in the initial and continuing cost increases. These increases have been a major factor in state and federal efforts to control health services costs, or at least limit what they will pay.

The large percentage of expenditures consumed by hospitals (see Figure 2.6) has caused most state and federal cost controls to be directed there. Historically, it was thought that hospitals were inefficiently managed and that excessive use of high technology, expensive tests, and treatments was the major cause of cost increases, especially in Medicare. Less time spent in hospitals was posited as reducing costs to the system; thus there was great emphasis on reducing admission rates and average lengths of stay. It has been suggested, however, that a policy of "single-mindedly emptying hospitals not only does not save any money, it might even add to total national health spending."[179] Continuing rapid increases in Medicaid expenditures generally, and for subacute and postacute services, such as nursing facilities and home health care, are likely to redirect and broaden cost-control efforts.

Sources and Uses of Funds in Health Care

This section describes sources and uses of funds in various parts of the U.S. health care system. Table 2.5 shows personal health care expenditures, by type of expenditure and source of funds, for

TABLE 2.4. NATIONAL HEALTH EXPENDITURE AMOUNTS, PERCENT DISTRIBUTION, AND AVERAGE ANNUAL PERCENT CHANGE, BY SOURCE OF FUNDS: SELECTED CALENDAR YEARS 1970-2007ᵃ

Item	1970	1980	1990	1992	1994	1996	1998	1999	2001	2003	2005	2007
									Projected			
Amounts in Billions												
National health expenditures	$73.20	$247.30	$699.50	$836.60	$945.70	$1,035.10	$1,146.80	$1,216.70	$1,384.10	$1,591.20	$1,841.00	$2,133.30
Private	45.5	142.5	415.1	478.1	521.8	552.0	606.4	649.6	746.6	860.3	992.3	1,145.90
Public	27.7	104.8	284.4	358.5	423.9	483.1	540.4	567.1	637.4	731.0	848.7	987.4
Medicare	7.7	37.5	112.1	141.4	169.8	203.1	231.1	241.2	267.8	306.2	356.1	415.6
Medicaid	5.3	26.1	75.4	106.4	131.0	147.7	165.5	175.6	203.2	238.7	283.6	337.0
Other	14.7	41.1	96.9	110.8	123.1	132.3	143.8	150.4	166.4	186.1	209.0	234.9
Total federal	17.8	72.0	195.8	257.0	304.1	350.9	393.8	412.5	461.3	527.9	612.6	712.9
Total state/local	9.9	32.8	88.5	101.6	119.8	132.2	146.6	154.7	176.1	203.1	236.1	274.5
Percent Distribution												
National health expenditures	100.0	100.0	100.0	100.0	100.0	100.0	100.0	100.0	100.0	100.0	100.0	100.0
Private	62.2	57.6	59.3	57.1	55.2	53.3	52.9	53.4	53.9	54.1	53.9	53.7
Public	37.8	42.4	40.7	42.9	44.8	46.7	47.1	46.6	46.1	45.9	46.1	46.3
Medicare	10.5	15.2	16.0	16.9	18.0	19.6	20.1	19.8	19.3	19.2	19.3	19.5
Medicaid	7.3	10.6	10.8	12.7	13.9	14.3	14.4	14.4	14.7	15.0	15.4	15.8
Other	20.1	16.6	13.8	13.2	13.0	12.8	12.5	12.4	12.0	11.7	11.4	11.0
Total federal	24.3	29.1	28.0	30.7	32.2	33.9	34.3	33.9	33.3	33.2	33.3	33.4
Total state/local	13.5	13.3	12.7	12.1	12.7	12.8	12.8	12.7	12.7	12.8	12.8	12.9
Average Annual Percent Change from Previous Year Shown												
National health expenditures	—	12.9	11.0	9.4	6.3	4.6	5.3	6.1	6.9	7.3	7.6	7.7
Private	—	12.1	11.3	7.3	4.5	2.9	4.8	7.1	7.2	7.2	7.5	7.5
Public	—	14.2	10.5	12.3	8.7	6.8	5.8	4.9	6.5	7.4	7.8	7.9
Medicare	—	17.2	11.6	12.3	9.6	9.4	6.7	4.4	5.9	7.4	7.9	8.2
Medicaid	—	17.3	11.2	18.8	11.0	6.2	5.9	6.1	8.1	8.5	9.1	8.9

	C1	C2	C3	C4	C5	C6	C7	C8	C9	C10	C11	C12
Other	10.8	8.9	6.9	5.4	3.7	4.3	4.6	5.4	6.0	5.8	6.0	6.0
Total federal	—	15.0	10.5	14.6	8.8	7.4	5.9	4.7	6.2	7.3	7.8	8.0
Total state/local	—	12.7	10.4	7.1	8.6	5.1	5.3	5.5	7.2	7.5	7.9	7.8
Gross domestic product (billions)	$1,035.60	$2,784.20	$5,743.80	$6,244.50	$6,947.00	$7,636.00	$8,384.10	$9,531.60	$10,469.00	$11,579.10	$12,865.50	
U.S. population (millions)[b]	214.8	235.1	260.0	265.3	270.4	275.3	280.2	287.2	291.7	296.1	300.5	
National health expenditures per capita	$341.00	$1,052.00	$2,691.00	$3,154.00	$3,497.00	$3,759.00	$4,093.00	$4,820.00	$5,456.00	$6,218.00	$7,100.00	
National health expenditures as a percentage of gross domestic product	7.10%	8.90%	12.20%	13.40%	13.60%	13.60%	13.70%	13.90%	14.50%	15.20%	15.90%	16.60%

Source: Health Care Financing Administration, Office of the Actuary. See www.hcfa.gov/stats/nhe-oact/tables/t17.htm.

[a]The health spending projections for 1998–2007 were based on the 1996 release of the National Health Expenditures (NHE). Data in subsequent releases of the NHE may not be consistent with these projections and should not be substituted for the 1996 historical estimates. Numbers and percentages may not add to totals because of rounding.

[b]July 1 Social Security area population estimates.

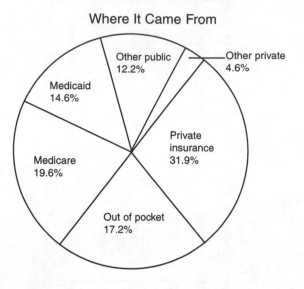

The U.S. Health Dollar, 1997

Where It Came From

Other public 12.2%

Other private 4.6%

Medicaid 14.6%

Private insurance 31.9%

Medicare 19.6%

Out of pocket 17.2%

Where It Went

Admin. & net cost 4.6%

Other 26.7%

Rx drugs 7.2%

Nursing facilities 7.6%

Hospital care 34.0%

Physicians' services 19.9%

Figure 2.6.   Sources and expenditures of U.S. health dollars. (From Office of the Actuary, National Health Statistics Group. Washington, DC: Health Care Financing Administration, 1998.)

1990 and 1997, with projections for 2007. During the period from 1990 to 1997, personal health care expenditures increased by more than 50%, with most of the increase funded from government sources. Figure 2.6 shows the source and use of the health dollar for 1997. Private (nongovernmental) sources continue to provide more than 50% of the funds for personal health care expenditures. The portion consumed by hospitals and nursing facilities is more than 40%, which targets them for cost-cutting efforts.

Table 2.6 shows annual percentage increases for various items on the CPI from 1969 to 1996. With few exceptions, the percentage for "All medical care items" has maintained steady, significant increases year after year, and almost always these increases have been consistently greater than those of "All items."

TABLE 2.5. PERSONAL HEALTH CARE EXPENDITURES, BY TYPE OF EXPENDITURE AND SOURCE OF FUNDS CALENDAR YEARS 1990, 1997, AND 2007 (PROJECTED)

Amount (billions)

Source of funds	TOTAL	Hospital care	Physician services	Dental services	Other professional services	Home health care	Drugs and other medical nondurables	Vision products and other medical durables	Nursing facility care	Other personal health care
1990										
Personal health care expenditures	$614.7	$256.4	$146.3	$31.6	$34.7	$13.1	$59.9	$10.5	$50.9	$11.2
Out-of-pocket payments	145.0	11.1	32.2	15.4	13.7	3.6	40.4	6.7	21.9	—
Third-party payments	469.6	245.4	114.2	16.2	21.0	9.5	19.5	3.7	29.0	11.2
Private health insurance	207.7	95.6	66.8	15.1	12.0	2.2	13.0	0.8	2.1	—
Other private	20.8	10.2	2.7	0.1	2.5	2.2	—	—	0.9	2.2
Government	241.1	139.6	44.7	0.9	6.5	5.1	6.5	2.9	25.9	9.0
Federal	177.0	105.4	35.6	0.5	4.3	4.1	3.1	2.7	15.8	5.4
Medicare	108.6	68.7	29.2	0.0	3.3	3.0	0.1	2.5	1.7	—
Medicaid	40.4	16.6	4.1	0.4	0.3	1.1	2.9	—	13.0	2.0
Other	28.0	20.1	2.2	0.1	0.7	—	0.1	0.2	1.0	3.5
State and local	64.2	34.2	9.1	0.4	2.2	1.0	3.4	0.1	10.2	3.6
Medicaid	31.0	12.9	2.9	0.3	0.2	1.0	2.1	—	10.1	1.5
Other	33.1	21.4	6.2	0.1	2.0	0.0	1.2	0.1	0.1	2.1
1997										
Personal health care expenditures	969.0	371.1	217.6	50.6	61.9	2.3	108.9	13.9	82.8	29.9
Out-of-pocket payments	187.6	12.4	34.1	23.9	24.6	7.0	53.0	6.8	25.7	—
Third-party payments	781.5	358.6	183.6	26.8	37.3	5.3	55.9	7.1	57.0	29.9
Private health insurance	313.5	113.0	109.1	24.3	18.9	3.7	39.9	0.5	4.0	3.6
Other private	35.6	17.2	4.3	0.2	4.8	3.9	—	—	1.6	3.6
Government	432.4	228.4	70.1	2.3	13.6	7.7	16.0	6.6	51.4	26.3
Federal	337.3	185.6	58.4	1.3	10.8	5.4	9.2	6.4	34.5	15.6
Medicare	208.9	123.7	46.4	0.1	8.8	2.8	1.0	6.0	10.1	—
Medicaid	91.1	36.2	9.3	1.1	1.0	2.6	7.8	—	22.6	10.4
Other	37.3	25.7	2.7	0.1	1.1	—	0.4	0.4	1.7	5.1
State and local	95.1	42.8	11.7	1.0	2.8	2.3	6.8	0.1	16.9	10.7
Medicaid	61.2	21.4	6.4	0.9	0.7	2.1	5.5	—	16.8	7.5
Other	33.9	21.4	5.3	0.1	2.1	0.1	1.4	0.1	0.1	3.3

(continued)

TABLE 2.5. *(continued)*

		Amount (billions)								
Source of funds	TOTAL	Hospital care	Physician services	Dental services	Other professional services	Home health care	Drugs and other medical nondurables	Vision products and other medical durables	Nursing facility care	Other personal health care
					2007 (Projected)					
Personal health care expenditures	$1,859.2	$649.4	$427.3	$95.2	$134.5	$66.1	$223.6	$23.3	$148.3	$91.4
Out-of-pocket payments	310.7	15.1	39.1	41.4	50.7	17.4	88.3	11.4	47.3	0
Third-party payments	1,548.4	634.3	388.2	53.8	83.8	48.7	135.3	11.9	101	91.4
Private health insurance	643.4	219	223.9	50	43.2	8.9	86.5	0.9	10.9	0
Other private	64.4	31.4	8.9	0.4	9	4.1	0	0	2.9	7.6
Government	840.6	383.8	155.5	3.4	31.5	35.7	48.8	11	87.2	83.7
Federal	656.4	325.3	126.1	2.1	23.7	30	29.2	10.7	60	49.2
Medicare	399.4	223.3	97.4	0.4	18.9	23.4	5.4	10.1	20.4	0
Medicaid	—	—	—	—	—	—	—	—	—	—
Other	—	—	—	—	—	—	—	—	—	—
State and local	184.2	58.5	29.4	1.3	7.8	5.7	19.6	0.2	27.2	34.5
Medicaid	317	86.7	39.3	2.6	4	12	39.3	0	63.2	69.9
Other	—	—	—	—	—	—	—	—	—	—

Source: Health Care Financing Administration, Office of the Actuary, National Health Statistics Group. See www.hcfa.gov/stats/nhe-oact/tables/t17.htm.

Notes: 0.0 denotes amounts less than $50 million. Medicaid expenditures exclude Part B premium payments to Medicare by states under buy-in agreements to cover premiums for eligible Medicaid recipients. Numbers may not add to totals because of rounding.

TABLE 2.6. CONSUMER PRICE INDEX, AVERAGE ANNUAL PERCENTAGE CHANGE, ALL URBAN CONSUMERS, 1969–1996

Year	All items	All medical care items	Physicians' services	Dental services	Hospital services	Medical care commodities	Prescription drugs	Internal and respiratory over-the-counter drugs
1969	5.5	8.2	7.0	7.2	13.6	0.9	1.3	1.0
1970	5.7	7.0	7.5	5.7	12.9	2.4	1.7	2.7
1971	4.4	7.4	7.0	6.4	12.3	1.7	0.0	3.8
1972	3.2	3.5	3.0	4.1	6.4	0.2	−0.4	0.9
1973	6.2	4.5	3.4	3.2	5.0	0.2	−0.2	1.1
1974	11.0	10.4	9.2	7.6	10.5	3.6	2.3	4.5
1975	9.1	12.6	12.1	10.4	17.1	8.3	6.2	10.7
1976	5.8	10.1	11.2	6.2	13.8	6.0	5.3	6.8
1977	8.5	9.9	9.3	7.6	11.5	6.5	6.1	6.9
1978	7.6	8.5	8.4	7.1	11.1	7.0	7.7	7.1
1979	11.3	9.8	9.1	8.3	11.3	7.1	7.8	7.4
1980	13.5	11.3	10.5	11.0	13.1	7.7	9.7	11.1
1981	10.3	10.7	11.0	8.3	14.9	11.0	11.4	12.4
1982	6.2	11.8	9.4	7.6	15.7	10.3	11.6	10.8
1983	3.2	8.7	7.8	6.8	11.3	8.6	11.0	7.5
1984	4.3	6.0	6.9	8.1	8.3	7.3	9.6	6.2
1985	3.6	6.1	5.9	6.2	5.9	7.2	9.5	5.4
1986	1.9	7.7	7.2	5.6	6.0	6.6	8.6	4.9
1987	3.6	6.6	7.3	6.8	6.9	6.7	8.0	5.3
1988	4.1	6.4	7.2	6.8	9.3	6.8	8.0	5.6
1989	4.8	7.7	7.4	6.3	11.5	7.8	8.7	6.1
1990	5.4	9.0	7.1	6.6	10.9	8.4	10.0	5.1
1991	4.2	8.6	6.0	7.4	10.2	8.2	9.9	4.5
1992	3.0	7.4	6.3	6.8	9.1	6.4	7.5	3.9
1993	3.0	5.9	5.6	5.3	8.4	3.7	3.9	3.3
1994	2.6	4.8	4.4	4.8	5.9	2.9	3.4	1.9
1995	2.8	4.5	4.5	4.9	5.0	1.9	1.9	0.7
1996	2.7	3.5	3.6	4.7	4.5	2.9	3.4	1.9

Source: U.S. Department of Labor, Bureau of Labor Statistics, 1997.

Table 2.6 also shows the average annual percentage change for various components that make up all medical care items. Hospital services have had significant increases since 1969. The contribution of physicians' services to all medical care items has been significant, even if they are less than hospital services. Data such as these have caught the attention of federal policy makers. DRGs, RUGs, and RBRVS have been their response.

Much of the cost of health services is borne by employers, and many have been instrumental in forming coalitions to find ways to control them. Coalitions bring together hospitals, physicians, employers, labor, insurers, and sometimes government to collect and exchange data and discuss how to finance and deliver health services in a community. Coalitions are discussed in Chapter 5.

Private Payment Under the Insurance Principle

The first insurer to write "sickness" insurance did so in 1847, but the insurance industry paid little attention to health insurance until after World War II. Contributing to this lack of interest was a perception that sickness and consequently paying for its treatment were too unpredictable to fit into then-extant actuarial concepts.

It was not until 1929 that Blue Cross showed it could be done. Blue Cross began when a group of schoolteachers made an agreement with Baylor Hospital in Dallas that it would provide hospital room and board and certain diagnostic services for a monthly fee. In 1932 the first citywide plan was established with a group of hospitals in Sacramento, California. The comparable plan for physicians' services became known as Blue Shield and was established in California in 1939. Hospitals fostered development of Blue Cross to enhance their patients' ability to pay the costs of hospitalization. After several mergers and reorganizations during the 1990s, there were 53 independent and 3 for-profit Blue Cross Blue Shield plans in the United States at the end of 1998, with 71.1 million subscribers.[180]

Private health insurance coverage grew rapidly during the 1940s and 1950s. It received a boost during World War II when wages and salaries were subjected to federal controls but fringe benefits were not. Commercial carriers began writing health insurance in substantial amounts, and by 1955 they had more insureds than Blue Cross. By 1981 more than 1,000 commercial insurance companies were writing health insurance in the United States.[181] Tables 2.7 and 2.8 present key health insurance statistics. Most private insurance coverage comes through the employment relationship. Table 2.7 estimates the number of people with and without health insurance, by source, for 1988–2002. The number of uninsureds is estimated to be more than 45 million by 2002. Some uninsureds are self-pay; many choose not to pay for insurance coverage at their employment or similar source; most would be medically indigent in the event of a major illness. The estimate does not, however, indicate how many uninsured cannot get care when needed. Table 2.8 shows that more than 185 million Americans had private (nongovernmental) health insurance coverage in 1995— 70.6% of the population. The data do not describe the extent of coverage and its adequacy to meet health needs.

Historically, Blue Cross was a community-rated (i.e., all insureds in the same geographic area pay the same rate) service plan, which paid providers pursuant to a contract. In contrast to service plans, indemnity insurance—the type usually written by commercial insurers—indemnifies (pays) the insured a fixed amount for each diagnosis or treatment. A variation of indemnification is assignment—the insured assigns the payment to the provider, who is paid directly. Service plan limits are expressed in days of care and services covered. Blue Shield paid participating physicians according to a fee schedule, which was payment in full and which had the effect of assignment. Nonparticipating physicians billed the patient, who is reimbursed per the fee schedule. Another difference between Blue Cross (and Blue Shield) and commercial carriers is that historically the former were not-for-profit corporations that prided themselves on low overhead costs in plan administration.

Government Programs

As noted, until 1965 the federal government concentrated on providing the wherewithal to support the private delivery of services; it financed little care. Direct services are provided to groups such as veterans and military personnel and Native Americans. State governments provide services for special health problems such as mental illness, tuberculosis, and mental retardation. States also operate general acute care hospitals that are part of academic health centers connected with state medical schools. Other HSOs, typically general acute care hospitals, are owned by local governments.

Table 2.5 shows increases in public (government) expenditures for health services. The federal government has sought to control the increase in expenditures through programs such as PROs, DRGs, RUGs, and RBRVS, which were described earlier. The states have sought to slow the growth in Medicaid expenditures by hospital preadmission screening, limiting hospital days available to any beneficiary, reducing what is paid for each day of care or each service, paying months or years after bills are submitted by the HSO/HS, requiring patients to pay larger copayments for

TABLE 2.7. PEOPLE WITH AND WITHOUT HEALTH INSURANCE, BY SOURCE, 1988–2002

Year	Total	Uninsured	Own job	Working spouse dependent	Dependent	Retirement	Nongroup	CHAMPUS or military	Medicaid	Dual eligible	Medicare
1988	241,154	30,627	67,523	18,087	59,565	3,135	12,058	5,305	14,469	3,376	27,009
1989	243,684	31,435	67,500	19,251	59,459	3,412	11,941	5,361	14,377	3,655	27,293
1990	246,190	32,005	68,195	19,695	59,578	3,447	12,556	5,170	14,033	3,693	27,819
1991	248,887	33,351	67,199	18,915	58,986	3,484	12,444	5,476	16,675	3,982	28,373
1992	251,435	34,195	68,390	19,360	58,081	2,001	12,069	5,532	18,858	4,274	28,664
1993	254,240	35,848	67,119	19,576	57,967	2,034	12,966	5,085	20,085	4,322	29,238
1994	259,753	38,184	70,133	18,183	57,145	2,598	11,027	4,676	21,559	4,156	29,092
1995	262,106	39,578	72,865	18,872	53,994	2,621	11,416	4,456	21,493	4,194	29,618
1996	264,465	40,992	73,257	18,513	53,157	2,380	11,075	4,231	22,480	4,231	30,149
1997	266,845	41,628	73,916	18,412	52,302	2,668	11,001	3,736	23,482	4,270	30,420
1998	269,247	42,541	74,581	18,040	51,157	2,692	11,963	3,500	24,501	4,308	30,963
1999	271,670	42,924	75,253	17,930	50,259	2,988	11,930	3,260	25,565	4,347	31,514
2000	276,383	44,221	76,282	17,965	49,749	3,041	11,070	3,040	26,809	4,422	31,784
2001	278,871	45,456	76,968	17,569	49,081	3,068	12,079	2,789	27,329	4,462	32,070
2002	281,381	45,584	77,661	17,446	48,398	3,377	12,104	2,532	28,419	4,502	32,359

Source: Lewin Group estimates, 1996.

TABLE 2.8. PEOPLE WITH PRIVATE HEALTH INSURANCE, BY TYPE OF INSURER, 1940–1996 (MILLIONS)

		Total insurance companies				
	All insurers[a]	Total no. of people	Group	Individual/ family	Blue Cross Blue Shield	Other plans
1940	12.0	3.7	2.5	1.2	6.0	2.3
1945	32.0	10.5	7.8	2.7	18.9	2.7
1950	76.6	37.0	22.3	17.3	38.8	4.4
1955	101.4	53.5	38.6	19.9	50.7	6.5
1960	122.5	69.2	54.4	22.2	58.1	6.0
1961	125.8	70.4	56.1	22.4	58.7	7.1
1962	129.4	72.2	58.1	23.1	60.1	6.9
1963	133.5	74.5	61.5	23.5	61.0	7.2
1964	136.3	75.8	63.1	34.0	62.1	6.8
1965	138.7	77.6	65.4	24.4	63.3	7.0
1966	142.4	80.4	67.8	24.9	54.3	6.6
1967	146.4	82.6	71.5	24.6	67.2	7.1
1968	151.9	85.7	74.1	25.3	70.1	7.3
1969	155.0	88.8	77.9	25.9	82.7	7.7
1970	158.8	89.7	80.5	26.7	85.1	8.1
1971	161.8	91.5	80.6	27.8	76.5	8.5
1972	164.1	93.7	81.5	29.1	78.2	8.1
1973	168.5	94.5	83.6	27.5	81.3	9.6
1974	173.1	97.0	85.4	28.8	83.8	11.1
1975	178.2	99.5	87.2	30.1	86.4	13.1
1976	176.9	97.0	86.8	27.0	86.6	14.9
1977	179.9	100.4	89.2	28.7	86.0	18.1
1978	185.7	106.0	92.5	36.1	85.8	21.5
1979	185.7	104.1	94.1	34.4	86.1	25.5
1980	187.4	105.5	97.4	33.8	86.7	33.2
1981	186.2	105.9	103.0	25.3	85.8	40.3
1982	188.3	109.6	103.9	29.4	82.0	48.2
1983	186.6	105.9	104.6	22.2	79.6	53.6
1984[b]	184.4	103.1	103.0	20.4	79.4	54.4[b]
1985	181.3	100.4	99.5	21.2	78.7	55.1[b]
1986	180.9	98.2	106.6	12.1	78.0	64.9[b]
1987	179.7	96.7	106.1	10.4	76.9	66.9[b]
1988	182.3	92.6	100.5	10.7	74.0	71.3[b]
1989	182.5	88.9	98.7	10.0	72.5	78.6[b]
1990	181.7	83.1	88.7	10.2	70.9	86.2[b]
1991	181.0	78.0	83.3	9.9	68.1	93.5[b]
1992	180.7	76.6	82.1	8.5	67.5	97.9[b]
1993	180.9	74.7	80.9	7.4	65.9	105.7[b]
1994	182.2	75.8	82.4	7.0	65.2	112.9[b]
1995	185.3	76.6	83.3	7.0	65.6	120.1[b]
1996	187.5	75.4	84.2	7.0	67.6	128.8[b]

From Health Insurance Association of America, *Source Book of Health Insurance Data, 1997–1998,* 39. Washington, DC: Author. Reprinted by permission.

Data Sources: Health Insurance Association of America; Group Health Association of America; Blue Cross Blue Shield Association.

[a]The data refer to the net total of people protected (i.e., duplication among people protected by more than one insuring organization or more than one policy providing the same type of coverage has been eliminated). They exclude hospital indemnity coverage included in prior years. The 1992 hospital indemnity count was 8.2 million for group and 5.4 million for individual policies.

[b]For 1984 and later, estimates of people covered by "other plans" have been developed by HIAA in the absence of other available data.

Note: Self-insured and HMOs includes people covered under ASO arrangements and MPPs. Some data were revised from previous editions. For 1975 and later, data include the number of people covered in Puerto Rico and U.S. territories and possessions. Data for 1978 and later have been adjusted downward because of new data on average family size. Data for 1987 and 1965 reflect the use of a revised HIAA survey form. Data for 1989 and 1990 reflect a change in methodology. Data split is available for years 1990–1994.

optional services, increasing eligibility standards, and decreasing the range of services in the program. Oregon developed a priority listing of services for which its Medicaid program will pay.

In addition, states lobbied for repeal of the Boren amendment (enacted in 1980), which required that states participating in Medicaid take into account the situation of hospitals, nursing facilities, and intermediate care facilities for people with mental retardation, which "serve a disproportionate number of low-income patients with special needs," when setting "reasonable and adequate" payment rates. Although the disproportionate share requirement was retained, the safeguard of reasonable and adequate payment for services provided under Medicaid was repealed by the Balanced Budget Act of 1997. The reasonable and adequate standard was replaced by a requirement that states "engage in a public notice-and-comment process when making rate changes." This new standard offers fewer protections to affected HSOs at a time when states will be pressing to reduce Medicaid costs. Nursing facilities will be especially hard hit by the change; Medicaid programs paid less than 15% of hospital care in 1995, but paid for almost 50% of nursing facility care.[182] Medicaid managed care organizations grew exponentially in the mid- to late 1990s, and payment to them will be affected by the Balanced Budget Act of 1997 as well. It will be several years before this new standard, and other provisions of the Balanced Budget Act, are clarified by regulations and litigation.[183]

For many services, Medicaid pays only a fraction of the cost to provide them. Reducing what Medicaid pays has several implications. Other payers must make up the difference or the HSO will go bankrupt. Government programs do not pay charges, nor does Blue Cross. Commercial insurers are almost certain not to pay charges, and indemnity plans have always paid only a fixed fee regardless of what the beneficiary is charged. It is only self-pay patients who must pay charges, and the small number of self-payers makes this increasingly infeasible.

As important, cost shifting raises basic questions of fairness. Should any payer pay less than costs for services? Medicare is a case more politically difficult than Medicaid. This is because Medicare is exclusively a federal program and Congress has been unwilling to cut benefits, although it has increased copayments and deductibles (Medicare Part A, hospitalization) and the insurance premium (Medicare Part B, physicians' treatment) several times since 1965. Medicare has been called an uncontrollable program, a statement that is true only because, politically, limiting coverage and benefits is virtually impossible. Once beneficiaries are eligible, all benefits are available. Meaningful cost savings can occur only if benefit levels are controlled—a politically unpalatable option.

TRENDS AND DEVELOPMENTS IN THE SYSTEM

This section identifies some of the changes occurring in health services and how they will affect HSO/HS managers. Efforts by state and federal governments to control their health services programs' costs will continue. The large component of fixed and semivariable costs will limit the savings that HSOs/HSs can achieve. Because hospitals consume such a large percentage of national health care expenditures, they will receive the most attention. Case-mix cost control through DRGs will cause hospitals to treat patients with the most remunerative diagnoses. There will be economic pressure to discharge patients as quickly as possible, perhaps earlier than clinically warranted. In addition, treating the less ill with alternative regimens and in HSOs such as ambulatory services leaves only the most ill in acute care hospitals, with the result that costs per patient day will increase. Unless hospitals close beds, discontinue services, and eliminate employees, the cost per case and the total cost of hospitalization will rise. Regardless, population increases will cause the total expenditures for health care to increase.

Regulation was the watchword of the late 1960s and early 1970s. The competitive environment that emerged in the late 1970s and early 1980s continued into the late 1990s, spurred by the failed Clinton health reform plan in 1993. Competitive pressures have increased, and public and private payers of medical services have become less willing to set payment levels high enough to save the inefficient. The 1980s witnessed large numbers of bankruptcies, mergers, and joint activities among HSOs/HSs. To enjoy the advantages of shared services, group purchasing, and access to capital without merger or acquisition, some HSOs joined strategic alliances. Many HSOs merged with or were acquired by a HS, which diminished their independence. Predictions in the early 1980s that the end of the decade would find a few national hospital systems, some large unaffiliated facilities, and few, if any, small freestanding hospitals proved incorrect. Nevertheless, fewer HSOs will be freestanding in the future.

Corporate restructuring gained wide acceptance in the early 1980s. This concept protected and enhanced the HSO's assets and reimbursement, as well as expanded its range of activities. Corporate restructuring has many complexities and results from state and federal efforts to control the HSO's income and expenses, as well as its freedom to establish services and facilities. Restructuring is addressed in Chapter 5.

Fragmentation and ultraspecialization of clinical staff will continue. As a result, the problems of acquiring, retaining, and managing human resources and their appropriate role in HSOs will be exacerbated. These issues are addressed in Chapter 11.

SUMMARY

This chapter provides background information about the U.S. health services system. The discussion of U.S. health services includes a conceptual framework of its health care and health services system, a brief history of its early development, and data and commentary about various components. The result is an understanding of the environment in which HSOs/HSs and their managers function. The system's enormity and complexity as well as the various elements are apparent. Readers are urged to keep this chapter in mind and reference it as necessary when reading the remainder of the book. Comprehensive awareness of the environment and its effect is a crucial dimension of knowledge for successful managers. In that sense, one can never know too much; this reinforces the need for lifelong learning and the stimulation provided by organized continuing education efforts.

The U.S. health services delivery system of the 21st century is likely to be very different from what it has been. Fewer services will be provided to inpatients in acute care hospitals, but those admitted will be more acutely ill. Higher intensity of illness will cause significantly higher hospital costs per case. Less need for inpatient care will result in hospitals' closing or converting to other uses. A common site of treatment will be the patient's home. Innovative relationships among various types of HSOs through HSs will deliver and finance health services in unique ways. The increase in the numbers and types of health services workers needed to support new technologies and services will raise salary costs. It is unlikely that health services costs will decrease, even as pressures to control them result in moderation of increases. Physicians will be increasingly fully integrated into HSOs, which are likely to be part of comprehensive, integrated HSs. These changes and challenges will require skillful and effective managers.

DISCUSSION QUESTIONS

1. What are the ramifications and implications for the health services system of the model developed by Blum? What are its strengths and weaknesses?
2. Select a disease problem and apply the PRECEDE-PROCEED model described in the chapter. How should HSO/HS governing bodies and managers use this model?
3. Describe and analyze the relationships among the various institutional and programmatic providers in the health services system.

4. Facilities and programs other than acute care hospitals are much more numerous and probably have a much greater effect on health status, yet the acute care hospital is the focal point of most of the attention that is directed at the health care system. Why has this occurred? What are the desirable and undesirable aspects of this attention from the standpoint of the acute care hospital provider and the consumer of health services?

5. The proliferation of the health professions continues unabated. What are the desirable and undesirable aspects of this fragmentation? If something should be done to slow or stop it, what should this be and how can it be achieved?

6. Highlight the changes in reimbursement to HSOs that have occurred since 1965. What forces in the general environment were most important in causing these changes? Sketch and defend a scenario that suggests the likely developments in reimbursement during the early 21st century.

7. Federally supported state health planning has risen and fallen since the passage of Medicare and Medicaid. Identify the advantages and disadvantages of statewide or areawide health planning from the standpoints of providers and consumers.

8. Describe how licensure, registration, and certification are different. What are the advantages and disadvantages of each from the standpoints of providers and consumers?

9. Resources consumed by the health services system have soared uncontrollably since the late 1960s. What factors contributed to these increases? Identify actions that have been taken, and identify what else might be done to control costs.

10. Identify the advantages and disadvantages of excess numbers of physicians and nonphysician clinicians to health services managers. What are the advantages and disadvantages to society?

CASE STUDY 1: GOURMAND AND FOOD—A FABLE[182]

The people of Gourmand loved good food. They ate in good restaurants, donated money for cooking research, and instructed their government to safeguard all matters having to do with food. Long ago, the food industry had been in total chaos. There were many restaurants, some very small. Anyone could call himself a chef or open a restaurant. In choosing a restaurant, one could never be sure that the meal would be good. A commission of distinguished chefs studied the situation and recommended that no one be allowed to touch food except for qualified chefs. "Food is too important to be left to amateurs," they said. Qualified chefs were licensed by the state with severe penalties for anyone else who engaged in cooking. Certain exceptions were made for food preparation in the home, but a person could serve only his own family. Furthermore, a qualified chef had to complete at least 21 years of training (including 4 years of college, 4 years of cooking school, and a 1-year apprenticeship). All cooking schools had to be first class.

These reforms did succeed in raising the quality of cooking, but a restaurant meal became substantially more expensive. A second commission observed that not everyone could afford to eat out. "No one," they said, "should be denied a good meal because of income." Furthermore, they argued that chefs should work toward the goal of giving everyone "complete physical and psychological satisfaction." For those people who could not afford to eat out, the government declared that they should be allowed to do so as often as they liked and the government would pay. For others, it was recommended that they organize themselves in groups and pay part of their income into a pool that would undertake to pay the costs incurred by members in dining out. To ensure the greatest satisfaction, the groups were set up so that members could eat out anywhere and as often as they liked, could have as elaborate a meal as they desired, and would have to pay nothing or only a small percentage of the cost. The cost of joining such prepaid dining clubs rose sharply.

Long ago, most restaurants would employ one chef to prepare the food. A few restaurants were more elaborate, with chefs specializing in roasting, fish, salads, sauces, and many other things. People rarely went to these elaborate restaurants because they were so expensive. With the establishment of prepaid dining clubs, everyone wanted to eat at these fancy restaurants. At the same time, young chefs in school disdained going to cook in a small restaurant where they would have to cook everything. The pay was higher and it was much more prestigious to specialize and cook at a really fancy restaurant. Soon there were not enough chefs to keep the small restaurants open.

With prepaid clubs and free meals for the poor, many people started eating their 3-course meals at the elaborate restaurants. Then they began to increase the number of courses, directing the chef to "serve the best with no thought for the bill." (Recently a 317-course meal was served.)

The costs of eating out rose faster and faster. A new government commission reported as follows: 1) Noting that licensed chefs were being used to peel potatoes and wash lettuce, the commission recommended that these tasks be handed over to licensed dishwashers (whose 3 years of dishwashing training included cooking courses) or to some new category of personnel. 2) Concluding that many licensed chefs were overworked, the commission recommended that cooking schools be expanded, that the length of training be shortened, and that applicants with lesser qualifications be admitted. 3) The commission also observed that chefs were unhappy because people seemed to be more concerned about the decor and service than about the food. (In a recent taste test, not only could one patron not tell the difference between a 1930 and a 1970 vintage but he also could not distinguish between white and red wines. He explained that he always ordered the 1930 vintage because he knew that only a really good restaurant would stock such an expensive wine.)

The commission agreed that weighty problems faced the nation. They recommended that a national prepayment group be established, which everyone must join. They recommended that chefs continue to be paid on the basis of the number of dishes they prepared. They recommended that Gourmandese be given the right to eat anywhere they chose and as elaborately as they chose and pay nothing.

These recommendations were adopted. Large numbers of people spent all of their time ordering incredibly elaborate meals. Kitchens became marvels of new, expensive equipment. All those who were not consuming restaurant food were in the kitchen preparing it. Because no one in Gourmand did anything except prepare or eat meals, the country collapsed.

QUESTIONS

1. Read and analyze the fable of Gourmand. How well does the allegory fit the U.S. health care system?
2. What is, and what should be, the role of the consumer in a health services system?
3. How do health services managers assist the United States in avoiding the fate of the Gourmandese?

CASE STUDY 2: WHERE'S MY ORGAN?

Organizations that support and encourage transplantation of human organs estimate that tens of thousands of people with end-stage renal disease who are now maintained on dialysis could resume a relatively normal life with a kidney transplant. The supply of cadaver kidneys, however, falls far short of the demand. To encourage people to sign organ donor cards and to encourage families to consent to organ donation, a Congressman introduced a bill to provide tax incentives for what is often called the "gift of life." Here, the gift is vascularized organs, including the heart, liver, pancreas, lungs, and kidneys.

Tax incentives are twofold: a $25,000 deduction per organ on the individual's last taxable year, plus a $25,000 exclusion per organ from estate taxes. To qualify, the organ must be in a condition suitable for transplantation. The same tax incentives would be granted if the donor is a dependent as defined by the federal tax code. As the Congressman stated when he introduced the bill: "Thus minors with significant income would reduce their family's tax liability with a posthumous donation that benefits both their loved ones and the loved ones of the recipient of the life-saving organ."

The Congressman noted, too, that enactment of his bill would result in significant cost savings to the federal government, which pays for the dialysis of people in end-stage renal failure under Medicare, for example. Assuming a 50% income tax bracket and an average of two organs per taxpayer, the deductions for 10,000 donors would reduce tax collections by $250 million. Renal dialysis is projected to cost the federal government almost $12 billion in fiscal year 2010.

QUESTIONS

1. Identify the issues that this proposal raises.
2. Choose to support or oppose the bill. Develop a set of arguments that justifies your position.
3. Develop an alternative proposal to the Congressman's that you believe would be more effective in encouraging organ donation.

APPENDIX*

MEDICARE AT A GLANCE

What Is Medicare and How Is It Financed?

Medicare is the nation's health insurance program for 34 million older adults and 5 million disabled people. Prior to the enactment of Medicare, fewer than 50% of all older Americans had health insurance. Today, virtually everyone ages 65 and older is insured by Medicare. Medicare beneficiaries comprise one in seven Americans, and this proportion is expected to grow to one in five by 2030, when the number of beneficiaries will exceed 76 million people.

Medicare consists of two parts: Hospital Insurance (Part A) and Supplementary Medical Insurance (Part B). Part A is financed mainly by a 1.45% payroll tax paid by both employees and employers. Revenue from the payroll tax is held in the Hospital Insurance Trust Fund and is used to pay Part A benefits. Part B is financed by both beneficiary premiums ($45.50 per month in 1999) and general revenue. Premiums cover approximately 25% of total Part B spending.

Most individuals ages 65 and older are automatically entitled to Medicare because they are eligible for Social Security payments. People under age 65 who receive Social Security cash payments because they are disabled become eligible for Medicare after a 2-year waiting period. People with end-stage renal disease are entitled to Part A regardless of their age. Part B is voluntary, but 95% of all Part A beneficiaries enroll in Part B.

Who Is Covered Under Medicare?

People who are eligible for Medicare often are described in homogeneous terms, yet health care needs and ability to afford care differ among the program's 39 million beneficiaries. Medicare covers a broad age spectrum, with 12% (4.7 million in 1996) under age 65 and another 12% age 85 or

*From The Henry J. Kaiser Family Foundation website, www.kff.org. Copyright © 1999; used by permission.

older. Nearly half of all beneficiaries have incomes below 200% of the poverty level ($15,480 for individuals, 1996).

Although many beneficiaries are in relatively good health, nearly one in three (29%) say their health is fair or poor, about one in four (23%) have problems with mental functioning, and one in five (20%) have difficulties with physical functioning.

Racial and ethnic minority Americans account for 16% of people on Medicare, a proportion that will double by 2025. African American and Latino beneficiaries are likelier than caucasians to have low incomes, serious health problems, and long-term care needs. Nearly 33% have incomes below poverty as compared with 10% of caucasians.

What Benefits Does Medicare Cover?

Medicare benefit payments were projected to be $212 billion in 1999, accounting for 12% of the federal budget and 22% of national spending for health services. Medicare finances 33% of all hospital services, 21% of physician services, and 1% of outpatient prescription drugs.

Medicare Part A finances approximately 53% of benefits, covering inpatient hospital services, skilled nursing facility (SNF) benefits, home health visits following a hospital or SNF stay, and hospice care. Inpatient hospital services are subject to a deductible ($768/benefit period in 1999) and a daily coinsurance beginning after the 60th day of a hospital stay. SNF care is limited to 100 days, subject to a prior hospitalization requirement, with coinsurance ($96/day in 1999) applied to Days 21–100. No copayments apply to home health services.

Medicare Part B accounts for 30% of Medicare benefits spending, covering physician and outpatient hospital services, home health visits not covered under Part A, annual mammography and other cancer screening, and other services such as laboratory procedures and medical equipment. After the $100 Part B deductible, a 20% coinsurance is required for almost all services. Over time, an increasing share of home health visits will be covered under Part B.

Managed care plans contract with Medicare to provide both Part A and B services to enrolled beneficiaries. Managed care accounts for 17% of benefit spending.

Gaps in Medicare: Implications for Beneficiaries

Medicare provides broad coverage of basic health care services, but it does not cover outpatient prescription drugs, has relatively high deductibles, and has no cap on out-of-pocket spending. To help with Medicare's cost-sharing requirements and to fill gaps in the benefits package, most beneficiaries carry supplemental insurance. In 1995, 33% had retiree health benefits, 25% owned Medigap policies, and 14% had Medicaid, the major public financing program for low-income Americans. Another 9% were enrolled in Medicare HMOs, which typically cover more generous benefits and have lower cost-sharing requirements.

Supplemental coverage varies by income level. Almost half of all poor beneficiaries (49%) have Medicaid assistance, compared with 12% of the near poor. One in six (16%) of those with incomes below twice the poverty level have no supplemental coverage, compared with 7% of higher income beneficiaries. More than half (52%) of the group with incomes twice the poverty level has retiree health benefits, twice the rate of the near poor.

Despite the prevalence of public and private supplemental coverage, beneficiaries face substantial out-of-pocket expenses. Medicare covers less than half of older adults' total health spending and is less generous than health plans that are typically offered by large employers. On average, older Americans spend 20% of their household income for health services and premiums. The most vulnerable spend an even higher percentage; those with incomes below the poverty level spend more than 33% of their income; those in fair/poor health spend more than 25%.

Lack of prescription drug coverage contributes to high out-of-pocket spending. More than 33% of all beneficiaries have no supplemental coverage to help pay for medications. In 1997 beneficiaries using prescription drugs spent an average of $440 out of pocket for their medications, with 10% of beneficiaries spending more than $1,200 annually.

Growth of Medicare Managed Care

Six million Medicare beneficiaries (16%) are enrolled in Medicare HMOs, more than four times the 1990 enrollment of 1.4 million. By 2009, enrollment in Medicare HMOs and other Medicare+Choice plans is expected to reach 14 million, accounting for 31% of all people on Medicare.

The Medicare+Choice program, established by the Balanced Budget Act of 1997 (BBA), expanded the range of private health plan options that is available to beneficiaries, although the availability of non–HMO private plan options is very limited, with one PSO participating in Medicare, and no PPOs or private fee-for-service plans offered.

Medicare Expenditures

Over the long term, per capita Medicare spending has grown at the same rate as has private insurance. However, the growth in total Medicare spending has slowed, increasing only 1.5% in 1998, and declining by a projected $1 billion (0.5%) in 1999. This slowdown is associated with changes enacted as part of BBA, delays in processing bills, and greater compliance with Medicare payment rules. BBA slowed growth in payments to providers and managed care plans, and increased beneficiary Part B premiums. Along with a strong U.S. economy, these spending reductions have extended the expected life of the Hospital Insurance Trust Fund from 2008 to 2015.

Although the slow spending growth will produce long-term savings, aggregate Medicare spending will continue to grow by a projected 8%/year to 2010 as a result of both the increasing number of Americans reaching retirement age and the continued rise in health care costs. By 2009, Medicare is projected to be 19% of federal spending.

Outlook for Medicare's Future

The Medicare program has broad public support because it offers health security to many older and disabled people. Yet the need for a long-term approach to program financing, improved benefits, and protections for people with low incomes remains an important issue to be addressed. Medicare is facing the challenge of financing and managing health care for the growing number of Americans who will rely on this program for health insurance protection.

MEDICAID AT A GLANCE

Medicaid is the nation's major public financing program for providing health and long-term care coverage to low-income people. In 1997, 40.6 million people—more than 1 in 7 Americans—were enrolled in Medicaid at a cost of $161.2 billion.

Authorized under Title XIX of the Social Security Act, Medicaid is a means-tested entitlement program financed by the state and federal governments and administered by the states. Federal financial assistance is provided to states for coverage of specific groups of people and benefits through federal matching payments based on the state's per capita income. The federal share ranges from 50% to 80% of Medicaid expenditures and averaged 56% in 1997.

Who Is Covered by Medicaid?

Although Medicaid was created to assist low-income Americans, coverage depends on several other criteria in addition to income. Eligibility is primarily for people who fall into particular "categories," such as low-income children, pregnant women, older adults, people with disabilities, and parents meeting specific income thresholds. Since the Temporary Assistance to Needy Families

(TANF) welfare reforms were implemented in 1996, Medicaid coverage is no longer automatic for families who receive cash assistance. Within federal guidelines, states set their own income- and asset-eligibility criteria for Medicaid, resulting in large state variations in coverage.

The diverse Medicaid population comprises

- 21.0 million children (1 in 4 U.S. children)
- 8.6 million adults in families
- 4.1 million older adults
- 6.8 million blind and disabled people

Adults and children in low-income families make up nearly 75% of Medicaid beneficiaries, but they account for only 25% of Medicaid spending. Older adults and people with disabilities account for the majority (65%) of spending because of their intensive use of acute and long-term care services.

Although Medicaid increasingly has been used to expand coverage to low-income people, in 1997 it covered less than 30% of nonelderly, low-income Americans with incomes below 200% of the poverty level. The State Child Health Insurance Program (CHIP) enacted in 1997 promises to extend coverage to many of the 8 million low-income uninsured children, but more than 17 million low-income adults will remain without coverage.

What Services Are Covered Under Medicaid?

Medicaid covers a broad range of services with nominal cost sharing because of the limited financial resources of its beneficiaries. Federally mandated services include

- Inpatient and outpatient hospital
- Physician, midwife, and certified nurse practitioner
- Laboratory and x-ray
- Nursing facility and home health care
- Early and periodic screening, diagnosis, and treatment (EPSDT) for children under age 21
- Family planning
- Rural health clinics/federally qualified health centers

States have the option to cover additional services and still receive federal matching funds. Commonly offered services include prescription drugs, clinic services, prosthetic devices, hearing aids, dental care, and intermediate care facilities for people with mental retardation (ICF/MR).

Of the $161.2 billion that Medicaid spent in 1997

- Acute care services were about half (53%) of total spending, with spending for managed care organization (MCO) premiums accounting for 18% of total acute care spending.
- Long-term care services were 37% of expenditures. Nationally, Medicaid pays for approximately 50% of all nursing facility care and 14% of all home health spending.
- Payments to Medicare for premiums accounted for 3% of total spending.
- Supplemental payments for hospitals with a disproportionately large population of indigent patients (DSH) composed roughly 10% of total expenditures.

How Is Care Delivered Under Medicaid?

As of June 1998, 16.6 million Medicaid beneficiaries were enrolled in managed care, a sixfold increase from 2.7 million in 1991. More than half of all Medicaid beneficiaries had been enrolled in managed care by June 1998. Medicaid managed care models range from HMOs that use prepaid capitated contracts to loosely structured networks that contract with selected providers for discounted services and use gatekeeping to control utilization.

States initially targeted low-income families for managed care enrollment, but efforts to enroll older adults or disabled beneficiaries are increasing. Under BBA, states have the authority to mandate managed care enrollment, except for certain children with special needs, Medicare beneficiaries, and Native Americans. In 1998 approximately 1 in 4 disabled Medicaid beneficiaries was enrolled in managed care, primarily in mandatory, capitated arrangements.

Long-term care is a major component of Medicaid. Although more than 75% of Medicaid spending for long-term care is on institutional services, Home- and Community-Based Services (HCBS) waivers are often used by states to deliver community-based care. Although all states have HCBS waivers, the population served remains small. States also have the option to provide dual eligibles (Medicaid/Medicare) with acute and community-based long-term care services under the Program for All-Inclusive Care for the Elderly (PACE).

Enrollee and Expenditure Growth

Medicaid enrollment rose dramatically in the early 1990s, peaking at 41.7 million beneficiaries in 1995. This growth was mostly attributable to expanded coverage of low-income pregnant women and young children and increases in the number of blind and disabled beneficiaries. However, from 1995 to 1997 enrollment declined, especially for low-income adults and children eligible for Medicaid based on receipt of cash assistance under welfare. These reductions may be related to state and federal changes in welfare and immigration policies.

Medicaid is a major budgetary commitment for the federal and state governments. In 1997 it accounted for more than 16% of the $969 billion in U.S. personal health expenditures and was the single largest source of federal funds to the states.

During the early 1990s, Medicaid expenditures grew nearly 30% annually due to a combination of health care inflation, state use of alternative financing mechanisms, and an increase in enrollment. Only a small fraction of spending growth was due to the expansions in coverage of low-income pregnant women and children.

Legislation that was enacted to limit the states' capacity to raise funds through provider taxes and to limit disproportionate share hospital payments played a role in slowing Medicaid spending growth in the late 1990s. From 1992 to 1995, growth in annual expenditures dropped to less than 10% and has nearly leveled off, rising only 3% annually from 1995 to 1997.

Since its enactment in 1965, Medicaid has improved access to health care for the poor, pioneered innovations in health care delivery and community-based long-term care services, and stood alone as the primary source of financial assistance for long-term care. As Medicaid struggles to meet multiple responsibilities under continued fiscal pressure, the program plays a critical role in providing acute and long-term care services to many of our nation's most vulnerable people.

NOTES

1. *Healthy America: Practitioners for 2005,* 55. Durham, NC: Pew Health Professions Commission, 1991.
2. Health Care Financing Administration. "Highlights: National Health Expenditures, 1998." *http://www.hcfa.gov/stats/NHE-OAct/hilites.htm,* March 21, 2000.
3. Health Care Financing Administration. "National Health Expenditures Projections, 1998–2008." *http://www.hcfa.gov/stats/NHE-Proj/proj1998/hilites.htm,* March 22, 2000.
4. Blum, Henrik L. *Expanding Health Care Horizons: From a General Systems Concept of Health to a National Health Policy,* 2nd ed., 34. Oakland, CA: Third Party Publishing, 1983.
5. Blum, Henrik L. *Planning for Health: Development and Application of Social Change Theory,* 96–100. New York: Human Sciences Press, 1974.

6. This discussion of the PRECEDE-PROCEED planning model is adapted from Daniel, Mark, and Lawrence W. Green. "Application of the PRECEDE-PROCEED Planning Model in Diabetes Prevention and Control: A Case Illustration from a Canadian Aboriginal Community." *Diabetes Spectrum* 8 (March/April 1995): 74–84; reprinted with permission.

7. Health Care Financing Administration. "Trends in Medicare Skilled Nursing Facility Utilization: CYs 1967–1994." *Health Care Financing Review,* Statistical Supplement (1996): 64.

8. Data from the National Center for Health Statistics, 1987 and 1988; and Thompson-Hoffman, Susan, and Inez Fitzgerald Storck. *Disability in the United States: A Portrait from National Data,* 37. New York: Springer-Verlag, 1991.

9. Bureau of the Census. "Resident Population of the United States: by Age and Sex," and "Resident Population of the United States: Middle Series Projections, 2035–2050." *http://www.census.gov/population/projections/nation/nas/npas3550.txt,* February 8, 1999.

10. Hospital Survey and Construction Act of 1946 (Hill-Burton Act), PL 79-725, 60 Stat. 1040 (1946).

11. Public Health Service. *Directory of Facilities Obligated to Provide Uncompensated Services, by State and City as of March 1, 1989,* I. Washington, DC: U.S. Department of Health and Human Services, 1989.

12. National Institutes of Health. "Institutes and Offices." *http://www.nih.gov/icd/,* March 22, 1999.

13. National Institutes of Health. "Biomedical Research at NIH: The NIH Budget." *http://Irp.info.nih.gov/BioResearch/budget.htm,* March 5, 1999.

14. Balanced Budget Act of 1997, PL 105-33, 111 Stat. 251 (1997).

15. Grimaldi, Paul L. "Medicare Part C Means More Choices." *Nursing Management* 28 (November 1997): 30.

16. Comprehensive Health Planning and Public Health Service Amendments Act of 1966, PL 89-749, 80 Stat. 1180 (1966); National Health Planning and Resources Development Act of 1974, PL 93-641, 88 Stat. 2225 (1974); Social Security Amendments of 1972, PL 92-603, 86 Stat. 1329 (1972).

17. Bureau of Labor Statistics. *Consumer Price Index, Average Annual Percentage Change, All Urban Consumers, 1969–1996.* Washington, DC: U.S. Department of Labor, 1997.

18. Tax Equity and Fiscal Responsibility Act of 1982, PL 97-248, 96 Stat. 324 (1982); Social Security Amendments of 1983, PL 98-21, 97 Stat. 65 (1983).

19. Hilzenrath, David S. "Health Benefits Costs' Jump Called Ominous: Easy HMO Savings Ending, Survey Suggests." *The Washington Post,* January 6, 1999, F3.

20. Agency for Health Care Policy and Research. "Equalizing Payments for Cesarean and Vaginal Deliveries Has Little Effect on Cesarean Rates." *Research Activities* 201 (February 1997): 2.

21. National Center for Health Statistics. *Health United States 1990,* 185. Washington, DC: U.S. Department of Health and Human Services, 1991.

22. Anderson, Gerard F. "In Search of Value: An International Comparison of Cost, Access, and Outcomes." *Health Affairs* 16 (November/December 1997): 164.

23. Hageman, Winifred M., and Richard J. Bogue. "Layers of Leadership: The Challenges of Collaborative Governance." *Trustee* 51 (September 1998): 20.

24. Strenger, Ellen Weisman. "The Road to Wellville." *Trustee* 49 (May 1996): 20–25.

25. Pickett, George E., and John J. Hanlon. *Public Health Administration and Practice,* 9th ed., 83. St. Louis: Times Mirror/Mosby College Publishing, 1990.

26. Seebach, Linda. "Alternative Therapy Eruption." *The Washington Times,* July 6, 1998, A14; Okie, Susan. "Widening the Medical Mainstream: More Americans Using 'Alternative' Therapies, Some Prove Effective." *The Washington Post,* November 11, 1998, A1.

27. National Center for Health Statistics. *Health United States 1998: Socioeconomic Status and Health Chartbook,* 288. Washington, DC: U.S. Department of Health and Human Services, 1999.

28. Desai, Kamal R., Gary J. Young, and Carol VanDeusen Lukas. "Hospital Conversions from For-Profit to Nonprofit Status: The Other Side of the Story." *Medical Care Research & Review* 55 (September 1998): 298–308.

29. "The Disturbing Trend of Not-for-Profit Hospital Conversions." *Health Letter* 12 (July 1996): 1–7. (Published by Public Citizen Health Research Group, Washington, DC)

30. "Images from the History of the Public Health Service." *http://130.14.74.3/exhibition/phs_history/139.html,* March 1, 1999.

31. Indian Health Service. "Fact Sheet." *wysiwyg://37/http://www.ihs.gov/AboutIHS/ThisFacts.asp,* March 24, 1999.

32. Department of Veterans Affairs. "Summary Report: Audits of VA–Medical School Affiliation Issues," January 29, 1997. *http://www.va.gov/oig/52/reports/1997/7R8-A99-026—medsch.htm,* February 19, 1999.

33. "Intermediate Care Facilities for the Mentally Retarded (ICFs/MR)." *http://www.ahca.org/info/icf.htm,* March 5, 1999.

34. Norback, Judith. *The Mental Health Yearbook/Directory 1979–80,* 200. New York: Van Nostrand Reinhold, 1979.

35. National Center for Health Statistics, *Health United States 1998,* 335.

36. Council of Teaching Hospitals and Health Systems. *COTH Activities and Member Services.* Washington, DC: Association of American Medical Colleges, February 4, 1999.

37. Council of Teaching Hospitals and Health Systems. *Council of Teaching Hospitals: Selected Activities Report—May 1990,* 1. Washington, DC: Association of American Medical Colleges, 1990.

38. Fisher, Karen S., and Melissa H. Wubbold. *Selected Activities Report: AAMC Council of Teaching Hospitals and Health Systems,* 83. Washington, DC: Association of American Medical Colleges, 1998.

39. Council of Teaching Hospitals and Health Systems. *About COTH Activities and Member Services.* Washington, DC: Association of American Medical Colleges, February 19, 1999.

40. Association of American Medical Colleges. *Integrated Academic Medical Center Hospitals.* Washington, DC: Association of American Medical Colleges, 1997. Criteria include a nonfederal, short stay, general hospital that has common ownership with a college of medicine or has certain connections with a medical school.

41. Bureau of Labor Statistics. "Employees on Nonfarm Payrolls by Industry." *ftp://146.142.4.23/pub/news.release/empsit.txt,* April 19, 1999.

42. Inglis, Brian. *Fringe Medicine,* 94–102. London: Faber & Faber, 1964.

43. American Osteopathic Association. *AOA Fact Sheet.* Chicago: American Osteopathic Association, January 1999.

44. Inglis, *Fringe Medicine,* 102–105, 111–113.

45. Peterson, Edward S., Anne E. Crowley, Joseph Rosenthal, and Robert Boerner. "Medical Education in the U.S. 1979–1980." *Journal of the American Medical Association* 244 (December 26, 1980): 2810–2823.

46. Jones, Robert F., Janice L. Ganem, Donna J. Williams, and Jack Y. Krakower. "Review of US Medical School Finances, 1996–1997." *Journal of the American Medical Association* 280 (September 2, 1998): 813–818.

47. Dunn, Marvin R., Rebecca S. Miller, and Thomas H. Richter. "Graduate Medical Education, 1997–1998." *Journal of the American Medical Association* 280 (September 2, 1998): 809–812.

48. Dunn, Miller, and Richter, "Graduate Medical Education, 1997–1998," 810.

49. Grumbach, Kevin, and Janet Coffman. "Physician and Nonphysician Clinicians: Complements or Competitors." *Journal of the American Medical Association* 280 (September 2, 1998): 825–826.

50. Weinstock, Matthew. "Specialists Are Back in Demand as 'Frenzy' for Primary Docs Subsides." *AHA News* 34 (September 7, 1998): 5.

51. "Pew Health Professions Commission." *http://www.futurehealth.ucsf.edu/pewcomm.html,* April 13, 1999.

52. Grumbach, and Coffman, "Physician and Nonphysician," 825.

53. Cooper, Richard A., Prakash Laud, and Craig L. Dietrich. "Current and Projected Workforce of Nonphysician Clinicians." *Journal of the American Medical Association* 280 (September 2, 1998): 788–794.

54. Grumbach, and Coffman, "Physician and Nonphysician," 825. One commentator has suggested that the oversupply of specialists is the result of "(G)overnment policies funding GME (graduate medical education) without regard for the changing dynamics of physician employment" (Ruhnke, Gregory W. "Physician Supply and the Shifting Paradigm of Medical Student Choice." *Journal of the American Medical Association* 277 [January 1, 1997]: 70).

55. Mundinger, Mary O. "Advanced-Practice Nursing—Good Medicine for Physicians?" *New England Journal of Medicine* 330 (January 20, 1994): 211–214; Scheffler, Richard M., Norman J. Waitzman, and John M. Hillman. "The Productivity of Physician Assistants and Nurse Practitioners and Health Work Force Policy in the Era of Managed Health Care." *Journal of Allied Health* 25 (Summer 1996): 207–217.

56. Association of University Programs in Health Administration. *Health Services Administration Education: Directory of Programs, 1999–2001,* 296. Washington, DC: Association of University Programs in Health Administration, 1999.

57. *Health Services Administration Education,* xiv.

58. Association of University Programs in Health Administration, *Health Services Administration Education.*

59. Omnibus Budget Reconciliation Act of 1987, PL 100-203, 101 Stat. 1330 (1987); American Hospital Association. *Professional Credentialing Statutes,* 1. Chicago: American Hospital Association, 1990.

60. American Dietetic Association. *Laws that Regulate Dietitians/Nutritionists.* Chicago: American Dietetic Association, 1999.

61. American Society of Clinical Pathologists. "About the ASCP." *http://www.ascp.org/general/about,* February 24, 1999.

62. Association of American Medical Colleges. *U.S. Medical School Finances: Part I and Part II, 1989–1990,* 2. Washington, DC: Association of American Medical Colleges, 1991.

63. Barzansky, Barbara, Harry S. Jones, and Sylvia I. Etzel. "Educational Programs in U.S. Medical Schools, 1997–1998." *Journal of the American Medical Association* 280 (September 2, 1998): 803–808.

64. National Center for Health Statistics, *Health, United States, 1990,* 169.

65. Liaison Committee on Medical Education. "Overview: Accreditation and the LCME." *http://www.lcme.org/overview.htm,* March 27, 1999.

66. Fisher, and Wubbold, *Selected Activities Report,* 156.

67. Buske, Lynda. "For the First Time, Men a Minority in Graduating Class." *Canadian Medical Association Journal,* 158 (1999): 568. (*http://www.cma.ca/cmaj/vol%2D158/issue%2D4/0568e.htm,* March 23, 1999)

68. American Osteopathic Association. *AOA Fact Sheet.* Chicago: American Osteopathic Association, February 1999.

69. In the early 1980s, some medical schools' admissions policies were redesigned to reverse a trend toward goal-oriented training in premedical education. For example, The Johns Hopkins University 1) allows juniors and seniors to integrate undergraduate and professional training, and 2) offers deferred admissions to accepted seniors. This relieves pressure associated with medical school admission and encourages pursuit of broader studies. (The Johns Hopkins University School of Medicine. *The FlexMed Program* and *The Senior Flexible Medical Option for Deferred Admissions.* Baltimore: The Johns Hopkins University School of Medicine, 1999.)

70. *Health Care Almanac,* 2nd ed., edited by Lorri A. Zipperer, 305. Chicago: American Medical Association, 1998.

71. American Board of Medical Specialties, Research & Education Foundation. *1998 Annual Report & Reference Handbook,* 122. Evanston, IL: American Board of Medical Specialties, 1998.

72. Department of Veterans Affairs. "A History of Veterans Healthcare," n/d., and "Summary Report: Audits of VA–Medical School Affiliation Issues." *http://www.va.gov/oig/52/reports/1997/7R8-A99-026—medsch.htm,* February 19, 1999.

73. Logan, Jane, and Billie Jean Summers. "The 'New' VA." *Tennessee Nurse* 60 (June 1997): 14–15.

74. Larson, Ruth. "Medical Advances Can Outpace Doctors: Retraining Not Enforced, Critics Say." *The Washington Times,* March 21, 1999, A1.

75. Rich, Spencer. "Report Questions Discipline by State Medical Units." *The Washington Post,* June 3, 1990, A17.

76. Public Citizen Health Research Group. "Ranking of State Medical Board Disciplinary Actions in 1997." Faxed personal communication, February 9, 1999; Public Citizen Health Research Group. "Health Group Names 16,638 Questionable Doctors." *http://www.citizen.org/Press/pr-qd1.htm.*

77. Personal communication, American Dental Association, February 22, 1999.

78. American Dental Association. *ADA Fact Sheets: Dentistry.* Chicago: American Dental Association, 1999.

79. American Dental Association. "About the ADA: Background on the American Dental Association." *http://www.ada.org/p&s/history/adaback.html,* February 19, 1999.

80. Personal communication, American Dental Association, "Licensure of Specialists," March 23, 1999.

81. Personal communication, American Dental Association, April 6, 1999.

82. American Podiatric Medical Association. "Podiatric Medicine: The Physician, the Profession, the Practice." *http://www.apma.org/podiat.html,* March 26, 1999.

83. Stanfield, Peggy S., and Y.H. Hui. *Introduction to the Health Professions,* 131. Boston: Jones & Bartlett, 1998.

84. Malone, Beverly L., and Geri Marullo. "Workforce Trends Among U.S. Registered Nurses" (American Nurses Association Policy Series). *http://www.nursingworld.org/readroom/usworker.htm,* March 24, 1999.

85. Moore, Amy Slugg. "The Way It Is Today." *RN* 60 (October 1997): 27–31. This article is the report of a survey of 2,000 nurses, with 857 respondents.

86. American Nurses Association. *The Nursing Shortage: Situation & Solutions,* 7, 8. Kansas City, MO: American Nurses Association, 1991.

87. Green, Jeffrey. "Increased Enrollment Difficult for Nursing Schools to Swallow." *AHA News* 27 (August 26, 1991): 1.

88. Greene, Jan, and Anne M. Nordhaus-Bike. "Where Have All the RNs Gone?" *Hospital & Health Networks* 72 (August 5 & 20, 1998): 78, 80.

89. American Association of Colleges of Nursing. "Nursing School Enrollments Lag Behind Rising Demand for RNs, AACN Survey Shows." *http://www.aacn.nche.edu/Media/enrl98wb.htm,* January 26, 1999.

90. Dunn, Philip. "More Areas Report Nursing Shortages, but Analysts Don't Foresee a Crisis." *AHA News* 34 (September 7, 1998). (*http://wwww.ahanews.com/CGI-BIN/SM40i.exe?docid=100.7293&%50assArticleId=12772,* April 5, 1999)

91. American Nurses Credentialing Center. "1998 Generalist Board Certification Catalog." *http://www.nursingworld.org/ancc/generlst/index.htm,* February 1999; American Nurses Credentialing Center. "1998 Advanced Practice Board Certification Catalog." *http://www.nursingworld.org/ancc/ap98/index/htm,* February 1999.

92. American Nurses Credentialing Center. *ANCC Certification* (pamphlet). Kansas City, MO: American Nurses Credentialing Center, 1991.

93. American Nurses Association. *ANA Certification Catalogue.* Kansas City, MO: American Nurses Association, 1983.

94. American Nurses Credentialing Center, *ANCC Certification.*

95. "Certified Nurses by Selected Practice Areas by State: October 1998." In *The Universal Healthcare Almanac,* edited by Linda L. Cherner, 98.4. Phoenix, AZ: Silver & Cherner, 1998.

96. Cooper, Richard A., Tim Henderson, and Craig L. Dietrich. "Roles of Nonphysician Clinicians as Autonomous Providers of Patient Care." *Journal of the American Medical Association* 280 (September 2, 1998): 795–802.

97. Skrzycki, Cindy. "Can Nurses Administer Anesthesia as Well as Doctors?" *The Washington Post,* February 20, 1998, G1.

98. Greene and Nordhaus-Bike, "Where Have All the RNs Gone?" 78, 80.

99. Stanfield and Hui, *Introduction to the Health Professions,* 147–148.

100. American Dietetic Association. *Laws that Regulate Dietitians/Nutritionists,* and *Fact Sheet: Registered Dietitian.* Chicago: American Dietetic Association, 1999.

101. American Society of Radiologic Technologists. "Who We Are." *http://www.asrt.org/who_we_are.htm,* March 22, 1999.

102. American Society of Radiologic Technologists. "Frequently Asked Questions." *http://www.asrt.org/FAQ.htm#FAXBack,* March 22, 1999.

103. Stanfield and Hui, *Introduction to the Health Professions,* 341–345.

104. American Academy of Physician Assistants. *Annual Census Data on Physician Assistants, 1997.* Alexandria, VA: American Academy of Physician Assistants, 1998.

105. Hooker, Roderick S., and James F. Cawley. *Physician Assistants in American Medicine,* 220. New York: Churchill Livingstone, 1997.

106. American Academy of Physician Assistants, *Annual Census Data.*
107. *Health Care Almanac,* 2nd ed., edited by Lorri A. Zipperer, 253. Chicago: American Medical Association, 1998.
108. Joint Commission on Accreditation of Healthcare Organizations. "State Legislative and Regulatory Activity." *http://www.jacho.org/about_je/govt.htm,* January 27, 1999.
109. "HCFA's New Proposed Conditions of Participation for Medicare Hospitals Emphasize Outcomes, Not Procedures." *Health Lawyers News* 2 (January 1998): 5–6.
110. O'Donnell, James W. "The Rise and Fall of Federal Support." *Provider* 13 (December 1987): 6.
111. Thomas, Constance. "Certificate of Need: Taking a New Look at an Old Program." *State Health Notes* 114 (June 1991): 1.
112. Thomas, "Certificate of Need," 1.
113. Piper, Thomas R. "1999 Relative Scope and Reviewability Thresholds of CON Regulated Services." Compiled by Piper from *American Health Planning Association 1999 National Directory of Health Planning, Policy and Regulatory Agencies,* 10th ed. Falls Church, VA: American Health Planning Association, 1999.
114. Cohen, Harold A. *Health Services Cost Review Commission.* Baltimore: Health Services Cost Review Commission, 1983.
115. Kent, Christina. "Twenty Years of Maryland Rate Regulation." *Medicine & Health* (Perspectives insert) 45 (August 19, 1991).
116. Parts of this section are adapted from Health Care Financing Administration. *History of Peer Review.* Washington, DC: Health Care Financing Administration, n.d. (unpublished report received December 1991).
117. Health Care Financing Administration. "PRO Results: Bridging the Past with the Future, September 1998, Executive Summary." *http://www.hcfa.gov/quality/3k1.htm,* March 26, 1999.
118. Ready, Tinker. "PROs Under Assault by Government, Consumers." *Healthweek* 4 (February 12, 1990): 6, 44–45.
119. Health Care Financing Administration. "Medicare Provider Analysis and Review (MEDPAR)." *http://www.hcfa.gov/stats/medpar.htm,* March 22, 1999.
120. Fries, Brant E., Gunnar Ljunggren, and Bengt Winblad. "International Comparison of Long-Term Care: The Need for Resident-Level Classification." *Journal of the American Geriatrics Society* 39 (January 1991): 12–13.
121. Meyer, Harris. "RUG Burn." *Hospital & Health Networks* 72 (June 5, 1998): 24–26.
122. HealthIQ. "IQToolkit(tm) Glossary: Definition for APG—Ambulatory Patient Groups." *http://www. healthiq.com/HealthcareResources/glossary/G25.htm,* March 30, 1999.
123. Meyer, Harris. "Prospective Payment Gets Legs." *Hospitals & Health Networks* 72 (August 5 and 20, 1998): 52.
124. Omnibus Budget Reconciliation Act of 1989, PL 101-239, 103 Stat. 2106 (1989).
125. Inlander, Charles B., and Michael A. Donio. *Medicare Made Easy,* 111. Allentown, PA: People's Medical Society, 1997.
126. Grimaldi, Paul L. "RBRVS: How New Physician Fee Schedule Will Work." *Health Care Financial Management* 45 (September 1991): 74.
127. "Has HCFA 'Broken Faith' with MD Fee Schedule?" *Medical Staff Leader* 20 (August 1991): 8.
128. "Has HCFA 'Broken Faith,'" 1.
129. Grimaldi, "RBRVS," 74.
130. Gosfield, Alice G. "Private Contracting by Medicare Physicians: The Pit and the Pendulum." *Health Law Digest* 26 (January 1998): 3–9.
131. Vanderkam, Laura R. "Seniors get 'huge win' on doctors consultations." *The Washington Times,* July 28, 1999, A9.
132. Koska, Mary T. "Hospitals: Begin Strategic Planning for RBRVS." *Hospitals* 65 (February 20, 1991): 28–30.
133. "News at Deadline." *Hospitals* 64 (November 5, 1990): 8.
134. Harris-Wehling, Jo, and Michael G.H. McGeary. "Medicare: A Strategy for Quality Assurance, IV: Medicare Conditions of Participation and Quality Assurance." *QRB* 17 (October 1991): 321.

135. Joint Commission on Accreditation of Healthcare Organizations. "Board of Commissioners." *http://www.jcaho.org/about _ jc/boc.htm,* January 27, 1999.

136. *http://www.jcaho.org/aboutjc/facts.html,* March 21, 2000.

137. Joint Commission on Accreditation of Healthcare Organizations. "Benefits of Joint Commission Accreditation" (photocopy sheet). Oakbrook Terrace, IL: Joint Commission on Accreditation of Healthcare Organizations, 1998.

138. Zeglen, Margaret. "Accreditation Requirements for ORYX: The Next Evolution in Accreditation." *Journal of AHIMA* 68 (June 1997): 20–22, 24–28, 30–31.

139. Joint Commission on Accreditation of Healthcare Organizations. "ORYX: The Next Evolution in Accreditation." *http://www.jcaho.org/perfmeas/oryx/oryx_qa.htm,* June 15, 1998.

140. American Hospital Association. "Quality and Accreditation Initiatives Update." *http://www.aha.org/quality/qualityupdate5-98.html,* March 2, 1999.

141. Joint Commission on Accreditation of Healthcare Organizations. "Sentinel Event Policy and Procedures," 1. *http://www.jacho.org/sentinel/se_pp.htm,* January 25, 1999.

142. Joint Commission on Accreditation of Healthcare Organizations, "Sentinel Event," 1–12.

143. American Osteopathic Association, "AOA Fact Sheet," January 1999.

144. American Osteopathic Association, *The People and Events that Shaped Our History: A Centennial Perspective, 1897–1997.* Chicago: American Osteopathic Association, 1997.

145. The order of letters, ISO, was chosen because it was not intended to be an acronym. ISO is a word, derived from the Greek *isos*, meaning "equal." This makes the connection between "ISO" and "standard" clear. Non–health care examples of standardization that benefit consumers worldwide are photographic film speed codes, telephone and banking cards, paper sizes, and symbols for automobile controls. (International Organization for Standardization. "Introduction to ISO." *http://www.iso.ch/infoe/intro.htm,* January 8, 1999.)

146. "Generic Management System Standards." *http://www.iso.ch/9000e/generic.htm,* February 10, 1999; "ISO 9000 and ISO 14000 in Plain Language." *http://www.iso.ch/9000/plain.htm,* February 10, 1999.

147. "The Three-Headed 'Ation' Beast: Certif*ication*, Regist*ration*, and Accredi*tation*." *http://www.iso.ch/9000e/ation.htm,* February 10, 1999; " 'ISO Certificates Don't Exist." *http://www.iso.ch/9000e/dontexis.htm,* February 10, 1999.

148. Community Health Accreditation Program, Inc. "What is CHAP?" (information sheet). New York: Community Health Accreditation Program, Inc., 1998.

149. Community Health Accreditation Program, Inc. "Description of CHAP Accreditation Program." *http://www.chapinc.org/chapdesc.htm,* February 16, 1999.

150. Community Health Accreditation Program, Inc. "The Community Health Accreditation Program (CHAP) Seeks Deeming Authority for Hospice Programs." *http://www.chapinc.org/pressc-081298.htm,* February 16, 1999.

151. Community Health Accreditation Program, Inc. "Description of CHAP Accreditation Program." *http://www.chapinc.org/chapdesc.htm,* February 1, 1999.

152. NCQA. "Accreditation '99." *http://www.ncqa.org,* January 25, 1999. NCQA. "Managed Care Organization Accreditation Status List." December 31, 1998.

153. NCQA. "Accreditation '99." *http://www.ncqa.org,* January 25, 1999.

154. American Accreditation HealthCare/URAC. *History of the American Accreditation HealthCare/URAC.* Washington, DC: American Accreditation HealthCare/URAC, 1998.

155. American Accreditation HealthCare/URAC. *States that Recognize American Accreditation HealthCare Commission/URAC Accreditation.* Washington, DC: American Accreditation HealthCare/URAC, 1998.

156. American Accreditation HealthCare/URAC. "Commission/URAC Issues 1,000th Accreditation Certificate" (press release). Washington, DC: American Accreditation HealthCare/URAC, March 4, 1998; American Accreditation HealthCare/URAC. "Commission/URAC Board Approves Development of Accreditation Standards for Case Management Programs" (press release). Washington, DC: American Accreditation HealthCare/URAC, January 30, 1998.

157. *Medical and Health Information Directory,* Vol. 1, 10th ed., edited by Lynn M. Pearce, 2901. Farmington Hills, MI: Gale Research, 1999.

158. Personal communication, American Medical Association, Chicago, February 16, 1999.

159. Personal communication, American Medical Association, Chicago, November 1991.
160. National Medical Association. "Why You Should Join." *http://www.nmanet.org/hq/membership/home.html,* February 16, 1999.
161. *Encyclopedia of Associations,* Vol. 1, 33rd ed., edited by Christine Maurer and Tara E. Sheets, 1498. New York: Gale Research, 1998.
162. Personal communication, American Hospital Association staff, January 1999.
163. *Medical and Health Information Directory,* 200.
164. *Encyclopedia of Associations,* 1444.
165. *Encyclopedia of Medical Organizations and Agencies,* 10th ed., edited by Lynn M. Pearce, 196. Farmington Hills, MI: Gale Research, 1999.
166. "Who We Are: Profile of the American Health Care Association." *http://www.ahca.org/who/profile.htm,* March 5, 1999.
167. *Medical and Health Information Directory,* 67.
168. "About AAHSA." *http://www.aahsa.org,* November 20, 1998.
169. "The American Association of Health Plans." *http://www.aahp.org/services/home_page_links/homelinks/about_aahp.htm,* April 13, 1999.
170. ACEHSA. "Corporate Sponsors." *http://monkey.hmi.missouri.edu/acehsa/sponsors.htm,* and *http://monkeyhmi.missouri.edu/acehsa/programs.htm#Following,* March 22, 1999.
171. Personal communication, Council on Education for Public Health, April 6, 1999.
172. Personal communication, International Association for Management Education, April 6, 1999.
173. National League for Nursing. "National League for Nursing History." *http://www.nln.org/info-history.htm,* February 19, 1999.
174. National League for Nursing Accrediting Commission. "Our Mission." *http://www.accrediting-comm-nlnac.org/homepagetext.htm,* March 22, 1999.
175. American Board of Medical Specialties, Research & Education Foundation, *1998 Annual Report.*
176. Larson, "Medical Advances Can Outpace Doctors," A1.
177. Koska, Mary T. "Specialty Board Proliferation Causes Confusion." *Hospitals* 63 (August 5, 1989): 58.
178. Health Care Financing Administration, "National Health Expenditures," March 22, 2000.
179. Reinhardt, Uwe E. "Spending More Through 'Cost Control': Our Obsessive Quest to Gut the Hospital." *Health Affairs* 15 (Summer 1996): 145–154. Reinhardt argues that the incremental cost of convalescent days in a hospital is much less expensive than care that is provided by alternative sources such as home health care. Thus, instead of reducing national health care costs, shifting care outside the hospital has actually added to them. It is noted that, despite severe reductions in inpatient stays from 1980 to 1995, total U.S. health spending increased by more than 50%.
180. Blue Cross Blue Shield Association. "1998 Year in Review." *http://www.bluecares.com/Newsroom/yearend/98yir.html,* February 24, 1999.
181. Health Insurance Association of America. *Source Book of Health Insurance Data, 1982–83,* 7. Washington, DC: Health Insurance Association of America, 1982–83.
182. Gardner, Jonathan. "Repeal of 'Boren Amendment' Raises Fears." *Modern Healthcare* 32 (August 11, 1997): 3, 14.
183. Clark, Lisa W. "The Demise of the Boren Amendment: What Comes Next in the Struggle Over Hospital Payment Standards Under the Medicaid Act?" *Health Law Digest* 26 (January 1998): 11–18.
184. From Lave, Judith R., and Lester B. Lave. "Health Care: Part I." *Law and Contemporary Problems* 35 (Spring 1970); reprinted by permission. Copyright 1970, 1971 by Duke University.
185. "Common Concerns: International Issues in Health Care System Reform." President's message in the annual report of The Commonwealth Fund, New York, 1998, p. 5, using 1998 Organization for Economic Cooperation and Development data.

SELECTED BIBLIOGRAPHY

American Board of Medical Specialties, Research & Education Foundation. *1998 Annual Report & Reference Handbook.* Evanston, IL: American Board of Medical Specialties, 1998.

American Hospital Association. *AHA Hospital Statistics.* Chicago: American Hospital Association, 1999.

Association of American Medical Colleges. *Council of Teaching Hospitals: Selected Activities Report—October 1998.* Washington, DC: Association of American Medical Colleges, 1998.

Barer, Morris L., Robert G. Evans, and Roberta J. Labelle. "Fee Controls as Cost Control: Tales from the Frozen North." *The Milbank Memorial Fund Quarterly* 66 (1988): 1–62.

Blum, Henrik K. *Expanding Health Care Horizons: From a General Systems Concept of Health to a National Health Policy,* 2nd ed. Oakland, CA: Third Party Publishing, 1983.

Blum, Henrik K. *Planning for Health: Development and Application of Social Change Theory,* 2nd ed. New York: Human Sciences Press, 1981.

Braddock, David, Richard Hemp, Susan Parish, and James Westrich. *The State of the States in Developmental Disabilities,* 5th ed. Washington, DC: American Association on Mental Retardation, 1998.

Bullough, Vern L., and Bonnie Bullough. *The Care of the Sick: The Emergence of Modern Nursing.* London: Croom Helm, 1979.

Green, Lawrence W., and Marshall W. Kreuter. *Health Promotion Planning: A Educational and Environmental Approach,* 2nd ed. Mountain View, CA: Mayfield Publishing, 1991.

Herzlinger, Regina E. *Market Driven Health Care: Who Wins, Who Loses in the Transformation of America's Largest Service Industry.* New York: Addison-Wesley, 1997.

Hooker, Roderick S., and James F. Cawley. *Physician Assistants in American Medicine.* New York: Churchill Livingstone, 1997.

Hsiao, William C., Peter Braun, Daniel Dunn, and Edmund R. Becker. "Results and Policy Implications of the Resource-Based Relative-Value Study." *New England Journal of Medicine* 319 (September 29, 1988): 881–888.

Inglis, Brian. *Fringe Medicine.* London: Faber & Faber, 1964.

Kozak, Robert J., and George Krafcisin. *Safety Management and ISO 9000/QS-9000: A Guide to Alignment and Integration.* New York: Quality Resources, 1997.

Lumsdon, Kevin, and Mark Hagland. "Mapping Care." *Hospital & Health Networks* 67 (October 20, 1993): 34–40.

Pickett, George E., and John J. Hanlon. *Public Health Administration and Practice,* 9th ed. St. Louis: Times Mirror/Mosby College Publishing, 1990.

Reinhardt, Uwe E. "Spending More Through 'Cost Control': Our Obsessive Quest to Gut the Hospital." *Health Affairs* 15 (Summer 1996): 145–154.

3

Concepts
of Organization
Design

*The fragmentation the patient faces is, of course, the direct
result of highly specialized providers operating within highly
complex organizational structures.*[1]

Management is defined as *the process, composed of interrelated social and technical functions and
activities, occurring within a formal organizational setting for the purpose of accomplishing predetermined objectives through the use of human and other resources.* An important element of this definition is that management occurs in a *formal organizational setting.* This means that organizing—or
building and maintaining the formal organizational setting—is a crucial function of managers. This
chapter focuses on the key concepts of organization design as they influence organizational structures. Chapter 4 builds on the design concepts that are contained in this chapter and presents several
types of health services organizations (HSOs). Chapter 5 extends the discussion of organization design to the level of health systems (HSs). How well managers carry out their organization design roles
is critical to how well their organizations perform.

Figure 3.1 shows that organization design begins by designating individual positions and progresses to large HSs, which integrate multiple separate organizations. The structure of all organizations begins with individual positions, which serve as the building blocks for workgroups, clusters
of workgroups, entire organizations, and systems of organizations.[2] Managers at all levels of HSOs/
HSs are involved in the organizing function. Senior managers are concerned more with broad aspects of organizing, such as authority and responsibility relationships, departmentation, coordinating components, and perhaps formation of systems of organizations. In essence, they are concerned
with how effectively the HSO/HS is structured to meet its objectives. Middle-level managers are
more concerned with organizing workgroups and clusters of workgroups. First-level managers are
more directly concerned with organizing individual positions; their tasks include job design, work
process flow, and work methods and procedures.

In their organizing function, managers build the formal organization, the structure conceptualized
and sanctioned by the HSO's/HS's senior managers and governing body. Coexisting with the formal or-

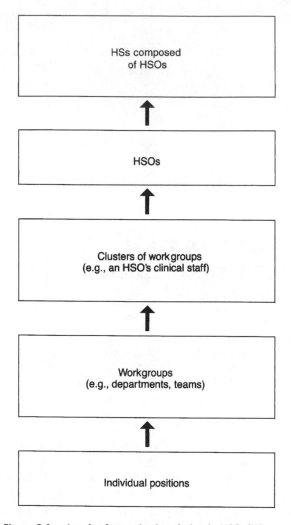

Figure 3.1.   Levels of organization design in HSOs/HSs.

ganization, however, is the informal organization. It exists because people working together invariably establish relationships and interactions outside the formal structure. Thus every HSO/HS has a formal structure developed by management and an informal structure that reflects the wishes and preferences of the staff. Aspects of both formal and informal organization designs are considered in this chapter.

It may be useful to review the comprehensive model of management for HSOs/HSs in Figure 1.7, which shows that conversion of inputs to outputs takes place in a formal organizational setting with structure, tasks/technology, and people elements. "Structure" includes formally designed arrangements such as authority-responsibility relationships; grouping work activities into departments; and coordination, communication, information, and control mechanisms. "Tasks/technology" is work specialization: job design, work processes, methods and procedures, and logistical and work flows. It also represents technological characteristics of the organizational setting, including equipment, cybernetics, and, to some degree, information/knowledge used by management and other personnel in performing their duties and tasks. It is only through people that work occurs. Managers accomplish work by integrating structure, tasks/technology, and people. In doing so they must contend with the dynamics of formal, informal, and individual behavior—positive and negative—including roles, perceptions, expectations, and values.

Organizing is necessitated by the desire for cooperation. When one considers the complexity of direct, support, and management work done in HSOs/HSs, and the diversity of the professional, technical, and support people who perform it, the need for cooperation is evident—a need that may be more important in HSOs/HSs than in any other type of organization. Even within a single unit, such as diagnostic radiology, a wide range of work is performed at many skill levels, and organizing this work is vital to overall effectiveness and efficiency, both of which concern the manager. An organization design is effective if it facilitates attaining the HSO's/HS's objectives; it is efficient if objectives are attained using minimum resources.

It is sometimes erroneously assumed that organization design is something managers do once, when a new organization is created, and then turn their attention elsewhere. Actually, organizing is continuous and ongoing and involves not only initial design but also routine redesign. There are a number of specific instances and circumstances in which HSO/HS managers are likely to find design changes necessary:

- The organization (HSO/HS) is experiencing severe problems. Indicators of inadequate performance may be presented to the manager from external reviews such as accreditation processes and customer satisfaction surveys or from internal reviews such as financial statements and clinical audits. These problems may be identified at varying levels within the organization, for example, for a particular position, a workgroup, a department, or a total organization.
- There is a change in the environment that directly influences internal policies. In some circumstances there may be major changes in the environment, such as prospective payment for hospital services, capitation payment for all health services that are received by a given population, or new policies regulating pharmaceuticals. These changes may require a redesign and refocusing of key organizational groups.
- New programs or product lines are developed. When an organization recognizes certain markets or product lines as high priority, an organization design change may be necessary to infuse resources into the new areas. Conversely, when old programs are to be dropped, new structural arrangements may be necessary.
- There is a change in leadership. New leadership may provide considerable opportunity to rethink the way in which the organization has been designed. New leadership tends to view the organization from a different perspective and may bring innovative ideas to the reorganization.[3]

DESIGN CONCEPTS IN BUILDING
FORMAL ORGANIZATION STRUCTURES

As has been noted, "Because of their natural affinity for contemporary things and ideas, it is difficult for some people to recognize the importance of old ideas and concepts. It would be a serious mistake, however, to overlook the historical roots of what we know about organization design."[4] Although they have been modified over the years, the key organization design concepts that guide the formal structure of most HSOs/HSs were developed by a group of general administrative theorists who worked early in the 20th century. Most influential among these theorists were Max Weber, a German sociologist, and Henri Fayol, a French industrialist. The writings of Weber[5] and Fayol[6] and their colleagues represent what have come to be called the classical concepts of organization design. Perhaps the durability of these concepts in strongly influencing contemporary HSOs/HSs attests to the wisdom in their conceptualization. As Williams and Huber noted,

Most organizations are strongly influenced by classical theory. Some of its assumptions are questionable and many of its principles are deficient; its assertions are too sweeping, and its application has often led to undesirable results. It is, nevertheless, a brilliant expression of organization

theory and a standard of reference which cannot be ignored or considered insignificant by theorist or practicing manager.[7]

Classical Concepts

Weber's Contributions to Design

Weber (1864–1920) is most often associated with the organizational form he termed *bureaucracy.* Weber thought that bureaucracy, in its pure form, represented an ideal or completely rational form of organization. The term *bureaucracy,* usually associated with large public-sector organizations, is used frequently to disparage such undesirable characteristics as duplication, delay, waste, low morale, and general frustration (characteristics sometimes termed *red tape*) found in many large organizations. In Weber's conceptualization, however, the term meant something very different. He used it to describe an organization structure based on the sociological concept of rationalization of collective activities. Weber abstracted the concept of an "ideal" organization from observing many actual organizations and combining them into his model of an ideal bureaucracy. This model became the basis for his theories about how work should be done in large organizations. The key features that Weber[8] believed were necessary if an organization were to achieve the maximum benefits of ideal bureaucracy included the following:

- A clear division of labor ensures that each task performed by employees is systematically established and legitimized by formal recognition as an official duty.
- Positions are arranged in a hierarchy so that each lower position is controlled and supervised by a higher one. The effect of this arrangement is a chain of command.
- Formal rules and regulations uniformly guide the actions of employees. In Weber's view a system of rules ensures a rational approach to organization design and a degree of uniformity and coordination that could not exist otherwise. The basic rationale for rules in Weber's model is that the manager uses them to eliminate uncertainty in the performance of tasks resulting from differences among individuals. Beyond this, he believed that rules and regulations provide continuity and stability to an organization.
- Impersonal relationships and avoidance by managers of involvement with employees' personalities and personal preferences; Weber believed this practice ensured that the bureaucrat did not permit emotional attachments or personalities to interfere with rational decisions.
- Employment should be based entirely on technical competence and protection against arbitrary dismissal. Employees in the ideal bureaucracy are selected using rigid criteria that apply uniformly and impersonally to each candidate. Criteria are based on objective standards for the job established by the officials of the organization. Promotions in the ideal bureaucracy are awarded on the basis of seniority and achievement.

Originally published in 1916, these characteristics of Weber's ideal bureaucracy continue to provide many important aspects of the design prototype for large contemporary organizations,[9] including HSOs/HSs.

Fayol's Contributions to Design

Like Weber, Fayol made contributions to organization design theory that remain fundamentally important in understanding the organization of contemporary HSOs/HSs. Fayol's contributions were primarily based on his identification of a set of "principles" of management. Table 3.1 is an abbreviated version of Fayol's 14 principles of management. Just as Weber's conceptualization of the ideal bureaucracy has significance in the design of today's organizations and systems, many of Fayol's observations remain relevant. As noted by Higgins,

*Virtually all organizations are still arranged according to the division of work using highly spe-
cialized labor, whether they are making . . . microchips or providing health care services. All organizations use the principle of authority; virtually all employ the unity of command concept;
and all use some degree of centralization versus decentralization, and the scalar chain.*[10]

Relevance of Classical Concepts

The work of Fayol, Weber, and other early general administration theorists, such as Luther Gulick
and Lyndall Urwick[11] and James Mooney and Alan Reiley,[12] remains relevant to the design of modern organizations, including HSOs/HSs. However, these classical concepts must be updated to reflect new information about how organizations are best structured to meet the present and future
needs of society as well as the needs of workers in them. The following sections present the most
important and relevant classical concepts of organization design, along with a contemporary perspective on each concept. The key classical concepts that remain relevant and important to managers
as they design and redesign their organizations and systems are 1) division of work, 2) authority and
responsibility relationships, 3) departmentation, 4) span of control, and 5) coordination.

Division of Work

Classical View

The classical theorists—and before them the economist Adam Smith, author of *The Wealth of Nations,* published in 1776[13]—recognized the potential benefits of division of work. Fayol considered
it first among his 14 principles of management (see Table 3.1). He and other classical theorists considered the division of work—or, as it is also known, the specialization of work—to be an important source of certain economic benefits. These economic benefits derived from the fact that

TABLE 3.1.   FAYOL'S 14 PRINCIPLES OF MANAGEMENT

1. *Division of Work:* This principle is the same as Adam Smith's "division of labor." Specialization increases
   output by making employees more efficient.
2. *Authority:* Managers must be able to give orders. Authority gives them this right. Along with authority,
   however, goes responsibility. Wherever authority is exercised, responsibility arises.
3. *Discipline:* Employees must obey and respect the rules that govern the organization. Good discipline is
   the result of effective leadership, a clear understanding between management and workers regarding the
   organization's rules, and the judicious use of penalties for infractions of the rules.
4. *Unity of Command:* Every employee should receive orders from only one superior.
5. *Unity of Direction:* Each group of organizational activities that has the same objective should be directed
   by one manager using one plan.
6. *Subordination of Individual Interests to the General Interests:* The interests of any one employee or group of
   employees should not take precedence over the interests of the organization as a whole.
7. *Remuneration:* Workers must be paid a fair wage for their services.
8. *Centralization:* Centralization refers to the degree to which subordinates are involved in decision making.
   Whether decision making is centralized (to management) or decentralized (to subordinates) is a question
   of proper proportion. The problem is to find the optimum degree of centralization for each situation.
9. *Scalar Chain:* The line of authority from top management to the lowest ranks represents the scalar chain.
   Communications should follow this chain. However, if following the chain creates delays, then cross-
   communications can be allowed if agreed to by all parties and superiors are kept informed.
10. *Order:* People and materials should be in the right place at the right time.
11. *Equity:* Managers should be kind and fair to their subordinates.
12. *Stability of Tenure of Personnel:* High employee turnover is inefficient. Management should provide or-
    derly personnel planning and ensure that replacements are available to fill vacancies.
13. *Initiative:* Employees who are allowed to originate and carry out plans will exert high levels of effort.
14. *Esprit de Corps:* Promoting team spirit will build harmony and unity within the organization.

From *Management,* 3/e by Robbins, ©1991. Reprinted by permission of Prentice-Hall, Inc., Upper Saddle River, NJ.

division of work enhanced individuals' proficiency in performing their work and thus improved the efficiency and effectiveness with which work could be performed. For example, in a contemporary context, an organ transplant team reflects a careful division of work among a group of people. Each member performs specialized work and becomes proficient in it. The team is excellent because the work of individual members is marked by excellence. The team is efficient because individual members are proficient at their work and contribute to the team's overall efficiency.

Technically, division of work means dividing the work of an organization into specific jobs, each consisting of specified activities.[14] The content of a job is determined by what the person doing it is to accomplish. For example, the job of pharmacist in a HSO/HS is defined by the activities a person in this position is expected to accomplish. These activities are different from those expected of someone with the job of nurse, vice president for professional affairs, dietitian, or chief information officer.

Much of the world's work, and certainly that performed in HSOs/HSs, is performed by people who are specialized in particular work through education and experience. Specialization of workers is a common way to divide work in these organizations because licensure and accreditation rules and policies require HSOs/HSs to employ people who have met specific licensure and certification requirements—in other words, to employ people who are properly credentialed for the work that they do. The work of health professionals is to some extent defined and to a large extent prescribed by licensure and certification requirements. Specialization, including but not limited to that which is documented by licensure or certification, implies expertise based on education and experience in the activities of a job. HSOs/HSs, more so than most organizations, are structured to accommodate the specialties of the people who work there.

Organizations, through the division of work, also encourage job or work specialization. Much specialization has a functional basis.[15] *Functionalization* is dividing the HSO's/HS's work based on functions to be performed. Division of work causes HSOs/HSs to be organized into numerous departments or units within which work is functionally similar but among which work is functionally dissimilar. For example, work in the dietary department is dissimilar from that in admitting. Within these departments, however, the work is functionally similar. Specializing has several advantages, including enhancing the HSO's/HS's ability to select, train, and equip people to do work by matching their activities with functions. In functionally specialized work, people often learn the job more quickly than if work is not specialized. This allows managers to achieve greater levels of control because they can more easily standardize functionally specialized work.[16]

Contemporary View

The classical theorists who developed the concept of the division of work saw it as an important, and at the time largely untapped, source of increased productivity. Examples of the potential economic benefits of work division and specialization abounded at the beginning of the 20th century. However, increased division of work has a negative side—people who perform specialized work may find it repetitive, monotonous, and unfulfilling. The proficiency and efficiency benefits of the division or specialization of work are real and they can be significant, but they must be balanced against negative consequences. Taken too far, the division of work can become dysfunctional.

In response, such contemporary developments as programs in cross-training (equipping people with skills and tools that permit them to perform more than one job), job enlargement (combining tasks to create a new job with broader activities), and job enrichment (expanding responsibilities so that work becomes more challenging and satisfying) are increasingly important in all types of organizations, including HSOs/HSs. For example, integrated patient care teams formed through job enrichment efforts involve each member in team decisions and the total care of patients. Cardiac rehabilitation teams can work together to diagnose, treat, rehabilitate, and provide extended care, as a team, from the point of patients' initial incidents through satisfactory recoveries.

Many jobs in HSOs/HSs include work that is tedious and narrow in scope. Those in transport, food preparation, and laundry are good examples. Such jobs can be enlarged readily and to good effect. Similarly, however, health professionals with relatively broad duties in their work also can benefit from job enlargement. Nurses with enlarged responsibilities often enjoy the new challenges. The best job enlargement and enrichment programs are consistent with the widely popular quality-of-work life (QWL) movement. Organizations initiate QWL programs to make the work environment more compatible with their employees' physical, social, and psychological needs at work.[17] The central purpose of QWL programs is to make work meaningful for people and to create an environment in which they can be motivated to perform and derive satisfaction from the results of their work.

Authority and Responsibility Relationships

Classical View

Another important classical organization design concept that is relevant for HSOs/HSs is the establishment of authority and responsibility relationships in performance of work. Growing directly out of the division of work in organizations is the need to assign the responsibility for and authority over the performance of the work. *Authority* is the power derived from a person's position in an organization. Sometimes called legitimate power, organizational authority permits managers to give orders and to expect that they be carried out as managers fulfill their directing function. *Responsibility* is the obligation to perform certain functions or achieve certain objectives and, like authority, is derived from one's position in the organization.

Classical theorists were obsessed with the concept of authority in organizations, viewing it as the glue that held organizations together. Furthermore, they believed that the rights attached to one's position were the only important sources of power or influence in the organization. The effect of this was to believe, as the classical theorists did, that managers were all-powerful in their organizations. This might have been true 100 years ago, but no longer. Now, authority is seen as just one element in the larger concept of power in organizations.[18]

Authority and responsibility are delegated downward in organizations or systems from higher levels of management to lower levels, resulting in a scaling or grading of levels of authority and responsibility. The authority and responsibility of a HSO/HS president are different from those of vice presidents, department heads, and individual employees. Vertical layers in an organization are the clearest evidence of this scalar process. As Higgins noted,

> The scalar chain simply defines the relationships of authority from one level of the organization to another. In the scalar chain, individuals higher up on the chain have more authority than those below them. This is true of all succeeding levels of management from top management to the first-level employee. The scalar chain helps define authority and responsibility and, thus, accountability.[19]

Classical theorists distinguished two forms of authority relationships: line authority and staff authority. As organizational concepts, "line" and "staff" are best understood as a matter of relationships. A line relationship is one in which a superior exercises direct authority over a subordinate. This is command authority and is represented by the chain of command in an organization. The chain of command in a HSO/HS is illustrated by the relationships among nurses on a unit to the nurse manager of the unit, to the nursing supervisor, to the vice president for nursing, and finally to the president of the HSO, and from there on up the ladder if the organization is part of a HS. Each person in this chain has the authority, by virtue of organizational position, to issue directives to and expect compliance from people who are lower in the chain.

Staff authority, in contrast, is advisory authority. Staff authority is expressed in the form of counsel, advice, and recommendations. A HSO's/HS's in-house lawyer/attorney occupies a staff position. This means that the attorney cannot dictate the terms of a sales contract between the HSO/HS and another organization acquiring it. However, based on expertise, the in-house attorney is expected to advise the HSO's/HS's line managers (chief executive officer and other senior officers involved in the sales decision, along with the governing body, in this instance) about language and terms in the contract.

Contemporary View

The most important contemporary developments in how authority and responsibility are viewed in organizations derive from broader views of power in organizations than the narrow perspective held by the classical theorists. There are numerous sources of power and influence in HSOs/HSs (this is discussed more fully in Chapter 15 in relationship to the power of leaders). The authority that derives from one's formal position is only one source of power. French and Raven[20] conceptualized interpersonal power with five distinct bases in organizations: legitimate, reward, coercive, expert, and referent. Only the first three bases derive from the manager's formal position.

Power that is derived from position in an organization is legitimate power. This formal authority resides in managers and exists because organizations find it advantageous to assign power to individuals so that they can do their jobs effectively. All managers have some legitimate power or authority based on position. Managers also have reward power, which is based on their ability to reward desirable behavior and stems from the legitimate power granted to managers. Because of their position, managers control rewards such as pay increases, promotions, and work schedules, and this buttresses legitimate power. Managers also have coercive power because of their position. It is the opposite of reward power and is based on the ability to punish employees or prevent them from obtaining desired rewards. By definition, these sources of power in organizations are restricted to managers. However, other sources of power that are not restricted to managers are quite important in HSOs/HSs, and the existence of these other sources often means that power and influence are spread beyond the organization's managers.

One of the most important sources of power in HSOs/HSs is expert power, which derives from possessing knowledge that is valued by the organization or system. Expert power is personal to the individual with the expertise. Thus it is different from legitimate, reward, and coercive power, which are prescribed by the organization, even though people may be granted such power because they possess expert power. For example, people with expert power often rise to management positions in their areas of expertise. It is also noteworthy that, in HSOs/HSs where work is highly technical or professional, expert power alone makes people powerful. For example, the power of physicians and other licensed independent practitioners is based on clinical knowledge and skills. Physicians with scarce expertise, such as transplant surgeons, have more expert power than do physicians whose expertise is more readily replaceable.

Some individuals arouse admiration, loyalty, and emulation to the extent that they gain the power to influence others. This referent power, sometimes called charismatic power, certainly is not limited to managers. In HSOs/HSs charismatic individuals wield considerable influence. As with expert power, referent power cannot be given by the organization as can legitimate, reward, and coercive powers.

The contemporary view of authority and responsibility in HSOs/HSs is that they remain key ·concepts, heavily influencing the organization design. However, the contemporary view expands on the classical idea and views authority as only one of several sources of power. In this larger context power is not limited to managers.

Another important contemporary development in the concept of authority and responsibility pertains to delegation. Almost without exception, classicists thought that decisions should be made at the lowest possible level in the organization and that this was compatible with good decisions. This means top-level managers should not make decisions on routine matters that could be handled at a lower level. A viewpoint typical of the classicists was that

> *One of the tragedies of business experience is the frequency with which men [business in 1939 was an almost exclusively male domain], always efficient in anything they personally can do, will finally be crushed and fail under the weight of accumulated duties that they do not know and cannot learn how to delegate.*[21]

The importance and logic of delegation was first expounded by the classicists. Contemporary managers now consider it an integral part of the question of how centralized or decentralized decision making in organizations should be. Decentralization is closely related to delegation, but it is also a philosophy of organization and management. Decentralization requires more than handing authority or responsibility to subordinates. Organizations discover that decentralizing requires carefully selecting which decision making to push down and which to hold at or near the top.

It is relatively simple to measure the degree of decentralization in an organization or system. For example, the greater the extent to which decisions are made lower in the management hierarchy, the greater the degree of decentralization. Also, if important decisions are made lower in the management hierarchy, the degree of decentralization is greater. For example, a HSO/HS manager's ability to commit to capital expenditures indicates the degree to which authority has been delegated. Another indication of decentralization is shown when less checking or gaining clearance is required for decisions that are made at lower levels. Decentralization is greatest when no check at all is required; decentralization is less when organizational superiors must be informed of the decision after it has been made, and still less if superiors must be consulted before the decision is made. The fewer people to be consulted and the lower they are in the management hierarchy, the greater the degree of decentralization.

Departmentation

Classical View

Every organized human activity—from a sandlot baseball game to the Human Genome Project—has two fundamental and opposing requirements: division of work to be performed on the one hand, and integration and coordination of the divided work on the other. The classical management theorists recognized the relationship between dividing work and the subsequent need to then coordinate divided work to achieve satisfactory results. They developed the concept of departmentation (sometimes called departmentalization) as an organization design concept that partially addresses these dual concerns. Departmentation, the grouping of work and workers into manageable units or departments, still heavily influences the design of modern organizations.

The classical view of departmentation is that it is a natural consequence of division and specialization of work. Because it is rational to specialize work, it is also rational to group similar workers into workgroups. In turn, these are grouped into clusters of workgroups until the organization has a superstructure (see Figure 3.1). The classicists Gulick and Urwick[22] noted four reasons for departmentation: purpose, process, persons and things, and place. Bases for departmentation have increased since their time, but the basic concept is largely unchanged. Mintzberg,[23] for example, suggested six bases for grouping workers into units and units into larger units:

1. *Knowledge and skills:* Workers are grouped by specialized knowledge and skills. For example, HSOs/HSs group surgeons in one department, pediatricians in another.

2. *Work process and function:* Workers are grouped by processes or functions performed. Departments of marketing or finance in HSOs/HSs are examples.
3. *Time:* Workers are grouped by when work is done. Typically, HSOs/HSs are 24-hour-a-day operations, in which some workers are grouped into day, evening, and night shifts.
4. *Output:* Workers are grouped by outputs, whether services or products. For example, many HSOs/HSs group workers by whether they produce inpatient or outpatient services.
5. *Client:* Workers are grouped by the clients or patients served. It is common for some HSOs/HSs to establish workgroups based on age or gender of patients, such as in geriatric and women's health programs.
6. *Place:* Workers are grouped by physical location. A HS might operate ambulatory clinics in downtown locations as well as in the city's suburbs.

A single HSO/HS may use all of these bases for grouping workers to design an effective organization.

No matter which basis is used, the act of grouping workers helps establish the means by which their work can be coordinated within the groups and with other workgroups. Mintzberg[24] suggested that grouping (or departmentation) has at least four important implications for workers and their organizations:

1. Grouping sets up a system of common supervision. Once workers are grouped, a manager can be appointed to coordinate and control the work of the group.
2. Grouping facilitates sharing resources. People in workgroups share a common budget, facilities, and equipment.
3. Grouping typically leads to common measures of performance. Shared resources on the input side and group-level objectives on the output side permit group members to be evaluated by common performance criteria. Common performance measures encourage group members to coordinate work.
4. Grouping encourages communication. Shared input resources and output objectives and close physical proximity encourage communication. This facilitates coordinating the work of group members.

HSOs/HSs use all six of the bases of departmentation discussed above, including departmentation by function, the basis most favored by the classical theorists. This basis for departmentation, reinforced by the specialized knowledge and skills of many workers, is clearly visible in HSOs/HSs. Nurses are in nursing service, pharmacists in the pharmacy, and so on. Even within departments, the departmentation concept is evident. For example, a large clinical laboratory (a result of functional departmentation) comprises even more functionally specialized workgroups, such as blood bank, chemistry, and hematology.

Contemporary View

One important contemporary development in the organization design of many HSOs/HSs is the increased focus on patients as the basis for departmentation or grouping. This is one result of the increased competition for patients among HSOs/HSs. A direct outgrowth of this phenomenon is a significant increase in grouping workers on the basis of patients. Geriatric and women's health programs abound, as do comprehensive cardiac care programs that are marketed specifically to corporate executives as HSOs/HSs seek to hold or build market share.

Another important contemporary development in organization design is the recognition by many HSOs/HSs that rigidly departmented organizational structures, no matter what the basis for departmentation, face significant problems of coordination across departments and other divisions of workers. The bureaucratic form, which stresses departmentation and hierarchy, works well in some circumstances but not in others. The bureaucratic form is effective in stable circumstances, but it is a disadvantage when flexibility in response to changing circumstances is more important. Organization designs that are more flexible—or, as some prefer to call them, more organic—work better in dynamic circumstances. As suggested by Gibson and Ivancevich,

> *The organic organization is flexible and adaptable to changing environmental demands because its design encourages greater utilization of the human potential. Managers are encouraged to adopt practices that tap the full range of human motivations through job design that stresses personal growth and responsibility. Decision making, control, and goal-setting processes are decentralized and shared at all levels of the organization. Communications flow throughout the organization, not only down the chain of command.*[25]

A good example of organic design occurs in the context of how HSOs/HSs respond to difficulties that are encountered in managing large-scale projects that require the skills of people in different departments or in situations in which patient care is enhanced by multidisciplinary teams. Project teams use groups of workers drawn from different departments to carry out specific projects or programs. Project teams do not replace the departmental structure. They are organic complements to the more mechanistic and bureaucratic functional departmental structure and eliminate some of its rigidity in certain circumstances.

A project team could be used to organize services for a comprehensive home health care program for people who are chronically ill. Team members are drawn from nursing, social services, respiratory therapy, occupational therapy, pharmacy, and physicians specializing in chronic disease. To market the program and to handle finance and reimbursement issues, expertise would be provided by team members drawn from the HSO's/HS's administration. A project manager would be named.

Project organization permits flexibility, enhances skill development, and enriches jobs for team participants, but it has a negative side. Project organization can cause ambiguity for workers who participate in a project with its own manager while holding a position in their home department, which has a different manager. Project organization is time consuming because it relies on extensive communication, often in face-to-face team meetings. Furthermore, good project managers are scarce. They must be knowledgeable in the area of the project's focus and possess good interpersonal skills. Managers who are accustomed to working in a departmented structure must adopt a new approach to the job to successfully manage projects. Management of project teams differs from managing departments along the dimensions illustrated by Table 3.2.

HSOs/HSs can use the project organization designs by superimposing these designs on their existing functionally departmented design. This can be done in a few areas, such as the home care program noted earlier, or for the whole organization. Figure 3.2 is a matrix design for a psychiatric hospital in which functional managers head departments and program or product line managers head major clinical programs or product lines. Notice that the individual worker depicted is a member of the nursing and the Alzheimer's disease programs.

Span of Control

Classical View

An organization design question of fundamental concern to classical theorists was how large to make groupings of workers. How many people should be grouped in a department, and on what basis was the decision made? In considering these questions, classical theorists developed the span-of-control concept, which remains an important concept in the design of HSOs/HSs. Span of control is defined as the number of subordinates reporting directly to a superior.

TABLE 3.2. DIFFERENCES IN DEPARTMENT AND PROJECT MANAGEMENT

Function	Department management	Project management
Planning	Repetitive with annual, monthly, weekly and daily issues that are similar from cycle to cycle	Single cycle of planning, broken into discrete phases
Communication	Clearly defined channels which emphasize chain of command and adherence to procedure	Must be more rapid, relies on both formal and informal channels; meetings are more frequent
Leadership	Generally hierarchical, multiple layers of administration	More streamlined; requires advocacy rather than administration for leadership
Roles and responsibilities	Clearly defined, supported by position descriptions, formal policy, and procedure documentation; social pecking order determined by job	Must be defined at the start of project and redefined as project progresses

From Stevens, George H. *The Strategic Health Care Manager*, 125. San Francisco, Jossey-Bass, 1991; reprinted by permission.

Classical theorists generally agreed that managers should have limited numbers of subordinates reporting directly to them, a pragmatic conclusion based on the need for managers to exercise control. Some theorists even specified numbers for the optimum span. For example, Urwick[26] specified six as the maximum span if the manager were to maintain close control. Davis[27] distinguished two types of span of control: executive and operative. Executive span refers to senior- and middle-level management positions, operative to first-level management positions. Davis judged that an effective executive span of control could vary from three to nine, while the operative span could have as many as 30 employees reporting directly to a first-level manager.

How an organization answers the span-of-control question significantly affects its design. As seen in Figure 3.3, smaller spans of control produce "tall" organizations and larger spans produce "flat" organizations. The tall and flat structures in Figure 3.3 have equal numbers of positions, but the tall structure has five levels and the flat one has three.

Complex HSOs usually have a tall pattern. The shape of HSs depends on whether they are horizontally or vertically integrated. The tall pattern of HSOs results from differentiation and specialization of numerous and varied departments (e.g., from the dietary department to the department of surgery) and the consequent need for limited spans of control. Less complex HSOs, such as clinics or small nursing facilities, have flatter structures. More important, even large HSOs have begun to flatten their structures as they seek efficiencies and cost reductions through reduced workforces, cuts that often have been concentrated in the middle-management ranks.

Contemporary View

The most important change has been the recognition that several factors determine the appropriate spans of control in an organization or system's design. In contemporary thinking about the span, several factors are taken into account, including[28]

- *Level of professionalism and training of subordinates.* Professionalized and highly trained workers (characteristics prevalent in HSOs/HSs) require less close supervision, which permits wider spans of control.
- *Level of uncertainty in the work being done.* Complex and varied work requires close supervision, compared with simple and repetitive work. Close supervision requires narrow spans of control.
- *Degree of standardization of work.* Standardized and routinized work—whether professional, such as in a pharmacy or laboratory, or work such as food preparation—requires less direct supervision; thus spans of control can be wider.

- *Degree of interaction required between managers and workers.* Work situations in which more interaction is needed between managers and workers require narrower spans of control because effective interaction takes time. Increasing the number of subordinates reporting to a manager exponentially increases the number of possible interactions between managers and subordinates because managers can interact with individuals and with combinations of individuals. The number of possible interactions between a manager and two subordinates, individually or in combination, is six. If the number of subordinates is five, potential interactions increase to 100; six subordinates mean 222 possible interactions between manager and subordinates.
- *Degree of task integration required.* If work done in a group is integrated or interdependent, a narrower span of control may be needed.

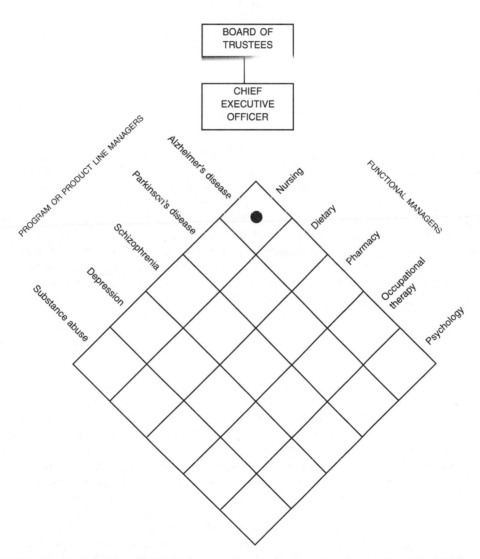

Figure 3.2.   A matrix design for a psychiatric hospital. (From Leatt, Peggy, Stephen M. Shortell, and John R. Kimberly. "Organization Design." In *Health Care Management: Organization Design and Behavior,* 4th ed., edited by Stephen M. Shortell and Arnold D. Kaluzny, 290. Albany, NY: Delmar Publishers, 2000; reprinted by permission.)

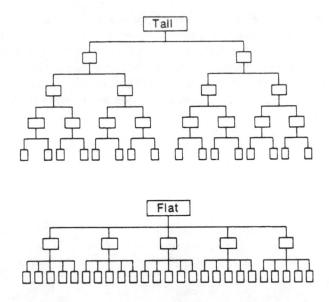

Figure 3.3.   Contrasting spans of control.

The contemporary view is that the classical concept of span of control is highly relevant to HSO/HS design. However, several contingencies must be recognized when applying it. Senior levels in a HSO/HS typically have narrow spans of control (e.g., a president may have five or six vice presidents). At levels at which work is more standardized and routinized, the spans can be much wider. Another factor is the nature of the work. It is easier to supervise 10 file clerks than five nurses. Also, the abilities and availability of managers must be taken into account. The training and personal qualities of some managers enable them to manage more subordinates than others, thus facilitating a broader span of control. Similarly, better training and higher potential for self-direction of subordinates reduce the need for relationships with management and increase the number of subordinates a manager can effectively supervise.

Coordination

Classical View

The classical theorists attributed great importance to the organization design concept of coordination. Chester Barnard, an influential classical theorist, went so far as to say that, in most circumstances, "the quality of coordination is the crucial factor in the survival of the organization."[29] Fayol's conceptualization was representative of how classicists viewed coordination. He defined it as "pulling together all activities of the enterprise to make possible both its working and success."[30] He believed that a well-coordinated organization had distinct characteristics: Each department works in harmony with other departments, each department knows the share of common tasks it must assume, and work schedules of all departments are integrated. He also thought that organizations are poorly coordinated for several reasons: People in each department may know little about what happens in other departments; by focusing too much on their departments, managers have difficulty thinking of the organization's general interest; and managers create barriers between their departments and other departments. Fayol called this last point creating "water-tight compartments," a concept now called "protecting turf." Fayol noted that failing to consider the organization's general interest, which he judged disastrous for an organization, "is not the result of preconcerted intention but the culmination of nonexistent or inadequate coordination."[31]

Classical theorists saw coordination as a way to link various parts of an organization and considered it a vital activity for managers. The early theorists saw coordination as consciously assembling and synchronizing different work efforts to function harmoniously in attaining organization objectives.[32] This view remains valid. Some authors use the term *integration* to express this concept. Lawrence and Lorsch, for example, defined integration as the process of achieving unity of effort among the various parts of an organization.[33] Coordination and integration have similar meanings and may be used interchangeably.

The classical definition of coordination has an important limitation when applied to coordination in contemporary HSOs/HSs. It pertains only to coordination within a HSO—an intraorganizational perspective. Increasingly important, with the development of HSs, is the issue of coordination among and between organizations—an interorganizational perspective. Coordination in the context of several organizations joined together in a HS is "the articulation of elements in a service delivery system so that comprehensiveness, accessibility, and compatibility among elements are maximized."[34]

Although much of what is known about intraorganizational coordination as it was conceptualized by the classicists applies to interorganizational coordination, important differences are examined in this section. It is important to note that the definition of coordination applies both to intraorganizational coordination within HSOs and to interorganizational coordination among HSOs in a HS. Thus coordination in HSOs/HSs can be described as activity that is intended to achieve unity and harmony of effort in pursuit of shared organizational objectives within a HSO or among the organizations participating in a HS.

Contemporary View

Coordination is a critical task for all managers in contemporary HSOs/HSs. It differs with the organizational levels of managers. Senior-level managers are concerned with coordination or integration of an entire HSO, and with interorganizational coordination between their organizations and others in the external environment. This latter responsibility is especially important when a HSO is part of a HS. Middle-level managers face significant challenges as they seek to coordinate the various clusters of workgroups that compose HSOs. First-level managers focus on coordination within their departments and, along with the middle-level managers to whom they report, between their departments or units and other parts of their HSO. Appropriate coordinating mechanisms differ from one organizational level to another, but their selection and use are important for all managers.

Central to understanding the importance of coordination to management success in HSOs/HSs is appreciating the high level of interdependence exhibited by these organizations and systems. Interdependence among the individuals and units within or among organizations varies with the structural complexity and objectives of organizations. There are three forms of interdependence: pooled, sequential, and reciprocal.[35]

Pooled interdependence occurs when individuals and organizational units are related but do not have a close connection. They simply contribute separately in some way to the larger whole. For example, a HS formed by geographically dispersed nursing facilities owned by a corporation may be linked largely in that each contributes to the overall success of the corporation, but they have little direct interdependence. Their activities are pooled to make the corporation more effective.

Sequential interdependence occurs when individuals and organizational units have a close and sequential connection. For example, patients admitted to a HSO can become the focal points for extended chains of sequentially interdependent activities. In an acute care hospital, for example, the admitting office admits patients and schedules them in the operating room if surgery is part of their care plan, notifies the dietary department of special needs, notifies the laboratory regarding tests, and so on. Most of what is done for the patients in HSOs/HSs is sequentially interdependent.

Reciprocal interdependence occurs when individuals and organizational units have a close relationship and the interdependence is bidirectional. For example, a vertically integrated HS with acute care and long-term care HSOs exhibits reciprocal interdependence. Long-term care beds are occupied by patients who are referred from acute care beds; the acute care unit depends on the long-term care unit as a place to which it can discharge certain patients. The acute care unit suffers if the long-term care unit cannot accept a patient. Conversely, the long-term care unit suffers if patients are not discharged to it from the acute unit. Furthermore, the long-term care unit may need to transfer patients back to the hospital when acute episodes of illness occur. The interdependence between these units is reciprocal because it clearly goes in both directions.

Typically, interdependence is greater as its form moves from pooled to sequential to reciprocal.[36] The higher the level of interdependence, the greater the need for managerial attention to coordination. HSOs/HSs, in general, exhibit very high levels of interdependence among their component parts, usually of the sequential or reciprocal forms. Thus the need for effective coordination usually is very great in these organizations and systems.

Mechanisms of Coordination

A wide variety of mechanisms are available to coordinate within and among HSOs/HSs. The success of these mechanisms varies with the situations in which they are applied. That is, the choices managers make from the menu of coordinating mechanisms are contingent on the situation in which coordination is pursued. Available mechanisms can be categorized in several different ways.

In the view of Litterer,[37] managers have three mechanisms available to achieve coordination. They can coordinate by using the organization's hierarchy or its administrative system, or through voluntary activities. Hierarchical coordination links various activities by placing them under a central authority. In a simple HSO this form of coordination is often sufficient. In larger, more complex HSOs and HSs, hierarchical coordination is more difficult. The chief executive officer is a focal point of authority, but one person cannot solve all of the coordinating problems in the hierarchy. Therefore, coordination through the hierarchical structure must be supplemented by other mechanisms.

The administrative system is a second mechanism to coordinate activities. Litterer noted that "A great deal of coordinative effort in organizations is concerned with a horizontal flow of work of a routine nature. Administrative systems are formal procedures designed to carry out much of this routine coordinative work automatically."[38] Work procedures such as memoranda with routing slips help coordinate operating units. For nonroutine and nonprogrammable events, administrative systems or techniques such as coordinating committees also may provide integration.

A third type of coordination, according to Litterer, is accomplished through voluntary action when individuals or groups perceive a need for coordination, develop a method, and implement it. In HSOs/HSs much of the coordination depends on the willingness and ability of individuals or groups to voluntarily integrate their activities with other organizational participants. Achieving voluntary coordination is one of the most important yet difficult problems for the manager. Voluntary coordination requires that individuals possess sufficient knowledge of organizational objectives, information about specific problems of coordination, and the motivation to do something about the problems. Fortunately, voluntary coordination in HSOs/HSs is facilitated by the professionalism of many of the staff. Although their example is the hospital, the point made by Georgopoulos and Mann applies to all HSOs/HSs:

> *The hospital is dependent very greatly upon the motivations and voluntary, informal adjustments*
> *of its members for the attainment and maintenance of good coordination. Formal organizational*

plans, rules, regulations, and controls may ensure some minimum coordination, but of them-
selves are incapable of producing adequate coordination, for only a fraction of all the coordi-
native activities required in this organization can be programmed in advance.[39]

Managers can facilitate voluntary coordination by providing individuals with knowledge of the organization or system's objectives and with information concerning specific problems of co-ordination. If coupled with the motivation to do something about coordination problems, voluntary coordination can easily occur. In part, such motivation stems from the professionalism of many HSO/HS workers. Their value systems, which are supportive of patients' welfare, facilitate volun-tary coordination.

Mintzberg[40] categorized the mechanisms of coordination that are available to managers as mu-tual adjustment, direct supervision, standardization of work processes, standardization of work out-puts, and standardization of workers' skills. Figure 3.4 illustrates these coordinating mechanisms.

- *Mutual adjustment*—This mechanism provides coordination by informal communications among those whose work must be coordinated. Like Litterer's voluntary actions noted earlier, work is coordinated by those performing it (see Figure 3.4a)
- *Direct supervision*—Like Litterer's hierarchical coordination, this mechanism coordinates work when someone takes responsibility for the work of others, including issuing instructions and monitoring actions (see Figure 3.4b).
- *Standardization of work processes*—This mechanism is an alternative coordinating mechanism that programs or specifies the content of work. HSOs/HSs can rather easily standardize many work processes through such actions as establishing standard admission and discharge proce-dures or standard methods of performing laboratory tests. Other standardization efforts are more complicated, such as those involving development of patient care protocols (see Figure 3.4c, work processes).
- *Standardization of work outputs*—This mechanism specifies the product or expected perfor-mance, with the process of how to perform the work left to the worker (see Figure 3.4c, outputs).
- *Standardization of workers' skills*—Standardization occurs when neither work processes nor output can be standardized. If standardization is to occur in such situations, it must be through worker training (see Figure 3.4c, input skills). This form is frequently found in HSOs/HSs, in which complexity does not allow standardization of work processes or outputs. Standardization of workers' skills and knowledge is an excellent coordinating mechanism. For example,

When an anesthesiologist and a surgeon meet in the operating room to remove an appendix, they
need hardly communicate; by virtue of their respective training, they know exactly what to expect
of each other. Their standardized skills take care of most of the coordination.[41]

Hage[42] provided yet another list of coordination mechanisms: programming, planning, cus-toms, and feedback. In using programming, organizations develop explicit rules and prescriptions (called programs) that define jobs and the sequence of activities for all jobs. Programming allows staff to learn and do their jobs and reduces the need for communication except for questions about interpreting a rule. Programming yields a result that is similar to Litterer's administrative system and is accomplished with rules, manuals, job descriptions, personnel procedures, promotion poli-cies, and the like. HSOs/HSs rely heavily, but not exclusively, on programming as a means of coordination.

Planning differs from programming. A plan delineates objectives that the organization or sys-tem hopes to achieve and the means to achieve them. Planning and programming can be combined. Programs are specific means to achieve the HSO's/HS's planned objectives. Planning as a coordi-

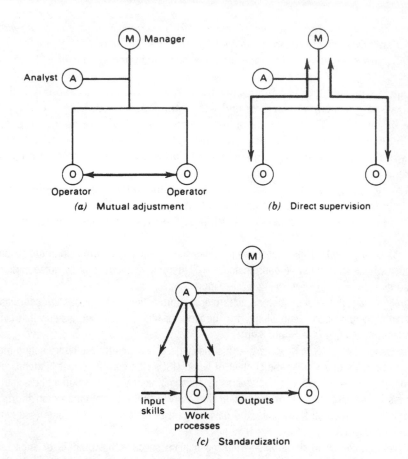

Figure 3.4.   Mintzberg's five coordinating mechanisms. (From *Structure in Fives: Designing Effective Organizations.* Mintzberg, Henry, 1983. Reprinted by permission of Prentice-Hall, Inc., Upper Saddle River, NJ.)

native mechanism is exemplified by the need for planning in one unit to be made part of the whole. For example, overall expansion plans must be considered in the human resources planning that occurs in nursing service, or the expansion plans of a health maintenance organization must take into account the unit that is responsible for physician recruitment and retention. No subunit plan should be made that does not contribute to the objectives set forth in the plans of the entire organization or system. Senior managers are responsible for ensuring that all managers understand organizational objectives. It is the joint duty of all managers to determine whether their plans are compatible with all of the other plans. To the extent that this is done, coordination is facilitated.

Customs are a frequently overlooked coordination mechanism, yet many managers rely heavily on them as coordination mechanisms. For example, it may be customary in a particular nursing facility to use the holiday season as an occasion to invite the families of residents into the facility for a meal and social interaction. Knowing of this custom permits departments to begin their preparations well in advance and facilitates the coordination of their contributions to its success. Customs based on a history of trial and error represent a distillation of good practice, but in complex HSOs/HSs they are not sufficient to meet the coordination challenge.

The final coordination mechanism in Hage's list, feedback, can indicate when a HSO/HS or some part of it is not functioning well. Properly designed feedback systems can trigger renewed efforts to coordinate work. Feedback often takes the form of written reports on operations and activities in organizations and systems, but it also includes the verbal exchanges that occur. All forms of effective communication include feedback, as is discussed in Chapter 17.

In addition to the coordination mechanisms identified by Litterer, Mintzberg, and Hage, there are a number of other effective mechanisms available to HSO/HS managers. In certain circumstances, committees can be very effective coordination mechanisms. Committees are frequently composed of members from a number of departments or functional areas for the specific purpose of coordination among them. Using committees for purposes of coordination is well established in HSOs/HSs. Of course, committees serve other purposes besides coordination; they may act in a service, advisory, informational, or decision-making capacity.

In contrast to committees, a single person can sometimes be an effective mechanism of coordination. Lawrence and Lorsch[43] found that well-coordinated organizations often rely on individuals, whom they term *integrators,* to achieve coordination. Successfully playing an integrator role depends more on having particular expertise than occupying a particular formal position. People are successful integrators because of specialized knowledge and because they represent a central source of information. Examples of effective integrators are found among individual nurses who provide significant coordination among various departments and subunits, particularly as they relate to patient care.

Coordination may be especially difficult in managing large-scale projects that require the skills of people from several different units or that incorporate multidisciplinary approaches to patient care. For example, in the earlier discussion about using matrix designs to organize services into a comprehensive home health care program for people who are chronically ill, the project manager would coordinate the work of the entire team. This person would play an important integrator role and would be key in achieving effective coordination within the project and between it and the other parts of the HSO in which it is embedded. When entire HSOs use the project organization design— creating a matrix design as shown in Figure 3.2—program or product line managers play integrator roles. This coordination mechanism will be increasingly important as HSOs/HSs adopt product line management orientations.

Other structural devices or organization design features also can help with problems of coordination. Cross-functional quality improvement teams (QITs) are useful mechanisms through which to achieve coordination in HSOs/HSs. Originally developed in Japan, QITs have gained widespread acceptance as a means of coordinating, especially at the operational level, in organizations and systems. This mechanism features small-group, problem-oriented meetings in which organizational participants focus on ways to improve quality and work processes. They result in improved communication and inspire more effective teamwork, both of which contribute directly to enhanced coordination. Cross-functional quality improvement teams rely on flow diagrams, nominal group processes, multicriteria decision making, cause-and-effect diagrams, and related problem-identification and problem-solving tools to improve communication, coordination, and ultimately the quality of work.

The contemporary view of coordination as an organization design concept is that it is vital to effective HSO/HS operation and performance and that managers can select from a lengthy menu of coordinating mechanisms: administrative system; committees; customs; direct supervision; feedback; hierarchy; integrators; matrix designs; mutual adjustment; planning; programming; project management through task forces or teams; standardization of work processes, outputs, or workers' skills; QITs; and voluntary action. Managers in HSOs/HSs use various combinations of these mechanisms to achieve coordination; usually several are used concurrently.

Depending on the circumstances that are inherent in different situations, various packages of these mechanisms can be appropriately tailored. For example, a senior-level manager concerned about how the responsibilities, roles, and performance of the departments in a HSO are coordinated might select one package of coordination mechanisms. The vice president for nursing services in the same organization, concerned about coordination within nursing service, might select a somewhat different set of mechanisms. The pharmacy director, concerned about coordination issues involved in the proper dispensing of pharmaceuticals, might select yet another set of mechanisms. A different package of coordinating mechanisms might be selected by the president of a HS who is concerned about coordinating the set of HSOs in the system.

Summary of the Classical Organization Design Concepts

The relationship of classical design concepts to the actual organizational structure of a HSO/HS is readily seen in the schematic representation known as an organization chart. For example, the prototype organization chart in Figure 3.5 shows the basic nature of the concept of division of work. Each unit in the chart represents a subdividing of work and suggests that staff in each unit specialize. The chart also suggests authority and responsibility relationships. The vertical dimension gen-

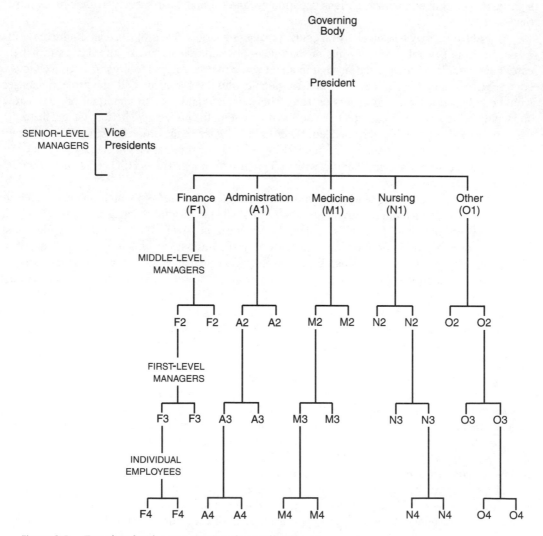

Figure 3.5.   Template for the organization charts of HSOs.

erally suggests who has authority over and responsibility for whom. People who are higher in the chart generally have authority over those who are lower in it. People on the same level have similar amounts of authority and responsibility. The chart also depicts groupings of people into units in the departmentation process. The chart permits easy assessment of a span of control simply by counting the people with a direct reporting relationship to a manager. Finally, the chart suggests who is responsible for coordinating parts of the HSO, although the coordinating mechanisms they might use are not apparent. With some variation, the application of these classical design concepts also helps explain the shape of systems comprising scts of organizations. Figure 3.6 shows a HS comprising a number of HSOs, both hospitals and long-term care facilities.

Of course, organizational structures built on the classical design concepts such as the ones shown in Figures 3.5 and 3.6 do not show entire organizational structures. Coexisting with this formal organization is an informal organization that is not visible in the organization chart.

DESIGN CONCEPTS IN INFORMAL ORGANIZATION STRUCTURES

Existing within the formal pattern of authority–responsibility relationships is another important pattern the informal organization. The formal organization is a planned and prescribed effort to establish relationships, and a great deal of management time and effort is spent establishing and maintaining it. The results include development of formal organization structures such as those depicted in Figures 3.5 and 3.6, and related job descriptions, formal rules, operating policies, work procedures, control procedures, coordinating mechanisms, compensation arrangements, and other ways to guide employee behavior. However, many interactions among members of an organization are not prescribed by the formal structure. Interactions and relationships that arise spontaneously from activities of members, but are not set forth in the formal structure, make up the informal organization. Formal and informal organizations coexist and are, in fact, inseparable. "The distinction between the formal and the informal aspects of organization life is only an analytical one . . . ; there is only one actual organization."[44]

The formal and the informal organizations together constitute the organizational setting in which work is performed in HSOs/HSs. The formal organization is characterized by prescribed authority–responsibility relationships, division of work and departmentation, and the hierarchical structure. The formal organization is the planned interrelationships of people, things, and activities. By contrast, the informal organization is characterized by dynamic behavior and activity patterns that occur within the formal organization structure as a result of people working with other people—their interaction and fraternization across formal structural lines. Managers must pay careful attention to both formal and informal aspects of organization design.

Nature of Informal Organizations

Keen awareness of and interest in informal organization design concepts stem from the Hawthorne studies of the 1930s.[45] These studies showed that informal organization is integral to the work setting. The informal organization arises from social interactions of people in an organization. Much of what managers know about the informal organization is based on the work of sociologists and social psychologists, who study groups and the behavior of people in groups.

A group is "two or more persons, who come into contact for a purpose and who consider the contact meaningful."[46] Group members depend on one another to achieve their objectives.[47] Thus groups have a purpose, although it may be implicit rather than stated, and there is interdependence among members. Groups in organizations can be classified as formal or informal. Formal groups are created intentionally by managers as a means of achieving organizational objectives. Examples of formal groups include committees, QITs, task forces, and project teams. In contrast, informal

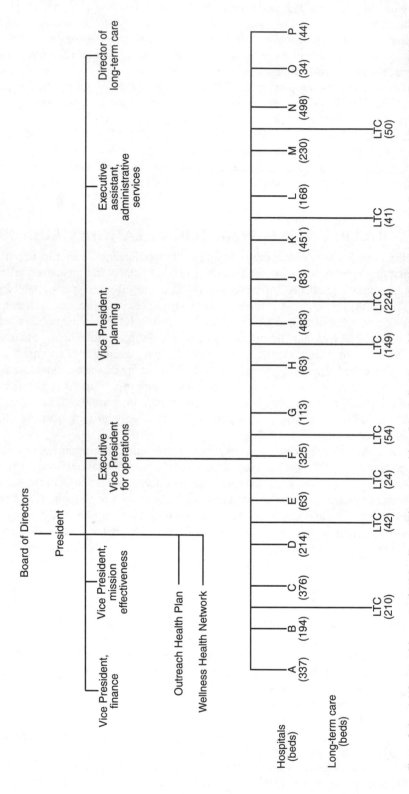

Figure 3.6. A HS comprising several HSOs. (From Kaluzny, Arnold D. "Centralization and Decentralization in a Vertically Integrated System: The XYZ Hospital Corporation." In *Strategic Alignment: Managing Integrated Health Systems*, edited by Douglas A. Conrad and Geoffrey A. Hoare, 125–132. Chicago: Health Administration Press, 1994; reprinted by permission.)

groups arise from spontaneous attractions among individuals seeking social reinforcement or other benefits of group membership. They seldom have stated organizational objectives and lack the assumption of permanence.

Managers should realize that the informal organization is inevitable. They can change any aspect of the formal organization because they created it. However, because the informal organization is not created by management, it is much less subject to management's preferences. As long as people are involved in formal organizations, there will be informal organizations, with both positive and negative consequences for the formal organization. To capitalize on the advantages and minimize the disadvantages of the informal organization, the manager must understand the informal organization and, therefore, must understand groups in the organization.

Why People Form Informal Groups

When one considers why a human being does anything, motivation is the starting point. As discussed in Chapter 16, people are motivated by whatever satisfies their needs. If the formal organization satisfied all of the needs of participants, there would be no informal organization. Informal groups come into being because members' needs are not fully met by the formal organization.

What needs does the informal organization satisfy? Interpersonal contacts within the informal organization provide relief from the boredom, monotony, and pressures of the formal organization. People in informal groups usually are surrounded by others with similar values, and this reinforces their value system. Another reason people join informal groups is that groups accord informal status, which may be nothing more than belonging to a distinct unit that is more or less exclusive. Informal group membership also provides a degree of personal security; the group member feels acceptance by peers as an equal and feels secure in their company. Group membership permits the individual to express views before sympathetic listeners. The group helps satisfy an individual's recognition, participation, and communication needs. The group member may even find an outlet for leadership drives. These important forms of satisfaction are available in the group—usually to a greater degree than in the formal organization.

Another important reason for group membership is to secure information. The grapevine—the flow of informal information detailed in Chapter 17—is a phenomenon known to all who participate in organizations. Suffice it to say that informal group membership gives members access to informal communication. The common denominator in all of these reasons for group membership is that they meet specific needs of members that are not fully met by the formal organization. Informal groups arise and persist in the organization because they perform desired functions for their members.

Leadership in Informal Groups

An important parameter of how informal groups function is leadership within the group, even if the leadership is unofficial or unsanctioned by the formal organization. Leaders of informal groups possess attributes that group members perceive to be critical to the satisfaction of members' needs. Group leaders embody values of the groups from which they come. Leaders perceive these values, organize them into a philosophy, and verbalize them to members and nonmembers. Finally, group leaders receive communications that are relevant to their groups and communicate the new information to them. In effect, leaders are information centers for informal groups.[48]

Informal group leaders emerge from within groups because they serve several functions. The leader not only initiates action and provides direction but also resolves differences of opinion on group-related matters and conflicts between or among the group's members. Furthermore, the leader communicates group values and feelings to nonmembers, such as representatives of the formal organization. The informal group leadership role is retained only if the role is performed well.

Stages of Group Development

Another important parameter of groups is how they are formed. Groups in workplaces, whether they are part of the formal organization (e.g., committees or QITs) or are informal groups, generally develop in discernable stages: forming, storming, norming, performing, and adjourning.[49]

In the forming stage the group is established by management in the case of formal groups or develops informally. Members become acquainted and learn about the tasks they are to perform or the benefits they might obtain from membership. The storming stage is characterized by real and potential conflict in the group. This must be sorted out before progress can be made, and sometimes the sorting out process is quite stormy.

In the norming stage the members begin to cooperate. Members establish the rules of conduct or norms. In the performing stage the members of the group are well organized and fully functional; they are concerned about the group and its performance, and are able to achieve results and deal with conflict effectively. The group dissolves in the final stage, adjourning (this stage is sometimes called dissolution). All groups eventually dissolve, because the reasons for which they were formed are no longer relevant, because the group no longer serves the needs of its members, or because the group can no longer deal effectively with new circumstances or conditions.

Managers should know the group's stage of development because their reaction to a forming group should be different from their reaction to a performing group. The most appropriate reaction to an adjourning group might be to ignore it because its days are numbered, unless the manager considers it to be a positive force in the organization and wishes to continue it.

Structure of Informal Groups

Another important variable in informal group formation and operation is the tendency to develop a complex structure of relationships. The structure of informal groups is determined by different status positions of members: group leader, primary group member, fringe group member, and out status. For example, Figure 3.7 shows the informal structure of a group of nine people working in one section of a HSO's clinical laboratory. The solid square in the center represents the group leader. Clustered around the leader are the other four members of the primary group. This close association is characterized by intense interaction and communication. The three people at the fringe are likely to be newcomers who are, in effect, being evaluated by the primary group and who may be-

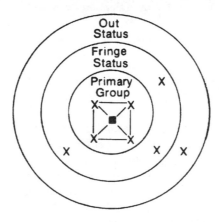

Figure 3.7.   Informal group structure.

come full members. If not accepted, they move to out status. One person is already in out status. This has profound behavioral effects if the person in out status wants to belong to the primary group. Belonging to the formal group of employees in the laboratory section is no subsititute for full membership in the informal group.

Positive Aspects of the Informal Relationships in HSOs/HSs

Because the informal relationships in HSOs/HSs are neither created by managers nor as controllable by them as is formal organization design, the informal relationships are sometimes viewed as problems by managers. These relationships can indeed cause problems for managers, but informal relationships can serve useful purposes as well. The primary benefit of informal relationships occurs when they blend with the formal organization to facilitate work.

Formal structures, policies, and other aspects of formal organization design can be too inflexible for a dynamic situation. Thus the more flexible and spontaneous characteristics of informal relationships are a great advantage if they permit or encourage deviations that contribute to organizational objectives. In emergencies, for example, the informal relationships that have been established in a HSO/HS may preserve the organization from the harm that would result from strict adherence to formal channels of communication or literal obedience to the rules and regulations governing who does what in the organization. There are several other potential benefits of informal relationships and arrangements in organizations.

Informal relationships can provide social values and stability to HSOs/HSs. For example, employee turnover, which can be caused by poor matching of people with jobs or by pragmatic reasons such as offers of better jobs or family-related moves, also can occur because new employees cannot become primary members of one or more informal groups. Group membership is a means by which employees achieve a sense of belonging and security. If an organization is cold and impersonal and informal interpersonal contacts are not encouraged or even permitted, new employees may seek employment elsewhere. Of course, informal group membership can be carried to such an extreme that the workplace becomes a social circle, to the detriment of the organization's effectiveness and efficiency. Good management avoids this extreme, however, and provides an atmosphere in which workers, through informal relationships, can meet human needs of acceptance and gregariousness.

Another potential advantage of informal relationships is that they can sometimes simplify managers' jobs. When there is informal group support, supervision may be more general than when such support is not available. Managers can delegate and decentralize more easily when informal groups are cooperative. The converse is true as well.

Managers who understand the reasons for informal relationships in the workplace will become better managers. They are more likely to improve their knowledge of the nature of people in general and subordinates in particular. They are more likely to realize that organizational performance can be affected by the workers' willingness to cooperate and be enthusiastic, and that means other than formal authority are necessary in developing worker attitudes that support effective performance.[50]

Another potential benefit of the informal relationships that exist within formal organization designs is their ability to provide an additional channel of communication. The so-called grapevine, or informal channel of communication, can enhance managers' effectiveness if they study and use it. Chapter 17 includes an in-depth discussion of informal communication in HSOs/HSs. Although grapevines permit the free flow of unfounded rumors, which can be destructive, managers can use them to relay certain information to employees quickly. Often, informal communications also can be used to determine the feelings and attitudes of employees on issues more effectively than can be done through formal communication channels.

Living with Informal Relationships in Organizations

The informal relationships and arrangements that exist within the formal design are a fact of organizational life in HSOs/HSs. Formal and informal aspects of organizations must be balanced if optimal performance and the attainment of objectives for individuals and for entire organizations are to be achieved. Attempts by managers to suppress informal relationships and arrangements can create destructive and dysfunctional situations. To protect themselves and to make their work situation acceptable, people typically resist what they perceive as autocratic management. The resistance often takes place within the context of informal relationships and arrangements. The resistance might exhibit itself in the form of such undesirable outcomes as work restriction, insubordination, disloyalty, and other manifestations of an antiorganization attitude.

The optimum situation occurs when the formal organization design can maintain suitable progress toward organizational objectives but simultaneously permits a well-developed pattern of informal relationships to exist. Attaining a balance between formal and informal aspects of organization design may be difficult, but managers can do two things to achieve it. First, they can seek to understand the informal relationships in their organizations and demonstrate their understanding and acceptance of these informal relationships. Particularly important in conveying acceptance is that managers minimize the negative effect of their actions on the often-fragile informal relationships. Second, managers can integrate the interests of the formal and informal aspects of organization design to the maximum extent. In so doing, managers should avoid actions through the formal organization that unnecessarily threaten or diminish the quality of informal relationships. In effect, blending the informal relationships and arrangements within organizations with their formal design elements helps establish the culture of the organization.

Organizational culture is the pattern of shared values and beliefs that becomes ingrained in the members of an organization or system over time and helps influence behaviors and decisions. A HSO/HS can establish an organizational culture that values excellence in patient care, for example. Strong organizational cultures invariably are built through both formal and informal organization design elements. Furthermore, understanding the informal relationships that people establish at work reflects the manager's recognition that people in organizations are not mechanistic—they are instead changing, complex, and social beings.

AN INTEGRATED PERSPECTIVE ON ORGANIZATION DESIGN

HSOs/HSs, from the simplest enterprise to large, complex systems, have five interrelated parts. Mintzberg[51] labeled them the strategic apex, the operating core, the middle line, the technostructure, and the support staff.

- The *strategic apex* consists of those who set the strategic direction of an organization. In HSOs/HSs this typically includes the governing body, the president, and perhaps the vice presidents.
- The *operating core* is composed of those who do the basic work of the organization or system. They convert inputs to outputs, the products and services of the organization or system. Physicians, nurses, technologists, therapists, and others who provide health services in a HSO/HS are examples.
- The *middle line* are middle- and lower-level managers who are located between the senior-level managers in the strategic apex and the people in the operating core. They are the middle of the organization or system's chain of command. Included are department heads and heads of other units and subdivisions. Examples include nurse managers and nursing supervisors and directors of pharmacy, laboratory, and dietetics.

- The *technostructure* consists of workers who help plan and control the basic work of the organization or system. The people in the technostructure affect the work of others; their role is to help standardize the work of the organization. Workers in the technostructure are removed from direct operations—from the operating work flow—but "they may design it, plan it, change it, or train the people who do it."[52] The technostructure in HSOs/HSs varies with size and complexity but can include industrial engineers, risk managers, and those who support efforts for continuous quality improvement because they help standardize work processes; strategic planners, budget analysts, and accountants because they help standardize outputs; and people who recruit and train workers because they help standardize the skills in the organization's or system's workforce.
- *Support staff* are those who provide indirect services. In Mintzberg's conceptualization they provide support to the organization or system's basic work, but they do not do the basic work. In HSOs/HSs these staff support the provision of health services but do not directly provide these services. Examples of support staff include people involved in fund-raising and development, legal counsel, marketing, public relations, finance, and human resources management. Support staff differ from people in the technostructure primarily in that support staff do not focus on work standardization.

Mintzberg diagrammed the five parts of organizations or systems as shown in Figure 3.8, and described that structure by saying that it

shows a small strategic apex connected by a flaring middle line to a large, flat operating core. These three parts of the organization are shown in one uninterrupted sequence to indicate that they are typically connected through a single line of formal authority. The technostructure and the support staff are shown off to either side to indicate that they are separate from this main line of authority, and influence the operating core only indirectly.[53]

Five Basic Organization Designs

In Mintzberg's view the structures of almost all organizations or systems can be included in one of five basic designs based on various configurations of the strategic apex, operating core, middle line, technostructure, and support staff. He labeled these design alternatives as the simple structure, the machine bureaucracy, the professional bureaucracy, the divisionalized form, and the adhocracy.[54] They are shown in Figure 3.9.

Simple Structure

As this design's name implies, it represents the simplest organization design. It has a strategic apex, which may be one person, such as the owner of a small enterprise, a physician in private practice, or the director of a small ambulatory care center. In addition, it has an operating core consisting of a group of workers. The middle line, technostructure, and support staff components are very small or missing.

Machine Bureaucracy

This design is characterized by a large, well-developed technostructure and support staff because there is great emphasis on work standardization and a focus on marketing and financial and operational control systems. Major decisions are made in the strategic apex, which features rigid patterns of authority. Spans of control are narrow, decision making is centralized, and the organization is functionally departmentalized. This design typifies manufacturing organizations, although some hospitals also exhibit elements of this design.

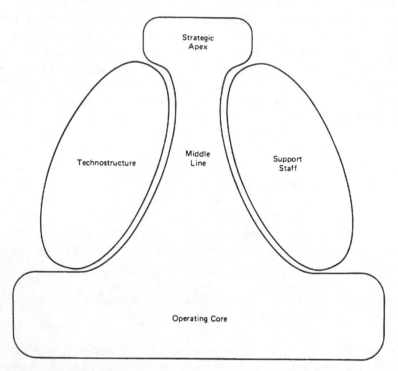

Figure 3.8.   Mintzberg's five basic parts of organizations. (From *The Structuring of Organizations,* by Mintzberg, ©1979. Reprinted by perission of Prentice-Hall, Inc., Upper Saddle River, NJ.)

Professional Bureaucracy

More typical, hospitals and other large HSOs, as well as universities and other professionally dominated organizations such as public accounting firms, are organized as professional bureaucracies. This form is characterized by an operating core that is composed primarily of professionals and that forms the heart of the organization; authority is decentralized to it. The technostructure is underdeveloped because work is done largely by professionals who do not need—indeed, do not permit—others to do their work. In larger professional bureaucracies, such as hospitals, support staff may be highly developed and diverse. This staff is needed to support the professionalized operating core.

Divisionalized Form

The divisionalized form of organization design has independent units that are joined by a shared administrative overlay. In contrast to other designs this form is characterized by a large, well-developed middle line because division managers are responsible for their divisions and may be given considerable decision-making latitude. Examples of divisionalized forms include corporations such as IBM, federal and large state governments, and HSs. Such HSs have become prevalent through corporate restructuring (creating several corporate entities to perform medical and nonmedical functions previously carried out by one corporation) and through active programs of merger and consolidation within the health care industry.

Adhocracies

The adhocracy, the fifth of Mintzberg's organization designs, is the most difficult of the five to describe or understand. It is both complex and nonstandardized. This form contradicts much of what

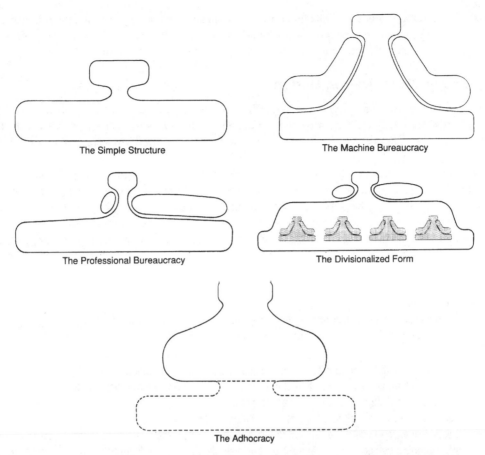

Figure 3.9. Mintzberg's five organizational configurations. (From *The Structuring of Organizations,* by Mintzberg, ©1979. Reprinted by permission of Prentice-Hall, Inc., Upper Saddle River, NJ.)

the classical design concepts described earlier dictate—hierarchical authority and control, standardization of work and workers, and strategic direction from the top level of the organization. Instead, adhocracies have "a tremendously fluid structure in which power is constantly shifting and coordination and control are by mutual adjustment through the informal communication and interaction of competent experts."[55]

The adhocracy form is complicated by the existence of two variations of this configuration: the operating adhocracy and the administrative adhocracy. In the operating adhocracy "the operating and administrative work blend into a single effort. That is, the organization cannot easily separate the planning and design of the operating work—in other words, the project—from its actual execution."[56] As shown in the solid line portion of the adhocracy diagram in Figure 3.9, "the organization emerges as an organic mass in which line managers, staff, and operating experts all work together on project teams in ever-shifting relationships."[57] By contrast, administrative work in an adminstrative adhocracy is sharply separated from operating work. This is shown by the dotted line operating core in the adhocracy diagram.

The adhocracy often takes the form of a matrix structure or project teams (see Figure 3.2) with emphasis on activities in both the operating core and technostructure. The power in adhocracies shifts between professionals and technical experts. This design can be a free-form structure with frequently changing job descriptions and a flexible concept of authority. HSOs/HSs might use ad-hocracy in multidisciplinary programs for elderly or chronically ill people or women, or in the research-oriented departments (e.g., oncology, genetics) in academic health centers.

Choosing an Organization Design

There is no magic formula by which managers choose an organization design. Furthermore, typical HSOs/HSs have many different designs embedded in them as various parts try to match structure to objectives, management philosophies, the preferences of their workers, and environmental pressures.

In a large and complex HSO, such as a teaching hospital, the dental clinic may have a simple structure, the clinical laboratory may be structured as a machine bureaucracy, and the medical and surgical nursing units may be professional bureaucracies. The hospital might be one of several hospitals that form a HS, with the system using the divisionalized form. Simultaneously, the hospital could have a project team of administrative experts in strategic management, marketing, finance, and information systems that, parallel to the team members' regular staff positions and structured as an adhocracy, operates as a consulting firm selling expertise to clients such as smaller hospitals and physician groups. Table 3.3 summarizes key structural elements and situations in which these design options might fit.

A leading management theorist, Peter Drucker, suggested that managers selecting an organization design evaluate the options against the following criteria:

- Clarity, as opposed to simplicity: The Gothic cathedral is not a simple design, but your position inside it is clear; you know where to stand and where to go. A modern office building is exceedingly simple in design, but it is very easy to get lost in one.
- Economy of effort to maintain control and minimize friction
- Direction of vision toward the product rather than the process, the result rather than the effort
- Understanding by each individual of his or her own task, as well as that of the organization as a whole
- Decision making that focuses on the right issues, is action oriented, and is carried out at the lowest possible level of management
- Stability, as opposed to rigidity, to survive turmoil, and adaptability to learn from it
- Perpetuation and self-renewal, which requires that an organization be able to produce tomorrow's leaders from within, helping each person develop continuously; the structure also must be open to new ideas[58]

SUMMARY

In carrying out the organizing function, managers build a formal organization structure. Coexisting with the formal structure is the informal organization, which is that set of interrelationships and interactions that occur among people in an organization but that lie outside the planned and sanctioned structure.

Formal organization structures are built on a set of organization design concepts, the roots of which can be traced back to general administrative theorists who lived early in the 20th century. Among them, Fayol and Weber made particularly important contributions to understanding the design of organizations. Their work and that of several of their contemporaries form what are called the classical concepts of organization design. Five of these concepts are examined: division of work and specialization, authority and responsibility relationships, departmentation, span of control, and coordination.

TABLE 3.3. KEY DIMENSIONS OF MINTZBERG'S FIVE ORGANIZATIONAL CONFIGURATIONS

Dimensions	Simple structure	Machine bureaucracy	Professional bureaucracy	Divisionalized form	Adhocracy
Key means of coordination	Direct supervision	Standardization of work	Standardization of skills	Standardization of outputs	Mutual adjustment
Key part of organization	Strategic apex	Technostructure	Operating core	Middle line	Support staff (with operating core in operating adhocracy)
Structural elements					
Specialization of jobs	Little specialization	Much horizontal and vertical specialization	Much horizontal specialization	Some horizontal and vertical specialization (between divisions and headquarters)	Much horizontal specialization
Training and indoctrination	Little training and indoctrination	Little training and indoctrination	Much training and indoctrination	Some training and indoctrination (of division managers)	Much training
Formalization of behavior—bureaucratic/ organic	Little formalization— organic	Much formalization— bureaucratic	Little formalization— bureaucratic	Much formalization (within divisions)— bureaucratic	Little formalization— organic
Grouping	Usually functional	Usually functional	Functional and market	Market	Functional and market
Unit size	Wide	Wide at bottom, narrow elsewhere	Wide at bottom, narrow elsewhere	Wide at top	Narrow throughout
Planning and control systems	Little planning and control	Action planning	Little planning and control	Much performance control	Limited action planning (especially in administrative adhocracy)

(continued)

TABLE 3.3. *(Continued)*

Dimensions	Simple structure	Machine bureaucracy	Professional bureaucracy	Divisionalized form	Adhocracy
Liaison devices	Few liaison devices	Few liaison devices	Liaison devices in administration	Few liaison devices	Many liaison devices throughout
Decentralization	Centralization	Limited horizontal decentralization	Horizontal and vertical decentralization	Limited vertical decentralization	Selective decentralization
Situational elements					
Age and size	Typically young and small	Typically old and large	Varies	Typically old and very large	Typically young (operating adhocracy)
Technical system	Simple, not regulating	Regulating but not automated, not very complex	Not regulating or complex	Divisible, otherwise like machine bureaucracy	Very complex, often automated (in administrative adhocracy), not regulating or complex (in operating adhocracy)
Environment	Simple and dynamic; sometimes hostile	Simple and stable	Complex and stable	Relatively simple and stable; diversified markets (especially products and services)	Complex and dynamic; sometimes disparate (in administrative adhocracy)
Power	Chief executive control; often owner managed; not fashionable	Technocratic and external control; not fashionable	Professional operator control; fashionable	Middle-line control; fashionable (especially in industry)	Expert control; very fashionable

The division of work refers to dividing the work of an organization into specific jobs having specific activities. For example, the job of pharmacist is defined by the activities that a person in this position is expected to accomplish. The corollary of division of work is the specialization of workers. As a result of the boredom and monotony that can accompany divided and specialized work, it is sometimes necessary to implement job enrichment programs to offset these negative consequences of specialization.

Growing directly out of the division of work is a need to assign responsibility for and authority over performance of work. This assignment occurs through the technical process of delegation. This results in scaling or grading the levels of authority and responsibility in the HSO. Also inherent in the authority structure of organizations is the distinction between line and staff authority. Line authority is command authority and follows the chain of command. Staff authority is advisory authority.

A natural consequence of division and specialization of work is departmentation, the grouping of jobs under the authority of one manager. Six bases for grouping workers are examined: knowledge and skills, work process and function, time, output, client, and place. The span of control concept is examined, with emphasis on the influence of span on the shape (tall or flat) of the organization or system. A number of contingency factors that help determine the proper span of control are discussed.

This chapter notes that rigidly applying the concepts of division of work, hierarchical authority, departmentation, and span of control results in mechanistic organization structures. Although these are appropriate structures in some circumstances, they are inappropriate in others. Therefore, such organic organization structures as project teams and matrix designs are considered as ways to reduce the rigidity of mechanistic designs.

The organization design concept of coordination is important in HSOs/HSs in which there is a high degree of division and specialization of work and functional departmentation coupled with a need to closely integrate the work. Several coordinating mechanisms are examined: the administrative system, committees, customs, direct supervision, feedback, hierarchy, integrators, matrix designs, mutual adjustment, plans, programming, project management through task forces or teams, standardization (of work processes, outputs, or workers' skills), QITs, and voluntary action.

The informal organization consists of relationships that occur spontaneously from the activities and interactions of staff in the organization but that are not set forth in the formal structure. To a large extent, the nature of small groups explains the informal organization. If the manager is to fully realize the positive benefits of an informal organization and simultaneously minimize its negative impact, then two things must be done: 1) the manager must understand the informal organization and accept it as a fact of organizational life; and 2) to the extent possible, the manager must integrate the interests of the informal organization with those of the formal organization.

Mintzberg's five organizational designs are used to integrate the discussion. They are variations of organizations' strategic apex, middle line, operating core, technostructure, and support staff. The five configurations are simple structure, machine bureaucracy, professional bureaucracy, divisionalized form, and adhocracy. Situations in which each form fits are considered.

DISCUSSION QUESTIONS

1. What are the major characteristics of Weber's ideal bureaucracy as an organization form?
2. Discuss the concept of departmentation and apply it to a hospital, a nursing facility, and a small freestanding ambulatory center.
3. Why is coordination so important for HSOs/HSs, and what are the mechanisms of coordination?
4. Discuss the relationships among span of control, delegation, and centralization-decentralization.

5. Discuss the characteristics of a matrix organization and how it differs from the "classical" functionally departmented organization.
6. Discuss the differences between a tall and a flat organization or system. Is one form better than the other? Why or why not?
7. Is decentralization better than centralization of authority and decision making?
8. Discuss why informal groups form. Identify their major characteristics.
9. Why is the function of organizing so important in HSOs/HSs?
10. Compare and contrast Mintzberg's five basic organizational configurations.

CASE STUDY 1: A NEW APPROACH ON THE NURSING UNITS

A number of problems existed at Horizon Hospital, a large psychiatric facility. Turnover among nursing personnel was much higher than is typical for psychiatric hospitals, and relationships between the nursing service and members of the professional staff organization (PSO) were unusually poor. Psychiatrists and clinical psychologists often complained that their patients received inadequate attention from nurses and that their orders were not fully and promptly followed.

The hospital president asked the vice president for nursing to recommend a course of action to resolve the problems. He developed a plan to restructure the nursing units using a matrix design (as in Figure 3.2). The vice president's plan included a new structure, reporting relationships, authority and responsibility relationships, and a timetable for implementing the matrix design.

The president was impressed with the plan and believed it might improve the situation. However, when she showed the plan to the chief of professional staff and several members of the PSO, she was told in no uncertain terms that they would oppose it and would do nothing to implement the change.

Puzzled by their reaction, the president called the vice president into her office to discuss the next step.

QUESTIONS

1. Why do you think the PSO members reacted as they did?
2. Is there anything inherently wrong with the matrix design? Is it inappropriate for psychiatric hospitals?
3. What should the president and vice president for nursing do now?

CASE STUDY 2: TROUBLE IN THE COPY CENTER

Janice Arnold, the new and ambitious administrative resident at the central office of Eastern Rehabilitation System, a HS comprising 22 rehabilitation hospitals in the eastern United States, was eager to make improvements in the organization of the system's central office. She found what she thought was a likely candidate for improvement in the system's copy center. She rolled up her sleeves when she found out by talking with the center's supervisor that, although turnover was very low, there was a great deal of dissatisfaction among the personnel in the copy center. The six people who ran the copying equipment were very close in age (mid-40s), all women, socialized with one another after working hours, and frequently discussed personal matters at work. Arnold regarded Ms. Kelly, the center's supervisor, as very capable, although she complained frequently that the center's employees were overworked and underpaid.

Arnold checked with other employers in the area and found that, among copy centers, Eastern Rehabilitation System had one of the lowest rates of pay for such employees in the region. When she approached the HS's vice president for administration on the matter of higher pay for the center's personnel, she was told it would be impossible to increase their pay at the present time.

Arnold set about to do what she could to help the center's employees in other ways. In order to even out the work, she proposed changing their work schedule. Instead of all six employees working the day shift, Arnold proposed having three of them work a night shift when many of the larger copying jobs could be run without too much interruption. To her surprise, neither the center's supervisor nor the six employees liked this idea. As a second idea, Arnold actually convinced the vice president for administration to hire a receptionist so that the center's employees could concentrate on running the copying machines. However, the receptionist was not given any cooperation by the center's other employees and soon resigned. Arnold felt certain that the center's supervisor was responsible for the other employees' not accepting the new receptionist. She requested that the vice president for administration ter-

things were worse in the copy center than when she started "reforming" it.

QUESTIONS

1. What do you think about Arnold's decisions and behavior?
2. Why did the copy center's employees react as they did?
3. Why did the center's employees not help the receptionist?
4. If you were the vice president for administration, what would you do?

CASE STUDY 3: ALTERNATIVE FACILITIES: NEW MINI-HOSPITAL RAISES HACKLES[59]

The following description of an attempt to establish a new type of health facility was reported in *American Healthline,* an Internet newsletter:

A Louisiana surgeon and entrepreneur is producing the test case for a year-old state law that permits a "basic health care facility." This new type of health care facility is "a cross between a day surgery center and a recovery care center" where simple surgeries can be performed and patients can stay for up to 72 hours. Dr. Joseph Bellina, who is building the $5 million facility that is expected to open in October, says he plans to charge 15%–30% less than area hospitals. Louisiana's new law may be the first in the nation to "marry treatment and recovery into a single institutional license." The special license will not require Bellina to provide costly emergency or intensive care or to have a 24-hour laboratory. Bellina said he will not treat Medicare patients, thus "removing the need to meet many costly accreditation standards."

Hot Spot
Bellina's planned facility has "infuriated local and state hospital groups and attracted interest from outside Louisiana." Many hospitals contend that Bellina should not be permitted to run a mini-hospital without meeting the proper requirements. "This is stuff that's not even recognized by HCFA [Health Care Financing Administration, the federal agency responsible for overseeing the Medicare program]," said Dino Paternostro of the Metropolitan Hospital Council of New Orleans. Clark Cosse of the Louisiana Hospital Association said, "You can't have half a hospital. Either you do it all the way or not at all. And if you don't have the mandated levels of care to stay open 24 hours a day, the patient will be in danger." Bellina said that he will transfer any

patients who experience postoperative complications to an area hospital. Hospitals also fear Bellina's facility will siphon off their self-paying and privately insured patients. People who are admitted for less than 72 hours make up "two-thirds of hospital business," said Cosse.

Will The New Breed Take Off?

Mary Grealy, senior Washington counsel for the American Hospital Association, predicted that new centers like these will not become players in the health care market because hospitals already provide similar services, such as skilled nursing and subacute care. "It's a niche of a niche market," she said. But Mark Mayo, executive director of the Illinois Freestanding Surgery Center Association, believes that the trend will grow. Illinois already grants a special license to allow recovery centers to keep patients up to 72 hours under special circumstances. Mayo added, "Texas, Connecticut, Missouri and Arizona grant similar licenses."

Barriers Ahead?

But whether Bellina will get to open the facility remains to be seen. The state Department of Health and Hospitals "will not license any new facility until a committee draws up appropriate regulations." Because the committee is composed largely of hospital interests, Rene Rosenson, administrator for the new facility, expects the committee will delay issuance of the regulations.

QUESTIONS

1. Sketch out an organization structure for this new type of health care facility.
2. What is the impact of the external environment on this proposed organization?
3. Would this facility be a good candidate for participating in a HS? Why?

CASE STUDY 4: "I CANNOT DO IT ALL!"

When Harold Brice was named president of Health Care, Inc., a health maintenance organization (HMO), he inherited a staff including vice presidents for marketing, finance, medical affairs, and professional services. Each executive was capable in many ways, and Health Care, Inc., was on a solid financial footing with bright prospects. It was located in an expanding community; a 15%–20% annual growth rate was projected for the next 5 years.

Within a few weeks of joining Health Care, Inc., Brice perceived a serious flaw with his vice presidents: None of them would make a decision, not even on rather routine matters such as personnel questions, choice of marketing media, or changing suppliers. This troubled him. Before long the situation seriously impeded his efforts to give thought to strategic plans for the HMO. To make matters worse, he found that the vice presidents routinely discussed their own problems among themselves, to the extent that a great deal of time was consumed in doing so. Yet even with all of this activity, the vice presidents frequently presented him with issues in their areas of responsibility and requested that he make the decision.

At a regular staff meeting, when every member of his staff had an issue requiring a decision, Brice finally lost his temper. Waving his arms in exasperation, he shouted (very uncharacteristic for him), "I cannot do it all! You are going to have to make these decisions yourselves."

The meeting broke up with the vice presidents looking very puzzled, and Brice realizing that he had to do something besides shout at them.

QUESTIONS

1. Is this an organization problem? What factors might be contributory?
2. In terms of the organizing function, what can Brice do?

CASE STUDY 5: THE SECRETARIES[60]

There are three secretaries in the business office of Pleasant Valley Nursing Center. The secretarial output proved to be a bottleneck in the smooth flow of work in the office. The secretaries had been assigned to various sections of the business office, and the office manager discovered that, when one secretary was overloaded with reports and other work, one or both of the other secretaries often had time on their hands. The peaks and valleys of the secretaries' workloads were usually in contraposition as follows:

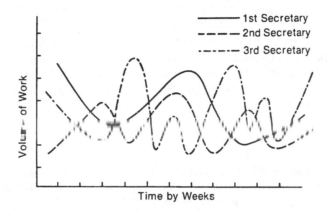

The business office manager decided to pool the work of these secretaries instead of assigning them to one section of the office. On Friday afternoon she called them into her office and explained the new idea. They made little comment. During the weekend, however, one of the secretaries called the business office manager and told her she was resigning, giving the customary 2 weeks' notice.

On Monday the other two secretaries spoke to the business office manager and told her they did not like the new plan. They were very concerned about the impact of the pooling arrangement on their work and on the perception other people who worked at Pleasant Valley would have of their job status. The business office manager pointed out that they would be performing exactly the same work as before, at the same rate of pay, with the same titles. The secretaries said that they had been aware of the overload situation but had not done anything about it because they had thought they were doing things the way that the business office manager wanted. The two secretaries then asked if they could work out a plan on their own.

Realizing that the pressure of her regular duties required her full attention, the business office manager shrugged her shoulders and told the secretaries to make their own arrangements. A replacement for the departing secretary arrived toward the end of that week.

Within a few weeks the three secretaries had devised a plan for synchronizing and interchanging work during rush periods. Although the plan looked very much like a pooled arrangement of work, the secretaries were satisfied with the arrangement. The business office manager was also satisfied because the workflow had been smoothed and efficiency increased.

QUESTIONS

1. Why did the secretaries react as they did?
2. Using concepts of informal organization, how could the business office manager have improved the process by which this change was initiated?
3. Is the new arrangement part of the formal or informal organization at Pleasant Valley? Why?

CASE STUDY 6: SOMEBODY HAS TO BE LET GO[61]

Ken was a senior vice president of one of the nation's leading quality consulting firms. In 4 years the makeup of the company had expanded from the founder, a secretary, 2 full-time trainers, and 4 part-time trainers to 125 full-time employees. Of these, 15 were full-time account executives, trainers with limited sales and customer service responsibility. About 70% of the company's revenues came from offering training courses on continuous quality improvement to clients. Revenues and profits had grown substantially, but early in the fourth year revenues dropped drastically as managed care cost-cutting pressures were felt throughout the health sector and expected sales from the company's largest client, a HS, failed to materialize.

Ken was assigned the task of determining what to do structurally. Losses were projected for this quarter, and the president and chairman of the board—the firm's founder—had decreed that members of the workforce who were not productive had to be let go. A target number of 25 people had been set. Ken had been placed in charge of a three-person task force and given 1 week to develop a plan, including the names of those to be fired and the timing of these personnel actions. The firings had to be completed within 3 weeks.

The company had grown so rapidly that it had not had time to complete job descriptions for any of the jobs in the company. It was common knowledge that a lot of people, including some account executives, were sitting around doing nothing a lot of the day. There had never been any evaluations of employees, other than those of the training staff.

At the end of the briefing session in which Ken was assigned this task, the president commented: "Good luck! You are going to need it."

QUESTIONS

1. If you were Ken, where would you start? How would you proceed?
2. How can you rationally make these choices?
3. What kind of organization design does this company need?

NOTES

1. Shortell, Stephen M., Robin R. Gillies, David A. Anderson, Karen Morgan Erickson, and John B. Mitchell. *Remaking Health Care in America: Building Organized Delivery Systems,* 2. San Francisco: Jossey-Bass, 1996.
2. Mintzberg, Henry. *The Structuring of Organizations.* Englewood Cliffs, NJ: Prentice-Hall, 1979; Mintzberg, Henry. *Structure in Fives: Designing Effective Organizations.* Englewood Cliffs, NJ: Prentice-Hall, 1983.
3. Leatt, Peggy, Stephen M. Shortell, and John R. Kimberly. "Organization Design." In *Health Care Management: Organization Design and Behavior,* 3rd ed., edited by Stephen M. Shortell and Arnold D. Kaluzny, 245. Albany, NY: Delmar Publishers, 1994.
4. Longest, Beaufort B., Jr. *Health Professionals in Management,* 137. Stamford, CT: Appleton & Lange, 1996.
5. Weber, Max. *The Theory of Social and Economic Organization.* Translated by A.M. Henderson and Talcott Parsons. New York: The Free Press, 1947.
6. Fayol, Henri. *General and Industrial Management.* Translated by Constance Storrs. London: Sir Isaac Pitman & Sons, 1949.
7. Williams, James C., and George P. Huber. *Human Behavior in Organizations,* 3rd ed., 270. Cincinnati, OH: South-Western Publishing Company, 1986.
8. Weber, *Theory of Social.*
9. Robbins, Stephen P., and Mary K. Coulter. *Management,* 6th ed. Upper Saddle River, NJ: Prentice-Hall, 1998.

10. Higgins, James M. *The Management Challenge: An Introduction to Management,* 42. New York: Macmillan, 1991.
11. Gulick, Luther, and Lyndall Urwick, Eds. *Papers on the Science of Administration.* New York: Institute of Public Administration, 1937.
12. Mooney, James D., and Alan C. Reiley. *Onward Industry: The Principles of Organization and Their Significance to Modern Industry.* New York: Harper & Brothers, 1931.
13. Smith, Adam. *The Wealth of Nations.* London: Dent, 1910.
14. Gibson, James L., and John M. Ivancevich. *Organizations: Behavior, Structure, Processes,* 9th ed. Homewood, IL: Irwin, 1996.
15. Newstrom, John W., and Keith Davis. *Organizational Behavior: Human Behavior at Work,* 9th ed., 321–322. New York: McGraw-Hill, 1993.
16. Holt, David H. *Management: Principles and Practices,* 3rd ed. Englewood Cliffs, NJ: Prentice-Hall, 1993.
17. Pierce, Jon L., and Randall B. Dunham. *Managing.* Reading, MA: Addison-Wesley, 1990.
18. Pfeffer, Jeffrey. *Power in Organizations.* Marshfield, MA: Pitman, 1981.
19. Higgins, *Management Challenge,* 253–254.
20. French, John R.P., and Bertram H. Raven. "The Basis of Social Power." In *Studies of Social Power,* edited by Dorwin Cartwright, 150–167. Ann Arbor, MI: Institute for Social Research, 1959.
21. Mooney and Reiley, *Onward Industry,* 39.
22. Gulick and Urwick, *Papers on the Science,* 15.
23. Mintzberg, *Structuring of Organizations,* 108–111.
24. Mintzberg, *Structuring of Organizations,* 106.
25. Gibson, James L., and John M. Ivancevich. *Organizations,* 540.
26. Urwick, Lyndall. *The Elements of Administration.* New York: Harper & Row, 1944.
27. Davis, Ralph C. *Fundamentals of Top Management.* New York: Harper & Row, 1951.
28. Barkdull, Charles W. "Span of Control—A Method of Evaluation." *Michigan Business Review* 15 (May 1963): 27–29; Steiglitz, Harry. *Organizational Planning.* New York: National Industrial Conference Board, 1966.
29. Barnard, Chester I. *The Functions of the Executive,* 256. Cambridge, MA: Harvard University Press, 1938.
30. Fayol, *General and Industrial,* 104.
31. Fayol, *General and Industrial,* 104.
32. Haimann, Theo, and William G. Scott. *Management in Modern Organizations,* 2nd ed., 126. Boston: Houghton Mifflin, 1974.
33. Lawrence, Paul R., and Jay W. Lorsch. "Differentiation and Integration in Complex Organizations." *Administrative Science Quarterly* 11 (June 1967): 1–47.
34. Alter, Catherine, and Jerald Hage. *Organizations Working Together: Coordination in Interorganizational Networks,* 87. Newbury Park, CA: Sage Publications, 1992.
35. Thompson, James D. *Organizations in Action.* New York: McGraw-Hill, 1967.
36. Bolman, Lee G., and Terrence E. Deal. *Reframing Organizations: Artistry, Choice, and Leadership.* San Francisco: Jossey-Bass, 1997.
37. Litterer, Joseph A. *The Analysis of Organizations,* 223–232. New York: John Wiley & Sons, 1965.
38. Litterer, *Analysis of Organizations,* 227.
39. Georgopoulos, Basil S., and Floyd C. Mann. "The Hospital as an Organization." *Hospital Administration,* 7 (Fall 1962): 57–58.
40. Mintzberg, *Structuring of Organizations*; Mintzberg, *Structure in Fives.*
41. Mintzberg, *Structuring of Organizations,* 6–7.
42. Hage, Jerald. *Theories of Organizations: Forms, Processes, and Transformations.* New York: Wiley-Interscience, 1980.
43. Lawrence and Lorsch, "Differentiation and Integration."
44. Blau, Peter M., and W. Richard Scott. *Formal Organizations,* 6. San Francisco: Chandler Publishing, 1962.
45. Roethlisberger, Fritz J., and William J. Dickson. *Management and the Worker.* Cambridge, MA: Harvard University Press, 1939.

46. Mills, Theodore M. *The Sociology of Small Groups,* 2nd ed., 2. Englewood Cliffs, NJ: Prentice-Hall, 1983.

47. Wexley, Kenneth A., and Gary A. Yukl. *Organizational Behavior and Personal Psychology,* 2nd ed. Homewood, IL: Irwin, 1983.

48. Scott, William G., Terence R. Mitchell, and Philip H. Birnbaum. *Organization Theory: A Structural and Behavioral Analysis,* 4th ed. Homewood, IL: Irwin, 1981.

49. Tuckman, Bruce W., and Mary Ann C. Jensen. "Stages of Small-Group Development Revisited." *Group and Organizational Studies* 2 (Summer 1977): 419–427; Gersick, Connie J.G. "Time and Transition in Work Teams: Toward a New Model of Group Development." *Academy of Management Journal* 31 (March 1988): 9–41.

50. Mondy, R. Wayne, Judith R. Gordon, Arthur Sharplin, and Shane R. Premeaux. *Management and Organizational Behavior,* 226. Boston: Allyn & Bacon, 1990.

51. Mintzberg, Henry. "Organization Design: Fashion or Fit?" *Harvard Business Review* 59 (January/February 1981): 103–116; Mintzberg, *Structuring of Organizations*; Mintzberg, *Structure in Fives.*

52. Mintzberg, *Structuring of Organizations,* 29.

53. Mintzberg, *Structuring of Organizations,* 20.

54. Mintzberg, *Structuring of Organizations*; Mintzberg, "Organization Design"; Mintzberg, *Structure in Fives.*

55. Mintzberg, "Organization Design," 111.

56. Mintzberg, "Organization Design," 112.

57. Mintzberg, "Organization Design," 112.

58. Drucker, Peter F. "New Templates for Today's Organizations." *Harvard Business Review* 52 (January/February 1974): 51.

59. As reported in *American Healthline: National Journal Daily Briefing,* August 6, 1998; reprinted by permission. (World Wide Web site http://www.cloakroom.com/ *Note:* This is a password-protected site that charges a subscription fee for its use.)

60. From Longest, Beaufort B., Jr. *Business Management of Health Care Providers.* Chicago: Hospital Financial Management Association, 1975; reprinted by permission.

61. Adapted from Higgins, James M. *The Management Challenge: An Introduction to Management,* 311. New York: Macmillan, 1991; reprinted by permission.

SELECTED BIBLIOGRAPHY

Alter, Catherine, and Jerald Hage. *Organizations Working Together: Coordination in Interorganizational Networks.* Newbury Park, CA: Sage Publications, 1992.

Bolman, Lee G., and Terrence E. Deal. *Reframing Organizations: Artistry, Choice, and Leadership.* San Francisco: Jossey-Bass, 1997.

Fayol, Henri. *General and Industrial Management.* Translated by Constance Storrs. London: Sir Isaac Pitman & Sons, 1949.

Gersick, Connie J.G. "Time and Transition in Work Teams: Toward a New Model of Group Development." *Academy of Management Journal* 31 (March 1988): 9–41.

Gibson, James L., and John M. Ivancevich. *Organizations: Behavior, Structure, Processes,* 9th ed. Homewood, IL: Irwin, 1996.

Gulick, Luther, and Lyndall Urwick, Eds. *Papers on the Science of Administration.* New York: Institute of Public Administration, 1937.

Hage, Jerald. *Theories of Organizations: Forms, Processes, and Transformations.* New York: Wiley-Interscience, 1980.

Holt, David H. *Management: Principles and Practices,* 3rd ed. Englewood Cliffs, NJ: Prentice-Hall, 1993.

Kaluzny, Arnold D. "Centralization and Decentralization in a Vertically Integrated System: The XYZ Hospital Corporation." In *Strategic Alignment: Managing Integrated Health Systems,* edited by Douglas A. Conrad and Geoffrey A. Hoare, 125–132. Chicago: Health Administration Press, 1994.

Lawrence, Paul R., and Jay W. Lorsch. "Differentiation and Integration in Complex Organizations." *Administrative Science Quarterly* 11 (June 1967): 1–47.

Leatt, Peggy, Stephen M. Shortell, and John R. Kimberly. "Organization Design." In *Health Care Management: Organization Design and Behavior,* 4th ed., edited by Stephen M. Shortell and Arnold D. Kaluzny, 274–306. Albany, NY: Delmar Publishers, 2000.

Longest, Beaufort B., Jr. *Health Professionals in Management.* Stamford, CT: Appleton & Lange, 1996.

Longest, Beaufort B., Jr., and James M. Klingensmith. "Coordination and Communication." In *Essentials of Health Care Management,* edited by Stephen M. Shortell and Arnold D. Kaluzny, 220–255. Albany, NY: Delmar Publishers, 1997.

Mintzberg, Henry. *The Structuring of Organizations.* Englewood Cliffs, NJ: Prentice-Hall, 1979.

Mintzberg, Henry. *Structure in Fives: Designing Effective Organizations.* Englewood Cliffs, NJ: Prentice-Hall, 1983.

Mondy, R. Wayne, Judith R. Gordon, Arthur Sharplin, and Shane R. Premeaux. *Management and Organizational Behavior.* Boston: Allyn & Bacon, 1990.

Mooney, James D., and Alan C. Reiley. *Onward Industry: The Principles of Organization and Their Significance to Modern Industry.* New York: Harper & Brothers, 1931.

Newstrom, John W., and Keith Davis. *Organizational Behavior: Human Behavior at Work,* 9th ed. New York: McGraw-Hill, 1993.

Pierce, Jon L., and Randall B. Dunham. *Managing.* Reading, MA: Addison-Wesley, 1990.

Porter, Michael E. *Competitive Advantage: Creating and Sustaining Superior Performance.* New York: The Free Press, 1985.

Robbins, Stephen P., and Mary K. Coulter. *Management,* 6th ed. Upper Saddle River, NJ: Prentice-Hall, 1998.

Roethlisberger, Fritz J., and William J. Dickson. *Management and the Worker.* Cambridge, MA: Harvard University Press, 1939.

Scott, W. Richard. "Managing Professional Work: Three Models of Control for Health Organizations." *Health Services Research* 17 (Fall 1982): 213–240.

Scott, William G., Terence R. Mitchell, and Philip H. Birnbaum. *Organization Theory: A Structural and Behavioral Analysis,* 4th ed. Homewood, IL: Irwin, 1981.

Shortell, Stephen M., Robin R. Gillies, David A. Anderson, Karen Morgan Erickson, and John B. Mitchell. *Remaking Health Care in America: Building Organized Delivery Systems.* San Francisco: Jossey-Bass, 1996.

Smith, Adam. *The Wealth of Nations.* London: Dent, 1910.

Stevens, George H. *The Strategic Health Care Manager.* San Francisco: Jossey-Bass, 1991.

Thompson, James D. *Organizations in Action.* New York: McGraw Hill, 1967.

Tuckman, Bruce W., and Mary Ann C. Jensen. "Stages of Small-Group Development Revisited." *Group and Organizational Studies* 2 (Summer 1977): 419–427.

Urwick, Lyndall. *The Elements of Administration.* New York: Harper & Row, 1944.

Weber, Max. *The Theory of Social and Economic Organization.* Translated by A.M. Henderson and Talcott Parsons. New York: The Free Press, 1947.

4

How Health Services Organizations Are Organized

"It is a pretty good zoo," said young Gerald McGrew, "and the fellow who runs it seems proud of it, too."[1]

This chapter describes common types of health services organizations (HSOs), including acute care hospitals, nursing facilities, ambulatory care organizations, hospice, managed care organizations, birth centers, and home health agencies. These HSOs may be freestanding or part of a delivery system. Following a brief historical sketch of each genre, information about functions, structure, governance, management, professional staff organization (PSO), caregivers and support staff, and licensure and accreditation is provided. The examples are paradigmatic of those types of HSOs. Chapter 5 provides a conceptual framework and examples of how such types of HSOs are organized into health systems (HSs).

The chapter begins with generic background about HSOs and how they are organized, including legal status; governing body (GB) role and functions, composition, and committees, and the relationship of the GB to senior management; managerial functions, qualifications, and relationships; and PSO credentialing, membership, privileges, discipline, and integration, as well as the problem of impaired clinicians.

BACKGROUND

Chapter 2 discussed the historical development of health services delivery, with hospitals prominent among delivery sites. Suffice it to say that voluntary governance, independent physicians, and underprepared management brought many HSOs—especially acute care hospitals—to the latter half of the 20th century with a convoluted, inefficient organization structure, much of which continues. The resulting triad is discussed later in this section.

Governing Body

Regardless of ownership, role, or other characteristics, all HSOs have a GB or its equivalent. These range from a GB as simple as one individual in a sole-proprietorship nursing facility, to the Central Office found in the Department of Veterans Affairs, to the complex arrangement found in an acute care hospital in an academic health (medical) center, to the GB of an integrated delivery system. The GB is the ultimate authority and decision maker for HSOs. It determines direction and evaluates progress toward objectives. Among the GB's most important tasks is selecting and evaluating the chief executive officer (CEO).

Chief Executive Officer

Although titles vary, all HSOs have a CEO. As HSOs have adopted the accoutrements of business enterprise, they have tended to use corporate titles such as president and executive vice president. GBs select and delegate authority to a CEO, who acts as its agent to organize inputs to achieve organizational objectives. For many reasons, including HSOs' legal relationships and the financial demands on them, GBs are being held to a higher level of legal and sometimes public accountability, and this necessitates a close and effective working relationship between CEO and GB. As with titles, this relationship is extraordinarily varied and may range from a CEO with great latitude in management decisions to a CEO with little independence. CEOs evaluate other managers; senior-level managers may be evaluated jointly by the GB and CEO.

Clinical Staff

By definition, HSOs have clinical staff who deliver health and health-related services. The makeup of clinical staff and how staff are organized vary markedly among HSOs, even within the same type. Broadly defined, clinical staff are all individuals who care for patients. Here, however, "clinical staff" refers to licensed independent practitioners (LIPs).[2] In most HSOs physicians are the clinically and economically most important LIPs. Increasingly, a HSO's clinical staff include nonphysician LIPs such as dentists, clinical psychologists, podiatrists, nurse-midwives, and chiropractors. In acute care hospitals and some other types of HSOs the clinical staff comprise a separate, unincorporated association with its own bylaws that organize these clinicians.

The association of clinical staff is commonly called the medical staff organization because historically it was composed almost exclusively of physicians. Increasingly, the term *professional staff organization* is more appropriate because it suggests the broad range of preparation and activities of members. Consequently, that term and the acronym PSO are used here. Nonhospital HSOs will likely use PSO or a synonym to designate their clinical staff. The varying levels of PSO self-governance are described later.

PSO members provide services themselves or order other HSO staff to do so. Relationships among PSO members depend on the setting and services being provided. In some HSOs, such as a physician group practice, the numbers of nonphysician providers may be equal to or greater than the number of physicians. The care in HSOs such as nursing facilities is chronic and custodial. Here, only intermittent physician contact is necessary, even though treatment by other LIPs and non-LIP caregivers such as registered nurses (RNs), licensed practical nurses (LPNs), and nursing assistants, who are not part of the PSO, is frequent. These caregivers are following either standing orders approved prospectively by the chief medical officer (CMO) or the PSO and applied to all patients of that type, or LIP-determined individual treatment orders. The presence of a PSO increases complexity greatly, but the HSO's work is impossible without its members.

The Triad

Historically, the GB, CEO, and PSO in an acute care hospital were known as a *triad* (group of three), but the term is rarely used in contemporary discussions. The triad remains common in acute care hospitals; variations of it are found in other types of HSOs, even though outwardly many have adopted a corporate structure, especially in the use of titles. The proportion of nonphysician LIPs is increasing, but physicians tend to be the predominant group on PSOs. The PSO members of many HSOs are independent contractors who use the HSO to treat their patients but have no employment relationship with it. This has major implications for the control function of management. The dual pyramid in Figure 4.1 suggests the triad.

The triad is inefficient and incompatible with the demands on contemporary HSOs, especially hospitals. Lack of a clear, effective reporting relationship between the PSO and either the GB or the CEO is confusing, and the trend is to streamline the structure and clarify accountability, thus further diminishing the triad. Ethical and legal pressures for this change are irresistible, as is the imperative of common sense management. The epitome of complexity is found in the academic health (medical) center.

LEGAL STATUS

Nongovernmental (privately owned) HSOs may be organized as sole proprietorships, partnerships, corporations, or a new form, limited liability companies. HSs are invariably organized as corporations. Various types of HSOs (and sometimes HSs) are owned by state and local (county, city, or special tax district) governments and are established by enabling legislation or incorporated like privately owned HSOs. Some HSOs/HSs are owned by the federal government; their legal status is based on federal legislation, and the states may not regulate them. Examples are Department of Veterans Affairs hospitals; U.S. Air Force, Army, and Navy hospitals; and U.S. Public Health Service clinics.

Sole-proprietorship HSOs have no special legal status; the term simply describes a business owned by one person. This form is rarely used today. Historically, a common example was a for-profit nursing facility.

Partnerships are voluntary contracts between two or more persons to engage in commerce or business. Partnerships may be general or limited. Whether general partnerships have special legal

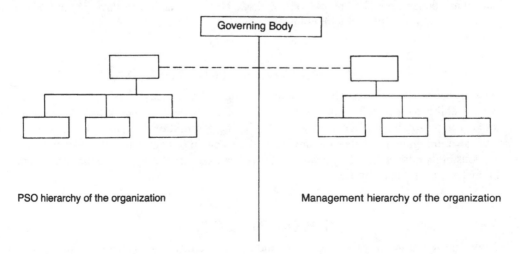

Figure 4.1.   Dual pyramid of the typical hospital.

status depends on state law. A common example of a general partnership is a physician group practice. "General" means that each partner is liable for the debts and errors of other partners. Limited partnerships have one or more general partners who are jointly and individually legally responsible for the partnership; the liability of "limited" partners is limited to the assets they have invested. Limited partnerships are commonly found in HSO/HS-physician joint ventures such as imaging centers or ambulatory surgery centers. Limited partnerships are established with state approval.

A common legal form for HSOs/HSs is the corporation, which the law recognizes as an artificial person. States allow physicians and other types of LIPs to organize special types of corporations called professional corporations, which are designated by "PC." Some states use "limited" (abbreviated Ltd.), to show the same status. On application and filing articles of incorporation, the state issues a charter that creates a corporation.

The limited liability company (LLC) is a hybrid that uses partnership and corporate principles. It is favored for HSOs and in some HS relationships because it offers owners the same protection from personal liability as incorporating, while treating the owners as partners for federal and state income tax purposes.[3]

Corporations may be organized not for profit or for profit; the advantages and disadvantages of each depend on the tax laws and the purposes for which the corporation is organized. Corporate charters are amended on application to, and approval by, the state. A corporation must develop bylaws that describe how it is organized to carry out its purposes, including definitions; meetings; elections; GB composition, committees, and officers; and roles of CEO, and PSO, if any. Bylaws are important because they guide governance and senior management. The charter and bylaws are the HSO's/HS's basic law, and all activities are subordinate to and must be consistent with them. An example is the PSO bylaws, which must be approved by the GB and must be consistent with the corporate bylaws.

The police powers discussed in Chapter 2 are almost exclusively a domain of state government, and HSOs/HSs are largely regulated by states. A common type of regulation is licensure, the specific application of which is discussed later. The state's police powers are delegated to local government, which regulates HSOs/HSs in the same way as non–health care organizations that carry on similar functions (e.g., storing, preparing, and serving food). Specialized regulatory activities apply to some types of HSOs. An example is control, storage, and use of radioactive materials or disposal of hazardous waste. Federal laws affect some of these areas, and enforcement occurs through federal and state cooperation. The "regulation" of HSOs/HSs that may occur through the financing of services should not be confused with police powers.

ORGANIZATION STRUCTURE

Weber suggested that an organization must prevent the idiosyncrasies of individuals from interfering with its ability to accomplish specific tasks.[4] This end is achieved by establishing a bureaucracy in which each person has a place and a set of tasks. The pyramid of the typical bureaucratic structure is shown in Figure 4.2. This structure is based on a chain of command that delegates authority and responsibility downward. Historically, larger HSOs were structured as bureaucracies; in this regard they have been joined by HSs.

GOVERNING BODIES

The health care environment is having a profound effect on GBs and will change them dramatically. Members can no longer be chosen as a way to honor them or because they might make financial contributions. Casual participation by GB members is a thing of the past. The pressures and need

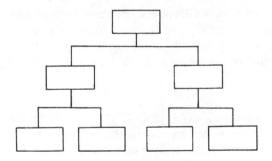

Figure 4.2.   Typical bureaucratic pyramid.

for GBs to be effective will increase, and this means recruiting people who understand health services, are prepared in business matters, and have backgrounds that are important to the HSO. Some HSOs pay GB members to attend meetings. This practice is common in business and may gain wider acceptance in health services as demands on time and the need for expertise increase. In the future many GB members will have no employment other than serving on GBs of noncompeting HSOs and HSs. Significant changes in GB structure and function can take place only when the CEO makes this a priority and the GB leadership is open to change.[5] The following discussion applies specifically to HSOs; it has general applicability to HSs, too, even though their governance is significantly more complex and is discussed in Chapter 5.

Role and Functions

The GB's first role is to establish the HSO's mission, vision, and objectives and review strategies formulated by senior-level managers to achieve objectives. All of this must be done within the context of organizational philosophy or values. The second role is to determine whether these goals and objectives have been achieved. To do so, GB members must have a general understanding of health services that is similar to that of the HSO's/HS's management.

The American Hospital Association's (AHA's) concept of GB roles and functions applies to all HSOs. The GB

1. Has the responsibility for organizing itself effectively, for establishing and following the policies and procedures necessary to discharge its responsibilities, and for adopting bylaws in accordance with legal requirements
2. Has the responsibility for selecting a qualified chief executive officer and for delegating to the chief executive officer the necessary authority to manage . . . effectively
3. Has the authority and responsibility for ensuring proper organization of the . . . [clinical] staff, and for monitoring the quality of care provided . . .
4. Has the authority and responsibility for monitoring and influencing public policies concerning the establishment and maintenance of appropriate external relationships
5. Has responsibility and authority, subject to the . . . charter, for determining the . . . mission and for establishing a strategic plan, goals, objectives, and policies to achieve that mission
6. Is entrusted with resources . . . and with the proper development, utilization, and maintenance of those resources
7. Has the responsibility and authority for the organization, protection, and enhancement of . . . human resources
8. Is responsible for the provision of health care education and research programs that further the . . . mission[6]

In meeting these responsibilities, GBs review operating statistics, budget performance, financial management performance, and capital planning. Patient survey results, employee attitude survey results, and morbidity and mortality data are further down the list.[7] Written bylaws, periodically reviewed and approved by the GB, set out the HSO's/HS's organization and guide activities.

Composition

Traditionally, many GB members of not-for-profit HSOs had skills that the organization needed but did not want to purchase. Business and community leaders, attorneys, and bankers were common, and such types are still found on GBs. At least in hospitals, people are likely to be members of GBs because their values are consistent with the organization's, they are community leaders and representatives, and they have strengths in strategic planning and establishing the organization's vision.[8] GBs of not-for-profit HSOs tend to be much larger than those of for-profit HSOs.

Historically, not-for-profit hospitals commonly excluded physicians from GB membership because they had potential conflicts of interest regarding resource allocation, capital equipment purchases, and quality of care. (Conflicts of interest are discussed in Chapters 13 and 14.) The contemporary view, however, encourages physician membership because it is generally believed that conflicts of interest are avoidable and that physicians bring vital clinical expertise to governance. Research that is done in hospitals—the results of which are readily extended to nonhospital HSOs—suggests that integrating physicians into management and governance enhances performance and helps align incentives.[9] Physicians are increasingly involved in governance and policy development in HSOs.[10]

GB members may be external or internal. External members are not employed by the HSO, but internal members are. External members include those described earlier (e.g., community leaders). Internal members typically include the CEO, chief operating officer (COO), CMO, and chief financial officer (CFO). The proportion of internal members is likely to grow as greater expertise is needed by GB members, even though this increases the probability of conflicts of interest.

Committees

Committees allow specialized, effective work when GBs are large (e.g., 100 or more members in some not-for-profit HSOs). Standing committees usually include executive, professional staff, human resources, quality evaluation, finance, planning, public relations and development, investment, capital equipment and expenditures, and nomination. Committees on quality improvement and ethics are additions made in the 1990s. Ad hoc (special) committees are established as needed.

Two committees are noteworthy. The executive committee is the most important because of its ongoing monitoring and review, activities especially important when GBs are large or meet infrequently. The executive committee receives reports from other committees, oversees policy implementation, and provides interim decision making. The executive committee is chaired by the chair of the GB; membership usually includes chairs of standing committees. CEOs should attend executive committee meetings.

The professional staff committee is responsible for the quality of clinical activities. It reviews PSO recommendations on appointments, reappointments, and clinical activities (privileges) and the performance of PSO members to determine whether privileges should be modified. Both tasks rely heavily on assistance from the PSO, from GB members who are experts, or from consultants. The HSO's ethical and legal obligations to protect patients from substandard care are ultimately met through GB review and approval.

The critical need for management, the PSO, and the GB to communicate and coordinate may be satisfied in several ways. One, the joint conference committee, is described in the section on acute care hospitals later in this chapter. Other means are to include members from each group on one another's committees and to send copies of minutes and reports to other committees. Figure 4.1

shows the dual pyramid typical of acute care hospitals and other types of HSOs and suggests the difficulty of communicating and coordinating. Chapter 5 addresses health systems governance.

Relationship to the CEO

The GB's responsibility to recruit, select, and evaluate the CEO has been noted. CEOs assemble and organize resources and develop the systems to carry out GB–approved programs and policies. CEOs also provide information to the GB so it can develop policy, monitor implementation, and oversee results.

The CEO's performance should be assessed regularly and systematically by the GB; specific recommendations should result from this process. Performance should be measured against predetermined objectives mutually identified and accepted by the CEO and GB. A traditional CEO assessment scheme using performance levels in specific accountabilities was developed by Harvey.[11] This approach requires negotiation and is a type of management by objectives with bilaterally established performance objectives. In addition, GBs always measure CEO performance (and that of senior-level managers) by negative developments. Consistent with the philosophy of W. Edwards Deming discussed in Chapter 9, GBs should not set objectives that CEOs must meet without giving them sufficient authority and resources. The four most common areas for hospital CEO evaluations are financial performance, vision/other leadership qualities, physician relations/integration, and fulfillment of the strategic plan.[12]

Employment contracts for CEOs and senior management are increasingly common in HSOs— a development that follows the pattern set elsewhere in the economy. These contracts set terms of employment, including severance.

CEOs walk a narrow line as they focus GB members' expertise and encourage interest, dedication, and enthusiasm, but simultaneously dissuade direct participation in internal operations. Figure 4.3 shows the appropriate relationships in a HSO hierarchy. When GB members intervene in operations, CEO authority is undercut and subordinates are frustrated and confused—conditions unlikely to enhance effectiveness or efficiency. Interference is forestalled by GB job descriptions and clarification of roles and activities by GB member orientation and education.

The CEO should be present at GB meetings and many are voting members. This raises the potential for conflicts of interest just as when PSO members serve on the GB. Evaluation of the CEO raises the issue most starkly. The views of the CEO always should be considered, but GB membership gives the CEO a weight that may be at variance with objective assessment and the HSO's best interests. Problems are lessened if CEOs are absent when issues of self-interest are considered, a practice that reduces but does not eliminate potential conflicts of interest. In addition to membership, professional and personal ties between the CEO and GB members may give the CEO excessive influence as well as lessen the objectivity of evaluations and decision making. Conversely, there are advantages when the CEO is a voting member of the GB. Two of the most important are enhanced communication and participation in policy development. A measure of prestige accrues to the CEO, but this is more a personal than an organizational advantage.

It also is important that the GB evaluate its own performance. First, it must demonstrate accountability for its actions and resource utilization. Discussions could begin by identifying how and where the GB adds value to the HSO/HS, beyond that contributed by management and staff. Once this is known, members can identify ways to use time, skills, and other resources more effectively to strengthen GB contributions. After selecting targets for improvement, the GB can identify criteria for monitoring progress and delineating steps to obtain and use feedback to ensure further improvement.[13]

MANAGEMENT

The work of HSO/HS managers is unmatched elsewhere in society. They are responsible for organizations that deliver unique personal services to ill or anxious people in complex settings, and

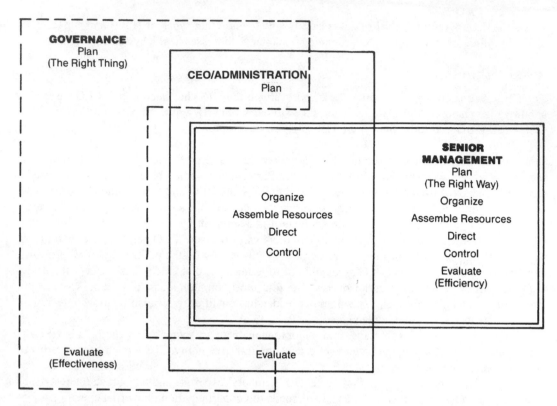

Figure 4.3.   A model of hospital governance, administration, and management. (From Henry, William F., and Vernon E. Weckwerth. "When Corporate Executives Serve as Hospital Trustees." *Trustee* 34 [June 1981]: 30; reprinted by permission. Copyright 1981, American Hospital Publishing, Inc.)

often in emotionally charged circumstances. In addition, the relationships that HSO/HSs have with professional staff through the PSO are unparalleled in other enterprises. All of this management work must be accomplished in a highly competitive, economically demanding environment.

Historically, various titles were used for chief managers in HSOs: administrator, director, CEO, president, and superintendent. This discussion uses CEO, a generic title applicable to HSOs of all types. Comments about the CEO usually apply to all senior-level managers in line positions.

Function

The CEO's basic task is managing inputs (human resources, material, technology, information, and capital) to achieve the outputs that are the HSO's/HS's objectives. Except in very small HSOs, CEOs delegate tasks and authority to subordinate managers. The ultimate responsibility (account-ability) to design, change, and operate an effective management structure to achieve the HSO's/HS's objectives is the CEO's, however, and cannot be delegated. It is the CEO whom the GB will hold accountable for failure, and perhaps reward for success.

The CEO manages the entire HSO/HS. Management was defined in Chapter 1 as a process composed of interrelated social and technical functions and activities (including roles) occurring in a formal organizational setting for the purpose of accomplishing predetermined objectives through utilization of human and other resources. This definition suggests four criteria that define the CEO's role. First is to create and meet a set of objectives. Second is to attain objectives effectively by op-timally allocating limited resources (inputs). A third criterion focuses on the staff—also an input—

through which managers accomplish work. The fourth criterion is that the HSO/HS must change over time. The theory and application of change are extensively treated in Chapter 12. CEOs continue to have the training, position, and authority that necessarily make them agents for change.[14]

Qualifications

There is no standard statement of a CEO's qualifications. Although directed to hospital CEOs, the Joint Commission on Accreditation of Healthcare Organizations (Joint Commission) expectation is instructive, if general: "The chief executive officer is competent and has the education and experience required for the size, complexity, [and] mission of the hospital, and the scope of services it provides."[15] Similar requirements are found for other types of HSOs accredited by the Joint Commission. The didactic and applied formal educational preparation of health services managers is described in Chapter 2.

Relationships

The highly complex staff relationships in HSOs/HSs arise from factors including the involvement in voluntary GB members in not-for-profit HSOs, lack of an employment relationship for most LIPs who provide medical treatment, and the technical and highly specialized functions of most staff. Such complexity and interrelationships make special demands on managers.

CEO and Senior Management

Larger HSOs/HSs are likely to divide the CEO's role into two parts. The CEO is primarily involved in GB and external relations, as well as planning, fund-raising, and undertaking capital projects. PSO relations may be on this list. The COO is responsible to the CEO for day-to-day operations. This division of responsibility helps meet increasingly complex demands. Universally found in the large HSO/HS is a CFO and a CMO. The CFO is an extension of the concept of controllership, with additional responsibilities for reimbursement, capital financing, and investment. The CMO may be known as the medical director, chief of staff, or vice president for medical affairs and is responsible for PSO relations, credentialing and privileges, and quality of clinical care. In the future, it is likely there will be a chief information officer (CIO) and chief quality officer (CQO). The CIO will be responsible for information services, and the CQO for continuous quality improvement.

The presence of both a CEO and a COO is problematic if their spheres of authority and responsibility are ill-defined. Confusion is certain if the CEO intervenes directly in matters for which the COO is responsible; unless there are emergencies, lines of authority and reporting relationships must be followed. The COO must be cognizant of GB reporting relationships so as not to bypass the CEO.

Below these senior-level managers are management layers that ultimately lead to staff who do the day-to-day work of the organization. The number of management layers in large health systems and major medical centers declined dramatically between 1985 and 1991; high-performing organizations had the fewest management layers.[16] This "flattening" of the organization is continuing.[17] Reducing layers of management is consistent with the views of leading management theorists such as Peter Drucker[18] about the desirability of flattening organizations and reflects the move toward employee empowerment that is advocated by Deming and others as described in Chapter 9.

ORGANIZING THE PROFESSIONAL STAFF

It is crucial to understand that the LIPs who treat and order treatment for patients are the engine that drives a HSO in service delivery activities. In most HSOs, patients must be admitted before treatment can be ordered and begun. No medical treatment can be rendered without express orders or standing orders that were approved prospectively. Acute care hospitals, for example, want physicians and other LIPs on their PSOs to admit patients, but, once a patient is admitted, the pressures of prospective payment (diagnosis-related groups [DRGs]) demand that treatment be efficient. Similarly, if a HSO's LIPs are salaried and an admission generates income, admission is encouraged. A HSO that receives no additional income when a patient is treated, however, will seek to minimize admission and treatment consistent with patient needs.

HSOs with a PSO have a relationship that is unique by conventional organizational standards. PSOs are likely to have bylaws, officers, a committee structure, and other characteristics that reflect the autonomy of physicians and other LIPs, who are often independent contractors in the HSO. Even when salaried, LIPs exhibit a high degree of independence and commonly have more allegiance to their professions and each other than to the HSO. Because of this independence and the technical content of clinical practice, GBs have historically exercised little direct control over the PSO.

History

Acute care hospitals have the most complex and highly developed PSO structures. This development paralleled the concentration of medical technology in hospitals in the late 19th century and the transfer of traditional physician–patient relationships to this new locus. The preeminence of the physician–patient relationship was reflected in the medical ethics of the American Medical Association (AMA), which was founded in 1847. AMA viewed fee for service (a fee paid to the physician by or on behalf of the patient) as vital to this relationship; as physicians hospitalized patients, this payment system followed. The hospital billed the patient separately for services it provided. Relationships or allegiances that interfered with physicians' judgments about what was best for their patients were unacceptable. Thus it was unethical for physicians to be salaried because employers might pressure physicians to act in ways that are contrary to the patients' best interests. AMA ethics allowed exceptions for physicians in the military, government, and industrial medicine and for physician-faculty in medical schools and teaching hospitals.

Treating private patients who paid a fee for service meant that physicians were independent contractors with limited loyalty to the hospital. This independence led physicians to believe they were accountable only to themselves (and their patients) or, at most, to peers. Private patients and independence supported a view among physicians that governance, management, and clinical practice were distinct; convergence and control occurred at the GB level. This basic view continues in HSOs with a PSO.

Professional Staff Organization

An acute care hospital's PSO is unique but also paradigmatic. The generic discussion that follows identifies general principles that may require modification to fit other HSOs.

Self-Governance

As evidence of the strong tradition of physician independence, PSOs continue to be largely self-governing. LIPs are part of the PSO whether they are salaried by the HSO or are fee-for-service LIPs. The PSO has its own bylaws, which must be approved by the GB. The bylaws are central to self-governance and identify officers, committees and their functions, categories of membership, the application process, the procedure for amending the bylaws, and a process for reviewing actions that are adverse to members. In addition, the PSO adopts rules and regulations that control clinical practice, which may be supplemented by even more detailed rules for clinical specialties, subspecialties, and departments. Hierarchically inferior (lesser) guidelines must be consistent with those that are superior.

Open or Closed

The PSO may be open, closed, or a combination of the two. This concept is highly developed in acute care hospitals but also affects other HSOs, such as nursing facilities and hospice. If a PSO is open, any qualified LIP (as defined in the PSO bylaws) is granted clinical privileges (with or without PSO membership) and may treat patients. If a PSO is closed, qualified LIPs (as defined in the PSO bylaws) may or may not be granted clinical privileges (with or without PSO membership), depending on the parameters put on the PSO by the PSO itself, as approved by the GB. Such parameters may include absolute size of the PSO or limits on the numbers in various specialties or types of LIPs. Most hospitals, for example, have a combination of an open and a closed PSO in that they close some clinical departments, such as anesthesia, clinical and anatomical laboratories, emergency medicine, and radiology, but grant privileges to any qualified surgeon or physician. Closing staffs, clinical departments, or both is justified on the grounds that it improves quality of patient care and enhances efficiency. When departments are closed, the HSO usually has entered into an exclusive contract with an individual physician or provider group, who are known as concessionaires. All LIPs who function under the terms of the contract must have clinical privileges delineated consistent with their licenses and demonstrated current competence.

Committees

In many ways hospital GB and PSO committee structures are parallel. The PSO is led by an executive committee whose members usually include the chairs of standing committees. Like its GB counterpart, the executive committee acts for the PSO and coordinates its activities. It provides continuity and enhances communication between the PSO and management. Major activities include implementing PSO policies, receiving and acting on reports and recommendations from PSO committees, making recommendations on PSO membership and clinical privileges, monitoring quality of care, and taking corrective action, including discipline. Other functional areas that must be managed and for which there may be committees include

> *Credentials*—reviews qualifications of clinicians for PSO membership and recommends specific privileges to executive committee; reviews continuing appropriateness of privileges
>
> *Surgical case review*—reviews justification for surgery; checks relationship between pre- and postoperative diagnoses
>
> *Medical records*—checks for timely completion of medical records; reviews clinical usefulness and adequacy of record for quality of care
>
> *Pharmacy and therapeutics*—develops formulary and monitors drug use and other therapeutics policies; may have special interest in antibiotics use
>
> *Utilization review*—reviews resource use in providing care, with special attention to length of stay and use of ancillary services
>
> *Quality assessment*—may be used instead of surgical case review and medical records committees, or may review pre- and postoperative reports, use of ancillary services such as radiology and laboratories, and condition of patient on discharge to determine appropriateness of treatment

Other common committees are infection control, blood use, risk management and safety, disaster planning, bylaws, and nominating. The CEO or a designee should attend all PSO meetings, including its committee meetings and related functional activities.[19]

In the future it is likely that there will be a PSO quality improvement committee that uses monitoring and assessment completed by its other committees to focus clinical process analysis and improvement activities. Continuous quality improvement is discussed in Chapter 9.

Clinical Departmentation

The extent and type of clinical departmentation (like its managerial counterpart) are determined by the HSO's size and activities. Nonhospital HSOs, such as health maintenance organizations (HMOs) and multispecialty group practices, have clinical departments. Nursing facilities and hospice have a medical director (CMO) but are unlikely to have a PSO. Small hospitals have only departments of medicine and surgery in their PSO. Larger hospitals typically add obstetrics-gynecology, pediatrics, and family practice. Departmentation expands from there to include clinical specialties or subspecialties as separate departments or sections within departments.

Clinical department heads are elected by department members or are appointed by administration; in either case they serve at the sufferance of the GB. Clinical managers may be paid or unpaid, although larger units and greater demands increase the likelihood that the HSO will pay a salary to a clinical manager who is not already an employee. If specialization warrants, divisions, sections, or both are established within departments. The upward chain of command goes to a physician, who is the CMO. Larger HSOs typically pay a salary to the CMO. Eventually, the line of authority reaches the GB. The CMO may report to the CEO, which is consistent with the accountability that the management structure should demand of the PSO. This reporting relationship is most likely if the CEO is also a clinician. It is least likely in a community hospital, where the CEO is rarely a clinician. HSOs must make and are making special efforts to develop the management skills of physician managers and to develop physician leaders.[20]

Managing the PSO

Working effectively with the PSO is problematic regardless of HSO type, ownership, or size. The greatest potential for control is found in Department of Veterans Affairs and military facilities, where PSO members are employees or under orders and the CEO has line authority over them. Here, too, however, LIPs generally and physicians especially have significant independence. Historically, GBs accepted the PSO's assurances that the quality of care was acceptable. More attention to ethics, greater malpractice liability, and medicine's somewhat tarnished image have changed HSO–patient relationships. There is a general sense among the public, reinforced by the courts, that HSO governance and management must be concerned about patient well-being and must take steps to ensure the competence of clinicians.

Credentialing

Credentialing LIPs is crucial to the quality of care and is done by the HSO with the help of the clinical staff or PSO. One approach that is applicable in a multiunit HSO or a HS is central credentials verification, with a multidisciplinary, uniform credentialing and privileging process carried out separately at each practice site.[21] Credentialing is essential for physicians because, unlike other LIPs, their licenses are unlimited. Only through the credentialing process are physicians' activities in HSOs made consistent with their demonstrated current competence. The activities allowed under the limited licenses of other LIPs may be narrowed even further by the HSO. The same credentialing process should be used for all LIPs (including physicians), whether or not they are eligible to be members of the PSO.

Credentialing has two parts. The first is to determine the applicant's PSO membership category, if the LIP is eligible for membership. The second is assessing the LIP's demonstrated current competence to determine what the applicant will be allowed (credentialed) to do—this is known as delineating and granting clinical privileges. PSO membership (and category) and the clinical privileges the practitioner may perform in the HSO are separate. The two-part process applies to initial appointment and to reappointment, which are different. PSO bylaws determine the content of the process and include due process safeguards for the applicant or reapplicant. PSO bylaws may provide that, in addition to physicians, all or only certain other types of LIPs may be members of the PSO, or the bylaws may have separate, nonmembership categories for nonphysician LIPs. Regardless, nonphysician LIPs may be precluded from serving on certain committees or holding PSO offices. Restrictions on committee membership and offices may apply to physicians in certain categories, too. Nonphysician LIPs who are members of the PSO are credentialed only to undertake specific clinical activities (privileges), just as are physicians. The nuances and variations are included in the bylaws, which have been developed by the PSO, subject to state law and approval by the GB.

Process

The credentialing process usually is organized and monitored by the CEO or a designee. Completed application files are referred to the PSO for credentials committee review, and this committee makes a recommendation to the PSO executive committee. The next level of review is the CMO and the president of the PSO. Final approval of recommendations lies with the GB, through its committee structure. Historically, GBs may have taken their responsibility to control PSO membership and credentialing more lightly than they should. Increased ethical and legal accountability have forced HSOs to be more attentive and not abdicate their responsibility to the PSO.

PSO Membership—Initial Appointment

The process and substance of initial application for PSO membership must be thorough, detailed, and comprehensive. Applicants should provide basic information that is used in a screening process: demographic data; details on postsecondary, professional, and postgraduate education; certificates of specialty and professional memberships; licenses; information about previously successful and current challenges to licenses, certifications, registrations, and PSO memberships; voluntary or involuntary limitations, reductions, or losses of clinical privileges or licenses, certifications, or registrations; a statement of physical and mental health indicating that the applicant has no disability that is inconsistent with privileges being sought[22]; an authorization allowing verification of information; and references. Screening saves HSO resources and the applicant's time if the applicant lacks the basic credentials for appointment.[23]

If the applicant meets the screening requirements, additional information is provided: details of all malpractice actions in the previous 5 years and evidence of continuous malpractice insurance coverage; a request for membership and privileges in the department in which the applicant desires to practice; a signed statement that the PSO bylaws and its rules and regulations have been read and will be met; and a statement that, if appointed, the applicant will provide or provide for the continuous care of patients for whom he or she is responsible.

It is prudent to require photographs of applicants; these are sent to references to verify that applicants are who they claim to be. The national data bank established by the Health Care Quality Improvement Act of 1986[24] (see Chapter 14) must be queried prior to both initial appointment and reappointment to determine whether there are adverse reports. Problems uncovered are investigated as necessary.

The burden of proof is the applicant's. Applicants must complete the process to the HSO's satisfaction, including all specific elements. No assumptions should be made. Rather, applicants must provide all information and documentation that the HSO requires. The applicant may choose character references. It is imperative, however, that the HSO choose which professional references to query because this is the only way to obtain complete, objective information about clinical competence. Questions asked of references must be answered to the HSO's satisfaction. No LIP should be allowed to undertake clinical activities until the application is complete in all respects and has been reviewed and approved. Prudence must be the watchword because things are not always what they seem.

The PSO may have several categories of membership. This is always true for acute care hospitals. Typically, these categories range from most involved (active) to least involved (honorary or emeritus). New members, except those in the consulting and honorary categories, often are given provisional appointments. This amounts to a probationary status and allows clinical performance to be monitored or reviewed. In the future, PSO membership categories for nonprovisional LIPs are likely to be fewer and include only active, courtesy, and emeritus, with the latter having no admitting or clinical privileges.[25]

In 1984 the Joint Commission adopted a medical staff standard that allowed hospitals to extend PSO membership to LIPs other than physicians and dentists. The changes were especially important for podiatrists, clinical psychologists, and nurse-midwives. Chiropractors also benefited from this change and from revisions in AMA's *Principles of Medical Ethics* that are noted in Chapter 13. A 1989 AHA survey found that hospital PSO bylaws allowed nonphysician LIPs to apply for membership; 67% of hospital PSOs accept podiatrists, 43% accept clinical psychologists, and 5% accept chiropractors. These percentages are significant increases from a similar study done in 1984.[26]

It bears repeating that membership and clinical privileges are separate. PSO bylaws may not allow nonphysician LIPs to be members; nonetheless, these LIPs may be granted clinical privileges consistent with their license or certification and demonstrated competence. Or, a physician appointed in the "honorary" membership category has no clinical privileges. In contrast, PSO members in the "active" category have significant clinical privileges, which may be temporarily suspended because of a disciplinary action.

PSO Membership—Reappointment

Typically, reappointment to the PSO occurs every 2 years. Reappointment is similar to initial appointment but has one very important difference: During the preceding appointment the HSO has monitored and evaluated the LIP's performance. This information is used in decisions regarding membership category and clinical privileges to be granted, if any, in the next appointment cycle. The following information should be provided by the reapplicant: name, current addresses, and telephone number; description of paid or unpaid affiliations with other HSOs and authorization to obtain performance indicators from them; successful or pending challenges to licenses, certifications, and registrations; voluntary or involuntary termination of PSO memberships or voluntary or involuntary limitations, reductions, or loss(es) of clinical privileges at another HSO; involvement in a professional liability claim since the previous reappointment; a statement of physical and mental health that the applicant has no disability inconsistent with privileges being sought[26]; continuing professional education; PSO activities, including attending PSO and committee meetings; and insurance coverage as specified in PSO bylaws.[27]

Clinical Privileges

Clinical privileges must be delineated (individually or by category) for all LIPs delivering care in the HSO, whether or not they are PSO members. Prudence demands that clinical activities be limited to the skills and qualifications that LIPs can initially demonstrate and continue to justify. In addition, the HSO must be able to support the LIPs' clinical activities.

By license, some LIPs are limited to performing specific clinical activities. For example, podiatrists are licensed to treat the foot and its related or governing structures by medical, surgical, or other means.[28] HSOs may restrict but may not expand what the state license allows LIPs to do. Categories of LIPs may be granted privileges as a group in the HSO. Physicians and dentists are granted privileges individually.

Privilege delineation comprises two elements. The first is determining the specific content of clinical privileges. The second is ongoing and systematic review of care delivered to determine whether changes in privileges, either increases or decreases, are justified. Clinical privileges should be specific to the HSO—a Joint Commission requirement for hospitals. Each procedure/activity may be listed on the application or reapplication forms, or there may be a general reference such as "internal medicine" with whatever limitations are appropriate for the level of qualification (e.g., board certification). The definition of a general term or category such as internal medicine must be found in the PSO bylaws or the PSO rules and regulations. Clinical privileges for nonphysician LIPs are handled similarly, although the privileges are more likely to be listed specifically. It is common and desirable that any special relationships of nonphysician LIPs to physicians be described in the grant of privileges or referenced in the PSO bylaws or the rules and regulations. Examples are nurse-midwives who practice with or are employed by obstetricians, or nurse-anesthetists who practice with or are employed by surgeons or anesthesiologists. Typically, privileges are granted on 2-year cycles, or as accrediting bodies require.

PSO Discipline

It may be necessary to take disciplinary action against a LIP with clinical privileges. Most often such action results from minor infractions of the PSO bylaws or their subsidiary rules and regulations. Sometimes, HSO policies are involved. More rare is that the quality of care rendered by the practitioner is judged deficient. Regardless, it may be necessary to act to protect patients or find ways to encourage appropriate behavior, which almost always involves a recommendation by a PSO committee. Depending on the matter, it may be necessary for the GB to review and approve the recommendation.

A common problem in hospitals is that LIPs do not complete medical records of discharged patients in the time limits that are set by the PSO rules and regulations. Such lapses diminish quality of care but usually pose no significant risk to patients. Verbal or written warnings are a typical first step in a disciplinary process. A continuing problem might result in temporary suspension of admitting privileges, which means that elective admissions are prohibited. LIPs whose admitting privileges are suspended usually take immediate steps to make records current.

PSO bylaws usually identify a variety of disciplinary options. In order of increasing severity, they are mandatory continuing or special medical education, letter of admonition, supervision, suspension of admitting or clinical privileges or both, censure, reduction of privileges, and termination of privileges. It may be appropriate to take two or more actions concurrently. The underlying motivation is to protect patients from deficient or inappropriate clinical treatment. Depending on the action, the affected LIP may be entitled to due process as set out in the PSO bylaws. If so, the PSO recommendation is reviewed and the GB makes the final decision. In situations in which risk of imminent harm to patients exists, the CEO or another senior official such as the medial director, acting for the GB, must take whatever action is necessary. The Health Care Quality Improvement Act of 1986 requires that actions that are adverse to clinical privileges for a period longer than 30 days must be reported to a national data bank.

Special Issues in Managing the PSO

Economic Credentialing

Competitive and reimbursement pressures force HSOs to be more efficient. This suggests the importance of judging LIPs by their economic performance, as well as by their clinical performance. Physicians vary widely in use of resources such as hospital admission and length of patient stay, diagnostic tests for outpatients, and types and duration of therapies. Decisions on such matters have major cost and revenue implications for HSOs. Patients should receive needed services—no more and no less. With few exceptions, such care is both high quality and efficient.

Judging economic performance, often called economic credentialing, means that, in addition to reviewing the quality of care, data are collected as to LIPs' economic effect on the HSO. Two criteria are useful: *volume of referrals* (typically, HSOs are interested in admissions [under non-capitated payment], generally; patients who are insured or private pay are preferred) and review of *practice patterns* to determine whether resources are used efficiently. The profiling that is necessary to undertake economic credentialing is possible because data systems enable HSOs/HSs to link cost and patient treatment information.[29] Using severity-adjusted data when comparing physician practice patterns minimizes potential unfairness that could arise if a physician treats patients who are significantly more ill.[30] Economic credentialing already is used in managed care and will become commonplace in all HSOs/HSs. Legal challenges are unlikely to be successful if the actions are not arbitrary and capricious and are consistent with corporate and PSO bylaws.[31]

Turf Conflicts

Conflicts as to what the various types of LIPs are allowed to do in HSOs result from professionalism, economics, and technology.[32] The ego of professionalism causes groups to enhance their training, which causes them to infringe on traditional clinical areas of other providers. The economics of reimbursement cause groups to gravitate toward more remunerative clinical activities. Also, new diagnostic and therapeutic technology can be applied by several types of LIPs. HSOs must have a means by which LIPs claiming expertise in new procedures or clinical activities are reviewed and receive (or are denied) clinical privileges to perform them. Self-reported competence is inadequate; independent verification is necessary. Chapter 6 describes how technological developments blur the lines that traditionally separated medicine and surgery, medical and surgical specialties and subspecialties, and nonphysician LIPs.[33] Such blurring causes turf conflicts that disrupt referral patterns and PSO relationships. The results can be negative for HSOs with independent LIPs on their staff. The economic dimensions of turf conflicts for the HSO include duplicating equipment, space, and staff to placate various LIPs, and the likelihood that disgruntled LIPs will sever their relationship with the HSO and treat patients elsewhere. Technology should not be acquired until there is agreement about its use.

Integration

Individual LIPs and the PSO as a whole perform technical services that must be integrated into a total effort if the organization is to achieve its objectives. Non–LIP managers neither deliver clinical services nor judge quality independently. They can and must, however, obtain the expert advice and technical assistance to make informed judgments about individual and aggregate PSO practice. This is what managers do when they judge the technical aspects of pharmacy or data processing, for example.

Historically, PSO members have had little involvement in managing the HSO. The exception has been clinical managers and PSO officers. In the 1990s, however, the value of their participation was recognized, and LIPs have become more involved in management decision making. Such interactions are good practice and are strongly recommended by accrediting bodies such as the Joint Commission. This has been termed the *conjoint medical staff*.[34] PSO members can be integrated into a HSO's managerial structure in several ways: They may join PSO, management, and GB committees; managers may ask them for advice formally and informally; and those who manage clinical departments or units are part of the management team. Some aspects of such relationships in a HSO are shown in Figure 3.5. Integrating clinical staff into HS management and governance also is key to high quality and low costs.

Clinical managers have a special place in an efficiently managed HSO because even small PSOs are divided into departments or sections based on clinical interest. Clinical managers perform all management functions. Although medical education and clinical practice teach physicians to think logically and to view problems systematically and consider their implications, these skills do not adequately prepare them as managers. Only competent clinical managers can further organizational objectives. Thus it is a matter of self-interest that the HSO ensures their competence. The presence of full- or part-time salaried clinical managers in a HSO allows even more involvement in management. When clinicians and managers understand each other's problems, enhanced communication and organizational effectiveness result, all of which enable HSOs/HSs to align incentives so as to deliver integrated services successfully.[35]

Licensing and Credentialing

Licensing and credentialing physicians and other clinicians are problematic. Legal issues regarding LIPs are discussed in Chapter 14. Suffice it to say that those who diagnose and treat patients in a state where they are not licensed violate that state's licensing laws. This occurs whenever telemedicine consultations cross state lines, for example. Using out-of-state "advice nurses" for off-hour consultations is a common example. Similarly, physicians and other LIPs who use electronic links to a HSO in which they are not credentialed violate credentialing standards of organizations such as the Joint Commission or the National Committee for Quality Assurance (NCQA). It is likely that credentialing issues will be resolved more easily than reconciling licensing requirements in the 50 states.

Impaired Clinicians

PSOs such as those in acute care hospitals have a less-than-enviable record of handling impaired LIPs, especially physicians. It has been common for clinical staff or the PSO to band together to prevent patient and public scrutiny. This human tendency may cause HSOs/HSs to be less than rigorous in meeting ethical and legal duties to patients, and even to staff. HSOs are morally (and perhaps legally) obliged to try to rehabilitate all impaired staff, including LIPs, whenever possible. This may not be done, however, in a way that puts patients at risk.

Its varied types and subtlety make impairment among caregivers hard to detect and document. Impairment may be physical, mental, or both and may result from aging, disease, or chemical dependency. Estimates in the early 1980s suggested that tens of thousands of physicians were impaired.[36] In the 1980s, 5%–17% of physicians in North America were estimated to be impaired.[37] In the 1990s it was estimated that 15% of physicians were impaired because of drug and alcohol addiction.[38] A survey of physicians found that 8% had abused or been chemically dependent on alcohol or drugs during their lives.[39] Some physicians, such as anesthesiologists, appear to be at higher risk than others.[40] Similar estimates of impairment of all types have been made for nonphysician caregivers; one survey of nurses found that 10% were addicted to at least one controlled substance.[41] Despite such data, few HSOs conduct drug testing, except for cause. Another type of impairment occurs when caregivers allow their clinical skills to become outdated. Regardless of cause, the HSOs in which these LIPs practice are ethically and legally bound to identify the problem and act in the patients' interests. Impairment may be identified through the risk management activities discussed in Chapter 10.

For reasons that are unclear, HSOs often fail to act when clinical practice is marginal; they may not even react vigorously when practice is clearly substandard. The HSO may fear legal action by the impaired clinician; perhaps HSO management finds the task distasteful. Members of the PSO should be even more interested in improving the quality of clinical practice than are management and the GB. Unless accountability mechanisms and authority that are available to management and the GB are defined and used, the problem will persist until a patient is harmed. Even then, action may not occur until it is stimulated by a lawsuit against the HSO. Inaction is a luxury that no HSO can afford.

ORGANIZATION OF SELECTED HSOs

The preceding information is background to discussing selected HSOs. Included in this discussion are acute care hospitals, nursing facilities, ambulatory care organizations, hospice, managed care organizations (MCOs), birth centers, and home health agencies (HHA). These are the most common types, but the list is by no means exhaustive of the variety of types that are, and will be, found in the health services system.

The discussion of each HSO uses the client title most often given to those whom the HSO serves. For example, hospitals use "patient," MCOs use "enrollee," nursing facilities use "resident," and HHAs use "client." Such titles indicate the relationship a type of HSO has, or seeks to have, with the people it serves and reflect the philosophical model implicitly or explicitly underlying that relationship. Three models of HSO interactions with the people they serve are shown in Table 4.1. The medical/hospital model is driven by high technology, is physician directed, and is designed for people with immediate acute health care needs. Treatment of disease is the principal goal. The nursing facility/social model is driven by basic principles of the psychosocial disciplines, is interdisciplinary team directed, and is designed for people with chronic, long-term physical and mental functional deficits. Quality of life is a major goal. The hospitality/hotel model is driven by marketing data that show client desires and satisfaction, is client directed, and is designed for people with personal care needs. Security and comfortable living arrangements are major goals.[42] Assisted living and continuing care retirement communities are examples, but these are not HSOs. Table 4.1 should be kept in mind as the types of HSOs are discussed.

Acute Care Hospitals

Hospitals have been present in various forms for millennia. Approximately 5,000 years ago Greek temples were the first, but similar institutions can be found in ancient Egyptian, Hindu, and Roman societies. These "hospitals" evolved from temples of worship and recuperation to almshouses and pesthouses and finally to places where medical "miracles" are daily occurrences.

Hospital is derived from the Latin *hospitalis*. Although well regarded early in their history, hospitals in the Middle Ages and later had unsavory reputations and primarily served the poor. This reputation improved only slowly, beginning in the middle of the 19th century. Until well into the 20th century, physicians provided charity care in hospitals but treated private (fee-for-service) patients at home. New medical technology made treatment efficacious, especially with surgical intervention, and this focused attention on acute care hospitals. Treatment of private patients brought acute care hospitals prestige and wide acceptance. This evolution was well underway by the 1920s as acute care hospitals became dif-

TABLE 4.1.   BASIC MODELS OF HSO INTERACTIONS WITH PEOPLE SERVED

Model	Attributes
Medical/hospital model	Principal goal: disease treatment Physician directed Acute care oriented Driven by high technology
Nursing facility/social model	Principal goal: quality of life Interdisciplinary team directed Chronic and long-term oriented Driven by psychosocial disciplines
Hospitality/hotel model	Principal goals: security and comfort Client directed Personal care needs oriented Driven by marketing data showing client needs and satisfaction

Adapted from Stryker, Ruth. "Characteristics of the Long-Term Care Model." In *Creative Long-Term Care Administration,* 3rd ed., edited by George Kenneth Gordon and Ruth Stryker, 17. Springfield, IL: Charles C Thomas, 1994.

ferentiated and specialized to organize and deliver an expanded scope of services. Many acute care hospitals were small and owned by physicians as a convenient way to hospitalize their patients.

Definitions and Numbers

By convention of common use, a community hospital is an acute care hospital that treats the public for general medical and surgical problems. The title is used whether the hospital is organized as not for profit or for profit. A community hospital has permanent facilities (including inpatient beds), continuous nursing services, and diagnosis and treatment through an organized PSO for patients with a variety of surgical and nonsurgical conditions. This is in contrast to special hospitals, which admit only certain types of patients or those with specified illnesses or conditions.

In 1946, 6,125 hospitals were registered with AHA. From a peak of 7,174 in 1974, the number declined to 6,649 in 1990, to 6,097 in 1997, and declined further to 6,021 in 1998.[43] This downward trend is likely to continue. Not all hospitals submit data or register with AHA, but estimates are made for them and are included in the annual AHA publication *Hospital Statistics,* an important data source. From 1980 to 1994 more than 800 hospitals closed; most were community hospitals.[44] More ⁙⁙⁙⁙ ⁙⁙ ⁙⁙⁙⁙⁙⁙ ⁙⁙ ⁙⁙⁙⁙ ⁙⁙⁙⁙ ⁙⁙⁙⁙,[17] ⁙⁙⁙⁙⁙⁙ ⁙⁙⁙⁙, ⁙⁙⁙⁙⁙⁙ ⁙⁙⁙⁙⁙⁙⁙, ⁙⁙⁙ ⁙⁙⁙⁙⁙⁙⁙ ⁙⁙⁙⁙⁙⁙⁙⁙ ⁙⁙⁙⁙ have been identified with hospital closures.[46] Another analysis found that some hospitals that closed were more efficient but had both low volumes and poor payer mix.[47]

The distribution of community hospitals by bed size in Table 4.2 shows that almost half have fewer than 100 beds. They tend to be isolated and need linkages to other hospitals through networks and voluntary associations, as well as the multiorganizational systems described in Chapter 5. Smaller hospitals are among those that are most in need of competent managers.

Classification

Hospitals are classified by length of stay, type of control, and type of service. Length of stay is divided into short term and long term. "Acute" (of short duration or episodic) is a synonym for short term. "Chronic" (of long duration) is a synonym for long term. The AHA defines short-term hospitals as having an average length of stay (ALOS) of less than 30 days, and long-term hospitals as having an ALOS of 30 days or more. More than 90% of hospitals are short term. Community hospitals are acute care (short term). Rehabilitation and chronic disease hospitals are long term. Psychi-

TABLE **4.2.** DISTRIBUTION OF COMMUNITY HOSPITALS[a] BY BED SIZE IN 1980, 1990, AND **1997**

No. of beds	No. of hospitals			Percent change (1990–1997)
	1980	1990	1997	
	5,830	5,384	5,057	–13.3
6–24	259	226	281	8.5
25–29	1,029	935	890	–13.5
50–99	1,462	1,263	1,111	–24.0
100–199	1,370	1,306	1,289	–5.9
200–299	715	739	679	–5.0
300–399	412	408	367	–10.9
400–499	266	222	185	–30.5
500+	317	285	255	–19.6

Source: American Hospital Association. *American Hospital Association Hospital Statistics, 1991–1992,* xxxvii. Chicago: American Hospital Association, 1991; and American Hospital Association. American Hospital Association Hospital Statistics, 1999. 10–25. Chicago: American Hospital Association, 1999.

[a]The AHA defines community hospital as all nonfederal, short-term general, and special hospital whose facilities and services are available to the public.

atric hospitals are usually long term. Some acute care hospitals have long-term care units to treat psychiatric illnesses, for example.

Type of service denotes whether the hospital is "general" or "special." General hospitals provide a broad range of medical and surgical services, to which are usually added obstetrics-gynecology; pediatrics; orthopedics; and eye, ear, nose, and throat services. "General" describes both acute and chronic care hospitals but usually applies to short-term hospitals. "Special" hospitals offer services in one medical or surgical specialty (e.g., pediatrics, obstetrics-gynecology, rehabilitation medicine, psychiatry) or in a discrete surgical procedure, such as hernia repair. Although special hospitals are usually acute, they also may be chronic. A leprosy (Hansen's disease) or tuberculosis hospital is an example of the latter. In 1997, 730 long-term, nonfederal, special hospitals of various types were AHA registered: psychiatric hospitals (587), institutions for people with mental retardation (14), hospitals for people with tuberculosis and other respiratory diseases (4), and long-term general and other special hospitals (125).[48]

A third classification divides hospitals by type of control or ownership into not for profit, for profit (investor owned), or governmental (federal, state, or local governments, or hospital authority). Figure 4.4 shows various types of hospital ownership. In 1997 there were 6,097 AHA-registered hospitals in the United States. Of these, 5,082 were community hospitals (nonfederal short-term general and other special hospitals), a decline of 577 from 1987. The 5,082 community hospitals included 3,000 nongovernmental not-for-profit (also called voluntary) hospitals (59%) with 591,000 beds, 797 investor-owned hospitals (16%) with 115,000 beds, and 1,260 hospitals owned by state or local governments (25%) with 148,000 beds. The difference between 6,097 and 5,082 (1,015) is federal and nonfederal psychiatric hospitals, federal general and other special hospitals, nonfederal institutions for people with mental retardation, tuberculosis and other respiratory disease hospitals, and long-term general and special hospitals.[49]

The acute care hospital field has a strong tradition of voluntarism; ownership is predominantly not for profit. During the late 19th and early 20th centuries, acute care hospitals became larger, more complex, and more costly. In addition to voluntarism, the increase in not-for-profit acute care hospitals resulted from favorable tax treatment and the federal Hill-Burton program (begun in 1946), which provided money for their construction.

Prior to passage of Medicare in 1965, investor-owned acute care hospitals had become virtually nonexistent. (Chapter 2 contains an appendix that provides a concise overview of the Medicare and Medicaid programs.) After passage of Medicare, investor ownership of community hospitals increased dramatically and stabilized in the 700–800 range.[50] In addition, investor-owned companies have management contracts with large numbers of hospitals.

New Types

During the 1980s and early 1990s, several states blurred the traditional definition of acute care hospitals by licensing new types of HSOs. The postoperative (postacute) recovery center, sometimes called a medical inn or recovery care center, is neither a traditional acute care hospital nor an ambulatory HSO. These HSOs provide a lower-cost alternative to hospitalization when a patient has undergone outpatient surgery and may need observation for 24–48 hours.[51] Some states also license a category of subacute facility whose level of service lies between an acute care hospital and a nursing facility. Given the excess beds in acute care hospitals and the availability of nursing facilities, it seems unlikely that these types of HSOs will gain a significant foothold in health services delivery.

Functions

Acute care hospitals diagnose and treat the sick and injured and, sometimes, the worried well. A patient's medical condition determines the care received and, to some extent, the type of hospital where it is provided. Care may be delivered on an inpatient or outpatient basis.

PRIVATE (NONGOVERNMENT) OWNERSHIP

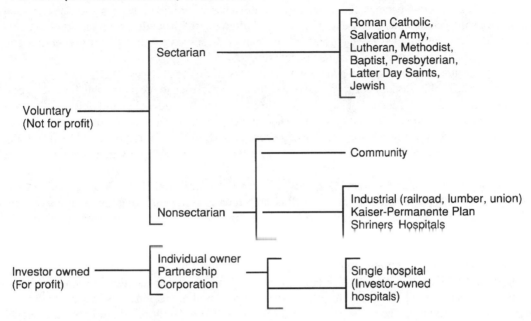

GOVERNMENT OWNERSHIP

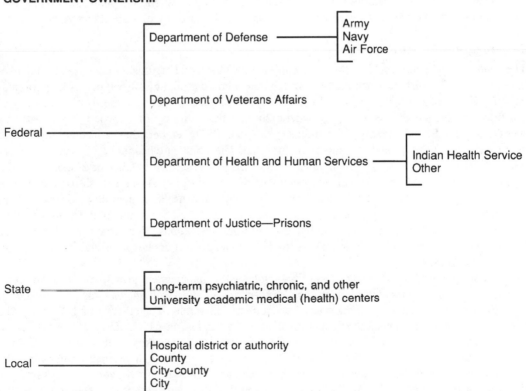

Figure 4.4. Hospital ownership.

A second function of acute care hospitals is preventing illness and promoting health. Examples include instructing patients about self-care after discharge, providing referrals to services such as home health, conducting disease screening, and holding childbirth education and smoking cessation classes. The competitive environment has caused hospitals to mix illness prevention and health promotion with generous amounts of marketing.

A third function is educating people who will work in health services. HSOs train many different types of health services workers who need clinical experience to receive a state license or certification from a professional society. Physician education in residencies and fellowships is a common example. Nursing assistants, medical social workers, and dietitians are other examples. In addition, master's-level health services management education usually requires field experience; managers are likely to have been an administrative intern, resident, or fellow in a hospital or other type of HSO.

A fourth function of acute care hospitals is research. Clinical trials for new drugs and devices come to mind first but are the least common. Research such as assessing utilization of intensive care units and determining why staff ignore universal precautions when treating patients in emergency departments is more common. One type of nonclinical research is to improve hospital processes through quality improvement activities such as administering patient satisfaction surveys, increasing efficiency in patient billing, and delivering supplies to nursing units more efficiently.

Acute care hospitals treat the sick and injured; emphasis on other functions depends on organizational mission and objectives. Hospitals have become involved in activities beyond traditional acute care—for example, home health services (58%), skilled nursing/long-term care (transitional care units [45%]), hospice (27%), and Meals on Wheels (17%).[52] In addition to diversification, Chapter 5 describes new relationships that are being developed among hospitals and other HSOs such as in integrated delivery systems to deliver services in innovative, more effective ways.

Organization Structure

The acute care hospital would be far less complex if it fit the usual organizational pyramid. Its management structure differs substantially from the bureaucratic model of other types of large organizations. These differences are caused by the unusual relationships between the formal authority of position represented by the managerial hierarchy and the authority of knowledge possessed by members of the PSO. In the typical community hospital, PSO members do not fit into the pyramid as do staff who work for and are paid by the hospital. The acute care hospital PSO includes physicians, dentists, and, increasingly, the other types of LIPs as described in Chapter 2. Except for administrative work, PSO members are usually not paid by the hospital. As a result, the organizational pattern is a dual pyramid with the managerial hierarchy and the PSO hierarchy side by side, as shown in Figure 4.1. Adding governance to management and the PSO results in the triad described earlier. Some acute care hospitals integrate the PSO into the organization structure, which means its members are likely to be salaried; Department of Veterans Affairs hospitals and military hospitals are examples.

A dual pyramid—two lines of authority—violates the management principle of unity of command, which contravenes a postulate of the classicist Henri Fayol. One line extends from the GB to the CEO and from there into the managerial structure and hierarchy. The other extends from the GB to the PSO. These two intersect in departments such as nursing, in which activities are both managerial and clinical, forming a matrix set of relationships. The complexity of this structure is illustrated by the fact that many hospital staff often have more than one immediate superior. For example, the work of nurses in clinical areas is directed by a head nurse, who is a first-level manager in a functional department (nursing), as well as by members of the PSO, usually physicians, in terms of specific orders for a patient. These directions may be contradictory because each group interprets objectives and the means of attaining them in terms of its own value systems and requirements.

Governance

Historically, hospital GBs included public-spirited business and financial leaders in the community. This pattern continues in the not-for-profit sector, where GB members are almost never paid for their service. In terms of what GB members should know, understanding the health care field, the local market, and the health care culture are considered to be more important than knowledge of finance, planning, quality, or legal issues, a shift over previous priority listings.[53] There has been a trend toward smaller, better qualified, and more active hospital GBs. Not-for-profit hospitals tend to have larger GBs. A typical large, not-for-profit community hospital GB has 18 members, including 1 inside director (usually the CEO [77% of hospitals]) and 3 PSO members.[54]

The extensive changes in the external environment described in Chapter 2 have caused GBs to be more closely scrutinized and have put them under greater pressure to perform. Proposals to increase GB member competence have focused on specialized seminars and continuing education. Such approaches are inadequate, and many hospitals will be better served by adopting the business enterprise model, in which directors are paid for their time and talent. Governance performance is but a matter of chance if GBs are ill prepared.

To facilitate communication and coordination among the GB, management, and the PSO, hospitals may have a joint conference committee (JCC) as a standing committee of the GB or the PSO. The JCC usually has few members; typically there are three from the GB and three from the PSO, with the CEO as a seventh member. Although the JCC has no line authority, it plays a major role in considering policy issues for the organization.

Management

Acute care hospitals are complex organizations with several levels of management. Figure 4.5 is the organizational chart of a community hospital that has reorganized into a small vertically integrated health care system that includes a hospital, a physician-hospital organization (PHO), home health services, a nursing facility (part of senior services), and several joint ventures. It uses corporate titles—a common development in hospitals since the 1980s. The chart suggests the dual hierarchy described earlier. The medical staff, the traditional name for the PSO, is shown as separate from the hospital, and there is no clear line or reporting relationship between it and the CEO. The senior vice president for medical affairs (CMO) reports to the hospital president and has numerous responsibilities related to PSO functioning. Some CMOs use the title "medical director." Departments and activities that provide direct patient care, clinical support, and administrative functions are identifiable from the titles. In addition, departments and units such as planning and marketing, development (fund-raising), and human resources perform a variety of essential staff functions.

One of the most important roles of a GB is to select and evaluate the CEO. The last major study of hospital governance showed that only 66% of responding hospitals formally evaluate the CEO; written evaluation criteria/objectives and economic performance (97%) and medical staff relations (96%) are the most important criteria used. Personal qualities are used by 85% of responding hospitals, and quality of care by 77%.[55] Hospital GBs that fail to link management to quality of care have a view that is woefully inconsistent with contemporary thinking and good practice. About 50% of hospital CEOs have employment contracts, a percentage that is likely to increase.[56]

Professional Staff Organization

The LIPs on the PSO, primarily its physicians, control all hospital admissions and, generally speaking, are key to a hospital's economic success. PSO members may be salaried, but overwhelmingly they are independent contractors, a fact that is especially applicable to community hospitals. Under traditional payment systems, revenue is generated for the hospital only if LIPs admit patients. However, if the hospital is part of a HS that is paid a capitated (fixed fee) payment, then the hospital

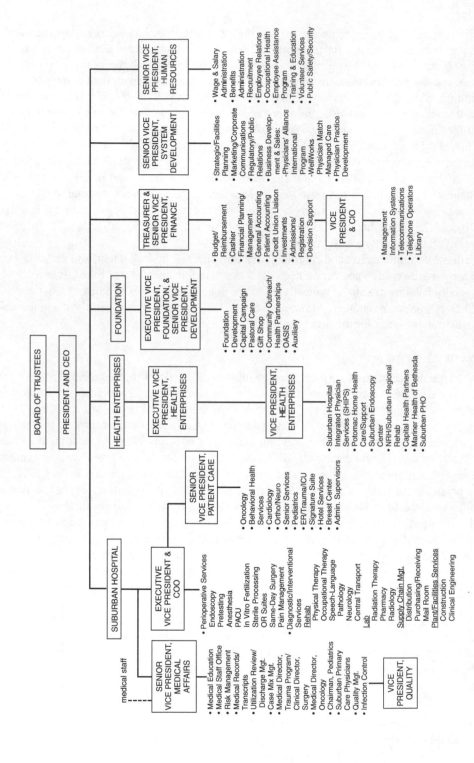

Figure 4.5. Organization chart of a vertically integrated health care system. (Reprinted by permission of the Suburban Hospital Healthcare System, Bethesda, MD.)

176

may be a cost center—each admission takes money from the pool. In that case the hospital must suboptimize its economic performance so that the economic performance of the whole system can be optimized.

Accredited hospitals have a highly structured PSO, which reflects good practice. As noted earlier, hospital PSOs are largely self-governing. They have bylaws that set out how the PSO is organized and detail officers, committees, and various processes, including appointment of members, credentialing, and discipline.

The CMO is central to effective coordination, communication, and management of the PSO. The CMO is usually employed full time in larger hospitals and part time in smaller hospitals. Smaller hospitals may have a volunteer CMO, often called the chief of staff. Other clinical managers include department chiefs or chiefs of service, who may be paid depending on the demands on their time. Consistent with the bylaws, clinical managers have significant autonomy in managing their departments, but they are accountable to the CMO for clinical and administrative matters.

Numerous researchers have sought to understand, analyze, and describe physicians in hospitals: Georgopoulos and Mann studied 41 community general hospitals,[57] Roemer and Friedman studied the relationship between the medical staff organization (the PSO) and hospital performance,[58] Neuhauser studied the relationship between managerial activities and hospital performance,[59] and Shortell and Evashwick studied factors of medical staff organization (PSO) structures and their relationships to one another and certain hospital characteristics.[60] A general conclusion reached by these researchers is that increasing physician participation in hospital management will enhance effectiveness and efficiency and improve the quality of patient care. Later discussions of hospital–physician relationships continue this theme while recognizing the need for hospitals and physicians to be both competitors and collaborators.[61] Physician involvement in governance appears to be associated with greater occupancy and higher operating margins, whereas financial integration was related to lower hospital operating costs.[62] Quality improvement, however, may be an example of a management function in which physicians are reluctant to participate because they distrust hospital management's motives, lack time, and fear that reducing variation in clinical processes will compromise their ability to meet individual patients' needs.[63] Similarly, greater physician-at-large (physicians without clinical privileges in the hospital) involvement in governance has led to a lower likelihood of hospital adoption of continuous quality improvement and total quality management (concepts discussed in Chapter 9) and to a lower degree of clinical involvement in the hospital's quality efforts.[64]

Perhaps no organizational problem facing hospitals is more significant than the need to develop an effective relationship among the GB, management, and the PSO. Numerous means have been suggested. One is to include physicians on the GB. Based on historical data, a GB is likely to have two or three physician members.[65] Another is to appoint nonphysician GB members to PSO committees. This is a relatively easy and politically painless way to coordinate goals. Much effort, cooperation, and patience will be required to develop policies and practices that simultaneously maintain the prerogatives of LIPs and the managerial integrity of the organization.

Caregiver and Support Staff

In 1999 almost 4 million people were employed in U.S. hospitals.[66] Numerous departments/units deliver clinical services: nursing, pharmacy, dietary services, radiology, and laboratories are common. In addition, there is a wide variety of support departments, including housekeeping, maintenance, security, business office, and admitting. Figure 4.5 suggests the range and activity of these various departments/units. The ratio of staff to patients in community hospitals is more than 3 to 1; in teaching hospitals it is much higher. In the future, sicker patients, shorter lengths of stay, and increasingly sophisticated treatment will likely result in even higher ratios of staff to patients. Chapter 11 notes that about 200 different types of positions are needed to staff a general acute care community hospital; more than 300 are necessary for a large teaching hospital. Registered nursing is the most common health occupation in hospitals.[67]

Hospitalists are a new type of physician provider. Typically, they are internists who limit their practice to the inpatient setting and who are employed by a medical group, hospital, or MCO.[68]

Licensure and Accreditation

Hospitals are licensed in all states and must meet those regulations and requirements. In most states Joint Commission accreditation meets licensure and other regulatory requirements in whole or in part. The Joint Commission hospital accreditation program accredited more than 5,100 U.S. hospitals in 1999.[69] Chapter 2 discusses the advantages of Joint Commission accreditation. In addition, various hospital programs and activities may be ISO 9000 certified or accredited by the Community Health Accreditation Program (CHAP) or others.

Future

Successful hospitals must compete for a declining amount of inpatient care and seize opportunities different from traditional activities. One strategy is to develop centers of excellence to diagnose and treat specific diseases; another is to focus on groups such as women or physical fitness and sports enthusiasts. These diagnostic and therapeutic services may be offered on either an inpatient or outpatient basis, with strong financial incentives for the least-costly site. Such initiatives reflect a trend toward market segmentation and boutique medicine. Common, too, are joint risk taking or joint ventures between hospitals and their PSOs and efforts to provide advances in patient convenience and patient-centered care.

Chapter 6 describes the increasing portability of technology and suggests some implications for hospitals. The most important implication is that PSO members will expand the nonhospital portion of their practices at the hospital's expense. Having both to cooperate and to compete with their PSOs puts hospitals in a difficult position. Extrapolating the trend of technological portability suggests significant changes for the inpatient portion of hospital services.

Hospitals, especially those in HSs, will compete with HMOs and preferred provider organizations (PPOs) by contracting directly with employers to provide services. By direct contracting, the hospital (or HS) controls utilization and performance and eliminates the middleman, such as the PPO, thereby reducing costs by reducing overhead. The perils of this strategy include financial risk; failure to understand case mix, utilization, and employer incentives; and inadequately managing the contract.[70]

Despite pressure from ambulatory providers, surveys of public perceptions about both emergency and outpatient care show a preference for hospital-linked care,[71] with a very strong preference for emergency services delivered in hospitals—91% of people surveyed received care there.[72] Of 27.7 million surgical and nonsurgical procedures performed in ambulatory surgery centers in 1994, 85% were performed in hospital-based settings and 15% in freestanding settings.[73] Notwithstanding this strong performance, hospitals will continue to be challenged by freestanding ambulatory providers.

There is speculation that the inpatient portion of acute care hospitals will be large intensive care units because only the most acutely ill patients will be hospitalized. If true, this prediction means staff-to-patient ratios and costs will increase, and the work of hospital managers will become even more complex.

Nursing Facilities

HSOs that serve frail elderly people, those with infirmities, and other people needing skilled care are referred to as nursing facilities. Saint Helena (250–330 A.D.) is credited with establishing one of the first homes for older people (*gerokomion*). "She was a wealthy, intelligent, Christian convert and mother of Constantine the Great. Like other early Christian 'nurses' who devoted their lives to the sick and needy, she gave direct care herself."[74] Many early American towns operated almshouses— or poorhouses, poor farms, or workhouses, as they were also known—for those who were "down on their luck" and who needed a sheltered environment. In the early 1900s affluent elderly people used privately owned boarding houses, and church-sponsored homes for older Americans emerged.[75]

The Social Security Act of 1935 included an Old Age Assistance program with minimal requirements to be met by the states. States could not make payments to residents of public facilities, and this further stimulated growth of small private board and care homes. Most nursing board and care homes were for profit and were operated by people without special training.[76] It was not until 1950 that every state licensed them.[77] In 1951 passage of the Kerr-Mills bill provided federal matching funds to states that met licensing and inspection requirements.[78]

Enactment of Medicare and Medicaid in 1965 placed major emphasis on delivery of skilled nursing care in nursing facilities. The law's positive effects included mandated relationships between hospitals and nursing facilities and improved medical care and supervision and therapies for residents. Negative effects included defining extended care to mean time-limited, posthospital treatment rather than continued care of older adults with physical and mental disabilities, basing the laws on the hospital/medical model, which emphasizes disease rather than functional competence, treatment rather than quality of living, regulations that viewed residents as a group rather than individuals, and the greatest problem—the emphasis on physical rather than emotional and mental needs.[79] As a hybrid of the health care models discussed in Table 4.1 to guide HSO interactions with the people they serve, Stryker suggested the residential model:

> *When health care is delivered in a residential setting, it incorporates client-driven decision making as much as possible in order to maintain the highest possible psychological and physical functioning. What is done for acute conditions in hospital settings is not appropriate for what is done for chronic conditions in long-term care settings. Provision of health care, attention to a quality living environment and as much client decision making as possible characterize both the residential model and long-term care model. The major difference between these two models is the amount and intensity of health care delivered. The long-term care model is expected to provide an increasing amount of health care, but it must not lose sight of its psychosocial goals.[80]*

The average size of nursing facilities and the number of beds increased dramatically after 1965.[81] Initially, federal regulations distinguished nursing facilities by the nursing care provided. Skilled nursing facilities (SNFs) provided the most nursing care. Intermediate care facilities (ICFs) provided nursing services in accordance with residents' needs and were available to residents to help them achieve and maintain the highest degree of function, self-care, and independence. Residential care facilities (RCFs) did not provide nursing care and were only a sheltered environment for which there was no federal payment. States may use a variety of titles for RCFs (such as assisted living), and it is common for various levels of care and services to be provided in different parts of the same facility.

Definition and Numbers

The Nursing Home Reform Act, part of the Omnibus Budget Reconciliation Act of 1987,[82] eliminated the distinction between SNFs and ICFs; beginning in 1991 both were called nursing facilities. The nomenclature, commonly used in place of "nursing homes," will continue to be confusing, however. The Nursing Home Reform Act also addressed training, continuing education, levels of professional and nonprofessional staffing, quality of life, and residents' rights and made numerous other changes, most of which have been judged successful.[83]

In 1999 there were 16,995 nursing facilities with more than 1.8 million beds. The average nursing facility has 107 beds. Most (66%) are owned for profit; 27% are not for profit, and 7% are government owned. In 1999 only 53,138 beds were certified Medicare-only; 608,070 had dual (Medicare and other use) certification; a little more than 1 million were Medicaid-only beds.[84] Nursing facilities must provide skilled services to be Medicare certified. Regardless, they may serve Medicaid and private-pay residents.

Many acute care hospitals operate what were historically called extended care facilities, which provide subacute care. They are now known as hospital-based nursing facilities; in 1999, 13% of nursing facilities were hospital based,[85] compared with 2% in 1990.[86] They function like nursing facilities but have fundamental differences. Hospital-based nursing facilities (subacute units) are likely to be smaller, have a shorter length of stay, and are more costly than freestanding nursing facilities, probably because of a higher cost staffing pattern and staffing mix.[87] Nonetheless, per diem costs in subacute units are estimated to be 40%–60% less than costs in acute care units.[88] These postacute services are important in the continuum of care.

The overwhelming majority of nursing facility services are funded by Medicare and Medicaid. Part A of Medicare covers long-term care services such as postoperative and posthospitalization care, including rehabilitation. Medicaid services are provided to state residents who meet financial and medical eligibility requirements.[89]

Functions

Federal regulations are important to nursing facilities, even though most are not Medicare certified. The Nursing Home Reform Act mandated that all Medicare-certified nursing facilities have a RN director of nursing; a RN on duty for 8 hours a day, 7 days a week; and a licensed nurse (RN, LPN, or licensed vocational nurse [LVN]) on duty around the clock. In addition, the law required sufficient nursing staff to provide nursing and related services to attain or maintain the highest practicable level of physical, mental, and psychosocial well-being of each resident.[90] An underlying purpose was to protect residents' rights by requiring individually focused care plans.

Nursing facility activities are organized into departments: clinical services, such as physician and dental care, nursing, and rehabilitation (occupational therapy [OT], physical therapy [PT], and speech-language pathology); clinical support services, such as laboratory, radiology, and pharmacy; and administrative services, such as housekeeping, laundry, and maintenance. The medical director (CMO) provides direct clinical care and coordinates private physicians and the work of committees in clinical areas. Beginning in 1990, Medicare-certified nursing facilities were deemed to meet Medicaid standards.[91]

Organization Structure

Depending on their size, nursing facility organization structures may be pyramidal (tall), with several levels of management, or flat, with few levels of management. Most nursing facilities are small and have few managers or levels of management between the administrator and staff. A large nursing facility, however, may have several levels of managers between the administrator and staff. These managers perform the typical line and staff functions such as general administration, financial management, and human resources management. An organization chart for a large not-for-profit nursing facility is shown in Figure 4.6.

Governance

Historically, small for-profit nursing facilities were sole proprietorships or partnerships, forms that are rare today. They are organized as for-profit corporations, which will have few directors, thus in effect combining governance and management functions. Larger, for-profit or not-for-profit nursing facilities are organized as corporations and have a GB that is likely to be called the board of di-

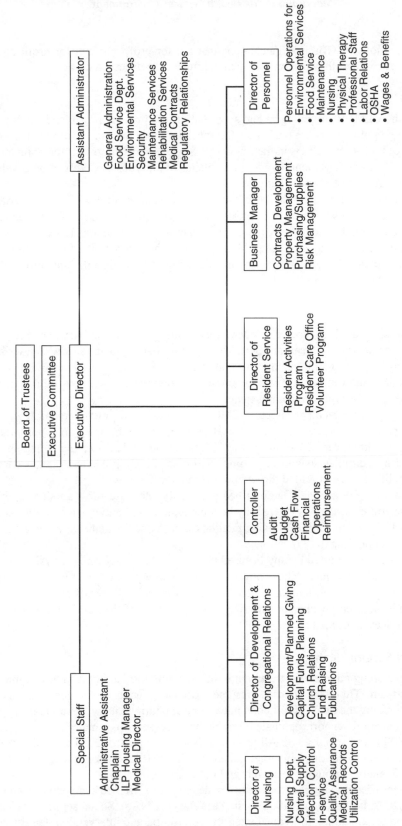

Figure 4.6. Organization chart for a large, not-for-profit nursing facility. (Reprinted by permission of the National Lutheran Home, Rockville, MD.)

rectors. The functions of GBs in organizations that are for-profit and not-for-profit corporations have few differences, and they perform the generic functions discussed earlier.

Management

In addition to the CEO, other managers and special skills are present as size and activities require. CEOs of nursing facilities that are part of a HS, especially those organized for profit, may have little independence and are not CEOs in the true sense. Such systems centralize many functions, most prominently financial management. In addition, policies of all types are likely to be developed centrally and promulgated to the operating units.

All states require that nursing facilities have a licensed administrator of record; variation in licensure requirements limits reciprocity. Most states, however, use the national licensure examination governed by the National Association of Board of Examiners for Nursing Home Administrators to test basic competencies among entry-level administrators. The examination focuses on patient care, personnel management, financial management, marketing and public relations, physical resource management, and laws, regulatory codes, and GBs.[92]

Professional Staff Organization

The PSOs of nursing facilities receiving federal funds must have written bylaws and rules and regulations, just as do acute care hospital PSOs. The content of such documents was described previously. PSOs may be open or closed, concepts that were described earlier. Compared with hospitals, far fewer LIPs are found in nursing facilities. Use of standing orders allows clinical activities to occur without a specific order from a physician.

Medicare requires a medical director (CMO), which is good practice regardless. The CMO may be full or part time and ensures that medical services are coordinated and appropriate, which includes providing direct care. In addition, the CMO is responsible for credentialing and privileging LIPs, ensuring compliance with regulations and disciplinary procedures, and reviewing and maintaining quality of care provided throughout the nursing facility.[93]

Practitioners are credentialed as described previously. Because most nursing facility care is chronic and uses little technology, there may be a perception that patients are at low risk and credentialing may be less demanding. Nursing facilities should use the acute care hospital model and be rigorous in credentialing.

Residents may be admitted by any licensed physician. Residents whose physicians have privileges may be attended by them. These physician services are paid by the resident, either directly or through a third-party payer, including Medicare and Medicaid. The staff of larger nursing facilities may include salaried physicians who supplement the role of the resident's private physician and provide services as needed.

Caregiver and Support Staff

The ideal in developing an effective treatment milieu in a nursing facility is to have a multidisciplinary geriatrics team. The team concept presumes that participants have specialized expertise in gerontology, including the fields of religion/ethics, clinical pharmacology, dental/oral hygiene, medicine, nursing, nutrition support, ophthalmology/podiatry/surgery, psychiatry/psychology, rehabilitation therapy (RT), and social work. All team members are expected to act as patient advocates.[94] These skills are likely to be found in larger nursing facilities. Regardless of internal capacity, all of these skills are available through consultants and volunteers.

Medicare-certified nursing facilities have a wide range of staff. Most are part of the nursing service, including RNs, LPNs, and certified nursing assistants (CNAs). Social services staff are part of intake/admissions, maintaining individual integrity, counseling and intervention, family support, interdisciplinary relations, and referral.[95] Activities coordinators use resident assessments to prepare individualized activities plans whose goals are to "enable the residents to continue their previous lifestyles, enjoying the same activities and leisure pursuits as they did at home . . . , both recreation therapy and activity services are goal-oriented and resident outcome-based."[96] The Nursing Home Reform Act required that Medicare-certified nursing facilities have an activities director and a dietitian. If justified by size, nursing facility staff may include PTs, OTs, speech-language pathologists, and pharmacists.

In 1995 more than 1.3 million FTE employees provided direct and indirect services to 1.5 million nursing facility residents. There were 52.7 FTE staff per 100 beds providing direct patient care in 1995, a ratio that has steadily increased since 1973. The ratio of employees providing nursing care was 51.6 FTEs per 100 beds. Nursing assistants and orderlies had the highest ratio (33.9/100 beds), followed by LPNs and RNs (10.5 and 7.3/100 beds, respectively).[97]

Licensure and Accreditation

Nursing facilities are licensed in all states and must meet applicable regulations and requirements. The Joint Commission has an accreditation program for nursing facilities, but they have no deemed status (as is the case with accredited hospitals under Medicare), and accreditation does not relieve nursing facilities of federal Medicare certification inspections.

Future

Pessimistic predictions of the future for nursing facilities suggest that inadequate reimbursement rates, costly demands of new federal regulations, and sicker residents may cause an economic crisis for them. Demographics support optimistic predictions, however, and suggest that rising demand for nursing facility beds and a more affluent elderly population are harbingers of a bright future. Because of the growing number of nursing facilities, many states apply certificate-of-need requirements to them; others are considering doing so.

Maintaining adequate staffing levels will challenge nursing facilities, especially with regard to technically skilled staff such as RNs and PTs, who have been in chronically short supply. Recruiting and retaining less-skilled employees such as CNAs will be a problem as well.

In 1993 about 25% of Medicare beneficiaries needed assistance in one or more activities of daily living or were in an institution.[98] The level of assistance is likely to increase as the U.S. population ages; this suggests strong future demand for nursing facilities. It is estimated that by 2020, approximately 52 million Americans, or more than 20% of the population, will be ages 65 and older. Of even greater importance in terms of care needs is that the number of people ages 80 and older is projected to double to 14 million by 2025.[99] The number of people needing nursing facility care during the next 30 years is expected to triple.[100] Such data suggest significant opportunities for management careers in nursing facilities.

Ambulatory Health Services

Ambulatory care is not a recent development in health services delivery. Throughout history it has been the most common type. New, however, is the growing proportion of services that are delivered to people who spend less than 24 hours in an ambulatory care facility. Ambulatory care may be defined as care delivered to people who go to a physician's office or other setting under their own recognizance, at a time and place they determine, receive care, and return home. Physicians' offices are the most likely setting for ambulatory services. In addition, ambulatory services have been available for decades in the emergency departments and outpatient clinics of acute care hospitals. Chapter 6 describes how technology increasingly allows significant diagnostic and therapeutic services to be provided to outpatients. From 1990 to 1996, outpatient (ambulatory) services were the fastest growing part of national health care expenditures.[101]

Ambulatory HSOs are a specialized type of HSO that are similar to one another in several respects but have different functions. Ambulatory HSOs provide a wide range of services. Comprehensive outpatient rehabilitation facilities, voluntary sterilization centers, renal dialysis centers, abortion clinics, family planning clinics, podiatric surgery centers, oral surgery centers, birth centers, HMOs, general purpose (same-day) ambulatory surgery centers, eye surgery centers, and dermatology surgery centers are examples of the myriad of different types.[102] Several are discussed in more detail later.

Many ambulatory health services operate as freestanding facilities. The definition of "freestanding" is elusive. AHA defines it as a facility not located on the hospital campus. The Joint Commission considers a facility to be part of a hospital when the hospital is legally responsible for its activities. The concept of freestanding is complicated further by state licensing practices, some of which give hospitals wide latitude to own and operate remote facilities under a single license. Other states require hospitals to hold licenses for both off-campus facilities and separately administered units (separate part facilities) within the hospital building.[103] Complexities are heightened when these considerations are added to the extraordinarily wide range of business affiliations, such as joint ventures, contractual relationships, and vertically and horizontally integrated systems, that might result in establishing an ambulatory HSO. The result is some uncertainty and disagreement about definitions and data.

Medical Group Practice

A medical group practice may be defined as the application of medical services by three or more physicians who are formally organized.[104] The earliest evidence of such an arrangement is found in ancient Egypt around 2500 B.C. in the presence of a whole collegium of doctors, probably all specialists.[105] Throughout the latter half of the 19th century, American surgeons often worked as collaborators in hospital "clinics."[106] One of the first large American multispecialty group practices was the Mayo Clinic, established in Rochester, Minnesota, after the Civil War.

The majority of medical group practices are owned by physicians.[107] In 1997 there were 184,000 FTE physicians in the 7,491 group practices that were members of the Medical Group Management Association, the predominant trade association for medical groups. This number included 3,842 single-specialty groups, 1,469 multispecialty groups, and 2,180 that were undesignated.[108] The predominance of single-specialty group practices continues a trend that began in the 1960s and mirrors the emphasis on specialization and the decline of general practice in medicine that has since been reversed. The most common single-specialty group practice in 1997 was orthopedics.[109]

The large number of formally linked physicians suggests that they recognize the many professional and economic advantages that are enjoyed by group practice, as well as the need for a survival strategy. Competitive and economic pressures will force small group practices to consolidate. In addition, affiliation with networks or integrated delivery systems will allow them to remain economically viable but retain the benefits of a largely independent group practice. Electronic linkages will be very important in this effort.[110] Notably, almost 40% of groups use treatment protocols (guidelines).[111]

Ambulatory Surgery Centers

"Surgicenter" and "same-day surgical center" are names often applied to ambulatory surgery centers (ASCs). The first freestanding ASC in the United States was established in Phoenix in 1970,[112] but hospitals have provided this service for decades. There were approximately 1,200 ASCs in 1989.[113] By 1999 the number had doubled, and more than 2,400 ASCs performed nearly 5 million procedures, the majority of which were ophthalmic, gynecologic, ear/nose/throat, orthopedic, general surgical, plastic, and podiatric. More than 50% of all surgery is performed on an outpatient basis, and is estimated to cost 30%–60% less than hospital inpatient surgery.[114] Overwhelmingly, ASCs are operated independent of either hospitals or HSs. Insurers and managed care providers encourage growth by contracting with ASCs; about 60% of ASCs have business agreements with HMOs and nearly 50% contract with a PPO.[115] It is notable, however, that 82% of outpatient surgery was performed in hospitals in 1990.[116] Rapid growth has occurred in the number of ASCs offering extended recovery care of up to 23 hours, or from 24 to 72 hours.[117] This greatly expands the types of procedures that can be undertaken in ASCs and makes them much more competitive with acute care hospitals.

In 1980 Medicare Part B was amended to include ambulatory surgery, and the regulations identified approximately 100 covered procedures. The list has been greatly expanded. In 1997 Medicare reimbursed for 2,200 ambulatory procedures, almost double the number in 1991.[118] The Health Care Financing Administration (HCFA) has established groups of procedures and pays for ambulatory surgery in a manner similar to the DRG system for hospitals.

Imaging Centers

In 1994 there were 2,151 diagnostic imaging centers, triple the number 10 years earlier. The highest volume of services were radiographs (x-rays) and mammographies, followed by exploratory and experimental scans. More than 22 million patients visited diagnostic imaging centers in 1994. The typical center performed 10,504 procedures per year. A major source of revenue for diagnostic imaging centers was managed care contracts.[119]

Organization Structures

The various types of ambulatory HSOs are organized similarly to typical HSOs, although the specifics vary widely.

Governance

Ambulatory HSOs are almost always corporations that can be organized for profit or not for profit. Physicians are commonly involved as owners-investors, which suggests that many ambulatory HSOs will be organized for profit. Regardless of ownership, the GBs of ambulatory HSOs set policy and evaluate performance of management and, ultimately, the practitioners. GB composition and size is a function of whether the ambulatory HSO is organized for profit or not for profit.

Management

Managers include a CEO, whose title is likely to be administrator, director, or clinic manager. Commonly, the CEO is a physician with special preparation in management. In such cases, a nonphysician administrator or business manager is typically hired to assist the CEO. The skills, knowledge, and abilities of ambulatory services managers include knowledge of health insurance product design, demographics for the service area, systems theory, physician availability, and Internet and management software; being a mentor and providing educational opportunities; and having sales and marketing skills.[120]

Ambulatory HSOs are likely to have flat organization structures with few managerial levels. Larger organizations will have intermediate-level managers as required. Depending on specific activities, the HSO may employ marketing and contract specialists who interact with a MCO if the ambulatory HSO is a preferred provider, for example. The CEO may also act as the CMO.

Professional Staff Organization

Ambulatory HSOs are unlikely to have the number of LIPs that would necessitate a PSO as in hospitals. If physicians are owners and employees, then a PSO is unnecessary. Physician-owners employ other LIPs who are likely to be credentialed less formally than in a hospital. There may be a committee to evaluate performance.

Caregiver and Support Staff

Caregiver staff may include a variety of types depending on the specific activities of the organization. Physician assistants, RNs, LPNs, nursing assistants, surgical assistants, laboratory technologists, and radiology technicians are common. Support staff include secretaries, receptionists, transcriptionists, billing and collections clerks, medical records technicians, and supervisory staff. Some nonphysician employees may have employment contracts. The ratio of FTE staff per FTE physician in multispecialty groups averages 4.63; the ratio in the best performing groups is as high as 5.37.[121]

Licensure and Accreditation

Licensure requirements for ambulatory HSOs vary widely, especially as to which types must be licensed and how affiliation with a hospital affects licensure and regulation. For example, 41 states require ASC licensure; ASCs that receive Medicare reimbursement must be Medicare certified.[122]

Joint Commission accreditation of ambulatory HSOs began in 1975; examples of the wide range of ambulatory care HSOs accredited include ambulatory surgery centers, freestanding emergency and urgent care centers, group medical practices, imaging centers, lithotripsy units, pain centers, primary care centers, sleep centers, and women's health centers.[123] The Accreditation Association for Ambulatory Health Care (AAAHC) also accredits virtually every type of ambulatory care HSO. Examples include dental group practices, college health centers, community health centers, HMOs, hospital-sponsored ambulatory care clinics, independent practice associations, occupational health services, office-based surgery centers and practices, and podiatry offices. AAAHC member organizations include groups such as the American Academy of Cosmetic Surgery, American College Health Association, Association of Freestanding Radiation Oncology Centers, Federated Ambulatory Surgery Association, National Association of Community Health Centers, and Outpatient Ophthalmic Surgery Society. AAAHC began accrediting in 1979 and in 1999 accredited more than 1,000 ambulatory HSOs.[124]

Future

Ambulatory HSOs have become a major force in delivering health services and have challenged more traditional providers for market share. Hospitals responded by developing on-campus outpatient centers rather than pursuing off-campus sites. Off-campus sites proved difficult to operate and manage and often were in conflict with hospitals' ongoing inpatient and outpatient operations.[125] The home health market offers excellent opportunities for multispecialty group practices, primarily because of the continuity of care they can offer and the potential for significant new referrals. Improved and more portable technology, improved drugs, increasing competition between hospitals and their LIPs, and consumer awareness and economics are likely to mean continued strong growth in the number, range, and medical complexity of services that are offered in ambulatory HSOs. "Hospital without beds," customer-oriented ambulatory HSOs will grow in number given that 90% of all cancer treatments are provided on an outpatient basis and the estimates that ultimately 85% of surgery will be performed in the same manner.[126]

Hospice

The modern hospice concept was developed in England by Dr. Cicely Saunders in the early 1960s, but its progenitors were found in India in the time before Christ.[127] Dr. Saunders's work was stimulated by the unsatisfactory conventional treatment of people with terminal illness. Her work led to the establishment of St. Christopher's Hospice near London in 1967.[128] The first U.S. hospice program was established in New Haven, Connecticut, in 1974.[129] Dr. Elisabeth Kübler-Ross is credited with stimulating the acceptance of the hospice in the United States.[130]

Function and Numbers

Hospice has a unique philosophy. Most HSOs use an allopathic philosophy as they intervene dramatically to return a patient to maximum functioning. Hospice, however, does not include therapeutic (curative) intervention even though there are efforts to maximize a patient's quality of life. Hospice provides a special kind of care for the dying; it

1. Treats the physical needs of patients *and* their emotional and spiritual needs
2. Takes place in the patient's home, or in a homelike setting
3. Concentrates on making patients as free of pain and as comfortable as they want to be so they can make the most of the time that remains to them
4. Considers helping family members an essential part of its mission
5. Believes the quality of life to be as important as the length of life[131]

Hospice philosophy contrasts sharply with the medical model. Historically, hospice focused on emotional support, comfort care, and pain control, and provided no artificial medical treatment, including hydration and nutrition. The philosophy is broader today, and it is common to do what is necessary to enhance quality of life without therapeutic (curative) intervention. Hospice is appropriate only when the patient is terminally ill and is no longer seeking active treatment. Hospice stresses patient autonomy and family involvement. In 1995, 60% of hospice patients had cancer, 6% had heart-related diagnoses, 4% had acquired immunodeficiency syndrome, 2% had Alzheimer's disease, 1% had renal diagnoses, and 27% had other diagnoses; the average length of stay was 61.5 days.[132]

Medicare has covered hospice since 1983. Core services required by Medicare include nursing care, physicians' services, and medical social services and counseling, services that must be routinely provided directly by hospice employees. Supplemental services that must be provided, but for which there is no additional reimbursement, include medical appliances and supplies (including drugs and biologicals), PT, OT, speech-language pathologist, home health aide, homemaker, bereavement counseling, and special modalities such as chemotherapy and radiation therapy.[133] Medicare hospice reimbursement is a per diem payment for one of four levels of care: routine home care, continuous care, general inpatient care, and respite care. Actual rates are adjusted annually.[134] In 1998 nearly 80% of all hospice were Medicare certified.[135] Receiving the Medicare hospice benefit requires a physician to certify a medical prognosis of a life expectancy of 6 months or less.[136]

If these requirements and other conditions of participation are met, the hospice benefit in Medicare Part A includes two 90-day periods, followed by unlimited subsequent periods of 60 days each.[137] Both home health care and inpatient hospice are covered. Generous reimbursement led to charges that the Medicare hospice benefit had significant fraud, waste, and abuse. The result was a model compliance plan developed by the Office of the Inspector General of HCFA.[138]

In addition to Medicare, hospice is covered by many Medicaid programs, private insurance, and some HMOs. In 1998 hospice care was covered by Medicaid in 42 states and the District of Columbia, as well as by 82% of managed care plans.[139] Unreimbursed hospice depends on community charitable support, a form of which is the volunteers who are an essential part of the hospice philosophy.[140]

In 1989 only 703 hospice programs (approximately 50%) were participating providers under Medicare's hospice certification program.[141] By 1998 there were 3,100 operational or planned hospice programs in the 50 states, the District of Columbia, and Puerto Rico. During the 1990s the average annual growth of hospice programs increased from about 8% to 17%. Hospice served about 495,000 terminally ill patients and their families in 1997.[142]

Models

There are several organizational models of hospice[143]:

1. *Hospital-based hospice units.* Hospice is a program or department of a hospital. These are sometimes called palliative care units.
2. *Hospital-based hospice team.* Caregivers go to hospital units and sometimes to nursing facilities or chronic-care hospitals. Hospice staff may coordinate all other services.
3. *Freestanding hospital-affiliated units.* These may be located in separate buildings but are affiliated with a specific hospital, usually a teaching hospital.
4. *Home health agency–based hospice.* Sometimes known as hospice without walls. Patients stay at home and receive care from homemakers, clergy, volunteers, social workers, nurses, and physicians.
5. *Freestanding facilities.* St. Christopher's Hospice is the prototype. Such a hospice provides the care and atmosphere needed for comfort and pain control, but no facilities for acute medical care.

A model that is potentially most efficient is coalition-based hospice, in which coordination and administrative support are provided to a group of HSOs such as HHAs and hospitals. In addition, HMOs, Blue Cross, and religious groups may own, sponsor, and operate hospice. Contracts expand relationships; a hospice may contract with a nursing facility for a residence when an individual has no caregiver at home, for example.

Organization Structure

As noted, hospice may be offered in a variety of ways. The sponsoring organization may be a corporation organized for profit or not for profit, although the former are rare. It is clear that hospice is a philosophy, not an institution or building.

The hospice organization structure is flat. Few managers or levels are needed because the hospice tends to be small and there are few staff, as compared with most types of HSOs. Below the director are a few supervisors and the staff. A large hospice has middle-level managers between the director and staff. These people perform the typical line and staff functions such as general administration, financial management, and human resources administration, with the latter especially concerned with recruiting and coordinating volunteers. Because reimbursement and patient service depend on staff providing direct services, hospice minimizes management staff.

Governance

The type of governance depends on whether the hospice is independent or dependent. An independent hospice has a GB similar to that of a freestanding organization. This means the GB has full authority and accountability and performs the generic functions described earlier. A dependent hospice may have a committee that provides guidance, or direction may simply be the responsibility of a member of the parent organization's management team. In the latter case the usual organizational relationships would be present.

Management

Because there are few staff, the hospice has few managers. Typically, there is a director, who may be a registered nurse or social worker, although people with master's-level management preparation are increasingly present. As the hospice movement grows in number and size, opportunities for managers will increase.

Caregiver and Support Staff

The interdisciplinary team described by McDonnell in the mid-1980s[144] continues to be key to the hospice concept.[145] The core team includes the attending and hospice physicians, a RN skilled in patient assessment and training in pain and symptom management, a social worker experienced in family counseling, spiritual counselors, and volunteers. Other team members include OTs, PTs, speech-language pathologists, music and art therapists, massage therapists, hypnotherapists, dietitians and nutritionists, psychologists, and a wide range of community resource providers. Not all types of staff are available daily. Special services might include enterostomal therapy, specialty medical evaluations, and mental health and bereavement counseling.

> *Every member of the hospice interdisciplinary patient care team recognizes the value of his or her own particular level of expertise, in either a professional or personal capacity, for meeting at least one aspect of a patient and family's needs with the awareness that each discipline relates with other disciplines in the delivery of the overall plan of care to the patient. This results in what is often referred to as "role blurring." . . . The strength of the interdisciplinary team . . . is that all members of the team have a common commitment to meet the patient's and family's needs, and this commitment supersedes the boundaries of their own disciplines.[146]*

Hospice makes heavy use of volunteers; more than 80% of the people involved in hospice care are volunteers.[147] A dependent hospice (part of a HSI/HS) is likely to have fewer staffing problems than an independent hospice. Using staff from an acute care hospital or HHA may raise problems of compatible philosophy, however, because the primary philosophy of hospice is palliation, not treatment.

Licensure and Accreditation

In 1998, 43 states licensed hospice, using widely varying requirements.[148] Absent licensure requirements, hospice are likely to be licensed in other categories, usually as HHAs or health facilities.[149] The Joint Commission had a separate accreditation program for hospice from 1983 to 1990, when it was incorporated into the home care accreditation program.[150] Standards for addressing the needs of dying patients also were developed and incorporated into the accreditation process for all health care settings beginning in 1992.[151]

CHAP has accredited hospice since 1989.[152] Its accreditation process is similar to the Joint Commission's, including application for survey, self-study, site visit, and CHAP review of the self-study and site visit. Standards emphasize organization structure and function, quality of services, resources, and long-term viability. The deemed status conferred by CHAP accreditation grants Medicare certification to a hospice without the need for routine Medicare inspections by state inspectors.[153] States that require licensure retain the responsibility of investigating complaints against a hospice despite deemed status through the Joint Commission or CHAP.

Future

Coverage of hospice under Medicare (and Medicaid in many states) was a significant step. There is no nationwide standard on the cost of inpatient hospice, but more than 90% of hospice hours are provided in a patient's home.[154] Home hospice appears to be cost effective, clinically appropriate, and in the patient's best interests. Hospice have yet to specifically address physician-assisted suicide, an issue that is certain to confront them.

The growth of hospice programs has been dramatic. Given U.S. demographics and a likely increased acceptance of hospice for the terminally ill, these programs are likely to achieve continued growth well into the 21st century. Bereavement support and respite care are likely to be increasingly important services provided by hospice.

Managed Care

The first "managed care" can be traced to HMOs, which earlier had been called prepaid group practice plans. The term *health maintenance organization* was coined in the early 1970s during the presidency of Richard M. Nixon and is reflected in the Health Maintenance Organization Act of 1973 (PL 93-222).[155] HMOs resulted from efforts to provide an alternative delivery system based on a unique philosophy about health services. The HMO philosophy stresses a close relationship between patients and physicians and a financial arrangement and preventive measures (compared with the acute treatment emphasized by traditional third-party coverage), and provides incentives to both insureds and providers to minimize expensive inpatient (hospital) treatment. Prepaid group practice plans and early HMOs usually employed physicians who were paid a salary. Enrollees paid a fixed premium that covered all services.

A unique aspect of early HMOs was that, unlike conventional HSOs, HMOs grouped hospitals, physicians, and other health services staff and providers into an "organization"—more accurately, an arrangement—that provided a full range of medical services to an enrolled population for a fixed, prepaid fee. Thus a HMO may have been a set of contracts—a virtual HSO, or an actual organization. It was clearly a forerunner of the PPO. According to Zelten, "the feature which most clearly differentiate[d] HMOs from existing health delivery and financing systems is the combination of delivery and financing within one organized system."[156] From the late 1980s to the mid-1990s, HMOs diversified their products to include point of service (POS) plans and PPOs. (Further discussion of MCOs as health systems can be found in Chapter 5.) POS plans allow HMO enrollees to seek care outside the network, usually with higher cost sharing in both deductibles and copayments.[157] Most HMOs view themselves as MCOs that offer an array of health plans and products, rather than as traditional, closed-ended HMOs.[158] More than two thirds of all HMOs are organized as for-profit corporations, and they have substantially more than half of all HMO enrollees.[159] In 1998, 85% of working Americans were enrolled in HMOs or another form of managed care,[160] compared with 29% in 1988.[161] Another way to state the impact of managed care is that, in 1998 the membership in managed care plans was 76 million and the industry's gross revenue was approximately $173 billion.[162]

Characteristics

HSOs (including HMOs) that provide managed care are commonly called managed care plans or organizations. MCOs have the following characteristics[163]:

1. Arrangements with physicians, hospitals, and other health care professionals to provide a defined set of health care services to members
2. Criteria and processes for selecting and monitoring health care providers
3. Programs and systems to gather, monitor, and measure data on health services utilization, physician referral patterns, and other quality performance measures
4. Incentives or requirements for members to use providers and procedures associated with the plan
5. Activities aimed at improving the health status of members
6. Incentives for providers to encourage the appropriate use of health care resources

The fifth characteristic is a way that managed care differs from traditional indemnity insurance, which pays set amounts to insureds who develop a specific illness or medical condition, and from service plans such as Blue Cross, which historically paid for inpatient hospital services regardless of costs. Conversely, MCOs provide services that keep patients in good health (e.g., annual physical examinations), detect illnesses or conditions (e.g., cancer screening), treat acute illnesses (e.g., hospitalization), and minimize complications from chronic ailments (e.g., home care)—all of which, it is argued, means that the MCO has implicitly made a commitment to keep the enrollee healthy. Opponents assert, however, that accepting a fixed fee encourages MCOs to enroll only healthy people and deny care to enrollees to keep costs down.[164]

Types

The six characteristics in the previous section provide a definition that is broad enough to include managed care Blue Cross Blue Shield plans and managed indemnity insurance plans, as well as HMOs. The organizations and arrangements that meet this definition run a gamut[165]:

Managed care organizations. *MCOs are entities that offer a HMO, PPO, or POS plan, or a combination of them. They can be owned by national managed care firms, physician groups, hospitals, commercial health insurers, Blue Cross Blue Shield plans, community cooperatives, private investors, or other organizations, both for profit and not for profit.*

Health maintenance organizations. *HMOs offer comprehensive health services to members for a fixed monthly fee by contracting with or employing physicians, hospitals, and other health professionals to provide services on behalf of enrollees. Ownership runs a gamut from national managed care organizations to Blue Cross Blue Shield to independent ownership. There are four basic models of HMOs.*

Staff-model. *Physicians and other health services providers are salaried employees who work only for that HMO and generally care only for that HMO's patients. Care is usually delivered at sites owned by the HMO.*

Group-model. *The HMO contracts on an exclusive basis with a large physician practice to provide comprehensive services to HMO enrollees. The HMO and group practice are separate organizational entities. The HMO pays the group, which pays the physicians.*

Independent practice association (IPA)-model. *The HMO contracts with individual physicians or groups of physicians to treat patients in their offices. These physicians are usually organized as solo practitioners or small group practices. IPA physicians may treat nonplan patients.*

Network-model. *A HMO that uses several contracting methods is often called a network-model HMO. The HMO contracts with several larger multispecialty groups or IPAs, rather than individual physicians or small practices. These groups or IPAs treat nonplan patients.*

Preferred provider organizations. *PPOs are networks of hospitals, physicians, and other health care providers that provide services for a negotiated fee. PPOs are often sold as an option (also known as a rider) to a traditional insurance plan. PPOs do not assume the financial risk of the health benefits being offered; risk is often assumed by the sponsoring organization, such as an insurance company, third-party administrator, or self-insured employer. PPOs do not perform many customary HMO functions, such as underwriting, utilization management, and review of quality. (Shouldice argued that a better name for PPOs is preferred provider arrangements because they are brokered arrangements between providers and purchasers of health services, the terms and conditions of which are specified by contract.[166])*

Provider sponsored organizations. *PSOs are MCOs that are owned or controlled by health care providers. Many of the original HMOs were and are provider controlled. PSO is a term that is used to describe the emerging provider organizations that are formed to directly contract (direct contracting) with purchasers to deliver services. Unlike IPAs and other provider groups, PSOs assume insurance risk for beneficiaries. PSOs are formed by organizations such as IPAs, physician-hospital organizations (PHOs), and integrated delivery systems (IDSs).*

MCOs have developed a wide variety of products. Table 4.3 compares closed-panel HMOs, exclusive provider organizations (EPO), open-access HMOs, POS plans, and open-access PPOs in terms of characteristics such as the role of the primary care physician, enrollees' cost sharing, access to specialists (a chronic source of complaints among MCO enrollees), and out-of-network coverage. In addition to the aspects identified in Table 4.3, managed care may have specialty "carve outs" (also called specialty or single-service networks) that offer specialized services such as prescription drugs,

TABLE 4.3.   MANAGED CARE PRODUCT COMPARISONS

	Role of PCP	Patient cost sharing	Access to specialists	Out-of-network coverage
Closed-panel HMO	Member required to select a PCP; PCP functions as a gate-keeper, managing and coordinating care and authorizing visits to specialists	Minimal copayment for office visit; 100% hospital coverage	Must have referral from PCP for coverage	No
EPO	Member not required to select a PCP; PCP does not function as a gatekeeper	Minimal copayment for office visit; 100% hospital coverage	Permits direct access to network providers	No
Open-access HMO	Member required to select a PCP; PCP functions as a gate-keeper, managing and coordinating care and authorizing visits to specialists	Higher copayment when self-referring to a specialist	Permits self-referral to network special-ists with higher copayment	No
POS plan	Member required to select a PCP; PCP functions as a gate-keeper, managing and coordinating care and authorizing visits for in-network coverage	Minimal copayment for in-network care; higher copayment and deductible for out-of-network coverage	Must have referral from PCP for in-network coverage; permits direct access to network providers with higher copayment	Yes
Open-access PPO	Member not required to select a PCP; PCP does not function as a gatekeeper	Minimal copayment in network; coinsur-ance and deductible for out-of-network coverage	Permits direct access to network providers	Yes

Adapted from Knight, Wendy. *Managed Care: What It Is and How It Works,* 34–35. Gaithersburg, MD: Aspen Publishers, 1998. PCP, primary care physician.

dental care, mental health, and vision care, and centers of excellence, or networks of tertiary facilities that provide complex procedures such as organ transplants or cancer therapies. Important considerations that affect managed care products include utilization review and reimbursement.

Health Maintenance Organizations

The genesis of HMOs was in prepaid group practice plans in the late 1920s and the early 1930s. Growth was slow because indemnity and service insurance coverage was widespread, people were reluctant to give up choice of physician, organized medicine opposed HMOs historically, and physicians preferred fee-for-service payment. Opposition by organized medicine resulted in *AMA v. United States,* the landmark antitrust case described in Chapter 14.[167]

In 1972 there were only 72 HMO plans with 4.5 million enrollees. Federal lawmakers' belief in the potential of HMOs stimulated the 1973 legislation that assisted start-up HMOs. By 1982, 265 HMOs had almost 11 million enrollees. In 1990 there were 35 million enrollees in 615 HMOs.[168] By 1998 there were more than 76 million enrollees in 651 HMOs.[169] HMO enrollment is concentrated in large metropolitan markets—more than 72% of enrollees were in markets with populations of 1 million or more; another 21% are in medium-sized markets (250,000–999,999 population). The large markets have an average HMO penetration of 36.9%, whereas the most heavily penetrated exceed 50%.[170] HMOs have reported declining profitability since 1994 and have expanded products such as open-ended or POS plans, Medicare, and Medicaid to improve their financial situations. The results have been mixed.[171]

Independent Practice Associations

The first of what became known as IPAs was begun in 1954 when the San Joaquin Foundation for Medical Care was established by fee-for-service physicians who were competing with the Kaiser Permanente prepaid group practice plan. In 1998 IPAs comprised 65% of all HMOs.[172] In the late 1980s and early 1990s they were the fastest growing type of HMO, especially among those that offered a POS option.[173]

IPAs are a distinct type of MCO that is usually developed to deliver services in conjunction with HMOs or PPOs. An IPA-model HMO is a common example. Some IPAs were established so that physicians could offer their services as a PPO to purchasers such as insurers or employers. Physicians' utilization patterns are reviewed when they apply to become part of an IPA to determine whether they are efficient resource users. Such review continues throughout the relationship.

Increasingly, IPA is a misnomer. IPAs are evolving from a predominantly loose association of independent physicians who contract with a HMO to a form that involves physicians in group practice. IPAs may even be organized around a group practice. A network model results from a HMO contracting with several multispecialty groups to serve a defined population of enrollees. A group model results if enrollees in a HMO are served exclusively by a medical group, and an IPA/network is present when a medical group uses its affiliated IPA to deliver care.[174]

Preferred Provider Organizations

PPOs are a development of the 1980s. Even more than a HMO, a preferred provider is a concept—to the extent that it can be a virtual organization—and not a specific type of HSO. A PPO may be an insurance company, a HMO, a hospital, a medical group practice, an ASC, or an IPA. Regardless, it is an organization, often a HSO or HS, that contracts with employers or enrollees. In turn, it may provide services directly or contract with independent physicians and other HSOs, such as hospitals, to provide services. The PPO concept is broad enough that an employer who offers employees medical services from specific providers with which it has contracts would meet the definition.

In the late 1980s PPOs as a group grew faster than HMOs (which also may be PPOs) because they are seen as a lower-cost alternative.[175] By the end of 1988 there were 691 PPOs with an estimated 18.3 million members.[176] During the 1990s the outlook for PPOs became less certain, however, primarily because their structure has been linked to indemnity insurance and discounted fee-for-service payments. These payment mechanisms are less likely to reduce utilization and costs enough to compete with more aggressively managed and more integrated managed care models. To this extent, PPOs may be a transitional phase through which individuals move from fee-for-service to HMO plans. However, to predict the demise of PPOs is premature, given that in 1997 there were 1,035 PPOs covering 89 million eligible employees. EPOs, a subset of PPOs, covered 3.1 million people in 1997.[177]

Payment

MCOs differ widely in how they pay providers, and most use several different types of reimbursement methods, even in the same market. Salaried physicians and other LIPs in staff-model HMOs are the easiest example. Hospitals may be paid by discounted fee-for-service, per diem or per case rates, DRGs, or capitation, whereas HHAs are usually paid using a per-hour or per-visit fee schedule. DRGs are used exclusively for hospitals; other payment methods, such as discounted fee-for-service, can apply to all providers. PPOs use discounted fee-for-service arrangements almost exclusively.[178] Table 4.4 shows how HMOs are likely to pay various providers: fees or discounted fee schedules, per diem rates, DRGs, capitation (including primary, specialty, multispecialty, hospital care, and full-risk capitation and risk pools or bonus arrangements), and relative value scales (including the McGraw-Hill unit value system, the resource-based relative value scale system, and the American Society of Anesthesiologists' relative value unit system for anesthesia procedures). In addition, MCOs pay based on case rates, per hour or per visit. MCOs are likely to carry a stop loss form of reinsurance that provides financial protection when medical expenses exceed a certain dollar amount or percentage of risk pool funds.[179]

Group- and staff-model HMOs often use salary or capitation payments or both; IPA-model HMOs may use combinations of individual and group capitation, modified fee-for-service arrangements, or both. In 1995 approximately 25% of physicians received some form of capitated payment for their patients.[180] HMOs may offer experience-rated indemnity plans that allow enrollees their choice of providers who are paid fee-for-service and by various types of coverage (e.g., deductibles, coinsurance). Hospitals are most likely to be paid per diem rates. Capitation is most common for primary care physicians in multispecialty groups and for solo or single-specialty practices. Specialty care physicians in multispecialty group settings and in solo or single-specialty practices are

TABLE 4.4.   METHODS OF PROVIDER REIMBURSEMENT (N = 266)

Method of reimbursement	No. of HMOs	Percentage of HMOs
Hospitals		
Fees or discounted fee schedules	187	70.6
Per diem rates	239	89.8
DRGs	128	48.9
Capitation	94	35.6
Primary care physicians		
Multispecialty group settings		
Fees or discounted fee schedules	114	48.5
Relative value scales	63	23.7
Capitation	165	70.2
Salary[a]	26	11.1
Solo or single-specialty practices		
Fees or discounted fee schedules	153	60.7
Relative value scales	82	32.5
Capitation	178	70.6
Salary	12	4.8
Specialty care physicians		
Multispecialty group settings		
Fees or discounted fee schedules	154	66.7
Relative value scales	76	32.9
Capitation	108	46.7
Salary[a]	18	7.8
Solo or single-specialty practices		
Fees or discounted fee schedules	187	75.7
Relative value scales	98	37.6
Capitation	96	38.9
Salary	8	3.2

From *HMO Industry Report 7.1*, 60. Reprinted by permission. © 1997, InterStudy.

[a]Respondents may have reported how the physician was paid by a group practice rather than how the HMO pays the multispecialty group.

most likely to be paid fees or discounted fee schedules. Some financial arrangements involve risk sharing. An example is a capitation arrangement in which the PHO, medical group network, or integrated delivery system is responsible for providing all covered services or contracting for them to be provided. Arguably, if a PHO, for example, understates the capitation payment, then the risks that are assumed are business risks that involve time, personal service, and perhaps income. In general, these risks do not threaten the capacity of the provider to deliver the promised product. Conversely, however, if those at risk must pay for services, rather than provide them, the lack of adequate finances will put enrollees in jeopardy of not receiving the services. States are beginning to treat risk-bearing health services delivery as an insurance product, thus subjecting it to significant regulation.[181]

Competition continues to blur the distinctions between managed care plans and traditional indemnity insurers. There is concern that, as occurred in the indemnity market in the 1980s, self-insuring HMO plans (e.g., PSOs) will erode the insurance function in the HMO market by taking people who are better health risks (their employees) out of the risk pool and leaving sicker people to pay higher premiums.[182]

Organization Structures

MCOs are so varied in how they may be organized that a comprehensive discussion is not possible here. What follows is information generally applicable to MCOs, including specific examples.

Governance

MCOs are corporations that can be organized for profit or not for profit. Both have GBs that set policy and evaluate overall performance. Figures 4.7 and 4.8 are sample organization charts for a HMO and a PPO, respectively.

Management

Managers include a CEO, whose title is likely to be executive director, administrator, or president. It is not unusual to find CEOs of MCOs who are physicians, often with management training. Smaller MCOs are likely to have flat organization structures with few management levels; those that are larger will have a taller hierarchical structure.

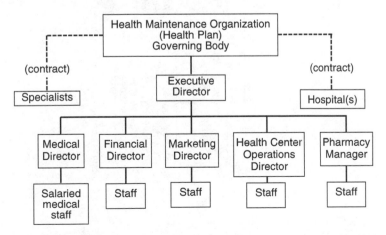

Figure 4.7.   Organization structure of a staff-model HMO. Solid lines, direct lines of authority/accountability; dashed lines, contractual relationships between the HMO and another party. (From Shouldice, Robert G. *Introduction to Managed Care*, 98. Arlington, VA: Information Resources Press, 1991; reprinted by permission.)

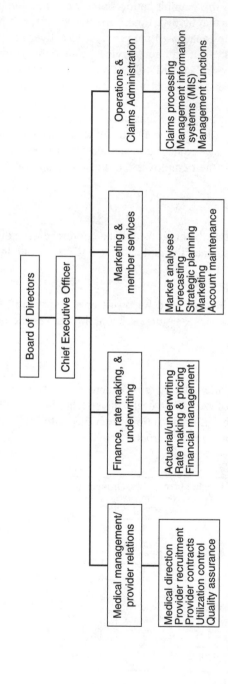

Figure 4.8. Typical PPO organization chart. (From Shouldice, Robert G. *Introduction to Managed Care*, 69. Arlington, VA: Information Resources Press, 1991; reprinted by permission.)

Other managers include those at the intermediate level, as required. Among the most important senior managers is the CMO, who is employed part or full time. As in other HSOs with CMOs, this position in managed care has clinical and administrative responsibilities. Monitoring efficient use of medical and hospital services (utilization review) is a primary activity. Other activities include quality assurance, recruiting clinicians, credentialing, disciplinary action, and developing and implementing policies and procedures related to medical services. Also, the CMO has a role in negotiating and managing provider contracts and in enrollee relations.

Professional Staff Organization

MCOs use various approaches to organizing the professional staff. They are unlikely to use the PSO model found in hospitals, however. The most tightly controlled is the staff-model HMO, in which physicians and other LIPs are employed and are screened and credentialed similarly to hospitals. The least controlled are MCOs with IPA characteristics. In the past, HMOs were unlikely to perform their own credentialing of LIPs; they relied on the credentialing done by affiliated or nonaffiliated hospitals. The numerous disadvantages of this approach, including issues of liability, stimulated MCOs to begin credentialing. In addition, accreditors such as NCQA began to require credentialing by the MCO. Using information provided by the LIP applicant, the credentialing process is likely to include primary source verification: licensure and board certification status, medical education and training, drug dispensing license, hospital admitting privileges, malpractice history and insurance coverage, and any sanctions under the Medicare and Medicaid programs.[183]

Relationships with physicians are established through contracts, which may be employment contracts or service contracts, depending on the type of MCO. Such contractual relationships should be contrasted with those in hospitals, where physicians are unlikely to be employees, use the hospital only to treat patients, and have no financial relationship with it. The least complex contract is found in a staff-model HMO, in which the plan hires practitioner and support staff in all categories and is their employer. Employed nonphysician LIPs may have employment contracts that specify duties and compensation. Support staff are unlikely to have contracts and will be employees at will.

Caregiver and Support Staff

Figures 4.7 and 4.8 suggest the variety of staff and skills that may be found in MCOs. The staff-model HMO employs the widest range of staff, from RNs and other staff who support the work of physicians and other LIPs, to marketers and contract specialists. The ratio of prepaid group practice staff to physicians is from four to five direct paramedical staff per physician, with the average usually on the lower side.[184]

Some PPOs are virtual MCOs because they deliver clinical services using contracts with providers and do not directly employ LIPs or clinical staff. The staff of such PPOs is concerned with finance, marketing, underwriting, and recruiting enrollees. Utilization review is central to maintaining financial viability and is likely found in all MCOs. The wide variety of organization structures means that few MCOs have staff and programs with identical characteristics.

Licensure and Accreditation

There is no specific licensure for MCOs, except to the extent that they must be licensed to perform an activity, such as delivering medical services as a specific type of HSO, or as the states regulate activities relating to insurance. About half of the states regulate the quality assurance activities of MCOs with standards for provider credentialing, member and physician grievance procedures, and medical practice standards used by the plan's quality assurance committee.[185] In addition, 1,100 state laws have been enacted since the mid-1970s that require MCOs to cover certain services in all health insurance contracts, including specific types of treatment (e.g., bone marrow transplants for breast cancer), services of a specific provider (e.g., chiropractic), expanding the categories that a plan must insure (e.g., same-sex couples, part-time employees), and specifying terms and conditions of coverage (e.g., same payments for mental and physical health services). The cumulative costs of multiple benefit mandates have been high.[186]

The Joint Commission accredits MCOs as part of its ambulatory care accreditation program. NCQA also accredits MCOs. Utilization management organizations and credentials verification organizations that support MCOs may be accredited by the American Accreditation HealthCare Commission (see Chapter 2).

Future

Despite their early presence in American health services and the boost that was given them by federal legislation, the number of HMOs has grown slowly. Contributing factors include consumer hesitance to give up choice of physicians and physician reluctance to relinquish autonomy and fee-for-service payment. Major efforts by employers and, to a lesser extent, beneficiaries to control costs will likely eliminate this reluctance in the 21st century, however.

Successful MCOs will have excellent management, will be diversified, and may or may not be legally constituted as HMOs. Many will be product lines of larger health management companies. A fourth generation of managed care may be emerging in which providers such as hospitals and physicians control an organization that includes peer review and utilization review, quality control with computerized monitoring of patient care data, cost control measurement, high standards of practice by LIPs and non-LIPs, and efficient administration in operating the organization as a business. This model is suggested in Figure 4.9.

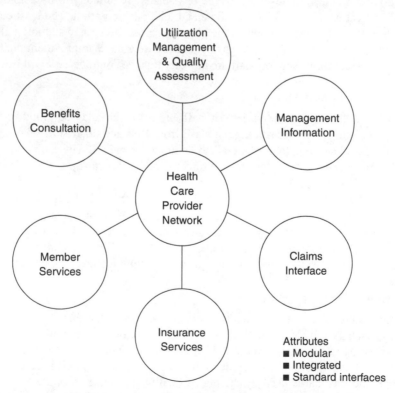

Figure 4.9.   Fourth-generation managed health care organization. (Reprinted with permission from the *Group Practice Journal.* Copyright ©1989 American Medical Group Association, July/August 1989.)

The evolution of managed care that began in the late 1980s gained momentum after the failed Clinton health care reform plan of the early 1990s. MCOs have established their importance among providers, payers, and employers who are eager to control health care costs. Winners in the managed care drama will be those plans—whatever their structure or acronym—that can document delivery of high-quality care in a cost-efficient manner.

Birth Centers

The childbirth education movement since the 1950s began with parents' efforts to regain responsibility and control of the birth experience. The freestanding birth center provides a holistic environment for the practice of midwifery and care of women anticipating medically uncomplicated childbirth.[187]

As late as 1900 fewer than 5% of births occurred in hospitals.[188] It was not until 1940 that half of all births occurred in hospitals, and by 1960 almost all births occurred in hospitals.[189] The movement toward "natural childbirth" was born about 1940.[190] This was the beginning of a small but determined effort to take normal childbirth out of the high-technology setting.

By the 1970s the thrust for natural childbirth, which had been a loosely organized cultural movement among middle-class women aimed at enhancing their experience in childbirth, acquired a social and political cast; women of all classes began to organize, educate one another, and try to change or avoid the professional and institutional structures that exerted such dominance over birth.[191]

In 1975 the Maternity Center Association of New York City opened a birth center that offered obstetrical and nurse-midwife care during labor and delivery in a homelike setting. This created a furor among obstetricians, and their professional organization issued a strong statement opposing out-of-hospital delivery as unsafe for mother and child.[192] Despite this opposition, birth centers flourished, stimulated in part by the increasing interest in alternative medicine.[193] Questions regarding safety remain unsettled, however.[194]

Definition and Numbers

Birth centers are places where healthy pregnant women receive prenatal care and deliver their babies with assistance. The principles for membership in the National Association of Childbearing Centers suggest the philosophy of birth centers: meeting standards of care and safety, not intervening in the process of natural childbirth, taking a personalized approach to the care of families, eliminating unnecessary cost, and seeking the participation of qualified midwives and physicians.[195] Births take place with minimal intervention in a comfortable, homelike environment. Some medical equipment and drugs, such as intravenous lines and fluids, oxygen, infant resuscitator, infant warmer, local anesthesia for repair of tears and episiotomies, and oxytocin to control postpartum bleeding, are available. Birth centers do not provide epidural anesthesia, have no intensive care unit, and do not transfuse blood. They do not induce labor with drugs; very few use electronic fetal monitoring. They provide neither meals nor newborn nursery. Birth centers do not perform operative obstetrics or caesarean sections.[196] Historically, mothers and infants were expected to be discharged within 24 hours,[197] but this policy has been modified by state and federal statutes.

Despite opposition, there were 150 birth centers nationwide by 1988,[198] with a slight decline to 145 in 1999.[199] The goal is natural childbirth, but women using birth centers do not avoid all interventions. Approximately 40% receive some analgesia or tranquilizing medication, 38% have artificial rupture of the amniotic membranes, and approximately 15% are transferred to a hospital.[200]

In 1996 there were 10,278 births at freestanding birth centers, which was less than 0.5% of all births in the United States. About half were attended by certified nurse-midwives (CNMs) and 20% were attended by other midwives.[201] Birth center deliveries are lower cost; the average cost of a 1-day birth center stay is approximately one third less than a 1-day hospital stay.[202]

Organization Structure

Governance

Birth centers may be organized as for-profit or not-for-profit corporations. Most are freestanding; some are attached to hospitals. Most are owned by nurse-midwives or physicians, which suggests they are organized as for-profit corporations. A few are not-for-profit centers.[203] The composition and number of GB members will vary by size and type of ownership.

Management

Birth centers are small HSOs and have a flat organization structure. The CEO is very likely to be a clinician, whether a CNM or a physician. Supervisory staff will depend on the number of staff and range of services.

Professional Staff Organization

CNMs are the primary caregivers. They are RNs with advanced training in midwifery, are certified by the American College of Nurse-Midwives, and are licensed as midwives in many states. Some states require a master's degree for licensure.[204] In 1999 there were more than 6,000 CNMs in the United States,[205] a substantial increase from the approximately 1,500 in 1988.[206] Birth centers may use a "co-management model of care" in which midwives handle most prenatal services, including family issues, education, and the emotional and social aspects of childbirth. This model has been endorsed by the American College of Obstetricians and Gynecologists.[207]

　　Obstetricians may be members of a birth center PSO. Their presence may be required by state law, but they will be on call as backup, regardless, and are available to accept transfers during pregnancy and labor. Birth center PSOs should have bylaws that prescribe their organization, requirements for membership, and delineation of privileges. Consulting obstetricians and pediatricians should have hospital privileges. Birth centers should have a relationship with a nearby hospital for transfer of women in labor who develop complications. Some states license midwives, who are trained laypeople but not RNs. Licensed midwives are unlikely to be on a birth center staff, however.

Caregiver and Support Staff

Compared with other types of HSOs, staffing in a freestanding birth center is of limited scope and complexity. Nursing assistants (who may be certified) assist the CNMs. Support staff include clerical staff, laboratory technologists, and housekeepers. Acute care hospitals provide back-up services in their emergency departments or obstetrics units. They are needed infrequently, however, because only low-risk pregnancies are treated in freestanding birth centers. Volunteers are common in birth centers and are important to the centers' mission and philosophy.

Licensure and Accreditation

Birth centers are regulated in 31 states and licensed in 6.[208] They are accredited by the Commission for the Accreditation of Freestanding Birth Centers, which was established in 1985 by the National Association of Childbearing Centers.[209] In addition, they are accredited by the Accreditation Association for Ambulatory Health Care and the Joint Commission.

Future

Although birth centers have developed a presence in many areas of the United States, they have achieved limited acceptance. This is regrettable because the National Birth Center Study concluded that

> *Few innovations in health service promise lower cost, greater availability, and a high degree of satisfaction with a comparable degree of safety. The results of this study suggest that modern*

birth centers can identify women who are at low risk for obstetrical complications and can care for them in a way that provides these benefits.[210]

Birth centers have an uncertain future. Despite modern origins, they remain few in number and provide services to small numbers of pregnant women. Birth centers will not disappear as a source of care for uncomplicated deliveries, but they are likely to care for fewer patients than their potential suggests.

Home Health Agencies

A program similar to a contemporary visiting nurse association (VNA) provided home health care in Philadelphia as early as 1842.[211] The first sustained effort for home health care in the United States, however, dates from 1893, when Lillian Wald established the Visiting Nurse Service of New York City, as part of the Henry Street Settlement services to the poor. By 1909 she had persuaded the Metropolitan Life Insurance Company to begin home nursing care for policyholders in New York City. The pilot project was so successful that it was adopted in many communities by other insurance companies in the 1920s.[212] Home health care in rural communities was pioneered as a visiting nurse service through the Red Cross.[213]

The first European program to provide services in the home was organized in Frankfurt, Germany, in 1892. A similar program for "home helps" followed in London in 1897.[214] Home help paraprofessional groups did not appear in the United States until the mid-20th century. Homemakers were the first, were often financed by welfare funds, and were available through some VNAs. Home health aides as a group were first included in the federal Kerr-Mills Medical Assistance for the Aged Act in 1960.[215] They were defined as health caregivers (similar to hospital aides) and were distinguished from homemakers.[216]

In 1947 the first hospital-based home health program was established at Montefiore Hospital in the Bronx, New York, to serve patients newly discharged from hospitals. It expanded traditional home nursing care and used an interdisciplinary team that coordinated physicians, therapists, aides, and social workers.[217]

Before Medicare took effect in 1966, most home health care was delivered by voluntary (not-for-profit) VNAs. Except in rural areas, few public agencies were involved. Nursing was the main service offered; homemakers and home health aides were sometimes available.[218] The mainstay of pre-Medicare home care agencies, the VNAs, decreased in number after 1966 because of the expense and risk to small entities of building the care components that were needed for Medicare eligibility.[219]

Definition and Numbers

Contemporary home health care is much more than skilled nursing services; it includes a wide array of services. HHAs are HSOs that primarily provide services including skilled nursing services by RNs and LPNs; PT, OT, and speech-language pathology; medical social work; and home health aides. HHAs may offer home hospice, home-delivered meals, Lifeline (telephone link with clients), and other supportive services. Services often use a multidisciplinary team approach and are commonly part of postacute hospital care.

Medicare defines home health care services as skilled, intermittent, and part time; ordered by a physician; and provided in the residence of the homebound client. Medicare Part A (hospital insurance) and Part B (supplementary medical insurance) cover home health care services without a deductible or coinsurance. If the client continues to meet all eligibility criteria, the number of visits is unlimited and prior hospitalization is unnecessary.[220] In 2000, Medicare payment for home health care services will change from cost-based, fee-for-service reimbursement to payment of a prospective rate for each episode of care, adjusted for patient case mix.[221] This change will require more physician involvement for HHAs to be successful.[222]

In 1997 the United States had nearly 15,069 HHAs, compared with 5,250 in 1986.[223] Three fifths of hospitals operate HHAs.[224] Five of every six highly integrated health systems included home health as a component in 1997.[225] The Balanced Budget Act of 1997 included an interim payment system (IPS) to control home health care expenditures and to provide a transition to prospective payment.[226] IPS resulted in significant reductions in home health care use. Between 1998 and 1999 average visits per patient decreased from 50 to 27; the average reimbursement per patient dropped from $3,384 to $1,844.[227] These unintended effects produced a 20% reduction in beneficiaries served and reduced expenditures by 40%. Individual HHAs that were unable to maintain costs within per-visit and per-beneficiary limits were devastated—more than 2,500 of the 10,500 Medicare-certified HHAs closed between 1997 and late 1999. Thousands of HHAs must repay large overpayments.[228]

By making home health care a medical adjunct to acute hospital services, Medicare changed it dramatically. Since the introduction of DRGs for hospital payment in 1983, home health care has been Medicare's fastest growing component and a major type of hospital diversification. In 1995 expenditures for HHA services exceeded $27 billion, of which Medicare spent $14.5 billion on 3.5 million patients. In 1989 Medicare spent less than one fifth of that amount on half as many beneficiaries. This explosive growth results primarily from cost-cutting efforts but also from shorter hospital stays; new, portable, high-technology equipment; and the growing elderly population.[229] However, despite heavy use and rapid growth, it is not clear that home health care shortens hospital stays:

> *Home health care visits are used primarily to provide long-term care. There is no evidence that services provided at home replace hospital services, and the dramatic geographic variation in home health utilization patterns suggests a lack of consensus about their appropriate use.*[230]

Functions

Skilled Services

To be Medicare certified, HHAs must provide part-time or intermittent skilled nursing services and at least one other therapeutic service—medical social work, OT, PT, speech-language pathology, or home health aide services. At least one qualifying service must be provided directly by agency employees.[231] States that require HHA licensure may have additional requirements concerning qualifying services. Nonskilled providers include home health aides, homemakers, chore workers, and personal care aides—in aggregate one of the most costly parts of home health care services. Other services may include medical supplies and equipment. Most providers use Medicare eligibility guidelines because a large percentage of their clients are Medicare beneficiaries. Many commercial insurance and managed care companies have adopted the Medicare guidelines as well.[232] Medicare regulations are becoming increasingly stringent, and requirements such as licensing or certification for nonprofessional staff and limitations on using independent contractors will increase costs and diminish the ability of smaller HHAs to deliver services, especially in rural areas.

Clients for skilled services are referred directly by or with concurrence of attending physicians, often through hospital discharge planners who identify a need for skilled services and assist the physician with the referral. Hospitals are a major source of referrals of people needing home health care, and this is a cause of concern for freestanding providers.

Private-Pay or Demand Services

Home health clients may pay privately for services because disability, illness, or the infirmities of age necessitate assistance in the activities of daily living, such as bathing and personal care. Although significant, such services are unlikely to be covered by public or private payment. In response, HHAs offer services such as general nursing care, specialties, and therapies; homemakers; companions; house cleaning services; and live-in care. Home health aides and homemaker staff often constitute the majority of employees in private-pay programs that offer such services.[233] This type of client is referred from various sources.

Home Medical Equipment

Another activity of home health services involves home medical equipment (HME), the generic category for respiratory therapy (RT) and durable medical equipment (DME).[234] RT equipment includes oxygen, oxygen concentrators, and associated apparatuses; humidifiers; nebulizers; ventilators; tracheostomy supplies; and the like. DME includes hospital beds, wheelchairs, bathroom aides, walkers, and the like. Third-party payment for HME usually requires a physician's order, and the recipient is subject to qualification guidelines. Medicare often imposes specific criteria for services, especially those with a history of abuse.[235]

Organization Structure

The HHA may be organized in several ways. It may be an independent organization, incorporated either for profit or not for profit. It may be in a dependent relationship with an acute care hospital (or other provider), either as a department or freestanding. Each arrangement has advantages and disadvantages.

The organization structure is likely to be flat, with a CEO, perhaps an associate, and department heads for various specialized activities such as skilled care (provided by RNs, LPNs, OTs, PTs, speech-language pathologists, and medical social services) and unskilled services such as those provided by home health aides. The management team also will include staff with financial, accounting, billing, and information systems expertise. The presence of marketing staff will reflect the increasing attention to marketing the HHA. Foci of marketing include insurers, employers, discharge planners, and case managers in acute care hospitals, as well as private physicians, all of whom are important sources of referrals, especially for non–hospital-affiliated home care agencies. Figure 4.10 presents an organization chart for a freestanding HHA.

Governance

Not-for-profit HHAs that are not hospital affiliated will have a separate GB. A HHA organized for profit may or may not have a GB. If a HHA is a sole proprietorship or a partnership, the owner(s) make(s) all decisions.

Hospital-affiliated HHAs may be freestanding, in which case they have a separate GB. If integrated as a hospital department, the HHA may report through the hospital hierarchy to the hospital GB (perhaps through a subcommittee). Sometimes, an advisory board with no line authority is used. Vertically integrated health services systems or diversified HSOs may have a variety of relationships with the HHA, including overlapping GB membership.

Management

As is typical in small HSOs, small HHAs have few managers beyond the CEO, who uses a title such as director or administrator. In small HHAs the CEO is usually responsible for operations and is also the clinical leader.[236] Larger HHAs have a CEO educated in management, who may have a clinical background. Large HHAs have characteristics and scalar relationships similar to those of large HSOs, and specialized functions are provided by staff; clinical coordinators, a financial officer, and marketing specialists are common. Special attention to reimbursement is important because of the distinct reimbursement and regulatory constraints governing home health care.

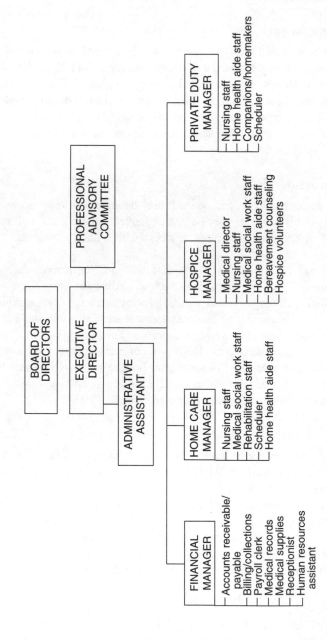

Figure 4.10. Organization chart of a freestanding home health agency.

Home health care is very different from the services provided by most HSOs. It is unique because practitioners work without direct supervision at many individual sites. This necessitates specialized mechanisms to organize staff and ensure quality of care.

Professional Staff Organization

HHAs have no PSO as such. Medicare-certified HHAs must have a clinical director who is responsible for the clinical coordination of services. Skilled care is ordered and directed by the attending physician. Medicare requires that plans of care be reviewed and signed by the physician at least every 62 days for patients to remain eligible for home health care[237]; this requirement is often applied to all clients of Medicare-certified HHAs. Academic medical education programs specific to home health care are rare, and few faculty have teaching or research experience in home health care services. The result is that physicians may be unaware of significant advances in home health services; this undoubtedly limits their effective use.[238] Family practice residencies may include home health care experiences.

Medicare-certified HHAs must have a group of professional personnel, often called the professional advisory committee, that is composed of at least one physician, one RN, and appropriate representation from other disciplines. This group's function is to establish and review annually the HHA's policies regarding scope of services, admission and discharge policies, medical supervision and plans of care, emergency care, clinical records, personnel qualifications, and program evaluation. At least one member of the group is neither an owner nor an employee of the HHA.[239]

Caregiver and Support Staff

The types of services provided suggest the staff. The Medicare requirement for at least one skilled service—skilled nursing, PT, or speech-language pathology—means RNs and LPNs, PTs, and/or speech-language pathologists will be part of a HHA. In addition, OTs, medical social workers, dietitians, and audiologists are typically found in a HHA. A variety of home care providers, including PT assistants, certified OT assistants, home health aides, homemakers, chore workers, and personal care aides are needed to offer a full range of services. PT assistants and certified OT assistants have degrees from technical colleges or junior colleges. Home health aides complete a program through technical schools to become certified. Homemakers, chore workers, and other personal care aides have little formal education and may not be high school graduates. Their activities are largely unskilled clinically but are an important source of service to and interaction with clients. They receive job-specific training. In 1997 it was estimated that HHAs employed nearly 800,000 people.[240]

Licensure and Accreditation

Most states license HHAs, in which case they must meet legal and regulatory requirements. As noted previously, only certified HHAs are eligible for Medicare reimbursement. The certification process is conducted for Medicare by state health departments.

Two organizations accredit HHAs, the Joint Commission and CHAP. (Both organizations' activities are discussed in Chapter 2.) By 1996 home care accreditation had become the Joint Commission's largest program.[241] Accreditation by either the Joint Commission or CHAP after an unannounced survey means the HHA has "deemed" status for purposes of Medicare.[242] In 1996 the Joint Commission and CHAP agreed to reduce duplicate on-site evaluations of HHAs in integrated organizations surveyed under the Joint Commission's Network Accreditation Program.[243] States that require licensure retain the responsibility of investigating complaints against HHAs despite deemed status through the Joint Commission or CHAP. The National Homecaring Council does not accredit HHAs, but its standards assist them to improve quality.

Future

Despite the tumultuous reimbursement environment, the need for home health care is almost certain to increase as the population grows older. In addition to the significant involvement by hospitals and HSs in home health care, it is likely that managed care will become increasingly important.[244] These two concepts are not mutually exclusive. Coupled with aggressive discharge planning, the availability of a HHA, whether hospital owned or not, allows acute care hospitals to reduce lengths of stay and maximize DRG income.

Physicians tend to prescribe therapies they know and use. Therefore, home health care, which historically was low technology and low cost, has become a service filled with high-cost services under Medicare. Use of high-technology diagnostic and therapeutic activities in home health care seems almost limitless: oximetry, glucometry, and portable kits to test drug levels; high-risk pre-natal monitoring, electrocardiography, portable radiology, and ultrasound; management of pressure sores and surgical wounds with healing problems; gastrointestinal drainage systems management[245]; and home infusion (including intravenous antibiotic, chemotherapy, or blood component infusion), parenteral or enteral nutrition, and phototherapy.[246]

Although high-technology services receive more attention, low-technology services that supplement Medicare-reimbursed home care, including companionship, housekeeping, respite care, transportation services, errand-running, shopping, and general security services, are fast-growing parts of private-pay care. This is reflected by the fact that home health aides and homemaker service staff often are the majority of employees in private-pay programs that provide ancillary services.[247]

Home health care expenditures were only 3.8% of total Medicare expenditures in 1987, but they were the most rapidly growing segment of Medicare in the late 1980s,[248] a trend that continued until the late 1990s.[249] Medicare payments for home health care increased from $2.1 billion to $19 billion between 1988 and 1997, primarily because the number of beneficiaries doubled and the number of visits tripled.[250] This rapid growth undoubtedly led to IPS, and the prospective payment system (PPS) that will follow. Success under PPS for HHAs will require careful analysis and reengineering of financial, operational, and patient care systems.[251] The significant changes in the home health industry will increase the opportunities for competent managers.

SUMMARY

This chapter begins by providing a basic, generic background about how HSOs are established and organized. The components of governance, management, and clinical staff are detailed. The roles and relationships among these three elements of the triad are described and analyzed, as are the difficulties this unique organization structure presents for managing the many types of HSOs that have it. Other special problems addressed include credentialing PSO members and dealing with impaired practitioners.

The chapter describes several types of HSOs in detail, including background; definitions and numbers; organization structure, including governance, management, PSO, and caregiver and support staff; licensure and accreditation; and their future. Space is insufficient to identify and describe the myriad of current HSOs or to suggest the potential new HSOs and organizational patterns that may be developed to meet future demands of health services delivery. Those presented run the gamut of the types of organizations that provide health services. They are paradigmatic and assist in understanding management and the organizational principles that apply.

DISCUSSION QUESTIONS

1. Identify the typical legal status of various types of HSOs. Why are they overwhelmingly organized as corporations? (Referring to Chapter 14 might be helpful.)

2. Describe the generic roles and activities of the GB, management, and PSO. Relate these roles and activities to HSO ownership.
3. Describe the triad. Identify the types of problems the triad causes using management terms and concepts. Suggest means to eliminate or minimize the problems.
4. Refer to the discussion of conflicts of interest found here and in Chapters 13 and 14. How do conflicts of interest arise in the roles and relationships of people in the triad?
5. Most types of HSOs have physicians and other LIPs whose credentials are reviewed before their membership on the PSO is approved and clinical privileges are delineated. Describe the credentialing process. How does it differ for an acute care hospital, a nursing facility, and an independent practice association–model HMO? Why?
6. What are the functions of a general acute care hospital? It has been defined as a health team. What other definitions are appropriate?
7. How does the typical general acute care hospital differ organizationally from the usual bureaucratic form? Why? Are these differences necessary?
8. How does the organization structure of a nursing facility differ from that of a general acute care hospital? Relate these differences to the ease or difficulty of managing each.
9. How can relationships between members of the typical PSO (or physicians and other LIPs, if there is no PSO) and management be improved to enhance organizational effectiveness? Why is this important?
10. Federal reimbursement for medical services provided in several types of HSOs was referenced in this chapter. Identify why federal reimbursement is important and the implications it has for managing these HSOs.

CASE STUDY 1: THE CLINICAL STAFF

You are the CEO of Bradley Hospital, a 400-bed voluntary, general acute care hospital. The recently elected president of the PSO has just told you that many members, but especially the physicians, are unhappy because they believe you are trying to control their activities. She stated, "We feel that hospital management should take care of the nonmedical areas and leave the practice of medicine where it belongs—in the hands of professionals."

QUESTIONS

1. How should you respond to the president of the PSO?
2. What arguments should you use to support your position?
3. Sketch an outline showing the appropriate relationship among the GB, management, and the PSO.

CASE STUDY 2: THE EMERGENCY DEPARTMENT

You are the CEO of Holbrook Hospital, which has an active emergency department (ED) with more than 60,000 visits annually. Historically, the department has been organized like that of most hospital EDs. Nursing staff report to nursing service; registration clerks, cashiers, and other clerks report to the admissions department; security officers report to the security department; residents who provide medical services report to various chiefs of departments such as internal medicine and surgery; and the crisis intervention social workers report to the department of social services.

You have just employed a full-time salaried physician as ED director. He has informed you that changes must be made if he is to do the job properly. The basic change is that all nursing service employees must report to him instead of nursing service. He has considerable experience in emergency medicine and has told you that this change will help employees feel a greater *esprit de corps* because they would be in one department rather than dividing their loyalties between the ED and their "home" department. The director believes that this change will promote efficiency, boost morale, and make coordinating work in the ED easier.

The director of nursing service is not pleased with the proposal. She has told you that, if the change is approved, the ED director should not expect nursing service to provide staff even in an emergency. For example, if an ED nurse does not report because of illness, the director will have to call in other ED nurses, rather than expect nursing service to move nurses from elsewhere in the hospital. At present, when ED needs more nurses, either because of absenteeism or sudden increased activity, nurses are pulled from various floors.

The director of nursing pointed out, too, that in the past nursing service, with help from the human resources department, has been responsible for recruiting and training ED nursing staff. If the change is made, she thinks the ED director should be responsible for these activities as well.

Currently, operating room (OR) nurses report to nursing service even though a salaried chief of surgery heads the department. The same is true in the intensive care unit (ICU), where nurses report to nursing service even though a salaried physician is head of ICU. These physicians are unconcerned that nursing employees report to nursing service because they retain responsibility for directing the nurses' professional activities.

QUESTIONS

1. Why does the ED director want nursing staff to have a line relationship to him?
2. What advantages and disadvantages would this line relationship have when compared with the pattern in the OR and the ICU?
3. Will this change accomplish the things the ED director claims (better *esprit de corps,* efficiency, morale, coordination)? Why? Why not?
4. What decision should you as CEO make? Why?

CASE STUDY 3: AUTHORITY RELATIONSHIPS

You were recently appointed CEO of Green Acres, a 300-bed nursing facility, after your predecessor retired. You found many problems. Your predecessor refused to delegate authority, and all 17 department heads report to you. You have been unable to determine the quality of their performance, but you believe that most will not meet your expectations. One reason for this belief is that, because the former CEO did not delegate, department heads could not develop their managerial skills. As a result, they now come to you for every decision, and you are asked constantly for permission to do the smallest things.

In contrast, the CMO functioned with such freedom that you are concerned that the facility will not be able to pass the next Joint Commission survey. Patient records are poorly organized and often unavailable, and there are no minutes of PSO committee meetings. Your philosophy is that members of the PSO should have considerable autonomy but that the GB is legally responsible for the facility and management, and the PSO must be a team if organizational objectives are to be met.

QUESTIONS

1. As the new CEO, what should you do? (Resigning is not an option!)
2. What priorities should you establish? Why?
3. What major problems do you face in making changes?

4. Would it be easier to solve these problems in a for-profit or in a not-for-profit organization? Why?

CASE STUDY 4: THE ORTHOPEDIC SURGERY GROUP PRACTICE

Your executive assistant prepared the following data about the 15-member orthopedic surgery group practice where you were recently appointed administrator.

1. *Membership status* in the PSOs at the 4 community hospitals where 15 of the members of the group admit patients for surgery:
   Active members: 6
   Associate members: 9
   TOTAL: 15
2. *Board certification:*
   Board certified: 8
   Eligible to take boards: 3
   Failed boards twice: 4
3. *Age distribution:*
   Average age: 59
   Range: 34–68
4. *Surgical procedures performed:*

Type	Year					
	1998	1999	2000 (proj.)	2001 (proj.)	2002 (proj.)	2003 (proj.)
Major	3,351	2,801	2,922	2,545	2,300	2,340
Minor	3,911	4,265	4,198	4,077	4,100	4,150
Total	7,262	7,066	7,120	6,622	6,400	6,490

QUESTIONS

1. Prepare an analysis of these data that will be given to the management committee of the group practice.
2. What recommendations will you make?
3. What additional data should you request?

CASE STUDY 5: THE RIGHT THING TO DO[252]

Mr. Sterling, CEO of University Hospital, leaned back in his chair and contemplated the document in his hands with mild disbelief. The "Executive Summary of the Hospice Inpatient Unit Feasibility Study" was concise and emphatic. All committee members had individually summarized their reasons for recommending establishment of a discrete inpatient hospice unit at the hospital. The summary noted, too, that if the hospital and/or its physicians failed to provide or disclose the hospice option to terminally ill patients, such action might constitute a harm that could be unethical or illegal. Failing to inform terminally ill patients about the option of hospice, whether located in or out of the hospital, was unacceptable to the committee.

   Professional perspectives included:

1. Hospital legal counsel—Disclosing the hospice option may be a tort in negligence because it fails to meet the duty owed by physicians to inform patients of alternative forms

of treatment. It could also be actionable as a breach of physicians' fiduciary duty to give patients information that is in their best interests to know.

2. Hospital physician-ethicist—Failing to disclose the hospice option could be judged as manipulating information, an external constraint on autonomous decision making. Failing to seek the greater balance of good over harm for the patient, as seen by the patient, is unethical.
3. Member of GB, known as board of trustees—Institutional policies and mission statements affirm the patient's right to self-determination. University Hospital is in an academic health center and well positioned for hospice care. Interorganizational relationships offer well-developed referral patterns; patient volume is sufficient to fill a hospice unit; and the trustees take pride in community perceptions that the hospital, and their role in it, is to provide innovative medical and nonmedical care.
4. Physician director, ICU—On reflection, recent increases in ethics consultations for ICU patients and their families were largely attributable to the many terminally ill patients inappropriately referred to ICU. Availability of an in-house hospice as a resource for patients, families, and physicians would reduce inappropriate referrals.

Mr. Sterling considered the recommendations. From his viewpoint there was financial risk in creating a discrete inpatient hospice unit, as well as in changing from income-generating, high-technology care to low-technology, palliative care with a possible reduction in reimbursement. However, he also realized that even if the hospice lost money, benefits might outweigh losses: as part of the hospital, the hospice would provide charitable or altruistic services to the community, thereby justifying its valuable tax-exempt status.

Mr. Sterling realized that he had an opportunity to do something that made sense medically, reduced legal risks, and met high ethical standards. He wondered, however, about the economic implications for the hospital and for some PSO members, especially those who treated many terminally ill patients. What was the right thing to do?

QUESTIONS

1. A large academic health center might be able to invest in an inpatient hospice unit. Could a medium-size community hospital do so? What are the implications of enhanced fundraising and/or public relations in this decision?
2. Even if a hospital lost money on an inpatient hospice unit, how does it contribute to the system, and what noneconomic factors are important? Can a HSO overlook the ethical and legal implications of disclosing this option to terminally ill patients?
3. Would your decision be different if ethical, legal, and medical factors supported establishing an inpatient hospice unit, but a number of physicians viewed it as an economic threat to their practices?

NOTES

1. Geisel, Theodor Seuss (Dr. Seuss). *If I Ran the Zoo,* 1. New York: Random House, 1950.
2. The Joint Commission on Accreditation of Healthcare Organizations defines LIP as "Any individual permitted by law and by the organization to provide care and services without direction or supervision, within the scope of the individual's license and consistent with individually granted clinical privileges." (Joint Commission on Accreditation of Healthcare Organizations. *Comprehensive Accreditation Manual for Hospitals, Refreshed Core, January 1998,* MS-15. Oakbrook, IL: Joint Commission on Accreditation of Healthcare Organizations, 1998.)

3. Nathanson, Martha Dale. *Home Health Care Answer Book: Legal Issues for Providers,* 33. Gaithersburg, MD: Aspen Publishers, 1995.

4. Weber, Max. *The Theory of Social and Economic Organizations,* 151–157. Translated by A.M. Henderson and Talcott Parsons. New York: The Free Press, 1947.

5. Kovner, Anthony R., Roger A. Ritvo, and Thomas P. Holland. "Board Development in Two Hospitals: Lessons from a Demonstration." *Hospital & Health Services Administration* 41 (Spring 1997): 98.

6. American Hospital Association. *Role and Functions of the Hospital Governing Board,* 1–4. Chicago: American Hospital Association, 1990. This statement is unchanged as of April 1999.

7. "Trustees in Transition." *Trustee* 51 (July/August 1998): 16.

8. "Trustees in Transition," 15.

9. Asplund, Jon. "Report Reveals Docs' Fears of Hospital Execs—and Vice Versa." *AHA News* 34:9 (March 9, 1998): 5.

10. Asplund, Jon. "Physician Relations." In *Leadership Report 1998: Key Issues Shaping the Future of Health Care,* edited by Alden Solovy, 181–184. Chicago: American Hospital Publishing, 1998.

11. Harvey, James D. "Evaluating the Performance of the Chief Executive Officer." *Hospital & Health Services Administration* 23 (Spring 1978): 5–21.

12. "Trustees in Transition," 17.

13. "Better Boards and Beyond." *Hospitals & Health Networks* 71 (April 5, 1997): 80, 82, 84.

14. Kovner, Anthony R. "The Hospital Administrator and Organizational Effectiveness." In *Organization Research on Health Institutions,* edited by Basil Georgopoulos, 373. Ann Arbor: Institute for Social Research of the University of Michigan, 1972.

15. Joint Commission, *Comprehensive Accreditation Manual,* MA-3.

16. *Health Care Competition Week* 8 (May 20, 1991): 1.

17. McConnell, Charles R. "Fattened and Flattened: The Expansion and Contraction of the Modern Organization." *The Health Care Supervisor* 17 (September 1998): 72–83.

18. Drucker, Peter F. "The Coming of the New Organization." *Harvard Business Review* 66 (January–February 1988): 45–53.

19. Lambdin, Morris, and Kurt Darr. *Guidelines for Effectively Organizing the Professional Staff.* Baltimore: Health Professions Press, 1999.

20. Asplund, "Physician Relations," 163.

21. Lumb, Eileen W., and Roger M. Oskvig. "Multidisciplinary Credentialing and Privileging: A Unified Approach." *Journal of Nursing Care Quality* 12 (April 1998): 36–43.

22. It is unclear whether the Americans with Disabilities Act of 1990 (PL 101-336, 42 U.S.C. § 12101 *et seq*) applies to nonemployed LIPs who practice in HSOs. Given the uncertainty, prudent HSOs will ask questions about mental and physical health status only after a conditional offer of appointment to the PSO has been made.

23. Lambdin and Darr, *Guidelines for Organizing,* 7–10.

24. Health Care Quality Improvement Act of 1986, PL 99-660, 100 Stat. 3784 (1986).

25. Lambdin and Darr, *Guidelines for Organizing,* 19–22.

26. "More Non-MDs Eligible for Med Staffs." *Trustee* 43 (November, 1990): 26.

27. Lambdin and Darr, *Guidelines for Organizing,* 14–16.

28. American Podiatric Medical Association. "Podiatric Medicine: The Physician, the Profession, the Practice." *http://www.apma.org/podiat.html,* March 26, 1999.

29. Ewell, Charles M. "Economic Credentialing: Balancing Quality with Financial Reality." *Trustee* 44 (March 1991): 12.

30. Kolb, Deborah S., Randall L. Hughes, and C. Edward Young. "Economic Credentialing." *Journal of Health Care Finance* 19 (Spring 1993): 58–67. Potential review criteria include length of stay and charges by DRG, severity-adjusted charges or length of stay, utilization review denials, bad debt/write-offs, cost of malpractice when hospital is a defendant, timeliness of medical record completion, and incident reports.

31. Riley, Donovan W. "Economic Credentialing of Physicians: New Criteria and Evaluation of Physicians." *Spine* 21 (1996): 141–146.

32. An excellent treatment of the issues of physician domain and turf conflicts is found in Bloom, Stephanie Lin. "Hospital Turf Battles: The Manager's Role." *Hospital & Health Services Administration* 36 (Winter 1991): 590–599.

33. Salant, Jonathan D. "Doctors, Nurses Wage Costly Lobbying Battle." *The Washington Times,* December 29, 1998, B9. This article describes the dispute between anesthesiologists and certified registered nurse-anesthetists (CRNAs) regarding a HCFA proposal to allow states to decide whether nurse-anesthetists can administer anesthesia without an anesthesiologist's supervision. (Currently, HCFA requires physician supervision when a nurse-anesthetist is used during surgery on a Medicare or Medicaid patient.) CRNAs earn about one third the salary of anesthesiologists, and HSOs and managed care plans will make greater use of them if the proposed regulations are adopted.

34. Griffith, John R. *The Well-Managed Healthcare Organization,* 4th ed., 673. Chicago: Health Administration Press/AUPHA Press, 1999.

35. Orlikoff, James E., and Mary K. Totten. "New Relationships with Physicians: An Overview for Trustees." *Trustee* 50 (July/August 1997): W1–W4.

36. Council on Mental Health of the American Medical Association. "The Sick Physician: Impairment by Psychiatric Disorders, Including Alcoholism and Drug Dependence." *Journal of the American Medical Association* 223 (February 5, 1973): 684–687; Teich, Jeffrey. "How to Bring the Impaired Physician to Treatment." *Hospital Medical Staff* 11 (September 1982): 8–14.

37. Jacyk, William. "Impaired Physicians: They Are Not the Only Ones at Risk." *Canadian Medical Association Journal* 141 (July 15, 1989): 147; Talbott, G. Douglas, and Karl V. Gallegos. "The Pilot Impaired Physicians Epidemiologic Surveillance System." *QRB* 14 (April 1988): 133.

38. Fugedy, James. "Should Hospitals Test Doctors for Drugs?" *The Washington Post,* Health, July 16, 1991, 14.

39. Perignon, Maria-Caroline. "This is Your Doc on Drugs." *The Wall Street Journal,* September 15, 1997, A20.

40. Montoya, Isaac D., Jerry W. Carlson, and Alan J. Richard. "An Analysis of Drug Abuse Policies in Teaching Hospitals." *Journal of Behavioral Health Services & Research* 26 (February 1999): 28–38.

41. Fiesta, J. "The Impaired Nurse: Who is Liable?" *Nursing Management* 21:10 (October 1990): 20, 22.

42. Stryker, Ruth. "Characteristics of the Long-Term Care Model." In *Creative Long-Term Care Administration,* 3rd ed., edited by George Kenneth Gordon and Ruth Stryker, 17. Springfield, IL: Charles C Thomas, 1994.

43. American Hospital Association. "1999 AHA Hospital Statistics." *http://www.aha.org/state_metro/trendanalysis/tahospstats.html,* February 25, 1999; American Hospital Association, "Fast Facts on U.S. Hospitals from *Hospital Statistics." http://www.aha.org/resource/newpage.html,* March 21, 2000.

44. Green, Jeffrey. "50 Community Hospitals Closed, 43 Opened in 1990." *AHA News* 27 (March 18, 1991): 1; Burda, David. "Hospital Closings Down." *Modern Healthcare* 24 (March 28, 1994): 3. The AHA stopped reporting hospital closure data in 1995. (Burda, David. "AHA to Drop Controversial Closure Report." *Modern Healthcare* 25 [June 5, 1995]: 2.)

45. Office of Evaluation and Inspection, Department of Health and Human Services. "Hospital Closure: 1996." *http://waisgate.hhs.gov/cgi-bin/wai...015564238+3+0+0&WAISaction=retrieve,* March 24, 1999.

46. " 'Chain Reaction' Blamed for Closure of 76 Hospitals in 1989." *AHA News* 27 (February 18, 1991): 2.

47. Cleverly, William O. "More Efficient Hospitals Are Closing." *Healthcare Financial Management* 47 (April 1993): 82.

48. American Hospital Association, "1999 AHA Hospital Statistics," 4.

49. American Hospital Association, "1999 AHA Hospital Statistics," 2–4.

50. American Hospital Association, "1999 AHA Hospital Statistics," 3.

51. Federated Ambulatory Surgery Association. "History and Growth of the Ambulatory Surgery Center Industry." *http://www.fasa.org/about_fasa.html,* March 26, 1999.

52. "What Hospitals Do." *AHA News* 35 (March 1, 1999): 6.

53. Pointer, Dennis D. "Governance 100 Survey: Membership Makeup of Hospital Boards Hasn't Changed Much—Yet." *Hospitals & Health Networks* 68 (June 5, 1994): 76.

54. Pointer, "Governance 100 Survey," 76.

55. Alexander, Jeffrey. *The Changing Character of Hospital Governance,* 15–16. Chicago: The Hospital Research and Educational Trust, 1990.

56. Alexander, *The Changing Character,* 13–14.

57. Georgopoulos and Mann. *Community General Hospital.* New York: Macmillan, 1962. (Cited in Shortell, Stephen M. "Hospital Medical Staff Organization: Structure, Process, and Outcome." *Hospital Administration* 19 (Spring 1974): 104.

58. Roemer and Friedman. *Doctors in Hospitals, Medical Staff Organization and Hospital Performance.* Baltimore: The Johns Hopkins University Press, 1971. (Cited in Shortell, Stephen M. "Hospital Medical Staff Organization: Structure, Process, and Outcome." *Hospital Administration* 19 (Spring 1974): 104.

59. Neuhauser, Duncan. *The Relationship Between Administration Activities and Hospital Performance* (Research Series No. 28). Chicago: University of Chicago Center of Health Administration Studies, 1971; Shortell, Stephen M. "Hospital Medical Staff Organization: Structure, Process, and Outcome." *Hospital Administration* 19 (Spring 1974): 104.

60. Shortell, Stephen M., and Connie Evashwick. "The Structural Configuration of U.S. Hospital Medical Staffs." *Medical Care* 19 (April 1981): 419.

61. Shortell, Stephen M. "The Medical Staff of the Future: Replanting the Garden." *Frontiers of Health Services Management* 1 (February 1985): 3–48; Shortell, Stephen M. "Revisiting the Garden: Medicine and Management in the 1990s" *Frontiers of Health Services Management* 7 (Fall 1990): 3–32.

62. Goes, James B., and ChunLiu Zhan. "The Effects of Hospital-Physician Integration Strategies on Hospital Financial Performance." *Health Services Research* 30 (October 1995): 507.

63. Blumenthal, David, and Jennifer N. Edwards. "Involving Physicians in Total Quality Management: Results of a Study." In *Improving Clinical Practice: Total Quality Management and the Physician,* edited by David Blumenthal and Ann C. Scheck, 229–266. San Francisco: Jossey-Bass, 1995.

64. Weiner, Bryan J., Stephen M. Shortell, and Jeffrey Alexander. "Promoting Clinical Involvement in Hospital Quality Improvement Efforts: The Effects of Top Management, Board, and Physician Leadership." *Health Services Research* 32 (October 1997): 491–510.

65. Alexander, *The Changing Character,* 17.

66. American Hospital Association. "Trend Watch: Hospital Employment Up in May." *AHA News* 35:22 (June 7, 1999): 2.

67. American Hospital Association. "Changes in Staffing Mix." *Emerging Trends* 14 (Summer 1998): 6.

68. *Research Activities* 226 (May 1999): 10–11.

69. Joint Commission on Accreditation of Healthcare Organizations, personal communication, January 26, 1999.

70. Gee, E. Preston, and Allan Fine. "Dealing Direct." *Hospital & Health Networks* 71 (August 20, 1997): 46–48.

71. Robertson, E. Marie. "Hospitals Still Hold the Lead in Emergency and Outpatient Care." *Health Care Competition Week* 6 suppl. (December 11, 1989): 7–10.

72. Robertson, E. Marie. "Hospitals, Doctors Losing Ground to Diagnostic Centers for Outpatient Care." *Health Care Competition Week* 8 suppl. (March 25, 1991): 1–2, 7–8.

73. Hall, Margaret Jean, Lola Jean Kozak, and Brenda S. Gillum. "National Survey of Ambulatory Care: 1994." *Statistical Bulletin-Metropolitan Life Insurance Company* 78 (July 18, 1997); "LEXIS-NEXIS Academic Universe." http://web.lexis-nexis.com/universe...d5=b6fbb5cc418a49ef59c9e5371ec166e, April 1, 1999.

74. Stryker, Ruth. "Historical Obstacles to Managing Organizations for the Aged." In *Creative Long-Term Care Administration,* edited by George Kenneth Gordon and Ruth Stryker, 3rd ed., 6. Springfield, IL: Charles C Thomas, 1994.

75. Stryker, "Historical Obstacles," 7.

76. American Nursing Home Association. *Nursing Home Fact Book, 1970–1971,* 3. Washington, DC: American Nursing Home Association, n.d.

77. American Nursing Home Association, *Nursing Home Fact Book,* 3.

78. American Nursing Home Association, *Nursing Home Fact Book,* 4.

79. Stryker, "Historical Obstacles," 8.

80. Stryker, "Characteristics," 18.

81. American Nursing Home Association, *Nursing Home Fact Book,* 5.
82. Omnibus Budget Reconciliation Act of 1987, PL 100-203, 101 Stat. 1330 (1987).
83. Marek, Karen Dorman, Marilyn J. Rantz, Claire M. Fagin, and Janet Wessel Krejci. "OBRA '87: Has It Resulted in Positive Change in Nursing Homes?" *Journal of Gerontological Nursing* 22 (December 1996): 32–40.
84. American Health Care Association. "National Data on Nursing Facilities." *http://www.ahca.org/who/profile4.htm,* January 22, 1999.
85. American Health Care Association. "National Data on Nursing Facilities."
86. Marion Merrell Dow, Inc. *Managed Care Digest: Long Term Care,* 12. Kansas City, MO: Marion Merrell Dow, Inc., 1991.
87. "Profile of Medicare Skilled Nursing Facilities." *Health Care Financing Review,* Medicare and Medicaid Statistical Supplement (1996): 70–71.
88. Gemignani, Janet. "A Big Niche for a Lower Notch of Care." *Business and Health* 15 (May 1997): 45–46.
89. American Health Care Association. "National Data on Nursing Facilities."
90. Harrington, Charlene, Helen Carrillo, Joe Mullan, and James H. Swan. "Nursing Facility Staffing in the States: The 1991–1995 Period." *Medical Care Research and Review* 55 (September 1998): 334–363.
91. Office of Information Analysis. *1990 HCFA Statistics,* 19. Baltimore: Health Care Financing Administration, 1990.
92. Singh, Douglas A., Leiyu Shi, Michael E. Samuels, and Roger L. Amidon. "How Well Trained Are Nursing Home Administrators?" *Hospital & Health Services Administration* 42 (Spring 1997): 102.
93. Levinson, Monte J., and Jonathan Musher. "Current Role of the Medical Director in Community-Based Nursing Facilities." *Clinics in Geriatric Medicine* 11 (August 1995): 343–358.
94. Rogers, Elizabeth L. "Physicians and the Long-Term Care Team." In *Medical Direction in Long Term Care: Clinical and Administrative Guide,* edited by Steven A. Levenson, 175. Owings Mills, MD: Rynd Communications, 1988.
95. Stryker, Ruth, and George Gordon. "Social Services in Long-Term Care." In *Creative Long-Term Care Administration,* edited by George Kenneth Gordon and Ruth Stryker, 3rd ed., 237–242. Springfield, IL: Charles C Thomas, 1994.
96. Selman, Catherine R., and Karen B. Land. "PPS: Why You Still Need Certified Activity Professionals." *Nursing Homes* 47 (November/December 1998): 44.
97. Strahan, Genevieve W. "An Overview of Nursing Homes and Their Current Residents: Data from the 1995 National Nursing Home Survey." *NCHS Advance Data* 280 (January 23, 1997): 5–6.
98. Feder, Judith, and Jeanne Lambrew. "Why Medicare Matters to People Who Need Long-Term Care." *Health Care Financing Review* 18 (Winter 1996): 99.
99. Williams, T. Franklin, and Helena Temkin-Greener. "Older People, Dependency, and Trends in Supportive Care." In *The Future of Long-Term Care: Social and Policy Issues,* edited by Robert H. Binstock, Leighton E. Cluff, and Otto von Mering, 51–52. Baltimore: The Johns Hopkins University Press, 1996.
100. Atkins, G. Lawrence, Vern L. Bengston, Robert H. Binstock, Christine K. Cassell, Linda K. George, and Vernon L. Greene. *Old Age in the 21st Century: A Report to the Assistant Secretary for Aging, U.S. Department of Health and Human Resources* (The Maxwell School, Syracuse, NY), 10. Syracuse, NY: National Academy on Aging, 1994.
101. Lake, Timothy. "Current Trends in Health Plan Payment Methods for the Facility Costs of Outpatient Care." *Journal of Health Care Finance* 25 (Winter 1998): 1–8.
102. Duggar, Benjamin C. "Ambulatory Surgery Facilities: Definition and Identification." *Journal of Ambulatory Care Management* 13 (February 1990): 2–3.
103. Duggar, "Ambulatory Surgery Facilities," 2–3.
104. Havlicek, Penny L. *Medical Groups in the U.S.,* 1. Chicago: American Medical Association, 1984. The definition of "medical group" will be affected by regulations that are being developed pursuant to the federal fraud and abuse amendments (Stark II), which are discussed in Chapter 14.
105. Sigerist, Henry E. *A History of Medicine. Vol. I, Primitive and Archaic Medicine,* 320. New York: Oxford University Press, 1951.

106. Madison, Donald L. "Notes on the History of Group Practice: The Tradition of the Dispensary." *Medical Group Management Journal* 37 (September/October 1990): 54.

107. Hoechst Marion Roussel. *Managed Care Digest Series: Medical Group Practice Digest,* 6. Kansas City, MO: Hoechst Marion Roussel, 1998.

108. Hoechst Marion Roussel, *Managed Care Digest Series: Institutional Digest,* 4. Kansas City, MO: Hoechst Marion Roussel, 1998. The American Medical Group Association had 119 group practice members with 37,000 physicians, Hoechst Marion Roussel, *Managed Care Digest Series,* 33.

109. Hoechst Marion Roussel, *Managed Care Digest Series,* 6.

110. McManis, Gerald L., Louis Pavia, Jr., F. Kenneth Ackerman, Jr., and Isabel Connelly. "Opportunities and Issues for Medical Group Practices." *MGM Journal* 43 (September/October 1996): 30, 34, 35, 36, 39, 108.

111. Hoechst Marion Roussel, *Managed Care Digest Series,* 13.

112. "Congratulations to Surgicenter on Its 20th Anniversary." *FASA Update* 7 (March/April 1990): 19.

113. Henderson, John A. "Surgery Centers Continue Making Inroads." *Modern Healthcare* 20 (May 21, 1990): 98–100.

114. Federated Ambulatory Surgery Association. "History and Growth of the Ambulatory Surgery Center Industry." *http://www.fasa.org/about_fasa.html,* March 26, 1999.

115. Henderson, John A. "Healthcare Providers Will Face Critical Issues in 1990's." *FASA Update* (November/December June 1990). 13.

116. Anderson, Howard J. "Outpatient Planning: Still More Art than Science." *Hospitals* 64 (December 20, 1990): 31.

117. Federated Ambulatory Surgery Association. "Recovery Care Centers." *http://www.fasa.org/recovery.html,* March 26, 1999.

118. Todd, Joanne M. "HealthSouth Acquisitions Throw Another Log on the Burning Market for Ambulatory Centers." *Health Care Strategic Management* 16 (August 1998): 14–17.

119. "For the Record." *Modern Healthcare* (December 4, 1995): 16. *http://web.lexis–nexis.com/univers...5=cf4a4dd9ccfec58d5b431431cb8f2a92,* April 5, 1999.

120. Hudak, Ronald P., Paul P. Brooke, Jr., Kenn Finstuen, and James Trounson. "Management Competencies for Medical Practice Executives: Skills, Knowledge and Abilities Required for the Future." *Journal of Health Administration Education* 15 (Fall 1997): 219–239.

121. "Managed Care Continues to Push Fee-for-Service Gross Collections Downward." *Health Care Strategic Management* 14 (December 1996): 7.

122. Federated Ambulatory Surgery Association, "History and Growth."

123. Joint Commission on Accreditation of Healthcare Organizations. "Ambulatory Care." *http://wwwa.jcaho.org/acr_info/ambcare.htm,* March 26, 1999.

124. Accreditation Association for Ambulatory Healthcare. "About AAHC." *http://aaahc.org/pros/about2.html#2,* April 1, 1999.

125. Henderson, "Surgery Centers," 99.

126. "The Cure for What Ails Health Care: Outpatient Facilities." *Building Design & Construction* 40 (January 1999): 11.

127. An excellent history of the development of hospice is found in Manning, Margaret. *The Hospice Alternative: Living with Dying.* London: Souvenir Press, 1984.

128. Davidson, Glen W. "Introduction." In *The Hospice: Development and Administration,* 2nd ed., edited by Glen W. Davidson, 2. Washington, DC: Hemisphere Publishing, 1985.

129. Mor, Vincent, David S. Greer, and Robert Kastenbaum. "The Hospice Experiment: An Alternative in Terminal Care." In *The Hospice Experiment,* edited by Vincent Mor, David S. Greer, and Robert Kastenbaum, 11. Baltimore: The Johns Hopkins University Press, 1988.

130. McDonnell, Alice. *Quality Hospice Care: Administration, Organization, and Models,* 4. Owings Mills, MD: National Health Publishing, 1986.

131. National Hospice Organization. "Hospice: A Special Kind of Caring" (pamphlet). Arlington, VA: National Hospice Organization, 1999.

132. National Hospice Organization. "Hospice Fact Sheet." Arlington, VA: National Hospice Organization, 1998.

133. Health Care Financing Administration. "Hospice Manual." *http://www.hcfa.gov/pubforms/21_hospice/ hsO-fw.htm,* March 25, 1999.

134. Kilburn, Linda H. *Hospice Operations Manual: Hospice for the Next Century,* 340–341. Dubuque, IA: Kendall/Hunt Publishing, 1997.

135. National Hospice Organization, "Hospice Fact Sheet."

136. "Part 418—Hospice Care, Subpart C—Conditions of Participation." Code of Federal Regulations, pt. 42, ch. IV. Washington, DC: Office of the Federal Register, 1998.

137. Jones, Diane H. "Issues & Trends Affecting the Nation's Hospices." *CARING* 16 (November 1997): 18.

138. Jones, "Issues & Trends," 14–16, 18, 20, 22, 24.

139. National Hospice Organization, "Hospice Fact Sheet."

140. Gardia, Gary. "Hanging on to the Spirit of Hospice in the Midst of Bottom Line Management." *American Journal of Hospice & Palliative Care* 15 (January/February 1998): 7–9.

141. Committee on Ways and Means, U.S. House of Representatives. "Overview of Entitlement Programs, 1990 Green Book: Background Material and Data on Programs within the Jurisdiction of the Committee on Ways and Means, 136. Washington, DC: U.S. House of Representatives, 1990.

142. National Hospice Organization, "Hospice Fact Sheet."

143. Burnell, George M. *Final Choices: To Live or to Die in an Age of Medical Technology,* 281–282. New York: Plenum, 1993.

144. McDonnell, *Quality Hospice Care,* 38–39.

145. Leland, June Y., and Ronald S. Schonwetter. "Advances in Hospice Care." *Clinics in Geriatric Medicine* 13 (May 1997): 381–401.

146. McDonnell, *Quality Hospice Care,* 39.

147. National Hospice Organization, "Hospice" (pamphlet).

148. National Hospice Organization, "Hospice Fact Sheet."

149. Beresford, Larry, private communication, January 25, 1991.

150. Joint Commission on Accreditation of Healthcare Organizations. *Joint Commission History.* Oakbrook, IL: Joint Commission on Accreditation of Healthcare Organizations, 1998.

151. Joint Commission on Accreditation of Healthcare Organizations. "Joint Commission Discontinues Hospice, Managed Care Accreditation Programs." *Perspectives* 10 (May/June 1990): 1.

152. Community Health Accreditation Program. "CHAP Accreditation" (information sheet). New York: Community Health Accreditation Program, 1990.

153. Community Health Accreditation Program. "What's New" (information sheet). New York: Community Health Accreditation Program, 1998.

154. National Hospice Organization, "Hospice Fact Sheet."

155. Health Maintenance Organization Act of 1973, PL 93-222, 87 Stat. 914 (1973).

156. Zelten, Robert A. *Alternative HMO Model* (Issue Paper no. 3), 2. Philadelphia: National Health Care Management Center of the University of Pennsylvania, 1979.

157. Zelman, Walter A. *The Changing Health Care Marketplace: Private Ventures, Public Interests,* 28. San Francisco: Jossey-Bass, 1996.

158. Gabel, Jon, Heidi Whitmore, Chris Bergsten, and Lily Pan Grimm. "Growing Diversification in HMOs, 1988–1994." *Medical Care Research and Review* 54 (March 1997): 101–117.

159. Zelman, *The Changing Health Care Marketplace,* 86.

160. "The Lowdown on HMOs." *Business and Health* 16 (October 1998): 12.

161. Knight, Wendy. *Managed Care: What It Is and How It Works,* 12. Gaithersburg, MD: Aspen Publishers, 1998.

162. Caldwell, Bernice. "Trends and Developments: MCO Administration, Plan, Design, Cost." *Employee Benefit Plan Review* 53 (February 1999): 28.

163. Knight, *Managed Care,* 22.

164. Knight, *Managed Care,* 39–40.

165. Knight, *Managed Care,* 24.

166. Shouldice, Robert G. *Introduction to Managed Care,* 2nd ed., 60. Arlington, VA: Information Resources Press, 1991.

167. AMA v. United States, 130 F. 2d 233 (D.C. Cir. 1942); affirmed 317 U.S. 519 (1943).

168. Marion Merrell Dow, Inc. *Managed Care Digest: Update Edition,* 7. Kansas City, MO: Marion Merrell Dow, Inc., 1990.
169. InterStudy's New HMO Industry Report." *http://www.hmodata.com/ir81pr.html,* February 18, 1999.
170. "InterStudy's New Regional Market Analysis." *http://www.hmodata.com/rma82pr.html,* February 18, 1999.
171. "InterStudy's New HMO Trend Report." http://www.hmodata.com/trprelease.html, February 18, 1999.
172. Hoechst Marion Roussel. *Managed Care Digest Series: HMO-PPO/Medicare/Medicaid Digest,* 13. Kansas City, MO: Hoechst Marion Roussel, 1998.
173. Zelman, *The Changing Health Care Marketplace,* 25.
174. Zelman, *The Changing Health Care Marketplace,* 23–28.
175. Henderson, "Healthcare Providers," 15.
176. Henderson, "Healthcare Providers," 18.
177. Hoechst Marion Roussel, *Managed Care Digest Series: HMO-PPO/Medicare/Medicaid Digest,* 65.
178. Knight, *Managed Care,* 99–100.
179. Knight, *Managed Care,* 102–116.
180. Remler, Dahlia K., Karen Donelan, Robert J. Blendon, George D. Lundberg, Lucian L. Leape, David R. Calkins, Katherine Binns, and Joseph P. Newhouse. "What Do Managed Care Plans Do to Affect Care? Results from a Survey in Physicians." *Inquiry* 34 (Fall 1997): 196–204.
181. Zelman, *The Changing Health Care Marketplace,* 242–248.
182. Gabel, Whitmore, Bergsten, and Grimm, "Growing Diversification," 101–117.
183. Knight, *Managed Care,* 92–93.
184. Shouldice, *Introduction to Managed Care,* 203.
185. Riley, T. "The Role of States in Accountability for Quality." *Health Affairs* 16 (May/June, 1997): 42.
186. Knight, *Managed Care,* 235.
187. Ernst, Eunice K.M. "Health Care Reform as an Ongoing Process." *Journal of Obstetric, Gynecologic, and Neonatal Nursing* 23 (February 1994): 129.
188. Wertz, Richard W., and Dorothy C. Wertz. *Lying-in: A History of Childbirth in America,* 133. New Haven, CT: Yale University Press, 1989.
189. Wertz and Wertz, *Lying-in,* 135.
190. Wertz and Wertz, *Lying-in,* 178.
191. Wertz and Wertz, *Lying-in,* 179.
192. Wertz and Wertz, *Lying-in,* 285.
193. Barnes, Denise. "Midwives: Special Delivery." *The Washington Times,* Metropolitan, October 21, 1998, C8–C9.
194. Waldenstrom, Ulla, Carl-Axel Nilsson, and Birger Winbladh. "The Stockholm Birth Centre Trial: Maternal and Infant Outcome." *British Journal of Obstetrics and Gynaecology* 104 (April 1997): 410–418. Research using an experimental design found that "(W)omen allotted to birth centre care had fewer interventions during their pregnancy, a longer labour, and a shorter postpartum stay than the women allotted to standard care. . . . However, the excess of perinatal deaths and infants with serious morbidity (at the centre) gives cause for concern" (pp. 416–417).
195. National Association of Childbearing Centers. "NACC Membership Benefits." *http://www.birthcenters.org/naccinaction/benefits.shtml,* March 24, 1999.
196. American College of Nurse-Midwives. "Having Your Baby with a Nurse-Midwife: What Birth Centers Are, What They Are Not." *http://www.acnm.org/focus/bc.htm,* March 25, 1999.
197. "Guidelines for Licensing and Regulating Birth Centers." *American Journal of Public Health* 73 (March 1983): 333.
198. Wertz and Wertz, *Lying-in,* 285.
199. National Association of Childbearing Centers, personal communication, April 5, 1999.
200. Wertz and Wertz, *Lying-in,* 285.
201. Ventura, Stephanie J., Joyce A. Martin, Sally C. Curtin, and T.J. Matthews. "Report of Final Natality Statistics, 1996." *Monthly Vital Statistics Report* 46 (June 30, 1998): 73.
202. American College of Nurse-Midwives. Press release, November 1992. *http://www.acnm.org/press/nbcs.htm,* March 25, 1999.

203. American College of Nurse-Midwives, "Having Your Baby."
204. American College of Nurse-Midwives. "Licensure as a Nurse-Midwife." *http://www.midwife.org/educ/fenmlice.htm,* April 5, 1999.
205. American College of Nurse-Midwives. "Certified Nurse-Midwives in Virginia." *http://www.acnm.org/press/SFVIRGIN.HTM,* March 25, 1999.
206. Wertz and Wertz, *Lying-in,* 285.
207. Bergman, Rhonda. "The Birthplace Boom." *Hospitals & Health Networks* 68 (December 5, 1994): 48.
208. National Association of Childbearing Centers. "State Regulations for Licensing Birth Centers." *http://www.birthcenters.org/healthcarepolicy/regs.shtml,* March 24, 1999.
209. Commission for the Accreditation of Freestanding Birth Centers. "Reach for Excellence through Accreditation." *http://www.birthcenters.org/faqbirthcenters/accreditation.shtml,* March 25, 1999.
210. Rooks, Judith P., Norman L. Weatherby, Eunice K.M. Ernst, Susan Stapleton, David Rosen, and Allan Rosenfield. "Outcomes of Care in Birth Centers: The National Birth Center Study." *New England Journal of Medicine* 321 (December 28, 1989): 1810.
211. Deloughery, Grace L. *History and Trends of Professional Nursing,* 8th ed., 102. St. Louis: Mosby, 1977.
212. Mundinger, Mary O'Neil. *Home Care Controversy: Too Little, Too Late, Too Costly,* 37. Rockville, MD: Aspen Systems Corporation, 1983.
213. Mundinger, *Home Care Controversy,* 38.
214. Spiegel, Allen D. *Home Healthcare: Home Birthing to Hospice Care,* 10. Owings Mills, MD: National Health Publishing, 1983.
215. Social Security Amendments of 1960 (Kerr-Mills Social Security Act), PL 86-778, 74 Stat. 924 (1960).
216. Mundinger, *Home Care Controversy,* 18.
217. Lerman, Dan. "The Home Care Controversy." In *Home Care: Positioning the Hospital for the Future,* edited by Dan Lerman, 1. Chicago: American Hospital Publishing, 1987.
218. Mundinger, *Home Care Controversy,* 39.
219. Mundinger, *Home Care Controversy,* 43.
220. National Association for Home Care. "Transition to PPS: The Interim Payment System for Medicare Home Health Services." Washington, DC: National Association for Home Care, 1997.
221. Meyer, Harris. "Home (Care) Improvement." *Hospitals & Health Networks* 71 (April 20, 1997): 40.
222. Soundappan, Appavuchetty, Terry Goodwin, Roberta Greengold, and Eugenia L. Siegler. "How to Get the Most Benefit from a Changing Home Health Care System." *Geriatrics* 52 (October 1997): 85.
223. Hoechst Marion Roussel. *Managed Care Digest Series: Institutional Digest,* 32. Kansas City, MO: Hoechst Marion Roussel, 1998.
224. Meyer, "Home (Care) Improvement," 40.
225. Hoechst Marion Roussel, *Managed Care Digest Series: Institutional Digest,* 39.
226. Balanced Budget Act of 1997, PL 105-33, 111 Stat. 251 (1997).
227. *Home Health Line,* 24,42 (November 5, 1999): 10; Egger, Ed. "The Home Care Crisis: Time To Abandon Ship?" *Strategic Management* 16 (December 1998): 1.
228. St. Pierre, Mary and William A. Dombi. "Home Health PPS: New Payment System, New Hope." *CARING* 19 (January 2000): 6; Blecher, Michele Bitoun. "Unhappy Landings." *Hospital & Health Networks* 72 (November 20, 1998): 26.
229. Gemignani, Janet. "Who'll Pay the Bill When Health Care Comes Home?" *Business & Health* 14: 6 (June 1996): 67.
230. Welch, H. Gilbert, David E. Wennberg, and W. Pete Welch. "The Use of Medicare Home Health Care Services." *New England Journal of Medicine* 335 (August 1, 1996): 324–329. In 1993, about 3 million Medicare enrollees received more than 160 million home health care visits.
231. Nathanson, Martha Dale. *Home Health Care Answer Book: Legal Issues for Providers,* 135. Gaithersburg, MD: Aspen Publishers, 1995.
232. Lerman, *Home Care,* 19.
233. Daniels, Kaye. "Start-Up Considerations for Private-Pay Home Care Programs." In *Hospital Home Care: Strategic Management for Integrated Care Delivery,* edited by Dan Lerman and Eric B. Linne, 253–254. Chicago: American Hospital Publishing, 1993; Daniels, Kaye. "Operational Considerations for

Private-Pay Home Care Programs." In *Hospital Home Care: Strategic Management of Integrated Care Delivery,* edited by Dan Lerman and Eric B. Linne, 263. Chicago: American Hospital Publishing, 1993.

234. Schulmerich, Susan Craig. "General Information." In *Home Health Care Administration,* edited by Susan Craig Schulmerich, Timothy J. Riordan, Jr., and Stephanie Taylor Davis, 15. Washington, DC: Delmar Publishers, 1996.

235. Lerman, *Home Care,* 27.

236. Anderson, Tim. "Priorities of Expertise: What Home Care Agencies Look for in Managers." *CARING* 8 (February 1989): 53.

237. Soundappan, Goodwin, Greengold, and Siegler, "How to Get the Most," 85.

238. Keenan, Joseph M., and James E. Fanale. "Home Care: Past and Present, Problems and Potential." *Journal of the American Geriatrics Society* 37 (November 1989): 1078.

239. Health Care Financing Administration, U.S. Department of Health and Human Services. "Condition of Participation: Group of Professional Personnel." *Code of Federal Regulations,* pt. 42, ch. 484, 16. Washington, DC: Office of the Federal Register, 1998.

240. Hoechst Marion Roussel, *Managed Care Digest,* 39.

241. Joint Commission on Accreditation of Healthcare Organizations, *Joint Commission History.*

242. Walden, Victoria. "A CHAP to Meet: The Community Health Accreditation Program." *Journal of Nursing Administration* 67 (November–December 1996). 35–50.

243. "Community Health Accreditation Program and Joint Commission Announce Cooperative Agreement." *Journal of Nursing Administration* 26 (December 1996): 4. The Joint Commission agreed to accept CHAP's accreditation process, findings, and decisions on HHAs when surveying integrated delivery systems and health plans.

244. Fazzi, Robert A., and Robert V. Agoglia. "Managed Care's Expectations: Final Results from a National Study." *CARING* 15 (January 1996): 10–14, 16.

245. Keenan and Fanale, "Home Care," 1077.

246. Schulmerich, "General Information," 15.

247. Daniels, "Operational Considerations," 263.

248. Short, Pamela Farley, and Joel Leon. *Use of Home and Community Services by Persons Ages 65 and Older with Functional Difficulties,* 4. Washington, DC: Agency for Health Care Policy and Research, 1990.

249. Montauk, Susan Louisa. "Home Health Care." *American Family Medicine* 58 (November 1, 1998): 1608–1614.

250. Grimaldi, Paul L. "Medicare Imposes New Caps on Postacute Care." *Nursing Management* 29 (November 1998): 10–12.

251. St. Pierre and Dombi. "Home Health PPS," 11.

252. Reprinted by permission of the author, Carolyn H. Longest.

SELECTED BIBLIOGRAPHY

Alexander, Jeffrey. *The Changing Character of Hospital Governance.* Chicago: The Hospital Research and Educational Trust, 1990.

Beresford, Larry. *The Hospice Handbook: A Complete Guide.* Boston: Little, Brown, 1993.

Binstock, Robert H., Leighton E. Cluff, and Otto von Mering, Eds. *The Future of Long-Term Care: Social and Policy Issues.* Baltimore: The Johns Hopkins University Press, 1996.

Conger, Jay A., David Finegold, and Edward E. Lawler, III. "Appraising Boardroom Performance." *Harvard Business Review* 76 (January–February 1998): 136–148.

Davis, Feather Ann. "Medicare Hospice Benefit: Early Program Experiences." *Health Care Financing Review* 9 (Summer 1988): 99–111.

Deloughery, Grace L. *Issues & Trends in Nursing,* 3rd ed. St. Louis: Mosby-Year Book, 1997.

Donaldson, Molla S. "The Importance of Measuring Quality of Care at the End of Life." *Hospice Journal* 13 (1 & 2 1998): 117–138.

Drucker, Peter F. "The New Productivity Challenge." *Harvard Business Review* 69 (November–December 1991): 69–79.

Drucker, Peter F. "The New Society of Organizations." *Harvard Business Review* 70 (September–October 1992): 95–104.

Drucker, Peter F. "The Theory of the Business." *Harvard Business Review* 72 (September–October 1994): 95–104.

Ernst, Eunice K.M. "Health Care Reform as an Ongoing Process." *Journal of Obstetric, Gynecologic, and Neonatal Nursing* 23 (February 1994): 129–138.

Gordon, George Kenneth, and Ruth Stryker, Eds. *Creative Long-Term Care Administration,* 3rd ed. Springfield, IL: Charles C Thomas, 1994.

Health Care Financing Administration, Department of Health and Human Services. "Conditions of Participation: Home Health Agencies." 42 CFR 484." *Federal Register* 54 (August 14, 1989): 33354–33373.

Hooyman, Nancy, and H. Asuman Kiyak. *Social Gerontology: A Multidisciplinary Perspective,* 4th ed. Needham Heights, MA: Allyn & Bacon, 1996.

"Hospice Care, Subpart C—Conditions of Participation—General Provisions and Administration." In *Code of Federal Regulations,* pt. 42, ch. 418. Washington, DC: Office of the Federal Register, 1998.

Jaffe, Carolyn, and Carol H. Ehrlich. *All Kinds of Love: Experiencing Hospice.* Amityville, NY: Baywood Publishers, 1997.

Kaye, Lenard W. *Home Health Care.* Newbury Park, CA: Sage, 1992.

Kilburn, Linda H. *Hospice Operations Manual: Hospice for the Next Century.* Arlington, VA: National Hospice Organization, 1997.

Knight, Wendy. *Managed Care: What It Is and How It Works.* Gaithersburg, MD: Aspen Publishers, 1998.

Kovner, Anthony R., Roger A. Ritvo, and Thomas P. Holland. "Board Development in Two Hospitals: Lessons from a Demonstration." *Hospital & Health Services Administration* 41 (Spring 1997): 87–99.

Lambdin, Morris, and Kurt Darr. *Guidelines for Effectively Organizing the Professional Staff.* Baltimore: Health Professions Press, 1999.

Leland, June Y., and Ronald S. Schonwetter. "Advances in Hospice Care." *Clinics in Geriatric Medicine* 13 (May 1997): 381–401.

Lerman, Dan, and Eric B. Linne, Eds. *Hospital Home Care: Strategic Management for Integrated Care Delivery.* Chicago: American Hospital Publishing, 1993.

Madison, Donald L. "Notes on the History of Group Practice: The Tradition of the Dispensary." *Medical Group Management Journal* 37 (September/October 1990): 52–54, 56–60, 86–91.

Nathanson, Martha Dale. *Home Health Care Answer Book: Legal Issues for Providers.* Gaithersburg, MD: Aspen Publishers, 1995.

Rivlin, Alice M., and Joshua M. Weiner. *Caring for the Disabled Elderly: Who Will Pay?* Washington, DC: The Brookings Institution, 1988.

Rorem, C. Rufus. *Non-profit Hospital Service Plans.* Chicago: American Hospital Association, 1940.

Ross, Austin, Stephen J. Williams, and Ernest J. Pavlock. *Ambulatory Care Management,* 3rd ed. New York: Delmar Publishers, 1998.

Saunders, Cicely, Mary Baines, and Robert Dunlop. *Living With Dying: A Guide to Palliative Care,* 3rd ed. New York: Oxford University Press, 1995.

Schulmerich, Susan Craig, Timothy J. Riordan, Jr., and Stephanie Taylor Davis. *Home Health Care Administration.* Washington, DC: Delmar Publishers, 1996.

Shortell, Stephen M. "The Medical Staff of the Future: Replanting the Garden." *Frontiers of Health Services Management* 1 (February 1985): 3–48.

Shortell, Stephen M. "Revisiting the Garden: Medicine and Management in the 1990s." *Frontiers of Health Services Management* 7 (Fall 1990): 3–32.

Shouldice, Robert G. *Introduction to Managed Care,* 2nd ed. Arlington, VA: Information Resources Press, 1991.

Sigerist, Henry E. *A History of Medicine. Vol. I, Primitive and Archaic Medicine.* New York: Oxford University Press, 1951.

Warzinski, Katherine V., and Ann Ward Tourigny. "Nursing Home Administrator Licensure: A History." *Journal of Long-Term Care Administration* 15 (Spring 1987): 6–10.

Weber, Max. *The Theory of Social and Economic Organizations,* 151–157. Translated by A.M. Henderson and Talcott Parsons. New York: The Free Press, 1947.

Wertz, Richard W., and Dorothy C. Wertz. *Lying-in: A History of Childbirth in America.* New Haven, CT: Yale University Press, 1989.

Zelman, Walter A. *The Changing Health Care Marketplace: Private Ventures, Public Interests.* San Francisco: Jossey-Bass, 1996.

5 How Health Systems Are Organized

If statistics are valid, integrated health care delivery and financing systems are spreading across the United States like kudzu in an untended southern garden.[1]

As discussed in Chapter 1, health services are provided through a variety of health services organizations (HSOs) and, increasingly, through two or more HSOs joined together in health systems (HSs). HSOs were defined as entities that provide the organizational structure within which the delivery of health services is made directly to consumers, whether the purpose of the services is preventive, acute, chronic, restorative, or palliative. The structures and functions of common types of HSOs are described and discussed in Chapter 4.

Chapter 1 also defines HSs as formally linked HSOs, which may include financing arrangements, joined together to provide more coordinated and comprehensive health services. This chapter describes the linking of HSOs into HSs, including the reasons for these linkages, the resulting HSs, and their management and governance. First, however, it is necessary to describe two overarching aspects of the phenomenon of HSOs linking to form HSs.

The first aspect is that not all linkages among HSOs are established for the purpose of creating HSs. Linking to form HSs is only one interorganizational relationship (IOR) that HSOs establish and maintain with other entities. The formation of HSs is best understood in the context of the larger phenomenon of HSOs relating to entities through a variety of IORs. In fact, there are three different and distinct types of IORs, as described in the next section. Each of the three types, however, is used by HSOs to manage some aspect of the interdependence between them and other entities. A HSO is interdependent with other entities that can affect it or that can be affected by it. As Figure 5.1 shows, HSOs maintain interdependent relationships with many other entities.

A second important aspect of the linking of HSOs into HSs is the wide variety of resulting HSs. They range from relatively simple arrangements—perhaps involving only two HSOs or one HSO and a physician group—to the other extreme, in which linkages among many HSOs result in a large, complex HS that is capable of providing a continuum of health services in its market. Allina

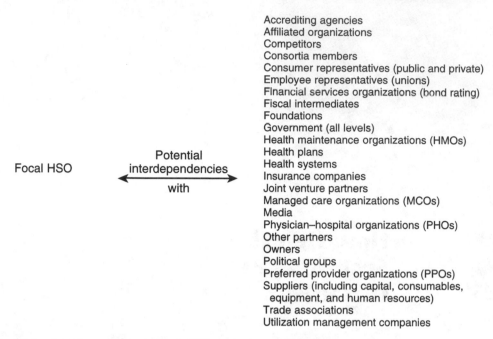

Figure 5.1.   Interdependencies between HSOs and other entities.

Health System,[2] for example, includes 20 hospitals and provides a continuum of services ranging from prevention to advanced inpatient and outpatient services, home care, long-term care, and hospice care. It is the largest HS in Minneapolis, accounting for more than 27% of hospital admissions in that city in 1998.[3]

Because of the different interdependencies between a HSO/HS and other entities, the IORs established to manage the interdependencies also differ. Discussed in the next section are three broad types of IORs, based on their purpose or use, with which HSOs/HSs are involved.[4] This discussion provides a contextual background for subsequent consideration of the formation, management, and governance of HSs.

INTERORGANIZATIONAL RELATIONSHIPS

As is generally true for organizations, the most prevalent type of IOR in which HSOs/HSs are involved is the market transactions between them and other entities. HSOs/HSs use market transactions to secure needed resources from suppliers and to ensure markets for their outputs. For example, a HSO/HS maintains an IOR with a supplier such as Baxter International, Inc.,[5] through which it purchases blood transfusion systems or heart surgery equipment. It can ensure markets for its services through IORs with insurance companies, managed care plans, employers, or groups of employers joined together in purchasing coalitions.

A second type of IOR occurs because HSOs/HSs *must* participate in linkages with certain entities such as federal or state regulatory agencies, fiscal intermediaries, bond rating services, utilization management companies, and unions with which they have collective bargaining agreements. Because the HSO/HS has no choice but to participate in these IORs, they can be labeled involuntary IORs. An example is the IOR that must be maintained between a HSO/HS operating in Pennsylvania and the Pennsylvania Department of Health's Bureau of Facility Licensure and Certification, which *licenses and verifies compliance with state and federal health and safety standards in supervised health care facilities as mandated by law, including hospitals, nursing homes, home health agencies, certain primary care providers, ambulatory surgical facilities, and intermediate care facilities for persons with developmental disabilities. The Department conducts regular on-site surveys to assure health, safety, sanitation, fire and quality of care requirements and identify deficiencies which may affect state licensure or eligibility for federal reimbursements under the Medicaid and Medicare programs.[6]*

The third type of IOR in which HSOs/HSs engage—the type through which HSOs establish HSs as well as accomplish other purposes—is voluntary IORs. These occur when HSOs/HSs voluntarily enter into a variety of linkages with other entities that are different from their market transactions. Voluntary IORs are established between or among entities for purposes of mutual benefit or gain and are used by HSOs/HSs to accomplish purposes such as enhancing their competitive positions by better meeting consumer expectations for delivery and coordination of care.[7] Voluntary IORs, ranging from the simplest to the most complex and extensive linkages, are generally referred to as alliances or strategic alliances (SAs)[8] as they are called in this chapter.

SAs are defined as "any formal arrangements between two or more organizations for purposes of mutual gain."[9] The arrangements are established through a variety of mechanisms including but not limited to the formation of HSs.[10] By definition, all HSs are SAs, although HSs range from simple to very complex; not all SAs, however, are HSs.

A taxonomy developed by Stein suggests that SAs form in three ways: Participants in a SA can pool resources, they can ally for some shared purpose, or they can link together through bonds of ownership or contractual relationships. The acronym PAL (*p*ool, *a*lly, *l*ink) is used by Stein to identify the three possibilities.[11] Later in this chapter, the structural attributes and characteristics of SAs are described more fully in terms of participants, purposes, and form.

The concept of integration[12] is vital to understanding the formation of SAs, including HSs. In this context, integration can be thought of as bringing together component parts to make a whole. A SA can involve little integration or a great deal of integration. For example, in a SA established between a single HSO and members of its professional staff organization, there is integration, but it is limited. In contrast, the Allina Health System described earlier involves extensive integration.

Linkages among HSOs in the form of SAs are pervasive in health services and are likely to continue to be established and maintained in the future.[13] Most hospitals, an important category of HSOs, are now "allied with other hospitals in their markets through . . . organizational linkages."[14] The American Hospital Association reports that in 1998, 3,556 of the nation's 5,015 community hospitals were in a system or network.[15] As Brown stated, "Hospitals, physicians, insurers, and managed care firms are networking, merging, and forming horizontally and vertically integrated organizations to finance and deliver health care."[16]

Thus HSOs/HSs participate in a variety of IORs—market transactions, involuntary IORs, and SAs—because they relate to many different interdependent entities, as shown in Figure 5.1. Management implications of the different types of IORs are considered later in the chapter. First, however, a closer look at SAs is taken, including the formation of HSs.

STRATEGIC ALLIANCES

A great variety of SAs have become commonplace in health services delivery and financing. Although there is debate about the evidence regarding significant benefits gained through integration,[17] there are several reasons for the pervasiveness of this activity in health services. There are several compelling reasons and pressures for HSOs to continue to integrate into SAs in health services.

Reasons to Ally

One reason for establishing SAs is no more complicated than the fact that, as the external environments facing many independent HSOs have grown increasingly difficult, turbulent, and challenging, these organizations have sought safety in the strength of numbers. Longest argued this as the basis for the formation of horizontal systems of hospitals as early as the 1970s. Referring to the HSs being formed then as "multihospital arrangements," he pointed out that "decision makers in participating hospitals believe that the formation of multihospital arrangements makes possible the achievement of a higher level of organizational stability than is available . . . when their organizations remain completely autonomous and independent."[18]

This rationale for establishing SAs is not limited to their formation in health services. It has been used to partially explain the larger phenomenon of alliance formation in business. As Ohmae noted, "Companies are beginning to learn what nations have always known—in a complex uncertain world, filled with dangerous opponents, it is best not to go it alone."[19]

The growth and pervasiveness of managed care is another reason, beyond this "circle the wagons" mentality, that continues to drive some integration in health services. The most extensively integrated HSs are found in markets with the greatest degree of managed care penetration,[20] for reasons discussed next.

Managed care, which is discussed extensively in Chapter 4, is an umbrella term encompassing several different types of organizations, collectively termed *managed care organizations* (MCOs), that integrate the financing and delivery of health services.[21] Typically, the term *managed care* refers to forms of health insurance coverage "that integrate financing and delivery, as well as the organizations (MCOs) that provide this coverage—health maintenance organizations (HMOs), preferred provider organizations (PPOs), and point-of-service (POS) plans."[22]

A HMO is

> *an organization interposed between providers and [payers] that attempts to "manage the care" on behalf of the health services consumer and [payer]. HMOs are responsible for both the financing and delivery of comprehensive health services to an enrolled group of patients.*[23]

A variation is the POS plan, which permits patients to "select network or nonnetwork physicians at the 'point of service,' usually with significant differences between network and nonnetwork care in terms of coinsurance or deductibles."[24] A PPO is a health plan in which patients "are given a financial incentive to use a 'preferred' network of providers, usually through differences in coinsurance or deductibles."[25]

In 1998 there were 651 HMOs in the United States, with more than 76 million enrollees.[26] Nearly two thirds of the HMOs offered POS options, and there were 1,035 operating PPOs in 1997.[27]

Greater managed care penetration and increased integration in health services both have occurred to a great extent simultaneously "in response to market pressures for cost containment and demands for value and accountability."[28] These pressures have been described as follows:

> *Both government and private purchasers of health care are demanding value (high quality at low cost) for their health care dollar. This is creating irresistible pressure on hospitals to change the way health care is organized and delivered. To provide the value that the market demands, hospitals and health care systems must integrate all of their many and diverse clinical and operational functions. This includes integration of physicians, clinical services, information systems, inpatient and outpatient access points, governance, quality improvement, and all parts of the health care continuum.*[29]

Increased integration, especially vertical integration as discussed later, has occurred because managed care has pressured the traditionally fragmented financing and delivery structures to transform into "rationally designed, integrated health care systems."[30] In effect, market pressures have stimulated the growth of managed care and integration, and more managed care has stimulated more integration. In combination, market pressures and increasing levels of managed care continue to exert significant pressure for increased integration in health services.

Other reasons for integration include the conviction among participants, especially in vertical integration, that it improves competitive position by adding value to their activities.[31] Integration offers HSOs/HSs opportunities to add value for their patients or consumers through provision of a coordinated continuum of care. For example, it has been demonstrated that a hospital's ownership of a nursing facility helps to ensure the "timely transfer of patients who are well enough to be discharged from acute care, but not well enough to be sent home."[32] Integration also adds value in other ways, such as by increasing participants' ability to manage financial risk, facilitating their access to capital, and helping them achieve cost reductions through consolidation and joint buying power.[33] In addition, as was noted at the outset of this section, many HSOs/HSs have integrated into SAs, at least in part, as a means of improving adaptive capability in the face of challenges.[34]

Approaches to Understanding SAs

SAs in their rich variety and diversity can be usefully examined from three interrelated perspectives: participants, purposes, and forms. Each approach is considered in the following sections, along with defined examples demonstrating how each perspective contributes to understanding SAs. Among the most important aspects of SAs, however, is that no matter who participates in them or for what purposes or what their specific form, alliances are established for strategic purposes and they are entered into voluntarily. Managers voluntarily enter into SAs because they believe that they can better achieve some organizational objective or improve some aspect of organizational performance.

SAs Categorized by Participants

Although integration in health services frequently is considered in terms of HSOs linking into HSs, the integrative activity through which SAs are established can begin with individuals. Individual physicians engage in integration when they form a group practice, which is "a formal association of three or more physicians, dentists, podiatrists, or other health professionals providing services, with income from the medical practice pooled and redistributed to the members of the group according to a prearranged plan."[35] Group practices, which are SAs, can in turn participate in many other alliances.[36] The extent and variety of integrative activity forming SAs, categorized by participants, can be understood in the following interactions between and among physicians, HSOs, and HSs.

Physician–Physician SAs

In addition to group practices, physicians can form other SAs, such as an independent practice association, a "legal entity composed of physicians who have organized for the purpose of negotiating contracts to provide medical services."[37] They also can form a physician-owned management services organization (MSO), a "legal corporation formed to provide practice management services to physicians."[38]

Physician–HSO/HS SAs

SAs are formed when physicians, as individuals or groups, are employed by, when their practices are owned by, or when they contract with HSOs/HSs. The popularity of HSO/HS ownership of physician practices as a SA—typically in the context of a highly integrated HS—has been mixed. Still, however, as Orlikoff and Totten noted,

> *A fully integrated health system model is often achieved by purchasing physician practices (and subsequent employment of those physicians) or by establishing a staff-model health maintenance*

organization, or HMO. This model promises the greatest opportunity for hospitals and physicians to respond together to the market, manage outcomes and rationalize resource allocation. While doctors still tend to favor a degree of autonomy over total integration with hospitals, continuing market pressure for effective cost control and the ability to demonstrate quality and performance are moving hospitals and physicians closer together.

Regardless of the relationship model selected, to be truly integrated, an integrated delivery system (IDS) must share risk and align incentives with its doctors.[39]

Other relationship models include HSOs/HSs and physicians forming HSO/HS–based MSOs, in contrast to those that are physician-only. The services that are provided to physicians by such MSOs typically include billing, information system acquisition and installation, staffing, staff training and development, managed care contract negotiation and compliance, and other office management functions.[40]

Physicians and a hospital can form a physician–hospital organization (PHO), defined as a "legal entity formed by a hospital and a group of physicians to further mutual interests and to achieve market interests."[41] PHOs play important roles in many other SAs because each combines physicians and a hospital into a single entity, making it easier to obtain contracts with health plans, employers, or purchasing coalitions.[42] PHOs form SAs with the entities with whom they contract. For example, SAs are routinely established between PHOs and HMOs.

MSOs and PHOs involving HSOs/HSs and physicians typically are organized as joint ventures. A joint venture is "a legal entity characterized by two or more parties who work on a project together, sharing profits, losses, and control."[43] Joint ventures between HSOs/HSs and members of their professional staff organizations, including ventures in which they set up diagnostic imaging facilities or establish surgicenters or urgicenters, are commonplace.[44] Joint ventures, which are widespread in health services, are discussed in more detail in a subsequent section.

HSO–HSO SAs

HSOs that are alike, such as groups of community hospitals or nursing facilities, can form horizontally integrated HSs (Figure 5.2). Alternatively, joining with dissimilar or other types of HSOs, they can form vertically integrated HSs (Figure 5.3). Horizontal integration is the formation of lateral relationships among like entities performing at the same functional level. Its purpose is "to improve the degree to which resources are used efficiently and to increase purchasing power and marketing and management capacity."[45] It "occurs when two or more separate firms, producing either the same services or services that are close substitutes, join to become either a single firm or a strong interorganizational alliance."[46]

Vertical integration, in contrast, is

coordinating, linking or incorporating within a single organization activities or entities at different stages of a production process—in health care the processes of producing and delivering patient care. These activities or entities would otherwise be completely independent, or would interact through arm's-length transactions.[47]

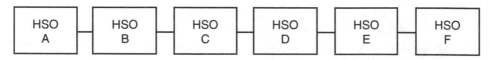

Figure 5.2.   Horizontally integrated HS. All HSOs in the HS perform at the same functional level: All are hospitals, nursing facilities, home health agencies, or the like.

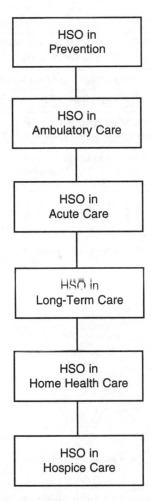

Figure 5.3.   Vertically integrated HS. The HSOs in the HS are performing at different functional levels: prevention, ambulatory care, and so forth.

Vertical integration can involve only two entities at different stages of the process of producing and delivering health services, or it may involve more entities at different stages. Although the terminology is not universally agreed on, the term *highly integrated HS* is increasingly reserved for situations in which a HS has integrated to the extent that it includes at least three or more stages of health services delivery and at least one systemwide contract with a payer. The highly integrated HS either owns or contracts with three or more stages of health services delivery, including at least one acute-care hospital; at least one physician component, such as a PHO or group practice; and at least one other stage, such as a HMO, nursing facility, home health agency, or surgery center. In addition, it has at least one systemwide contract with a payer, which can be an employer or employer coalition, a traditional insurer, a MCO, or a government entity.[48] Figure 5.4 shows the continuing growth in the formation of vertically integrated HSs, including growth of those that are highly integrated, which increased from 228 in 1997 to 266 in 1998.

Increasingly, when people talk of integrated health care, they mean highly integrated HSs. These HSs are difficult to establish and maintain. Satinsky identified eight key factors in the success of HSs by summarizing the research on HSs, the views of consultants who have facilitated HS formation, and representatives of HSs.[49] These factors are listed in Table 5.1, along with HSs that

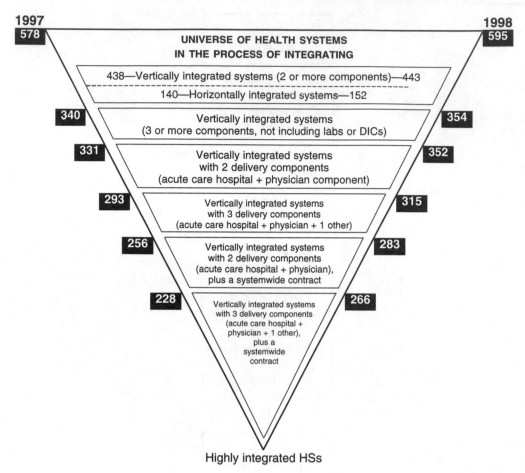

1997
578

1998
595

UNIVERSE OF HEALTH SYSTEMS
IN THE PROCESS OF INTEGRATING

438—Vertically integrated systems (2 or more components)—443
140—Horizontally integrated systems—152

340

354

Vertically integrated systems
(3 or more components, not including labs or DICs)

331

352

Vertically integrated systems
with 2 delivery components
(acute care hospital + physician component)

293

315

Vertically integrated systems
with 3 delivery components
(acute care hospital + physician + 1 other)

256

283

Vertically integrated systems
with 2 delivery components
(acute care hospital + physician),
plus a systemwide contract

228

266

Vertically integrated systems
with 3 delivery components
(acute care hospital +
physician + 1 other),
plus a
systemwide
contract

Highly integrated HSs

Figure 5.4.   HSs in the process of integrating. (Adapted from Hoechst Marion Roussel. *Managed Care Digest Series: Integrated Health Systems Digest,* 5. Kansas City, MO: Hoechst Marion Roussel, 1999; used with permission.)

exemplify each. A philosophical commitment to systems integration is a key factor that is consistent with the view expressed by Orlikoff and Totten. They believe that the managers and members of governing bodies (GBs) who lead successful highly integrated HSs "have a vision that the whole [HS] is greater—and different from—the sum of its parts."[50]

The most highly integrated HSs combine under a unified approach, either through ownership or contractual relationships, all of the major components of the delivery system—physicians, hospitals, and other facilities as shown in Figure 5.3, as well as health plan services. Most of the highly integrated HSs in existence and under formation "contract with multiple health plans without owning or being owned by any one."[51] Many do, however, own a health plan. For example, the University of Pittsburgh Medical Center (UPMC) Health System is a highly integrated health care delivery system primarily serving the region of western Pennsylvania through a network of hospitals and other HSOs. The system also owns UPMC Health Plan, a managed care insurance company, as well as all or parts of HMOs serving Medicaid- and Medicare-eligible populations.[52] Similarly, the Henry Ford Health System primarily serves southeastern Michigan through a network of six hospitals with nearly 2,000 beds, more than 35 other health care facilities, and approximately 1,800 physicians. The system's Health Alliance Plan provides managed care and health insurance to more than 570,000 members.[53]

TABLE 5.1. KEY SUCCESS FACTORS IN HSs, WITH EXAMPLES

Success factor	HSs with proven track records
Philosophical commitment to systems integration	Advocate Health Care (IL); Henry Ford Health System (MI)
Clarity of purpose and vision	Baylor Health Care System (TX); Copley Health System (VT)
Strong physician leadership	Fairview Hospital and Healthcare Services (MN); Friendly Hills HealthCare Network (CA); Henry Ford Health System (MI); North Shore Medical Center (MA)
Alignment of financial incentives and rewards that recognize system performance	Samaritan Health System (AZ)
Customer focus on purchasers; enrollees; system components; legal, regulatory, and accrediting agencies; and communities	Appalachian Regional Healthcare (KY, VA, WV); Carolinas HealthCare System (NC, SC); Group Health Cooperative (WA); Laurel Health System (PA)
Information systems and technology that support systems goals and operations	Advocate Health Care (IL); Allina Health System (MN); Graduate Health System (NJ, PA)
Ongoing emphasis on quality improvement	Harvard Pilgrim Health Care (New England); Henry Ford Health System (MI); Lovelace Health System and Presbyterian Healthcare Services (NM)
Focus on creating market-driven value	Dartmouth-Hitchcock Health System–Northern Region (New England); Henry Ford Health System and Mercy Health Services (MI)

Adapted from Satinsky, Marjorie A. *The Foundation of Integrated Care: Facing the Challenges of Change*, 73. Chicago: American Hospital Publishing, reprinted by permission.

The highly integrated HSs are also called IDSs, organized delivery systems (ODSs), or integrated delivery networks (IDNs). Whatever the name, the highly integrated HSs are distinguished by the fact that each "provides or arranges to provide a coordinated continuum of services to a defined population and is willing to be held clinically and fiscally accountable for the outcomes and the health status of the population served."[54]

A critical aspect of HSs is that the establishment of formal linkages between or among HSOs can be made through ownership arrangements, or they can be based on contractual relationships, establishing what have come to be called virtual HSs.[55] This distinction also is termed ownership-based integration and contractual-based integration.[56]

Whether HSOs in a HS are linked through ownership or, alternatively, through contracts, has led to use of the terms *health networks* to refer to situations in which the linkages are contractual and *health systems* to refer to situations in which the ownership of the assets of the linked HSOs is unified.[57] Others have made a similar distinction between linked HSOs, dividing them into two groups, with one group characterized as loosely coupled alliances that have two or more owners (corresponding to health networks) and the other as tightly coupled alliances that have single owners (corresponding to HSs).[58]

To summarize, SAs can usefully be considered in terms of their participants. Physician–physician SAs are commonplace. Physician–HSO/HS alliances are another category, as are those that are HSO–HSO. SAs also can be categorized and usefully considered according to their purpose, as is discussed next.

SAs Categorized by Purpose

When HSOs/HSs participate in SAs, they do so for one or more specific purposes.[59] Common, although not the only, purposes for alliance activity are cost reduction and revenue enhancement. Group purchasing organizations (GPOs), for example, are SAs formed for the purpose of gaining purchasing power as a means of reducing the participants' costs of certain supplies. An example of such a SA is AmeriNet, a national GPO founded by a consortium of regional GPOs. This alliance is one of the nation's largest GPOs, with a membership in excess of 8,200 HSOs/HSs, representing more than 324,000 beds located in all 50 states.[60] It negotiates on behalf of its members to obtain volume discount contracts with suppliers to provide its members with favorable pricing, terms, and conditions. Its product and service agreements include administrative services, diagnostic imaging, environmental services, information and technical services, IV solutions and supplies, laboratory supplies, medical supplies, nutrition supplies, pharmacy supplies, plant engineering, office supplies, and surgical supplies.

A typical example of a SA that is formed for the purpose of revenue enhancement is a PHO, described in the previous section as a legal entity formed by a hospital and members of its professional staff to further their mutual interests. The typical purposes of forming PHOs are to seek contracts with managed care plans or to sponsor a surgery center, an imaging center, or some other business venture.[61]

Other purposes for which SAs can be formed, at least in part, include the ability of alliances to enhance the participants' capacity to innovate and adapt to environmental threats, to experience organizational learning, and to make quality improvements.[62] For example, SAs such as Harvard Pilgrim Health Care[63] in Massachusetts, Henry Ford Health System[64] in Michigan, and Lovelace Health Systems[65] in New Mexico have been cited for their ability to help HS participants make quality improvements.[66] Kraatz has shown that organizations that face threatening environmental changes, as many HSOs/HSs do, may significantly increase their chances of successfully adapting by forging SAs that provide informational benefits and opportunities for mutual learning among participants.[67]

SAs, as noted earlier, also can be formed as ways for participants to stabilize themselves in uncertain environments or to maintain and enhance their competitive positions. Hospitals, for example, have been especially prone to pursue SAs as a means of positioning themselves to compete more effectively for managed care contracts. Luke, Olden, and Bramble pointed out that hospitals, by aligning with other hospitals in their local markets, gain certain advantages in a managed care environment.[68] They argued that many hospital SAs provide their members with important advantages because the alliances are able to negotiate for contracts that cover whole communities. SAs also give participants greater "mass and leverage,"[69] providing them with strength in their negotiations with managed care companies that might otherwise pit one hospital against others in negotiations based on price.

To summarize, in addition to considering SAs in terms of who participates in them, they can be usefully considered in terms of their purposes, including cost reduction and revenue enhancement; increased capacity to innovate and adapt to environmental threats; the advantages of organizational learning that can accompany participation in an alliance; opportunities to enhance quality; and the increased likelihood that participants might stabilize themselves, enhance their competitive positions, or both in uncertain environments. These are important purposes from the viewpoint of HSOs/HSs, and some SAs fulfill more than one.

Although considerations of SA participants and the purposes for which SAs are pursued are important in understanding them, neither fully explains the forms that the alliances might take. Form as a third basis for categorizing and considering SAs is discussed in the next section.

SAs Categorized by Form

No matter who participates in them or what their purpose, SAs can take many different organizational forms. Choice of form is related to participants and purposes but also to dimensions of SAs such as their importance and the need for permanence of the IORs that they are established to serve.[70] Some IORs are of critical importance to participants; others are of less importance. Some IORs are intended to be of short duration, others are entered into for the long term. Often, enduring relationships are necessary if SA participants are to achieve important shared strategic objectives. Form also is shaped in part by whether SA participants adopt limited or what are called loose coupling arrangements or develop more extensive, tightly structured arrangements.

HSO/HS managers considering a SA have options about form in a continuum from simple to complex. The options described in this section include co-opting, loose coupling or coalescing, and mergers and consolidations.

Co-opting

At the simplest end of the continuum, a HSO/HS can absorb limited elements or components of interdependent entities into itself. Thompson labeled such arrangements co-opting.[71] Other than market transactions, co-opting is the most flexible and easiest to implement of all SAs, two advantages that make it a pervasive form of alliance.

The most basic form of co-opting occurs when one entity appoints a representative from another interdependent entity to a position within itself. For example, a HSO/HS that wishes to improve ties to the community it serves might add community representatives to an advisory panel to help guide decision making and gain support. Similarly, a HMO that is concerned about quality may find advantages in adding members of the clinical staff to its GB.

A somewhat more complex but still relatively simple co-opting form through which to establish a SA is contract management. Also known as outsourcing, contract management is an administrative arrangement whereby a HSO/HS arranges for a firm that specializes in a particular area such as dialysis, clinical equipment maintenance, waste management, housekeeping, laundry, or food service to manage its corresponding department under contract.[72] In these arrangements, contractors perform the day-to-day management of departments or other units or functions of a HSO/HS under terms specified in the contract.

Loose Coupling or Coalescing

Moving along the continuum of organizational forms for SAs from relatively simple to more complex, one finds IORs in which participants "coalesce"[73] or couple themselves loosely[74] into SAs in forms such as joint ventures, partnerships, or consortia. The central feature of these coalesced or loosely coupled SAs is the partial pooling of resources by two or more entities to pursue defined objectives.

Loosely coupled or coalesced SAs link interdependent and mutually responsive organizations and systems in ways that preserve their legal identities and most of their functional autonomies. These relationships are bound by ties that are stronger than those in market transactions or in the simplest IORs, such as co-opting or contract management, but are less binding and extensive than those in ownership arrangements.

When SAs are not based on formal ownership arrangements but behave as if they are, they are called virtual SAs. Such alliances exhibit many of the characteristics of a true organization (shared goals, mutual dependency, task subdivision and specialization, bureaucratic structures, and formal coordinating and control mechanisms), but they lack ownership linkages among participants. They rely instead on contractual relationships.

For example, a virtual SA can be formed by an acute care hospital, a large multispeciality group practice, a nursing facility, and an insurance carrier creating IORs among themselves based on contractual agreements to collaborate in designing, producing, and marketing a managed care product. In such an arrangement the four organizations forming the SA continue to operate independent of one another in accomplishing other, perhaps mutually exclusive, objectives. However, the collaborative activity may have significant strategic importance to the participating organizations, including survival.[75] In this example the interdependencies among participants in the SA are managed through IORs that avoid the restrictions and diminution of autonomy and identity that are associated with such ownership arrangements as acquiring or merging with other interdependent entities.

Another example of a partial pooling of resources among organizations participating in a SA to pursue specific objectives can be seen in a decision by three health care quality oversight organizations. The American Medical Accreditation Program (AMAP), the Joint Commission on Accreditation of Healthcare Organizations (Joint Commission), and the National Committee for Quality Assurance (NCQA) established a coordinating body, the Performance Measurement Coordinating Council (PMCC).[76]

PMCC is a coalesced or loosely coupled organization. The participants who coalesced into this SA have the shared objectives of directing PMCC to make performance measurement more efficient and coherent across all levels of the health care system and to more efficiently provide meaningful information to health care purchasers, providers, and consumers.

The desirability of forming PMCC and pursuing certain objectives through it grows from the overall objectives of the three participating organizations. AMAP, which is sponsored by the American Medical Association, sets standards for and seeks to improve the performance of individual physicians. The Joint Commission sets standards for and supports performance improvement in HSOs/HSs. It evaluates and accredits almost 20,000 HSOs/HSs, including hospitals, HSs, and organizations that provide home care, long-term care, and behavioral health care, as well as laboratory and ambulatory care services. NCQA measures and reports on the quality of the care that is provided by the nation's MCOs. More than 75% of HMO enrollees are in health plans that have been reviewed by NCQA. NCQA also manages the Health Plan Employer Data and Information Set (HEDIS), the performance measurement tool used by more than 90% of the nation's health plans.

Given the similarities in function and objectives and the relationships among the work of the participants, it is easy to understand why they view the PMCC strategic alliance as a way to jointly address specific performance measurement objectives. PMCC's objectives include creating a common process by which performance measurement development efforts will be prioritized, reaching consensus on a set of desired attributes for performance measures, and adopting a common framework for evaluating new measures.[77]

Joint ventures are a prevalent type of loosely coupled SA for HSOs/HSs. As noted earlier, a joint venture is an IOR that is characterized by the presence of a contract or agreement and a legal entity through which participants pursue some activity in which they share costs, revenues, and control. Some joint ventures are organized as limited liability companies (LLCs), as discussed in Chapter 4. However, joint ventures involving HSOs/HSs and physician members of their clinical staff typically are limited partnerships, a different type of legal entity. The HSO/HS is the general partner and physicians are limited partners. The general partner usually invests the bulk of the capital and usually is the managing partner. Limited partners invest far less capital, sometimes insignificant amounts, a fact that has caused problems with the Internal Revenue Service for some not-for-profit HSOs/HSs. The primary reason to involve physicians in joint ventures, however, is not the capital they bring to the enterprise. The key reasons are that this ties them more closely to the HSO/HS and that they provide referrals to the health services delivery activity that is the purpose of the joint venture; or, in the case of a medical office building (usually on the HSO's/HS's campus), physicians rent space from the limited partnership and locate their practices there. Efforts to tie physicians who are independent contractors into the HSO/HS are known as bonding. Well-conceived and well-executed joint ventures may help HSOs/HSs improve their profitability or market position, and perhaps even physician relations.

In addition to joint ventures involving a HSO/HS and members of its professional staff, other joint ventures are undertaken between HSOs/HSs. One example is a joint venture formed in 1996 between Columbia/HCA Healthcare Corporation, a for-profit entity, and the Arlington Health Foundation, a not-for-profit entity, to establish the for-profit Columbia Arlington Healthcare System LLC. The purpose of the joint venture was to manage several northern Virginia hospitals, including Arlington Hospital and Reston Hospital Center. This SA formed between entities with different tax-exempt statuses, however, dissolved in 1999 because the Internal Revenue Service questioned whether the Arlington Health Foundation could keep its charitable status while owning half of the for-profit joint venture.[78]

Mergers and Consolidations

Extensive ownership arrangements are found at the most complex end of the continuum of forms that alliances can take. Some involve changes in ownership of entire HSOs/HSs through mergers or consolidations. A merger results when one (or more) HSO/HS is absorbed by another, which retains its name and identity. Consolidation occurs when two or more HSOs/HSs dissolve and are unified in a new legal entity.

The most complex SAs are formed through the establishment of ownership-based highly integrated HSs. As noted earlier, these SAs seek to link the components of health services delivery and, in some cases, financing in ways that more efficiently and effectively meet the health services needs of the populations they serve. The specific forms that HSs take are idiosyncratic; each is unique. However, the objectives of the integrative activity involved in forming highly integrated IISs—whether through ownership, contract, or a combination—are rather uniformly established as[79]

- Acceptance of financial risk and the ability to contract based on a single signature
- Capability to manage the different components of risk among the different providers
- Development of a strong central GB (discussed later) that has earned support from all HS components
- Increased physician leadership and participation in management
- Information systems capable of integrating financial, operational, clinical, and management data and delivering them in an appropriate and timely manner
- Coordination to ensure a smooth transition of patients along the continuum of care
- Improvements in outcomes of care and quality of services
- Accountability for the health status of enrollees
- Assumption of responsibility for managing the total health of the enrolled population

These interconnected objectives are shown in Figure 5.5. As this figure illustrates, the process of integration can begin at any of a number of points—either one at a time or several simultaneously—as objectives for integration are pursued. The figure also shows that a particular HS may be closer to achieving effective integration in one objective than in others. For example, a HS might be quite far along in centralizing governance but at the same time have made relatively little progress toward the goal of involving physicians in leadership roles.

Figure 5.5 does not rank the objectives of integration as to importance. However, other investigators argue that clinical integration is the most important aspect of integration.[80] Clinical integration is defined by Shortell and his colleagues as "the extent to which patient care services are coordinated across people, functions, activities, processes, and operating units so as to maximize the value of services delivered."[81] They also pointed out that clinical integration "includes both horizontal integration (the coordination of activities at the same stage of delivery of care) as well as vertical integration (the coordination of services at different stages)—for example, between acute care and post acute care."[82] Clinical integration, at the operational level, includes concern for continuity and coordination

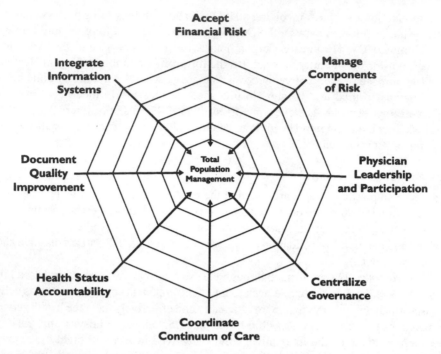

Figure 5.5.   Objectives of integration. (Adapted from Hoechst Marion Roussel. *Managed Care Digest Series: Integrated Health Systems Digest,* 2. Kansas City, MO: Hoechst Marion Roussel, 1999; used with permission.)

of care as well as "disease management, good communication among caregivers, smooth transfer of information and patient records, elimination of duplicate testing and procedures, and efficient use and management of resources."[83] Conrad noted that "administrative and organizational-managerial integration is a necessary complement to the clinical integration of patient care, but it is the latter that is crucial to achieve a viable vertically integrated regional health system."[84] Kittredge noted that

> *to be truly successful in managing the care of the large population it seeks to serve, an integrated delivery system must establish as its long-term goals the measurable improvement of the outcomes of care and experience of the patients it serves and the ability to successfully provide healthcare for a market price. . . . What's required to achieve this goal is the clinical integration of the system.*[85]

Summary

SAs can begin with voluntary IORs such as one HSO/HS appointing a representative from another to a position within itself, perhaps to a seat on its GB. The continuum of SA forms, with increasing complexity, moves from this relatively simple form to contract management or outsourcing to IORs in which participants coalesce or couple themselves loosely into alliances based on the partial pooling of their resources to pursue common objectives. These SAs might be more virtual than real in the sense that they are based more on contractual relationships than ownership. They move through joint ventures, which are SAs that are characterized by the presence of contracts or agreements and a legal entity that pools only limited interests through ownership, to SAs in which the ownership of entire HSOs/HSs is involved. The most complex end of the continuum is HSs, especially highly integrated HSs. The complexity of highly integrated HSs varies in terms of whether they are established through ownership or contractual arrangements.

The Future of SAs: A New Health Services Ecosystem

Whether examined from the perspective of participants, purposes, or forms, the trend is toward more integration between and among HSOs/HSs. Furthermore, the trend is toward increased formation of highly integrated HSs, the most extensive form of integration in health services. In a quite imaginative and descriptive analogy, Orlikoff and Totten[86] compared the trend toward more integration in health services, especially in the form of highly integrated HSs, to a forest ecosystem (an ecosystem is simply a community of organisms within their environment). They noted that in the forest, the source of all life is the sun. The plants that inhabit the forest have a simple objective: to position themselves to absorb as much sunlight as possible. Plants that cannot acquire enough sunlight by position must ensure their existence by evolving mechanisms to survive on diminished energy from the sun. They become niche players in the forest ecology. Plants, in their pursuit of sunlight, seek to block the rays of the sun from their competitors.

Using this oversimplified forest ecosystem as an analogy for the health services ecosystem, Orlikoff and Totten suggested that the source of all life in the health services ecosystem is those who pay for health services (Figure 5.6). Payers are not the same as insurers; instead, payers are the employers, Medicare and Medicaid programs, and individuals who actually pay for the costs of health services. In the Orlikoff-Totten analogy, just as plants in the forest attempt to position themselves as close as possible to the sun, the participants in the health services ecosystem have the basic objective of positioning themselves as close as possible to their source of life: the payers. As is shown in Figure 5.6, the participants in the health services ecosystem in the best positions to thrive are the most highly integrated HSs; the less-integrated participants—freestanding HSOs and independent physicians—have less desirable positions.

Among the emerging advantages that may be of increasing importance to highly integrated HSs is their ability to directly contract with purchasers. Direct contracting occurs through "an agreement between a purchaser (e.g., employer, union health and welfare fund) and providers to render care to employees and/or retirees without the involvement of an insurer or health plan."[87] Purchasers may turn to direct contracting as a means of avoiding some of the costs that are associated with purchasing health benefits through insurers or health plans and as a means of gaining more control over the health care services being purchased.[88] For example, some business purchasing coalitions have chosen to contract directly with health care services providers. Maxwell and colleagues reported that "American Express, 3M, General Mills, and other employers participating in the Twin Cities (MN) purchasing coalition, the Buyers Health Care Action Group (BHCAG), have created a system of direct contracting with exclusive provider groups."[89] They pointed out that in this approach, "large provider groups composed of physicians and clinics compete for the enrollment of the participating companies' employees."[90] Employers in Orlando, Florida, also have contracted directly with hospital-based integrated HSs to provide comprehensive health care services to their employees.[91]

With this background on the nature of SAs, which have been categorized by participants, purpose, and form, attention turns to managing in SAs, especially in the HSs formed through this activity.

MANAGING SAs

All SAs require effective management to flourish. However, just as SAs differ in terms of participants, purposes, and forms, their management differs. It is useful to review the discussion of managerial competencies in Chapter 1, where it is noted that the important clusters of knowledge and skills that make up managerial competencies are 1) conceptual, 2) technical managerial/clinical, 3) interpersonal/collaborative, 4) political, 5) commercial, and 6) governance. This section uses these competencies as a framework and highlights how they pertain to managing in SAs, especially HSs.[92]

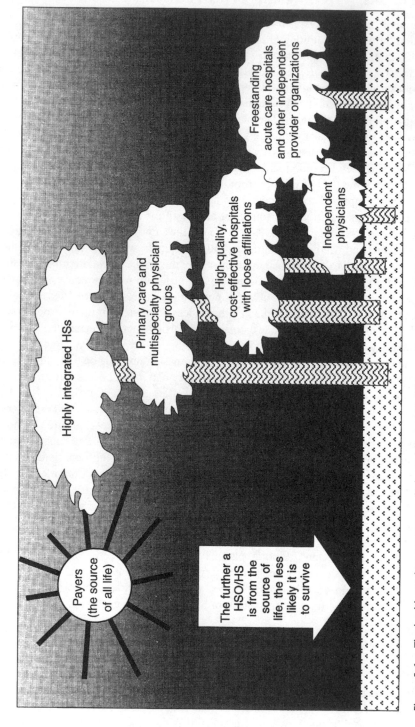

Figure 5.6. The health services ecosystem. (Adapted from Orlikoff, James E., and Mary K. Totten. *The Future of Health Care Governance: Redesigning Boards for a New Era, 5.* Chicago: American Hospital Publishing, 1996; used with permission.)

Conceptual Competence in Managing SAs

The knowledge and skills that compose the conceptual competence needed by managers to envision the place and role of a HSO in the larger society can be magnified many times when applied to a complex SA such as a HS. This competence is necessary, however, if managers involved in SAs are to visualize and understand both the IORs within the alliances and the places of entire alliances in their larger settings. Furthermore, SAs are always works in progress, as are the separate entities participating in them. Typically, their structures and operations are changed continually, and, as noted in Chapter 1, each change expands the notion of an adequate level of conceptual competence.

Apart from organizational and operational complexities, managers in HSs face new or expanded conceptualizations of mission. When missions change, everything about organizations and systems, including their organizational cultures, also may change. The missions of HSs differ from those of their component organizations, although, as discussed in Chapter 8, the missions are interrelated. Furthermore, as HSOs join other organizations in HSs, managers face new and more complex conceptualizations of their own managerial roles as well as the roles of other managers with whom they work. In particular, they are more likely to share their leadership responsibilities with physicians. As has been noted, "success in integrated health care absolutely requires physicians in leadership positions."[93]

In HSs senior-level managers must shift their concepts of managerial success from advancing individual HSOs and achieving incremental improvements in the health of individuals. They must focus on the more complex attainment of synergistic levels of integration among sets of HSOs and perhaps other entities to enhance the health status of the defined populations that their HSs serve. At middle and first-line levels, managers must meet new conceptual challenges entailed in meshing their units with demands imposed by larger systems. They may need to suboptimize performance of their unit to optimize the system's performance.

The more extensive and demanding conceptual challenges of increasingly integrated health services significantly broaden the notion of conceptual competence for managers. To achieve success, managers working within HSs and other types of SAs must be more creative and able to synthesize ideas into new forms and patterns. They must be creative in adapting their domains to constantly evolving circumstances as alliances change by maturing or disintegrating. These managers will increasingly rely on information, often from disparate sources, to build frameworks, concepts, and hypotheses about the future of their units, organizations, or systems. They will be required to identify and evaluate options for solving ever more complex challenges and to select among them. To succeed in HSs managers must[94]

- Seek harmony in interactions within the HS
- Balance analysis (the examination of parts of the HS) with synthesis (seeing the parts as a whole)
- Focus on seeing the whole picture of the HS with all of its parts, large and small
- Emphasize patterns of change over time rather than static snapshots of activity or behavior
- Pursue root causes of performance problems to avoid symptomatic responses
- Focus on integration, interconnectedness, and interrelationships within the HS

Technical Managerial/Clinical Competence in Managing SAs

As with conceptual competence, the technical managerial/clinical competence that is required of managers in more complex SAs is generally more extensive than needed for an independent HSO. As noted in Chapter 1, all senior-level managers in HSOs/HSs need to possess both a degree of clinical and significant management expertise. However, this increases, especially on the clinical side, in integrated situations in which SAs are formed among entities that are involved in diverse aspects of clinical care.

In highly integrated HSs, for example, senior-level managers lead their systems in providing continua of health services to defined populations. In doing so managers face difficult work imperatives requiring new or expanded competencies as they assess health needs in the populations they serve and measure performance as improvements in the health status of their client populations; as they use population-based data to determine appropriate system or network size and configuration in terms of primary and specialty providers, acute care and nursing facility beds, home health, hospice, and related components of the continuum of service; and, perhaps, as they assume financial risk for the provision of services.

Interpersonal/Collaborative Competence in Managing SAs

The essence of the interpersonal competence of managers, in any setting, is knowing how to motivate people, communicate visions and preferences, handle negotiations, and manage conflicts. In addition to the traditional interpersonal competence that is required of managers in independent HSOs when HSOs integrate into SAs, especially in the more complex HSs, two elements of interpersonal knowledge and skills become important. Together, these elements form collaborative competence.

The first element in collaborative competence is the ability to partner, which is creating and maintaining multiparty organizational arrangements, negotiating complex agreements and contracts that sustain these arrangements, and producing mutually beneficial outcomes through such arrangements.[95] The second element of collaborative competence, closely related to but distinct from partnering ability, is the ability to manage within the context of a HS. This context is different from an independent HSO and requires different decisions and actions by managers.

A partnering skill that is crucial to success in establishing and maintaining effective HSs is the ability of managers to develop shared cultures. In this context, culture is the pattern of shared values and beliefs that become ingrained in the HS participants over time and that influence their collaborative behaviors and decisions. A senior manager in one HS noted,

> *Nothing is more important to the long-term success of integrated systems than developing a culture. We have to do it or we won't survive. Without it, we won't be able to stand the pressures and develop the team approach we need.*[96]

Collaborative competence also may mean establishing not only new mission statements and associated organizational objectives but also new types of missions and objectives that fit the HS's needs and toward which others can be led. In independent HSOs organizational objectives typically pertain to success in meeting volume, revenue, market share, and narrowly specified quality targets. In HSs organizational objectives at the system level pertain to enhancing the health status of a defined population and integrating functionally diverse organizations.

For the senior managers of HSs the core interpersonal/collaborative management challenge is to convince the senior managers of the system's component organizations not to view success in terms of "advancing individual organizational priorities and favorably positioning the organization within the wider system"[97] but to consider the system's broader vision, values, and objectives. They must suboptimize individual unit performance to optimize performance of the whole system. For managers at all levels of a HS's component HSOs, the challenge is adjusting their mindsets regarding success and helping subordinates do the same. These adjustments in thinking are made more challenging by perceptions and habits ingrained during years of pursuing narrower definitions of success.

In the context of independent HSOs, conflict management responsibilities primarily involve managers in resolving issues of intrapersonal conflict (within a person), interpersonal conflict (between or among individuals), intragroup conflict (within a group), or intergroup conflict (between or among groups). Increased levels of integration among HSOs as they form SAs, especially the more complex HSs, have added managing conflicts between and among the organizations participating in a SA to this list of substantial traditional conflict management responsibilities.

As integration levels increase, senior-level managers become involved in interorganizational conflict. Integration of providers at different points in the patient services continuum brings into proximity disparate organizations, especially when HSs are linked with insurers or health plans. Conflicts are unavoidable, and the knowledge and skills that are useful in managing them effectively are imperative. Interpersonal/collaborative competence is required of senior-level managers in all HSOs, but it is even more complex and important in HSs.

Political/Commercial Competencies in Managing SAs

Managers in SAs must possess political and commercial competencies. Political competence in any setting is defined as the dual capability to accurately assess the impact of public policies on the manager's domains of responsibility and to influence policy making at state and federal levels.[98] Commercial competence, in any setting, is the ability of managers to establish and operate value-~~~~~~ of these competencies differs in the situations that are created by the formation of SAs. The competencies are no more or less important than for the manager of an independent HSO, but the context in which they are applied is different.

Political competence in the context of a SA such as a HS requires successful interactions with more policy decisions and with more policy makers than is typical for an independent HSO. Contrast the numbers and variety of policy decisions that are relevant for a single, independent community hospital with those of relevance to a large, highly integrated HS.

Similarly, commercial competence in any setting is based on knowledge and associated skills in identifying markets and positioning a HSO/HS in its markets, and in establishing product/service strategies that enhance the HSO's/HS's ability to compete effectively. Increasingly, commercial success for HSOs/HSs involved in alliance formation is determined by their ability to contract with health plans to provide a package of integrated services, and, in some cases, to contract with employers to provide services directly to their employees. Indeed, the ability to enter into such contracts is one of the principal motives in forming many SAs.

As HSs are formed to deliver a continuum of health services under managed care contracts, they must develop the following characteristics to achieve commercial success[99]:

- Some level of clinical coordination, not just administrative or financial coordination, among organizations in the HS
- A focus by at least some HS actors, most likely primary care physicians, on performance of the HS as a whole
- Achievement of some level of physician integration (commitment of physicians to the HS) at least among primary providers
- A focus on primary care and prevention
- A minimum geographic and service breadth
- Development of sophisticated information systems
- A capacity to improve and compete on quality

In HSs that are the most integrated—where delivery and financing are integrated—the determinants of commercial success expand to include not only those noted previously but also marketing the system directly to consumers. Premiums and covered lives become crucial aspects of commercial success. No matter where along the spectrum of integration a SA is found, however, the commercial competence of its managers is increasingly important.

Governance Competence in Managing SAs

Finally, as also noted in Chapter 1, governance competence is important for managers in all HSOs/HSs. This competence becomes even more important in SAs, especially in HSs, in which the vast majority of chief executive officers (CEOs) are members of GBs and in which other senior-level managers, such as chief financial and chief medical officers, also are typically internal members of a HS's GB.

This competence also is important because it is difficult to separate what occurs under the rubric of governance from what occurs in the context of strategic management. Consequently, effective senior-level managers must be knowledgeable about management and governance. Furthermore, managers in SAs must possess governance competence so that they can assist others with direct governance responsibilities to do a better job. This includes providing development programs for members of GBs. It also may mean simplifying governance structures as HSs develop. As has been noted, "Byzantine board structures are an all-too-common by-product of hospital and health system mergers. While multiple boards and committees can facilitate communication, trust and community linkages, health systems often pay a high price to keep so many trustees involved."[100] Important aspects of governance in HSs are discussed in the next section.

GOVERNANCE IN HSs

This discussion of governance applies, at least in part, to many SAs. However, it focuses specifically on governance in vertically integrated HSs, the most complex form of SA.[101] Understanding governance in HSs requires an appreciation of the fact that because HSs are wholes made up of parts, their governance involves three sets of issues: 1) issues of governance of the whole (the HS), 2) issues of governance of the various parts or component HSOs of the HS, and 3) issues that arise between the two levels of governance. The question of who governs what (or who controls what) is relatively straightforward in independent HSOs (as discussed in Chapter 4), but it is more complicated in integrated situations. In general, the more organizationally complex the HS, the more complex its governance.

Centralized Versus Decentralized Governance Structures

The most basic governance issue in HSs is whether governance is centralized or decentralized.[102] The centralized governance structure model, sometimes referred to as a corporate or system board model, centralizes governance control in a single GB that exercises direct control over all of the component HSOs in the system (see Figure 5.7). Component HSOs may have advisory bodies, but these bodies have no legal or fiduciary authority; there is only one GB for the HS.

A second model, the decentralized governance structure, sometimes referred to as the parent holding company model, decentralizes governance control and shares it among the system GB and separate subordinate GBs, often at the level of component HSOs or entities. "Probably the biggest single asset of this arrangement is that it provides the opportunity to push selected governance functions down to the level where they can be fulfilled with a greater sensitivity to the distinctive circumstances faced by system components."[103]

In a decentralized model (see Figure 5.8) the parent or system GB retains defined authority over the subordinate GBs, but governance responsibilities within the HS are divided and shared among the system-level and component-level GBs according to an agreed-on plan. A key responsibility of the system GB in a decentralized governance structure is oversight and coordination of subordinate GBs. This can be difficult to accomplish when the various GBs have differences in viewpoints or philosophies that create dynamic tension between them, often with the HS's CEO caught in the middle. For example, the parent GB may have a futuristic vision, whereas the subor-

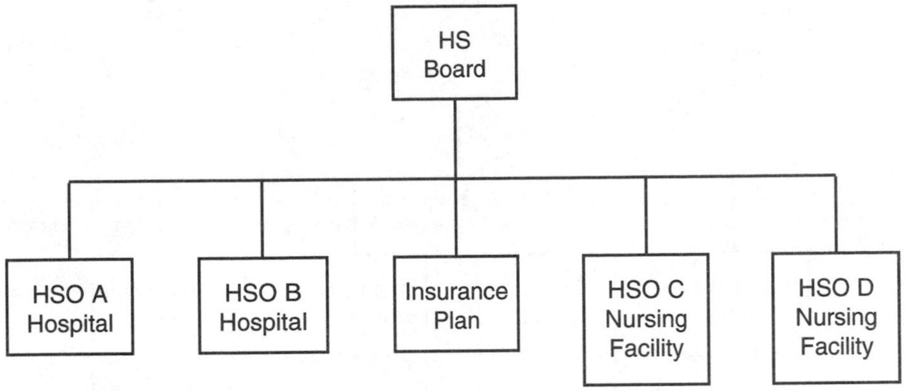

Figure 5.7. Centralized governance structure.

clients. GBs may focus more on [illegible] operational or financial concerns. These conflicts can occur even when some of the subordinate GB members serve on the HS's GB. CEOs may be able to avoid or minimize this conflict and the discontinuities it causes by insisting that their GBs help them develop a shared vision through the strategic plan.[104]

In decentralized HSs subordinate boards can be structured along organizational, regional, or functional lines.[105] In a decentralized HS that structures its subordinate boards organizationally, as is shown in Figure 5.8, there is a system board, and each component HSO of the HS is overseen by its own GB. When subordinate boards are structured regionally, each subordinate board oversees a particular market or geographic region where the HS operates. When subordinate boards are structured functionally, each oversees groupings of system components that perform similar functions (e.g., physician groups, hospitals, insurance companies). Figure 5.9 shows systems in which subordinate boards are structured regionally or functionally. Finally, Figure 5.10 illustrates a very complex governance structure in which a HS combines all three ways of structuring its subordinate boards. In this model the HS board oversees a functional board (the insurance company board), as well as regional boards that, in turn, oversee organizational boards within the regions.

Orlikoff compares the advantages of the centralized and decentralized models as follows.[106] In a centralized governance structure in a HS decisions can be made more quickly, the time that

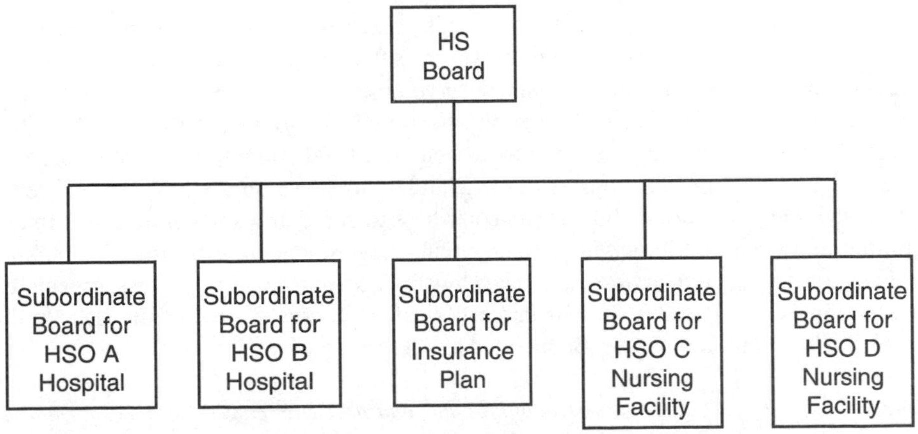

Figure 5.8. Decentralized governance structure.

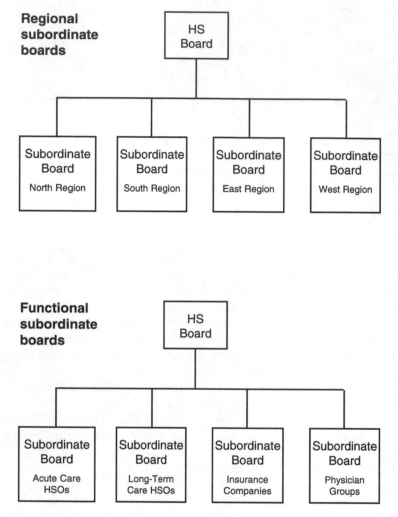

Figure 5.9. Decentralized governance structures with regional or functional subordinate boards.

managers must spend on governance interactions is minimized, and the system GB is encouraged to focus on strategic issues. Offsetting this, however, is the fact that a centralized governance structure limits the number of stakeholders that can serve on the GB. The advantages of the decentralized governance structure include that it permits the system GB to push details to subordinate GBs, subordinate GBs may be closer to and can focus better on local community or HSO issues, and decentralization permits a greater number of stakeholders to serve on a HS's GBs. Offsetting this, however, is the fact that multiple boards can contribute to confusion and conflict over roles and responsibilities and even to gridlock in extreme circumstances, can consume significant amounts of management time in GB interactions, and may slow the decision-making process, especially if subordinate GBs insist on focusing on their interests at the expense of those of the HS. On this latter point, which is a common problem, Bader cited a recent example:

> *Several years ago a California system of hospitals and physician enterprises confronted a jet-powered competitive market with a Model-T governance structure. The hospitals and physicians had joined up to gain system advantages. But, wary of losing control, individual-entity boards*

had retained enough power to put local interests ahead of system priorities. So the hospitals con-
tinued old habits of competing for patients instead of seeking system efficiencies and supporting
investments to help the system as a whole vie for managed care business. "This multitude of local
boards prohibited us from making planning or policy decisions on any reasonable basis that re-
flected all the areas we served," one board members says. Although the need to restructure gov-
ernance was clear, there was one barrier: "The autonomy these boards felt was very important
to them," the trustee says.[107]

Composition of the GB

Closely related to the issue of centralized versus decentralized governance structures in HSs is the
issue of the composition of the GB. A HS's GB can be composed of representative members, nonrepresentative members, or a combination.[108] Representative members of a HS's centralized corporate GB are selected because of their relationship to a particular component HSO of the system.
Nonrepresentative members are not directly aligned with, nor do they represent the specific concerns of, any particular system component HSO. Most often, representative members of a system-

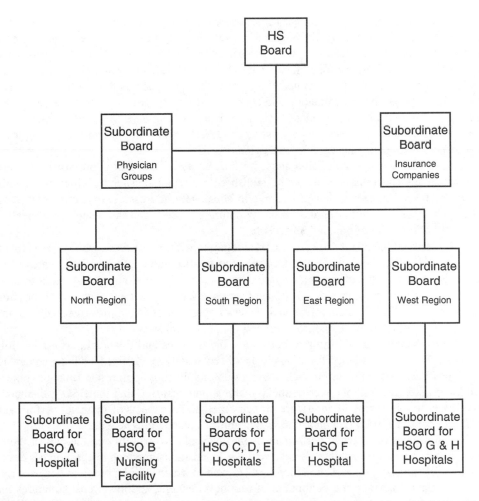

Figure 5.10.   Complex governance structure combining organizational, regional, and functional bases of structuring subordinate boards.

level GB are the CEOs or members of the GBs of the component HSOs. One obvious consequence of representative GBs is that, as the HSs they govern grow, the size of the GB also will grow, perhaps to an unmanageable size.

Governance Responsibilities

In addition to the fact that governance issues of control differ in integrated situations, various governance responsibilities are met differently. In both independent HSOs and HSs those who govern have five responsibilities to which they must attend, albeit differently, if they are to fulfill their obligations to stakeholders, including the owners or shareholders in for-profit situations.[109]

First, GBs are responsible for formulating organizational ends. That is, they are responsible for establishing a vision for the HSO/HS, from which a mission and associated organizational objectives grow. As noted earlier in the discussion of the conceptual competence of senior-level managers in SAs, the missions of HSs differ from those of any of their component HSOs. In a highly integrated HS, for example, the mission emphasizes enhancement of the health status of a defined population rather than reducing illness in individuals. Those who govern in integrated contexts must think very broadly and positively about health.

Second, GBs have a responsibility to ensure suitable performance from senior-level managers. The steps that are involved in fulfilling this responsibility typically include selecting the CEO, specifying performance expectations, and periodically appraising the CEO's actual performance.[110] This is not an easy task in integrated health care. As Ummel, reflecting on the difficulties faced by those who seek to build highly integrated HSs, noted, "it is obvious that the health care industry has not been through massive consolidation and restructuring before. Amateurish moves, setbacks, and missed opportunities are commonplace."[111] More than anything else, these difficulties reflect the fact that many senior-level managers and members of GBs of HSs are not very far along the learning curve of how to create highly integrated HSs.

Third, GBs are responsible, ultimately, for the quality of care that is provided. The legal responsibilities of GBs in this area are well established[112] and include such activities as credentialing members of the PSO; seeing that procedures to adequately address quality, utilization, and risk management issues are in place; and assessing both the process and the outcomes of health care, increasingly at the level of populations in HSs.

Concern about the quality of care is a traditional imperative for those who govern HSOs. The emergence of HSs, however, affords GBs new opportunities and challenges in this area of governance responsibility. The integration of various providers of care along a continuum of care presents unprecedented opportunities for the application of new algorithms, guidelines, or pathways toward improved clinical outcomes, as well as new opportunities for improved service quality and improved levels of customer satisfaction among the populations served.

GBs also bear responsibility in a fourth area, the finances and financial performance of their HSOs/HSs. This responsibility traditionally has been widely recognized in independent HSOs, where it has been concentrated on such activities as establishing appropriate financial objectives; maintaining adequate controls over financial matters; and ensuring that the HSO's financial obligations, including investing its funds, are properly met. These aspects of financial performance responsibility continue in HSs, even as the responsibility expands into new areas.

Certain aspects of financial performance and financial responsibility on the part of those who govern are especially different in integrated settings. In situations in which integration has developed to the point of single-signature contracting by a HS, and in which enough progress has been made in clinical outcomes management, continuum-of-care development, and lower cost structures for episodes of care, the HS is positioned to reap the financial benefits of large-scale, unified selling. That is, they are positioned to garner more managed care contracts with insurers and other payers and to obtain such contracts under more favorable terms, such as multiyear agreements and fair rates.

As HSs develop and mature, they also may successfully pursue commercial and Medicare risk contracting. With the assumption of risks comes significant opportunities for financial gain by the HSs. The potential financial benefits inherent in unified selling opportunities and in risk contracting represent significant new opportunities—and challenges—in the area of GBs' responsibilities for financial performance.

The fifth area of GB responsibility is one for self. That is, those who govern are responsible for doing so in an effective and efficient manner. Fulfilling this responsibility includes establishing and maintaining appropriate bylaws to guide the governance process, selecting GB members who can serve the HSO/HS well and seeing that they do, and ensuring that processes for evaluating GB performance and for member development are in place and properly functioning. The differences here between independent HSOs and HSs are mostly those of scope and complexity, although, as noted earlier, when HSs have a number of boards, there are significant challenges involved in having them work together well.

SELECTED TECHNICAL ISSUES IN MANAGING IORs

Among a number of important technical issues involved in understanding and managing the IORs that HSOs/HSs engage in, three are especially important: the use of negotiation in managing them, the special case of managing involuntary IORs with regulators and others, and corporate diversification and restructuring. These issues are discussed here because they may be critical to successful management of certain IORs.

Negotiations in Managing IORs

Critical to success in establishing and maintaining effective IORs in many situations are the abilities of managers to establish contracts or agreements and to conduct the negotiations that lead to them. Effectively managing all IORs—whether market transactions, involuntary IORs, or SAs—relies, at least in part, on establishment of and adherence to the terms of contracts between or among participants. Contracts, in turn, rely on effective negotiations between or among the parties involved.

Negotiation (also called bargaining) is a process through which the parties decide what each will give and take in their transactions. In negotiation the parties attempt to agree on a mutually acceptable outcome. Negotiations follow one of two approaches: cooperative, or win–win; and competitive, or win–lose. Given the expectation for ongoing relationships among the participants in negotiations, as typically is the case in negotiations within IORs, the use of cooperative approaches whenever possible is important. The main idea in win–win negotiations is for all parties to gain. Such negotiations have been called distributive in nature and rely on the parties' taking a problem-solving approach rather than a competitive approach.

Distributive negotiations must be built on a foundation of trust. This is especially important in the context of the negotiations that occur within SAs. In fact, at higher levels of integration, trust among senior-level managers is necessary for true partnerships to be established and maintained. For some managers, the ability to trust others or to engender trust may represent new skills.

Contracts, which are described more fully in Chapter 14, are widely used in SAs, as well as in IORs that are formed for the purpose of conducting market transactions and in the involuntary IORs that are formed with regulators and other entities. They provide essential guidelines for performance in all IORs. Contracts usually are negotiated agreements between parties for the exchange of future performance. They can rest simply on the faith and belief that each party will perform as agreed or, more rigorously, on specific terms that can be evaluated by third parties and that are the basis for damages if performance by either or both of the parties to the contract is unsatisfactory.

IORs that are guided by contracts may entail only an agreement for products or services, or they may be a complex agreement between a HS and a HMO, for example, to provide certain services to a defined population. Contracts permit HSOs/HSs to establish stable and predictable (but interdependent) relationships with federal and state governments as they purchase services for Medicare or Medicaid recipients and with health plans and commercial insurers for various types of reimbursement. They also permit employment and use of a workforce and orderly acquisition of other inputs.

The most important skills in developing effective contracts or agreements are negotiating skills. Technically, negotiation is "the process whereby two or more parties attempt to settle what each shall give and take, or perform and receive, in a transaction between them."[113] In negotiating, the parties in IORs seek agreement on a mutually acceptable outcome. Typically, at least two sources of conflict must be resolved: 1) dividing resources—the so-called tangibles of negotiation, such as which party will receive how much money, goods, or services in exchange for what consideration; and 2) resolving psychological dynamics and satisfying personal motivations of the leaders of organizations and systems that are involved in the negotiations. The latter aspects are so-called intangibles of negotiation and can include such variables as appearing to win or lose, competing effectively, or cooperating fairly. Negotiations between interdependent entities such as those that might occur between a Blue Cross plan and a HSO/HS sometimes hinge more on the intangibles than the tangibles.

As noted earlier, negotiations between interdependent parties are cooperative or competitive. The negotiating approach is a function of several variables. Optimal conditions for a cooperative negotiating approach include the following[114]:

- Both sides have tangible goals of obtaining a specific settlement that is fair and reasonable.
- Sufficient resources are available in the situation so that both sides can attain their tangible goals, more resources can be attained, or the problem can be redefined so that both sides can actually "win."
- Both sides believe that it is possible for them to attain their goals through the negotiation process.
- Both sides have intangible goals of establishing a cooperative relationship within which they can work together toward a settlement that maximizes their joint outcomes.

Optimal conditions for competitive negotiations include the following[115]:

- Both sides have tangible goals of obtaining a specific settlement in which they each get as much as possible.
- The resources available in the situation are insufficient for both sides to attain their goals, or their desire to get as much as possible makes it impossible for one or both to actually attain their goal(s).
- Both sides perceive that it is impossible for both of them to attain their goals.
- Both sides have intangible goals of beating the other, keeping the other from attaining its goals, perhaps even humiliating the other, or refusing to make concessions in their negotiating positions.

Whether interdependent parties are engaged in cooperative or competitive negotiation, the process tends to proceed in distinct phases.[116] First, there is a preparation phase, during which both sides assess the nature of their interests, establish their own goals and priorities and try to guess those of the other side, and determine the negotiating approach that they plan to use. Second, there is an entry phase in which the sides make initial contact with each other; establish an agenda, rules, and procedures for the negotiation; and present their initial goals and priorities. The third phase, elaboration and education, is characterized by each side learning more about its opponent's stated goals and priorities and elaborating on its own initially stated goals and priorities in light of what is learned. The fourth phase, bargaining, is the heart of the negotiating process and entails attempts by both sides to challenge their opponent's goals and logic, defend their own, search for ways to make compromises and trade-offs, and invent alternative solutions. The final phase of the negotiating process is closure, during which both sides seek to arrive at a basic agreement, consolidate the issues into a package, record the agreement in mutually satisfactory language, and begin planning for the implementation of the agreement.

Table 5.2 outlines tactics that can be used in both cooperative and competitive negotiations in each of the phases of the process. Often, negotiations are neither purely cooperative nor competitive, requiring a mixture of the tactics for successful results.

Unique Aspects of Managing Involuntary IORs

Some of the most important interdependencies for HSOs/HSs are with regulatory agencies such as state licensing agencies or the federal Health Care Financing Administration, or their interactions with private-sector organizations such as fiscal intermediaries and bond rating services. These interdependent relationships cannot be legally managed through market transactions, nor are they managed through the voluntary IORs or SAs discussed earlier, although these relationships do sometimes stimulate the creation of voluntary IORs. For example, a primary reason for forming a SA among HSOs/HSs with a common regulatory agency is to share expertise and thus achieve a stronger position in dealing with the regulator and its regulations. This phenomenon is not unique to health services. Regulation in any industry encourages consolidation among the regulated to develop counterregulatory expertise and power.

TABLE 5.2. TACTICS IN COMPETITIVE AND COOPERATIVE NEGOTIATIONS

Phase of negotiation	Competitive tactics	Cooperative tactics
Preparation	Set specific goals, bottom lines, and opening bids; develop firm positions and competitive tactics to attain those goals at the expense of the other.	Develop general goals and broad objectives; cultivate good options; cultivate good relations of trust and openness with opponent to promote effective problem solving.
Entry-problem identification	State the problem in terms of the organization's preferred solution; publicly disguise or misrepresent organization needs and goals; do not let the other side know what is really important.	State the problem in terms of the underlying needs of both sides; represent organization's needs accurately to the other side; listen carefully to understand their needs.
Elaboration or education	Disclose only the information necessary to support the organization's position and have the other side understand it; hide possible vulnerabilities and weaknesses.	Disclose all information that may be pertinent to a problem, regardless of whose position it supports; expose vulnerabilities in order to protect them in the joint solution.
Bargaining	Include false issues, dummy options, or options of low priority in order to trade them away for what your side wants; make an early public commitment and stick to it.	Minimize the inclusion of false or dummy issues and stick to the major problems and concerns; avoid early and public commitments to preferred alternatives in order to give all options full consideration.
Closure	Maximize own utility while not caring about the other's; overvalue concessions to other; undervalue achieved gains; use "nibbling" strategy of taking issues off the table as favorable settlements are achieved.	Maximize solutions that have joint utility; be honest and candid in disclosing preferences; use "nothing is ever final until all issues are settled" strategy.

Adapted from Greenberger, David, Stephen Strasser, Roy J. Lewicki, and Thomas S. Bateman. "Perception, Motivation, and Negotiation." In *Health Care Management: A Text in Organization Theory and Behavior,* 2nd ed., edited by Stephen M. Shortell, Arnold D. Kaluzny, and Associates, 134. Albany, NY: Delmar Publishers, 1988.

Managers use a variety of mechanisms to manage involuntary IORs. Just as contracts and the negotiations on which they are built are vital to managing market transactions and SAs, the establishment of rules and procedures to guide relationships between regulators and regulated HSOs/HSs in involuntary IORs is essential to managing these relationships. Negotiating skills are equally important in establishing rules and procedural guidelines in involuntary IORs as in developing contracts in market transactions or the contracts and other agreements in SAs.

Reliance on rules and procedures makes litigation one of the most important and frequently used mechanisms in managing involuntary IORs.[117] Regulatory decisions can be appealed to the courts, which are sensitive to procedural errors or infringement of due process rights. Regulators who overlook requirements for notice, public hearings, or the opportunity for full consideration of issues invite litigation. Regulators may lack resources for proper legal representation, or sometimes they must rely on state legal staff without expertise in health matters. Another factor that facilitates the litigation strategy is that some standards that are used by regulators are not substantiated by analysis or fact and thus are vulnerable to judicial scrutiny.

Although distasteful to many, cultivating supportive relationships with the executive and legislative branches and with state and federal regulatory agencies can be effective protection against overly enthusiastic or even dutiful regulators. It is no accident that HSOs/HSs routinely place prominent public officials and politically connected private citizens on their GBs, that physicians are among the most generous political campaign contributors, or that well-connected consultants flourish in and around Washington, D.C., and state capitals.

A mechanism drawn from textbooks on negotiating, sometimes called the "loaf-and-a-half"[118] approach, involves a regulated HSO/HS initially seeking more than it expects or wants to obtain from the regulator. For example, by enlarging a building project for which state approval is sought, the regulated HSO/HS gives the regulator the opportunity to "play hardball" and force a scaling back of a project without actually jeopardizing what the HSO/HS really wants. A common variation of this strategy is to offer regulators something they want (e.g., a commitment to provide care for indigent patients) to obtain approval.

Because regulated HSOs/HSs with the support of politically powerful constituencies are less vulnerable to adverse regulatory decisions, HSO/HSs cultivate powerful constituencies as a means of protecting themselves from regulators. The constituency may be based on religion, ethnicity, geography, or another common bond. Regulated HSOs/HSs sometimes are one another's constituents, and they trade regulatory approval opportunities.

Other mechanisms for managing interdependence that are unethical, illegal, or both—at least, they can be used that way—include data overload of the regulator. An advantage that HSOs/HSs frequently have over their regulators is their technical expertise and the ability to assemble and manipulate large volumes of data. When challenged, regulated HSOs/HSs may flood the agency with technical data that justify their position or simply obscure the issues.

Another well-worn but effective mechanism that some HSOs/HSs use with their regulators, which also can lead to unethical or illegal activity or both, is to attempt to buy them off with promises of attractive jobs. For example, U.S. Patent Office examiners often become patent attorneys in private practice. A few years of experience with the Federal Communications Commission are excellent training for lawyers seeking positions with law firms specializing in communications law. Organizations in health services know this strategy, too. Regulators, particularly those in state agencies, often go to work for large HSOs/HSs or in their associations. Usually, these are legitimate and appropriate transfers of knowledge and experience. However, sometimes the jobs repay a debt that was incurred in transactions between regulators and the regulated.

Finally, although clearly illegal and unethical, deception is possible in relationships between regulators and the regulated. The cost and scope of projects can be understated. Pertinent data can be fabricated or falsified. Regulated activities can be altered, obscured, or concealed. The complexity of regulated activities in HSOs/HSs, the turnover of regulatory staff, and the difficulty that government agencies have in coordinating their programs can prevent close scrutiny of regulated HSOs/HSs and encourage cheating.

The most important mechanism for managing involuntary IORs, as well as market transactions and SAs, may well be establishment of and adherence by all parties to contracts and other formal rules and procedures for guiding the relationships. This is supported by reliance on the courts when disputes arise about the rules or their application.

Corporate Restructuring and Corporate Diversification

Another important technical aspect of how HSOs/HSs seek to manage their interdependencies, with significant historical and continuing relevance, is corporate restructuring and corporate diversification. Corporate restructuring by a HSO/HS is defined as creating two or more corporate entities to perform functions that were previously performed by one corporation. Corporate restructuring has been used since the 1970s by hospitals to overcome problems inherent in their traditional corporate structure. For example, hospitals restructured in the mid-1970s to establish foundations that sheltered endowment funds so that they could not be used to reduce reimbursements from the Medicare program. During the late 1970s and early 1980s, many hospitals established subsidiaries to bypass state certificate-of-need regulations. These motives are no longer relevant for most hospitals, but, since the mid-1980s, many have used restructuring through diversification to generate revenue from new sources.

Corporate diversification is the process by which a HSO/HS such as a hospital "broadens the sources of revenue-generating activities and services through the establishment of corporations, foundations, and joint ventures to provide services, such as home care, primary care, and long-term care."[119] Diversification and other organizational strategies are discussed in Chapter 8.

Figure 5.11 shows two examples of restructuring. In the first example, a hospital corporation forms a related foundation whose purpose is to benefit the hospital by engaging in revenue-generating activities. In the second example, a holding company is established that holds controlling interest in the hospital and other corporate entities.

Diversification is a process through which HSOs/HSs add to existing product/service mixes, enter new markets, or both with existing or new products/services or both. It has been pursued almost without exception in the hope that new activities would provide new income to offset declines in revenue from traditional sources. For hospitals, this has primarily been inpatient activities. Revenue enhancement and profitability are the most important reasons to diversify, but there are other motives[120]:

- *Community service*—Health care needs might go unmet without a HSO/HS diversifying to respond to the need.
- *Innovation*—Being at the cutting edge of new products/services gives HSOs/HSs an advantage in identifying emerging business opportunities.
- *Risk management*—HSOs/HSs can minimize financial risk by spreading it among several activities and markets.
- *Professional staff relations*—Diversifying into services that the professional staff want to provide or have available to patients (e.g., substance abuse treatment) is a way to improve relationships with them.

There are two basic types of diversification: concentric and conglomerate. Concentric diversification is that in which different but related and complementary products/services are added to the HSO's/HS's existing set of products/services. Conglomerate diversification is that in which products/

Example I

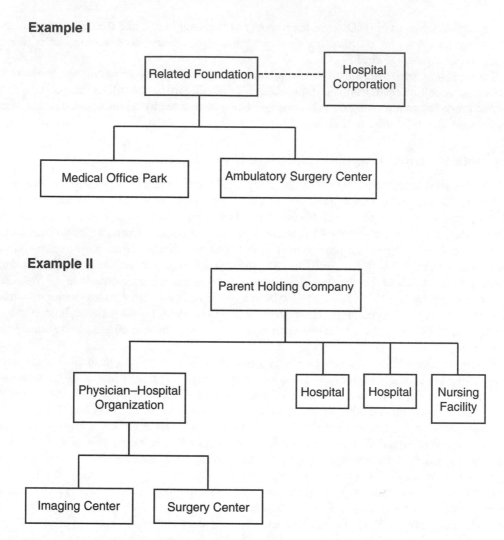

Example II

Figure 5.11.   Two examples of corporate restructuring: a related foundation (I) and a parent holding company (II).

services that are unrelated to the HSO's/HS's principal business or core products/services are added to the portfolio. With limited exceptions, almost all diversification by HSOs/HSs is concentric.

Concentric diversification in general entails developing or acquiring products/services to complement existing ones, expanding sales to current markets, and/or penetrating new markets. Characteristically, in pursuing such diversification a HSO/HS remains close to its competencies.[121] Because health services involve unique competencies that often are protected by licensure and professional dominance and are rarely substitutable, it is not surprising that most diversification in HSOs/HSs is concentric. This proclivity for concentric diversification distinguishes HSOs/HSs from organizations elsewhere in the economy, where diversifying within present competencies may be less important.

Related or concentric diversification can be achieved through internal development or acquisition. Opportunities for product/service diversification through internal development or acquisition are limited only by the products/services that the diversifying HSO/HS does not offer. Prominent examples of product/service diversification by acute care hospitals, for example, include outpatient therapeutic services such as chemotherapy and radiation therapy, outpatient diagnostic services such as magnetic resonance imaging, and outpatient health promotion services such as health screening and fitness centers. In addition, hospitals can add an array of inpatient services to expand their products/services. Examples are rehabilitation, psychiatric, obstetrical, pediatric, or trauma services.

Often, the objective of concentric diversification is to enter new markets for existing or new products/services. Many of the product/service diversifications noted previously allow this. For example, adding obstetrics or pediatrics may open new population groups to other hospital services. Services that target older adults, such as adult day services, home-delivered meals, home medical equipment, and in-home skilled nursing services, are examples of the opportunities that can be derived by serving a new population group.

Diversification to reach new markets often means establishing satellite primary care or urgent care centers to serve as sources of new customers, both for the new center and through referral to existing services. In this instance vertical integration is coupled with diversification. Diversification also may include establishing new patient referral patterns for existing services to enhance market share. This widely used strategy is based on redefining markets. One such redefinition involves the flow of patient referrals, which in the past went almost exclusively from routine care to specialty care. This meant teaching hospitals were the prime beneficiaries. As consumers and payers become more price sensitive, however, high-cost providers such as teaching hospitals must refer routine cases to less-expensive settings. HSOs/HSs that recognize this change and develop appropriate referral arrangements can expand markets for current and new products/services.

Although restructuring, especially when associated with diversification, continues to be pursued by many HSOs/HSs, others have reconsidered their earlier restructuring activities. Some have actually moved to simplify corporate organizations and relationships, except those occurring within the context of the formation of SAs. Reconsidering the wisdom of corporate restructuring and diversification reflects a changed environment, confused lines of authority that result from some arrangements, management that was often ill prepared for the demands of a restructured organization, different views of vision and objectives among some in management and governance, high overhead costs, diversification into activities that did not support the HSO's/HS's original mission, risk to tax-exempt status (discussed in Chapter 14), and damage to community image.[122] Hospitals simplified corporate structures—or resimplified them—because they saw several potential advantages[123]:

- Reducing the administrative expenses that come with multiple corporations and multiple GBs
- Cutting subsidiary losses in some cases
- Divesting businesses that no longer fit with the organization's mission and strategies
- Permitting a stronger focus on the hospital's core business
- Avoiding challenges to the hospital's tax-exempt status

SUMMARY

HSOs/HSs are interdependent with many other entities and seek to manage the interdependencies through IORs of three basic types discussed in the chapter: market transactions, involuntary IORs, and SAs. HSOs integrating into HSs occurs within the broader process of forming SAs.

SAs are defined as "any formal arrangements between two or more organizations for purposes of mutual gain."[124] The reasons that they form and the relationship of the process of integration to SAs, including the formation of HSs, are discussed. SAs in their rich variety and diversity are examined from three interrelated perspectives: who participates in them, their purposes, and their forms. Each approach is considered, along with defined examples, because each perspective contributes to understanding SAs.

The clusters of knowledge and skills that make up managerial competencies that are needed to manage SAs, especially HSs, are discussed. The competencies considered are 1) conceptual, 2) technical managerial/clinical, 3) interpersonal/collaborative, 4) political, 5) commercial, and 6) governance. In an extended discussion of governance in HSs centralized and decentralized models of governance structure are considered.

In the final section, four important technical issues involved in understanding and managing the IORs that HSOs/HSs engage in are discussed: negotiations in managing IORs, the special case of managing involuntary IORs with regulators and others, corporate restructuring, and diversification.

DISCUSSION QUESTIONS

1. Briefly distinguish among market transactions, involuntary interorganizational relationships, and strategic alliances as categories of mechanisms through which HSOs/HSs link with interdependent entities.
2. Discuss the reasons for HSOs to become involved in integrative activity.
3. Discuss strategic alliances in terms of who participates in them.
4. Discuss strategic alliances in terms of the purposes for which they are formed.
5. Discuss strategic alliances in terms of their forms.
6. List and discuss the managerial competencies that are needed in managing strategic alliances.
7. Define and give an example of vertical integration in health services.
8. List and briefly describe the seven strategies that regulated organizations use to deal with their regulators.
9. Describe joint ventures. Outline an approach that an acute care hospital could use in developing a joint venture with physician members of its clinical staff.
10. Discuss governance in HSs.

CASE STUDY 1: TEXAS HEALTH–BAYLOR: NETWORKS AGREE TO MEGA-MERGER[125]

Baylor Health Care System and Texas Health Resources signed a definitive agreement yesterday to combine operations under a single, $3.4 billion umbrella—a hospital network next to which area rivals will "pale in size." The move to establish the not-for-profit Southwest Health System concludes more than a year of negotiations between the two largest not-for-profit hospital chains in North Texas and brings together 24 hospitals and 40 clinics, home health centers, senior centers and retirement centers, creating the nation's seventh-largest hospital system.

The agreement combines Harris Methodist Health System, Arlington Memorial Hospital Foundation, Presbyterian Healthcare Resources, and Baylor University Medical Center. The Harris Methodist Health Plan was left out of the deal, as Texas Health Resources has been working to offload (sell) the debt-plagued plan through negotiations with Blue Cross and Blue Shield of Texas.

Spring Cleaning

Douglas D. Hawthorne, president and CEO of Texas Health Resources, explained that the Harris Methodist Health Plan "doesn't fit into the new company's mission," and notes that negotiations to sell the 300,000 member plan to Blue Cross and Blue Shield of Texas will likely conclude in March. "We're pretty far down the road," said Hawthorne. The *Ft. Worth Star-Telegram* reports that the Harris plan posted "record losses" of $13.7 million during the third quarter as enrollment plummeted.

More recently, "a company memo says that the Harris plan lost $37.2 million during the first 10 months of 1998." Baylor CEO Boone Powell noted that the affiliation "would be more appropriate" without the health plan, but indicated that the systems have designed a backup plan if Blue Cross leaves the negotiating table. In such a situation, Texas Health Resources would continue to exist, "but it would hold only the health plan and it liabilities," and transfer its other assets to Southwest.

Doctors on Board

The *Ft. Worth Star-Telegram* reports that physicians are supporting the merger in part because they have had input from the beginning. In fact, in order to guarantee input as talks went forward, a few doctors in 1997 created a working group called the Physician Alliance, a group that "might eventually create one of the largest organized physician groups in the country; the Southwest system would have 4,800 doctors across North Texas." Baylor and Texas Health Resources executives have "sought the physicians out for their participation." Dr. Thomas Russell explained, "We were told explicitly by the institutions that if the physicians did not support the affiliation between THR and Baylor, it would not happen."

Charity Care?

The *Dallas Morning News* reports that large employers and area health plans are cautiously eyeing the affiliation, which will have to tackle the as yet "unresolved" issues of savings and charity care. The deal is subject to approval, and while Texas Health Department records indicate that both partners "have always exceeded state requirements for charity care," the network would have to lay out a plan for continuing such care and improving operating efficiency.

Leadership

Under the agreement, Hawthorne, president and CEO of Texas Health Resources, will take the helm at Southwest and serve as the network's president and CEO. J. Andy Thompson, board chair of Texas Health Resources, will serve as chair of the Southwest board, and Powell, president and CEO of Baylor Health Care System, will serve as chair of Southwest's chief executive officer's council, created to advise Hawthorne.

"There are going to probably be some big changes," said John Gavras, president of the Dallas-Ft. Worth Hospital Council. He said, "I know that everyone has been preparing for it. But, obviously, preparing for the Super Bowl and playing the Super Bowl are two different things."

QUESTIONS

1. Discuss the possible reasons for this merger.
2. Discuss the challenges of managing Southwest Health System.
3. What are the options for the governance of Southwest Health System? What governance structure do you recommend? Why?

CASE STUDY 2: HARD TIMES[126]

Robin Wood Medical Center is experiencing problems and posted large losses for three consecutive years. It is located in a deteriorating neighborhood on the edge of a sprawling city with enough—some say far too many—hospital beds. The not-for-profit hospital is the largest employer in its area and serves a large share of the area's old and poor residents, many of whom do not own or drive cars. The community relies heavily on the hospital. Among its services, Robin Wood operates adult day services and other popular programs for older adults, a regional neonatal intensive care unit, a large kidney dialysis center, community clinics, and a busy emergency room. It loses money on all of these services except the dialysis center.

Managed care plans have become common in the region, and have more than 30% of the commercial insurance market. Because of its high costs, Robin Wood has lost many of those patients. In addition, several insurers have announced plans to start Medicare HMOs, and the state has passed legislation that will shift Medicaid recipients to managed care. This is not good timing for a hospital struggling—and so far failing—to control its costs.

Despite the poor financial picture, longtime CEO Joan Morgan has the support and confidence of Robin Wood's governing body (GB). Many GB members have served 10 years or longer and know that Morgan presided over years of expansion and strong financial margins. At a recent GB meeting she was asked to pursue affiliations with other hospitals for Robin Wood.

MetroCare, a large health system that owns two hospitals in the area, has made an offer to buy Robin Wood. Morgan thinks the price may be too low. MetroCare's chairman and CEO also have made promises to Morgan, offering her a generous severance and consulting agreement if she persuades her GB to approve a merger with their system. The two men have made it clear that they plan to close the hospital and transfer only a fraction of the staff to other sites. They have given no assurance that Robin Wood's services will be continued near the hospital's current location.

Morgan also has approached two other hospitals in the city, but they recently have entered into their own merger talks. Executives from the two facilities have told Morgan that they cannot consider deals with Robin Wood until those discussions come to a conclusion. Morgan worries that MetroCare's offer may be the only affiliation possible.

QUESTIONS

1. As a manager, what are Morgan's obligations to the hospital? The community?
2. How should Morgan weigh the ethical issues concerning the hospital's survival versus the survival of its vital services?
3. What are the ethical implications of MetroCare's offer for the hospital versus its financial promises to Morgan?
4. What should Morgan do?

CASE STUDY 3: COMMUNITY HEALTH PLAN[127]

The CEO of Community Health Plan (CHP) had been approached by a community group from "north of the river." This area of the city was economically depressed and had lost many of its privately owned HSOs and physicians to the suburbs over the past several decades.

"North of the river" seemed to be in a downward vortex with no apparent bottom in sight. Increasing numbers of uninsured patients there meant that remaining HSOs were less able to continue serving the area. The large city-owned hospital had made several ill-fated attempts to serve "north of the river" with a clinic system, but its efforts had been scandal ridden. The system was a political football with little credibility.

The representatives from "north of the river" were community leaders, none of whom appeared to have any political ambitions. They seemed genuinely willing to do whatever they could to assist in delivering high-quality health services "north of the river." They proposed that CHP establish and staff three storefront clinics in the area. The community leaders stated that they would organize volunteers to remodel the facilities and work in clerical capacities.

The CEO was describing the proposed activity to the CHP executive management committee, which included members of governance, managers, and physicians and others from clinical areas. In making the presentation, the CEO stressed the CHP's historical role in providing health services to those in need, its not-for-profit status, and its continuing modest surplus. The members listened patiently, but the minute the CEO was finished all of them seemed to speak at once.

Several were opposed and made the following points about the suggested venture:

- "North of the river" was the city's responsibility. Providing care to the needy was not something a small, not-for-profit health plan should attempt.
- CHP had a primary obligation to enhance benefits for its enrollees rather than get involved in new schemes. There were numerous services that several of their physicians and many plan members had requested.
- The modest surplus that the plan had accumulated over several years would quickly evaporate. The chief financial officer noted they were expecting an increase in reinsurance premiums in the next quarter.
- If CHP pulled the city's political chestnuts out of the fire by providing even stop-gap assistance, the city would never get its house in order and develop the system needed "north of the river."

Several spoke in favor of working "north of the river."

- Helping the "north of the river" community was the right thing to do. The people there deserved health services. It was noted that CHP's own start had come about when several physicians in the community had fought the prevailing attitude among their peers about prepaid practice.
- Those opposed were putting dollars ahead of people's health. They must be willing to assist people who are less fortunate.
- CHP's members would support such an initiative if it were properly explained to them.
- The positive publicity would further CHP's interests by increasing the number of enrollees.

It seemed to the CEO this was a no-win situation. The organizational philosophy was not well developed, and the proposal was a major step, but it seemed that something should be done to assist the people "north of the river." The executive committee members were raising points that merited analysis.

QUESTIONS

1. Identify the management issues and the ethical issues in the case. Which are the most important? Why?
2. Outline three alternatives that could be used to assist the community "north of the river." Choose the one that you think is best and identify its negative and positive aspects.
3. What interorganizational linkages are used in each of the alternatives identified in Question 2? Are these significant in choosing the "best" alternative?
4. Develop an implementation plan for the alternative that you chose in Question 2.

CASE STUDY 4: DOES IT MAKE SENSE?[128]

The following comments came from an executive in the medical equipment rental business:

"One particularly lucrative area for hospital diversification, designed to make it less dependent on inpatient revenues from third parties such as Blue Cross, has been the medical equipment rental market. Third parties, and particularly Medicare, have up until now focused on inpatient

cost controls and have provided fairly comfortable ceilings in terms of payments. A crutch that costs $65, for example, can be rented to a discharged patient for $17 a month. Where else can the cost of a capital investment be recovered in less than 4 months?

"This may seem like a nickel-and-dime candy store operation, and many administrators have ignored it because of this. On the average, a discharged hospital patient referred to one of these operations rents three to four different pieces of equipment (bed, respirator, and so on) in addition to consumables, such as oxygen, producing an average gross income per referral of as much as $5,000. These referrals have come often at the price of some holiday candy for the social workers."

"Many hospitals are now getting a bigger piece of the action, setting up their own subsidiaries to provide these supplies to patients or entering into joint ventures with particular suppliers, from which a moderate-sized hospital might expect to generate a two or three million dollar surplus per year.

QUESTIONS

1. What type of diversification would this be for a hospital?
2. What interorganizational linkages might be needed to ensure success for a hospital that is entering the equipment rental field?

CASE STUDY 5: AMERICAN HOSPITAL ASSOCIATION'S POLICY ON COMMUNITY ACCOUNTABILITY WITH CHANGES IN THE OWNERSHIP OR CONTROL OF HOSPITALS OR HEALTH SYSTEMS[129]

Preamble

Communities are facing many changes in their health system, including changes in its ownership and control. In all cases, the reason for and outcome of these changes should better serve the sick and improve the health of the community through a more efficient and effective health system.

For communities to understand these changes, it is important that hospitals and health systems making changes in ownership or control balance the health needs of the community with the needs of the organization for adaptation. The American Hospital Association has drafted these principles to help hospital executives, trustees, communities, and government officials more clearly define roles and expectations.

Principles for Changes in Ownership or Control

Hospitals and health systems are important resources for their communities. When planning a change in ownership or control, hospital leaders should educate and inform their communities—including medical staff and employees—in a timely manner of the objectives for the change, the process being followed, and the opportunities for community comment.

The core values of a hospital or health system are defined by its mission, including emphasis on its role of caring for the sick and improving community health. Board decisions with regard to changes of ownership or control should be made within the mission of caring for the sick and improving community health.

Boards of trustees have the fiduciary responsibility for our nation's hospitals and health systems. In making decisions about hospital ownership or control, boards should emphasize the future health care needs of the community and determine the best organizational arrangements for meeting those needs. Boards also are responsible for assuring the community that conflicts of interest are disclosed and private inurement is avoided.

Where the organization changing ownership or control holds charitable assets, the board should protect the value of those assets and ensure that the assets continue to improve the health of the community. Where necessary, the board should seek judicial approval of decisions to amend the assets' original charitable purpose or redefine the community for which they may be used.

Public accountability for ownership and control decisions is a board responsibility. Any state oversight of board actions should be limited and follow a clear and timely process which recognizes the Board's responsibility to make a decision on ownership or control and assures the public that the Board has followed an appropriate process in making its decision(s).

The federal role in changes in ownership should be limited to existing tax, anti-trust, Medicare reimbursement, and corporate disclosure requirements. Federal officials should not substitute their judgment for that of the board or the state oversight.

Guidelines for Hospitals/Health System Leaders When Changing Ownership or Control

Preamble

Changes in ownership or control present challenges for hospital and health system leaders. Perhaps most important is the challenge of community accountability—balancing the needs of the community for patient care and health improvement with the needs of the organization for adaptation. These voluntary guidelines have been prepared by the American Hospital Association to help hospital and health system leaders—trustees, executives, and physicians—meet this challenge.

Boards are encouraged to adopt these guidelines as policy for their institution/system before considering any proposal to change ownership or control.

Guidelines

I. *Regularly listen to the community and identify its future health improvement needs*

Work with the community to identify its health needs and the resources that are available to improve the health of the community and to meet its needs for health services.

Ensure that there is a plan for the provision of care to the underserved in the community as well as the continuation of other essential community services.

II. *Before considering a change in ownership or control*

Identify your organization's values and goals in advance of considering an ownership change.

Know any legal limitations of your organization's certificate of incorporation, articles of organization, or charter that may restrict consideration of alternatives.

Adopt criteria for evaluating any change in ownership or control before examining proposals.

Conduct a study to assess various options for change that may be available to your organization and your community. The study should examine your market and understand the changes that may affect your organization's ability to continue to fulfill its mission.

III. *Carefully evaluate proposed changes in ownership or control*

Evaluate proposals using community health improvement needs, your organization's values and mission, the protection and use of community assets, and organizational financial viability.

Encourage compatibility in values and philosophy by favoring changes that reflect shared missions, visions, and strategies.

Develop a communication plan that involves and informs all constituencies, including medical staff and employees.

Understand thoroughly the terms of the proposed transaction and of all collateral arrangements.

IV. Protect the value of the community's assets

Obtain a valuation, by a party not involved in the transaction, of charitable assets being converted or restructured to ensure reasonable value is received or used in structuring the transaction.

Identify financial incentives which may influence the views of trustees and executives involved in proposing and evaluating any change in ownership or control.

Disclose all conflicts of interest, offers of future employment, future remuneration, or other benefits related to the transaction.

Prohibit private inurement or personal financial gain by employees or trustees of any not-for-profit entity that is involved in the transaction.

Control and administer any foundation or charitable trust that is created by the transaction separate and distinct from the restructured health care organization.

Ensure that a foundation, charitable trust, or community payment created from transaction continues to serve an appropriate health need or charitable purpose of the community.

Require any foundation resulting from the change in ownership to provide regular reports to the community on how it improves community health.

V. Educate and inform your community about the changes taking place

Work with your community to increase understanding of the issues that are involved in the change of ownership or control, the evaluation and decision-making process involved in the transaction, and how the transaction will benefit the community.

Disclose publicly the terms of an agreement to transfer control or ownership once a letter of intent (or memorandum of understanding) is signed.

Provide an opportunity for public comment on the transaction before it is final.

Inform the appropriate state official, usually the attorney general, of the terms of a transaction once a letter of intent (or memorandum of understanding) is signed.

QUESTIONS

1. Why might a HSO's/HS's GB consider not following some of these guidelines? What would the consequences be?
2. Which aspects of these guidelines pertain to the roles of GBs? Which to senior managers?

CASE STUDY 6: BOARD EFFECTIVENESS[130]

This questionnaire is designed to test whether GBs are hampered by some typical pitfalls that prevent board effectiveness. Read the statements, and then answer the two questions posed about each one at the end.

1. Our board has representatives from various constituencies, such as our medical staff and subsidiary organizations, and the role of these board members is to represent the issues and interests of their community.
2. Our board agenda materials for each meeting include our organization's mission statement, and we refer to the mission frequently during our decision-making processes.

3. During board meetings, we spend the majority of our time reviewing what happened at committee meetings and approving the actions taken by our committees, and little time remains for discussion of strategic issues.
4. Our board's agenda materials consist primarily of management reports and committee minutes.
5. Our board has a clearly articulated process for removing dysfunctional board members.
6. Our board has performance standards that we use at least annually to review the performance of each board member.
7. Our trustees have a clear understanding of the roles of the board(s) and board committees of our organization and little, if any, duplication exists among those boards and committees.
8. Job descriptions exist for each of our boards, for trustees, and for board officers.
9. Our board members understand the role of the board on which they serve and its relationship to management, the medical staff, and other physician organizations in our system.
10. All board members participate in an orientation and continuing education and evaluation process that not only introduces them to health care, their board, and the system of which it is a part but also identifies and explains the governance culture—the way we do things on our boards.

QUESTIONS

1. What pitfall (problem or issue) is this statement designed to identify?
2. What steps should be taken to ensure that the pitfall (problem or issue) does not arise and hamper board effectiveness?

CASE STUDY 7: HOW TO TURN AN INTIMIDATING GOVERNMENT BUREAUCRACY INTO A PARTNER AND ALLY[131]

John Aaron, CEO of Crop Genetics International, had just left a boisterous hearing on Capitol Hill that had left him feeling as bleak as the late-winter Washington weather. The hearing had been called to investigate the questionable testing procedures of Advanced Genetic Sciences, Inc., which apparently had injected a test bacterium into 45 fruit trees at its corporate headquarters without Environmental Protection Agency (EPA) approval. Aaron recognized that his own company's future could be gravely affected by the outcomes of that meeting. His company, only 5 years old, was embarking on genetic-engineering projects for plants that were every bit as significant as McCormick's reaper had been to the food industry. But the products of his company's research, and that of other companies like his, could be so destructive if unanticipated consequences emerged that government was understandably cautious, even antagonistic, about unprofessionally conducted activities.

Aaron knew that his company's efforts would always be professional. But salable products were at least 5 years away for ongoing research and design, and he wanted to ensure that his firm's products had a chance to reach the marketplace.

It was then that Aaron decided on an unusual strategy. He reasoned that it was not necessary that business and government be enemies. He asked himself, "Why not turn government into an ally and partner?" Furthermore, he thought, "Why not consider environmental activists as a fourth branch of government?" He decided to make government relations the primary business of his firm for the immediate future.

Aaron believed deeply in what he was doing, and apparently so did others. For example, one of his company's probable products could significantly reduce the level of chemical fertilizers used each year, thus helping reduce fish and bird kills and potential food-chain problems for human beings. He assembled a team of key former government officials to aid him in his quest. The team's members included

- William D. Ruckelshaus, twice former director of EPA
- Douglas M. Costle, head of EPA during the Carter administration
- Robert M. Teeter, a prominent Republican pollster who would eventually become cochairman of the George H. Bush presidential transitional team
- Elliot L. Richardson, the Nixon administration's former attorney general, who has held a number of other federal posts

The "team" met in brainstorming sessions for which participants received $4,000 per day plus certain stock options. These sessions produced a list of obstacles that Aaron might face and strategies for overcoming them. The sessions also provided valuable insight into the workings of government and how a company could best work its way through the bureaucratic maze. The result? Crop Genetics became the first genetics firm to make it through the first round of regulator hoops without being delayed or stalled.

QUESTIONS

1. What is your assessment of the strategy that Crop Genetics International used to manage its relationship with EPA?
2. What other strategies might it have used?

NOTES

1. Satinsky, Marjorie A. *The Foundations of Integrated Care: Facing the Challenges of Change,* vii. Chicago: American Hospital Publishing, 1998.
2. Allina Health System. *http://www.allina.com/.*
3. SMG Marketing Group Inc. *Integrated Health Care 100 Directory.* Chicago: SMG Marketing Group Inc. and AHA Press, 1999.
4. Longest, Beaufort B., Jr. "Interorganizational Linkages in the Health Sector." *Health Care Management Review* 15 (Winter 1990): 17–28.
5. Baxter International, Inc. *http://www.baxter.com/.*
6. Pennsylvania Department of Health. "Health Care Facilities." *http://www.health.state.pa.us/,* September 3, 1999.
7. Satinsky, *The Foundations of Integrated Care*; Robinson, James C. "The Changing Boundaries of the American Hospital." *The Milbank Quarterly* 72 (Summer 1994): 259–275.
8. Zajac, Edward J., and Thomas A. D'Aunno. "Managing Strategic Alliances." In *Essentials of Health Care Management,* edited by Stephen M. Shortell and Arnold D. Kaluzny, 328–354. Albany, NY: Delmar Publishers, 1997.
9. Zajac and D'Aunno, "Managing Strategic Alliances," 330.
10. The Advisory Board Company. *The Grand Alliance: Vertical Integration Strategies for Physicians and Health Systems.* Washington, DC: The Advisory Board Company, 1993; D'Aunno, Thomas A., and Howard S. Zuckerman. "A Life Cycle Model of Organizational Federations: The Case of Hospitals." *Academy of Management Review* 12 (1987): 534–545; Kaluzny, Arnold D., and Howard S. Zuckerman. "Strategic Alliances: Two Perspectives for Understanding Their Effects on Health Services." *Hospital & Health Services Administration* 37 (Winter 1992): 477–490; Longest, "Interorganizational Linkages"; Luke, Roice D., James W. Begun, and Dennis D. Pointer. "Quasi-firms: Strategic Interorganizational Forms in the Health Care Industry." *Academy of Management Review* 14 (January 1989): 9–19; Provan, Keith G. "Interorganizational Cooperation and Decision Making Autonomy in a Consortium Multihospital System." *Academy of Management Review* 9 (1984): 494–504; Sofaer, Shoshanna, and Robert C. Myrtle. "Interorganizational Theory and Research: Implications for Health Care Management, Policy, and Research." *Medical Care* 48 (Winter 1991): 371–409; Zajac, Edward J. *Organizations, Environments, and Performance: A Study of Contract Management in Hospitals* [dissertation].

Philadelphia: University of Pennsylvania, 1986; Zajac, Edward J., Brian R. Golden, and Stephen M. Shortell. "New Organizational Forms for Enhancing Innovation: The Case of Internal Corporate Joint Ventures." *Management Science* 37 (1991): 170–184; Zajac and D'Aunno, "Managing Strategic Alliances."

11. Stein, Barry A. "Strategic Alliances: Some Lessons from Experience." In *Partners for the Dance: Forming Strategic Alliances in Health Care,* edited by Arnold D. Kaluzny, Howard S. Zuckerman, and Thomas C. Ricketts, III, 19–62. Ann Arbor, MI: Health Administration Press, 1995.

12. Coddington, Dean C., Keith D. Moore, and Elizabeth A. Fischer. *Making Integrated Health Care Work.* Englewood, CO: Center for Research in Ambulatory Health Care Administration, 1996.

13. Hoechst Marion Roussel. *Managed Care Digest Series: Integrated Health Systems Digest.* Kansas City, MO: Hoechst Marion Roussel, 1999; Bazzoli, Gloria J., Stephen M. Shortell, Nicole Dubbs, Cheeling Chan, and Peter Kralovec. "A Taxonomy of Health Networks and Systems: Bringing Order Out of Chaos." *Health Services Research* 33 (February 1999): 1683–1717.

14. Barton, Phoebe Lindsey. *Understanding the U.S. Health Services System,* 218. Chicago: Health Administration Press, 1999.

15. American Hospital Association. *Hospital Statistics, 2000.* Chicago: Health Forum, 2000.

16. Brown, Montague. "Mergers, Networking, and Vertical Integration: Managed Care and Investor-Owned Hospitals." *Health Care Management Review* 21 (Winter 1996): 29.

17. Goldsmith, Jeff C. "The Illusive Logic of Integration." *Health Forum Journal* 37 (September–October 1994): 26–31; Satinsky, *The Foundations of Integrated Care*; Conrad, Douglas A., and Stephen M. Shortell. "Integrated Health Systems: Promise and Performance." *Frontiers of Health Services Management* 13 (Fall 1996): 3–40.

18. Longest, Beaufort B., Jr., "A Conceptual Framework for Understanding the Multi-Hospital Arrangement Strategy." *Health Care Management Review* 5 (Winter 1980): 17.

19. Ohmae, Kenichi. "The Global Logic of Alliances." *Harvard Business Review* 89 (March–April 1989): 143–154.

20. Shortell, Stephen M., and Kathleen E. Hull. "The New Organization of the Health Care Delivery System." In *Strategic Choices for a Changing Health Care System,* edited by Stuart H. Altman and Uwe E. Reinhardt, 101–148. Chicago: Health Administration Press, 1996.

21. Gold, Marsha, Ed. *Contemporary Managed Care: Readings in Structure, Operations, and Public Policy.* Chicago: Health Administration Press, 1998; Burns, Lawton R., Gloria J. Bazzoli, Linda Dynan, and Douglas R. Wholey. "Managed Care, Market Stages, and Integrated Delivery Systems: Is There a Relationship?" *Health Affairs* 16 (November/December 1997): 204–218.

22. Gold, Marsha, and Robert Hurley. "The Role of Managed Care 'Products' in Managed Care 'Plans.' " In *Contemporary Managed Care: Readings in Structure, Operations, and Public Policy,* 47. Chicago: Health Administration Press, 1998.

23. Ginter, Peter M., Linda M. Swayne, and W. Jack Duncan. *Strategic Management of Health Care Organizations,* 3rd ed., 6. Malden, MA: Blackwell, 1998; see also American Association of Health Plans. "Network-Based Health Plans Definition." *http://www.aahp.org,* February 1, 1999.

24. Gold and Hurley, "The Role of Managed Care," 49.

25. Gold and Hurley, "The Role of Managed Care," 49.

26. "InterStudy's New HMO Industry Report." *http://www.hmodata.com/ir81pr.html,* February 18, 1999.

27. Hoechst Marion Roussel. *Managed Care Digest Series: HMO-PPO/Medicare/Medicaid Digest.* Kansas City, MO: Hoechst Marion Roussel, 1999.

28. Burns, Bazzoli, Dynan, and Wholey. "Managed Care," 205.

29. Orlikoff, James E., and Mary K. Totten. *The Future of Health Care Governance: Redesigning Boards for a New Era,* 3. Chicago: American Hospital Publishing, 1996.

30. Dowling, William L. "Strategic Alliances as a Structure for Integrated Delivery Systems." In *Partners for the Dance: Forming Strategic Alliances in Health Care,* edited by Arnold D. Kaluzny, Howard S. Zuckerman, and Thomas C. Ricketts, III, 140. Chicago: Health Administration Press, 1995.

31. Conrad and Shortell, "Integrated Health Systems."

32. Lehrman, Susan, and Karen K. Shore. "Hospitals' Vertical Integration into Skilled Nursing: A Rational Approach to Controlling Transaction Costs." *Inquiry* 35 (Fall 1998): 304.

33. Connor, Robert A., Roger D. Feldman, Bryan E. Down, and Tiffany A. Radcliff. "Which Types of Hospital Mergers Save Consumers Money?" *Health Affairs* 16 (November/December 1997): 62–74; Conrad and Shortell, "Integrated Health Systems."

34. Shortell, Stephen M., Ellen M. Morrison, and Bernard Friedman. *Strategic Choices for America's Hospitals: Managing Change in Turbulent Times.* San Francisco: Jossey-Bass, 1990; Longest, "Interorganizational Linkages."

35. O'Leary, Margaret R. *Lexikon,* 337. Oakbrook Terrace, IL: Joint Commission on Accreditation of Healthcare Organizations, 1994.

36. Coddington, Moore, and Fischer, *Making Integrated,* 14–21.

37. Ginter, Swayne, and Duncan, *Strategic Management,* 6.

38. Ginter, Swayne, and Duncan, *Strategic Management,* 6.

39. Orlikoff, James E., and Mary K. Totten, "New Relationships with Physicians: An Overview for Trustees" [workbook insert]. *Trustee* 50 (July/August 1997).

40. Orlikoff and Totten, "New Relationships."

41. O'Leary, *Lexikon,* 614.

42. Burns, Lawton R., and Darrell P. Thorpe. "Physician-Hospital Organizations: Strategy, Structure, and Conduct." In *Integrating the Practice of Medicine: A Decision Maker's Guide to Organizing and Managing Physician Services,* edited by Ronald B. Connors, ch. 17. Chicago: AHA Press, 1997.

43. O'Leary, *Lexikon,* 413.

44. Blair, John D., Charles R. Slaton, and Grant T. Savage. "Hospital-Physician Joint Ventures: A Strategic Approach for Both Dimensions of Success." *Hospital & Health Services Administration* 35 (Spring 1990): 3–26.

45. O'Leary, *Lexikon,* 366.

46. Conrad and Shortell, "Integrated Health Systems," 7.

47. Dowling, "Strategic Alliances," 141; for further discussion of vertical integration, see Conrad, Douglas A., and William L. Dowling. "Vertical Integration in Health Services: Theory and Managerial Implications." *Health Care Management Review* 14 (Fall 1990): 9–22.

48. Hoechst Marion Roussel. *Managed Care Digest Series: Integrated Health Systems Digest.*

49. Satinsky, *The Foundations of Integrated Care.*

50. Orlikoff, James E., and Mary K. Totten. "Systems Thinking in Governance" [workbook insert]. *Trustee* 52 (January 1999): 2.

51. Robinson, James C. "Physician-Hospital Integration and the Economic Theory of the Firm." *Medical Care Research and Review* 54 (March 1997): 6.

52. University of Pennsylvania Medical Center. *http://www.upmc.edu/,* February 2, 1999.

53. Henry Ford Health System. *http://www.henryfordhealth.org/,* February 2, 1999.

54. Shortell, Stephen M., Robin R. Gillies, David A. Anderson, Karen Morgan Erickson, and John B. Mitchell. *Remaking Healthcare in America: Building Organized Delivery Systems,* 7. San Francisco: Jossey-Bass, 1996.

55. Robinson, James C., and Lawrence P. Casalino. "Vertical Integration and Organizational Networks in Health Care." *Health Affairs* 15 (Spring 1996): 7–22.

56. Bazzoli, Shortell, Dubbs, Chan, and Kralovec, "A Taxonomy."

57. Bazzoli, Shortell, Dubbs, Chan, and Kralovec, "A Taxonomy."

58. Clement, Jan P., Michael J. McCue, Roice D. Luke, James D. Bramble, Louis F. Rossiter, Yasar A. Ozcan, and Chih-Wen Pai. "Strategic Hospital Alliances: Impact on Financial Performance." *Health Affairs* 16 (November/December 1997): 193–203.

59. Zajac and D'Aunno, "Managing Strategic Alliances," 337–340.

60. AmeriNet. *http://www.amerinet-gpo.com/,* January 26, 1999.

61. Dowling, "Strategic Alliances," 139–175.

62. Kraatz, Matthew S. "Learning by Association? Interorganizational Networks and Adaptation to Environmental Change." *Academy of Management Journal* 41 (December 1998): 621–643; Zajac, Golden, and Shortell. "New Organizational Forms"; Prahalad, C.K., and Gary Hamel. "The Core Competence of the Corporation." *Harvard Business Review* 68 (May–June, 1990): 79–82.

63. Harvard Pilgrim Health Care. *http://www.harvardpilgrim.org/.*

64. Henry Ford Health System. *http://www.henryfordhealth.org/.*

65. Lovelace Health Systems. *http://www.lovelace.com/.*

66. Satinsky, *The Foundations of Integrated Care,* 73.

67. Kraatz, "Learning by Association?"

68. Luke, Roice, Peter C. Olden, and James D. Bramble. "Strategic Hospital Alliances: Countervailing Responses to Restructuring Health Care Markets." In *Handbook of Health Care Management,* edited by W. Jack Duncan, Peter M. Ginter, and Linda E. Swayne, 86. Malden, MA: Blackwell, 1998.

69. Luke, Olden, and Bramble, "Strategic Hospital Alliances," 86.

70. Pointer, Dennis D., James W. Begun, and Roice D. Luke. "Managing Interorganizational Dependencies in the New Health Care Marketplace." *Hospital & Health Services Administration* 33 (Summer 1988): 167–177.

71. Thompson, James D. *Organizations in Action.* New York: McGraw-Hill, 1967.

72. Sunseri, Reid. "Outsourcing Loses Its 'Mo.' " *Hospital & Health Networks* 72, 22 (November 20, 1998): 36–40.

73. Thompson, *Organizations in Action.*

74. Weick, Kenneth. "Educational Organizations as Loosely Coupled Systems." *Administrative Science Quarterly* 21 (March 1976): 1–19; Zuckerman, Howard S., and Thomas A. D'Aunno. "Hospital Alliances: Cooperative Strategy in a Competitive Environment." *Health Care Management Review* 15 (1990): 21–30; Pointer, Begun, and Luke, "Managing Interorganizational."

75. Pointer, Begun, and Luke, "Managing Interorganizational."

76. Information on PMCC can be found on each of the participants' websites: National Committee for Quality Assurance, *http://www.ncqa.org*; Joint Commission on Accreditation of Healthcare Organizations, *http://www.jcaho.org*; American Medical Accreditation Program, *http://www.ama-assn.org/amap.*

77. Joint Commission on Accreditation of Healthcare Organizations. "News Release." Oakbrook, IL: Joint Commission on Accreditation of Healthcare Organizations, January 29, 1999.

78. Hilzenrath, David S., and Michael D. Shear. "Hospital Alliance in N. Va. to End." *The Washington Post,* January 29, 1999, E01.

79. Adapted from Hoechst Marion Roussel. *Managed Care Digest Series: Integrated Health Systems Digest,* 2–3.

80. Shortell, Gillies, Anderson, Erickson, and Mitchell, *Remaking Healthcare,* 152–226.

81. Shortell, Gillies, Anderson, Erickson, and Mitchell, *Remaking Healthcare,* 30.

82. Shortell, Gillies, Anderson, Erickson, and Mitchell, *Remaking Healthcare,* 30.

83. Satinsky, *The Foundations of Integrated Care,* 15.

84. Conrad, Douglas A. "Coordinating Patient Care Services in Regional Health Systems: The Challenge of Clinical Integration." *Hospital & Health Services Administration* 38, 4 (Winter 1993): 492.

85. Kittredge, Frank D. "What Is Clinical Integration and Why Is It So Important?" *The Bristol Review* (a publication of The Bristol Group, Boston) (October 1996): 1.

86. Orlikoff and Totten, *The Future of Health Care Governance,* 3–4.

87. Satinsky, *The Foundations of Integrated Care,* 262.

88. Hanson, Elizabeth, Susan Marsh, and Christopher H. Coulter. "Direct Provider Contracting: One Employer's Experience." *Benefits Quarterly* 15 (First Quarter 1999): 37–41.

89. Maxwell, James, Forrest Briscoe, Stephen Davidson, Lisa Eisen, Mark Robbins, Peter Temin, and Cheryl Young. "Managed Competition in Practice: 'Value Purchasing' by Fourteen Employers." *Health Affairs* 17 (May/June 1998): 224.

90. Maxwell, Briscoe, Davidson, Eisen, Robbins, Temin, and Young, "Managed Competition," 224.

91. John Snow, Inc. *Health Benefits Purchasers: Orlando, Report to the Florida Agency for Health Care Administration and the Robert Wood Johnson Foundation.* Boston: JSI, 1996.

92. This discussion is adapted from Longest, Beaufort B., Jr. "Managerial Competence at Senior Levels of Integrated Delivery Systems." *Journal of Healthcare Management* 43 (March/April 1998): 115–135.

93. Coddington, Dean C., Keith D. Moore, and Elizabeth A. Fischer. "Physician Leaders in Integrated Delivery." *Medical Group Management Journal* 44, 5 (September/October 1997): 90.

94. Orlikoff and Totten, "Systems Thinking in Governance."

95. Miles, Raymond E., and Charles C. Snow. "Twenty-First Century Careers." In *The Boundaryless Career: A New Employment Principle for a New Organizational Era,* edited by Michael B. Arthur and Denise M. Rousseau, 261–307. New York: Oxford University Press, 1996.

96. Coddington, Moore, and Fischer, *Making Integrated,* 119.

97. Schneller, Eugene S. "Accountability for Healthcare." *Healthcare Management Review* 22 (Winter 1997): 45.

98. Longest, Beaufort B., Jr. *Seeking Strategic Advantage Through Health Policy Analysis.* Chicago: Health Administration Press, 1997; Longest, Beaufort B., Jr. *Health Policymaking in the United States,* 2nd ed. Chicago: Health Administration Press, 1998.

99. Zelman, Walter A. *The Changing Healthcare Marketplace: Private Ventures, Public Interests.* San Francisco: Jossey-Bass, 1996.

100. Bader, Barry S. "Weight Loss: A Painless Approach to a Sleeker Governance Model." *Trustee* 56 (April 1997): 14.

101. This discussion is adapted from Longest, "Managerial Competence," 127–130.

102. Pointer, Dennis D., Jeffrey A. Alexander, and Howard S. Zuckerman. "Loosening the Gordian Knot of Governance in Integrated Health Care Delivery Systems." *Frontiers of Health Services Management* 11 (Spring 1995): 3–37.

103. Pointer, Alexander, and Zuckerman, "Loosening the Gordian Knot," 17–18.

104. Koska, Mary T. "CEOs Make the Most of Trustees' Business Acumen." *Hospitals* 64 (June 5, 1990): 27–30.

105. Orlikoff, James E. "Ensuring Board Effectiveness: It Could Be as Simple as Changing Your Board Structure." *Healthcare Executive* 13 (September–October 1998): 12–16.

106. Orlikoff, "Ensuring Board Effectiveness."

107. Bader, "Weight Loss," 12.

108. Pointer, Alexander, and Zuckerman, "Loosening the Gordian Knot."

109. Pointer, Alexander, and Zuckerman, "Loosening the Gordian Knot."

110. Charan, Ram. *Boards at Work: How Corporate Boards Create Competitive Advantage,* 151–178. San Francisco: Jossey-Bass, 1998.

111. Ummel, Stephen L. "Pursuing the Elusive Integrated Delivery Network." *Healthcare Forum Journal* 40 (March/April, 1997): 13.

112. Molinari, Carol, Laura L. Morlock, Jeffrey A. Alexander, and Charles A. Lyles. "Hospital Board Effectiveness: Relationships Between Governing Board Composition and Hospital Financial Viability." *Health Services Research* 28 (August 1993): 358– 377.

113. Rubin, Jeffrey Z., and Bert R. Brown. *The Social Psychology of Bargaining and Negotiation,* 2. New York: Academic Press, 1975.

114. Adapted from Greenberger, David, Stephen Strasser, Roy J. Lewicki, and Thomas S. Bateman. "Perception, Motivation, and Negotiation." In *Health Care Management: A Text in Organization Theory and Behavior,* edited by Stephen M. Shortell and Arnold D. Kaluzny, 2nd ed., 129. New York: John Wiley & Sons, 1988.

115. Adapted from Greenberger, Strasser, Lewicki, and Bateman, "Perception, Motivation, and Negotiation," 129.

116. Adapted from Greenberger, Strasser, Lewicki, and Bateman, "Perception, Motivation, and Negotiation," 131.

117. This and other mechanisms described here are adapted from Altman, Drew, Robert Greene, and Harvey M. Sapolsky. *Health Planning and Regulation: The Decision-Making Process,* 26–31. Ann Arbor, MI: AUPHA Press, 1981.

118. Altman, Greene, and Sapolsky, *Health Planning,* 28.

119. O'Leary, *Lexikon,* 218.

120. Coddington, Dean C., and Keith D. Moore. *Market-Driven Strategies in Health Care,* 114–115. San Francisco: Jossey-Bass, 1987.

121. Byars, Lloyd L., and Leslie W. Rue. *Strategic Management.* New York: McGraw-Hill, 1996.

122. Johnsson, Julie. "Hospitals Dismantle Elaborate Corporate Restructurings." *Hospitals* 65 (July 5, 1991): 45.

123. Johnsson, "Hospitals Dismantle," 41.

124. Zajac and D'Aunno, "Managing Strategic Alliances," 330.

125. Adapted from *American Healthline,* January 27, 1999; reprinted with permission.

126. Excerpted and adapted from "Ethics & the CEO." *Hospitals & Health Networks* 72 (January 20, 1998): 29; reprinted by permission.

127. Adapted from Darr, Kurt. *Ethics in Health Services Management,* 3rd ed., 80–81. Baltimore: Health Professions Press, 1997; reprinted by permission.
128. Adapted from Smith, David B., and Arnold D. Kaluzny. *The White Labyrinth: A Guide to the Health Care System,* 2nd ed., 172–173. Ann Arbor, MI: Health Administration Press, 1986; reprinted by permission.
129. Approved by the American Hospital Association Board of Trustees, Chicago, on July 19, 1997; reprinted with permission.
130. From Orlikoff, James E., and Mary K. Totten. "Systems Thinking in Governance" [workbook insert]. *Trustee* 52 (January 1999): 4; reprinted by permission.
131. Adapted from Higgins, James M. *The Management Challenge: An Introduction to Management,* 482–483. New York: Macmillan, 1991 (based on Finnegan, Jay. "All the President's Men." *Inc.* [February 1989]: 44–54); reprinted by permission.

SELECTED BIBLIOGRAPHY

The Advisory Board Company. *The Grand Alliance: Vertical Integration Strategies for Physicians and Health Systems.* Washington, DC: Advisory Board, 1993.

American Hospital Association. *Hospital Statistics, 2000.* Chicago: Health Forum, 2000

Bader, Barry S. "Weight Loss: A Painless Approach to a Sleeker Governance Model." *Trustee* 56 (April 1997): 12–16.

Barton, Phoebe Lindsey. *Understanding the U.S. Health Services System.* Chicago: Health Administration Press, 1999.

Bazzoli, Gloria J., Stephen M. Shortell, Nicole Dubbs, Cheeling Chan, and Peter Kralovec. "A Taxonomy of Health Networks and Systems: Bringing Order Out of Chaos." *Health Services Research* 33 (February 1999): 1683–1717.

Blair, John D., Charles R. Slaton, and Grant T. Savage. "Hospital-Physician Joint Ventures: A Strategic Approach for Both Dimensions of Success." *Hospital & Health Services Administration* 35 (Spring 1990): 3–26.

Brown, Montague. "Mergers, Networking, and Vertical Integration: Managed Care and Investor-Owned Hospitals." *Health Care Management Review* 21 (Winter 1996): 29–37.

Burns, Lawton R., Gloria J. Bazzoli, Linda Dynan, and Douglas R. Wholey. "Managed Care, Market Stages, and Integrated Delivery Systems: Is There a Relationship?" *Health Affairs* 16 (November/December 1997): 204–218.

Burns, Lawton R., and Darrell P. Thorpe. "Physician-Hospital Organizations: Strategy, Structure, and Conduct." In *Integrating the Practice of Medicine: A Decision Maker's Guide to Organizing and Managing Physician Services,* edited by Ronald B. Connors, ch. 17. Chicago: AHA Press, 1997.

Charan, Ram. *Boards at Work: How Corporate Boards Create Competitive Advantage.* San Francisco: Jossey-Bass, 1998.

Clement, Jan P., Michael J. McCue, Roice D. Luke, James D. Bramble, Louis F. Rossiter, Yasar A. Ozcan, and Chih-Wen Pai. "Strategic Hospital Alliances: Impact on Financial Performance." *Health Affairs* 16 (November/December 1997): 193–203.

Coddington, Dean C., Keith D. Moore, and Elizabeth A. Fischer. *Making Integrated Health Care Work.* Englewood, CO: Center for Research in Ambulatory Health Care Administration, 1996.

Coddington, Dean C., Keith D. Moore, and Elizabeth A. Fischer. "Physician Leaders in Integrated Delivery." *Medical Group Management Journal* 44, 5 (September/October 1997): 85–90.

Connor, Robert A., Roger D. Feldman, Bryan E. Down, and Tiffany A. Radcliff. "Which Types of Hospital Mergers Save Consumers Money?" *Health Affairs* 16 (November/December 1997): 62–74.

Conrad, Douglas A. "Coordinating Patient Care Services in Regional Health Systems: The Challenge of Clinical Integration." *Hospital & Health Services Administration* 38 (Winter 1993): 491–508.

Conrad, Douglas A., and William L. Dowling. "Vertical Integration in Health Services: Theory and Managerial Implications." *Health Care Management Review* 14 (Fall 1990): 9–22.

Conrad, Douglas A., and Stephen M. Shortell. "Integrated Health Systems: Promise and Performance." *Frontiers of Health Services Management* 13 (Fall 1996): 3–40.

D'Aunno, Thomas A., and Howard S. Zuckerman. "A Life Cycle Model of Organizational Federations: The Case of Hospitals." *Academy of Management Review* 12 (1987): 534–545.

Ginter, Peter M., Linda M. Swayne, and W. Jack Duncan. *Strategic Management of Health Care Organizations,* 3rd ed. Malden, MA: Blackwell, 1998.

Gold, Marsha, Ed. *Contemporary Managed Care: Readings in Structure, Operations, and Public Policy.* Chicago: Health Administration Press, 1998.

Goldsmith, Jeff C. "The Illusive Logic of Integration." *Health Forum Journal* 37 (September–October 1994): 26–31.

Hanson, Elizabeth, Susan Marsh, and Christopher H. Coulter. "Direct Provider Contracting: One Employer's Experience." *Benefits Quarterly* 15 (First Quarter 1999): 37–41.

Hilzenrath, David S., and Michael D. Shear. "Hospital Alliance in N. Va. to End." *The Washington Post,* January 29, 1999, E01.

Hoechst Marion Roussel. *Managed Care Digest Series: HMO-PPO/Medicare/Medicaid Digest.* Kansas City, MO: Hoechst Marion Roussel, 1999.

Hoechst Marion Roussel. *Managed Care Digest Series: Integrated Health Systems Digest.* Kansas City, MO: Hoechst Marion Roussel, 1999.

Kaluzny, Arnold D., and Howard S. Zuckerman. "Strategic Alliances: Two Perspectives for Understanding Their Effects on Health Services." *Hospital & Health Services Administration* 37 (Winter 1992): 477–490.

Kaluzny, Arnold D., Howard S. Zuckerman, and Thomas C. Ricketts, III, eds. *Partners for the Dance: Forming Strategic Alliances in Health Care.* Chicago: Health Administration Press, 1995.

Kittredge, Frank D. "What Is Clinical Integration and Why Is It So Important?" *The Bristol Review* (October 1996): 1.

Kraatz, Matthew S. "Learning by Association? Interorganizational Networks and Adaptation to Environmental Change." *Academy of Management Journal* 41 (December 1998): 621–643.

Lehrman, Susan, and Karen K. Shore. "Hospitals' Vertical Integration into Skilled Nursing: A Rational Approach to Controlling Transaction Costs." *Inquiry* 35 (Fall 1998): 303–314.

Longest, Beaufort B., Jr. "Interorganizational Linkages in the Health Sector." *Health Care Management Review* 15 (Winter 1990): 17–28.

Longest, Beaufort B., Jr. *Seeking Strategic Advantage Through Health Policy Analysis.* Chicago: Health Administration Press, 1997.

Longest, Beaufort B., Jr. *Health Policymaking in the United States,* 2nd ed. Chicago: Health Administration Press, 1998.

Luke, Roice, Peter C. Olden, and James D. Bramble. "Strategic Hospital Alliances: Countervailing Responses to Restructuring Health Care Markets." In *Handbook of Health Care Management,* edited by W. Jack Duncan, Peter M. Ginter, and Linda E. Swayne, 81–116. Malden, MA: Blackwell, 1998.

Miles, Raymond E., and Charles C. Snow. "Twenty-First Century Careers." In *The Boundaryless Career: A New Employment Principle for a New Organizational Era,* edited by Michael B. Arthur and Denise M. Rousseau, 261–307. New York: Oxford University Press, 1996.

Ohmae, Kenichi. "The Global Logic of Alliances." *Harvard Business Review* 89 (March–April 1989): 143–154.

O'Leary, Margaret R. *Lexikon.* Oakbrook Terrace, IL: Joint Commission on Accreditation of Healthcare Organizations, 1994.

Orlikoff, James E. "Ensuring Board Effectiveness: It Could Be as Simple as Changing Your Board Structure." *Healthcare Executive* 13 (September–October 1998): 12–16.

Orlikoff, James E., and Mary K. Totten. *The Future of Health Care Governance: Redesigning Boards for a New Era.* Chicago: American Hospital Publishing, 1996.

Orlikoff, James E., and Mary K. Totten. "New Relationships with Physicians: An Overview for Trustees." *Trustee* [workbook insert] 50 (July/August 1997).

Orlikoff, James E., and Mary K. Totten. "Systems Thinking in Governance." *Trustee* [workbook insert] 52 (January 1999).

Pointer, Dennis D., Jeffrey A. Alexander, and Howard S. Zuckerman. "Loosening the Gordian Knot of Governance in Integrated Health Care Delivery Systems." *Frontiers of Health Services Management* 11 (Spring 1995): 3–37.

Pointer, Dennis D., James W. Begun, and Roice D. Luke. "Managing Interorganizational Dependencies in the New Health Care Marketplace." *Hospital & Health Services Administration* 33 (Summer 1988): 167–177.

Robinson, James C. "The Changing Boundaries of the American Hospital." *The Milbank Quarterly* 72 (Summer 1994): 259–275.

Robinson, James C. "Physician-Hospital Integration and the Economic Theory of the Firm." *Medical Care Research and Review* 54 (March 1997): 3–24.

Robinson, James C., and Lawrence P. Casalino. "Vertical Integration and Organizational Networks in Health Care." *Health Affairs* 15 (Spring 1996): 7–22.

Satinsky, Marjorie A. *The Foundations of Integrated Care: Facing the Challenges of Change.* Chicago: American Hospital Publishing, 1998.

Schneller, Eugene S. "Accountability for Healthcare." *Healthcare Management Review* 22 (Winter 1997): 38–48.

Shortell, Stephen M., and Kathleen E. Hull. "The New Organization of the Health Care Delivery System." In *Strategic Choices for a Changing Health Care System,* edited by Stuart H. Altman and Uwe E. Reinhardt, 101–148. Chicago: Health Administration Press, 1996.

Shortell, Stephen M., Ellen M. Morrison, and Bernard Friedman. *Strategic Choices for America's Hospitals: Managing Change in Turbulent Times.* San Francisco: Jossey-Bass, 1990.

Stein, Barry A. "Strategic Alliances: Some Lessons from Experience." In *Partners for the Dance: Forming Strategic Alliances in Health Care,* edited by Arnold D. Kaluzny, Howard S. Zuckerman, and Thomas C. Ricketts, III, 19–62. Ann Arbor, MI: Health Administration Press, 1995.

Ummel, Stephen L. "Pursuing the Elusive Integrated Delivery Network." *Healthcare Forum Journal* 40 (March/April, 1997): 13–19.

Zajac, Edward J., and Thomas A. D'Aunno. "Managing Strategic Alliances." In *Essentials of Health Care Management,* edited by Stephen M. Shortell and Arnold D. Kaluzny, 328–354. Albany, NY: Delmar Publishers, 1997.

Zajac, Edward J., Brian R. Golden, and Stephen M. Shortell. "New Organizational Forms for Enhancing Innovation: The Case of Internal Corporate Joint Ventures." *Management Science* 37 (1991): 170–184.

Zelman, Walter A. *The Changing Healthcare Marketplace: Private Ventures, Public Interests.* San Francisco: Jossey-Bass, 1996.

Zuckerman, Howard S., and Thomas A. D'Aunno. "Hospital Alliances: Cooperative Strategy in a Competitive Environment." *Health Care Management Review* 15 (1990): 21–30.

6 Health Care Technology

Some technologies increase costs. Some technologies decrease costs. And some technologies do both. Some raise costs in the short run, but save dollars over the full course of treatment; others lower costs by moving care to nonhospital settings, but increase costs overall because care is more accessible and used more often. How technology affects costs depends on the technology, where it is used, and—above all—on how the concepts of costs and benefits are defined. Indeed, that is the challenge.[1]

The advancement and diffusion of technology are among the most controversial developments in the provision of health care. Technological innovations have given health services providers the means to diagnose and treat an increasing number of problems and illnesses. The same advances have been criticized, however, for their effect on the practice of medicine and on national health care expenditures, which increased from almost $27 billion in 1960 to more than $1.1 trillion in 1998 and are projected to be $2.2 trillion in 2008.

The dramatic rise in health care costs since 1950 is partly related to the proliferation of new technologies; the increased use of existing tests and procedures, including attendant specialized staff; and financing of the innovations. The purchase price of technology has a minimal effect on health care costs. In 1993, for example, expenditures for technology, defined as ranging from advanced diagnostic products and implantable devices to major capital equipment and routine medical supplies, totaled only 5.1% of health care spending.[2]

That part of the rise in health care costs that is attributable to the use of technology is uncertain. Estimates have been as high as 70%.[3] There seems to be a consensus that approximately 50% of the rise in total health care expenditures results from the use of new technologies and the overuse of existing ones.[4] An analysis of Health Care Financing Administration (HCFA) data shows, however, that from 1980 to 1990 new technologies contributed only 15% to the total increase in health care spending.[5]

Health economists conceptualize the issues in various ways. One theory examines the impact of technology on acute care hospital costs as measured by discrete units such as the labor and nonlabor inputs of using technology. A second theory analyzes the costs that are associated with specific acute care hospital-based technologies. A third theory examines the impact of technology on treating specific conditions and types of illnesses through time. A fourth theory measures the impact of technology on total health care expenditures. It is generally agreed that technology has increased the intensity of resources that are used to treat individual cases and that this has increased costs. Increased intensity also has resulted from the introduction of new technologies used on new categories of patients, in addition to the use of existing technologies in new ways. The exact contribution of technology—new procedures, capabilities, and products—and its use to health costs cannot be determined, but clearly it is a major contributor.

Medical technology can be defined as "any discrete and identifiable regimen or modality used to diagnose and treat illness, prevent disease, maintain patient well-being, or facilitate the provision of health services."[6] This broad definition includes biologicals and pharmaceuticals; high technology such as positron emission tomograph (PET) scanners; low technology such as laboratory tests; facilities such as intensive care units; specific procedures such as endoscopy, laparoscopy, and coronary artery bypass; clinical and management information and control systems for health services organizations/health systems (HSOs/HSs) and affiliated organizations; and managerial technologies such as how care is organized and provided (e.g., home health care or other types of providers, such as physician assistants or nurse practitioners).

A useful typology categorizing medical technologies by their characteristics is shown in Table 6.1. These technologies continue to be available predominantly in acute care hospitals. The increasing portability of technology, however, allows it to be delivered in nonhospital and outpatient settings; the economic implications for acute care hospitals are enormous. Portability has not lowered total costs. On the contrary, home health services are the fastest growing segment of Medicare,

TABLE 6.1.   TYPES OF MEDICAL TECHNOLOGIES

Type	Examples
Diagnostic	CT scanner
	Fetal monitor
	Computerized electrocardiography
	Automated clinical labs
	MRI
	Ambulatory blood pressure monitor
Survival (lifesaving)	Intensive care unit
	Cardiopulmonary resuscitation
	Liver transplant
	Autologous bone marrow transplant
Illness management	Renal dialysis
	Pacemaker
	PTCA (angioplasty)
	Stereotactic cingulotomy (psychosurgery)
Cure	Hip joint replacement
	Organ transplant
	Lithotripter
Prevention	Implantable automatic cardioverter-defibrillator
	Pediatric orthopedic repair
	Diet control for phenylketonuria
	Vaccines for immunization
System management	Medical information systems
	Telemedicine

From Rosenthal, Gerald. "Anticipating the Costs and Benefits of New Technology: A Typology for Policy." In *Medical Technology: The Culprit Behind Health Care Costs?* (Publication No. [PHS] 79-3216), 79. Washington, DC: Department of Health and Human Services, 1979, as updated.

which suggests that demand for health services is virtually limitless—only the location of its delivery changes.

Another way to describe medical technology is based on charge to the user. Technologies such as laboratory tests, radiographs (X rays), and other ancillary services, which typically cost less than $100, are considered low cost as compared to high-cost magnetic resonance imaging (MRI) scans and organ transplantation, which range from $600 to $30,000–$200,000 and beyond, respectively. The controversy over increasing costs focuses on high-cost technologies, but inexpensive technologies raise similar concerns because they are used in high volume and may be labor intensive. Data from the 1950s and 1960s show that the primary cost-raising changes were rapid increases in the use of low-cost ancillary services, such as laboratories and X rays, which are commonly called "little ticket" technologies. Data from the 1970s and 1980s, however, show that the use of little ticket technologies hardly changed but that several new and expensive "big ticket" technologies came into common use, raising costs considerably.[7] Sometimes, new technology is a hybrid—its use reduces treatment costs, but the resulting higher volume increases total costs for a treatment. Laparoscopic cholecystectomy is an example.[8]

Rather than classify technologies by cost, it is more useful to focus on the value obtained by their use, which can be done by emphasizing cost-effectiveness and clinical guidelines that reduce variation.[9] Despite differences in how technologies are described, development and use of technology will continue. It is important to examine the factors behind this trend and its effects on the health care system and on individual HSOs and HSs.

HISTORY AND BACKGROUND

The technology of modern allopathic (Western) medicine can be traced to the end of the 19th century and the advent of efficacious surgery. The most significant developments in diagnosing, treating, and managing disease, however, date from the 1950s, concomitant with the increasing prominence of the National Institutes of Health (NIH). Growth of NIH was sparked by the renewed interest in curing disease, which was in turn prompted by new knowledge in the basic sciences. By the 1950s immunizations to prevent infectious diseases such as polio and influenza and drug therapies to treat noninfectious conditions such as pernicious anemia, diabetes, gout, and hyperthyroidism were readily available. It was hoped that new technologies could be developed to cure or prevent chronic and life-threatening diseases such as cancer, heart disease, and stroke.

Acute care hospitals are especially quick to add technology. No acute care hospital reported having MRI in 1984; by 1988, 10.6% had MRI.[10] The speed of generalizing this technology is astounding—in the late 1980s a MRI unit cost $1.5 million to buy and $200,000 to install[11]; the cost in 2000 for a 1.5-Tesla MRI (the most powerful version available) is $1.8–$2.2 million.[12] In 1991 the ability to measure and map sources of electrical activity in the heart, the neuromuscular system, and especially the brain was substantially enhanced with the introduction of magnetic source imaging (MSI). Computerized tomography (CT) and MRI diagnose pathologies that leave lesions, but MSI provides important supplemental information. MSI units cost $2 million.[13] Acute care hospitals are likely to make this technology available to remain competitive and because their physicians expect access to the new diagnostic information that MSI provides. Laparoscopic surgical techniques may hold the record for rapidity of diffusion—nearly 100% of hospitals and surgeons adopted them the first year that they were available.[14] Acute care hospitals are slow to abandon old (established) diagnostic technology when newer technology could replace it[15] or to substitute a newer, lower cost treatment for an older one, however.[16] Such inertia is explained largely by the practice patterns and preferences of physicians, as well as by other clinical treatment and support staff. Hence, acute care hospitals have a large financial investment in newly acquired equipment and in the high maintenance costs of established equipment.

TYPES OF TECHNOLOGIES

Definitive (Curative, Preventive) Technologies

Technologies are definitive when they cure or prevent a central disease agent or mechanism.[17] Some, such as vaccines or antibiotics, are relatively inexpensive, even considering the costs of research and development. Some, such as surgical intervention for acute appendicitis, are more expensive but curative. Other definitive technologies, such as monitoring and screening programs, may or may not be expensive, depending on the cost of finding a true positive. Figure 6.1 shows the availability of clinical management and definitive technologies for several conditions.*

Halfway (Add-On) Technologies

Overwhelmingly, medical technologies are "halfway" or "add-on" technologies, which can range from inexpensive interventions such as feeding tubes to treatments costing several hundred thousand dollars, such as the historic iron lung that was used to treat polio victims. Unlike other fields, innovations in health care usually add to or generate new costs while achieving something not previously possible. Research in cancer, heart disease, and stroke has yielded primarily halfway technologies to diagnose and manage disease rather than cure it. New treatments produced by the "war" on cancer dating from the early 1970s have been disappointing; lower mortality reflects primarily changing incidence or early detection.[18] Transplants and grafts are halfway technologies that improve the health status of a few individuals but add considerably to costs. In 1995 there were 11,816 kidney, 3,924 liver, 2,316 heart, 1,027 pancreas/islet cell, 871 lung, and 68 heart-lung transplants. In addition, 44,652 cornea, 450,000 bone, and 5,500 skin grafts were performed.[19]

Halfway technologies have improved the diagnosis of brain diseases. CT and MRI scans show the brain's structure. Brain electrical activity mapping enhances the study of brain waves. Blood circulation, energy consumption, and chemical neurotransmitter systems are measured with single-photon emission computerized tomography (SPECT), PET scans, and functional magnetic resonance imaging (fMRI).[20] Each technology improves a clinician's ability to diagnose an abnormality, and the technologies are used in addition to, not instead of, each other. Another halfway technology is transesophageal echocardiography (TEE), which uses an ultrasound transducer mounted on a gastroscope to obtain images of the heart. It is recommended that acute care hospitals with cardiac surgery services have TEE and perhaps establish a dedicated ultrasound system to use it.[21] Figure 6.2 suggests the uses of penetrating radiation for imaging and treating disease.

Deferral Technologies

Some technologies slow the progression of disease and may even dramatically improve a patient's condition. Nevertheless, the improvement is of short duration and repeat treatments are required. Surgical treatment of coronary artery disease is an example. Coronary artery bypass grafting (CABG) is an expensive procedure that many patients must have repeated every 5–7 years. The development of coronary angioplasty provided a simple, less invasive procedure costing a fraction of bypass surgery; its use grew rapidly. The data, however, show no decline in bypass surgery. It is thought that after repeat angioplasties, bypass surgery is needed anyway. Thus angioplasty defers the need for bypass surgery but does not eliminate it, while adding considerable costs.[22]

---

*Progress in providing effective therapy differs widely for different conditions. For example, prevention, cure, and control have been attained for many infections. Many congenital malformations can be corrected by surgery, and high blood pressure can be effectively controlled. For conditions lacking definitive therapy, sophisticated technologies have been developed to replace or supplement the structure and function of affected organs. These technical triumphs should be regarded as pseudosolutions of value to current patients but not really directed toward the underlying causes and cures that must ultimately be developed for the benefit of future generations.

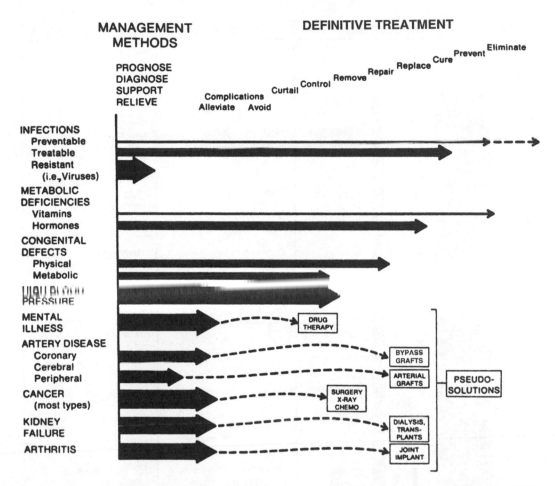

Figure 6.1.   Advances in medical technology. (From Rushmer, Robert F. "Technological Resources for Health." In *Introduction to Health Services,* 2nd ed., edited by Stephen J. Williams and Paul R. Torrens, 298. New York: John Wiley & Sons, 1984; reprinted by permission.)

Competing Technologies

Technologies that compete may have similar results but very different costs. An example is two thrombolytic (blood clot–dissolving) agents, streptokinase and tissue plasminogen activator (t-PA [Genentech's Activase]). In the mid-1990s streptokinase cost $400 per dose and t-PA cost $2,400. Research reported in 1994 comparing the two found that t-PA saves one more life per 100 patients treated than does streptokinase—a cost of $200,000 per life saved.[23] Such a difference raises cost–benefit issues, except, obviously, for the patient whose life is saved.

Cost-Saving Technologies

Few new technologies prevent disease either for individuals or populations (e.g., vaccines that protect future generations). Nonetheless, many reduce costs, especially when compared to old technologies that are used to treat the same disease. Examples include arthroscopy, implantable infusion pumps, laparoscopic and endoscopic procedures, and lasers. These technologies may be halfway or deferral therapies, but, if they replace more costly treatments or those of lesser quality, the result will

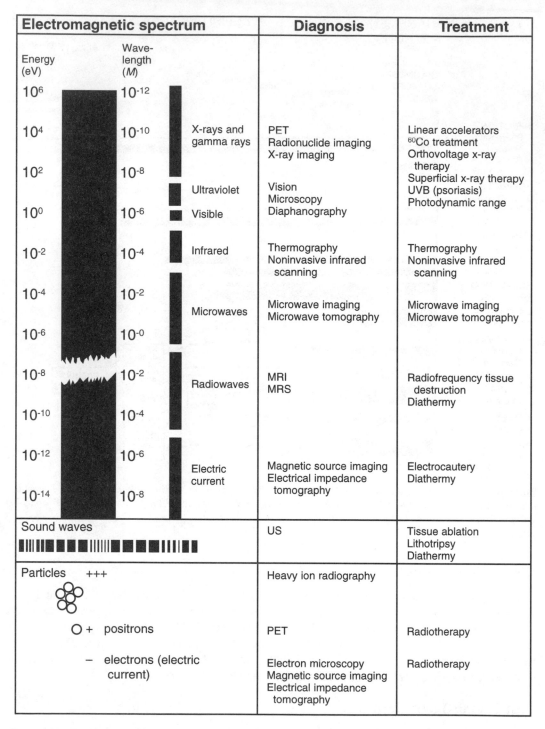

Electromagnetic spectrum			Diagnosis	Treatment
Energy (eV)	Wave-length (M)			
10^6	10^{-12}			
10^4	10^{-10}	X-rays and gamma rays	PET Radionuclide imaging X-ray imaging	Linear accelerators ^{60}Co treatment Orthovoltage x-ray therapy
10^2	10^{-8}	Ultraviolet	Vision Microscopy Diaphanography	Superficial x-ray therapy UVB (psoriasis) Photodynamic range
10^0	10^{-6}	Visible		
10^{-2}	10^{-4}	Infrared	Thermography Noninvasive infrared scanning	Thermography Noninvasive infrared scanning
10^{-4}	10^{-2}	Microwaves	Microwave imaging Microwave tomography	Microwave imaging Microwave tomography
10^{-6}	10^{-0}			
10^{-8}	10^{-2}	Radiowaves	MRI MRS	Radiofrequency tissue destruction Diathermy
10^{-10}	10^{-4}			
10^{-12}	10^{-6}	Electric current	Magnetic source imaging Electrical impedance tomography	Electrocautery Diathermy
10^{-14}	10^{-8}			
Sound waves			US	Tissue ablation Lithotripsy Diathermy
Particles +++			Heavy ion radiography	
O + positrons			PET	Radiotherapy
— electrons (electric current)			Electron microscopy Magnetic source imaging Electrical impedance tomography	Radiotherapy

Figure 6.2.   Penetrating radiation in imaging and treating disease. (From Lentle, Brian, and John Aldrich. "Radiological Sciences, Past and Present." *Lancet* 350 [July 26, 1997]: 281; reprinted by permission.)

be lower costs and better outcomes for the patient and the health services system. Costs and benefits are defined broadly and include hospitalization and sick days avoided, early return to work, reduced pain and discomfort, and short- and long-term quality of life. Assessing a technology must include these dimensions.[24] A laparoscopic technology that increases quality while reducing total costs is the port-access system that enables surgeons to perform heart surgery without "cracking" the patient's sternum (breast bone). Specially designed catheters, surgical instruments, and imaging equipment are used. Patients avoid the trauma and pain of having their chests opened and are hospitalized only 3–5 days as compared with 8–12 days using open-heart techniques; also, they can return to work within 2 weeks as compared with 8–12 weeks after open-heart surgery. In addition, the risk of infection and other complications is greatly reduced.[25] An estimated 20% of the 350,000 patients who undergo bypass surgery annually are candidates for less invasive procedures.[26] The potential savings in dollars, pain, and discomfort, as well as the increase in quality, are obvious.

EFFECTS OF TECHNOLOGY ON HEALTH STATUS

Although halfway and deferral technologies improve diagnosis and management of many diseases (e.g., a CT scan may prevent or shorten a hospital stay and save other resources), the effect on health status is uncertain. The modest increase in average life expectancy from 1966 (at the inception of Medicare and Medicaid) to 1997 of only 2.8 years suggests that advances in medical technology have had little effect on longevity. An average American's life expectancy is expected to increase only 1.1 years by 2025.[27]

Alarming is the negative change in disability-free years, which are projected to decline by 7.3 years for a male born in 1964. The decrease in disability-free years may have resulted from the neglect of public health.[28] It has been suggested that increased longevity may result from technological progress but not be reflected in standard health status statistics, such as life expectancy, until well into the future.[29] Since 1968, death rates from coronary artery disease have declined by 63% and death rates from strokes by 62%.[30] Such declines generally are attributed to technology; it is possible, however, that true cause-and-effect relationships are only partly known.[31]

Trying to credit technology with changes in health status indicators such as morbidity and disability raises other problems. It is paradoxical that, by saving a life or preventing disease, technology increases the likelihood of morbidity and disability. Similarly, health promotion such as smoking cessation may actually increase health care costs in the long term.[32] This means, of course, that the results of technology and prevention are a double-edge sword; the quality of life is improved by reducing morbidity and mortality, but costs for long-term debilitating disease may be increased. A new body of data is developing, however, indicating that people with lower health risks because of better health habits have less lifetime disability, as well as less disability at any given age.[33]

The development of two definitive technologies was stimulated by the risk of blood-borne diseases such as human immunodeficiency virus (HIV) and hepatitis B and C. One, a blood substitute to carry oxygen to the tissues and carbon dioxide back to the lungs, is expected to be available at a cost that is comparable to natural blood.[34] The other, a blood plasma-scrubbing technology that removes viruses, has received preliminary approval from the Food and Drug Administration (FDA).[35] The advantages of avoiding blood-borne diseases are obvious.

FORCES AFFECTING DEVELOPMENT AND DIFFUSION OF TECHNOLOGY

Medical Education and Practice

Among the most important factors encouraging the development and diffusion of technology after World War II were changes in medical training and the practice of medicine. Biomedical research funded by NIH stimulated medical schools to investigate specialized areas of medicine, which led to the growth of specialty departments within academic medical centers. Increasingly, medical school graduates went on to postgraduate training and then to practice in a medical specialty.

In 1970, 40.9% of physicians were primary care physicians, defined by the American Medical Association to include the general specialties of family practice, general practice, internal medicine, obstetrics-gynecology, and pediatrics. By 1980, 39.8% were primary care physicians; by 1990, the number was 34.7%. In 1996, 34.0% of physicians were classified as primary care, which means that almost two thirds of U.S. physicians were specialists.[36] Beginning in the 1970s, federal legislation sought to address the imbalance between primary care and specialization; in the late 1980s specialty societies and boards began reconsidering the number of residencies to be offered in the various specialties. Decisions of third-party payers, including the federal government but especially managed care organizations and health maintenance organizations (HMOs), have added impetus to reduce the relative number of specialists. It is generally believed that a ratio of two thirds primary care physicians to one third specialists is desirable—just the opposite of the current ratio.

Historically, specialization meant that physicians were trained to use technology. Not surprisingly, they expected to have the same technologies in their practices. This desire to have state-of-the-art technology available and to use it as necessary, despite the cost, is called the technological imperative. Evidence of the technological imperative is most apparent in acute care hospitals and explains the proliferation of highly specialized technology in that setting. From the late 1960s to the late 1980s plant assets in community hospitals rose rapidly. By 1989 the 50th percentile of net property, plant, and equipment was almost $96,000 per bed.[37] A decrease in beds and an increase in acuity of patient illness contributed to a significantly increased ratio of assets per bed. The need to attract and retain physicians exaggerates the interest in having various technologies and increases the pressure to acquire, operate, maintain, and ensure their safe use. The growth rate of capital expenditures decreased from 1992 to 1995; continued small declines are expected.[38]

The almost universal presence of technology should not suggest that it is applied similarly nationwide. There is wide geographic variation in the treatment that is given to patients with the same diagnoses.[39] These variations range from hospitalization rates and lengths of stay to treatment regimens such as whether patients with coronary artery disease are treated with risk factor modification (diet, exercise) and medication to reduce the frequency and severity of angina (chest pain) or receive percutaneous transluminal coronary angioplasty (PTCA) or CABG.[40]

The cost implications of choosing different treatment regimens are significant and increase the controversy. A 1983 NIH study found that CABG was a commonly overused procedure; it was estimated that 25,000 of the 200,000 CABG procedures performed annually could be eliminated without jeopardizing patient care.[41] A more recent evaluation concluded that "surgical therapy improves prognosis in high-risk patients, but the advantage over medical therapy declines with longer follow up."[42]

In early 1991 the Department of Health and Human Services (DHHS) contracted with four acute care hospitals to provide CABG to Medicare patients on a fixed-fee (global payment) basis that included physician and hospital costs. Rates paid were 5%–30% lower, depending on the site.[43] With savings exceeding $35 million, the pilot CABG program is considered successful and has been expanded to include more sites and other cardiac procedures, as well as hip and knee replacement. Although pilot hospitals' volumes did not increase, their financial margins did, probably because of greater efficiency.[44] Such efforts will increase as HCFA seeks further reductions in Medicare spending. Interestingly, the reputation of coronary artery bypass surgeons among peers may be less closely associated with the quality of their work than with the number of procedures done (patient volume).[45] The relationship between the number of procedures and the quality of outcomes is shown by studies of other physicians and applies to hospitals as well.[46]

Another form of variation in the application of technology is that physicians who have practiced longer than 15 years have significantly more inappropriate hospital admissions.[47] Beyond the application of technology is the question of treatment outcomes. Data show significant variation in mortality rates for some diagnoses by geographic region.[48]

Wide variation in practice patterns raises doubts about medicine's scientific certainty and whether low-technology, less interventionist, and less expensive treatment might not be as effective as high-technology, more interventionist, and more costly treatment. Understanding physician practice patterns and variation, as well as determining efficacy, will enable HSOs/HSs to deliver more efficient and effective medical services.

Reimbursement

Third-Party Payment

Central to the diffusion of technological advances into medical practice and the existence of the technological imperative has been the availability of third-party reimbursement. In traditional fee-for-service medical practice, decisions to use new technologies usually are made by individual physicians based on findings that the technology yields benefit with a low probability of harm. Unlike in other industries, innovations in medical technology have been judged not primarily on the basis of performing some function better or more efficiently but rather on whether they will yield a benefit to individual patients. Similarly, decisions to reimburse for new technologies have been based on the acceptance and use of those technologies by physicians. Manufacturers' prices for new technologies, particularly drugs and devices, tend to be high in order to recover research and development costs. Provider charges are high to compensate for the skill and expertise that are involved in learning and offering a technology, as well as recovering the capital costs of acquiring it. Historically, once established in the reimbursement system, these charges have tended to remain high even after initial costs have been recovered.[49]

Ensured payment for tests and procedures under cost-based reimbursement allowed HSOs to acquire technology, knowing that the costs of capital investment and operation would be met. Historically, there were few incentives to evaluate the cost-effectiveness of new technologies, and acquisition of technology was, and continues to be, stimulated by the need for HSOs/HSs to attract both physicians and patients. Changes in public health care funding and the growth of managed care suggest, however, that proper and timely reimbursement for new technology is no longer ensured.[50]

Like federal efforts, payers such as health plans control costs through disease management programs and utilization review of high-cost diagnoses and treatments. For example, utilization management caused a 40% reduction in unnecessary imaging by primary care physicians.[51] One study found that enrollees of not-for-profit health plans and HMOs had less access to three laser technologies than was available in for-profit and indemnity plans.[52] If this is true for access to technology in general, such findings have major implications for the diffusion of technology as well as for the costs of health services.

Diagnosis-Related Groups

In late 1983 the payment for Medicare patients in acute care hospitals was changed from cost-based reimbursement to a prospective payment system based on diagnosis-related groups (DRGs). (The details of DRGs were discussed in Chapter 2.) As noted, the incentive for hospitals under this payment method is to do less, not more, which is the opposite of retrospective, cost-based reimbursement. Reimbursement is calculated using average cost per case. This formula should create an incentive to carefully evaluate technology, use it more efficiently, and select cost-saving technologies when possible.

It was thought that acute care hospitals providing a service infrequently would be unable to compete with those providing it frequently. Theoretically, the latter group has lower average unit costs. It was thought, too, that because the costs of using technology were not reimbursed separately, acute care hospitals would have few incentives to adopt a new technology that increases per-case cost by adding new operational expenses. It appears, however, that acquisition and use of technology by acute care hospitals is unchanged. It may be that only when Medicare payments are reduced further will the effect of DRGs on technology be felt.

Congress continues to try to reduce Medicare costs, primarily by reducing the DRG payment. It appears that those who feared the DRG system would stifle the diffusion of new technology and adversely affect patient care were wrong; those who predicted that an acute care hospital's need to be competitive and maintain admissions levels would necessitate acquiring technology were correct. Regardless, the long-term influence of DRGs on acute care hospitals and their use of technology remains to be seen. The real effect of DRGs may not match what was intended.[53]

Health Care Financing Administration

In the late 1980s HCFA began applying more uniform and stringent standards by which to judge the appropriateness of technology use. In early 1989 HCFA issued proposed regulations to define for the first time the criteria "reasonable" and "necessary," words used in Medicare to describe technology and procedures for which it will pay.[54] In defining reasonable and necessary, the final regulations rely heavily on FDA categorizations by requiring that technology and procedures be safe, effective, and noninvestigatory.[55]

States often underfund Medicaid (state-managed programs for the indigent that receive significant federal monies), and this makes it noteworthy that considerable resources are devoted to transplants. The federal Early and Periodic Screening, Diagnosis, and Treatment Program requires that states provide "medically necessary" services, which is interpreted to mean bone marrow, liver, heart, and lung transplants to people younger than 21 years of age. In 1997 Medicaid in more than half of the states provided bone marrow, liver, and heart transplants to adults; almost half provided lung transplants. Some states put monetary limits on each type of transplant covered.[56]

The Public

A third force influencing the diffusion of technology has been the public who benefited from it. The practice of highly technical and specialty-oriented medicine, coupled with widely publicized advances in medical care, fostered patients' expectations that a technology is available to diagnose and treat every problem and that quality medical care necessarily involves extensive technology. Polls consistently show that a majority of the public is willing to pay for much of the increase in health services and to spend what is needed to improve and protect the health of Americans.[57] Thus patients economically protected by third-party reimbursement share their physicians' expectations that all possible technologies should be available. Given this context, limiting the use of technology threatens the autonomy of patients and providers, an issue that is increasingly present in managed care.

Competitive Environment

Competition is an increasingly important fourth force in the diffusion of technology. There is competition among HSOs/HSs, between physicians and HSOs/HSs, among physician specialties, and between physicians and nonphysician providers. Acute care hospitals, and to a lesser extent other types of HSOs, compete by acquiring and offering advanced technology and by shifting services to outpatient settings, which have lower costs for and offer greater convenience to users. The increasing portability of biomedical equipment allows physicians to compete with HSOs, especially acute care hospitals, which were the historic repository of high technology. Finally, technological innovations disrupt the traditional demarcations of medical specialties, causing them to compete.

Technology permitting health services to be moved from inpatient to outpatient settings includes improved anesthesia that allows quicker return to consciousness with few aftereffects; better analgesics for pain relief; and minimally invasive procedures such as laser surgery, endoscopy, and laparoscopy.[58] In 1987 the number of outpatient visits surpassed the number of inpatient days.[59] Of the 38.4 million combined total outpatient and inpatient surgical and nonsurgical procedures performed in 1994, 18.8 million, or 49%, were performed during ambulatory surgery visits.[60] As noted earlier, minimally invasive surgical techniques are revolutionizing cardiovascular surgery. They allow surgeons to even operate on a beating heart and may someday allow outpatient cardiovascular surgery.[61] The next large shift in delivery sites will be into home health services, already the fastest growing portion of Medicare.

New technology, much of it less costly to buy and operate, coupled with the efforts to limit the use of specialists, is blurring the traditional lines of physician specialties and is causing fierce competition among them. Ultrasound, lasers, laboratories, and mammography are examples of these new technologies. A 1988 study by the American College of Radiology found that 60% of imaging studies were done outside the acute care hospital by nonradiologists.[62] This development has major implications for the specialties involved, as well as for HSOs/HSs, and has the potential to increase costs to the system. Physicians are less constrained by regulations such as certificates of need (CONs), which means that establishing an imaging center, for example, is a matter of raising capital and finding a location. Alleged abuses resulting from physician ownership of HSOs providing diagnosis and treatment caused state and federal governments to regulate self-referrals, which are defined as physicians sending patients to HSOs in which they have an ownership interest.

Competition is touted as a means of reducing costs. There is evidence, however, that costs in geographic areas with competition among HSOs are higher than those in noncompetitive areas. One study found that average costs per admission were 26% higher in the most competitive markets than in acute care hospitals with no competitors within 16 miles.[63]

RESPONSES TO DIFFUSION AND USE OF TECHNOLOGY

As HSOs/HSs acquired technology, issues of cost, benefit, and safety emerged. It became clear that diffusion and use of technology were only partially based on cost–benefit or cost-effectiveness considerations. Existing technological capabilities often were ignored or discounted. In addition, the hazards associated with a technology were inadequately understood. These concerns were the focus of federal laws to improve premarket evaluation of medical devices and influence acquisition and use of technologies, particularly in acute care hospitals. Amendments to the Food, Drug, and Cosmetic Act; legislation providing for professional standards review organizations (PSROs) (followed by peer review organizations [PROs]) and CONs; and establishment of the congressional Office of Technology Assessment (OTA) and DHHS's National Center for Health Care Technology (NCHCT) were the result, both of which were later defunded.

Table 6.2 shows several of the public and private organizations that ensure the safety and efficacy of technology. Amendments to the federal Food, Drug, and Cosmetic Act in 1976 and 1990 gave FDA a greatly enhanced role in monitoring manufacturers and investigating devices linked to patient death or serious injury or illness.[64] State authorities are concerned with staff and patient safety—one of the traditional police powers of the state described in Chapter 14—and may require the licensure of practitioners who use equipment and the approval of types of equipment by a national testing laboratory and regular inspections, especially of radiation sources such as X-ray equipment. Private organizations have been important in producing consensus standards. Among them are the National Fire Protection Association, which has developed standards on design and use of facilities and some biomedical equipment, and the Joint Commission on Accreditation of Healthcare Organizations (Joint Commission), whose standards govern equipment maintenance

TABLE 6.2.   BIOMEDICAL EQUIPMENT REGULATION

Authority	Federal	State	Profession
	Food and Drug Adminstration (FDA)	Department of public safety/public health	JCAHO, NFPA, etc.[a]
Objectives	Manufacturer quality	Personal safety	Hospital quality
Standards	FDA specifications	National testing laboratory	JCAHO accreditation manual, NFPA codes, etc.

[a]JCAHO, Joint Commission on Accreditation of Healthcare Organizations; NFPA, National Fire Protection Association.

and management. Some standards affecting technology in HSOs have been established by court decisions.

Public Sector Activities

Food and Drug Administration

Although FDA has been involved in premarket approval of drugs since 1962, evidence of the safety and efficacy of other medical technologies was not required. The Medical Device Amendments of 1976 to the Food, Drug, and Cosmetic Act extended FDA's premarket approval process to medical devices, divided into three classes. The most stringent regulation (Class III) applies to devices that support life, prevent health impairment, or prevent an unreasonable risk of illness or injury. Manufacturers must obtain FDA approval before such devices may be marketed, a procedure that requires evidence of safety and efficacy.[65] FDA control of marketing new drugs and devices has been criticized as unnecessarily impeding the introduction of technological innovations because of the time and money that are required to conduct clinical trials and obtain licensing. In the late 1980s pressure on FDA from those wanting rapid access to new drugs to treat acquired immunodeficiency syndrome (AIDS) caused reconsideration of its review processes, especially those applying to drugs that were potentially beneficial in treating fatal illnesses.

Legal liability for HSOs/HSs increased when the Safe Medical Device Act of 1990 codified the need to report device-related serious injuries and death to the manufacturer and, in the case of death, to FDA. FDA defines "medical device" broadly; there are significant penalties for failing to report. A checklist form is recommended to guide incident investigation.[66]

Notably, FDA has not published medical device standards. Furthermore, it neither requires inspection of devices nor licenses repair technicians. Inspection is left to providers and is reviewed by voluntary groups such as the Joint Commission. Absent licensure, voluntary certification programs such as those of the International Certification Commission and the Association for the Advancement of Medical Instrumentation ensure a technician's competence.[67]

PSROs and PROs

A general history of PSROs and how they were replaced by PROs beginning in 1984 is included in Chapter 2. In terms of medical technology, PSROs were established in 1972 as part of federal and state efforts to control health care costs by regulating the acquisition of new technology and reducing its use by utilization review. PSROs sought to ensure that Medicare (and Medicaid) services were "medically necessary, met professional standards of care, and were provided in the most economical setting possible consistent with quality care."[68] Initially, review focused on the appropriateness of acute care hospital admission and length of stay. Later, services provided also were reviewed.

PSRO effectiveness was hampered by Medicare's interpretation of "reasonable and necessary." This concept usually means that a procedure that is no longer experimental and is accepted by the local community is deemed reasonable and necessary. PSROs determined indications for use.[69]

PROs have a similar role regarding the use of technology. They review the validity of diagnostic and procedural information provided by hospitals; the completeness, adequacy, and quality of care provided; and the appropriateness of admissions patterns, discharges, lengths of stay, transfers, and services furnished in outlier cases. As a condition of receiving payment under Medicare, acute care hospitals must have a contract with a PRO.[70] Decisions of the PRO are ordinarily binding as to reimbursement.

Certificate of Need

States enacted CON and Section 1122 laws pursuant to the National Health Planning and Resources Development Act of 1974 (PL 93-641),[71] which required that acquisition of technology (and construction) by acute care hospitals be approved. Amendments in 1981 and regulations in 1984 increased dollar limits. In the 1980s a philosophical shift at the federal level toward increased competition greatly reduced support for regulatory efforts such as CONs. Diminished federal support reduced state interest. As noted in Chapter 2, by 1997, 39 states had some type of CON program.

CON and health planning legislation assumed that the availability of technology invites use and potential abuse and that its cost is paid by all health care system users. CT scanners became controversial because of wide availability and improper overuse. In the 1990s MRI and cesarean sections became a focus. These examples illustrate the problem inherent in the assumption underlying CON legislation, that quality health care can be provided without the extensive use of technology. This assumption conflicted with societal expectations that available, appropriate technology be used.

There were several criticisms of CON legislation because it

1. Gave no attention to low-cost technologies, whose high-volume use can significantly affect costs; electronic fetal monitoring is an example of a widely used, low-cost technology whose capital cost excluded it from CON review[72]
2. Did not consider the operating costs that are associated with installing and using technology, which typically exceed capital costs in a few years
3. Decreased competition; regulating acute care hospital services and types of technology eliminated a major incentive to compete
4. Focused on acute care hospitals, while increasingly portable technology allowed freestanding HSOs to become ubiquitous
5. Did not consider the role of professional staff in acquiring and using technology, as well as its importance in attracting and retaining physicians

Underusing high technology can be avoided by requiring that existing equipment meet certain use levels before new units are approved.[73] Many metropolitan areas in the United States have more MRIs than all of Great Britain or France.[74]

Private Sector Activities

Joint Commission

Various public and private organizations have established mandatory and voluntary standards, respectively, that determine how HSOs/HSs manage biomedical equipment. Among the most important is the Joint Commission, whose standards typically require three levels of effort: 1) corrective maintenance to repair broken equipment, 2) preventive maintenance to ensure reliability, and 3) management to ensure cost-effectiveness. Level 3 covers planning and procedure development, user education, and participation in technology assessment, equipment acquisition, risk management, and safety committees, as appropriate.[75] As noted in Chapter 2, some acute care hospitals have abandoned Joint Commission accreditation in favor of complying with the federal "Conditions of Participation" that are applied by state inspectors.

ISO 9000

The International Organization for Standardization has created a set of standards, known as ISO 9000, that organizations may voluntarily adopt to help them meet or exceed their customers' needs and expectations. Distilled to their essence, the principles of ISO 9000 are that high-quality service results only from a well-planned, well-documented, and well-executed quality management system. ISO 9000 is not quality control, but quality assurance, which embraces planning and implementing systems designed to ensure that quality requirements are met.[76] The history of ISO standards was discussed in Chapter 2; their application is addressed in Chapter 10. The increasing use of ISO 9000 standards in HSOs and greater congruence with Joint Commission standards will diminish the importance and singularity of Joint Commission accreditation.

Tort Law

Concomitant with greater regulation of medical technology has been the application of more demanding liability standards. Strict liability has been applied to HSOs, and they may be liable for defects in devices that are unknown to the manufacturer. HSOs may be responsible for going beyond the maintenance recommendations of the manufacturer, if necessary; they must alert the FDA about experience contrary to that reported by the manufacturer.[77] This area of the law will evolve, almost certainly toward more demanding and costly standards for HSOs.

TECHNOLOGY ASSESSMENT

Technology assessment evaluates the safety, efficacy, cost, and cost-effectiveness of technology and identifies ethical and legal implications, both in absolute terms and by comparison with competing technologies.[78] The Institute of Medicine of the National Academy of Sciences estimated that in 1983 only 2.9% of national health expenditures were spent on technology assessment.[79] Relative expenditures for technology assessment were declining, and it was estimated that, in 1988, the budgets of the most prominent technology assessment programs, added to related activities of industry and exclusive of clinical trials, totaled approximately $50 million.[80] In 1995 the United States had 53 health technology assessment programs and activities, the vast majority of which were in the private sector.[81] A 1995 survey found that from 1 day to 3 years were needed to perform a technology assessment. The cost ranged broadly from $1,000 to $10 million per assessment, the latter reported by the medical industry manufacturers.[82]

Figure 6.3 uses an input–process–outcome sequence to show technology assessment. These general methods include randomized clinical trials, evaluating diagnostic technologies, series of consecutive cases, case studies, registers and data bases, sample surveys, epidemiological methods, surveillance, quantitative synthesis methods (meta-analysis), group judgment methods,[83] cost-effectiveness and cost–benefit analyses, and mathematical modeling. Often forgotten but important are the social and ethical issues of technology assessment.[84]

Public Sector Activities

In 1995 public sector technology assessment efforts included seven federal agencies (including the congressional OTA) and three state agencies (in Minnesota, New York, and Oregon). From 1974 to late 1995 OTA helped Congress understand and plan for the policy implications of applying technology by studying the efficacy of specific medical procedures, uses of health education, and quality of medical care.[85] OTA was abolished in late 1995 primarily as a cost-cutting measure.[86]

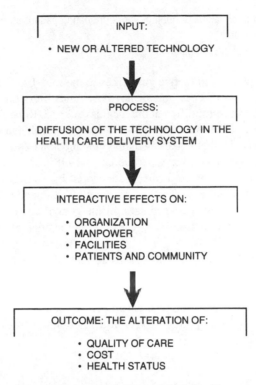

Figure 6.3. Technology assessment methods measure the impact on health care in an input-process-outcome sequence. (From *Health Policy*, 9 Glasser, Jay H., and Richard S. Chrzanowski, "Medical Technology Assessment: Adequate Questions, Appropriate Methods, Valuable Answers," 269, [1988], with permission from Elsevier Science.)

Concern about the proliferation of medical technology and its benefits, costs, and risks caused Congress to enact the Health Services Research, Health Statistics, and Health Care Technology Act of 1978 (PL 95-623).[87] The National Center for Health Care Technology was established in the Public Health Service of DHHS as a clearinghouse for information on medical technology, the safety and efficacy of new technologies, and their cost-effectiveness. NCHCT was to advise HCFA as to cost-effectiveness, appropriateness, and medical validity of various technologies that might be reimbursed by Medicare and Medicaid.[88] NCHCT was defunded in 1981, however, and its role was transferred to the Office of Health Technology Assessment (later called the Center for Health Care Technology) of the National Center for Health Services Research,[89] which was reauthorized in 1987 as the National Center for Health Services Research and Health Care Technology Assessment (NCHSRHCTA).[90]

In 1989 the Agency for Health Care Policy and Research (AHCPR) was established in the Public Health Service to replace NCHSRHCTA. AHCPR was reauthorized in 1999 as the Agency for Healthcare Research and Quality (AHRQ) and became the lead federal agency on quality research. AHRQ's strategic goals are to

- Support improvements in health outcomes
- Strengthen quality measurement and improvement
- Identify strategies that improve access, foster appropriate use, and reduce unnecessary expenditures
- Improve the quality of health care
- Promote patient safety and reduce medical errors

- Advance the use of information technology for coordinating patient care and conducting quality and outcomes research
- Establish an office of priority populations[91]

AHRQ's efforts to develop clinical practice guidelines in the mid-1990s failed because physicians saw them as a threat. As a consequence, the agency now funds literature reviews to develop practice recommendations that can be modified at the local level.[92] AHRQ collaborated with the American Medical Association and the American Association of Health Plans to establish a National Guideline Clearinghouse (NGC) that makes available guidance on treating specific conditions. The Internet website established by NGC was operational in 1998 and provides access to guidelines from public and private organizations.[93] Projects sponsored by AHRQ's Center for Organization and Delivery Studies are studying the effects of mergers on efficiency, insurance portability, and consumer prices, and the impact of managed care on integrated networks.[94] Increased funding in 1998 improved AHRQ's ability to disseminate research findings that affect the financing, organizing, and delivery of health care.[95]

AHRQ's role in technology assessment focuses on federal interests, but its recommendations have considerable impact because they are followed by other third-party payers. The lack of comprehensive federal activities led to the conclusion that "(T)he United States is thus out-of-step with much of the developed world where government-linked agencies have been established with responsibility for providing advice to policy-makers at the national or regional level."[96] This observation continues to be true.

Private Sector Activities

The majority of the 53 technology assessment programs and activities in existence in 1995 were private initiatives. They included 12 academic/not-for-profit organizations (often affiliated with major teaching hospitals); 11 health insurance companies (including managed care entities); 8 health professional societies; 5 hospitals or hospital chains; 4 consulting firms; and 3 medical industry manufacturers. In addition, there are an unknown number of private sector efforts that assess technology or aid potential users and purchasers in decision making.[97] Results produced in the private sector are likely to be available to general users only for a fee. Although these results are free of the pitfalls of publicly sponsored efforts, this fee requirement will slow dissemination of knowledge about technology.

Summary

It is clear that neither the public nor the private sector has set a high priority for assessing health care technology. This is difficult to understand, especially given that hundreds of billions of dollars are spent annually in a health services system that is driven to a large extent by technology. The modest efforts described above cannot develop the information that is needed to assist HSOs/HSs in making decisions about acquiring technology and using it efficiently and effectively. In addition, the information about a technology that is available may take some effort to find. The lack of a technology information clearinghouse and the absence of assistance in understanding and assessing technology must be decried. Developing a generic prototype for technology assessment by communities and HSOs/HSs should be a national priority.

HSO/HS TECHNOLOGY DECISION MAKING

Assessment of technology at the operating level is very different from that done by national public or private groups. Among the most important differences is that, when machine- and chemical-based technologies become generally available to HSOs/HSs, questions of safety and efficacy have been answered by FDA. At the operating level, the safety and efficacy of new surgical techniques or innovative uses of already-approved machine- and chemical-based technologies, however, have few controls, most of which are applied by the HSO/HS. It is somewhat less than reassuring to note that a 1992 survey by the American Hospital Association (AHA) found that only 20% of acute care hospitals have formal technology assessment committees.[98]

Criteria used by the HSO/HS to assess technology include appropriateness for the patient population; financial feasibility, cost-effectiveness, useful life, and operating costs; availability of trained technical personnel, expert physicians, and support services; availability of back-up technologies (e.g., open-heart surgery if a coronary angioplasty fails); and availability of reimbursement.[99] Nonexotic technologies and replacement equipment should be scrutinized in the same manner. Furthermore, it is important to evaluate new technology 6–12 months after introduction to determine its performance level and the effect on the quality of patient care.[100]

In general, physicians are regarded as technically qualified to make decisions about acquiring technology, and HSOs/HSs have given them great deference in making decisions about it. Furthermore, it is believed that a high level of technology is essential to attracting and retaining physicians.

Review and Planning

Cost-containment pressures, increased legal liability, and competition have caused HSOs/HSs to reassess how they make decisions to acquire and use technology and to ensure safe operation and maintenance. One approach establishes annual review and financial planning processes for medical technologies that are separate from other capital expenditure decision making. This is crucial for financial planning because many major technologies become obsolete sooner than the useful life that is estimated for depreciation purposes. As a result, depreciation and replacement allowances rarely meet the costs of newer technology. If the rate of technological innovation and diffusion increases, this problem will become more pressing. One example is the CT scanner, which sold for approximately $300,000 in 1973 with an estimated life of 5 years. Improved scanners costing more than $700,000 were available in 4 years.[101] In 1990 prices for CT scanners ranged from $195,000 to $1.6 million.[102] By 1998 the price was $2 million.[103] Similarly, the cost of fluoroscopes with image intensifiers rose from $40,000 in 1965 to $200,000 in 1977.[104] In 1990 fluoroscopic units for cardiac catheterization cost as much as $600,000.[105] By 1998 their cost ranged from $600,000 to $2.3 million.[106]

All HSOs/HSs should develop a strategic technology plan to guide technology acquisition, professional staff development, and market strategies. The plan should assess emerging medical technology in a near- and longer term time frame and identify niches where the HSO/HS should focus staff development and market strategies.[107]

Financing Technology

Acute care hospitals have had the most capital- and technology-intensive physical plants. Historically, acute care hospitals have had an annual capital equipment budget of several million dollars; technology had been financed out of internal funds and gifts because most capital equipment purchases were relatively small.[108]

In an era of diminished funding, successful executives must be creative to meet the costs of technology. Technology may be financed from current revenue, reserves, or charitable donations; by borrowing; or through joint ventures or venture capital. Other strategies have been suggested: 1) merge interests with physicians and other HSOs and develop complementary plans to minimize duplication of expensive technology; 2) obtain manufacturer support for development, training, and maintenance of technology; 3) become a demonstration site for manufacturers; and 4) become a service center for other providers.[109]

Evaluating and Acquiring Technology—TEAM

A methodology to improve decision making about technology was developed by AHA and the Center for Health Services Research at the University of California, Los Angeles, in the late 1970s. The Technology Evaluation and Acquisition Methods (TEAM) assessment organized a review process, determined participation, and developed criteria. It addressed four common problems that acute care hospitals faced in evaluating and acquiring technology: 1) treating requests for medical technology similar to requests for other capital expenditures, 2) absence of multidisciplinary staff participation in planning and evaluation of technology requests, 3) sporadic and unorganized physician participation in acquisition decisions, and 4) reliance on the same staff members who requested technology to assess its need and feasibility.[110]

In TEAM, the governing body and chief executive officer (CEO) established a policy to ensure that requests for technology were compatible with the HSO's/HS's mission statement and strategic plan. TEAM used an interdisciplinary standing committee to conduct mini-assessments and make recommendations for each proposed technology regarding need and use; impact on staffing, space, and supply; impact on patient care; vendor and product evaluation; and financial impact.[111] TEAM was not developed further by AHA.

Newer Alternatives to TEAM

Chief Technology Officer

Another approach to managing technology is appointment of a chief technology officer (CTO) to administer the HSO's/HS's technology base and translate the CEO's vision and planning into programs.[112] To accomplish this goal, Heller argued, the "line managers of technology" (chiefs of clinical pharmacy, clinical engineering, and information systems) should report directly to the CTO.[113] In practice, appointing a CTO, like TEAM, has had limited acceptance. The reason may be that both affect well-established responsibilities of senior managers, and technical support information flows up the organization only when solicited. Appointing a CTO has the additional difficulty of finding someone with appropriate qualifications.

Technical Support Committee

An alternative to TEAM or a CTO that has less impact on recognized modi operandi is to establish a standing technical support committee that provides technical recommendations to senior management and resolves day-to-day technical problems.[114] The committee's strength lies in making decisions about acquiring technology, which requires answering questions about the costs of acquisition, maintenance, and replacement. The committee is chaired by a senior manager, and membership includes managers of plant operations, clinical engineering, medical physics, information systems, and risk management and safety. Tasks are to

1. Coordinate and maintain strategic technology planning compatible with the strategic plan
2. Coordinate Joint Commission–mandated "environment of care" plans and programs
3. Provide technical recommendations for technology assessment and equipment acquisition
4. Ensure equipment effectiveness
5. Identify, secure funding for, and monitor problem reporting and correction

By design the committee has no clinical members. Its recommendations present technologically acceptable options; clinicians make their choices as users. Finally, such a committee goes far to maintain continuity of purpose and improve communication about biomedical equipment at the implementation level.

Multidisciplinary Technology Assessment Committee

The multidisciplinary technology assessment committee approach is the broadest of those discussed in this section. The multidisciplinary technology assessment committee draws on the organization's strengths and employs three phases.[115] Phase I is evolving the capital planning process to include the essential elements of technology assessment. The flow diagram in Figure 6.4 shows this evolution. The committee established in Phase I uses a multidisciplinary approach that emphasizes physician participation and applies assessment criteria to technology in the context of the organization's mission, vision, and strategic plan. Phase II includes a technology inventory and postacquisition evaluation of technology. In Phase III the committee develops a strategic technology plan, which includes identifying new technologies that meet service area and competitive needs. In all three phases the committee can function as decision maker or advisory body. Assuming that the technology meets the predetermined criteria, the committee performs an in-depth analysis and asks questions such as: Does it work? Is it safe? Is it an improvement over existing technology? Will it have organizationwide impact? What is its cost? Is it cost-effective? What are its potential effects on patient and community? Are there risk management and legal liability effects? Are there regulatory issues? Will it assist in a managed care environment? What are its potential social, ethical, and political effects? Is it needed urgently?[116]

Summary

Despite a paucity of assistance, HSOs/HSs must be able to assess technology. In addition to the literature, private services and the various public and private groups mentioned above are sources of information about technology. Hospital systems have more resources to develop methods for technology assessment. The criteria used by one system are like those that are recommended for freestanding HSOs: the technology's value to patients, system, and third-party payers; overall cost-effectiveness; fit with present technologies; and influence on finances in the next decade.[117]

MANAGING BIOMEDICAL EQUIPMENT IN HSOs/HSs

The technology discussed in this section is commonly called biomedical equipment. It is used to diagnose, treat, monitor, and support a patient, as shown in Table 6.3. Although some equipment is expensive (e.g., radiology scanners), most biomedical equipment is small and low cost. In total, however, this equipment is a major resource and has significant potential to consume resources. For instance, large acute care hospitals carry an inventory of between 5,000 and 15,000 pieces of equipment. Clearly, the complexity, abundance, and decentralization of this equipment places a substantial burden on management and on the training and management of those who operate and maintain it. In 1996 total expenditures for service and support of high-technology equipment in HSOs were estimated at more than $10 billion, with projections for continued increase.[118]

The staggering growth in the amount and complexity of biomedical equipment, coupled with greater legal liability for its defects and malfunction, necessitate considering biomedical equipment as one element in a complicated system that includes staff, internal environment, technology, organization, and external relations.[119] The matrix in Table 6.3 shows that all elements may potentially interact. For instance, certain equipment supports a surgical process, and vice versa. Equipment use depends on availability of trained staff, standard operating procedures, and staff credentialing and acceptance of new technology. Use is also a function of external factors such as availability and receptiveness of patients, certification of staff by professional societies, and regulations governing the safety and efficacy of the technology.

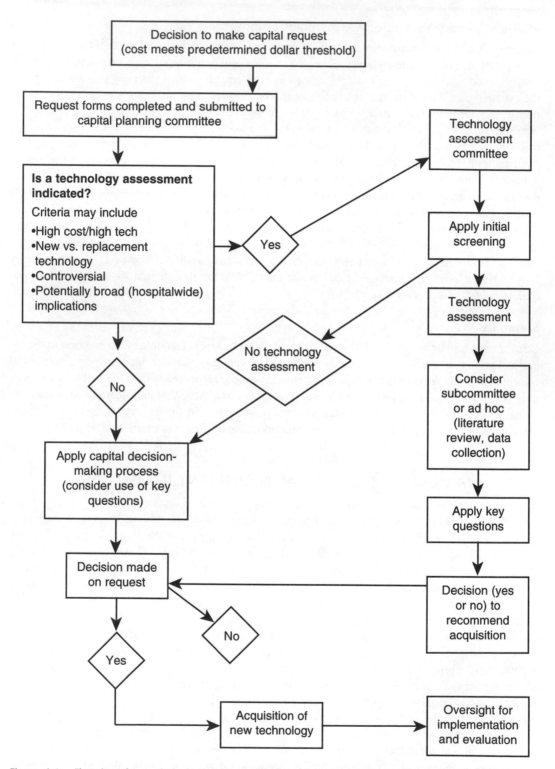

Figure 6.4.   Flowchart for capital planning and technology assessment. (From Uphoff, Mary Ellen, Thomas Ratko, and Karl Matuszweski. "Making Technology Assessment Count." *Health Measures* 2 [March 1997]: 22; reprinted by permission.)

TABLE 6.3. BIOMEDICAL EQUIPMENT CATEGORIES WITH EXAMPLES

Diagnostic	Therapeutic	Monitoring	Support
Body potentials	Resuscitation	Patient	Communication
Blood flow	Prosthetic and orthotic	Environment	Management
Chemical composition	Surgical support		Maintenance and testing
Radiant energy	Special treatment		Teaching
	Radiant energy		Records and statistics

Systems Engineering

A consideration in selecting biomedical equipment has been whether the proposed equipment can be integrated with existing equipment, people, processes, and environment to provide a safe and effective system under both normal and contingency conditions. Figure 6.5 suggests these relationships. This integration requires technical expertise, especially if it involves multiple units of programmable equipment from several manufacturers or when facility modifications are necessary. This "systems engineering" may be completed by HSO staff with the appropriate skills, by consultants, or by the manufacturers of the equipment.

Managing computerized biomedical equipment is much more complex because it is likely to be part of a HSO's information system. As a result, more elements of the organization are affected; among the most important elements are the governing body, managers, and clinicians. Other areas that may be affected are fiscal affairs, plant maintenance and operations, clinical engineering, risk management and safety, quality assessment and improvement, materials management, and information systems.

Organization

External Standards

HSOs/HSs that are accredited by the Joint Commission must establish and maintain a safe and effective medical equipment management plan.[120] Standards from the *Comprehensive Accreditation Man-*

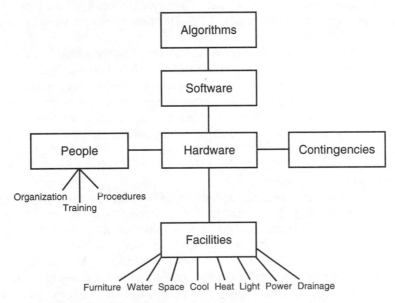

Figure 6.5. Systems engineering components.

ual for Hospitals are paradigmatic of those affecting other types of HSOs. The plan, which should be evaluated annually, must focus on safety in the environment of care and include processes for

1. Selecting and acquiring equipment
2. Establishing the criteria for identifying, evaluating, and inventorying equipment before use
3. Assessing and minimizing the clinical and physical risks that are associated with equipment through inspection, testing, and maintenance
4. Monitoring and acting on equipment hazard notices and recalls
5. Monitoring and reporting serious incidents involving equipment
6. Reporting and investigating equipment management program problems, failures, and user errors

The plan also should establish

7. An equipment orientation and education program
8. Performance improvement standards that include, for instance, the level of staff participation in equipment management
9. Emergency procedures in the event of equipment failure
10. How an evaluation of the medical equipment management plan's objectives, scope, performance, and effectiveness will occur

Joint Commission surveys determine whether the equipment management processes are appropriate and followed. Staff must receive orientation and education about the equipment's capabilities, limitations, special applications, and basic operation and maintenance, as well as emergency procedures and reporting problems. Furthermore, surveyors interview staff to assess their understanding of the equipment that they use and what is required of them.

Service

HSOs/HSs have four basic options for maintaining and servicing biomedical equipment: 1) a facility-based biomedical engineering and management information systems (MIS) support and service department; 2) a combination of facility-based service and subcontracted service from equipment manufacturers or independent service companies; 3) expanding facility-based biomedical and MIS service departments to provide service to other HSOs/HSs to achieve economies of scale; and 4) outsourcing of maintenance, repair, and technical support.[121]

Many HSOs/HSs and virtually all large acute care hospitals have biomedical or clinical engineering departments with biomedical equipment technicians to perform equipment maintenance and management functions within staffing limitations. Historically, biomedical engineering included equipment research and development, maintenance, and management support. As equipment proliferated and manufacturers became more active in research and development, however, biomedical engineering became the umbrella term for three subspecialties—bioengineering for research, medical engineering for development, and clinical engineering for integrating and servicing equipment. Nevertheless, many HSOs/HSs have kept the umbrella title, biomedical engineering, for their clinical engineering departments.

In larger HSOs/HSs with substantial equipment inventories, clinical engineers may be added to provide systems engineering and a higher level of equipment management. The scope of a clinical engineering department's functions is depicted in Table 6.4. Responsibility for some biomedical equipment may be vested in other departments, however. For instance, central supply may inspect and repair under contract some devices that are used throughout the HSO—intravenous pumps and suction equipment are in this category. Similarly, clinical departments such as anesthesiology, respiratory therapy, or radiology may prefer to manage their own equipment because of its specialized nature.

TABLE 6.4. CLINICAL ENGINEERING FUNCTIONS

1. Development and integration of new systems
   Planning
      System concept and design
      Facility, equipment, and interface diagrams
      Manufacturing and test specifications
      Cost estimates
      Operational and maintenance procedures
   Purchasing
      Sales literature files
      Sales quotations
      Buying decisions
   New installation
      Contractor liaison
      On-site installation and checkout support
   Training
      Scheduled nurse/technician training courses
      Educational seminars
   Evaluation
      specimen performance
      statistics
      cost-effectiveness
	2. Operation, maintenance, and calibration
	   Alignment and calibration
	   Pre-operation preparation and checkout
	   Routine performance/safety checks
	   Equipment operation
	   Failure repairs
	   Incoming quality control inspection and test
	   Spare parts inventories
	   Schematic, instruction book, and reference library
	   Operational improvements
	3. Medical research and development support
	   Proposal development
	   New equipment design and construction
	   Model shop operation
	   Evaluation testing

From Shaffer, Michael J., Joseph J. Carr, and Marian Gordon. "Clinical Engineering—an Enigma in Health Care Facilities." *Hospital & Health Services Administration* 24 (Summer 1979): 81; reprinted by permission. © 1979, Foundation of the American College of Healthcare Executives.

Organizationally, clinical engineering normally reports to an assistant administrator or to the director of plant operations or materials management. This chain can create a communication gap between the department and equipment users. Rarely, however, does clinical engineering report to upper management or the professional staff organization.

Figure 6.6 shows an organizational model in which the clinical departments perform setup and checkout and use their own biomedical equipment, and the administrative departments undertake management, inspections, and repairs. A critical care technician group is shown. Its purpose is to store, provide, and check out biomedical equipment that is used by several clinical departments in order to conserve equipment, ensure procedural consistency, and bridge the gap between clinical departments and clinical engineering. Arterial pressure and cardiac output monitors and aortic balloon pumps used in special care units are examples of equipment for which critical care technicians are responsible.

Fiscal constraints and increasing cost pressures from managed care have forced many HSOs to downsize their clinical engineering departments or to use external sources such as independent or manufacturer service organizations. One survey of acute care hospital CEOs found that 67% are outsourcing clinical engineering services and that 88% are satisfied with the results.[122] In addition, service providers are moving from basic reactive repair and maintenance to value-added services such as consultation and customized, project-oriented services. This change has given rise to multivendor servicing (MVS), which means that one company takes responsibility for servicing the equipment from other manufacturers as well as consolidating contracts, reducing costs, and providing one source of accountability.[123] In the mid-1990s, for example, 60% of General Electric's (GE) profits came from MVS. GE selects and services its biomedical equipment and that of other manufacturers for a major hospital system, an arrangement that makes it both advisor and vendor.[124]

In addition, service workloads have been reduced by improved equipment reliability, troubleshooting by substituting circuit boards, and eliminating preventive maintenance that has little effect on failure rates.[125] In many cases it may be impossible to materially change mean time between failures. Such equipment is replaced before failure.[126] These factors, in conjunction with manufac-

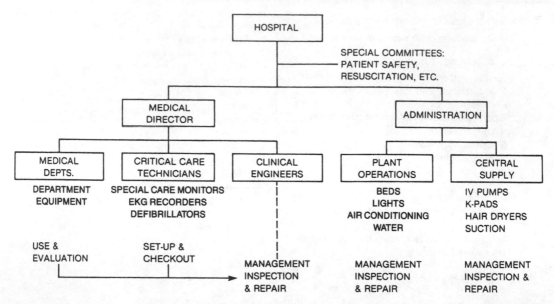

Figure 6.6. Organization of biomedical equipment. (From Shaffer, Michael J. "Managing Hospital Biomedical Equipment." In *Hospital Organization and Management,* 4th ed., edited by Kurt Darr and Jonathon S. Rakich, 283. Baltimore: AUPHA/National Health Publishing, 1989; reprinted by permission.)

turer offerings such as corrective maintenance contracts that range from complete to partial after-sales support, built-in diagnostics, and manufacturer-provided remote online failure diagnosis, enable HSOs/HSs to employ less-skilled technician and engineer staff. As a consequence, more experienced technician and engineer staff believe that their future opportunities lie in consulting, manufacturing, and independent service organizations.[127] This may make them a vanishing resource in HSOs. Indeed, there has been a change from data dominance, which provides information for reasoning and calculation, to knowledge dominance that is based on practical experience and learning. These clinical information systems may increase the need for systems engineering in the HSO/HS. Shaffer argues that the survival of clinical engineering in hospitals will depend primarily on how well it supports clinical information systems and only secondarily on its ability to support the equipment–management interface for administration.[128]

ELECTRONIC HEALTH INFORMATION SYSTEMS

Most computer applications in health services are and have been business related, such as finance and administration. Clinical applications became and will become more common with the growth of computing power and storage capability. As with other technical areas, executives need not be expert in information technology but will need help from someone who is. Information technology assists in four areas[129]:

1. Process management—redesigning processes to make them seamless and more efficient
2. Care management—expert systems and other ways to assist clinicians, some of which are described below
3. Demand management—especially useful in integrated systems to attract physicians, employers, health plans, and enrollees, as well as to direct patients to the least-intensive setting able to meet their needs
4. Health management—essential to store and retrieve risk assessment information, genetic profiles, family health histories, and similar data that predict and prevent disease, a use that is especially important in a capitated payment system

Information technology is addressed in detail in Chapter 10. Of the total information technology applications in HSOs/HSs, the subset that is used for clinical purposes is the focus of this section.

Electronic applications in health (clinical) information have developed at the national, regional (community), and enterprise levels. This discussion addresses the latter two levels, which have the most significant impact on HSOs/HSs. The regional-level electronic applications are known generally as community health information networks (CHINs), although there have been variants. Enterprise information networks, or corporate intranets, emphasize the internal applications of medical records but also link delivery sites that are part of a system.

Health information networks date from the 1960s, when the National Library of Medicine initiated an online bibliography, academic medical centers experimented with telemedicine, and the first internal patient information networks were established. Later developments included computerized links among pharmaceutical manufacturers, wholesalers, retail stores, and payers; hospitals and suppliers; and hospitals and fiscal intermediaries who processed Medicare claims.[130] In 1998 it was estimated that there were 10,000 medical-based websites; in addition, the Internet is used widely to connect service providers for clinical information interchange.[131]

Regional Level CHINs

A CHIN is broadly defined as an information technology–based network that links all health care stakeholders in a community to maximize the health of residents.[132] Stakeholders include providers, payers, schools, community agencies, patients, and residents. This contrasts with the discussion later in this chapter of enterprise information networks or corporate intranets, whose focus is on an electronic medical record (EMR) that links associated providers such as clinics, physician offices, and hospitals. An EMR is a necessary but not sufficient part of a CHIN.

A largely failed variant of CHINs was the community health management information system (CHMIS), whose purpose was not only to create a data network (the purpose of CHINs) but also to establish and make available to the public a data repository that routinely measured the cost and quality of care that was provided by competing providers in a community. In the early 1990s a private foundation was the chief financial sponsor of seven CHMIS initiatives, five of them statewide.[133] The CHMIS's difficulties were tied to the failure of health care reform, decline in fee-for-service practice, development of data clearinghouses, rise of managed care, development of Internet technology, and limited ability to charge transaction fees.[134] "The idea of bringing together all of the stakeholders in a community to build one great health network was bold. But it required so much cooperation in such a large undertaking that it seemed to many people in health care to be less practical than more narrowly conceived network-building efforts."[135]

Goals and Activities of CHINs

As noted earlier, CHINs seek to maximize health for all people in the community, as the terms are broadly defined. A CHIN serves its community best when it goes beyond financing of health services, and information is used for clinical, educational, research, and management purposes.[136] These goals are like those of a CHMIS, except that a CHIN does not necessarily have a commitment to make community-level health data public.[137] Figure 6.7 depicts the types of information links that are typical of a CHIN.

The Chemung Valley Health Network in Elmira, New York, is a community-based, Internet-supported health network that provides a central hub for health information.[138] Its goal is to show that patients connected to the Internet are more knowledgeable about and participate in their own care, and that physicians connected to the Internet are more knowledgeable and provide more coordinated and efficient care.

The Chemung Valley CHIN links 10 physicians offices and two area hospitals with patient information and provides a method to transfer information to other providers or institutions to facili-

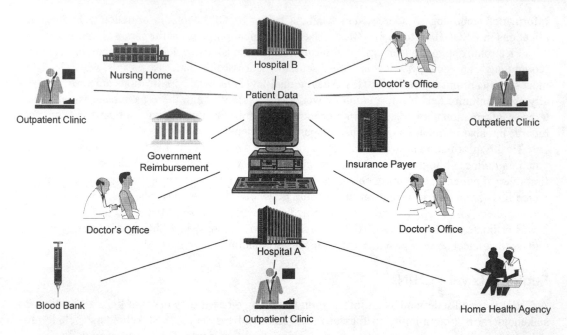

Figure 6.7.   Example of health care data links. (From Sheldon I. Dorenfest & Associates, Ltd.; reprinted by permission.)

tate coordination of services. The CHIN also maintains an Internet website where residents can obtain information about health, social, employment, and economic services, programs, and opportunities in the community. The website allows health providers to supply information, resources, and referrals to the public. In addition, the Internet provides nationally available health assessment tests and general health information.[139]

Problems of Implementing CHINs

Financial, political, legal, and technical issues have slowed the development of CHINs. Health information networks have long faced formidable barriers because they are complex and costly, are believed to threaten privacy, and have been resisted by professional groups and institutions. The health sector has been slow to adopt common data dictionaries and standards for electronic data exchange; physicians, hospitals, and insurers have been slow even to use e-mail and other network services that do not require structured data.[140] Basic to CHINs is sharing information, which is largely incompatible with a competitive environment. Some applications of CHINs that might serve enterprise information networks are providing electronic eligibility determination, precertification, and referral services. CHINs cannot function absent an EMR that is generally available at any point of service; this continues to be a significant obstacle.[141]

Future of CHINs

The future of CHINs will be a function of how closely their organizational, political, and practical incentives can be aligned with those of stakeholders.[142] The negative view is that the term *CHIN* has gone out of fashion in much of the industry, especially as it involves communitywide participation, protracted planning, and closed computer systems. The commonplace networks are limited to business partners, proprietary, quick to develop, narrowly focused, and based on open systems. This analysis concludes that the more a health information network has required community participation and information sharing, the less rapidly it has developed. Thus enterprise networks have developed furthest and CHMIS least.[143]

The positive view is that boundaries of organizations are ambiguous and constantly changing, and even those that are affiliated with different plans need to communicate. In addition, the market is likely to favor enterprise information networks that offer wider connections (including services on the Internet), and, unless there is monopolistic control, the broader networks will prevail.[144]

Enterprise Level—EMRs

Despite several decades of effort and billions of dollars spent by hospitals and other HSOs/HSs, the EMR remains an elusive goal for most providers.[145] The promise is enormous. For example, the medical record system at Wishard Memorial Hospital and the University of Indiana Medical Center has electronic records for 1.4 million patients, including 6 million prescription records, hundreds of thousands of narrative documents, 200,000 electrocardiograph tracings, millions of physician orders entered annually, and 100 million coded patient observations and laboratory results. This EMR system includes all diagnoses, orders, encounters, and dictated notes, as well as various pieces of clinical information from selected clinical sites. Even this extensive effort does not eliminate some paper records—physicians continue to make handwritten notes about hospital and clinic visits, most of which are not included in the EMR.[146]

Despite significant applications, a great deal of work remains to be done. The ultimate development of a computer-based patient record system that includes decision support functions as well as record-keeping functions is unrealized.[147]

Advantages of EMRs

There are numerous advantages to maintaining medical records in an electronic format. EMRs facilitate moving information contained in, or to be put into, the medical record. Internally, the need to move paper records around the organization is eliminated. Externally, the delivery of services at multiple sites is facilitated because all providers have access to the same medical information, something that is not possible with a paper record. A second advantage of EMRs is reduced offline storage and retrieval costs. Providers currently devote significant space and cost to storing paper records. Third, EMRs improve the quality and coherence of the care process. For example, the logistics problems of paper records—lost, unavailable when needed, difficulty finding information in them, illegibility—are largely solved.[148] A fourth advantage is that clinical guidelines and care pathways can be automated to positively affect physician behavior and care processes. One study found that computer-assisted decision support program reminders using local clinician-derived practice guidelines improved antibiotic use, reduced associated costs, and stabilized the emergence of antibiotic-resistant pathogens.[149] Fifth, EMRs support research and quality improvement. Both are data driven, and ready access to information in the medical record greatly facilitates them. Integrated EMR systems could be used to reduce variation in clinical processes and outcomes, thus lowering costs.[150] A sixth benefit of EMRs is that readily available data ease reporting of all types.

Problems of Establishing EMRs

A major problem facing EMRs is that literally dozens of electronic data sources are found in the typical HSO/HS; the most significant problem is in acute care hospitals. The number of such sources grew considerably with the ready availability of personal computers and increasingly powerful, inexpensive memory chips. Internal clinical information systems such as those in laboratories, pharmacies, emergency departments, and radiology typically are different and cannot "talk" to one another, nor can they interface with administrative and support areas such as admission and discharge, patient billing, scheduling, risk management, and medical transcription. External systems such as those in physicians' offices, commercial pharmacies, freestanding affiliated outpatient units and surgicenters, home health agencies, and CHINs store information that would facilitate the effective and efficient delivery of services were it available when needed. Both internal and external systems are rife with duplicate information, all of which is obtained and stored at significant cost to the HSO/HS and inconvenience and frustration to the consumer.

Obtaining an interface among these various clinical systems, especially those that are internal to the HSO/HS, is key to realizing many of the advantages of an EMR. The interface problems are solvable with interface standards available. "Standards provide the bridges to the many islands of electronic patient data so that the data can be inexpensively combined into an electronic medical record."[151] A remaining problem is capturing physician information inexpensively in a coded or structured form so that it is compatible with electronic storage. It is unlikely that this problem will be solved soon, and it will be necessary to continue using a mix of coded and free-text information.[152]

Confidentiality, privacy, and consent raise significant issues regarding EMRs. Confidentiality concerns may cause HSOs/HSs to control patient information so tightly that the advantages of EMRs are lost. For example, administration may determine that only the ordering physician can gain access to test results. This will cause problems when nurses or on-call colleagues need test results, or in an emergency.[153] "Family charts" result from compiling the medical records of family members. Although this makes family practice more efficacious, it raises issues of privacy and consent.[154]

For most patients, electronically linking internal medical record information is unlikely to raise confidentiality concerns. Paper records are subject to the same issues of misuse as are electronic records. In fact, paper records are potentially more subject to inappropriate use than are EMRs, for which access codes and audit trails can be established. For some patients, however, the mysteries of electronic formats may create a greater psychological issue than do paper records.

The efficiencies that are achieved by linking external data sources benefit providers and insurers, but ultimately accrue to the advantage of consumers. Consumers are much more likely to be concerned, however, about confidentiality and privacy issues as health information and data sets from external sources are linked. Beyond the reality is the psychological discomfort of knowing that comprehensive data banks contain personal, even embarrassing, information and that the potential exists for misuse. Confidentiality and privacy concerns, as well as the legal issues of consent and wrongful release of information, may cause such restrictions on the use of information in EMRs that many of their advantages will be lost.[155] In addition to dedicated electronic or hard-wired links, communication among providers can occur over the Internet, which has adequate available or announced security tools to alleviate confidentiality concerns.[156]

The efficiencies to be realized with EMRs are unlikely to come from reductions in support staff. The results of implementing EMRs in family practice residency programs did not decrease the need for support staff.[157] This finding is consistent with results from other clinical and nonclinical applications of computers.

Gauging patient reaction to increased computer use by physicians must be judged within the context that computers are ubiquitous. Concerns that patients may have less confidence in physicians who use computers as part of an expert system or to search for reference information regarding diagnosis and treatment during a consultation probably are unfounded.[158] Similarly, patients do not seem to believe that physicians who use computers are paying inadequate attention to them; apparently, patients support physicians' use of computers.[159] In fact, it is likely that patients increasingly will interpret failure to use computers in consultations and treatment as practicing something less than state-of-the-art medicine.

Summary

Paper medical records continue to be the norm. Progress toward EMRs will continue, but only slowly and at great cost. The ultimate EMR promises to retrieve whatever patient data are needed to perform tasks such as outcomes analysis, utilization review, profiling, and costing, abilities that are of special interest to CEOs at hospitals and managed care organizations.[160] Integrating the EMR with information retrieval systems to support diagnosis and treatment is a highly desirable, perhaps an essential, extension of medical records in an electronic format.

TELEMEDICINE

The National Library of Medicine divides telemedicine into three areas: aids to decision making, remote sensing (transmitting data and educational materials among sites), and collaborative arrangements for remote, real-time management of patients.[161] It is estimated that 25% of U.S. health services providers use telemedicine.[162] Clinical applications include radiology, dermatology, cardiology, psychiatry, emergency medicine, pathology, obstetrics and gynecology, and orthopedics. Table 6.5 shows various types of telemedicine interactions.

The prototype of telemedicine was the telephone consultation between physicians; more recently, facsimile machines are being used for electrocardiograms and medical records. Newer technologies include interactive television. For example, physicians use digital cameras in their offices to obtain images of a patient's retinas and transmit them to an image-reading center for the diagnosis of retinal disorders.[163] In addition to clinical consultation, telemedicine has significant uses for administrative support and education. Many applications do not, however, require two-way, full-motion video. Still images are used for radiology and pathology, in which "store and forward" technologies transmit static images or video clips to remote storage devices for later retrieval, review, and consultation.[164] Telemedicine can be used when physical barriers prevent ready transfer of medical management information between patients and providers[165]; monitoring patients at home is an example.

Managed care plans were early users of telemedicine, but, as the technology becomes ubiquitous, its advantages as a means of marketplace differentiation will diminish. Military hospitals are at the forefront of using telemedicine to serve personnel in remote locations where it is impossible to provide advanced technology, physician specialists, and other highly trained clinical staff.[166] Telemedicine offers opportunities for U.S. providers to consult and assist in providing health care to patients worldwide.

Five issues are unresolved in telemedicine[167]:

1. Clinical expectations and medical effectiveness (Much of the information about the clinical effectiveness of telemedicine is anecdotal.)
2. Matching technology to medical needs (Inconvenience of interactive technology is a major obstacle to widespread use. Rural practitioners may lack support technologies.)
3. Economics of telemedicine (Telemedicine equipment costs hundreds of thousands of dollars, plus thousands in maintenance. Health plans may not pay for telemedicine, and HCFA is reluctant to increase consultations.[168])
4. Legal and social issues (Remote licensure and liability must be addressed, as must the social and political issues relating to access to telemedicine. [Chapter 14 discusses the legal aspects of telemedicine.])
5. Organizational factors (Organizations must address issues surrounding telemedicine prospectively and specifically.)

Telemedicine continues to be an essential element in health services delivery in the 21st century, and significant growth is certain. Managers must enable their HSOs/HSs to participate in it fully.

TABLE 6.5. THE SPECTRUM OF CLINICAL TELEMEDICINE INTERACTIONS[a]

Purpose	Mode of interaction	Types of information transferred	Minimum bandwidth requirements[b]	Typical applications
Diagnostic or therapeutic consultation	Real-time, one-way or two-way interactive motion video	Voice, sound, motion video images, text, and documents	Moderate to high	Telepsychiatry and mental health applications, remote surgery, interactive examinations
	Still images or video clips with real-time telephone voice interaction	Voice, sound, still video images or short video clips, text	Low to moderate	Multiple medical applications, including dermatology, cardiology, otolaryngology, orthopedics
	Still images or video clips with text information; "store-and-forward," with data acquired and transmitted for review at a later date	Sound, still video images or short video clips, text	Low	Multiple medical applications, including dermatology, cardiology, otolaryngology, orthopedics
Medical education	One-way or two-way real-time or delayed video	Voice, sound, motion video images, text, and documents	Moderate to high	Distance education and training
Case management or documentation	Transfer of electronic text, image, or other data	Text, images, documents, and related data	Low to high	Community health information networks, medical record management

From Perednia, Douglas A., and Ace Allen. "Telemedicine Technology and Clinical Applications." *Journal of the American Medical Association* 273 (February 8, 1995): 484; reprinted by permission.

[a] Omits telemedicine consultations performed using the telephone alone.

[b] Bandwidth is the transmission capacity of a telecommunication link. Conventional telephone lines have relatively little carrying capacity (low bandwidth). High-capacity lines are required to transmit large amounts of information (e.g., images) rapidly.

FUTURE DEVELOPMENTS

Biomedical Equipment

Some see cost containment as slowing biomedical equipment manufacture and use. Conversely, some predict that competition among health care networks will encourage the purchase of advanced equipment and the availability of new procedures. Decentralized facilities are likely to contain state-of-the-art biomedical equipment, but with little standby equipment and few spare parts. This necessitates increased reliability and speed of repair to minimize downtime.

These developments suggest that attitudes will change

1. From performing maintenance because it is required to performing maintenance because it saves money
2. From purchasing based on price to purchasing based on life cycle cost
3. From biomedical service as a part of maintenance to managing technology as part of managing health care
4. From a focus on technology to a focus on information[169]

As technology continues to advance, HSO/HS managers must ensure that equipment is appropriate, complies with regulations, performs correctly, and is used properly. A major challenge will be achieving an interface between and among all of the elements. Only if various types of technology can "talk" to one another will maximum benefit be realized. In addition, organizations will expect to get more from their equipment; this means that portability and a good fit with the environment will be important.[170]

Clinical Support and Information Systems

Computer and communication technologies have supported the development of artificial intelligence; microprocessor and computer- and robot-assisted diagnosis and treatment; general applications of expert systems to integrate computers and machines; the Internet and intranets; and local area, wide area, and community health information networks, all of which give health care providers direct access to knowledge and information. In addition to the National Guideline Clearinghouse noted earlier, current operational and experimental uses of the Internet include online patient registration, interactive question-and-answer services for disease management, dissemination of HMO guidelines to member physicians, and e-mail. In 1997 it was reported that 176 sites on the Internet contained information on subjects such as consumer health information, support groups, physician specialties, disease tracking and reporting, physician recruitment, and long-term care facilities.[171] One manufacturer reported that its medical products group receives 20,000 visits (hits) to its website weekly for product information and service advice.[172]

Increasingly, physicians will use computerized scoring systems to determine the statistical effectiveness of treatments for critical care patients. One method uses a point system for age, seven morbid conditions that affect short-term mortality, and 16 physiologic variables that reflect values for vital signs, laboratory tests, and neurologic status.[173] Another expert system determines the optimum location of a health care facility using demographic surveys and factors such as anticipated financial, operational, and clinical performance; competing institutions; access roads; and ambulance support.[174] Most important, standards have been developed to transfer medical images and patient information, which brings medicine closer to the ultimate goal of a universal paperless electronic patient record.[175]

The Internet offers tremendous potential to centralize medical information in a website that is managed by the patient, with controlled access, including read-only protection. Providers could view and download information in the record as needed; entries would be made following treatment. Giving all providers access to the same database could greatly improve efficiency and efficaciousness.

Medical Technology

Developments in tissue and genetic engineering, gene therapy, artificial organs and tissues, implantable computer chips and "smart" wafers, nanotechnology (microscopic machines and molecular-level tools), and minimally invasive and bloodless surgery have only begun to affect medicine in what is likely to become a cascade of change. Advances in pharmaceutical research, including use of robo-chemistry—the science of applying computerization on a large scale to drug molecule research—will speed the basic research and development of medications.[176] Allopathic (traditional Western medicine) practice will be supplemented by holistic and nontraditional medicine, including chiropractic, homeopathy, naturopathy, and osteopathy; aroma-, music-, and massage therapies; biofeedback and visualization techniques; therapeutic touch; and Eastern medical theories, prominent among which are acupuncture, Chinese herbal remedies, and ayurvedic medicine. In sum, these developments promise to revolutionize medicine, including where and how services are delivered.

SUMMARY

This chapter examines the effect of technology on health care, especially HSOs/HSs and delivery systems. The technological imperative is a prominent reality at the macro and micro levels. A variety of initiatives, usually federally stimulated, have sought to control costs and guide organizations in effective and efficient use of high-cost technology. Often forgotten, however, is the aggregate financial effect of wholesale use of individually inexpensive technology. Although it seems unlikely, capitation may succeed in controlling acquisition and use of technology even as prospective payment failed to do so. Health services providers must be able to manage the technology necessary to retain physicians and offer high-quality care.

Effective managers are boundary scanners. Medical technology is a critical aspect of this activity. Various public and private organizations can assist managers in learning about new developments and providing information about existing technology. There is no substitute, however, for managers possessing basic knowledge about technology of all types.

The general framework of this chapter should be considered in combination with Chapters 13 and 14. Problem solving by health services managers requires understanding and analyzing legal, ethical, and technological components. These seemingly disparate elements may be present in Byzantine combinations—their dynamics and interactions add great complexity to the manager's job. Basic to this dynamic is that the law may be inadequately developed to deal with new technology; furthermore, in many instances ethics and the law disagree on the "best" course of action. This tension provides contradictory guidance for decision makers. Nonetheless, the pragmatic reality is that decisions must be made and actions taken.

DISCUSSION QUESTIONS

1. Describe the impact of medical technology on HSOs/HSs and the costs of health services. Link the theories of distribution of scarce lifesaving technology that are described in Chapter 13 and the problems that HSOs/HSs experience in managing medical technology.
2. Identify the effects of various payment mechanisms on the development of new medical technology. What are the likely effects on use? What are the implications for patient care?
3. The increasing portability of technology makes it available outside traditional HSOs, which poses special problems for acute care hospitals. Identify the advantages and disadvantages from the standpoint of the HSO and the patient.

4. Trends suggest significant consumer interest in alternatives to traditional medicine. These include the low- or no-technology treatment found in holistic medicine, wellness care, and disease prevention. Suggest the implications for society and traditional HSOs.

5. The control of development and generalization of medical technology is fragmented. Identify control points and suggest ways to improve them. Distinguish the private and public sectors.

6. Technology is present in HSOs/HSs because physicians ask for it and patients expect it. Describe changes in the external environment that affect availability and application of technology. Describe management's role in assessing technology.

7. The electronic medical record promises to revolutionize the delivery of health services. Identify the advantages and disadvantages for the patient and for providers.

8. The internal management of biomedical equipment poses several problems for managers. How do managers involve clinical staff to solve these problems? Identify types of equipment that managers can purchase without involving clinical staff.

9. Competition is a major force in health services, and marketing may be crucial to HSO/HS success. What are the relationships between marketing and acquisition and application of medical technology? Give examples from your experience or the literature.

10. Little attention usually is paid to nonclinical technology such as financial data systems, but such technology can dramatically affect HSO/HS costs and effectiveness. Identify the types of nonclinical equipment and their effects on managing HSOs/HSs. What links are there between clinical and nonclinical technologies?

CASE STUDY 1: THE FEASIBILITY OF BEAM

Brain electrical activity mapping (BEAM) is a technology for imaging the brain. It significantly improves the physician's ability to localize an abnormality. In response to increased demands for this procedure from staff radiologists and local neurologists and reports in the literature of the usefulness of BEAM testing, Metropolitan Hospital has decided to investigate the possibility of acquiring access to BEAM testing. Two options are lease or purchase. A third option is to ask nearby County Hospital to share its recently acquired BEAM machine.

A major unknown is uncertainty about the future of reimbursement. It is likely that Medicare DRG payments will be reduced. In addition, other third-party payers are requiring more stringent review of new technologies.

Because of the reimbursement issues and major expenditures involved, the governing body chair asked the CEO to form a committee and evaluate each option, including forgoing access to BEAM testing. The assessment will permit a final decision between BEAM and a proposed addition to the intensive care unit, a project that is supported strongly by the surgical staff and that has already been delayed twice.

The governing body would prefer to delay this decision until reimbursement is better understood, but several attending physicians think that BEAM testing is critical to their practices and have stated that, although they prefer the nursing staff at Metropolitan, they will be forced to admit certain patients to County to use BEAM. A rumor has just surfaced that several prominent physicians want to develop a consortium to purchase and operate BEAM and other diagnostic equipment in a professional office complex that is under construction.

QUESTIONS

1. Propose the membership of a committee that will be assigned to assess the need for BEAM testing and the option to be selected.

2. What types of information should be presented to the governing body in the committee's final report?

3. What political and economic complications are present in the decision-making process?
4. How should these complications be addressed? Be specific in identifying the sequence of steps.

CASE STUDY 2: "WHO DOES WHAT?"

When she purchased, installed, and staffed the single-photon emission computerized tomography (SPECT) camera at a cost of more than $500,000, Andrea Berson thought it was one of the most difficult things she had done as chief operating officer (COO) at Sinai Hospital. Looking back, however, it could pale by comparison with the problem looming on the horizon. The SPECT camera's three-dimensional visualization of the heart makes it an exquisite diagnostic tool. Cardiologists commonly perform biplanar (two-dimensional) nuclear cardiology studies in their offices, but SPECT's high cost virtually precludes its use in offices.

Sinai has an exclusive contract with a radiology group to perform all inpatient radiology services. Four members of the group are board certified in nuclear medicine and credentialed for SPECT. Several cardiologists who refer patients to Sinai have expressed grave concerns about the quality of readings of SPECT scans done by two of these four radiologists. When SPECT scans are done on their patients, these cardiologists want privileges to read the scans at Sinai. If their request is denied, then they threaten to refer patients for SPECT scans as well as other diagnostic radiology workups to a competing hospital.

The radiologists learned of the cardiologists' request and sent Berson a letter stating that they expect her to meet the terms of their exclusive contract. The letter stated that the radiologists who are board certified in nuclear medicine do high-quality work and have the training, experience, and proven capability to read SPECT scans. The letter emphasized that such a change would adversely affect the quality of patient care because the technologies involved in two- and three-dimensional scans are very different and reading SPECT scans requires unique skills. In addition, granting these privileges to cardiologists would violate established relationships and cause other, unspecified disruptions. Berson suspected there just might be an economic reason as well.

The problem in radiology reminded Berson of the turf war between interventional radiologists and surgeons about using lasers and the turf war over which specialties should perform laparoscopic surgery. As she reread the letter, Berson mused about the course of modern medicine. It had reached the point at which many conditions could be diagnosed and treated without a scalpel. She thought briefly about Dr. McCoy, the "Star Trek" physician who had only to pass a small, handheld device over someone to make a diagnosis. Is that where we're headed, she wondered?

"But, enough of science fiction," she said to herself. "How do I solve yet another turf battle without too many casualties, not the least of whom could be me?"

QUESTIONS

1. Identify the quality-of-care issues. How are they similar to, but different from, the economic issues?
2. What information should Berson possess to understand the facts and issues? To whom should Berson turn for advice?
3. Develop three options that Berson could use. Identify and justify your choice of the best.
4. Identify three other quality/economic controversies that occur among institutional or personal health services providers.

CASE STUDY 3: "LET'S 'DO' A JOINT VENTURE"

Five years ago a consortium of churches established Arcadia Continuing Care Community (Arcadia) as a not-for-profit, tax-exempt corporation. Located in the tidewater region of eastern Virginia near a major naval base, Arcadia had 200 independent living apartments and a 20-bed nursing facility. Arcadia featured indoor and outdoor recreational activities and emphasized maximum independence for residents in a supportive, caring environment.

By 1990 poor management had brought Arcadia to the brink of bankruptcy. It was rescued by a large loan from the consortium and put under professional management. Arcadia was soon on firm financial footing, and the board of directors determined that its services should be diversified. Arcadia developed a respite care program to provide weekend and day services for dependent older adults and give relief to family members. It also established a home hospice program.

The board hired a consultant to assist in strategic planning. Based on market analyses and community assessments, the consultant suggested several new programs. First on the list was a rehabilitation center. The consultant noted the absence of outpatient rehabilitation services in the area, that rehabilitation logically extended existing services (including respite care and residential services), and that reimbursement was adequate. Start up costs, including leasing space and equipping and staffing a rehabilitation center, were estimated at $500,000. The board was enthusiastic, but it had less than $100,000 for a new venture. Arcadia was leveraged (mortgaged) to the maximum and there was no ready source of new capital.

As the board grappled with this question, the consultant suggested a joint venture with a physiatry group located 35 miles away. The consultant proposed that they pool their capital and establish a for-profit subsidiary to offer rehabilitation services. A telephone call to the physiatrists group showed it was interested in the proposal.

QUESTIONS

1. Critique what Arcadia is doing in terms of the technology that it has considered and is considering. Include both the positive and negative aspects.
2. Identify additional compatible activities that Arcadia could undertake. Be specific as to how they fit.
3. Identify the benefits and risks of forming a joint venture with the physiatry group.
4. What is the role of Arcadia's managers, especially the CEO, in these activities?

CASE STUDY 4: "WHY CAN'T YOU KEEP MY LAB RUNNING?!"

Brent Jackson's assistant, Mark, had just buzzed and told him Dr. Farrington was calling. Jackson tensed as he picked up the telephone. This isn't going to be pleasant, he thought. Farrington directed the pulmonary function laboratory and always seemed to be on the telephone complaining about one piece of equipment or another. The technician from Gateway Hi-Tech had not come as promised, and now Farrington had to cancel a procedure that was scheduled for the next morning. This time Farrington didn't threaten to have Jackson fired—which he had done before. It was clear, however, that his patience was at an end. Something had to be done about equipment repair and maintenance.

Five years earlier Jackson joined Medical Associates, Inc., a large multispecialty group practice, as a strategic planner and marketer. After 2 years he was promoted to a job with line management responsibility. His work was exemplary and he was asked to manage several other areas and departments. When Jackson became responsible for biomedical equipment management there were two staff: a clinical engineer and a technician. The engineer left a few months later, and recruiting for the past 18 months had been unsuccessful. The technician was well trained and worked hard, but there was too much to do. Jackson estimated that there were about 300 pieces of diagnostic and therapeutic equipment, representing at least 200 different types. Some, such as the piece of equipment in Farrington's laboratory, were serviced under contract. In Jackson's experience, however, such contracts were expensive and service often was unreliable. In addition, Jackson knew that there were many activities, such as the evaluation of new equipment, training of staff, and preventive maintenance, that received little attention.

Farrington's complaints seemed to be only the tip of the iceberg. Jackson wasn't really sure where to start, but he knew something had to be done.

QUESTIONS

1. Develop a statement of the problem facing Jackson.
2. What alternative solutions are available to Jackson? Which would you choose? Why?
3. List the advantages and disadvantages of using contract equipment maintenance and repair companies.
4. Identify the steps that Jackson should take if he chooses to develop a comprehensive in-house medical equipment management program.

CASE STUDY 5: "ISN'T THERE A BETTER WAY?"

Alice Smith hated saying no to requests for new technology, but as vice president for clinical services at Community Hospital it was an unfortunate fact of her professional life. Smith had just shown Dr. Madeline Jones to the door of her office; she knew Jones was very unhappy. Jones, the acting chief of anesthesiology, had asked Smith to authorize $2,500 to modify an anesthesia machine. Although well educated and articulate, Jones was unable to explain how the modification would 1) save money for the hospital and/or 2) measurably enhance patient care (the quality of surgical outcomes). Smith almost always asked these questions, and she could not believe that there was anyone on the clinical staff or in the hospital who did not know that.

As Smith sat down, she thought about how her response to Jones would be viewed by the members of the professional staff, many of whom would hear the latest news about the "ogre" in administration by day's end. Smith knew that she already had a reputation for being hard-nosed. She didn't mind that. Smith feared, however, that hostility was increasing among professional staff, especially the physicians, and that it would spill over into other relationships.

The outcomes of Smith's discussions with various physician managers differed widely. Some did their homework and could answer her questions; their equipment requests were usually granted. Smith knew that this was seen as favoritism, but that simply was not true.

The intercom buzzer broke Smith's reverie. She knew that there had to be a better way to make equipment-related decisions.

QUESTIONS

1. Develop a statement of the problem facing Smith.
2. Identify the positive and negative aspects of the situation that Smith has allowed and encouraged to develop.
3. Assume that Smith wants to enhance the ability of physicians to articulate their equipment requests. What steps should she take? With whom should she work most closely?
4. What are the positive and negative aspects of enhancing the clinical staff's ability to articulate their equipment requests? What other group(s) would benefit from the same assistance?

NOTES

1. Samuel, Frank E., Jr. "Technology and Costs: Complex Relationship." *Hospitals* 62 (December 5, 1988): 72.
2. Littell, Candace L., and Robin J. Strongin. "The Truth About Technology and Health Care Costs." *IEEE Technology and Society Magazine* 15 (Fall 1996): 11.
3. Stevens, William K. "High Medical Costs Under Attack as Drain on the Nation's Economy." *The New York Times,* March 28, 1982, 50.
4. Newhouse, John P. "An Iconoclastic View of Health Cost Containment." *Health Affairs* 1993 (12, Suppl.): 152; Bucy, Bill. "'Star Trek' Medical Devices Not So Far Out in the Future." *The Business Journal* 13 (January 29, 1996): 23.
5. Littell and Strongin, "The Truth About Technology," 12.
6. Perry, Seymour, and M. Eliastam. "The National Center for Health Care Technology." *Journal of the American Medical Association* 245 (June 26, 1981): 2510–2511.
7. Scitovsky, Anne A. "Changes in the Costs of Treatment of Selected Illnesses, 1971–1981." *Medical Care* 23 (December 1985): 1345–1357; Showstack, Jonathan A., Mary Hughes Stone, and Steven A. Schroeder. "The Role of Changing Clinical Practices in the Rising Costs of Hospital Care." *New England Journal of Medicine* 313 (November 7, 1985): 1201–1207.
8. Chernew, Michael, A. Mark Fendrick, and Richard A. Hirth. "Managed Care and Medical Technology: Implications for Cost Growth." *Health Affairs* 16 (March/April 1997): 196–206.
9. Shine, Kenneth I. "Low-Cost Technologies and Public Policy." *International Journal of Technology Assessment in Health Care* 13 (1997): 562–571.
10. Souhrada, Laura. "Biotechnology, Cost Concerns Dominate in 1989." *Hospitals* 63 (December 20, 1989): 32.
11. Russell, Louise B., and Jane E. Sisk. "Medical Technology in the United States: The Last Decade." *International Journal of Technology Assessment in Health Care* 4 (1988): 275. By way of context, the most rapid generalization of new technology is probably the diagnostic X ray (radiograph). Discovered by German physicist Wilhelm Roentgen in 1895, it was only months before radiographs were in general use. Such rapid generalization was possible because scientists worldwide had similar apparatuses and made them available to clinicians. The chest X ray continues to be the most common radiological procedure. (Lentle, Brian, and John Aldrich. "Radiological Science, Past and Present." *Lancet* 350 [July 26, 1997]: 280–285.)
12. "ECRI White Paper Makes Predictions on Equipment and Device Purchases." *Health Industry Today* 58 (May 1995): 6–7.
13. Biomagnetic Technologies, Inc., San Diego, California, personal communication, July 22, 1998.
14. Chernew, Fendrick, and Hirth. "Managed Care and Medical Technology."
15. Eisenberg, John M., J. Sanford Schwartz, F. Catherine McCaslin, Rachel Kaufman, Henry Glick, and Eugene Kroch. "Substituting Diagnostic Services: New Tests Only Partly Replace Older Ones." *Journal of the American Medical Association* 262 (September 1, 1989): 1196–1200.
16. Shine, Kenneth I. "Low-Cost Technologies and Public Policy." *International Journal of Technology Assessment in Health Care* 13 (1997): 563–564.
17. Kennedy, Donald. "Health Care Costs and Technologies." *Western Journal of Medicine* 161 (October 1994): 424–425.
18. Bailar, John C., III, and Heather L. Gornik. "Cancer Undefeated." *New England Journal of Medicine* 336 (May 29, 1997): 1569. From 1990 to 1995, the annual number (incidence rate) of new cancer cases fell slightly but steadily. This suggests an ebbing of the disease, not because of improved treatments but because of changing lifestyles, earlier detection, and more aggressive treatment of precancerous conditions. (David Brown. "New Cancer Cases Decline in U.S." *The Washington Post,* March 13, 1998, A1.)
19. Bureau of the Census. *Statistical Abstract of the United States, 1997,* 134. Washington, D.C.: U.S. Department of Commerce, Economics and Statistics Administration, 1997.
20. "Schizophrenia Update—Part I." *Harvard Mental Health Letter* 12 (June, 1995). Because fMRI allows imaging of soft tissue and concentrations of substances, scientists have been able to track human thought and emotion. ("Mapping Thought Patterns." *Biomedical Instrumentation & Technology* 31 [March/April 1997]: 111–112.)

21. "ECRI White Paper."

22. Kennedy, Donald. "Health Care Costs."

23. Day, Kathleen. "Two Drugs, Two Prices Spark a Battle." *The Washington Post,* September 16, 1994, D1, D3.

24. A useful discussion of the process is found in Glasser, Jay H., and Richard S. Chrzanowski. "Medical Technology Assessment: Adequate Questions, Appropriate Methods, Valuable Answers." *Health Policy* 9 (1988): 267–276.

25. Ramage, Michelle. "New Devices Emphasize Less Trauma to Body and Billfold." *The Business Journal* 41 (January 20, 1997): 59.

26. Carrington, Catherine. "Finding a Gentler Way to Mend the Heart." *Health Measures* 2 (March 1997): 35–36, 41.

27. Reischauer, Robert D. "Should We Raise the Medicare Eligibility Age?" *The San Diego Union-Tribune,* July 16, 1997, B5, B7.

28. Massaro, Thomas A. "Impact of New Technologies on Health-Care Costs and on the Nation's Health." *Clinical Chemistry* 36 (B) (1990): 1613.

29. Zeman, Robert K. "Medicine: I'll Take High Tech." *The Washington Post,* August 16, 1983, A17.

30. Moore, Thomas J. "Look at the Mortality Rates; the 'War on Cancer' Has Been a Bust." *The Washington Post,* July 23, 1997, A23.

31. The significant decline of atherosclerosis (deposition of plaque on artery walls, an important factor in coronary artery disease) since the 1960s has been attributed to use of broad-spectrum antibiotics, particularly tetracycline, to cure other bacterial infections. Bacteria such as *Chlamydia pneumoniae* and *Bacteroides gingivalis* have been linked to atherosclerosis, as have viruses such as cytomegalovirus, which can be treated but cannot be cured. (Mason, Michael. "Could You Catch a Heart Attack from a Common Germ?" *Health* 11 [November 21, 1997]: 90, 92–94.)

32. Health care costs for smokers at a given age are as much as 40% higher than those of nonsmokers. In a population in which no one smoked, the (health care) costs would be 7% higher for men and 4% higher for women. If all smokers quit, health care costs would be lower at first, but after 15 years they would be higher. Over the long term, complete smoking cessation would cause a net increase in health care costs. (Barendregt, Jan J., Luc Bonneux, and Paul J. van der Maas. "The Health Care Costs of Smoking." *New England Journal of Medicine* 337 [October 9, 1997]: 1052–1057.)

33. Vita, Anthony J., Richard B. Terry, Helen B. Hubert, and James F. Fries. "Aging, Health Risks, and Cumulative Disability." *New England Journal of Medicine* 338 (April 9, 1998): 1035–1041.

34. Ross, Philip E. "Brewing Blood." *Forbes* 160 (November 17, 1997): 168.

35. Gillis, Judith. "Technology Cleans Donated Blood." *The Washington Post,* April 25, 1998, D1.

36. Randolph, Lillian. *Physician Characteristics and Distribution in the U.S.: 1997–1998,* 9. Chicago: American Medical Association, 1998.

37. "The Comparative Performance of U.S. Hospitals." In *Health Care Investment Analyst,* 84. Baltimore: Deloitte & Touche, 1990.

38. Cleverly, William O. *The 1997–98 Almanac of Hospital Financial & Operating Indicators,* 180. Columbus, OH: The Center for Healthcare Industry Performance Studies, 1998.

39. The Center for Evaluative Clinical Services, Dartmouth Medical School. *The Dartmouth Atlas of Health Care in the United States.* Chicago: American Hospital Publishing, 1998.

40. The Center for Evaluative Clinical Services, Dartmouth Medical School, *The Dartmouth Atlas,* 115.

41. Cohn, Victor. "Study Says Some Coronary Bypasses Are Unneeded." *The Washington Post,* October 27, 1983, A5.

42. Killip, Thomas. "Twenty Years of Coronary Bypass Surgery." *New England Journal of Medicine* 319 (August 11, 1988): 368.

43. "Medicare CABG Centers Chosen." *Health Policy Week* 20 (February 4, 1991): 1–2.

44. Weissenstein, Eric. "HCFA to Expand CABG Project, Add Others." *Modern Healthcare* 26 (February 5, 1996): 18–19.

45. Hartz, Arthur J., Jose S. Pulido, and Evelyn M. Kuhn. "Are the Best Coronary Artery Bypass Surgeons Identified by Physician Surveys?" *American Journal of Public Health* 87 (October 1997): 1645–1648.

46. Squires, Sally. "In Angioplasty, Experience Counts: Study Finds Higher Rate of Complications Among Doctors Who Perform Few of These Procedures." *The Washington Post,* Health, November 19, 1996, 11.

47. Agency for Health Care Policy and Research. "Longer-Practicing Physicians May Hospitalize More Patients Unnecessarily." *Research Activities* 136 (December 1990): 3.

48. Goodwin, James S., Jean L. Freeman, Daniel Freeman, and Ann B. Nattinger. "Geographic Variations in Breast Cancer Mortality: Do Higher Rates Imply Elevated Incidence or Poorer Survival?" *American Journal of Public Health* 88 (March 1998): 458–460.

49. Bunker, John P., Jinnet Fowles, and Ralph Schaffarzick. "Evaluation of Medical Technology Strategies: Effects of Coverage and Reimbursement." *New England Journal of Medicine* 306 (March 11, 1982): 622–623.

50. Kaden, Raymond J. "Ensuring Adequate Payment for New Technology." *Health Care Financial Management* 52 (February 1998): 46–50, 52.

51. Appleby, Chuck. "MRI's Second Chance." *Hospitals* 69 (April 20, 1995): 40–42.

52. Steiner, Claudia A., Neil R. Powe, Gerard F. Anderson, and Abhik Das. "Technology Coverage Decisions by Health Care Plans and Considerations by Medical Directors." *Medical Care* 35 (1997): 472. A contrasting view of technology availability in fee-for-service insurance compared with HMOs is found in Ramsey, Scott D., and Mark V. Pauly. "Structural Incentives and Adoption of Medical Technologies in HMO and Fee-for-Service Health Insurance Plans." *Inquiry* 34 (Fall 1997): 228–236.

53. Russell and Sisk, "Medical Technology in the United States," 280–282.

54. "Medicare Program: Criteria and Procedures for Making Medical Services Coverage Decisions That Relate to Health Care Technology. Proposed Rule. 42 CFR Parts 400 and 405." *Federal Register* 54 (January 30, 1989): 4302–4318.

55. "Section 405.201(a) (1). Subpart B—Medical Services Coverage Decisions That Relate to Health Care Technology." *Code of Federal Regulations,* pt. 42, ch. IV, 42. Washington, D.C.: Office of the Federal Register, October 1997.

56. *Medicaid Organ Transplant and Experimental/Investigational Services Survey.* Helena: Montana Department of Public Health & Human Services, 1997.

57. Newhouse, "An Iconoclastic View," 164–165. A 1982 survey found that 51% of respondents were unwilling "to limit the opportunities for people to use expensive modern technology"; another 14% were uncertain. Most respondents were willing, however, to consider changes in the health care system that might reduce costs, such as having routine illnesses treated by a nurse or a physician's assistant rather than by a doctor, and going to a clinic at which they would be assigned any available doctor instead of seeing their own private doctor. (Reinhold, Robert. "Majority in Survey on Health Care Are Open to Changes to Cut Costs." *The New York Times,* March 29, 1982, A2, D11.)

58. Kozak, Lola Jean, Margaret Jean Hall, Robert Pokras, and Linda Lawrence. "Ambulatory Surgery in the United States, 1994." *Advance Data* 283 (March 14, 1997): 3. (National Center for Health Statistics, Centers for Disease Control and Prevention, U.S. Department of Health and Human Services)

59. Robinson, Michele L. "Turf Battle Rocks Radiology." *Hospitals* 63 (November 5, 1989): 47.

60. Kozak, Hall, Pokras, and Lawrence, "Ambulatory Surgery in the United States, 1994," 1.

61. Carrington, "Finding a Gentler Way."

62. Robinson, "Turf Battle Rocks Radiology."

63. Robinson, James C., and Harold S. Luft. "Competition and the Cost of Hospital Care, 1972 to 1982." *Journal of the American Medical Association* 257 (June 19, 1987): 3241–3245.

64. Medical Device Amendments of 1976, PL 94-295, 90 Stat. 539 (1976); Safe Medical Device Act of 1990, PL 101-629, 104 Stat. 4511 (1990).

65. Russell and Sisk, "Medical Technology," 271.

66. Sloane, Elliot B. "Subacute: New Equipment, New Maintenance Concerns." *Nursing Homes* 44 (October 1995): 27.

67. Sloane, "Subacute: New Equipment," 24.

68. Lashof, Joyce C. "Government Approaches to the Management of Medical Technology." *Bulletin of the New York Academy of Medicine* 57 (January–February 1981): 40–41.

69. Lashof, "Government Approaches," 41.

70. Committee on Ways and Means, U.S. House of Representatives. *1998 Green Book Appendix D. Medicare Reimbursement to Hospitals.* Washington, D.C.: U.S. House of Representatives, 1998.

71. National Health Planning and Resources Development Act of 1974, PL 93-641, 88 Stat. 2225 (1974).

72. Cohen, Alan B., and Donald R. Cohodes. "Certificate of Need and Low Capital-Cost Medical Technology." *Milbank Memorial Fund Quarterly* 60 (Spring 1982): 307–328.

73. Brice, Cindy L., and Kathryn Ellen Cline. "The Supply and Use of Selected Medical Technologies." *Health Affairs* 17 (January/February 1998): 17. An example is Pennsylvania, where MRIs more than doubled between 1988 and 1993, to a total of 187 machines. Many were underused; now MRIs must operate at 85% of capacity before additional units are approved.

74. Appleby, "MRI's Second Chance."

75. Shaffer, Michael J. "Managing Hospital Biomedical Equipment." In *Hospital Organization and Management,* 4th ed., edited by Kurt Darr and Jonathon S. Rakich, 273. Baltimore: AUPHA/National Health Publishing, 1989.

76. Kantner, Rob. "ISO 9000—Quality Standards." *Global Opportunity* (1995): 62–66. (ISO is a nickname [a variant of *isos,* a Greek word meaning equal], and is not an acronym for the International Organization for Standardization.)

77. Burroughs, John T., and Carl R. Edenhofer. "Product Liability Actions in Medical Negligence: The Barrier Is Breaking." *Journal of Legal Medicine* 4 (June 1983): 218–229.

78. Perry, Seymour. "Technology Assessment in Health Care: The U.S. Perspective." *Health Policy* 9 (1988): 318.

79. Institute of Medicine, Committee for Evaluating Medical Technologies in Clinical Use. *Assessing Medical Technologies, 9,* 37. Washington, D.C.: National Academy Press, 1985.

80. Perry, Seymour, and Barbara Pillar. "A National Policy for Health Care Technology Assessment." *Medical Care Review* 47 (Winter 1990): 408.

81. Perry, Seymour, and Mae Thamer. "Health Technology Assessment: Decentralized and Fragmented in the US Compared to Other Countries." *Health Policy* 40 (1997): 181.

82. Perry and Thamer, "Health Technology Assessment," 182.

83. A concise discussion of consensus development conferences is found in Jacoby, Itzhak. "Update on Assessment Activities: United States Perspective." *International Journal of Technology Assessment in Health Care* 4 (1988): 100–101.

84. Institute of Medicine, *Assessing Medical Technologies,* 9, 70–175.

85. Office of Technology Assessment, United States Congress. *The OTA Health Program.* Washington, D.C.: Office of Technology Assessment, 1989.

86. Bimber, Bruce. *The Politics of Expertise in Congress,* 69. Albany: State University of New York Press, 1996.

87. Health Services Research, Health Statistics, and Health Care Technology Act of 1978, PL 95-623, 92 Stat. 334 (1978).

88. Perry, "Technology Assessment," 320.

89. Perry and Thamer, "Health Technology Assessment," 194.

90. National Center for Health Services Research and Health Care Technology Assessment. *Program Profile: Office of Technology Assessment,* 2. Washington, D.C.: U.S. Department of Health and Human Services, 1988.

91. *http://www.ahrq.gov/news/profile.htm#strgoals,* April 2, 2000.

92. Greene, Jan. "An Agency for Change." *Hospitals & Health Networks* 71 (October 20, 1997): 68, 70.

93. Agency for Health Care Policy and Research. "AHCPR to Collaborate with AMA and AAHP to Develop a National Guideline Clearinghouse." *Research Activities* 205 (June 1997): 16.

94. Greene, "An Agency for Change."

95. Cassil, Alwyn. "Once-Maligned Agency Poised for Pivotal Role in Advancing Medicine." *AHA News* 34 (February 16, 1998): 3.

96. Perry and Thamer, "Health Technology Assessment," 196.

97. Perry and Thamer, "Health Technology Assessment," 181.

98. Uphoff, Mary Ellen, Thomas Ratko, and Karl Matuszewski. "Making Technology Assessment Count." *Health Measures* 2 (March 1997): 18.

99. Perry, "Technology Assessment," 323.

100. Carrington, Catherine. "Community Hospitals Balance Progress and Costs." *Health Measures* 2 (March 1997): 9.

101. Sanders, Charles A. "Taming the Technological Tiger." *Trustee* 31 (March 1978): 24.
102. *Health Devices Sourcebook—The Hospital Purchasing Guide,* B 457. Plymouth Meeting, PA: ECRI, 1990.
103. *Health Devices Source Book, 1998,* B 517. Plymouth Meeting, PA: ECRI, 1997.
104. Sanders, "Taming the Technological Tiger."
105. *Health Devices Sourcebook,* B 407.
106. *Health Devices Sourcebook, 1998,* B 456.
107. Coile, Russell C., Jr. "The 'Racer's Edge' in Hospital Competition: Strategic Technology Plan." *Healthcare Executive* 5 (January/February 1990): 22.
108. Anderson, Howard J. "Survey Identifies Technology Trends." *Medical Staff Leader* October (1990): 30–33.
109. Miccio, Joseph A. "The Migration of Medical Technology." *Healthcare Forum Journal* September/October (1989): 24.
110. McKee, Michael, and L. Rita Fritz. "Team Up for Technology Assessment." *Hospitals* 53 (June 1, 1979): 119–122.
111. American Hospital Association. "Trustee Development Program: The Board's Role in the Planning and Acquisition of Clinical Technology." *Trustee* 32 (June 1979): 17 55.
112. Lodge, Denver A. "Someone Must Guide Technology Acquisition." *Modern Healthcare* 22 (December 7, 1992): 21.
113. Heller, Ori. "The New Role of Chief Technology Officer in U.S. Hospitals." *International Journal of Technology Management* (Special Issue on the Strategic Management of Information and Telecommunications Technology) 7 (1992): 455–461.
114. Shaffer, Michael D., and Michael J. Shaffer. "Technical Support for Biomedical Equipment and Decision Making." *Hospital Topics* 73 (Spring 1995): 35–41.
115. Uphoff, Ratko, and Matuszewski, "Making Technology Assessment Count," 22.
116. Uphoff, Ratko, and Matuszewski, "Making Technology Assessment Count," 24.
117. Souhrada, Laura. "System Execs Overcome Barriers to Tech Assessment." *Hospitals* 63 (August 5, 1989): 39.
118. Blumberg, Donald F. "Evaluating Technology Service Options: Technology Services for Healthcare Organizations." *Healthcare Financial Management* 51 (May 1997): 72.
119. Heller, "The New Role of Chief Technology Officer."
120. Joint Commission on Accreditation of Healthcare Organizations. "Standard EC.1.8: Medical Equipment." In *Comprehensive Accreditation Manual for Hospitals, Refreshed Core, January 1998,* EC-14. Oakbrook Terrace, IL: Joint Commission on Accreditation of Healthcare Organizations, 1998.
121. Blumberg, "Evaluating Technology Service Options," 72–74, 76, 78–79.
122. Solovy, Alden. "No, You Do It." *Hospitals & Health Networks* 70 (October 20, 1996): 40–46.
123. Kasti, Mohamad S. "The Future of Clinical Engineering Practice: ACCE's Vision 2000." *Biomedical Instrumentation and Technology* 30 (November/December 1996): 490–495.
124. Spears, Jack. "Justice vs. GE: Two Sides to Every Story." *Healthcare Technology Management* 7 (October 1996): 5.
125. Keil, Ode R. "Accreditation and Clinical Engineering." *Journal of Clinical Engineering* (July–August 1996): 258–260.
126. Keil, Ode R. "Is Preventive Maintenance Still a Core Element of Clinical Engineering?" *Biomedical Instrumentation & Technology* 29 (July/August 1997): 408–409.
127. Ridgeway, Malcolm. "Changes in Industry Bring Opportunity." *Health Technology Management* 7 (October 1996): 48.
128. Shaffer, Michael J. "The Reengineering of Clinical Engineering." *Biomedical Instrumentation & Technology* 31 (March/April 1997): 178.
129. Lando, MaryAnn. "Information Technology 101: What Every CEO Needs To Know." *Healthcare Executive* 13 (May/June 1998): 16–20.
130. Starr, Paul. "Smart Technology, Stunted Policy: Developing Health Information Networks." *Health Affairs* 16 (May–June 1997): 94.
131. Menduno, Michael. "Prognosis: Wired." *Hospitals & Health Networks* 72 (November 5, 1998): 2–30, 32–35.

132. Duncan, Karen A. "Evolving Community Health Information Networks." *Frontiers of Health Services Management* 2 (Fall 1995): 5–41.
133. Starr, "Smart Technology, Stunted Policy," 96.
134. Starr, "Smart Technology, Stunted Policy," 99.
135. Starr, "Smart Technology, Stunted Policy," 100.
136. Duncan, Karen A. "CHINs in the Context of an Evolving Health Care System." In Proceedings of the AMIA Fall Symposium, 1995, 604–607.
137. Starr, "Smart Technology, Stunted Policy," 101.
138. Zeidman, Cara. "Chemung Valley Health Network: The Development of a Community Health Information Network." *Journal of Nursing Care Quality* 11 (June 1997): 5–8.
139. Zeidman, "Chemung Valley Health Network," 7.
140. Starr, "Smart Technology, Stunted Policy," 91.
141. Duncan, "CHINs in the Context," 605.
142. Duncan, "CHINs in the Context," 605–607.
143. Starr, "Smart Technology, Stunted Policy," 101–102.
144. Starr, "Smart Technology, Stunted Policy," 102–103.
145. Electronic medical record is used here. Some literature uses electronic health or patient record, reflecting a greater focus on prevention, wellness, and holistic medicine, which are likely to receive more attention in the future.
146. McDonald, Clement J. "The Barriers to Electronic Medical Record Systems and How to Overcome Them." *Journal of the American Medical Informatics Association* 4 (May/June 1997): 214.
147. Cacy, Jim, Frank Lawler, Nancy Viviani, and Donna Wells. "The Sixth Level of Electronic Health Records: A Look Beyond the Screen." *M.D. Computing* 14 (January–February 1997): 46–49. This article contains a frank discussion of major implementation problems of an EMR in a department of family and preventive medicine.
148. McDonald, "The Barriers to Electronic," 213–221.
149. Pestotnik, Stanley L., David C. Classen, R. Scott Evans, and John P. Burke. "Implementing Antibiotic Practice Guidelines Through Computer-Assisted Decision Support: Clinical and Financial Outcomes." *Annals of Internal Medicine* 124 (May 15, 1996): 884–890.
150. Tierney, William M., J. Marc Overhage, and Clement J. McDonald. "Demonstrating the Effects of an IAIMS on Health Care Quality and Cost." *Journal of the American Medical Informatics Association* 4 (March/April [Supplement] 1997): S41–S46.
151. McDonald, "The Barriers to Electronic," 218.
152. McDonald, "The Barriers to Electronic," 219–220.
153. Potts, Jerry F. "Electronic Medical Records: More Information but Less Access?" *Postgraduate Medicine* 101 (February 1997): 31–32.
154. Potts, "Electronic Medical Records," 35.
155. Potts, "Electronic Medical Records," 36.
156. McDonald, "The Barriers to Electronic," 218.
157. Swanson, Todd, Julie Dostal, Brad Eichhorst, Clarence Jernigan, Mark Knox, and Kevin Roper. "Recent Implementations of Electronic Medical Records in Four Family Practice Residency Programs." *Academic Medicine* 72 (July 1997): 611.
158. Gardner, Martin. "Information Retrieval for Patient Care." *British Medical Journal* 314 (March 29, 1997): 350–353.
159. Swanson, Dostal, Eichhorst, Jernigan, Knox, and Roper, "Recent Implementations."
160. McDonald, "The Barriers to Electronic," 219.
161. McMenamin, Joseph P. "Telemedicine: Technology and the Law." *For the Defense* 39 (July 1997): 13.
162. Campbell, Sandy. "Will Telemedicine Become as Common as the Stethoscope?" *Health Care Strategic Management* 15 (April 1997): 1.
163. "Ophthalmic Imaging Network Premiers." *Biomedical Instrumentation & Technology* 31 (March/April 1997): 111.
164. Campbell, "Will Telemedicine Become," 1, 20–23.

165. Perednia, Douglas A., and Ace Allen. "Telemedicine Technology and Clinical Applications." *Journal of the American Medical Association* 273 (February 8, 1995): 483.

166. "Balancing Hospital Productivity, Health Care Utilization and Medical Expenditures." *Health Care Strategic Management* 15 (March 1997): 12.

167. Perednia and Allen. "Telemedicine Technology," 483–488.

168. HCFA has estimated that Medicare will pay $2.7 billion over 5 years if telemedicine consultations are available to rural America; supporters of telemedicine assert the estimate is too high (*Inside HCFA* January 22 [1998]: 16 [newsletter]).

169. Zambuto, Raymond P. "Current Health Care Trends and Their Impact on Clinical Engineering." *Biomedical Instrumentation & Technology* 31 (May/June 1997): 233–234.

170. Sandrick, Karen. "Interview with John E. Abele." *Hospitals & Health Networks* 70 (January 5, 1996): 28–30.

171. Jaklevik, Mary C. "Internet Technology Moves to Patient Care Front Lines." *Modern Healthcare* 26 (March 11, 1996): 47–50.

172. Hewlett-Packard. "Catch the Wave: You, Too, Can Surf the Net." *Probe* (Spring 1996).

173. Higgins, Thomas L., "Severity of Illness Indices and Outcome Prediction: Development and Evaluation." In *Textbook of Critical Care*, 4th ed., edited by Ake Grenvik, Stephen M. Ayres, Peter R. Holbrook, and William C. Shoemaker, 1639–1685, Philadelphia: W.B. Saunders, 2000.

174. "Inforum" brochure, Nashville, TN, 1994.

175. Steven, Peter. "All Roads Lead to the Electronic Patient Record." *Healthcare Technology Management* 7 (December 1996): 33–35.

176. Moukheiber, Zina. "A Hail of Silver Bullets." *Forbes* 161 (January 26, 1998): 76–81.

SELECTED BIBLIOGRAPHY

Bimber, Bruce. *The Politics of Expertise in Congress.* Albany: State University of New York Press, 1996.

Blumberg, Donald F. "Evaluating Technology Service Options: Technology Services for Healthcare Organizations." *Healthcare Financial Management* 51 (May 1997): 72–74, 76, 78–79.

Capuano, Mike. "Technology Acquisition Strategies for Clinical Engineering." *Biomedical Instrumentation & Technology* 31 (July/August 1997): 335–357.

Carrington, Catherine. "Community Hospitals Balance Progress and Costs." *Health Measures* 2 (March 1997): 35–36, 41.

Chandler, Kevin R. "Investing in the Future: High-Tech Solutions for Quality Improvement." *Quality Progress* 31 (July 1998): 65–69.

Chernew, Michael, A. Mark Fendrick, and Richard A. Hirth. "Managed Care and Medical Technology: Implications for Cost Growth." *Health Affairs* 16 (March/April 1997): 196–206.

Cromwell, Jerry, Debra A. Dayhoff, and Armen H. Thoumaian. "Cost Savings and Physician Responses to Global Bundled Payments for Medicare Heart Bypass Surgery." *Health Care Financing Review* 19 (Fall 1997): 41–57.

Daar, Judith F., and Spencer Koerner. "Telemedicine: Legal and Practical Implications." *Whittier Law Review* 19 (Winter 1997): 3–28.

Duncan, Karen A. "Evolving Community Health Information Networks." *Frontiers of Health Services Management* 12 (Fall 1995): 5–41.

Duncan, Karen A. *Health Information and Health Reform: Understanding the Need for a National Health Information System.* San Francisco: Jossey-Bass, 1994.

Frize, Monique, and Michael Shaffer. "Clinical Engineering in Today's Hospital: Perspectives of the Administrator and the Clinical Engineer." *Hospital & Health Services Administration* 36 (Summer 1991): 285–305.

Heller, Ori. "The New Role of Chief Technology Officer in U.S. Hospitals." *International Journal of Technology Management* (Special Issue on the Strategic Management of Information and Telecommunications Technology) 7 (1992): 455–461.

Kaden, Raymond J. "Ensuring Adequate Payment for New Technology." *Health Care Financial Management* 52 (February 1998): 46–50, 52.

Kasti, Mohamad S. "The Future of Clinical Engineering Practice: ACCE's Vision 2000." *Biomedical Instrumentation & Technology* 30 (November/December 1996): 490–495.

Leeming, Michael N., and John V. Fulginiti. "Validity and Clinical Engineering Indicators." *Biomedical Instrumentation & Technology* 31 (January/February 1997): 33–42.

McDonald, Clement J. "The Barriers to Electronic Medical Record Systems and How to Overcome Them." *Journal of the American Medical Informatics Association* 4 (May/June 1997): 213–221.

Newhouse, Joseph P. "An Iconoclastic View of Health Cost Containment." *Health Affairs* 12 (1993 Supplement): 152–171.

Perednia, Douglas A., and Ace Allen. "Telemedicine Technology and Clinical Applications." *Journal of the American Medical Association* 273 (February 8, 1995): 483–488.

Perry, Seymour, and Barbara Pillar. "A National Policy for Health Care Technology Assessment." *Medical Care Review* 47 (Winter 1990): 401–417.

Perry, Seymour, and Mae Thamer. "Health Technology Assessment: Decentralized and Fragmented in the US Compared to Other Countries." *Health Policy* 40 (1997): 177–198.

Pestotnik, Stanley L., David C. Classen, R. Scott Evans, and John P. Burke. "Implementing Antibiotic Practice Guidelines Through Computer-Assisted Decision Support: Clinical and Financial Outcomes." *Annals of Internal Medicine* 124 (May 15, 1996): 884–890.

Ramsey, Scott D., and Mark V. Pauly. "Structural Incentives and Adoption of Medical Technologies in HMO and Fee-for-Service Health Insurance Plans." *Inquiry* 34 (Fall 1997): 228–236.

Randolph, Lillian. *Physician Characteristics and Distribution in the U.S.: 1997–1998,* 9, 11. Chicago: American Medical Association, 1998.

Shaffer, Michael D., and Michael J. Shaffer. "Technical Support for Biomedical Equipment and Decision Making." *Hospital Topics* 73 (Spring 1995): 35–41.

Shaffer, Michael J. "The Reengineering of Clinical Engineering." *Biomedical Instrumentation & Technology* 31 (March/April 1997): 177–178.

Starr, Paul. "Smart Technology, Stunted Policy: Developing Health Information Networks." *Health Affairs* 16 (May–June 1997): 91–105.

Steiner, Claudia A., Neil R. Powe, Gerard F. Anderson, and Abhik Das. "Technology Coverage Decisions by Health Care Plans and Considerations by Medical Directors." *Medical Care* 35 (May 1997): 472–487.

Sykes, Dianne, and William Alex McIntosh. "Telemedicine, Hospital Viability, and Community Embeddedness: A Case Study." *Journal of Healthcare Management* 44 (January/February 1999): 59–71.

Tierney, William M., J. Marc Overhage, and Clement J. McDonald. "Demonstrating the Effects of an IAIMS on Health Care Quality and Cost." *Journal of the American Medical Informatics Association* 4 (March/April [Supplement] 1997): S41–S46.

Uphoff, Mary Ellen, Thomas Ratko, and Karl Matuszewski. "Making Technology Assessment Count." *Health Measures* 2 (March 1997): 18, 22, 24.

Zambuto, Raymond Peter. "Current Health Care Trends and Their Impact on Clinical Engineering." *Biomedical Instrumentation & Technology* 31 (May/June 1997): 228–236.

Managerial Tools and Techniques

7

Managerial Problem Solving and Decision Making

We try to make management decisions that, if everything goes right, will preclude future problems. But everything does not always go right, and managers therefore must be problem solvers as well as decision makers.[1]

Health services organizations and health systems (HSOs/HSs) are vibrant entities in a fluid environment. The management model in Figure 1.7 reflects this dynamism. HSOs/HSs convert inputs (such as human resources, materials and supplies, technology, information, and capital) into outputs (individual and organizational work results) to achieve objectives—work results such as delivering health services, educating, or researching. HSO/HS managers produce that conversion when they integrate structure, tasks/technology, and people. In doing so, they are accountable for allocating and using resources and for the outcomes.

Anticipating and preventing problems or solving them when prevention fails are traditional management tasks. The new paradigm includes continuous improvement of quality, a proactive approach that assumes that all processes can be improved and that managers must create the environment and give employees the tools to make improvement possible.

Like the introductory quote, this chapter distinguishes problem solving from decision making. A problem-solving model is developed and the factors influencing managerial problem solving and decision making are discussed. The benefits of various group problem-solving strategies are identified, and the use of teams in quality improvement is discussed. A model assists in determining when group rather than individual problem solving is more effective.

PROBLEM ANALYSIS AND DECISION MAKING

A manager's work revolves around the elements of problem solving–problem analysis and decision making. Problem analysis includes recognizing and defining circumstances that require action (a decision) and implementing and evaluating the alternative that is chosen. Chapter 1 identifies decision making as a managerial function, defined as choosing among alternatives.[2] "Choosing" is key and defines decision making. Simply put, decision making involves two steps: identifying and evaluating alternatives, and choosing an alternative.

Decision making is integral to all management functions, activities, and roles. For example, planning involves making decisions (choosing), whether senior-level managers are formulating strategy or middle-level managers are implementing programs. Decisions about the management function of organizing range from establishing authority–responsibility relationships to designing work systems, procedures, and flows, and from structure–task–people relationships to making job assignments. In the staffing function, managers decide about numbers of staff and their pay, training, and performance appraisal. In leading, motivating, and communicating, managers choose the most effective management style and when, where, and to whom information is imparted.

When managers control, they compare individual and organizational work results with predetermined expectations and standards and decide whether results can be improved or standards can be increased. This means making decisions about what type of information to collect and report and which monitoring systems should be used to measure and compare HSO/HS conversion activities and outputs with expectations and standards. Managers also decide which managerial roles to adopt, choosing among the interpersonal roles of figurehead, liaison, and influencer; the informational roles of monitor, disseminator, and spokesperson; and the decision roles of change agent, disturbance handler, resource allocator, and negotiator. Figures 1.2 and 1.4 show the interrelationship of decision making to other management functions and to managerial roles, respectively.

Types of Decisions

Three types describe most of the manager's decisions: 1) ends–means, 2) administrative-operational, and 3) nonprogrammable-programmable.

Ends–Means

Ends decisions determine the individual or organizational objectives and results to be achieved. Means decisions choose the strategies or programs and activities to accomplish desired results. For example, a decision to emphasize quality and productivity improvement (means) accomplishes the organizational objectives of enhanced quality of care and service, higher patient or customer satisfaction, and better resource use (ends). Ends are shown as the output component of the management model in Figure 1.7. Decisions about ends are inherent in strategic planning, which includes formulating objectives. Health systems may make these decisions at the corporate level. Greater specificity is found in a department's ends–means decision making, which reflects its objectives and the operational programs that contribute to the HSO's/HS's overall mission.

Administrative-Operational

Many administrative decisions that are made by senior-level executives significantly affect the HSO/HS and have major implications for resource allocation and utilization. Policy decisions are a synonym for administrative decisions. Examples include deciding whether to finance facility construction or renovation using debt, recognize a union without demanding a certification election, hire hospital-based physicians, contract for laundry services, reduce the capital equipment budget, or participate in an integrated system of HSOs. In contrast, operational decisions are made about day-to-day activities by middle- and first-level managers. Operational decisions include deciding whether to purchase noncapital equipment, reassign staff, modify work systems, and modify job content.

Nonprogrammable-Programmable

Nonprogrammable decisions are novel, unstructured, and significant.[3] Examples are whether to expand facilities; add, close, or share services; seek Medicare certification of skilled beds; restructure the organization or align with a network of HSOs; acquire a clinical information system; or add a family practice residency program. Such decisions occur infrequently. Programmable decisions are repetitive and routine; procedures and rules are used to guide them.[4] Patient admitting, scheduling, and billing and inventory and supply ordering procedures are examples.

Overlap of Decision Types

The Venn diagram in Figure 7.1 shows that the three decision types overlap—decisions may include parts of each. For example, merging with another HSO or establishing a satellite urgent care center or primary care preferred provider organization is a "means" decision because it is a strategy to achieve the organization's objectives. Furthermore, it is an administrative decision because it involves a major commitment of resources, compared with a primarily operational decision about day-to-day activities. Finally, the decision is nonprogrammable because it is unique and occurs infrequently.

MANAGERIAL PROBLEM SOLVING

Managers are problem solvers. Problems may be unstructured or structured; complex or simple; major or minor; urgent or nonurgent; and may involve varying degrees of cost, risk, and uncertainty. Problem solving involves a series of steps that are "characterized by intentional reasoning about what the problem is and what the solution should be,"[5] the result of which is to make the current state more closely match the desired state.[6] Using terminology from the management model, problem solving causes change so that actual HSO/HS results or outputs more closely align with those desired. The process by which managers solve problems includes

- Selecting and analyzing a situation that requires a decision
- Developing and evaluating alternative solutions to address the situation
- Choosing an alternative (this step is sometimes called decision analysis)
- Implementing the alternative
- Evaluating the results after implementation

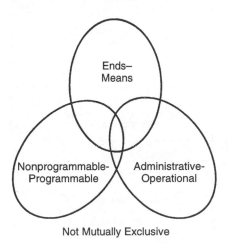

Not Mutually Exclusive

Figure 7.1. Types of decisions.

Figure 7.2 shows the relationships among problem solving, problem analysis, and decision making. The terms *problem solving* and *decision making* often are used interchangeably but are not synonymous. All problem solving involves decision making (i.e., choosing among alternatives), but not all decision making involves problem solving.[7] The distinction is that problem solving includes problem analysis–predecision situation assessment and postdecision implementation and evaluation. The discussion here is relevant to both problem solving and decision making, and they are distinguished as necessary.

Managers perform a series of steps when undertaking either problem analysis or decision making. As with all processes there are variables, conditions, and situations that influence the approach, manner, and style that are used. Problem-solving skills are crucial to managerial success; there are situations in which being an effective problem solver is more important than is communication or interpersonal relationships skills, which is not to diminish their importance, generally. It does mean, however, that problem solving is fundamental to everything that a manager does and to effective managerial performance.

Briefly described, a manager is a problem solver and decision maker. The role of problem solving in managerial effectiveness was demonstrated by a large Canadian study involving 4,000 HSO managers from hospitals, nursing facilities, community health centers, and medical clinics; 2,500 were chief executive officers (CEOs). Almost all of the managers identified problem solving, along with decision making, to be among their most important activities.[8] A major finding from research involving 524 U.S. hospital CEOs was the need to improve the process of problem solving. Areas ranked highest were external stakeholder (community) relations, business and finance, medical care and medical staff, and staff.[9]

PROBLEM-SOLVING PROCESS AND MODEL

Problem solving is a process by which managers analyze situations and make decisions that cause organizational results to be more like those desired. Prospective problem solving anticipates organizational results that are more or less desirable. Retrospective problem solving identifies and corrects previous causes of deviation from desired results. Concurrent problem solving occurs in HSOs/HSs that are committed to a philosophy of continuously improving quality and productivity.

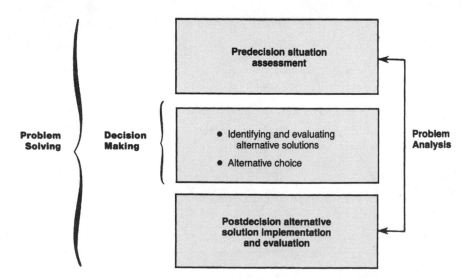

Figure 7.2.   Problem solving and decision making.

Conditions that Initiate Problem Solving

Another way to classify problem solving is by conditions that initiate it.[10] Figure 7.3 shows the conditions and corresponding approaches to problem solving. These are

- Opportunity/threat (prospective—might)
- Crisis (immediate—will)
- Deviation (retrospective—has/is)
- Improvement (concurrent—seek)

Opportunity problem solving is prospective and anticipatory. It occurs when a favorable internal or external circumstance enables the HSO/HS to achieve or enhance desired results.[11] For example, technology and consumer expectations permit an acute care hospital to offer obstetrics services at a birth center. Developing the program involves problem analysis, which consists of predecision assessment and postdecision evaluation. The outcome is organizational results (new service) that align more closely with desired results, including improved patient service and satisfaction and increased revenue.

Threat problem solving also is prospective and anticipatory but is the converse of opportunity problem solving. Threats may be internal or external and, if left unaddressed, may cause future results to be less than what is desired. For example, not responding to a competitor's aggressive marketing program might cause loss of market share.

Crisis problem solving is immediate. It responds to a current or predictable threat. Failing to act promptly will cause untoward results, such as a decline in near-term performance. Examples of crisis problem solving are a local natural disaster, a strike by unionized employees, bypass equipment malfunction during surgery, or a sudden reduction in Medicaid payments. Loss of an essential employee may be a crisis.

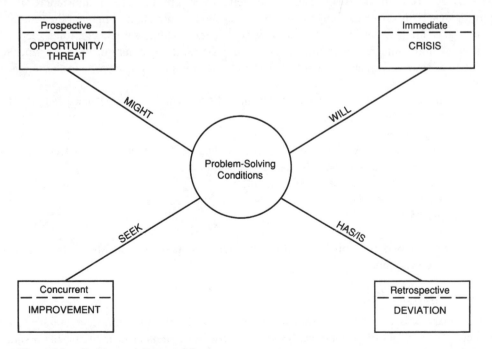

Figure 7.3.   Problem-solving conditions.

Deviation problem solving is retrospective and occurs when actual and desired results differ. Even small deviations may indicate large problems that must be resolved.

Improvement problem solving is concurrent and reduces future deviation problem solving. The perspective, mindset, and process of continuous improvement differ from other problem-solving conditions in two important ways. First, continuous improvement is rooted in a philosophy that further improvement is always possible and management's job is to support these efforts. This leads to continuously examining processes and seeking ways to improve them. Second, analysis is concurrent, broad based, and organizationwide and focuses on inputs and the conversion process. The management model in Figure 1.7 shows this relationship. In improvement problem solving, managers and staff are problem seekers who systematically seek opportunities for improvement.[12]

The condition of deviation is specifically referenced in the problem-solving process model that is depicted in Figure 7.4, but the model is generic and is applicable to all problem solving except that conducted under the condition of improvement, where problem analysis differs. Historically, managers engaged most frequently in problem solving under conditions of deviation[13] and less frequently under conditions of crisis.[14] The contemporary emphasis on continuous quality improvement (CQI), which is undertaken without a condition of deviation, is likely to make CQI the most common type of problem solving. Chapter 9 details improvement problem solving.

The strategic planning model shown in Figure 8.5 focuses on external opportunities and threats. Its elements, however, are like those of traditional problem solving, which makes the skills readily interchangeable. External and internal environment assessment, strategy choice, and implementation are comparable to problem identification, alternative selection, and implementation and evaluation, respectively.

Problem-Solving Activities

Middle- and senior-level managers spend most of their time solving problems. The results of these efforts affect allocation and use of resources as well as work product. The circumstances surrounding problem solving are often complex, unstructured, and nonroutine, thus making the task difficult and time consuming. Sometimes the situation is beyond the manager's direct control. Except for the condition of improvement, the process is essentially the same regardless of problem type, scope, time involved, intensity of analysis, or the conditions that initiate it. Basic problem solving includes

1. Problem identification: recognizing the presence of a problem (including gathering and evaluating information), and stating the problem
2. Making assumptions
3. Developing tentative alternative solutions and selecting those to be considered in depth
4. Evaluating alternative solutions by applying decision criteria
5. Selecting the alternative that best fits the criteria
6. Implementing the solution
7. Evaluating results

These steps are shown in Figure 7.4, and the numbers in that figure correspond to those noted in the following discussion.

Problem Analysis [1]

Problem analysis is divided into problem recognition and definition and developing a problem statement. The product of problem analysis is the problem statement. It is the problem statement about which assumptions are made in Step [2].

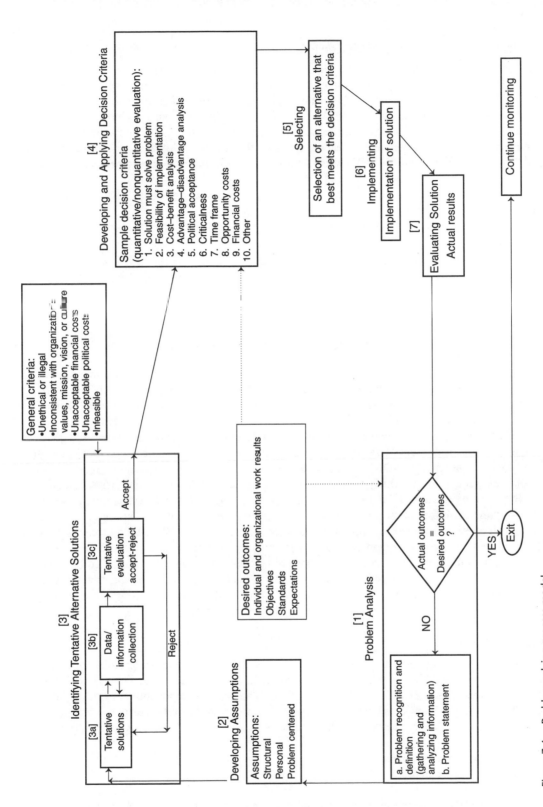

Figure 7.4. Problem-solving process model.

323

Problem Recognition and Definition

Problem solving under the condition of deviation begins when actual results are inconsistent with desired results and the manager determines that this constitutes a problem that is in need of a solution. Examples of desired results are 1) organizationwide objectives such as quality of patient care, better client services, or financial solvency; 2) departmental objectives such as increasing customer satisfaction, reducing staff turnover, decreasing surgical infection rates, eliminating mislabeled laboratory specimens and radiograph retakes, or minimizing budget variances; or 3) improving the work of an individual employee. Whether negative deviation indicates the presence of a problem depends on whether it is common cause variation or special cause variation, a statistical quality control concept that is discussed in Chapter 9. Similarly, positive special cause variation (deviation) should be studied so it can be incorporated into the process.

Applying the theory of problem recognition is not easy. Problem recognition

> *rarely occurs as a completely discrete event. In practice the process occurs through various time intervals (from seconds to years), amidst a variety of ongoing activities and in different ways depending on both situational and individual factors. At times, the process of problem recognition is automatic; at other times, it involves conscious effort. Often, it is a highly objective phenomenon resulting in problem descriptions that most anyone would agree on. At other times it is definitely a subjective process, where the nature of a problem description varies from individual to individual.*[15]

Problem recognition occurs in three stages. The first is gestation/latency, in which some cue or triggering event indicates a potential problem. The second is categorization, in which managers become aware that something is wrong but cannot fully describe it. Diagnosis is third, which involves efforts to obtain the information that will provide greater certainty in problem definition.[16]

Often, symptoms clutter and confuse and make it difficult to recognize a problem and define its parameters. More experienced and expert managers tend to be better problem solvers because they have superior problem recognition and definition skills. Asking the right questions, recognizing limits, and being sensitive to identifying and interpreting cues are skills gained only with experience.

Problem recognition and definition includes gathering, systematically evaluating, and judging the importance of information from sources such as routine reports and data, interviews and observation, information from workgroups, and customer feedback.[17] In unstructured or complex situations circumstantial evidence and deductive reasoning are helpful. Exclusionary thinking may be used to "rule out" problems. Once conclusions are reached, the problem is classified by type, nature, and scope. This recognition-definition stage is formative because subsequent actions, especially developing alternatives, are derived from it.[18] Ending the problem definition stage too soon may result in a low-quality solution or in solving the wrong problem.[19]

Problem Statement

The problem statement puts what is learned during the definition stage into a brief description of the problem to be solved. Usually, one sentence is sufficient. Good problem statements have four parts: 1) an invitational stem, 2) an ownership component, 3) an action component, and 4) a goal component.[20] A sample problem statement, "In what ways can we improve system response time to reduce how long marketing analysts must wait for an answer to an inquiry?," contains the four parts:

- In what ways can (stem)
- we (owner of problem)
- improve (action)
- response time to reduce how long marketing analysts must wait for an answer to an inquiry? (goal)[21]

The invitational stem "In what ways can we . . . ?" encourages a divergent response, rather than the more narrow "How . . . ?" Divergent means thinking in different directions or searching for a variety of answers to a question that may have many right answers.[22]

The problem statement should have other attributes as well. Ideally, the problem definition phase has identified the root cause, which is reflected in the problem statement. If the problem statement reflects only a symptom, then the problem must be "solved" again and again. A clinical simile is the symptomatic relief that aspirin gives flu sufferers; they feel better, but the cause is uncured. Sometimes, the root cause of the problem cannot be determined, or, even if the root cause is known, resources may be insufficient to solve it. Occasionally, it is politically infeasible to solve the root cause. There may be many reasons why addressing symptoms is the only realistic choice. Doing so, however, must be seen for what it is—a temporary, expedient solution.

The problem statement should be narrow enough so that solving it lies within the problem solver's authority, resource limits, and the like, but not so narrow that only the symptoms are "treated." For example, certain employees seem to be taking too many coffee breaks. A narrow problem statement focuses on the employees. A somewhat broader problem statement addresses coffee breaks or breaks in general. An even broader problem statement, but one that is not too broad, identifies the ef-fi̇ ḣ ṁ̇ ṁ̇ ṁ̇ḟ ḋ̇ṁ̇ ṁ̇ ṁ̇ ṁ̇ ṁ̇ḋ̇ḋ̇ ṀṀ̇ Ṁ̇ḋ̇ḋ̇. ḟ̇ḋ̇ḋ̇ṁ̇ḋ̇ ṁ̇ ṁ̇ ṁ̇ṁ̇ṁ̇ ṁ̇ ṁ̇ ṁ̇ ṁ̇ ṁ̇ ṁ̇ ṁ̇ ṁ̇, ṁ̇ḋ̇ ṁ̇ root cause.

The breadth of the problem statement also determines the clarity of direction that is given the problem solver. Narrow problem statements identify clearly what problem needs solving but risk addressing only a symptom. Overly broad problem statements may leave the problem solver without clear direction—no understanding of the first step. Sometimes problems are amorphous or lack specificity, especially as to knowing where to start. Organizational malaise or morale problems are amorphous. Here, problem solvers must cast their nets widely and engage in several iterations of problem solving—from the very broad to the more narrow and specific—before the problem is identified. Iterative problem solving also is known as heuristic problem solving.

The psychological stimulus that is provided by an action orientation should not be underestimated. Problem statements include positive goals but also may include limitations. The problem statement regarding coffee breaks described earlier could be "In what ways can I(we) solve the problem of excessive coffee breaks by staff so as to maximize use of staff resources, but without damaging morale?" Here, a limitation in the solution is avoiding damage to morale.

There is more than one correct way to state a problem, but doing it well requires thought and the patience to prepare more than one iteration. The importance of developing a problem statement lies in the discipline of reducing thoughts to writing and the advantages of a written document in communicating to others who are working to solve the problem. As the great American educator, John Dewey, stated, "A question well put is half answered."[23]

Facts and Reasoning

A fact can be defined as an actuality, certainty, reality, or truth. Facts are highly prized and provide the firmest grounding for problem solving and decision making. Some facts are objectively verifiable. Many "facts" are subject to dispute, however, unless they result from an operational definition. Deming stressed the importance of operational definitions.[24] Objectively verifiable facts or facts that are based on the same operational definition take precedence over all other types of information.

Once facts have been identified, two other issues arise. One is the weight to be given to them. Obviously, some facts are more important than others, and people who share problem-solving responsibilities must understand how facts are weighted. A second issue is that facts are subject to judgment and interpretation. For example, a tape measure will gauge a room's dimensions. Whether the room is large enough for a job that needs to be done is a matter of opinion. The fact that the room has seating does not answer the question of how comfortable the seating is. Decision makers must be able to separate fact from judgment, interpretation, and opinion and not allow them to merge.

Rarely are facts sufficient to solve a problem, however. One way for problem solvers to overcome this deficit is through inductive and deductive reasoning. Inductive reasoning moves from the single event or fact to a conclusion or generalization based on that event. Inductive reasoning allows one to conclude that the fact of a painted wall means that there was a painter. Deductive reasoning uses the facts of related or similar events to reach a conclusion. A kind of deductive reasoning is used in criminology when circumstantial evidence is used to prove a person's guilt, despite lack of direct evidence from a witness. Circumstantial evidence is based on inferences (deductions) that are drawn from facts. A deduction from finding room after room with half-painted walls is that the work of the painter(s) is undone.

Developing Assumptions [2]

The problem statement developed in problem analysis [1] is the focus of the next step, developing assumptions [2]. Assumptions never take the place of facts. When facts are insufficient, however, problem solvers use inductive and deductive reasoning to make assumptions. Only in the most unusual circumstances should problem solvers make assumptions that are unsupported by logic because doing so means that they were determined capriciously, which is certainly not a basis for good management. Most often, assumptions are based on extending what is known. For example, if every time a nurse is fired there are rumors that the nurses will unionize, deductive reasoning tells us that the same thing is likely to happen next time. This, then, is a logically supportable assumption.

Assumptions have a significant effect on the choice and quality of the solution and, as a result, on the quality of problem solving. In general, assumptions are of three types: structural, personal, and problem centered.[25]

Structural assumptions relate to the context of the problem. In a sense they are boundary assumptions: The problem lies within (or outside) a manager's authority; additional resources are (or are not) available to solve the problem; other departments cause the problem; or the problem is caused by an uncontrollable external factor—high unemployment in the service area means fewer people have employer-based health insurance to pay for elective procedures. Some of these examples may be facts, depending on the situation.

Personal assumptions are conclusions and biases that managers bring to the problem. They often are based on experience. Managers may have a high or low tolerance for the risk and uncertainty inherent in changes that invariably result from problem solving. A manager who previously worked in HSOs/HSs in which problem solving was equated with blame may be risk averse and may make assumptions about the problem or alternatives that cause selection of low-risk solutions. Also, assumptions may be made about the likely reaction of superiors, subordinates, or stakeholders to potential solutions. Personal biases, two of which are anchoring and escalating commitment, also may affect problem solving. Anchoring occurs when the individual "chooses a starting point (an 'anchor'), perhaps from past data, and then adjusts from the anchor based on new information."[26] An inaccurate anchor causes flawed analysis. The personal bias of escalating commitment means that a manager is unwilling to admit a previous mistake. Managers whose decisions have become a problem "tend to be locked into a previously chosen course of action."[27]

Problem-centered assumptions cover a wide range, including perceived relative importance of the problem, degree of risk posed by the problem, and how urgently a solution is needed. Other problem-centered assumptions include economic and political costs, the degree to which subordinates or superiors will accept solutions, and the likelihood of success if a solution is implemented.

It is important to emphasize that the three types of assumptions affect the decision maker and the problem-solving process differently. Assumptions differ in at least two ways: qualitatively and in the amount of control that decision makers have over them. For example, a structural assumption that no funds are available to solve a problem profoundly affects the solutions that can be considered, and there may be little or nothing the decision maker can do to remedy the lack of funds. A personal assumption in which the decision maker recognizes an aversion to risk can be overcome to some extent, even though the decision maker may remain less willing to accept certain solutions or continues to be reluctant to experience higher levels of discomfort. Problem-centered assumptions are likely to involve more judgment, which often is based on the decision maker's experience, hunch, or intuition, than are structural assumptions.

In summary, making assumptions is necessary to most problem solving. Decision makers must use caution in formulating and accepting assumptions because, if this is done poorly, assumptions can limit the scope of problem solving or even preclude identifying the best solution.[28]

Identifying Tentative Alternative Solutions [3]

Once the manager has recognized, defined, and analyzed the problem, established its cause(s) and parameters, prepared a problem statement [1], and made assumptions [2], tentative alternative solutions are developed [3]. In Figure 7.4 this step includes identifying tentative alternative solutions [3a], collecting data/information [3b], if necessary, and evaluating the merits of each tentative alternative [3c] for an initial accept–reject decision. The initial accept–reject decision uses general criteria such as whether the tentative solution is unethical or illegal; is inconsistent with organizational values, mission, vision, and culture; has unacceptable financial or political costs; or is infeasible. If no tentative alternatives meet these general criteria, the step is repeated. Unique, nontraditional, and creative tentative solutions are identified more readily if structural, personal, and problem-centered assumptions are not overly restrictive.

Identifying tentative solutions is very important because it consumes more resources than any other problem-solving activity and because, if creativity occurs, it must occur here.[29] It is in the tentative alternative loop that creativity is important.[30] Although the terms often are used synonymously, *creativity*—defined as imagination and ingenuity—should be distinguished from the narrower concept of *innovation,* defined as changing or transforming.[31] Figure 7.5 shows this distinction.

Several categories or tactics that can be used to identify ideas for solutions have been described.[32] Regrettably, most do not suggest creativity as a source. "Ready-made" tactics assume that organizations have a store of fully developed solutions—a situation in which solutions wait for problems. "Search" tactics identify solutions from available ideas. Proposals are elicited and compared to identify solutions that seem viable. A "design" tactic seeks a custom-made solution—an opportunity for creativity.

Several factors influence the time and resources that are devoted to the tentative alternative solution loop. Most important are the quality and precision of the initial problem definition and the

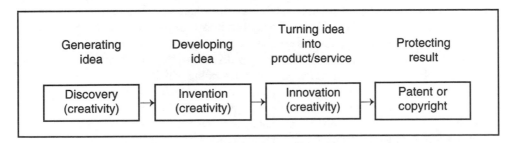

Figure 7.5.   Differentiation of discovery/invention/innovation. (Adapted from Cougar, Daniel J. *Creative Problem Solving and Opportunity Finding,* 18. Danvers, MA: Boyd & Fraser, 1995; reprinted by permission.)

restrictiveness of assumptions. Others include sophistication of the HSO's/HS's information systems, availability of data, and the degree to which the problem is structured. Unstructured problems are more complex, involve many variables, and take longer to solve than problems that are simple, relatively obvious, or narrowly defined.

The tentative alternative solution loop has two hazards. Some managers spend excessive time and resources seeking the optimal solution when another solution is acceptable. In addition, extensive attention to activities in the loop and reiteration may be an excuse for not taking action. "I need more information" may be an excuse to procrastinate and make no decision.[33]

Developing and Applying Decision Criteria [4]

The alternatives that met the general criteria applied in the tentative alternative solution loop [3] are now ready for formal assessment. To select the best of several alternatives, managers must develop decision criteria that allow alternative solutions to be evaluated and compared [4]. The decision criteria include those in the "Desired Outcomes" cell in the center of Figure 7.4: individual and organizational work results, objectives, standards, and expectations. At least three other decision criteria usually are applied: effectiveness of the alternative in solving the problem, feasibility of implementation, and acceptability of the alternative based on objective and subjective analyses.[34]

Alternatives that are not effective in solving the problem should be rejected. Examples are alternatives that solve only part of a problem, address only symptoms, or are not permanent. Exceptions may be necessary, however. For example, if the need for action is critical, then it may be appropriate to select and implement a less-than-effective solution because the consequences of doing nothing or waiting for a better solution are worse.

The feasibility of implementing an alternative is the second common criterion. Alternatives that are infeasible will be rejected in the tentative alternative solution loop. Those that survive may be implemented to varying degrees in terms of effort; structural boundaries and constraints; dependence on other people, departments, or both; and costs. Managers are less likely to select an alternative that depends on people and departments beyond their control. This is especially true if high political costs are associated with forcing implementation.

The third common criterion judges the effective use of resources, including quantitative (objective) cost–benefit analysis and assessment of nonquantitative (subjective) advantages and disadvantages. Lowest cost should not be a sole criterion—costs *and* benefits of alternatives must be considered, as should the opportunity costs of doing nothing. Objective evaluation means quantifying costs and benefits and should be attempted, despite the difficulty of estimating some data. Subjective evaluation means understanding advantages and disadvantages that may be impossible to quantify but cannot be ignored. Both types of assessment should be considered when evaluating and comparing alternatives. If an alternative is costly but the problem solver concludes that subjective considerations are more important, then a rational decision has been made.

Some decision criteria are likely to be more important than others in a given situation; several methods may be used to differentiate them. One method rank orders decision criteria using decision-maker judgments. Another method divides criteria into "mandatory" (must be met) and "wanted." A solution that does not meet a "mandatory" criterion is discarded. "Wanted" criteria are weighted by degree of desirability. The resulting weighted scores determine which solution is selected.[35] A third method assumes that all decision criteria are equally important (which is unlikely) and judges how closely or well each alternative meets them and assigns a numerical value. The highest total determines which alternative is chosen. A decision matrix is an excellent tool for arraying and comparing decision criteria and solutions. Table 7.1 presents a sample decision matrix.

The virtues of numerically weighting decision criteria include forcing decision makers to compare and evaluate them and providing a basis for discussion in group decision making. It is impor-

TABLE 7.1. DECISION MATRIX FOR EVALUATING ALTERNATIVE SOLUTIONS[a]

Decision criteria	Alternative solution 1	Alternative solution 2	Alternative solution 3
Must meet these requirements			
1. Solution effectively solves the problem	3	5	5
2. Feasibility of implementation	5	3	5
3. Cost–benefit analysis	5	5	3
4. Advantage–disadvantage analysis	3	3	5
Want to meet these requirements			
5. Political acceptability	1	3	3
6. Criticalness	1	3	5
7. Time frame	1	3	5
8. Opportunity costs	5	1	3
9. Monetary costs	3	5	5
Total score	27	31	39

Conclusion: Alternative solution 3 accepted.
Adapted from Arnold, John D. *The Complete Problem Solver: A Total System for Competitive Decision Making*, 62. New York: John Wiley & Sons, 1992.
[a]Key:
5 = Solution *fully* meets decision criterion.
3 = Solution *partially* meets decision criterion.
1 = Solution *fails* to meet decision criterion.

tant that the numbers are understood to be the results of judgments by decision makers, judgments that could be challenged by reasonable people. This basis in subjectivity means that the numbers are, at best, approximations. This must be borne in mind during analysis.

As noted earlier, this step is sometimes called decision analysis. Most often decision makers have several alternative solutions that can be used; it is a matter of determining which one best (fully or partially) meets the decision criteria. There are, however, other variations of decision analysis. Sometimes, there is only one solution and a yes–no, accept–reject decision must be made. Here, the analysis compares the proposed solution to a reasonable (perhaps idealized) model of what could or should be done to determine whether the proposal is acceptable. At other times there are no alternatives, and the decision maker must decide how to accomplish a desired result. Here, the first step is to clearly define the objectives. Then, a set of components that will most feasibly and effectively meet those objectives is selected from all of the available components.[36]

Selecting, Implementing, and Evaluating the Alternative Solution [5, 6, and 7]

Almost always a manager selects an alternative (makes a decision) [5] and implements it [6]. This does not end problem solving, however. The effects of the intervention (change) must be monitored [7] to determine whether they are consistent with desired results [1]. If they are, then the problem is solved. If they are not, then the problem-solving cycle begins again, perhaps fine-tuning the alternative implemented, reconsidering alternatives previously rejected, or developing new ones. Furthermore, solving one problem often causes others. For example, decreasing average length of stay has implications for revenue; thus another problem arises. Implementation and evaluation must be planned. Evaluation, especially, often is neglected—busy managers turn to new problems, assuming that the solution selected and implemented is effective. This may or may not be the case, but it is especially problematic when the root cause is unsolved. Evaluation should be part of implementation. Data collection must be specific, especially as to who is responsible for it, and built into process and outcome monitoring.

Implications for the Health Services Manager

Problem solving is a major responsibility of health services managers. When done effectively, resource allocation and consumption are superior and results are more consistent with those desired. Managers' skills in problem solving, including decision making, are directly reflected in the quality of solutions and interventions.

FACTORS INFLUENCING PROBLEM SOLVING AND DECISION MAKING

Problem solving and decision making do not occur in a vacuum; many factors shape how they are performed, the style that is used, and the outcome. Figure 7.6 shows three groups of factors: 1) attributes of the problem solver, 2) nature of the situation, and 3) characteristics of the environment.[37] These affect all steps of problem solving and decision making.

Problem-Solver Attributes

Experience, Knowledge, and Judgment

Among the most important attributes affecting problem solving are the experience, knowledge, and judgment of the decision maker. The training, knowledge, and experience of clinical staff such as physicians, nurses, and pharmacists are essential to high-quality patient care and are attributes that are recognized by licensing and certification. Health services managers are formally educated in graduate programs and informally educated through continuing education and in-service training. Their education is tempered and tested in administrative residencies and by initial work experience. Knowledge and experience are not sufficient, however. Sound judgment must be added to the mix to achieve effective problem solving. Sometimes, intuition and hunches are important.

Perspective, Personality, and Biases

The problem solver's perspective and personality influence problem solving and decision making. Decision-maker biases were discussed in the previous section on assumptions and warrant further attention here.

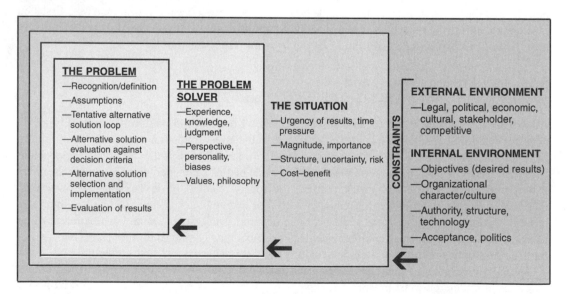

Figure 7.6.   Factors influencing problem solving and decision making.

Perspective determines how the problem solver views a problem or situation. Problem solvers with narrow perspectives (tunnel vision) and who think vertically rather than horizontally approach problems differently and are likely to make lower-quality decisions.[38] The conclusions and biases that were discussed in the section on personal assumptions are extensions of perspective. Perspective is the manager's general outlook; however, biases also affect problem solving, and making assumptions allows a decision maker to understand their effect on a specific situation.

Personality traits such as temperament, aggressiveness, self-centeredness, self-assurance, and self-confidence, as well as demeanor (introvert or extravert) and tolerance for risk, change, uncertainty, or instability, influence how managers solve problems and the quality of their decisions. Nonassertive, introverted, procrastinating people who are averse to risk and fearful of change are likely to make assumptions or select solutions that limit the range of problem solving. Such managers are less creative in the tentative alternative solution loop, stay in it longer as they search for the best solution (or implicitly hope the problem will dissipate), and make compromises or less bold decisions. Often, such people are reactive and must be forced to act. Conversely, proactive people take the initiative, anticipate problems, manage events rather than being managed by them, and get the job done. This type of manager is more inclined to make difficult, bold, progressive, or nontraditional decisions.

Values and Philosophy

Values and philosophy influence problem solving in two ways. Personal morals and ethics affect assumptions and define acceptable alternatives. Those that are inconsistent with the problem solver's value system are excluded. Managers with a self-centered personal ethic make decisions that provide short-term and self-serving benefit but that may be inconsistent with or even detrimental to the long-term good of the HSO/HS. A personal philosophy includes views on politics and policy issues, as well as on leadership and motivation. The manager's personal philosophy and values can limit the alternatives considered and influence the approach to problem solving.

The Situation

The circumstances and facts of a problem influence the problem-solving process and outcome. Those identified in Figure 7.6 are the urgency of results, time pressure, magnitude and importance of the problem, degree of structure, uncertainty, and risk, and costs versus benefits.

Urgency of Results and Time Pressures

Sometimes immediate decisions are required because delay is costly. Trauma or medical crises are examples. An impending work stoppage, a major initiative by a competitor, or inadequate cash flow requires action more quickly than do other situations because such problems have significant consequences. They necessitate rapid use of the tentative alternative solution loop and an evaluation process that is likely to be less thorough. In situations with little time pressure, such as problem solving under conditions of opportunity, noncrisis deviation, or improvement, problem solvers use a decision style that involves consultation, collecting more information, and thoroughly evaluating alternatives.

Magnitude and Importance

The problem's magnitude and importance directly affect the time, energy, and resources spent in assessing it and making a decision. For example, administrative decisions warrant greater attention and more intense evaluation than do operational decisions. The cost implications of resource commitment and opportunity costs of delay are other measures of importance.

Problems with high cost or resource commitment (e.g., those being addressed under conditions of opportunity or improvement) justify spending more time and collecting more information in the tentative alternative solution loop than do low-cost problems. The same is true for unstructured problems. A potential hazard for managers is that resources such as time consumed to find the best solution may approach or exceed the cost consequences of the problem. It is senseless to spend $15,000 on staff time for feasibility studies and collection of nonroutine data to solve a medical records storage problem when old records can be stored offsite. Obviously, the cost of developing alternatives must not exceed the benefits of the one that is selected. Conversely, a freestanding HSO in financial distress would appropriately spend more time and resources evaluating an acquisition offer by a HS.

Structure, Uncertainty, and Risk

From a problem-solving perspective, structure is the clarity of the situation—the degree to which the scope and nature of problem and alternatives are precise.[39] Ends–means, administrative, and non-programmable decision situations are less structured than are operational or programmable situations. Problems regarding equipment and material, job design, and process flow are more structured than are those with behavioral dynamics or with external stakeholders and competitors. Risk is a function of certainty. A problem that is certain is one for which the manager has complete information and can predict the outcomes of alternative solutions. Less information means greater risk because even carefully derived estimates have a degree of uncertainty. For example, certainty of negative results approaches 100% if mismatched blood is transfused. Certainty is much less than 100% if the problem-solving process determines that establishing a freestanding family practice center will provide inpatient referrals to a hospital. The more unstructured and uncertain the situation, the greater the time spent and resources allocated and the more participative the problem-solving and decision-making processes are likely to be.

Cost–Benefit

Ultimately, problem solving means selecting an alternative, which will be based partly on quantitative cost–benefit or nonquantitative advantage–disadvantage criteria, or both. Many problems are suited to cost–benefit analysis: What equipment most improves productivity and decreases patient waiting time? Which new service will increase revenues most? Will more nursing staff (cost) decrease length of stay (benefit)? Sometimes costs and benefits cannot be measured, or nonquantitative criteria may be more important. In fact, an alternative should be chosen only when both quantitative and nonquantitative decision criteria are used. Excluding either diminishes the quality of the decision.

The Environment

The HSO's/HS's environments influence managerial problem solving by imposing variables that management may be unable to control, affecting the feasibility of alternatives, and constraining implementation of the solution selected.

External

Legal, political, economic, cultural, stakeholder, competitive, and similar external forces are always present. A requirement to obtain a certificate of need for facility expansion or a new service constrains alternatives. High local unemployment with loss of employer-paid health insurance adversely affects revenues and increases bad debts. Unfunded federal mandates and regulations constrain health systems with a managed care component. Changes in Medicare and Medicaid payments may limit the organization's ability to add technology and equipment.

Internal

Environmental factors within the HSO/HS affect problem solving more directly. Organizational objectives restrict alternatives that can be considered. Influential but less precise is organizational character/culture—the embedded and permeating values and beliefs. Each organizational culture is unique. It may be creative or traditional, assertive or restrained, proactive or reactive, friendly or distant. Such characteristics influence problem solving. Managers in a reactive, tradition-bound culture are unlikely to select bold solutions. Similarly, managers in an action-oriented culture tend to act quickly, with less preparation. Finally, any alternative that is considered must be consistent with the organization's character/culture.

As managers apply decision criteria to the alternatives, they must consider implementation, which is affected by an array of factors ranging from resource availability to organizational commitment. Noteworthy factors are authority, structure, and technology. An alternative whose implementation is beyond the scope of the manager's authority may not be feasible. The president of the professional staff organization has no authority to change the HSO/HS information system; the CEO has no authority to discharge a patient.

Organizational configuration (structure) may make implementing one alternative infeasible; absence of a technology may eliminate another. For example, physical plant layout may preclude changing patient care work flow, union contracts may constrain job definition and design, or the computer system may not allow online connection to nursing units.

Another influence that is essential to successfully implementing an alternative is acceptance by superiors, peers, and subordinates. A decision to decrease inpatient length of stay by reducing turnaround time for diagnostic testing will be difficult to implement if those who read and interpret tests are resistant. Involving others in problem solving is influenced by how important their acceptance is to implementation. Moreover, organizational politics influence problem solving and its results. The degree of informal influence, conflict, and competition among factions may cause a manager to negotiate, collaborate, compromise, or "satisfice" (find a workable, if imperfect, solution) when solving problems.

Implications for the Health Services Manager

Problem-solver attributes, the nature of the situation, and the environment influence problem solving—how it is done, the time and resources consumed, and quality of the decision. These influences are not mutually exclusive, and one may supersede or preempt others. An urgent situation can force the manager who usually seeks input, develops a range of alternatives, and does extensive evaluation to act quickly and unilaterally.

Health services managers should recognize and be sensitive to the factors that affect problem solving, change their methods as appropriate, modify and mitigate detrimental influences when possible, and learn to cope with those factors that cannot be changed. Doing so will improve the quality of problem solving.

UNILATERAL AND GROUP PROBLEM SOLVING

In meeting their accountabilities for resource allocation and utilization, managers may solve problems and make decisions unilaterally, or they may involve superiors, peers, or subordinates on a continuum from minimal or consultative to group participation. Both methods have advantages and disadvantages. Consultative problem solving is intraorganizational in a freestanding HSO and interorganizational in a HS. Chapter 13 discusses the ethical aspects of problem solving and decision making.

Unilateral problem solving is efficient, whereas group problem solving raises overhead costs considerably.[40] Unilateral action avoids groupthink (extreme group conformity) and risky shift, which are negative aspects of group problem solving. Anchoring and escalating commitment are more likely in unilateral than group decision making.

Groups exert social pressure to conform and concur with decisions. Groupthink occurs when

> *team members: discount warnings about what others (competitors) may do; fail to examine criti-*
> *cal and underlying assumptions; stereotype others; put heavy pressure on dissenters; self-censor;*
> *share an illusion of unanimity; and stop the flow of information contrary to the group's position*
> *through self-appointed mindguards.*[41]

Others have observed that "Groupthink has been a primary cause of major corporate- and public-policy debacles. And although it may seem counterintuitive, . . . the teams that engaged in healthy conflict over issues not only made better decisions but moved more quickly as well."[42] The Watergate political scandal of the 1970s is the classical example of political groupthink.[43] The phenomenon of risky shift is a hazard of group problem solving. It occurs because the diffused responsibility of a group encourages acceptance of riskier decisions than would be acceptable to one person who is responsible for a decision.[44]

As a general rule, however, group problem solving produces better-quality solutions. The reasons are numerous. Multiple perspectives and more information and experience are brought to bear. Knowledgeable staff, especially subordinates, can help define a problem and identify tentative alternative solutions. Involving staff with process knowledge is essential to successful quality improvement. Group problem solving results in consideration of more alternatives because overly restrictive assumptions are likely to be challenged. Furthermore, involving others enhances acceptance and facilitates implementation because those involved take ownership and usually are more committed to implementation. Finally, group problem solving heightens communication and coordination because those involved in implementation have greater knowledge about the solution and the process that produced it.

The benefits of employee participation in problem solving and decision making are well documented in the behavioral science literature. Involved employees identify with the HSO/HS and its actions. Kaluzny's model of involvement and commitment has two foci that are especially useful in quality improvement.[45] First, senior-level managers must rethink problem-solving activities to increase the roles, responsibilities, and authority of middle-level managers. Second, middle-level managers must rethink superior–subordinate relationships so that greater involvement of subordinates in problem solving will increase their commitment to HSO/HS objectives. Staff participation in complex decisions adds expertise, which facilitates work unit performance and enhances commitment to the organization.[46]

Group Problem-Solving and Quality Improvement Techniques

Certain conditions must exist for group problem solving to be effective. First, a climate of openness must permit the free expression of ideas; the focus must be on reaching solutions rather than fault finding.[47] Second, participation must be legitimate—subordinates involved in problem solving must believe that managers are truly interested in the group's reasonable recommendations. This is called "empowering" because subordinates actually influence decisions.[48] Problem solving based on staff expertise about their work will result in better solutions; greater employee involvement and commitment to the HSO/HS will lead to higher motivation, morale, and job satisfaction.[49] Given the opportunity, employees can contribute significantly to solving problems.

Quality Circles

A failed group problem-solving method that held significant promise for improving productivity and quality in health services delivery was quality circles, which were especially common in nursing.

Quality circles are a parallel-structure approach to involving employees in problem solving. A parallel structure is one that is separate and distinct from the regular, ongoing activities of an organization and, as such, operates in a special way. In quality circle programs, groups are composed of volunteers from a work area who meet with a special type of leader and/or facilitator for the purpose of examining productivity and quality problems.[50]

For quality circles to be effective, senior-level management had to be committed to both the process and its outcomes. Staff time and employee training in problem solving were some of the substantial resources required. Management had to be willing to act on appropriate recommendations. It is generally believed that quality circles failed because management did not make a commitment to them, and this suggested that their efforts were unimportant.

Other Group Formats

Quality circles were one type of group problem solving. Ad hoc task forces may be formed to solve significant organizationwide problems or to address unstructured, major problems under conditions of opportunity or threat. Focus group teams[51] or quality improvement teams can be used. These teams may be departmental or cross-functional. As the name suggests, departmental teams are active in processes exclusive to a department, much as were quality circles. Cross-functional teams improve processes or undertake other quality improvement initiatives that span the organization and hierarchical levels. Chapter 9 provides detail on quality improvement teams. Finally, managers should encourage problem solving by subordinates, and assist them as necessary. This may involve one or several subordinates in a group; it need not be formalized or institutionalized, as are quality circles and quality improvement teams.

PROBLEM-SOLVING AND DECISION-MAKING STYLES

The manager's problem-solving and decision-making styles may involve individuals or groups. Style is influenced by the problem's nature and importance, how clearly it can be defined, and whether acceptance by organization members is key to implementation.

Involving Others—A Conceptual Model

A conceptual model of problem-solving/decision-making styles developed by Vroom is useful in determining the degree and conditions of involvement by others.[52] The five problem-solving and decision-making styles shown in Table 7.2 specify subordinate involvement, but they also are applicable to peers and superiors. Each style describes a different degree of subordinate involvement.[53] Style AI is unilateral (autocratic)—subordinates are not involved in predecision assessment or choosing the solution. AII is a variant of AI—subordinates only provide information. Managers using consultative styles CI or CII elicit and consider subordinates' opinions. GII is a group style that involves subordinates fully, and the manager accepts the group's decision. There are situations in which the quality of a decision and its acceptance by subordinates are enhanced with group problem solving. The styles and model in Figure 7.7 also are discussed in Chapter 15.

Situational Variables (Problem Attributes)

The situational variables influencing style are characterized by the seven different problem attributes (*a–g*) at the top of Figure 7.7. The problem-solving style outcomes in Figure 7.7 have capital letter notations AI, AII, CI, CII, or GII. The first four problem attributes, *a–d*, denote the importance of decision quality and acceptance by others. The last three problem attributes, *e–g*, moderate the effects of subordinate participation on quality and acceptance (*a–d*). The seven problem attributes in Figure 7.7 are repeated in Table 7.3, along with diagnostic questions requiring yes-or-no answers.

TABLE 7.2. MANAGEMENT PROBLEM-SOLVING AND DECISION-MAKING STYLES

AI	The manager solves the problem or makes the decision unilaterally, using information available at that time.
AII	The manager obtains necessary information from subordinate(s), then develops and selects the solution unilaterally. Subordinates may or may not be told what the problem is when the manager gets information from them. Subordinates provide necessary information rather than generating or evaluating alternative solutions.
CI	The manager shares the problem with relevant subordinates individually, getting their ideas and suggestions without bringing them together. The manager's decision may or may not reflect the subordinates' contribution.
CII	The manager shares the problem with subordinates as a group, obtains their ideas and suggestions, and then makes the decision that may or may not reflect the subordinates' contribution.
GII	The manager shares the problem with subordinates as a group. Together they generate and evaluate alternatives and attempt to reach agreement (consensus) on a solution. The manager's role is much like that of chairperson—not trying to influence the group to adopt a particular solution. The manager is willing to accept and implement any solution supported by the group.

Situations and Styles

Answers to the diagnostic questions for the seven problem attributes in Table 7.3 produce 14 possible situations, which are identified as 1–14 in Figure 7.7. Each is linked with the appropriate problem-solving/decision-making style AI–GII. Vroom assumes that managers wish to minimize the time that is required to solve a problem; thus each style is the most restrictive for that set of problem attributes. For example, a manager with Situation 1 could use Styles AII, CI, CII, or GII, but they require more time. Therefore, the problem attributes suggest that AI is appropriate and saves time compared with less-restrictive styles.

Using the Model

The manager assesses the situation by examining problem attributes *a–g* and answering the questions "yes" or "no." The model indicates which decision style (AI–GII) is most appropriate. The following discussion analyzes the branching for Situations 1, 2, 3, 11, 12, 13, and 14 to show how managers could use the model.

Situations 1, 2, and 3

Situations 1, 2, and 3 assume that there is no decision quality requirement [a]. The presence of several obvious, relatively meritorious alternatives implies that the decision maker has sufficient information [b] to solve the problem unilaterally. Thus the problem must be relatively structured [c]. If subordinate acceptance of the decision is not critical to implementation [d], the manager is correct in using unilateral Style AI for Situation 1 (1-AI in Figure 7.7). If subordinate acceptance is critical to implementation, Attribute *e* is evaluated. If subordinates are likely to accept the unilateral decision, the manager can use Style AI for Situation 2 (2-AI in Figure 7.7).

If subordinates are unlikely to accept the manager's decision, as in Situation 3, the Style GII is appropriate (3-GII in Figure 7.7) because participation increases acceptance. Also, the manager is indifferent as to which alternative solution is chosen because there is no quality requirement and all are relatively meritorious [a].

Situations 11, 12, 13, and 14

Situations 11, 12, 13, and 14 assume that there is a quality requirement [a], meaning that alternatives are not equally acceptable because one is more rational. Situations 11, 12, 13, and 14 also assume that the manager has insufficient information to make high-quality decisions [b] and that the problem is not structured [c].

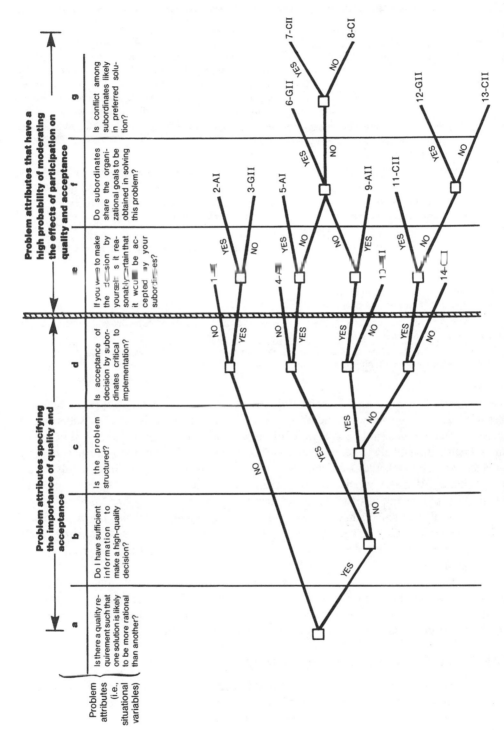

Figure 7.7. Problem-solving and decision-making style model. (Adapted from Vroom, Victor H. "A New Look at Managerial Decision Making." *Organizational Dynamics* 1 [Spring 1973]: 66–80; reprinted by permission. © 1973. American Management Association, New York. All rights reserved.)

TABLE 7.3.   PROBLEM ATTRIBUTES USED IN THE PROBLEM-SOLVING AND DECISION-MAKING STYLE MODEL (FIGURE 7.7)

Problem attributes	Diagnostic questions
a. Importance of the quality of the decision	Is quality requirement such that one solution is likely to be more rational (better) than another? (Another way of discerning the quality is: If the alternatives are *not* equally meritorious—some are or can be much better than others—there is a quality requirement.)
b. Extent to which the decision maker possesses sufficient information/expertise to make a high-quality decision unilaterally	Do I have sufficient information to make a high-quality decision?
c. Extent to which problem is structured	Is problem structured? (Does decision maker know what information is needed and where to find it?)
d. Extent to which acceptance or commitment of subordinates is critical to effective implementation	Is acceptance of decision by subordinates critical to effective implementation?
e. Prior probability that a unilateral decision will receive acceptance by subordinates	If decision is made unilaterally, will it probably be accepted by subordinates?
f. Extent to which subordinates are motivated to attain organizational goals as represented in objectives explicit in statement of problem	Do subordinates share organizational goals to be obtained in solving problems?
g. Extent to which subordinates are likely to be in conflict over preferred solutions	Is conflict among subordinates likely to occur in preferred solutions?

Adapted from Vroom, Victor H. "A New Look at Managerial Decision Making." *Organizational Dynamics* 1 (Spring 1973): 66–80; reprinted by permission. © 1973. American Management Association, New York. All rights reserved.

If the attribute of subordinate acceptance [*d*] is critical to implementation, then the manager determines whether subordinates would be likely to accept a unilateral decision [*e*]. If subordinates would accept a unilateral decision, then Style CII is appropriate for Situation 11 (11-CII in Figure 7.7). If subordinates are unlikely to accept a unilateral decision (i.e., the answer to Attribute *e* is no), then the manager assesses whether subordinates share the organizational goals met by solving the problem—Attribute *f*. If the answer is yes, Style GII is appropriate (12-GII in Figure 7.7). Group involvement is appropriate because the acceptance that is critical to implementing the alternative is enhanced. Because all participants have the same goals, the group cannot make a decision that is different from the decision the manager would have made. However, if the answer to Attribute *f* is no (i.e., subordinates do not share the organizational goals met by solving the problem), then Style CII is appropriate for Situation 13 (13-CII in Figure 7.7).

If the attribute of subordinate acceptance [*d*] is not critical to implementation, then the consultative Style CII is appropriate for Situation 14 (14-CII in Figure 7.7). Here, sharing the problem with subordinates and obtaining their ideas and suggestions provide information that the manager needs, yet the decision that is made need not reflect subordinates' influence.

Implications for the Health Services Manager

The problem-solving and decision-making style model in Figure 7.7 is an algorithm to assist in selecting the decision style that is appropriate for different conditions. Although linked here to the degree of subordinate involvement in problem solving, analyses of peer or superior involvement could use the same model. In addition, it is important to remember that individual, situational, and environmental variables influence decision style. Vroom's model provides a systematic way to determine the involvement of others in decision making and how that involvement affects the quality of the solution and the success of implementation.

SUMMARY

This chapter focuses on managerial problem solving and decision making in HSOs/HSs. Problem solving is continuously undertaken by managers to make outcomes of organizational activities consistent with desired results. Problem solving and decision making are distinguished, and types of managerial decisions are described. Figure 7.4, the hub of this chapter, presents the problem-solving steps of analyzing the problem, developing assumptions, identifying tentative alternative solutions, developing and applying decision criteria, selecting an alternative, and implementing and evaluating results. The attributes of each step and the implications for the manager are discussed.

Several factors influence the problem-solving process and quality of outcome: characteristics of the problem solver, such as experience and values; elements of the situation, such as the urgency of taking action and costs–benefits; the HSO's/HS's external environment, such as legal constraints and competition; and the HSO's/HS's internal environment, including objectives and culture.

Group problem solving is discussed. The participation of employees enhances the quality of defining and solving problems and increases their commitment. The problem-solving and decision-making style model includes questions that assist in determining levels of group involvement.

Skill in problem solving and decision making is critical. If health services managers understand the process, are aware of factors that influence it, and assess the appropriateness of subordinate, superior, or peer involvement, the quality of their decisions will be enhanced.

DISCUSSION QUESTIONS

1. Explain why decision making is a distinct management function and why it is linked to all other management functions. Identify the three managerial decision classifications and give examples of each.
2. What conditions initiate problem solving? Discuss how problem solving under the condition of improvement is related to problem solving under the condition of opportunity.
3. How are problem solving and decision making related? What predecision and postdecision activities are inherent in problem solving? What are the steps of problem solving?
4. Using the problem-solving process model in Figure 7.4, discuss and give examples of
   a. How assumptions affect problem solving
   b. Positive and negative results that can occur in the tentative alternative solution loop
   c. Why both quantitative and nonquantitative criteria are important when evaluating and choosing an alternative
5. Distinguish facts and assumptions. Give examples of the role of inductive and deductive reasoning in making assumptions.
6. Identify the factors that influence problem solving. Describe three situations and indicate which factors were influential in shaping the outcome.
7. What are the advantages of group problem solving? List reasons why it is critical to the success of organizationwide quality improvement. Describe a situation from your experience in which the phenomenon of groupthink occurred.
8. Identify the types of problem-solving and decision-making styles. Use Figure 7.7 and Table 7.3 to describe situations that show the following styles: AI, CI, and GII.

CASE STUDY 1: THE NURSING ASSISTANT

You are the supervisor on the day shift at a 100-bed nursing facility. In one 20-bed unit, the workload relative to other units has been very heavy for the past month. In that unit you observed family members of a bedbound resident turning the resident. When asked why they were doing that, one of the family members said, "Nursing assistant Johnson told us that the staff is too busy. If we want our father turned we have to do it ourselves, or wait 3 or 4 hours before the staff could help." On several occasions in the past week, you saw Johnson sitting in the utility room for what seemed to be long periods of time.

QUESTIONS

1. Identify the facts present in this case.
2. State the problem.
3. Make assumptions of the three types described in the chapter. List them in order of declining certainty.
4. Develop five solutions that should be considered. Which one should be chosen? Why?

CASE STUDY 2: THE NEW CHARGE NURSE

You are a third-shift (11:00 P.M. to 7:00 A.M.) nurse supervisor to whom several charge nurses report. Charge nurses are responsible for a nursing unit during evening and night shifts. Six months ago you promoted Sally Besnick to be one of the charge nurses on that shift. Six months before she was promoted, Besnick had earned a bachelor of science in nursing (B.S.N.) from an out-of-state university. She is the same age as the five registered nurses (R.N.) she supervises, all of whom graduated from a diploma program at a local hospital. Diploma programs emphasize much more "hands-on" experience than do B.S.N. programs. Sally is the only B.S.N. charge nurse who reports to you.

Besnick received the same in-service training in supervision as the other charge nurses, but there are major problems on her unit. Morale among her staff is low, absenteeism is high, and not all of the administrative work on the unit is getting done. There are no indications that the quality of care on her unit is below acceptable levels, however. You think Besnick's main difficulty is that she cannot control, lead, discipline, or correct her subordinates. She seems easygoing; her subordinates call her "Soft Sally" behind her back. They feel they can deliver technically better patient care than she can.

Besnick is personable and well liked by the other charge nurses and by you. She socializes with them after hours and has made it a point to participate in American Nurses Association professional activities, just like the other charge nurses. She and her husband just bought a new house in town after renting for the year she has worked at the hospital. They adopted a baby 2 months ago.

You are concerned that, if you demote Besnick, Besnick's pride will be hurt and she will quit. You do not want to lose a good R.N., especially one with a B.S.N.

QUESTIONS

1. Develop a problem statement. Identify several tentative alternative solutions.
2. Which solution is best? Why?
3. Describe how you would implement the solution chosen. How would you evaluate the results?

CASE STUDY 3: PREFERRED PROVIDER ORGANIZATION

You are the senior vice president and chief operating officer of Mercy Hospital, a 400-bed acute care hospital and medical center. The president of Mercy Hospital asked you to investigate what she thinks is a problem and to identify alternatives to solve it. The hospital's inpatient days, occupancy rate, ancillary services work units, and outpatient visits have been declining for a year; the president's estimate is at least 10% in each category. The president thinks that the cause is competition from a health maintenance organization (HMO) that was established a year ago and from two investor-owned freestanding emergency centers that opened 6 months ago. The two other hospitals in Lincoln City, a town of 300,000, have not done anything differently this year compared with the past. Uncollectible accounts have increased for them as well.

You know that the professional staff organization membership has changed little over the period, Mercy Hospital enjoys good media and stakeholder relations, there have been no quality problems, and Mercy's inpatient and outpatient charges are about 5% less than the other two hospitals. It seems that inpatient days and outpatient visits should have increased since the hospital completed a building expansion 6 months ago, especially because it added space to the outpatient department. In fact, it was completed ahead of schedule and under budget. The area's 13% unemployment rate allowed contractors to accelerate construction because skilled workers were readily available.

You are perplexed as to why there seems to be a problem. To your knowledge, the HMO has a contract with only one major manufacturer, whose employees and dependents represent fewer than 4% of the hospital's business.

You must submit your recommendation to the president in 2 weeks. You are considering calling a meeting of your subordinates, who include the vice president of patient care services (nursing service), two operations vice presidents, and the vice president of human resources. Two other individuals who report directly to the president could be invited to attend the meeting—the vice president for professional staff liaison and the chief financial officer. Your subordinates are united in purpose and it is easy to work with them. The two who report to the president see things differently from the way in which you do. They look at problems as they affect their areas of responsibility, not the hospital as a whole, and they do not always cooperate with you.

You have been thinking about recommending the formation of a preferred provider organization (PPO) under whose auspices the hospital would contract with solo and group practice fee-for-service physicians to provide inpatient and outpatient services at a contracted discounted rate. This program would be marketed to local businesses. You believe this arrangement would increase patient volume. In fact, as you think about it, you wonder if you need to hold that meeting.

QUESTIONS

1. Use the information in Figure 7.7 and Tables 7.2 and 7.3 to identify the problem-solving and decision-making style that you should use in solving the problem. Should the meeting be held? Why? Be prepared to discuss why you selected a particular style.

2. Assume that you unilaterally made a decision and recommended the PPO alternative to the president. Use the problem-solving model (Figure 7.4) to identify the activities that were not done or were not done well, and why.

CASE STUDY 4: THERE ARE HOURS AND THERE ARE HOURS

You are the vice president for support services at Sunrise Nursing and Rehabilitation Center. Frances "Frankie" Hammerman, the full-time coordinator of volunteers, reports to you. She has held that position for 6 months after working 10 years as a social worker in the social services department. Hammerman works alone and is responsible for recruiting, training, assigning, and monitoring the work of about 130 volunteers at the center.

Full-time center employees work 40 hours a week. Everyone, including managers, completes a time card biweekly. About a month ago, you took note of the fact that, whenever you called Hammerman after 2:00 P.M., you were connected with her voice mail. Although she called early the next working day, something seemed amiss. Out of curiosity, you reviewed her time cards for several months and noticed that she had entered 40 hours each week.

You asked Hammerman to meet with you. You are pleased with her work and began the meeting by telling her so. She was composed when you mentioned the apparent discrepancy between her time cards and availability. Without embarrassment, Hammerman tells you that she is efficient and her daily work is complete in less than 6 hours. She thought about slowing her pace and staying at her desk a full 8 hours, but she considered this dishonest. Hammerman believes that showing 8 hours worked each day on her time card is okay because she accomplishes the work of 8 hours in less time. Thus, when she is finished for the day, she goes home.

You reacted calmly, but with a sense of bewilderment—you have never heard such an explanation. Your first thought was to fire Hammerman because her actions seem blatantly dishonest.

QUESTIONS

1. State the problem.
2. Identify the facts in this case. What assumptions should be made?
3. Develop five alternative solutions.
4. Develop a set of decision criteria that should be used.

NOTES

1. Hayes, James L. In *The Manager's Book of Quotations,* edited by Lewis D. Eigen and Jonathan P. Siegel, 107. New York: American Management Association, 1989.
2. Drucker, Peter F. *An Introductory View of Management,* 396. New York: Harper's College Press, 1977; Pearce, John A., III, and Richard B. Robinson, Jr. *Management,* 62. New York: Random House, 1989.
3. Simon, Herbert A. *The New Science of Management Decision,* rev. ed., 46. Englewood Cliffs, NJ: Prentice-Hall, 1977.
4. Pearce and Robinson, *Management,* 63–64.
5. Gallagher, Thomas J. *Problem Solving with People: The Cycle Process,* 9. New York: University of America Press, 1987.
6. Vroom, Victor H., and Arthur G. Jago. *The New Leadership: Managing Participation in Organizations,* 56. Englewood Cliffs, NJ: Prentice-Hall, 1988.
7. Higgins, James M. *The Management Challenge: An Introduction to Management,* 70–71. New York: Macmillan, 1991.
8. Hastings, John E.F., William R. Mindell, John W. Browne, and Janet M. Barnsley. "Canadian Health Administrator Study." *Canadian Journal of Public Health* 72, suppl. 1 (March/April 1981): 46–47.
9. American College of Hospital Administrators. *The Evolving Role of the Hospital Chief Executive Officer.* Chicago: The Foundation of the American College of Hospital Administrators, 1984.
10. Cowan, David A. "Developing a Process Model of Problem Recognition." *Academy of Management Review* 11 (Spring 1986): 763–764.
11. Gallagher, *Problem Solving,* 77; Pearce and Robinson, *Management,* 65.
12. Postal, Susan Nelson. "Using the Deming Quality Improvement Method to Manage Medical Record Department Product Lines." *Topics in Health Record Management* 10 (June 1990): 36.
13. Cowan, "Developing a Process," 764.
14. Nutt, Paul C. "How Top Managers in Health Organizations Set Directions That Guide Decision Making." *Hospital & Health Services Administration* 36 (Spring 1991): 67.
15. Cowan, "Developing a Process," 764.
16. Cowan, "Developing a Process," 766.
17. Andriole, Stephen J. *Handbook of Problem Solving: An Analytical Methodology,* 25. New York: Petrocelli Books, 1983.

18. Nutt, "How Top Managers," 59.

19. For a discussion on problem definition, see Chow, Chee W., Kamal M. Haddad, and Adrian Wong-Boren. "Improving Subjective Decision Making in Health Care Administration." *Hospital & Health Services Administration* 36 (Summer 1991): 192–193.

20. Evans, James R. *Creative Thinking in the Decision and Management Sciences,* 104. Cincinnati: South-Western, 1991.

21. Couger, Daniel J. *Creative Problem Solving and Opportunity Finding,* 184. Danvers, MA: Boyd & Fraser, 1995.

22. Couger, *Creative Problem Solving,* 113.

23. Dewey, John. *How We Think: A Restatement of the Relation of Reflective Thinking to the Educative Process,* 108. Boston: D.C. Heath, 1933.

24. "There is no true value of any characteristic, state, or condition that is defined in terms of measurement or observation. Change of procedure for measurement (change in operational definition) or observation produces a new number. . . . There is no true value for the number of people in a room. Whom do you count? Do we count someone that was here in this room, but is now outside on the telephone or drinking coffee? Do we count the people that work for the hotel? Do we count the people on the stage? The people .... the ...... visual .... people, you come up with a new number." (Deming, W. Edwards. *The New Economics for Industry, Government, Education,* 2nd ed., 104–105. Cambridge, MA: MIT-CAES, 1994.)

25. A useful discussion of problem-solving constraints, including assumptions, is found in Chapter 3 of Brightman, Harvey J. *Problem Solving: A Logical and Creative Approach.* Atlanta: Business Publication Division, College of Business Administration, Georgia State University, 1980.

26. Chow, Haddad, and Wong-Boren, "Improving Subjective Decision Making," 194.

27. Chow, Haddad, and Wong-Boren, "Improving Subjective Decision Making," 202.

28. Chow, Haddad, and Wong-Boren, "Improving Subjective Decision Making," 192.

29. Nutt, Paul C. "The Identification of Solution Ideas During Organizational Decision Making." *Management Science* 39 (September 1993): 1071.

30. An excellent discussion of techniques for generating solutions is found in Chapter 8 of Couger, *Creative Problem Solving.*

31. Couger, *Creative Problem Solving,* 18.

32. Nutt, "The Identification of Solution Ideas," 1072.

33. Etzioni, Amitai. "Humble Decision Making." *Harvard Business Review* 67 (July–August 1989): 125.

34. Pearce and Robinson (*Management,* 75) describe these criteria as: Will the alternative be effective?, Can the alternative be implemented?, and What are the organization consequences?, respectively.

35. Kepner, Charles H., and Benjamin B. Tregoe. *The New Rational Manager,* 94–99. Princeton, NJ: Kepner-Tregoe, 1981.

36. Kepner and Tregoe, *The New Rational Manager,* 103–137.

37. Good discussions of problem solving and factors influencing problem solving are found in Ackoff, Russell L., *The Art of Problem Solving.* New York: John Wiley & Sons, 1978; Ivancevich, John M., James H. Donnelly, Jr., and James L. Gibson. *Management Principles and Functions,* 4th ed. Homewood, IL: Irwin, 1989; Kepner and Tregoe, *The New Rational Manager;* and Nutt, "How Top Managers."

38. Brightman, *Problem Solving,* 83–84.

39. Vroom and Jago, *The New Leadership,* 56.

40. Vroom and Jago, *The New Leadership,* 28.

41. Brightman, Harvey J. *Group Problem Solving: An Improved Managerial Approach,* 51. Atlanta: Business Publishing Division, College of Business Administration, Georgia State University, 1988. Pages 63–69 discuss techniques for overcoming groupthink.

42. Eisenhardt, Kathleen M., Jean L. Kahwajy, and L.J. Bourgeois, III. "How Management Teams Can Have a Good Fight." *Harvard Business Review,* 75, 4 (July–August 1997): 85.

43. Ways, Max. "Watergate as a Case Study in Management." *Fortune* 88 (November 1973): 196–201. (Watergate is the residential and commercial complex in Washington, D.C., that housed the Democratic National Committee during the 1972 presidential election campaign. Operatives of the [Republican] Committee to Re-elect the President [Richard M. Nixon] were arrested there during a failed burglary. The

political stonewalling, resulting scandal, and Nixon's resignation are collectively called "Watergate." The problem-solving process and mindset of the people who were involved exemplify groupthink.)

44. Higgins, *The Management Challenge,* 87.
45. Kaluzny, Arnold D. "Revitalizing Decision Making at the Middle Management Level." *Hospital & Health Services Administration* 34 (Spring 1989): 42.
46. Kaluzny, "Revitalizing Decision Making," 45.
47. Crosby, Bob. "Why Employee Involvement Often Fails and What It Takes to Succeed." In *The 1987 Annual: Developing Human Resources,* edited by J. William Pfeiffer, 179. San Diego, CA: University Associates, 1987.
48. Crosby, "Why Employee Involvement," 181.
49. Kahn, Susan. "Creating Opportunities for Employee Participation in Problem Solving." *Health Care Supervisor* 7 (October 1988): 39.
50. Lawler, Edward E., III, and Susan A. Mohrman. "Quality Circles: After the Honeymoon." In *The 1988 Annual: Developing Human Resources,* edited by J. William Pfeiffer, 201. San Diego, CA: University Associates, 1988.
51. Dailey, Robert, Frederick Young, and Cameron Barr. "Empowering Middle Managers in Hospitals with Team-Based Problem Solving." *Health Care Management Review* 16 (Spring 1991): 55.
52. Vroom, Victor H. "A New Look at Managerial Decision-Making." *Organizational Dynamics* 1 (Spring 1973): 66–80.
53. See also Vroom, Victor H., and Philip W. Yetton. *Leadership and Decision-Making.* Pittsburgh: University of Pittsburgh Press, 1973; Vroom and Jago, *The New Leadership.*

SELECTED BIBLIOGRAPHY

Ackoff, Russell L. *The Art of Problem Solving.* New York: John Wiley & Sons, 1978.

Andriole, Stephen J. *Handbook of Problem Solving: An Analytical Methodology.* New York: Petrocelli Books, 1983.

Arnold, John D. *The Complete Problem Solver: A Total System for Competitive Decision Making.* New York: John Wiley & Sons, 1992.

Brightman, Harvey J. *Problem Solving: A Logical and Creative Approach.* Atlanta: Business Publishing Division, College of Business Administration, Georgia State University, 1980.

Brightman, Harvey J. *Group Problem Solving: An Improved Managerial Approach.* Atlanta: Business Publishing Division, College of Business Administration, Georgia State University, 1988.

Chow, Chee W., Kamal M. Haddad, and Adrian Wong-Boren. "Improving Subjective Decision Making in Health Care Administration." *Hospital & Health Services Administration* 36 (Summer 1991): 191–210.

Couger, Daniel J. *Creative Problem Solving and Opportunity Finding.* Danvers, MA: Boyd & Fraser, 1995.

Cowan, David A. "Developing a Process Model of Problem Recognition." *Academy of Management Review* 11 (Spring 1986): 763–776.

Dailey, Robert, Frederick Young, and Cameron Barr. "Empowering Middle Managers in Hospitals with Team-Based Problem Solving." *Health Care Management Review* 16 (Spring 1991): 55–63.

Dewey, John. *How We Think: A Restatement of the Relation of Reflective Thinking to the Educative Process.* Boston: D.C. Heath, 1933.

Drucker, Peter F. *An Introductory View of Management.* New York: Harper's College Press, 1977.

Eisenhardt, Kathleen M., Jean L. Kahwajy, and L.J. Bourgeois, III. "How Management Teams Can Have a Good Fight." *Harvard Business Review* 75, 4 (July–August 1997): 77–85.

Etzioni, Amitai. "Humble Decision Making." *Harvard Business Review* 67 (July–August 1989): 122–126.

Evans, James R. *Creative Thinking in the Decision and Management Sciences.* Cincinnati, OH: South-Western, 1991.

Fabian, John. *Creative Thinking & Problem Solving.* Chelsea, MI: Lewis Publishers, 1990.

Gallagher, Thomas J. *Problem Solving with People: The Cycle Process.* New York: University of America Press, 1987.

Kaluzny, Arnold D. "Revitalizing Decision Making at the Middle Management Level." *Hospital & Health Services Administration* 34 (Spring 1989): 39–51.

Kirton, Michael J., Ed. *Adaptors and Innovators: Styles of Creativity and Problem-Solving.* New York: Routledge, 1989.

Newman, Victor. *Problem Solving for Results.* Aldershot, England: Gower Publishing, 1995.

Nutt, Paul C. "Flexible Decision Styles and the Choices of Top Executives." *Journal of Management Studies* 30 (September 1993): 695–721.

Nutt, Paul C. "How Top Managers in Health Organizations Set Directions that Guide Decision Making." *Hospital & Health Services Administration* 36 (Spring 1991): 57–75.

Nutt, Paul C. "The Identification of Solution Ideas During Organizational Decision Making." *Management Science* 39 (September 1993): 1071–1085.

Simon, Herbert A. *The New Science of Management Decision,* rev. ed. Englewood Cliffs, NJ: Prentice-Hall, 1977.

Vroom, Victor H. *Work and Motivation.* San Francisco: Jossey-Bass, 1995.

Vroom, Victor H., and Arthur G. Jago. *The New Leadership: Managing Participation in Organizations.* Englewood Cliffs, NJ: Prentice-Hall, 1988.

8 Strategic Planning and Marketing

"Cheshire Puss, . . . would you tell me, please, which way I ought to go from here?"
"That depends a good deal on where you want to get to," said the Cat.
"I don't much care where—" said Alice.
"Then it doesn't much matter which way you go," said the Cat.
"—so long as I get somewhere," Alice added as an explanation.
"Oh, you're sure to do that," said the Cat.[1]

As the opening quotation indicates, Alice did not know where she wanted to get to, and the Cheshire Cat responded, "Then it doesn't much matter which way you go." Without planning, where a health services organization (HSO) or health system (HS) is to get to (i.e., objectives to be accomplished) is unclear, and the way to get there (i.e., strategies to achieve the objectives) is unknown or at best haphazard. Planning provides direction and order for HSO/HS activities. If they do not know where they are going, HSOs/HSs usually will end up somewhere they do not want to be.

In Chapter 1 planning is described as a technical managerial function that enables HSOs/HSs to decide prospectively what the organization is to do—charting a course for the future. Planning enables organizations to deal with the present and anticipate the future.[2] It involves deciding what to do; when, where, and how to do it; and for what purpose. Planning also was described as a primary function—a precursor—because the other management functions of organizing, staffing, directing, controlling, and decision making are predicated on the most important outcomes of planning: objectives, strategies, and operational programs. Thus planning is a fundamental function of management.

Strategic planning and one of its elements, marketing, are the primary focus of this chapter. Through an understanding of the strategic planning process, it is possible to answer questions such as, How can the HSO/HS anticipate future demands and adapt to its environment, whether accommodating or hostile? How are objectives (i.e., desired outputs) of a HSO/HS established, and what influences their formulation? How does the HSO/HS develop and choose specific strategies and operational programs to accomplish objectives? How should the HSO/HS make structure, tasks/ technology, and people arrangements, and allocate resources to meet present and future demands, and to provide quality output with satisfied customers?

This chapter begins with foundation material, including a definition of planning and a discussion of planning characteristics and planning outcomes. Sections on the HSO planning environment and health services marketing follow. A comprehensive HSO/HS strategic planning model that integrates marketing is presented and analyzed; classifications and examples of strategies are given. The importance of and a model for interacting with stakeholders in a strategic context follows. Finally, the importance of public policy issues and how HSOs/HSs can shape the external environment is presented within the context of a strategic issues management life cycle model.

PLANNING DEFINED

Planning has been described in various ways. Pearce and Robinson consider it "determining the direction of a business by establishing objectives and by designing and implementing strategies necessary to achieve those objectives."[3] Planning is an orderly process that gives organizational direction, helps the organization prepare for change,[4] and helps it to cope with uncertainty. Planning involves deciding what to do and how to do it, as well as anticipating the future, which implies contending with the environment[5] and preparing for the future.[6]

Each description of planning incorporates at least one distinct attribute of planning. First, planning can be considered futuristic because it anticipates what will be required of the HSO/HS in the future and how this will be accomplished. When managers think systematically about the future and plan for contingencies, they greatly reduce the chance of their organization being unprepared. Second, planning involves decision making because determining what is to be done and when, where, how, and for what purposes requires that alternatives be evaluated, decisions made, and resources allocated. All of this results in a clearer sense of organizational direction and enhanced effectiveness. Finally, planning is dynamic and continuous—planned organizational activities are affected by future events and internal and external environmental forces. Consequently, continuous environmental surveillance and adaptive change are attributes of planning.

Incorporating these attributes, planning is defined as anticipating the future, assessing present conditions, and making decisions concerning organizational direction, programs, and resource deployment. The process of planning—how it is done—consists of a series of activities that include assessing present information about the organization and its environment; making assumptions about the future; evaluating present objectives, developing new ones, or both; and formulating organizational strategies and operational programs that will accomplish objectives when implemented.

PLANNING AND THE MANAGEMENT MODEL

When related to the management model in Figure 1.7, the importance of planning is evident. Planning enables HSOs/HSs and managers to deal with their external environment—their immediate health care environment and the larger general environment. Thus planning reduces uncertainty, ambiguity, and risk. By anticipating trends, and at times proactively influencing environmental forces, HSOs/HSs are more prepared for and able to respond to the myriad forces that affect them. Environmental forces that affect HSOs/HSs and the planning process are presented in Chapter 2.

Planning forces managers to focus on outputs. All organizational activity is directed toward accomplishing objectives, which are the ends, desired results, or outputs to be attained by the HSOs/ HSs and their units. From outputs, input needs are determined.

Planning enables managers to develop priorities and make better decisions about conversion design as well as allocation and use of resources. Integration of structure, tasks/technology, and people converts inputs to outputs. By identifying and focusing on objectives and formulating strategies and operational programs to achieve them, managers can design appropriate conversion processes and systems. These include some of the organizational arrangements that are presented in Chapters 3 and 4 and initiatives such as continuous quality improvement (CQI) and work process design/redesign, described in Chapter 9. The function of decision making and its importance to the HSO's/HS's planned conversion of inputs to outputs are presented in Chapter 7.

As managers initiate organizational activity to accomplish predetermined objectives through chosen strategies and operational programs, they do so through people; Chapters 11 and 15–17 focus on this important input resource.

Finally, planning is the foundation for resource allocation and control. It enables the HSO/HS to measure progress and determine whether expected results are being achieved. The control process described in Chapter 10 involves establishing standards for resource use and monitoring organizational activity. Criteria for measuring progress are based on objectives derived through planning.

PLANNING CHARACTERISTICS

Planning often is characterized by type and time frame, the individuals who plan, and the various approaches used in planning. A typology of these characteristics is presented in Figure 8.1.

Type of Planning

Type of planning refers to level (strategic/operational) and scope (broad/narrow). Strategic planning in HSOs/HSs is performed at the senior management level with input from other organization members, including those of the professional staff organization who hold leadership positions.[7] The governing body (GB) exercises oversight to ensure that the strategic planning process is in place and accomplished appropriately.[8] Strategic planning is all-encompassing in scope and concerned with environmental assessment; it addresses the elements of organizational objective and strategy formulation. Conversely, operational planning in HSOs/HSs is more narrow and limited than strategic planning and is performed at lower levels of the organization. Operational planning is subservient to, is derived from, and must be in harmony with strategic planning. Included are establishing subobjectives along with operational programs, policies, and procedures in units of the organization that may encompass groups of departments or individual departments.

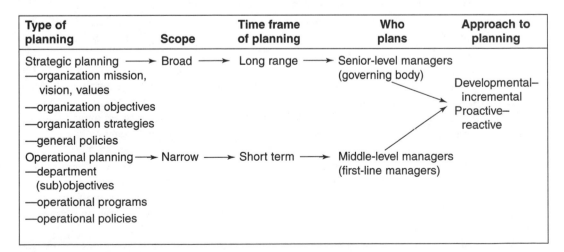

Figure 8.1. Planning characteristics.

Time Frame of Planning and Who Plans

Time frames of planning vary. Strategic planning is long range and encompasses multiple years. Operational planning is usually short term, with a time frame of 1 year or less. The GB and senior-level management are responsible for strategic planning in HSOs/HSs. The GB is responsible for setting the HSO's/HS's direction—its mission and objectives. Senior-level management has significant input in formulating organization objectives and is charged with developing and implementing organizational strategies to accomplish them; this is considered part of management work. The GB's role generally does not include originating strategy.[9] It is responsible, however, for ensuring that strategic proposals brought to it by senior-level management are properly prepared and are consistent with the HSO's/HS's mission as well as its responsibilities to stakeholders.

Middle-level managers also plan; it is part of their management work. In general, they are concerned with short-term operational planning and design and implementation of programs, policies, and procedures in their area of responsibility. This most often occurs at the level encompassing multiple departments. Finally, department managers and first-level supervisors also perform the management work of planning, usually in relation to specific operations or activities such as estimating workload, scheduling work activity, and allocating resources for which they have responsibility.

Approach to Planning

The many approaches to planning are described here as opposites. Individual–committee, systematic–ad hoc, and quantitative–nonquantitative describe how planning is done and are self-explanatory. Others, such as developmental–incremental and proactive–reactive, merit further attention.

Developmental–incremental planning refers to the degree of autonomy. Organizational settings or environments with fewer constraints, precedents, restrictions, and conventions can exploit developmental planning, which is characterized by bold, new, innovative, and nontraditional planning outcomes, especially organizational strategies. An industrial sector that is associated with developmental planning is personal computers and the Internet. Here, product lines change quickly, markets and uses are evolving, conventions and traditions are not fixed, and organizational rigidity is minimal. For-profit health systems have led the way in developmental planning, in part because there are fewer restrictions on the GB and senior-level management in setting organizational direction and there is greater autonomy in developing strategy. Many contemporary not-for-profit HSO/HS organizational structures, vertical integration and diversification strategies, and interorganizational linkages had their genesis in these for-profit systems. As some restrictions and conventions have been ameliorated in the health services sector, particularly through deregulation and greater emphasis on competition as public policy, not-for-profit HSOs/HSs have experienced greater autonomy and consequently are now more developmental in their planning.

Incremental planning is the opposite of developmental planning. It is characterized as less bold, less innovative, and more traditional. It may occur because of internal or external restrictions or because limited managerial autonomy has been granted by the GB. Some settings may be conducive to developmental planning, but incremental planning still may occur when managerial perspective is characterized by a limiting mindset, emphasis on short-term goals, narrow assumptions, and desire to avoid risk—attributes that also can restrict problem solving, as presented in Chapter 7. Incremental planning also may occur and be quite appropriate in a relatively slow-changing environment; in contrast, developmental planning often is most appropriate in a fast-changing environment. Incremental planning involves marginal as opposed to major changes in direction, thrust, and strategy. It can be characterized as mechanistic, versus the more creative developmental planning, or as "satisficing"—doing well enough but not necessarily as well as possible.

Another planning approach is proactive–reactive. Proactive planning is overt, systematic, formalized, and anticipatory. It involves not only anticipating the future but also intervening and influencing environments—making things happen and shaping events in the best interests of the

HSO/HS. Reactive planning, as the opposite of proactive, is default planning. It responds to events, is nonsystematic, and certainly is not anticipatory.

Often, proactive planning takes on some of the attributes of developmental planning. Managers who are proactive will make things happen, do things differently—perhaps innovate boldly. Reactive planners are followers. They tend to have the attributes of incremental planning—doing things differently on the margin yet very much the same centrally, altering and modifying activities because of the actions of others (competition) or environmental forces rather than shaping forces and causing others to react. More important, proactive–reactive planning is a major element in strategic planning relative to process and perspective. The treatment of HSO/HS strategic planning here advocates and presumes a proactive approach.

PLANNING OUTCOMES

Items that traditionally are considered to be outcomes of planning are organizational mission; objectives; and strategies and unit operational programs, policies, and procedures (see Figure 8.1).

Mission

All HSOs/HSs have a mission, which usually is stated explicitly. A mission statement identifies, in broad terms, the purposes for which the organization exists. It specifies the unique aim of the organization. For example, a HSO's/HS's mission is significantly different from that of an automobile manufacturer. The elements of a mission are as follows: Who are we? What are we? Why do we exist? Who is our constituency?[10] Mission statements "state the organization's purpose and reasons for existence" and "describe what the organization does and for whom."[11] In general, they include a specification of the organization's basic service, primary market, and technology or method of delivery.[12]

The statement of mission usually is accompanied by the HSO's/HS's vision—a strategic view of the future direction and "a guiding concept of what the organization is trying to do and to become."[13] The articulated vision becomes a vehicle to communicate to all constituents the future desired state of the HSO/HS.[14] In addition, there usually is an expression of the HSO's/HS's core values that are guiding principles in its conduct. Thus the mission, strategic vision, and values reflect a philosophy about the organization and its role in health services delivery. They are "the foundation on which the rest of the strategic planning process is built"[15] and are the basis for all other organizational planning, and are determined by the GB. Missions seldom change. However, when they do change, the change may result from accomplishment. For example, the March of Dimes's original mission was the elimination of polio, which was achieved; its contemporary mission is to combat arthritis and birth defects.[16] In single HSOs or highly developed systems a single mission statement prevails. In new or loosely coupled HSs each component entity may have a mission statement that eventually must be blended into the HS's overall mission as the HS matures.

Figure 8.2 presents the mission, vision, and values statement for Upper Chesapeake Health (UCH). UCH's mission is to maintain and improve health (basic service) of the people in its community (primary market) through an integrated health delivery system (method of delivery) that provides high-quality care to all. UCH's strategic vision is to become the preferred integrated health care system creating the healthiest community in its region (guiding principle). Furthermore, the core values held by UCH are excellence, compassion, integrity, respect, responsibility, and trust. Similarly, the mission of the American Diabetes Association is "to prevent and cure diabetes and to improve the lives of all people affected by diabetes." Its vision is "to make an everyday difference in the quality of life for all people with diabetes."[17]

Objectives

Objectives are statements of the results that the HSO/HS seeks to accomplish. In the context of the management model in Figure 1.7 they also are HSO/HS outputs. They are the ends, targets, and de-

---

Upper Chesapeake Health

Mission

Upper Chesapeake Health is dedicated to maintaining and improving the health of the people in its communities through an integrated health delivery system that provides high-quality care to all. Upper Chesapeake Health is committed to service excellence as it offers a broad range of health care services, technology, and facilities. It will work collaboratively with its communities and other health organizations to serve as a resource for health promotion and education.

Vision

The Vision of Upper Chesapeake Health is to become the preferred, integrated health care system creating the healthiest community in Maryland.

Values

Excellence—We constantly pursue excellence and quality through teamwork, continuous improvement, customer satisfaction, innovation, education, and prudent resource management.
Compassion—People are the source of our strength and the focus of our mission. We will serve all people with compassion and dignity.
Integrity—We will conduct our work with integrity, honesty, and fairness. We will meet the highest ethical and professional standards.
Respect—We will respect the worth, quality, diversity, and importance of each person who works with or is served by Upper Chesapeake Health.
Responsibility—We take responsibility for our actions and hold ourselves accountable for the results and outcomes.
Trust—We will strive to be good citizens of the communities we serve and build trust and confidence in our ability to anticipate and respond to community and patient needs.

Figure 8.2.   Mission, vision, and values statement of Upper Chesapeake Health. (From Upper Chesapeake Health. "Mission, Vision, Values." *http://www.uchs.org/about/mission.html*, April 2000; reprinted by permission.)

sired results toward which all organizational activity is directed. Most objectives are explicit, but some are implied. There are primary and secondary organization objectives—those to be accomplished by the organization as a whole—and subobjectives for particular differentiated units (i.e., divisions or departments of the organization).

Overall organization objectives are established by the GB or, in the case of HSs with differentiated subsidiary entities, entity objectives may be established by senior-level management with ratification by the GB. Often expressed in broad terms, organization objectives, when accomplished, result in mission fulfillment. Thus they are derived from and reflect the mission. In their classic study of hospitals, Georgopoulos and Mann describe organization objectives as follows: "The chief objective of the hospital is, of course, to provide adequate care and treatment to its patients. . . . A hospital may, of course, have additional objectives including its own maintenance and survival, organizational stability, and growth."[18] Henry Ford Health System is a network of six hospitals with nearly 2,000 beds and more than 35 other health care facilities including ambulatory care satellites, nursing facilities, and home health agencies. The system's health plan has more than 570,000 enrollees.[19] Two of its stated objectives are 1) to provide efficiently managed, clinically effective, high-quality health care; and 2) to be a research leader with a national research reputation.[20]

Typical HSO/HS objectives are listed in the management model in Figure 1.7. Included are patient care and customer service; quality improvement; appropriate costs relative to quality; organizational survival and fiscal integrity; social responsibility and responsiveness to stakeholders; education, training, and research; and reputation. They are the outputs of the input-conversion process. Organization objectives seldom change, but emphasis does change. In that way, a particular objective that once was secondary may become primary. Survival becomes the foremost organization objective for a HSO/HS facing deteriorating market share, declining census and clinical staff, and insolvency.

Subobjectives are ends and results to be accomplished by various units of a HSO/HS. They provide direction for managers and employees and are subsidiary to overall organization objectives. Figure 8.3 shows the hierarchical relationship between overall organization objectives and subobjectives for an integrated HS and a single HSO. In the case of the HS—which, for example, may be composed of a hospital, a managed care organization (MCO), and a nursing facility—each of these differentiated subsidiary entities that offer different services to different customers can have their own objectives set by the subsidiary's senior-level management. However, these objectives must be consistent with the system's overall objectives and mission. Subobjectives, in the case of the single HSO or subsidiary entities of a HS, are those that are pertinent to a specific unit or department. Typically, they are jointly formulated by middle- or first-level managers or both subject to senior-level management approval. They are derived from and must be consistent with subsidiary entity objectives in the case of a HS or overall organization objectives in a single HSO. Accomplishment of subobjectives at lower levels of the HSO/HS will result in accomplishing overall organization objectives. At times, a conscious decision may be made to suboptimize subsidiary entity or unit objectives if doing so will enable the HS to accomplish overall organization objectives. For example, a HSO medical director may seek to accomplish a unit objective of providing the "best medical education in the world," to the detriment of HSO fiscal survival. In this instance, suboptimization (i.e., something less, such as achieving the "best medical education in its class of peer facility programs") would be appropriate.

Objectives that state realistic, attainable, and measurable results are critical to HSOs/HSs for the following reasons:

1. They enable the organization and managers at various levels to focus attention on and initiate work toward specific ends.
2. They provide prioritizing criteria for decision making about services and programs.[21]
3. They facilitate efficiency, particularly in allocating and using resources.
4. They give employees a uniform sense of direction that results in greater organization stability.
5. Knowledge of intended results is critical to formulating strategies to accomplish organization objectives and operational programs to achieve subobjectives.
6. They become criteria to be used in the control process when actual results (outputs) are compared with desired results (objectives).

Organizational Strategies and Operational Programs

Organizational strategies are broad, general programs that are selected and designed by HSOs/HSs to accomplish their objectives. Strategies are long-term major patterns of activity requiring a substantial commitment of resources. *Strategy* is the term that is traditionally reserved to describe the means (way) of accomplishing organization objectives. Examples of strategies include changing the scope of services, perhaps by specializing (adding a catheterization laboratory or an open heart surgery unit); diversification (establishing a for-profit medical office building subsidiary); and for-

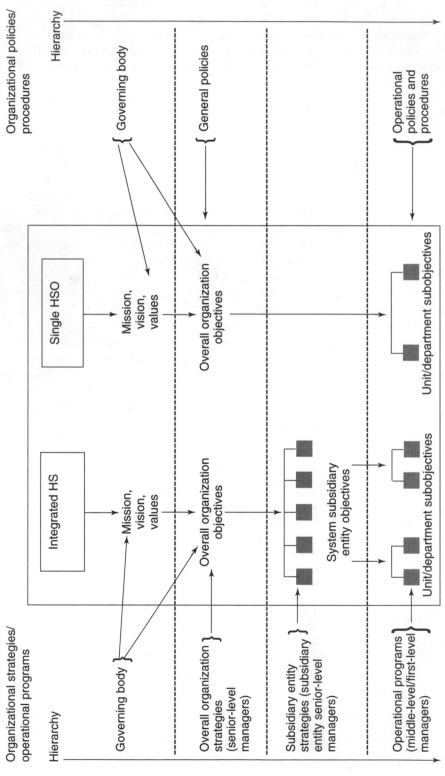

Figure 8.3.   Hierarchy of objectives, strategies, and policies, and operational programs and procedures.

ward or backward integration (expanding service area through a satellite family practice center or converting acute care beds to rehabilitation beds). Strategy formulation and implementation are the responsibility of senior-level management in HSOs/HSs. As presented in Figure 8.3, senior management formulates and implements overall organizational strategies to achieve objectives with oversight by the GB. In the case of an integrated HS, senior-level managers in subsidiary entities formulate and implement strategies for their entity to accomplish entity objectives. However, they must support the system's objectives.

Conversely, operational programs are the specific, planned activities of individual HSO/HS units or departments; their scope is less broad and global than that of organizational strategies and they are subsidiary to them. Just as all HSOs/HSs have a hierarchy of objectives, they also have a hierarchy of ways to accomplish them. As indicated in Figure 8.3, organizational strategy is the means to accomplish the HSO's/HS's overall organization objectives (and HS subsidiary entity objectives); operational programs are the subcomponents of strategies that accomplish HSO/HS unit (departmental) subobjectives.

Policies and Procedures

Policies are officially expressed or implied guidelines and systems for behavior, decision making, and thinking for organization members. Policies help organizations attain objectives and thus must be consistent with those objectives and with the HSO's/HS's mission. Policies are classified as general and operational. The former apply to the entire organization or system and are formulated by senior-level management; the latter apply to a specific unit or department and are formulated by department managers to be consistent with general policy.

Procedures guide actions for specific situations. Unlike policies, which are guidelines to thinking, behavior, and decision making, procedures prescribe specific actions. In general, they are expressed as a sequence of steps that are involved in a task. For example, there are procedures for patient admission and discharge, requisition of supplies, ordering tests, sterilizing equipment, processing patient records, and reporting unsafe conditions or incident reporting of untoward events affecting patients.

General and Operational Policies

Familiar general policies governing the personnel/human resources management function are compensation, terms of employment, and on-the-job behavior. Examples are "we are an equal opportunity employer," "whenever possible, promotion will be from within," and "our organization's compensation levels are competitive with those in the community." Other examples of general policies are "all patients will receive care regardless of ability to pay," "all employees are expected to ethically discharge their responsibility to patients/customers and each other," "capital equipment expenditures over $25,000 must have prior senior management approval," and "life support for the terminally ill will be maintained unless the patient has an advance directive indicating otherwise."

Operational policies for departments are subsidiary to general policies and must be consistent with them. A personnel/human resources department operational policy might be to continuously update the compensation system's pay grades and rate ranges to remain competitive with similar HSOs/HSs in the area. A nursing service policy might be replacing licensed practical nurses with registered nurses to increase the intensity of nursing care as vacancies occur through attrition.

Characteristics of Good Policies

Good policies are not easy to develop and implement. To be effective, a policy must be clear and appropriate and must serve to guide the ways in which organizational activities are carried out. Good policies have several characteristics.[22]

First, policies and their impact must be well thought out before they are formalized and must be in harmony with objectives. Policies whose negative effects have not been considered can be detrimental. For example, a professional staff organization policy of ordering a full laboratory workup for all newly admitted patients may have a noble (or defensive) purpose but may be inconsistent with the organization's objective of quality care at reasonable costs.

Second, policies must be flexible so they can be applied to typical as well as unique situations. Inflexible policies diverge from their intended purpose of providing guidelines for behavior and decision making. Situations may be encountered by a department head, supervisor, or employee that require judgment and atypical action. At times, managers appropriately deviate from policy—for example, not recording an employee's tardiness when delay was caused by an uncontrollable circumstance such as severe inclement weather.

Third, policies must be ethical and legal and reflect the values of the HSO/HS. A policy that permits employees to accept high-value gifts from suppliers may be legal, but it may be inconsistent with an integrity value.

Fourth, to be effective a policy must be clear, communicated, understood, and accepted by those to whom it applies. A clear and communicated policy on sexual harassment informs employees how they must and how they must not behave. Acceptability implies that organization members consider the policy to be reasonable, legitimate, and fair. Policies that display unwarranted favoritism toward certain employee groups or those that appear to be arbitrary and with no sound purpose will be resisted or possibly ignored.

Fifth, to serve their purpose, policies should be consistent with each other. They also should be consistent throughout the organization except when special and legitimate circumstances warrant differences. Unfounded inconsistency among policies and in application and enforcement of them is confusing and can cause disharmony, employee dissatisfaction, frustration, and perhaps litigation, and will detract from accomplishing objectives. Inconsistencies are most likely to occur among operational policies of various departments. Finally, to serve their intended purpose, policies must be continuously reevaluated and changed as necessary.

HSO/HS PLANNING ENVIRONMENT

HSO/HS planning, especially strategic planning, must occur in the context of the external environment. HSOs/HSs and their managers are affected by the external environment, and they must anticipate, predict, or make assumptions about its future configuration and the effect on them. Several environmental forces affecting HSOs/HSs are shown in the management model in Figure 1.7. The general environment includes ethical/legal, political, cultural/sociological, economic, and ecological forces. The HSO's/HS's health care environment includes public policy (regulation, licensure, and accreditation), competition, health care financing (public and private), technology, health research and education, health status, and public health activities. For good or ill, these forces always affect what HSOs/HSs do and how they do it.

The post–World War II health services environment was rather unobtrusive until the early 1980s. This was an era of expansion in capacity and growth in demand. The environment was relatively stable and predictable. Role clarity existed for HSOs/HSs. Risk was low. Proactive HSOs/HSs grew, those that were efficient thrived, and even the inefficient survived.

Since the mid-1980s, the health services environment has changed, becoming more turbulent and hostile. Most important, however, it is less certain. HSOs and HSs are less insulated. They are buffeted by fast-paced and changing external forces. The changes wrought by high technology and new diagnostic and treatment procedures are breathtaking. Societal, consumer, and third-party payer assertiveness and demands for greater accountability are accelerating.[23] Power is shifting from providers to purchasers and consumers of care. Public and private sector initiatives to control costs are intensifying, and this heightens financial risk for HSOs/HSs. These forces are contributing to intense and at times cutthroat competition among providers. Some of the results have been the formation of new financing and delivery arrangements, such as MCOs, health maintenance organizations (HMOs), and preferred provider organizations (PPOs); joint ventures; mergers and consolidations; and strategic alliances and integrated delivery systems (IDSs). Brown observed that more not-for-profit hospitals are being sold, often to for-profit enterprises, and that some Blue Cross plans are evolving into commercial enterprises driven, in part, by profit and stock values.[24] (MCOs are described in Chapter 4, and the other delivery forms are discussed in Chapter 5.)

As environmental turbulence gained momentum in the late 1980s, accelerated into the 1990s, and continues in the 21st century, HSOs/HSs are pursuing initiatives to contain the impact of external forces, decrease uncertainty, and lessen their risk. Recognizing that the rules of the game have changed, senior-level managers realize that their organizations no longer have guaranteed demand for their services from traditional constituencies, nor are they guaranteed a right to survive. Several proactive responses to environmental forces are 1) embracing the philosophy of CQI (see Chapter 9); 2) increased recognition and prominence of marketing; and 3) undertaking formalized, systematic strategic planning to enhance competitive position, including that of strategic issues management. Health services marketing is an environmental link to and integral part of strategic planning; strategic issues management is linked to strategic planning as a way of influencing public policy issues related to health services.

HEALTH SERVICES MARKETING—AN ENVIRONMENTAL LINK

HSOs/HSs have engaged in marketing-like activities for years.[25] Examples include public relations, liaison with and information dissemination to patients and other stakeholders, promoting the organization's image and services, donor/fund development, identification of new services to meet patient needs, aggressive recruitment and retention of physicians and other staff, patient origin studies, and patient satisfaction surveys.[26]

Marketing in HSOs/HSs has changed significantly in the past few decades. It is no longer viewed as a segregated, stand-alone activity that consists of disseminating information about types of services and products and their quality, or gathering information about patient/customer satisfaction. Informed individuals do not construe marketing only as advertising and selling, with the implication that physicians and patients will use the HSO's/HS's facilities only when there is a substantial promotional effort. It is not the artificial creation of demand for services.[27] Marketing in HSOs/HSs is properly consumer focused,[28] as is the case with CQI.[29] Market-oriented HSOs/HSs "are characterized by a concerted effort to collect, share, and respond to consumer information."[30] The contemporary perspective of marketing is that it is a designed process, integrated with other HSO/HS activities, in which the organization identifies and satisfies the needs and wants of stakeholders—especially patients/customers and clinical staff, as well as the community at large—so that the HSO/HS can accomplish its objectives and fulfill its mission. Kotler and Clarke, for example, observe that marketing is "a central activity of modern organizations. To survive and succeed, organizations must know their markets, attract sufficient resources, convert these resources into appropriate products, services, and ideas, and effectively distribute them to various consuming publics."[31]

Marketing is an integral part of strategic planning.[32] In fact, "because planning and marketing are both directed at keeping the organization responsive to its external environment, their activities interrelate and overlap."[33] It is impossible to plan strategically without including an assessment of the market (external) environment through a marketing audit and integrating both the information obtained and the marketing function with strategic planning.[34] The link between health services marketing and strategic planning is best understood with a base of knowledge in the marketing concept, marketing audit, and elements of marketing (Figure 8.4).

Marketing Concept

Authorities agree that the central concept of marketing is that of a voluntary exchange of something of value. The buyer receives something of value (a product or service) from the seller—the HSO/HS—in exchange for something of value. "The marketing concept holds that achieving organizational goals depends on determining the needs and wants of target markets and delivering the desired satisfactions more effectively than competitors do."[35] Consummation of exchange requires that sellers/providers create and make available, and that buyers/consumers locate and choose, services and products. Extended, this notion of exchange results in the marketing concept—a process by which HSOs/HSs seek to determine the wants and needs of prospective consumers and satisfy them with services or products.[36] Applying the basic marketing concept, health services marketing can be defined as "the analysis, planning, implementation, and control of carefully formulated programs designed to promote voluntary exchanges of values with target markets with the purpose of achieving organizational objectives."[37]

Marketing involves designing the HSO's/HS's services and products in response to the target market's needs and desires and using effective pricing, communication, and distribution to provide high-quality and better services or products. Figure 8.4 shows several important components of this definition. First, identifying needs, wants, and desires of target markets implies that HSOs/HSs know who their customers are. Second, identifying wants and needs leads to creating new or realigning existing services and products—those that meet and exceed customer expectations—rather than creating them first and then searching for customer needs. Third, the HSO/HS must engage in certain activities to facilitate the exchange of services and products. These are identified in Figure 8.4 as the elements of marketing. Information that leads to the development of organization marketing programs and activities is derived from the marketing audit.

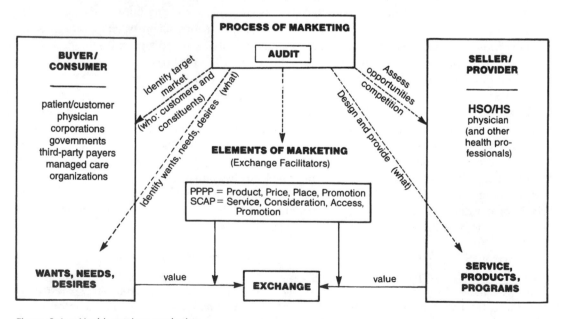

Figure 8.4.   Health services marketing.

Marketing Audit

The marketing audit is the systematic evaluation of the HSO's/HS's marketing situation. It includes 1) identifying target markets and their needs, identifying opportunities, and assessing competition through environmental surveillance; 2) evaluating present service mix or product line[38] relative to identified target market needs; and 3) modifying exchange facilitators so they are consistent with HSO/HS strengths and weaknesses and facilitate exchange.[39] Table 8.1 presents informational elements typically addressed in the marketing audit for a HSO/HS.

Target Market

Environmental assessment identifies present and potential target markets for the HSO/HS—potential purchasers of services as well as those who may influence purchase decisions on behalf of patients/customers. Included in this assessment is identification of their present and future needs, wants, and desires. In health services the traditional view is that the consumer in the exchange process is the patient. However, there are others who may intervene and influence who buys what service, for what price, and where, thus functioning as customers.[40] For example, physicians not only control patient admission to hospitals and, sometimes, nursing facilities but also review the services that are provided. Third-party payers, in particular government, large corporations, and MCOs, influence the prices of services. Regulation influences directly or indirectly the type and intensity of services provided through accreditation, licensure, quality assessment, and reimbursement mechanisms. Self-insured corporations influence where customers receive service by advocating alternatives such as HMOs and PPOs, and, through purchasing power, also can influence type, scope, and price charged for services. Consequently, HSO/HS marketing must seek to satisfy wants and needs of patients as well as to identify, recognize, address, and satisfy the wants and needs of others (i.e., customers) who influence the purchasing decision. Facility and staff support is important in building and retaining clinical staff. Cost and quality control are important in satisfying governmental and corporate payers. Depth and breadth of services are important in satisfying community needs.

Product Line/Service Mix

A marketing audit identifies the HSO's/HS's service area and evaluates its attributes, the needs of specific target markets, the satisfaction of present customers,[41] and the extent of competition. Such information allows the service mix (scope and intensity) and product lines to be expanded, reduced, realigned, or focused. Service areas can be large or small and are defined geographically. A general acute care hospital is likely to have a service area encompassing the community and its environs; a tertiary hospital service area may encompass a large region. Target markets can be classified by type of care (preventive, acute/short term, chronic/long term, rehabilitative); service (medical and surgical, obstetrics and gynecology, oncology); age (gerontology, pediatrics); income level; or type of payer (self-pay, commercial, managed care, public). Assessment information from the marketing audit reveals gaps in the service mix or product line, potential target markets, competitive and other marketplace threats to the HSO/HS, and whether special opportunities exist.

As target markets change, as competition and technology intensify, and as health service needs, preferences, and attitudes shift and change, HSOs/HSs need to evaluate and realign their mix of services, products, and programs. Such realignment must be consistent with the organization's capabilities and strengths and may include expansion or elimination of services under conditions of downsizing. For example, a competitor's introduction of an urgent care center or the formation of a HMO in the service area may require reassessment of the target market, plans for how to reach that market, and changes in services. Decline in birth rates may mean reevaluating the scope of the obstetrics service with the possible aim of redirecting resources to other services. New technology may suggest the need to introduce new or expanded services. Identified opportunities may lead to

TABLE 8.1.   QUESTIONS FOR A HSO/HS MARKETING AUDIT

I.   **Marketing Environment**
    A.   Constituents
        1.   Who are the organization's major constituents, and which should be targets of marketing activities?
        2.   What are the geographic, demographic, psychosocial, and usage/participation characteristics of each target market?
        3.   Should the various markets be segmented, and if so, how?
        4.   What are the needs that each market and segment is seeking to satisfy?
        5.   What attitudes do the markets and segments have toward the organization and its competitors (i.e., what do they know and how do they feel)?
        6.   What is the level of satisfaction of each user/supporter group? What factors contribute to satisfaction and dissatisfaction?
        7.   How do people in the various target markets make the decision to use or support the organization?
        8.   Does the health organization use resources and expertise available in the community, such as universities and business leaders?
    B.   Competition
        1.   Who are the organization's direct and indirect competitors?
        2.   What are the product/service, price, distribution, and promotion strategies of the competition?
        3.   What are the marketing strengths and weaknesses of each competitor (i.e., in terms of price, products and services offered, distribution, promotion, image, rate of growth, relationships with markets)?
        4.   What is the objective position of the organization vis-à-vis the competition (i.e., how is it similar and different)?
    C.   Social, Technological, Professional, and Legal Constraints
        1.   How are developments and trends in the following areas affecting the organization's activities?
            a.   State of the economy?
            b.   Demography of the marketing territory?
            c.   Activities of consumer groups?
            d.   Reimbursement policies of third-party payers?
            e.   Technological innovations?
            f.   Professional educational and certification requirements?
            g.   Planning, regulatory, and support activities of the local, state, and federal governments?
            h.   Changes in human values and lifestyles?

II. **Marketing Mix**
    A.   Services
        1.   What are the core services offered by the organization? What ancillary or peripheral services are provided?
        2.   Are the employees and volunteers who deliver the services properly trained, motivated, and evaluated?
        3.   What is the cost, revenue, and demand situation of each service? Are some services over- or underused?
        4.   What are the strengths and weaknesses of each program? Are there services that should be changed, eliminated, or added?
        5.   How are quality and effectiveness evaluated?
        6.   Are there satisfactory procedures for handling complaints?
        7.   Are the names given to different services or programs appropriate, descriptive, and appealing?
    B.   Access and Delivery
        1.   Are services offered at appropriate geographic locations (i.e., at a fixed site, temporary or mobile facilities, or in-home)?
        2.   Would it be advantageous to the public and to the health (services) organization to offer a service in a different or additional location?
        3.   Are services offered at times of the day, week, and year that are compatible with user needs?
        4.   Are facilities easily reached by public and private transportation? Is there sufficient parking? Access for people with disabilities?
        5.   Does the environment in which a service is offered convey a suitable atmosphere (e.g., of relaxation, warmth, efficiency)?
        6.   Does the organization cultivate referral agents?

(continued)

TABLE **8.1.** *(continued)*

C. Price
    1. What considerations determine pricing policies? Cost? Demand? Return on investment? Competition? Reimbursement requirements?
    2. What is the elasticity of demand for different services?
    3. Is price used as a competitive weapon? Is it used to manipulate demand (i.e., to increase or decrease service usage)?
    4. How does the organization's pricing structure compare with the competition?
    5. Do users see price as a cue for quality? Do they see price as being in line with value?
    6. What groups are most sensitive to price (users, referral agents, third-party payers, physicians, regulators, competitors)?
    7. Are quantity, seasonal, prompt payment, or other discounts offered? If price is adjusted to consumer income, does the sliding scale need revision?
    8. What are the psychological costs of using each service (e.g., in terms of anxiety, travel and waiting time, disruption of routine, red tape, coping with unfamiliar people and procedures, physical pain, personal abuse, loss of face or self-image, loss of control over one's life, demand for commitment, physical or mental exertion)?
D. Promotion
    1. Public Relations
        a. Is there a formal public relations program?
        b. Are there annual statements of goals, objectives, and strategies for the public relations program?
        c. Are public relations efforts appropriately distributed among various internal and external target publics, including employees, volunteer groups, the medical staff, referral agents, patients, donors, the community, and the media?
        d. Does the organization have a policy for dealing with negative publicity?
        e. How is the effectiveness of the public relations effort measured?
        f. Is the public relations function adequately coordinated with other marketing activities?
    2. Advertising and Incentives
        a. Does the organization use paid or public service advertising for recruiting, fund-raising, or promoting services?
        b. How big is the advertising budget and how is it set?
        c. Are specific objectives set for the advertising program, and is it evaluated in terms of those objectives?
        d. Are the advertising media appropriate in terms of the organization's resources and coverage of the target market?
        e. Does the advertising copy communicate effectively?
        f. Is the tone of the advertising congruent with the organization's desired image?
        g. Does or should the organization use a paid or volunteer advertising agency?
        h. Does the organization make effective use of such incentives as premiums or gifts, health fairs, diagnostic screenings, contests, and so on? Are the incentives compatible with the image of the organization?
    3. Personal Selling
        a. Does the organization use a paid or voluntary sales force for fund-raising or selling services?
        b. If so, is this sales force properly organized, trained, motivated, rewarded, and evaluated?
        c. Is the sales force large enough to achieve the organization's objectives?
        d. Is management used effectively to sell the organization?

Adapted from Schlinger, Mary Jane. "Marketing Audits for Health Organizations: A Practical Guide." *Hospital & Health Services Administration* 26 (Special Issue II, 1981): 38–41; reprinted by permission. © 1981, Foundation of the American College of Healthcare Executives.

a hospital offering wellness and employee assistance programs to large corporations, pharmacy services to nursing facilities, and home health services to discharged patients or residents.

Elements of Marketing—The Four Ps and SCAP

Figure 8.4 presents the elements of marketing that facilitate and make possible the exchange between consumer and seller. The marketing literature identifies them as the four Ps: product, price, place, and promotion.[42] A more appropriate classification for health services is SCAP: service, consideration, access, and promotion.[43]

Service

As HSOs/HSs plan and implement programs to bring about voluntary exchange between customer and provider, it is presumed that target markets and their needs and wants have been identified and that the present service mix has been evaluated through the marketing audit. Such information causes the organization to respond. Services are realigned (existing services are modified or new ones are introduced) to satisfy the needs, preferences, and expectations of consumers, stakeholders, or both. Included are actual care rendered or product delivered, as well as amenities, physical decor and comfort, and patient satisfaction with staff. In the context of CQI all aspects of customer interaction with the HSO/HS are included in the concept of service and quality.

Consideration

Consideration is the value (price) given for the product or service. When price is paid directly by consumers, it may be a barrier to service. When price is not paid directly by consumers, they may be indifferent to cost, which may not be important in the exchange decision. The trend toward deductibles and copayments for third-party coverage has made patients (consumers) more price conscious. In competitive environments HSOs/HSs are recognizing the price sensitivity of large self-insured corporate customers and managed care insurers and are bundling and pricing services nontraditionally; PPOs are an example. Beyond actual dollar cost, consideration also includes intangibles such as patient anxiety, inconvenience, waiting time, and the psychological value of service based on image and reputation, which affect the purchase-exchange decision.[44]

Access

In exchange, access—the ease of obtaining service, including the location and hours of operation—is important. Freestanding or satellite ambulatory care and family practice centers and mobile screening units are examples of methods to enhance access and expand geographic market area. Group practices that extend weekday hours and are open on weekends do so to enhance access as well as competitive position.

Promotion

Awareness is an important component in facilitating exchange in HSO/HS marketing. Customers or their intermediaries must be informed about services (type, scope, quality) that are offered, where and when, and for what consideration. Through promotion, HSOs/HSs not only convey such information but also suggest a reputation or image that is analogous to brand identification for products.

Criticism about health services marketing has been directed at promotion; some view advertising as artificially creating demand. This criticism is inconsistent with the marketing concept.[45] Promotion is the legitimate and necessary dissemination of information about service, consideration, and access so that consumers can make more informed purchase decisions.

Ethics and marketing as related to the issue of service expansion or contraction are addressed in Chapter 13. Certainly HSOs/HSs must be responsive to stakeholders, especially patients and payers. They are social enterprises with explicit and implicit responsibilities, however; they can only carry out their mission if they remain solvent. As stated in Chapter 13, "No margin, no mission!" The marketing audit gathers information about target market and stakeholder needs, external environment, and the HSO's/HS's circumstances relative to the environment and competition. Choice of organizational strategies that may expand or contract services and products is recommended by senior-level management and approved by the GB, just as are decisions about price, as in the case of the amount of uncompensated care that the organization will absorb. These decisions must include ethical considerations and be consistent with the HSO's/HS's mission and responsibility to society.

HSO/HS STRATEGIC PLANNING

Strategic planning is overt, anticipatory, and long term. In the case of single HSOs its perspective embraces the whole organization rather than single departments or units; in the case of HSs it embraces both the subsidiary (component) entities and the system as a whole. Strategic planning is both externally and internally oriented and involves assessment of the HSO/HS vis-à-vis its environments.[46] An integral part of strategic planning is health services marketing, particularly the marketing audit, which facilitates environmental linkage. Strategic planning is the process concerned with 1) formulating the overall objectives of the HSO/HS, and 2) developing organizational (or HS subsidiary entity) strategies and the derived operational plans to achieve them. It is an ends–means process in which objectives are ends to be achieved and strategies are means—the ways to accomplish them.

Objectives were defined previously and examples were given. Organizational strategies were described as the HSO's/HS's long-range, major patterns of activity requiring a substantial commitment of resources. It is appropriate to expand that definition here and add that strategies are the unified, comprehensive plans (means) that capitalize on the HSO's/HS's strengths, take advantage of external opportunities, seek to reduce or overcome threats, and mitigate weaknesses. They are the means (way) to achieve objectives. The discussion of the components of strategic planning that follows is linked to the HSO/HS strategic planning model presented in Figure 8.5 and addresses each element in turn. Components are referenced by number.

The components of strategic planning presented in Figure 8.5 are formulating objectives [I], strategic assessment [II], and strategy choice [III]. Subsequent to choosing one or more strategies, program implementation [IV] occurs through operational planning, resource allocation, and conversion. Finally, HSO/HS managers control [V] by monitoring and evaluating outputs to determine whether the strategies chosen and implemented result in objectives being accomplished. Discussion in this chapter focuses on the first three components of Figure 8.5. The latter two are treated in Chapters 3, 4, and 10, among others.

FORMULATING OBJECTIVES [I] IN STRATEGIC PLANNING

All HSOs/HSs have objectives. On occasion, objectives are reprioritized and new ones added. As the ends, targets, and desired outputs, they are the focus of organizational activity. As presented in Figure 8.5, objectives [I] influence selection criteria for strategy choice [IIIc]. If specific strategies are likely to accomplish objectives when implemented, then several of the choice criteria have been met.

The GB formulates overall HSO/HS objectives with input and assistance from senior-level management. Objectives reflect the organization's mission, the formulation of which is affected by organizational culture, influence of stakeholders, and values/ethics of the choice (i.e., decision) makers.[47]

Organizational Culture

As discussed in Chapter 1, organizational culture is the ingrained pattern of shared beliefs, values, and assumptions that is acquired by organization members over time. Culture is the legacy—what the organization is and what it stands for—that permeates the HSO/HS. It is known to and hopefully shared by all. Culture shapes the acceptable behavior of members and depicts the desired nature of relationships between the organization and its stakeholders. Objectives must be consistent

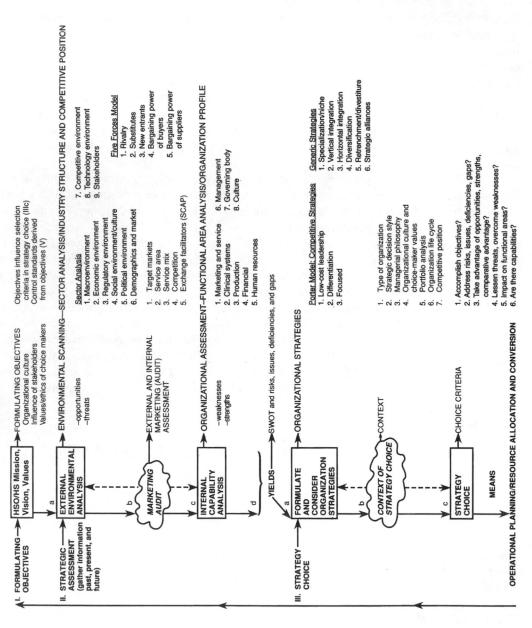

FORMULATE OBJECTIVES AND STRATEGIES

I. FORMULATING → HSO/HS Mission, → FORMULATING OBJECTIVES
   OBJECTIVES   Vision, Values   Organizational culture
                                        Influence of stakeholders
                                        Values/ethics of choice makers

   Objectives influence selection
   criteria in strategy choice (IIIc)
   Control standards derived
   from objectives (V)

II. STRATEGIC → EXTERNAL → ENVIRONMENTAL SCANNING—SECTOR ANALYSIS/INDUSTRY STRUCTURE AND COMPETITIVE POSITION
    ASSESSMENT   ENVIRONMENTAL
    (gather information   ANALYSIS   –opportunities
    past, present, and   –threats
    future)   a

    Sector Analysis   7. Competitive environment
    1. Macroenvironment   8. Technology environment
    2. Economic environment   9. Stakeholders
    3. Regulatory environment
    4. Social environment/culture   Five Forces Model
    5. Political environment   1. Rivalry
    6. Demographics and market   2. Substitutes
                                       3. New entrants
    1. Target markets   4. Bargaining power
    2. Service area   of buyers
    3. Service mix   5. Bargaining power
    4. Competition   of suppliers
    5. Exchange facilitators (SCAP)

                  b
              MARKETING
                AUDIT → EXTERNAL AND INTERNAL
                         MARKETING (AUDIT)
                         ASSESSMENT

                  c → INTERNAL → ORGANIZATIONAL ASSESSMENT—FUNCTIONAL AREA ANALYSIS/ORGANIZATION PROFILE
                      CAPABILITY
                      ANALYSIS   –weaknesses
                                  –strengths

    1. Marketing and service   6. Management
    2. Clinical systems   7. Governing body
    3. Production   8. Culture
    4. Financial
    5. Human resources

                  d → } YIELDS → SWOT and risks, issues, deficiencies, and gaps

III. STRATEGY → FORMULATE → ORGANIZATIONAL STRATEGIES
     CHOICE   AND
                  CONSIDER
                  ORGANIZATION
                  STRATEGIES
                  a

    Porter Model: Competitive Strategies   Generic Strategies
    1. Low-cost leadership   1. Specialization/niche
    2. Differentiation   2. Vertical integration
    3. Focused   3. Horizontal integration
                                             4. Diversification
                                             5. Retrenchment/divestiture
                                             6. Strategic alliances

                  b
              CONTEXT OF → CONTEXT
              STRATEGY CHOICE

    1. Type of organization
    2. Strategic decision style
    3. Managerial philosophy
    4. Organizational culture and
       choice-maker values
    5. Portfolio analysis
    6. Organization life cycle
    7. Competitive position

                  c → STRATEGY → CHOICE CRITERIA
                      CHOICE

    1. Accomplish objectives?
    2. Address risks, issues, deficiencies, gaps?
    3. Take advantage of opportunities, strengths,
       comparative advantage?
    4. Lessen threats, overcome weaknesses?
    5. Impact on functional areas?
    6. Are there capabilities?

                      MEANS →

OPERATIONAL PLANNING/RESOURCE ALLOCATION AND CONVERSION

364

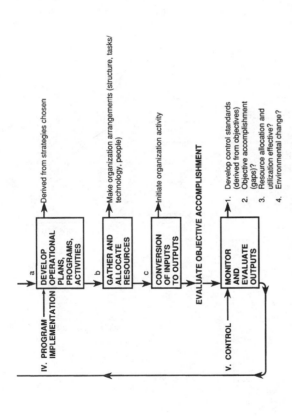

IV. PROGRAM IMPLEMENTATION

a → Derived from strategies chosen

DEVELOP OPERATIONAL PLANS, PROGRAMS, ACTIVITIES

b → Make organization arrangements (structure, tasks/technology, people)

GATHER AND ALLOCATE RESOURCES

c → Initiate organization activity

CONVERSION OF INPUTS TO OUTPUTS

EVALUATE OBJECTIVE ACCOMPLISHMENT

V. CONTROL

MONITOR AND EVALUATE OUTPUTS

1. Develop control standards (derived from objectives)
2. Objective accomplishment (gaps)?
3. Resource allocation and utilization effective?
4. Environmental change?

Figure 8.5. HSO/HS strategic planning model. (SWOT, strengths, weaknesses, opportunities, and threats.)

with mission and culture. Objectives that are inconsistent with the mission must be changed. A culture that is incompatible with the mission and mission-oriented objectives must be changed.

Stakeholders

Stakeholders are individuals, groups, or organizations affected by the HSO/HS who may seek to influence it and its objectives. In Chapter 1 three types of stakeholders were identified: internal; interface (e.g., the GB); and external stakeholders, such as third-party payers and the community at large. Stakeholder groups and subgroups have interests and demands that conflict, and each seeks to influence the HSO's/HS's priorities and objectives.[48] With the rise of HSs, "innovative governance structures that are responsive to internal and external stakeholder needs are particularly important as health care organizations join together to form integrated delivery systems/networks (IDS/Ns)."[49] Figure 8.6 presents a stakeholder map for an IDS/N (i.e., HS) and the GB's relationship to the stakeholders. It is the GB's responsibility to balance stakeholder demands and ensure that they are compatible with the organization's mission. Balancing requires maintaining ethical values and social responsibility and preventing inappropriate stakeholder demands from predominating.[50]

Values and Ethics

Establishing new objectives or modifying present objectives requires choice. It is the GB that makes this choice. Just as culture and stakeholders influence objectives, so too do the values and ethics of those who make the choice.

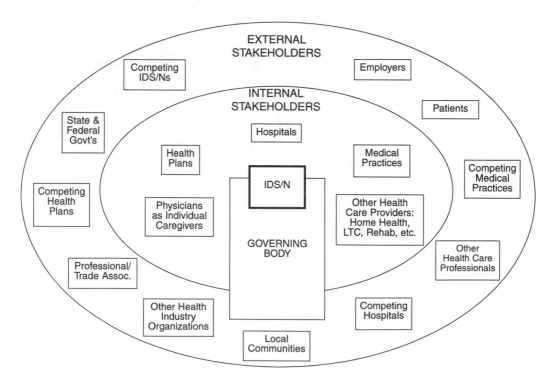

Figure 8.6.   Stakeholder map of an IDS/HS. (From Savage, Grant T., Rosemary L. Taylor, Timothy M. Rotarius, and John A. Buessler. "Governance of Integrated Delivery Systems/Networks: A Stakeholder Approach." *Healthcare Management Review* 22 [Winter 1997]: 7; reprinted by permission.)

Comments

HSO/HS objectives change for many reasons. New GB members with different values may influence the organization's direction. Other influences include emergence of new, more powerful stakeholders, and change brought about internally or imposed externally by forces such as competition, regulation, or public policy issues. For example, the primary objective of Columbia/HCA, a large, integrated, for-profit system, in the mid-1990s was growth; in the late 1990s its primary objective was survival. Finally, accomplishing objectives or a change in mission results in a need to reformulate objectives. For example, new medications and treatment for tuberculosis closed many sanitariums and altered the missions of those that remained.

STRATEGIC ASSESSMENT [II] IN STRATEGIC PLANNING

Strategic assessment [II] is the heart of strategic planning. It essentially involves gathering and evaluating information about the past and present and making assumptions about the future. The two major elements shown in Figure 8.5 include external environmental analysis [IIa] and internal capability analysis [IIc]. The marketing audit [IIb] facilitates both. The yields or results of assessment [IId] include identifying internal organizational strengths and weaknesses and external environmental opportunities and threats (called SWOT analysis), as well as risks, issues, and deficiencies confronting the HSO or HS. As observed by others in the business sector, principal assessment activities in strategy formulation include

> *identifying opportunities and threats in the company's environment and attaching some estimate of risk to the discernible alternatives. Before choice can be made, the company's strengths and weaknesses should be appraised together with the resources on hand and available. Its actual or potential capacity to take advantage of perceived market needs or to cope with attendant risks should be estimated as objectively as possible.*[51]

External Environmental Analysis [IIa]

Environmental scanning to identify external threats and opportunities is critical to strategy formulation and choice. Threats in the environment are events that may adversely affect the HSO/HS. Examples include competition and new forms and place of service delivery; change in third-party reimbursement; change in target market demographics and health status; new technologies; changes in accreditation, regulation, and licensure; and status of the economy.

Opportunities are favorable or advantageous circumstances in the external environment that may benefit the HSO/HS. They include change in demographics and service patterns; decline in primary care physicians in a rural area, which enables a hospital to open a family practice center; alteration of a reimbursement policy to cover preadmission testing; and changes in federal law. In part, opportunity evaluation includes a market assessment of present services and gaps (heart disease, trauma, perinatology) in service and clientele served.

Sector Analysis

Sector analysis is one way to perform environmental assessment: Threats and opportunities are identified and competitive position is assessed. Figure 8.5 [II] presents several important sectors[52]:

> *Macroenvironment:* "includes major trends and events taking place outside the specific environment in which the organization operates, e.g., the global economy, industry trends, national economic indicators," business cycle, unemployment (loss of third-party health insurance).

Economic environment: "includes trends, events, and economic indicators that are specific to the marketplace in which the organization operates; also included in this area is an assessment of the growth, strength, and impact of managed care arrangements in the delivery of health care services in the marketplace."

Regulatory environment: "includes recent or expected changes in the myriad of regulations that directly affect the organization," including that of local, state, and federal government.

Social environment/culture: "includes issues such as public health status of the marketplace, [and] health impacts of generalized social behaviors such as poor diet, sexually transmitted disease, smoking, [and] substance and alcohol abuse"; also includes cultural factors such as respect or disrespect for authority, attitudes of employees about work, sexual mores, personal ethics, and societal attitudes such as those regarding abortion.

Political environment: "includes factors such as recently enacted or pending legislation at the local, state, and federal levels"; health care as an actual or perceived right; public policy and federal responsibility for health care.

Demographics and market: includes demographic changes and trends in the marketplace, such as changes in service area composition or target market; age (Medicare), income (Medicaid), location, and patient–payer mix; demand for services.

Competitive environment: includes defining and assessing existing competitors who provide similar services to the HSO/HS; the extent of rivalry; and the HSO's/HS's competitive position in the marketplace, such as barriers to entry, threat of new entrants, potential for substitute services and products, and the strengths and weaknesses of other buyers/sellers and the organization's strength as a buyer/seller (see next section).

Technology environment: "includes assessment of recent advances in pharmaceuticals, genetics, and high-tech equipment, as well as the knowledge base, skills, and talents of the organization's workforce pools"; also includes medical education and research, cost, and pace of technology infusion.

Stakeholders: includes identifying and understanding stakeholder power and influence, their relative importance to the HSO/HS, and the demands they place on it.

Industry Structure and Competitive Position: Porter's Five-Forces Model

The classical model for evaluating an industry's structure and an organization's competitive position within it was developed by Porter.[53] It consists of five forces: 1) rivalry among competing sellers; 2) the extent to which other organizations provide substitute services/products; 3) the potential for new entrants in the marketplace; 4) the bargaining power (i.e., strength) of buyers; and 5) the bargaining power of sellers. Figure 8.7 presents the relationship of these five forces driving industry competition, which is particularly appropriate in analyzing the competitive position of HSOs/ HSs in the health services industry.

Rivalry

Rivalry among competing sellers characterizes their jockeying for position through tactics such as price competition, service, and product attributes, including quality, promotion, and image (i.e., brand identification). The aim is to achieve an advantageous competitive position. "Rivalry can range from friendly to cut throat, depending on how frequently and how aggressively companies undertake fresh moves that threaten a rival's profitability,"[54] and can result in both offensive and defensive responses by the rival. The attributes of rivalry follow[55]:

1. Rivalry is strong when competitors are numerous and relatively evenly balanced in size. Hospitals in a large metropolitan area are likely rivals; a single HSO in a market area is geographically more insulated from competition.

2. Rivalry intensifies when demand decreases or slows and competitors attempt to increase their market share. Similarly, it intensifies even if there is no change in demand but significant excess capacity is present, such as an oversupply of hospital beds in an area.

3. Rivalry is strong when the service or product is undifferentiated or there are low switching costs. The more one particular HSO/HS differentiates its services (i.e., brand identification, image, quality) or causes high switching costs to exist for customers, the more insulated it will be from competitors. Contracting to provide services to an external managed care insurer, or a captive (i.e., subsidiary) MCO in the case of an integrated HS, increases patient/customer switching costs by locking them in.

4. Rivalry increases when fixed costs are high and the service is perishable. Trauma centers are an example: If they are not used, then the fixed costs remain and no revenue is generated. The same logic and analysis holds for excess hospital beds.

5. Rivalry increases when exit barriers are high and it costs more to discontinue the service or go out of business than to compete. Some HSOs have high exit barriers; acute care hospitals are an example. Their high fixed plant and equipment costs can preclude exit, as might other noncost factors such as sense of community responsibility.

6. Rivalry can intensify when acquisitions, mergers, or consolidations of HSOs occur. For example, when a weak HSO is acquired (or merged/consolidated) by another from outside the area and the acquiring HSO launches aggressive and well-funded initiatives to increase market share of the acquired HSO, rivalry with others in the area is likely to intensify.

Substitutes[56]

The existence of or potential for substitute services/products can increase competitive pressures for organizations and pose a threat to their competitive position. The threat "is strong when substitutes are readily available and attractively priced, buyers believe substitutes have comparable or better features, and buyers' switching costs are low."[57] Potato chips and pretzels; Coke and Pepsi; Scotts

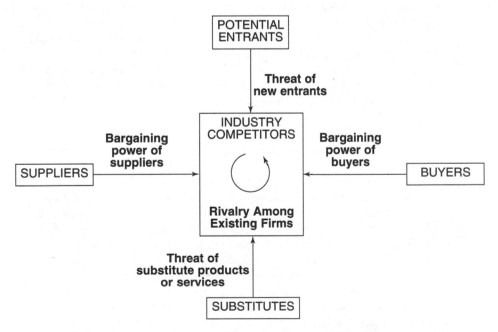

Figure 8.7. Forces driving industry competition. (From Porter, Michael E. *Competitive Strategy: Techniques for Analyzing Industries and Competitors,* 4. New York: The Free Press, 1980; reprinted by permission.)

Company and Green Thumb lawn care services can be substitutes. In health services, providers delivering measurably lower quality care are no substitute for those that are delivering high-quality care. However, there are instances when open heart surgery and angioplasty can be substituted. A HSO/HS offering one but not both services is exposed to competition. Similarly, receiving a flu shot at a public health clinic versus a physician's office and purchasing a generic drug versus a brand-name drug can be considered substitutes, with the latter in both instances being more expensive.

Potential for New Entrants

New entrants bring more capacity for the service or product, and thus greater competition. In health services, new entry urgicenters compete with hospital-based emergency departments for non–life-threatening care; new freestanding ambulatory care imaging and surgery centers compete with acute care hospitals; managed care insurers compete with indemnity insurance companies. The entry of new competitors is affected by barriers to entry, and competitiveness threats are fewer when barriers are high. Barriers are numerous [58]:

1. *Capital requirements and economies of scale.* High capital requirements and associated fixed costs drive the need for economies of scale, that is, the need to achieve high volume to lower the average cost of a service. The inability to obtain capital or the inability to achieve economies of scale and break even within a reasonable time will decrease the likelihood of new entry, as in the case of a competitor building a new hospital. In comparison, the opening of an outpatient surgery center has relatively low capital requirements and could achieve economies of scale and break even more quickly.
2. *Service differentiation* forces potential competitors to allocate large amounts of resources to overcome an existing HSO's/HS's advantage relative to quality, stature, reputation, and image. It would be difficult for a potential new entrant to succeed in matching or exceeding the high quality and stature of the internationally renowned Mayo Clinic, Cleveland Clinic, or Memorial Sloan-Kettering Cancer Center.
3. *Switching costs* that are high lock in buyers/patients and are a barrier to new entrants. The lower that switching costs are, the easier it is for competitors to enter markets. In a geographical area with a large indemnity plan–insured population there are lower switching costs for insured people, and thus a lower barrier for a new service provider/entrant than when a larger percentage of the population is enrolled in managed care. To succeed under the latter condition, the new entrant would need to convince the managed care insurer to contract with it to eliminate patient switching costs.
4. *Government policy* can be a barrier to entry. In the past, certificate-of-need legislation tended to preclude competitors from entering markets and offering certain health care services. Regulation and licensure, such as that for nursing facility beds, restricts entry.

Bargaining Power of Buyers [59]

The competitive strength of buyers in an industry ranges from weak to strong. Buyers have strength if what they purchase is undifferentiated, switching costs are low, they purchase in large volume, there are many suppliers, and the buyer has the potential to backward integrate and produce the seller's service itself. In health services the bargaining power of IDSs, multi-institutional systems under single ownership, and strategic alliances is increased relative to single HSOs because of the volume of purchases.[60] Similarly, a managed care insurer has increased bargaining power over independent HSOs and single licensed independent practitioners when contracting (i.e., buying) services because of the number of insured enrollees it can direct to or exclude from them. Managed care insurers command discounts from providers for services they purchase.

"Health plans and providers coexist in a complex buyer-seller relationship."[61] It is a reciprocal relationship; when the bargaining power of one weakens, it is strengthened for the other. A tension exists. Brown indicates, "sellers of service are bundling products [to enhance their supplier bargaining power] while buyers, including managed care firms, seek to unbundle. That tug of war will continue for the near term."[62]

An example of this positioning to gain competitive advantage is that many IDSs form their own provider-sponsored (i.e., subsidiary) MCO to market the health insurance product (i.e., plan) to the public and to large employers. By capturing enrollees and directing them to the system's acute care facility and network of licensed independent practitioners, the HS decreases the bargaining power of competitor MCOs as well as increasing its own bargaining power.

Bargaining Power of Suppliers [63]

The bargaining power of suppliers in an industry also ranges from weak to strong. Suppliers' bargaining power is strong when there are few competitors, the service is differentiated, buyers' switching costs are high, substitutes are few, suppliers' costs are lower than those of other suppliers, and the supplier has the potential to produce the buyers' services itself. To the extent that these conditions are not present, the bargaining power of the supplier is lessened. As in the earlier example, an independent acute care hospital in a competitive market has weak supplier power relative to a MCO. Conversely, its power may be greater if its services are appreciably differentiated from others based on attributes such as quality, reputation, experience, technology, or composition and skills of the clinical staff. Also, vertical integration augments the firm's internal (supplier-buying) power. [64] Vertically integrated health systems and regional multi-institutional HSs have greater (buying) bargaining power with their suppliers as well as (supplier) bargaining power with buyers of their services, such as MCOs.

Another example of altering the buyer/supplier power relationship is alliances between a hospital and physician–hospital organization (PHO). [65] PHOs are generally joint ventures with shared hospital–physician ownership. They provide a mechanism for the hospital and physicians to contract with MCOs to provide services. Thus, "they may increase the negotiating clout of their individual members with managed care organizations." [66] In addition, PHOs are a vehicle for risk sharing among providers and for the hospital and physicians to cooperate on utilization management and quality improvement. [67]

Marketing Audit [IIb]

The marketing audit is a systematic evaluation of target markets and their needs. It is an environmental link, and such evaluation facilitates strategic planning environmental analysis. To examine target markets means evaluating many of the environmental components of sector analysis. Consequently, market-specific information pertaining to service area, target market, competition, and appropriateness of exchange facilitators (SCAP) is an integral part of strategic planning.

Internal Capability Analysis [IIc]

Internal capability analysis [68] is assessing the HSO's strengths and weaknesses and drawing inferences about comparative advantage or, as some call it, distinctive competence. The analysis focuses on the HSO's/HS's functional areas and results in an organization profile. Examples of organizational strengths include referral patterns, reputation for quality, cost efficiency, technology, qualifications and stature of clinical staff and other professionals, resource (financial) availability, range and types of services and products provided, a cohesive culture, and proactive management. In addition, management skills (technical, human, and conceptual), roles (interpersonal, informational, and decisional as well as those of designer, strategist, and leader), and competencies (conceptual, technical managerial/clinical, interpersonal/collaborative, political, commercial, and governance) can be strengths. Weaknesses may include deficiencies in any of these elements; shortage of capital; outdated physical plant and equipment; hostile labor environment; poor quality/reputation; aging or decreasing numbers of physicians; or reactive management.

Functional area analysis is one method by which systematic internal capability analysis can be performed to identify strengths and weaknesses and to provide an organization profile. Among the functional areas analyzed are[69]

> *Marketing and service:* "includes analysis of the characteristics of current patients, such as payer source, acuity, demographics, origin and destination; referral sources; review of the current level of usage of services or product lines offered; channels or mechanisms for service delivery; promotional techniques; and success rate with each"; also includes target markets, reputation, specialization, image, barriers to market entry, breadth and depth of service, market share, access, and quality of clinical staff.
>
> *Clinical systems:* "includes evaluation of output measures of volume and quality; level of technology available; level of technology needed; and skills and knowledge base of clinicians"; also includes patient management control; skills, age and composition of medical staff; and status of clinical delivery CQI initiatives.
>
> *Production:* includes design of work processes and methods; cost of production; quality of outcomes; tasks–technology–people relationships; work scheduling and idle capacity; and equipment and facility size, capacity, and age.
>
> *Financial:* "includes evaluation of the availability and use of capital funds; use of operating revenues; ratio analysis; budget variances, and internal control mechanisms"; also includes patient-payer mix, leverage, financial reserves, accounting and billing systems, and earnings or residuals.
>
> *Human resources:* "includes evaluation of the skill levels in technical areas; availability of appropriately prepared personnel; recruitment and retention track record"; also includes quality of personnel skills, attitudes, compensation, stability of employment, productivity, commitment to CQI, and labor relations.
>
> *Management:* "includes evaluation of the number of levels; strength of each level as a whole and the individuals in that level"; also includes organizational structure and linkages; assessment of skills, roles, competencies, leadership and effectiveness of managers; and managers' perspective, experience, values, ethics, and philosophy.
>
> *Governing body:* includes the composition, strength, skills-knowledge, cohesiveness, commitment, oversight, and support to the HSO/HS and to the fulfillment of its mission.
>
> *Culture:* In addition to the functional area analysis, assessment of the organization's culture is important because it affects the functional areas. Assessment includes the organization's values and ethics; cohesiveness of the culture; philosophy about CQI, customers, and employees; and compatibility of culture with mission.

Awareness of a HSO's/HS's strengths in all functional areas and its culture permits conclusions to be drawn about comparative advantage and the ability to implement strategies chosen. Some of these conclusions identify the organization's particular skills, where it excels compared to other organizations, and how it can be differentiated. Is the HSO/HS the lowest cost provider? Does it provide the highest-quality service? Does it have the best reputation? Is it committed to CQI and customer satisfaction? Is it on the cutting edge of technology application? Comparative advantage is a barrier to entry that others must overcome to compete. Information about comparative advantage, strengths, and weaknesses allows consideration of organizational strategies that capitalize on the first two and mitigate the latter.

Yields [IId]

As depicted in Figure 8.5, the systematic appraisal and evaluation of a HSO/HS through external environmental analysis [IIa] and internal capability analysis [IIc] identifies external threats and opportunities facing the HSO/HS as well as internal organizational strengths and weaknesses. Conclusions can be drawn about the organization's comparative advantage and competitive position. In the literature this is referred to as SWOT analysis (strengths, weaknesses, opportunities, and threats). It enables managers to identify risks facing the HSO/HS, issues confronting it, organizational deficiencies, and gaps in objectives that are the difference or discrepancy between actual and desired results.[70] Objective gaps are identified in the control [V] portion of Figure 8.5. Are objectives being met, and will they be met in the future? The degree to which a gap exists, or is likely to exist, along with identification of SWOTs, risks, issues, and performance deficiencies, influences what strategies are considered, chosen, and implemented.

Table 8.2 presents issues for strategic and managed care planning. It consists of a series of questions that require both external and internal assessment for a HSO/HS that is considering entering the managed care market with its own MCO. The essence of the questions and issues examined incorporates, in general, a SWOT analysis as well as assessment of the HSO's/HS's competitive position.

STRATEGY CHOICE [III] IN STRATEGIC PLANNING

Figure 8.5 indicates that strategy choice includes formulation of organizational strategies on consideration [IIIa] and choice of one or more strategies relative to selection criteria [IIIc]. Both are done within a particular context [IIIb].

Formulate and Consider Organization Strategies [IIIa]

At any given time, an array of organization strategies can be identified, evaluated, chosen, and concurrently implemented by HSOs/HSs to achieve objectives. Seldom does a HSO/HS implement only one strategy; it usually implements a combination of them. Strategies are extensively discussed in the literature, which uses several typologies or classifications, two of which are described here: 1) Porter's classification of competitive strategies and 2) the classification of generic strategies (see Figure 8.5 [IIIa]).

Porter's Competitive Strategies

In his analysis of competitive strategy Michael E. Porter developed three categories: the low-cost leadership strategy, the differentiation strategy, and the focused strategy.[71] A HSO/HS that pursues a low-cost leadership strategy seeks to reach a broad market of buyers with services or products that are of equal or higher value/quality at prices lower than those of competitors. To sustain this strategy, the HSO/HS must continuously seek to drive down costs while maintaining or enhancing quality. As discussed in Chapter 9, CQI, reengineering, and strategic quality management—in which quality is linked to the strategic planning process—are initiatives that can lead to increased quality, productivity improvement (i.e., cost-effectiveness relative to quality), and enhanced competitive position.

The differentiation of services/products is a strategy in which the HSO/HS sets its services/products apart from those of other HSOs/HSs as it seeks to reach a broad or, even in some cases, a narrow market. Differentiation can be in the form of providing more features or amenities (birthing suites), paying greater attention to customers' needs, ensuring high value (quality relative to cost), or delineating perceived or actual image/reputation.

A focused strategy is one in which a HSO/HS selects a particular market segment—a narrow market niche—in which customers are appreciably different, fewer competitors are present, and it possesses a distinct advantage such as lower costs. Often, focused strategies are coupled with differentiation or low-cost leadership.[72]

All three competitive strategies are used singularly or in combination in health services. For example, a pediatric hospital uses a focused strategy, investor-owned chains often use a low-cost strategy, and tertiary hospitals use differentiation.

TABLE 8.2.   ISSUES FOR STRATEGIC AND MANAGED CARE PLANNING

Questions	Sample strategic issues (general)	Sample managed care issues
Where are we today?	• What is our overall market position? • Who are our competitors? • What is happening to our utilization? • What is happening to overall utilization in the market? • What are the strengths and weaknesses of our medical staff? Service scope? Geographic coverage?	• What are our current interactions with MCOs? • How much of our revenue is derived from managed care contracts? • How much penetration have PPOs and HMOs achieved in our market? • What are the key elements that MCOs are looking for in their contract negotiations? • Are there provider-sponsored MCOs in the market?
What is the future likely to look like?	• Will the market be dominated by several major systems of affiliated hospitals? Which ones? • What do we expect to happen to inpatient and outpatient utilization? • What are the growth areas of health care in the future? Do we have a role to play in these areas? • What kinds of relationships will successful providers have with physicians?	• How much penetration will MCOs command in our market over the next few years? • Will Medicaid adopt a managed care approach? Will managed care for Medicare take off in the market? • How much risk sharing will MCOs demand from hospitals? From physicians? • Will capitation become a dominant form of payment in our market? Over what time period? • What impact will MCOs have on use of our services? • Will MCOs in our market seek to employ physicians directly?
Where do we see ourselves fitting in?	• What components of the continuum of care do we want to provide or control directly? • Do we need to affiliate with other providers? What are our goals in such an arrangement? • Should we pursue some form of integration with our physicians? Do we need to acquire local practices?	• Do we need to have an ownership position in an MCO? • How do we want to "package" our services to appeal to MCOs? • How do we want to structure our changes to appeal to MCOs?
How do we get there?	• What are the resource requirements (facility, information systems, people, and capital) needed to achieve our desired position? • What specific actions need to be taken? Along what timetable? Who is responsible?	• What actions need to be taken to achieve our desired relationship with MCOs? What is the appropriate timetable? Who is responsible for implementation? • What resources are required? • What organizational changes are necessary? • What behavioral changes must be made by the organization and its employees?

From Horowitz, Judith L. "Using Strategic Planning to Address Managed Care Growth." *Healthcare Financial Management* 49 (April 1994): p. 24; reprinted by permission.

Classification of Generic Strategies

Another typology of strategies is that composed of traditional generic strategies (see Figure 8.5 [IIIa]):

- Specialization/niche by service/product, by market, or both
- Vertical integration, both forward and backward
- Horizontal integration

- Diversification, both concentric (related or complementary) and conglomerate (unrelated)
- Retrenchment (downsizing) or divestiture
- Strategic alliances (joint ventures, mergers and consolidations)

Figure 8.8 presents the relationship between vertical and horizontal integration.

To categorize, describe, and classify organizational strategies, two important points must be made. First, the categorization of strategy is always relative to the frame of reference of the HSO/HS—that is, its core services and products. For example, an acute care hospital adding a full-line family practice center would be categorized as related diversification (i.e., not a core service); if the center were freestanding in a different geographic or market area it also would be categorized as vertical integration (i.e., closer to the consumer–forward; downstream). However, in the case of a physician group practice, adding a related service such as a laboratory or dietary counseling services to its family practice center to provide a full line of services would be horizontal integration (i.e., related to its core service and the same point in production). The second point is that HSOs/HSs seldom choose and implement only one strategy; it is common for multiple organizational strategies to be implemented concurrently.

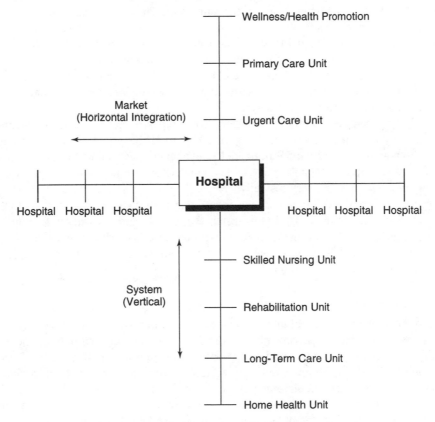

Figure 8.8.   Vertical and horizontal integration combination strategy. (Adapted from Ginter, Peter M., Linda M. Swayne, and W. Jack Duncan. *Strategic Management of Health Care Organizations,* 3rd ed., 203. Malden, MA: Blackwell, 1998; reprinted by permission.)

Specialization/Niche

Specialization is an organizational strategy in which HSOs/HSs have a core focus on or emphasize selected services or products, often based on disease or acuity of illness. Some hospitals, for example, are known for their specialization in oncology, organ transplantation, and cardiac surgery; nursing facilities specialize in long-term care; hospice specialize in the care of people who are terminally ill. A niche strategy involves focusing on a service area, such as the inner city, or a target market, such as outpatients. A HS specialization strategy might involve the HS's organizations focusing on rehabilitation or acute care services. Both strategies are essentially the same as the Porter "focused" strategy and usually are implemented in tandem—as in the case of a pediatric hospital that specializes by type of care (neonatal) and has a niche in a specific target market (children)—and may involve differentiation based on low-cost, high-technology leadership.

Vertical Integration

As discussed in Chapter 5, the organizational strategy of vertical integration occurs when a HS operates at more than one point on a chain of production, distribution, or both.[73] Conrad and Dowling describe vertical integration as a "broad range of patient care and support services operated in a functionally unified manner."[74] Brown and McCool define vertical integration as adding upstream or downstream services.[75] Vertical integration involves linking dissimilar services/products through ownership or contracts.[76] An extreme case of the latter is the virtual organization, in which organizations are integrated by contract only, not by ownership. The concept of vertical integration is generally based on patients' acuity of illness, which can range from acute to chronic. Examples of forward integration (i.e., downstream) for an acute care hospital would be involvement in a HS featuring ambulatory care, satellite family practice clinics, wellness promotion,[77] and freestanding fitness centers.[78] Backward integration (i.e., upstream) would include long-term care and rehabilitation as well as acquired home health agency services.[79]

In its industry study the Health Care Advisory Board reported on 566 vertically integrated systems. In 1996 they included 38% of U.S. hospitals, 16% of HMOs, 14% of physician clinics, 9% of outpatient treatment centers, and 5% of home health agencies, as well as 11,234 physician practices owned or managed by hospitals.[80] These data indicate that vertical integration, as a strategy, is extensively pursued in health services delivery.

Integration also may occur in nonservice areas—that is, in factors of production that involve make/buy decisions (i.e., upstream).[81] In this instance it is backward integration. Examples are the development or acquisition of businesses that provide contracted housekeeping or information system services for the HSO/HS, or those that supply or manufacture generic pharmaceuticals, prosthetic devices, and intravenous solutions.[82]

Horizontal Integration

In contrast to the strategy of vertical integration, horizontal integration occurs when HSOs expand its core services or products at the same point in the production process and in the same part of the industry. In the case of a system it would be "lateral relationships among like entities."[83] Horizontal integration usually is done to round out core service/product lines and to enter new markets with existing types of services. Horizontal integration may be achieved through internal development, acquisition, or merger. An acute care hospital that adds coronary bypass surgery to its existing core surgical services or that builds a suburban acute inpatient hospital is horizontally integrating. Multihospital systems or nursing facility chains, in which member facilities offer the same core services, are horizontally integrated, and they most often use this strategy to reach new markets and to achieve economies of scale for support and management services, enhance access to capital, and lower overall organization risk.

Horizontally linked HSOs/HSs may be closely coupled through ownership or loosely coupled through affiliations or alliances. An example of a geographically dispersed, horizontally integrated, for-profit health system is Beverly Enterprises. In 1997 it owned 632 nursing facilities in 31 states. Beverly also had vertical integration components of 30 transitional hospitals and hospice and 32 outpatient clinics.[84]

Diversification

Diversification is an organizational strategy in which HSOs/HSs add new services or products, enter new markets, or both where neither is directly related to its core services and products.[85] Diversification usually is defined relative to 1) the HSO's/HS's traditional main line of business, core services, or both; and 2) whether the activity is related or unrelated.[86] For acute care hospitals, diversification includes adding new noninpatient care services/products, such as industrial medicine, women's medicine, and wellness programs; nonacute care services, such as rehabilitation and substance abuse and behavioral treatment; or both.[87]

There are two types of diversification: concentric and conglomerate. Concentric diversification occurs when different but related health care services and products are added to the existing core of services. This may be done to increase revenues or to enhance competitive position and reach new target markets. Depending on the frame of reference (i.e., the HSO's/HS's core services and position on the "stage of illness" scale), concentric diversification also may constitute forward or backward integration. For example, an acute care hospital that diversifies into long-term care by converting acute care beds also is engaging in vertical integration[88]; establishing a freestanding diagnostic center also is vertical integration. One way of classifying strategy as vertical integration or diversification is intent relative to patient flow. If the purpose is to control patient flow, such as an acute care hospital acquiring physician practices, then this strategy can be classified as vertical integration. If the purpose of acquiring a skilled facility is to enter a growth market and not controlling patient flow from the hospital, then this strategy can be classified as concentric diversification.[89]

The second form of diversification is conglomerate diversification. Here a HSO/HS produces non–health-related products or services that are unrelated to the HSO's/HS's principal business or core services. An example is a hospital providing laundry or computer services to other organizations; investing in real estate, such as shopping centers, homes, or apartments; or providing catering services. Concentric diversification is the most common form for HSOs/HSs; few engage in conglomerate diversification.

Retrenchment/Divestiture

A strategy of retrenchment, or downsizing, involves reducing the scope or intensity of products and services, partial withdrawal from a market area, or decreasing capacity in terms of facilities, equipment, or staff. A divestiture is eliminating a group of services or products, complete withdrawal from a market area, or closing facilities. In highly competitive markets in which the HSO/HS has no comparative advantage or in instances in which demand has decreased, it may implement a strategy of retrenchment—in extreme cases, divestiture. The more commonly implemented strategy is retrenchment. This reduces losses, permits reallocation of resources to more promising services, and, in extreme cases, enables the organization to survive. Declining birth rates caused some hospitals to downsize obstetrics; high levels of uncompensated care led others to close (retrench/divest) trauma centers; and low inpatient occupancy rates caused still others to reduce the number of acute care beds (retrenchment) while converting those beds to long-term or rehabilitative care (both vertical integration and concentric diversification).

Strategic Alliances

Joint ventures, mergers, and consolidations are strategic alliances (SAs) that represent prevalent strategic arrangements in health services delivery (see Chapter 5). For the most part SAs are of recent origin (mid- to late 1990s) and represent an organizational strategy that usually is coupled with one or more of those previously described: Joint ventures can be coupled with vertical and horizontal integration, for example. SAs arise from mutual need and a willingness among the organizations to share knowledge, capabilities, risks, and costs; to leverage innovation; and to take advantage of complementary strengths and capabilities. "Such alliances are designed to achieve strategic purposes not attainable by a single organization, providing flexibility and responsiveness while retaining the basic fabric of participating [i.e., independent] organizations."[90] These linked organizations may be those with common religious preferences, those that are geographically distributed, or those that may be vertically linked.[91]

Combination Strategies

HSOs/HSs will generally implement multiple strategies concurrently. For example, Henry Ford Health System is both vertically (backward and forward) and horizontally integrated; it also specializes/niches and differentiates certain services.

Another example of a system that pursued vertical and horizontal integration, concentric diversification, and retrenchment/divestiture concurrently is Columbia/HCA. Formed in 1994 with the merger between Columbia Healthcare and the Hospital Corporation of America, the new system, Columbia/HCA, in 1996 owned or operated 343 hospitals (i.e., horizontal integration), some as joint ventures; 550 home health agencies and 186 nursing facilities (i.e., backward integration); 136 outpatient surgery centers (i.e., forward integration); and 131 psychiatric units (i.e., specialization/ niche). Aggregate revenues were $20 billion. It sought to enhance competitive position in particular markets, sometimes closing duplicate facilities (i.e., divest, retrench) in that market; exclusively contracting with physicians, purchasing physician practices, or both (i.e., vertical integration); and developing a nationally recognized brand identification (i.e., differentiation). The ultimate in vertical integration was its proposed acquisition of Blue Cross Blue Shield of NE Ohio to channel its 1 million subscribers to Columbia/HCA hospitals. Suit was brought by the state's attorney general to block this acquisition. A subsequent federal investigation of irregular billing practices led to a change in Columbia/HCA senior-level management, eventual abandonment of the strategy to differentiate the system with national branding,[92] and divestiture of some hospitals, resulting in less horizontal integration. As reported in 1998, there was planned divestiture of three hospital divisions with approximately 100 hospitals, some surgical centers, and the corporation's home health segment.[93]

Context of Strategy Choice [IIIb]

The range of alternative organizational strategies considered and those eventually selected is greatly influenced by the context in which strategy choice is made. Although there are other classifications of context, the focus here is on those identified in Figure 8.5 [IIIb] and Figure 8.9. They are

- Type of organization
- Strategic decision style
- Managerial philosophy
- Organizational culture and choice-maker values
- Portfolio analysis
- Organization life cycle
- Competitive position

Type of Organization

Type of organization refers to self-image and how the HSO/HS adapts to the environment, competitors, and customers. Organization types may be described as defender, prospector, or reactor.[94] A de-

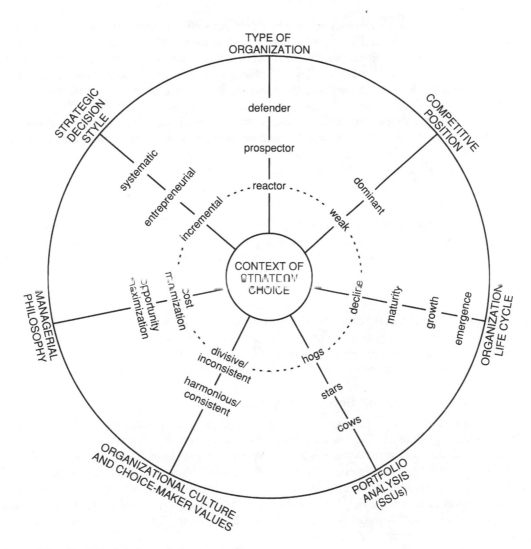

Figure 8.9.   Context of strategy choice.

fender organization seeks to maintain the status quo and stability; it is not innovative. In general, such HSOs/HSs vigorously protect what they have, such as a niche or specialized service/product domain. Prospector organizations occasionally redefine markets, seek new target markets, seize the initiative, and capitalize on opportunities; they are proactive, tending to be innovative and at the forefront of applying new technologies. Reactor organizations may not have a clear sense of direction and are "seriously out of stride with environmental or competitive change."[95] They are passive and usually stir to action only in a crisis or when external environmental forces cannot be ignored.

Strategic Decision Style

Strategic decision style describes the process by which organizational strategic alternatives are formulated and evaluated and decisions are made. It can be classified as systematic, entrepreneurial, or incremental.[96] A systematic strategic decision style is proactive. It involves comprehensive external and internal analysis; understanding interrelationships of threats, opportunities, strengths, and weaknesses; considering all strategic alternatives; and selecting an organizational strategy on the basis of rational criteria. Entrepreneurial strategic decision style has been described as "gut feel," hunch, or intuition. It in general does not include full and comprehensive strategic assessment, only selected review; thus it is more accurately described as a style in which strategic decisions are made carefully but quickly. In mature HSOs/HSs and industries entrepreneurial decision style is, in general, inappropriate. However, it may be appropriate for emerging or even mature HSOs/HSs in a turbulent, fast-changing environment, especially if windows of opportunity close rapidly, thus making quick decision making an imperative. Incremental strategic decision style is in general reactive and usually involves change at the margin. Sometimes it means simply muddling through.[97] It is a piecemeal approach to strategy choice and does not include comprehensive, systematic strategic assessment or reviewing and evaluating a full range of strategies.

Managerial Philosophy

Managerial philosophy in the context of strategy choice is best described as a continuum that ranges from opportunity maximization to cost minimization. The former is a proactive, prospector, systematic/entrepreneurial perspective. It implies that organizational strategies are chosen to take advantage of opportunities and capitalize on strengths. Cost minimization as a philosophy implies conservatism. It may be consistent with a defender HSO/HS but is certainly found in a reactor HSO/HS. It focuses on how to "save a buck" without considering opportunity costs. Organizations are never entirely at one end of the continuum but usually are closer to one end or the other. Other similar descriptive terms are aggressive-innovative versus lethargic-conservative or risk taking versus risk averse. HSOs/HSs that are opportunity maximizers, aggressors-innovators, and risk takers usually consider and choose different strategies than those at the other end of the continuum.

Organizational Culture and Choice-Maker Values

Organizational culture and the values of decision makers (choice makers) are contextual variables that affect the choice of strategies. Organizational culture is a continuum from harmonious to divisive, and the values of choice makers can be consistent or inconsistent with culture. Cultural disarray—perhaps caused by splintered factions, internal hostility, and a lack of cohesion, mutual support, and shared beliefs—leads to divisiveness in the organization. Under such circumstances it may be impossible to gain the commitment of participants to implement complex strategies and weather the resulting organizational change.[98] Mismatching culture and strategy translates into implementation difficulties. This restricts the range of realistic strategies.

As Bower and colleagues observe, "strategy is a human construction; it must in the long run be responsive to human needs. It must ultimately inspire commitment. It must stir an organization to successful striving against competition. People have to have their hearts in it."[99] HSOs/HSs with strong, cohesive cultures and values shared by managers and staff can prospect, be more opportunistic, and successfully implement a wider range of organization strategies than those with a divisive culture and managerial values at variance with the culture. As Digman observes, "What a business is able to accomplish may be determined as much, if not more, by its culture than its strategic plan. Strategies are only as good as the culture that exists to encourage and support them."[100]

Portfolio Analysis

Portfolio analysis is borrowed from marketing and describes and categorizes resource-producing or resource-consuming services and products. The typical nomenclature is cows, hogs, and stars.[101] Cows are services or product lines that yield more than they consume; hogs consume more than they yield; and stars, if nurtured, will evolve from embryonic resource consumers into cows. Portfolio analysis of services or product lines could determine that pharmacy and radiology are cows, obstetrics is a hog, and sports medicine is a star. Organizations with a preponderance of cows and stars are in a better position to prosper and have greater latitude in strategy choice than those with a preponderance of hogs. Portfolio analysis is important to strategy formulation and choice because it allows choice makers to recognize the cows, hogs, and stars of their organization and how alternative strategies may change the ratio of these three categories.[102]

Another variable that affects the context of strategy choice is strategic business unit or, as applied in health services, strategic service unit (SSU) analysis.[103] This type of segmentation is like portfolio analysis except that "SSU" generally refers to identifiable, relatively autonomous organizational units with distinct services and product lines that are offered to distinct target markets.[104] SSUs have reasonable control over their activities, are separate from other SSUs, compete with external groups for market share, and have their own revenues and costs.[105] Each differentiated subsidiary unit in a vertically integrated HS is a separate SSU. Pegels and Rogers observe that a vertically integrated HS that owns two hospitals, a HMO, and a nursing facility could segment them into four SSUs.[106] As conveyed in Figure 8.3, SSUs are important to the context of strategy choice because distinct and even different strategies may be chosen and implemented for each.

Organization Life Cycle

Organization life cycle refers to the stage of development of an organization. Conceptually, organization life cycle borrows from theories of aging for human beings and product life cycle as applied in marketing. All organizations go through stages of emergence, growth, maturity, decline, and perhaps regeneration, although time spans vary. Figure 8.10 presents this concept graphically, and Table 8.3 describes the stages of the organization life cycle as applied to industrial organizations.

It is important to note that external or internal events (changing technology, competition) can increase or decrease the slope of the life cycle curve, lengthen or shorten its line, and enable the HSO/HS to regenerate from one stage (maturity) to another (growth) or accelerate from one stage (maturity) to another (decline). Depending on where the HSO/HS is in its life cycle, the context of strategy choice differs. HSOs/HSs in the growth stage may choose aggressive, expansionary-type strategies such as forward and horizontal integration and concentric diversification. They are likely to be prospectors and opportunity maximizers. Those in decline likely will be forced to retrench, minimize cost, and perhaps pursue niche strategies.

Competitive Position

The feasible set of organizational strategies that a HSO/HS can consider is partially predicated on its competitive position. Barriers to market entry, threat of new entrants (competitors), availability of substitute products or services, and the HSO's/HS's strength as a seller or buyer are attributes of com-

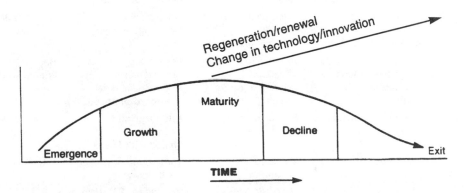

Figure 8.10.   Life cycle of a HSO/HS.

TABLE 8.3.   LIFE CYCLE OF AN ORGANIZATION

Emergence	There is almost invariably a shortage of liquid assets, a need to create consumer demand, and a need to expand production to meet this demand. Administrative processes are loosely defined and a flexible use of labor reduces dependence on more costly specialized personnel.
Growth	A point is reached where major refinancing becomes necessary and there may be some acquisitions as well. Extensions are made to the basic product line and overseas markets are evaluated. At the same time as new plants and machinery are purchased, control systems are strengthened and formal personnel policies instituted.
Maturity	Initially investments produce high returns, but over time higher unit production costs and overhead cut in. There is a tendency to become very conservative in marketing and to sacrifice opportunities. Unit production costs are increasingly affected by declining economies of scale and obsolescence of equipment. Conformity rather than individuality is rewarded and labor problems increase.
Regeneration	If regeneration occurs, it may be internal or external. Internally a company may divest itself of unprofitable subsidiaries, sell off assets, resort to rigid cost cutting, reduce labor use, and close some production lines. There is an attempt to reverse the decline in sales and profits of existing products and introduce new, profitable products. External regeneration may involve sacrificing a controlling interest, merger, being completely acquired, or government assistance.
Decline	As internal reserves are depleted, external financing becomes more difficult. The company is selling products that few want at excessive prices. Equipment becomes obsolete, production costs skyrocket, key personnel leave, and labor becomes increasingly militant.

From Steiner, George A., John B. Miner, and Edmund R. Gray. *Management Policy and Strategy,* New York: Macmillan, 1986; reprinted by permission. Copyright © 1986 Macmillan Publishing Co.

petitive position. Table 8.4 presents a strength of competitive position (from dominant to weak)– service/product life cycle (from embryonic to aging) matrix that suggests strategic behavior for each cell. These behaviors are determined by the strength of the HSO's/HS's competitive position and the position of its services in the product life cycle.[107] A HSO/HS with a mature service in a dominant position, such as acute inpatient care, would seek to hold its market share and grow with the industry. One in a weak competitive position, but with a growth service such as cardiac surgery, could choose to make a substantial resource commitment (turnaround) to strengthen competitive position or abandon that service and redirect resources.

TABLE 8.4.   COMPETITIVE POSITION/PRODUCT LIFE CYCLE MATRIX

Strength of competitive position	Life-cycle stage			
	Embryonic	Growth	Maturity	Aging
Dominant	Hold position All-out push for share	Hold position Hold share	Hold position Grow with industry	Hold position
Strong	Attempt to improve position All-out push for share	Attempt to improve position Push for share	Hold position Grow with industry	Hold position or harvest
Favorable	Selectively attempt to improve position Selective or all-out push for share	Attempt to improve position Selective push for share	Custodial or maintenance Find niche and attempt to protect it	Harvest Phased withdrawal
Tentative	Selectively push for position	Find niche and protect it	Find niche and hang on Phased withdrawal	Phased withdrawal or abandon
Weak	Up or out	Turnaround or abandon	Turnaround or phased withdrawal	Abandon

From Digman, Lester A. *Strategic Management: Concepts, Decisions, and Cases,* 2nd ed., 221. Homewood, IL: BPI/Irwin, 1990; reprinted by permission.

Strategy Choice [IIIc]

In choosing organizational strategies, the major context variables that influence choice are type of organization, strategic decision style, managerial philosophy, organizational culture and choice-maker values, portfolio analysis, organization life cycle, and competitive position. The specific criteria that are used in selecting strategies are presented in Figure 8.5 [IIIc]. Some of these criteria are, Will the organizational strategy accomplish objectives? Will the strategy address risks, issues, deficiencies, and gaps? Will the strategy take advantage of opportunities in the environment and capitalize on HSO/HS strengths and comparative advantage? Will the strategy lessen threats and overcome weaknesses? In addition, attention must be given to the effect that the organizational strategy selected will have on functional areas of the HSO/HS. That is, considering strengths and weaknesses, is it feasible? Does the organization have the capacity—financial resources, managerial systems and human resources, and productivity and conversion processes—necessary to implement the strategy successfully? If so, implementation is the next step. This is depicted in Figure 8.5 [IV].

As presented in Figure 8.5, once organizational strategies are chosen, operational plans, programs, and activities are developed for units or segments of the organization [IVa]. As depicted in Figure 8.2, they are derived from the strategies and must be consistent with them. It is necessary to gather and allocate resources and make organizational arrangements concerning structure, tasks/technology, and people so that, when all are integrated, inputs are converted to outputs (see Figure 8.5 [IVb and IVc]). Finally, after implementing the strategy or strategies, it is necessary to control. Results must be monitored and evaluated (see Figure 8.5 [V]) to determine whether objectives are being accomplished and whether resource allocation and utilization are effective. If not, the process begins again (Figure 8.5 [I]). In fact, strategic planning is a process that never ends. There is a reciprocal relationship between strategy formulation and implementation. Both are concurrent and continuous. Even though present strategy(ies) may result in a HSO/HS achieving its objectives, strategic assessment must continue to monitor environments with respect to whether and how they are changing and what the HSO's/HS's response should be.

STAKEHOLDERS AND STRATEGIC PLANNING

Stakeholders, such as those identified in Figure 8.6, can affect HSO/HS strategic planning in two ways: 1) they can influence formulation of organization objectives, and 2) they can be important, even critical, to the successful implementation of strategy. Consequently, "the identification, assessment, and diagnosis of stakeholder relationships . . . should be fully integrated into the organization's strategic planning process."[108] Relative to strategy implementation, a useful model has been developed that suggests tactics for interacting and negotiating with stakeholders based on two conditions: potential threat and potential for cooperation.[109]

Figure 8.11 presents the HSO/HS tactics of collaborate, subordinate, compete, and avoid negotiating. They are predicated on 1) whether the "substantive outcome," such as implementing a diversification or forward integration strategy, is important; and 2) whether the HSO's/HS's "relationship outcome" with stakeholders, such as maintaining friendly relations and cooperation, is or is not important. Depending on the HSO's/HS's priorities, interaction tactics with stakeholders are suggested. These four tactics appear in the "organizational contingencies" part of the expanded model in Figure 8.12. Adding the element of "stakeholder contingencies" expands the possible HSO/HS tactics for interacting with stakeholders. Questions such as, "Can HSO/HS management ensure stakeholder acceptance?" and "Will likely stakeholder coalitions be acceptable to the organization?" must be answered. For example, if a substantive outcome such as vertical integration is important to the HSO/HS and the relationship outcome with the stakeholder is important, a collaborative tactic (C1) is suggested. Furthermore, if HSO/HS management can ensure stakeholder acceptance of the

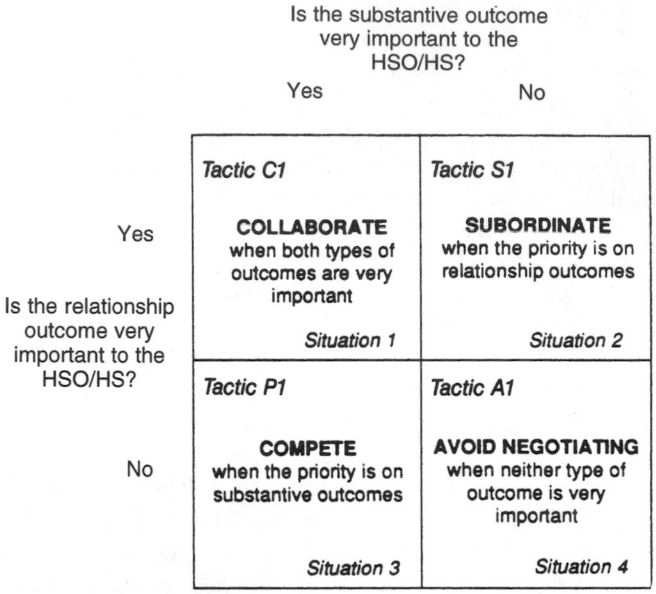

Is the substantive outcome
very important to the
HSO/HS?

Yes   No

	Is the substantive outcome very important to the HSO/HS?	
	Yes	**No**
Is the relationship outcome very important to the HSO/HS? **Yes**	*Tactic C1* **COLLABORATE** when both types of outcomes are very important *Situation 1*	*Tactic S1* **SUBORDINATE** when the priority is on relationship outcomes *Situation 2*
No	*Tactic P1* **COMPETE** when the priority is on substantive outcomes *Situation 3*	*Tactic A1* **AVOID NEGOTIATING** when neither type of outcome is very important *Situation 4*

Figure 8.11.   Selecting outcome-focused negotiation tactics. (Adapted from Blair, John D., Grant T. Savage, and Carlton J. Whitehead. "A Strategic Approach for Negotiating with Hospital Stakeholders." *Health Care Management Review* 14 [Winter 1989]: 17; reprinted by permission of Aspen Publishers, Inc., © 1989.)

strategy and the stakeholder is not likely to form a coalition that is acceptable to the HSO/HS, then either a cautious collaborative tactic (C2) or respectful competitive tactic (P2) is suggested.

This model assists strategic planning because it allows senior-level management to assess systematically the potential threat to or cooperation with the organization's stakeholders. In addition, it indicates how to interact with stakeholders who may have an impact on implementing these strategies.

STRATEGIC ISSUES MANAGEMENT

Discussion to this point has focused on strategic planning as related to creating a more favorable match between the HSO/HS and its external environment. The emphasis traditionally has been on changing/adapting the organization and its strategies to meet the demands of the environment to enhance its competitive position. Strategic issues management (SIM), which is a logical extension of HSO/HS strategic planning, is a systematic process that focuses on influencing the external environment so that it is more favorable to the organization.[110] That is, SIM involves proactively influencing and affecting public policy issues versus simply reacting and adapting to them.

In the management model in Figure 1.7, HSOs/HSs interface with the external environment, which includes the health care environment as well as the general environment. In both, public policy issues take on significance because HSOs/HSs must respond to them reactively when regulations/legislation are imposed (adaptive) or proactively (influence) in framing the debate and shaping the outcome. With the latter response, HSOs/HSs strategically seek to affect the external environment to be more favorable or less unfavorable to them by influencing the course and pace of externally imposed change.

Some characterize SIM as "political strategy."[111] This is not to imply that SIM, with its political dimension, is bad. Quite the contrary, failure by HSO/HS senior-level managers to proactively

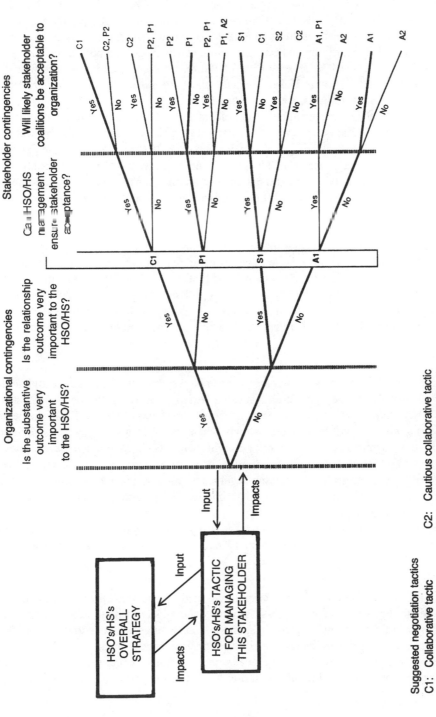

Figure 8.12. Selecting and refining stakeholder negotiation tactics. (Adapted from Blair, John D., Grant T. Savage, and Carlton J. Whitehead. "A Strategic Approach for Negotiating with Hospital Stakeholders." *Health Care Management Review* 14 [Winter 1989]: 19; reprinted by permission of Aspen Publishers, Inc., © 1989.)

influence public policy issues related to health services would be abdication of their political, strategist, and informational roles; nonapplication of their political competency; and not fulfilling their responsibility to defend the interests of their organizations (see also Chapter 17). For HSOs/HSs, "survival depends as much on an ability to anticipate and influence the public policy issues that arise in the sociopolitical environment as the competitive issues that arise in the economic environment."[112] Reeves argued that identifying and acting on policy issues requiring political action is essential for HSO/HS success, and it is an extension of the external environmental scanning that occurs with strategic planning.[113] Large IDSs, alliances, and trade associations usually are better positioned than are single HSOs to influence many issues.

HSOs/HSs are not insulated from external stakeholders and public policy issues. Government is a large purchaser of services and is a major stakeholder with legislative and regulatory power that affects HSOs/HSs. National health planning in the 1970s and early 1980s and prospective payment for Medicare beneficiaries are examples. (See Chapters 2 and 14 for regulation and legislation issues in health services.) Community groups and patients are another constituency. Access to health care, its cost, and scope of services issues are often raised to a level of public policy. Managed care restrictions exemplified by gatekeepers, physician gagging (contractual prohibitions against publicly criticizing the MCO), restrictive network specialist referral, and "drive-through" baby delivery (quick discharge) are examples of issues that rose to the level of political debate in health care federal legislation in the late 1990s. As a large payer of health care, the business community also has a significant stakeholder interest in the outcomes of HSOs/HSs. Finally, MCOs are external stakeholders that have enhanced strength of buyer power relative to independent HSOs because of their ability to direct patients to or away from specific HSOs and to ratchet down prices.[114] All of these groups may initiate public policy that may be favorable or unfavorable to HSOs/HSs.

Issue Life Cycle

Public policy issues are those that "arise when a gap exists between public expectations and actual organization performance and when public disagreement exists concerning the best solution for closing that gap."[115] With few exceptions the issue concerns broad types of HSOs/HSs or the health services industry as a whole. Issues may emerge slowly when only a limited number of stakeholders are affected by the performance (i.e., outcome), as with hepatitis C. They may emerge quickly when an outcome is highly visible, as with thalidomide, or a critical number are affected, as with AIDS or patients' rights in managed care. An issue becomes politicized when the public, special interest groups, or other stakeholders generate sufficient interest of legislators or regulators to place the issue onto the political agenda.[116]

Table 8.5 presents a public policy life cycle model and suggests strategies depending on the stage of the issue.[117] The issue life cycle stages are anticipatory, emergence, enactment, and implementation.

Anticipatory

The anticipatory stage is prevention and building political capital, and it is basically preissue. By means of goodwill strategies to strengthen relations with stakeholders through outreach services, donations, and support of professional associations, and by means of assessment strategies such as environmental scanning of customers' needs, the HSO/HS will enhance its image and ability to ask these groups for support on an issue should the need arise. "By anticipating public policy issues hospital managers are better prepared to take action early that has the potential to avoid or shape legislation."[118]

Emergence

Once an issue emerges, strategies focus on communication and stakeholder building by providing information to shape the parameters of the issue and to influence the outcome by presenting the

TABLE 8.5. PUBLIC POLICY ISSUES LIFE CYCLE

Stage	Strategies
Anticipatory	Good will strategies
	Corporate donations
	Community outreach
	Assessment strategies
	Environmental scanning
Emergence	Communication strategies
	Constituency building
	Advocacy advertising
	Press releases
	Formal organizational
	communications
Enactment	Information strategies
	Expert witnesses
	Personal visits to legislators
	Technical reports
	Political strategies
	Lobbying
	PAC contributions
	Trade associations
Implementation	Compliance strategies
	Negotiation
	Litigation
	Legislative relief
	Noncompliance

From Bigelow, Barbara, Margarete Arndt, and Melissa Middleton Stone. "Corporate Political Strategy: Incorporating the Management of Public Policy Issues into Hospital Strategy." *Health Care Management Review 22* (Summer 1997): 56; reprinted by permission.

HSO's/HS's position. During anticipation and emergence stages, the HSO/HS may have the opportunity to close the performance gap, alter or modify stakeholder expectations so that the issue becomes moot, or align with critical constituents to enhance political support.[119]

Enactment

During or close to the enactment stage, when public policy issues are resolved via legislation or regulation, the HSO/HS can employ two types of strategies—1) information strategies, such as expert witnesses, position papers, and visits to legislators, and 2) political strategies, such as lobbying, political action committee contributions, or trade association intervention—to shape the outcome. One proactive initiative may include providing legislators with sample legislation through a trade association.[120]

Implementation

Once legislation is enacted or regulations promulgated, the range of strategies narrows. The organization can negotiate for legislative relief or exemption, may choose to alter the outcome through amending legislation, or may litigate. The posture at this stage is reactive.

Factors that Can Affect Public Policy Issues

The implications of the public policy issues life cycle model for HSO/HS managers is that, as an issue moves through the stages, managers lose discretion because the range of options narrows. There is greater latitude in containing or stopping an issue in the anticipatory or emergence stage than in the implementation stage. Another implication, just as in the organization life cycle model, is issue path. An issue may follow the normal path through each successive stage; it may be unidirectional—stopped or taken off the table, interrupted, or some stages may be skipped; or it may be recursive by cycling back and forth between stages or be enduring. Recursive issues are seemingly unresolvable or so complex that broad-based consensus on resolving them is difficult to achieve. An example is Medicare solvency.[121]

Factors that can affect public policy issues through the life cycle stages and the paths they take are presented in Table 8.6. It presents a typology of issue evolution and the impact of various factors on the paths that issues take. The factors are facts, stakeholders, other issues, and the scope of the issue.

Facts can affect an issue's evolution by defusing or recasting it, as in the case of mammogram screening being recommended less frequently for women in some age groups. Another example is that of litigation by states' attorneys general resulting in the release of tobacco companies' internal documents indicating that they suppressed studies on the harmful effects of smoking. Forced release of documents caused the issue to gain prominence rapidly after many years of stonewalling and public denial by the tobacco companies.

Stakeholders have different values, perceptions, agendas, and influence. Some stakeholders are more aware of issues than others; some are likely to be involved sooner, later, or at different stages of the issue; and some may be engaged or disengaged as the issue moves through the life cycle stages.[122]

Other issues are always present and are in various stages of their life cycle. They compete for the attention of the public and legislators. "The emergence of new issues may abort or stall the development of existing issues, or as with facts, recast existing ones."[123]

Scope of the issue can influence its path. Those issues that are bounded and relatively easy to define, with general consensus among stakeholders on resolution, may quickly move through the

TABLE 8.6.   A TYPOLOGY OF ISSUE EVOLUTION: IMPACT OF FACTORS ON PATHS

	Facts	Stakeholders	Other issues	Scope of issue
Normal	Additional facts do not interfere with evolution	Stakeholder actions do not interfere with evolution	Other issues do not interfere with evolution	Issue bounded, amenable to resolution in some specified arena
Unidirectional				
Stopped	New facts emerge that render it a nonissue	Stakeholder actions successful at stopping issue	Other issues usurp attention	Issue bounded
Interrupt	Same as stopped; new facts emerge that reintroduce issue	Same as stopped; issue regains salience for stakeholders	Same as stopped; other issues resolved or stopped, attention returns to original	Issue bounded, amenable to resolution in some specified arena
Skip	Crisis occurs or new facts emerge that galvanize attention	New stakeholders enter that press issue forward	Outcomes of other issues push issue along path	Issue becomes well defined quickly
Recursive				
Cyclical	New facts cause a reinterpretation of issue or reassessment of positions	Stakeholders entering and exiting cause issue to move backward and forward	Other issues act similarly to new facts	Issue is not well bounded, subject to reinterpretation, shifting positions
Enduring	New facts constantly entering and altering face of issue	Same as cyclical	Other issues act similarly to new facts	Issue is not bounded

From Bigelow, Barbara, Liam Fahey, and John Mahon. "A Typology of Issue Evolution." *Business and Society* 32 (April 1993): 25; reprinted by permission.

life cycle stages. If it is a win–win situation, the issue may even skip stages. However, those issues that are not relatively bounded, or of such significance that they are not easily resolved, may cycle between stages or be enduring. Bigelow, Fahey, and Mahon observed that

> *health care, for example, has been an issue for seventy years. The face of the issue has changed as quality, access, and cost have competed for primacy. However, even with primacy accorded to cost, the issue has not been resolved despite "resolutions" in the form of business coalitions, legislation, and community action. Rather than marking the end of an issue, each of these actions is better understood as a stage in a continuing (cyclical-enduring) life cycle.*[124]

Implications

Strategic management is not just adapting to the environment but also changing it. Senior-level managers are transformational leaders who have a vision of where the HSO/HS should be, how to achieve a favorable competitive position, and how to communicate it to others. Similarly, they have a responsibility and it is legitimate for them to defend their organization from inappropriate intrusion by stakeholders or government. Engaging in strategic issues management to affect public policy issues, as well as being aware of the issue life cycle and the impact of factors that can affect an issue's path, can aid senior-level managers as they fulfill their various managerial roles.

As observed by Reeves, "political influence is like money. It can be spent, invested or saved." The question to ask is, "is the issue significant enough to . . . spend political resources?"[125] Among the criteria for answering this question are[126]

1. Is the issue consequential to the HSO/HS and worth spending political capital on?
2. Is favorable intervention possible by the HSO/HS at the particular stage of the issue's life cycle?
3. Are the available intervention strategies acceptable, legal, and consistent with the organization's mission, vision, values, and culture and professional ethics?
4. Can the strategies be feasibly implemented?
5. Will the cost–benefit results be acceptable?
6. Is this the best way to achieve the goal?

SUMMARY

This chapter discusses planning with specific focus on strategic planning and its integral component, marketing. Planning is a managerial function defined as anticipating the future, assessing present conditions, and making decisions concerning organizational direction, programs, and resource deployment. The results of planning answer questions of what to do, when, where, how, and for what purpose. Planning is linked to the management model. It helps HSO/HS managers cope with environments; reduce uncertainty, ambiguity, and risk; focus on outputs, develop priorities, design conversion processes, and allocate resources; and control to ensure that organization objectives are accomplished.

Planning characteristics addressed include type of planning, time frame and who plans, and approaches to planning. Figure 8.1 details these classifications. Outcomes of planning are discussed. Included are mission, which is the foundation for all planning, overall organization objectives (unit subobjectives), strategies and derived operational programs, and policies and procedures. Figure 8.3 presents their relationships for a single HSO and a HS.

Another major section of the chapter focuses on health services marketing and its link to strategic planning. The concept of marketing means determining the needs, wants, and desires of target markets and designing programs, services, and products to satisfy them. The marketing audit identifies and assesses target needs and wants along with elements of marketing to facilitate exchange between buyer/consumer and seller/provider. The traditional elements of marketing (product, price, place, and promotion) are recast and presented in the health services context as service, consideration, access, and promotion (SCAP).

The next section focuses on HSO/HS strategic planning: 1) formulating HSO/HS objectives, and 2) identifying, evaluating, choosing, and implementing organizational strategies and operational programs to accomplish objectives. Organizational strategies are defined as long-term patterns of activities requiring substantial commitment of resources; they are the means by which organization objectives are accomplished. Organizational culture and values of choice makers are discussed.

A HSO/HS strategic planning model is presented in Figure 8.5. The strategic assessment component [II] includes external environmental analysis [IIa], which identifies threats and opportunities; internal capability analysis and organization profile [IIc], which identifies weaknesses and strengths; and the marketing audit [IIb], which links them. In addition, industry structure and competitive position is discussed centering on the five forces model of competition consisting of rivalry, substitutes, new entrants, and bargaining power of buyers and suppliers. The results of strategic assessment yield information [IId] about the HSO's/HS's SWOTs, risks, issues, deficiencies, and objective gaps.

The strategy choice component of the strategic planning model in Figure 8.5 [III] addresses three elements: formulation and consideration of strategies [IIIa], strategy choice [IIIc], and the context of strategy choice [IIIb]. Two typologies of strategies are reviewed. First, Porter's model of competitive strategies consisting of low-cost leadership, differentiation, and focus is presented. Second, the generic organizational strategies discussed are classified as specialization/niche, vertical and horizontal integration, diversification, retrenchment/divestiture, and strategic alliances. For both typologies of strategies, examples are given and application to HSOs/HSs is made. In review of the context of strategy choice, the following components are examined: type of organization, strategic decision style, managerial philosophy, organizational culture and choice-maker values, portfolio analysis, organization life cycle, and competitive position.

Stakeholders such as those identified in Figure 8.6 can affect HSO/HS strategic planning by influencing the formulation of objectives and strategies, as well as the success of strategy implementation. A model is presented (Figures 8.11 and 8.12) that enables senior-level managers to identify the importance of a stakeholder and suggests tactics for interacting with it.

Finally, strategic issues management (SIM) is cast as a logical extension of HSO/HS strategic planning. SIM enables the organization to proactively seek to influence public policy issues so that the external environment is more favorable to it. SIM is a legitimate and appropriate activity for senior-level managers. The public policy issues life cycle is presented, along with a typology of issue evolution and impact of factors on the paths a public policy issue may take.

DISCUSSION QUESTIONS

1. Define planning. How is it related to the management model (see Figure 1.7)?
2. Identify and describe the characteristics of planning.
3. Identify the outcomes of planning and discuss how they are interrelated. Why are all outcomes based on mission? What are the typical elements included in mission, vision, values?
4. Identify and describe each of the five forces in Porter's model of competition.
5. What is health services marketing? Identify and discuss the elements of marketing.
6. Define strategic planning. Be prepared to discuss the strategic assessment components identified in Figure 8.5. How does the marketing audit relate to strategic assessment?
7. Identify and give examples of Porter's three competitive strategies and the generic organizational strategies for HSOs/HSs. How does context of strategy choice affect consideration and selection of strategy? Give examples.
8. Identify a HSO or HS with which you are familiar. Describe a situation in which the substantive and relationship outcomes were important to the organization and a C1 tactic with a stakeholder was suggested (refer to Figures 8.11 and 8.12).

9. Managed care has become a public policy issue. Identify the issue life cycle model stages. At what stage is this issue? Based on Table 8.6, what has been the path of the managed care issue and what factors have influenced its path?

CASE STUDY 1: HOSPITAL MARKETING EFFECTIVENESS RATING INSTRUMENT[127]

Complete the following instrument. Choose a hospital, other health services organization, or health system with which you are familiar. Circle the one most appropriate answer (A, B, or C) for each question below.

CUSTOMER PHILOSOPHY

1. How does the HSO/HS view its markets?
   A. Management thinks in terms of serving patient needs based on the facilities and clinical staff currently available.
   B. Management attempts to offer a broad range of health services, performing all of them well.
   C. Management thinks in terms of serving the needs of well-defined patient and physician segments that offer to the HSO/HS the best prospect for long-term growth and financial return.
2. What is the status of the HSO's/HS's publicity, promotion, and community education programs?
   A. There is limited activity in this area.
   B. The HSO/HS has a number of programs in this area, but coordination among them is limited.
   C. The HSO/HS has a well-coordinated program of information and community outreach efforts, all under the guidance of one staff member.
3. How does the HSO/HS attract and retain the clinical staff?
   A. Primary responsibility for selection and attraction of staff resides with current staff members.
   B. The HSO/HS relies essentially on specific incentives such as high salaries or special equipment to attract new members.
   C. As part of the planning and coordination process, the HSO/HS has developed a comprehensive system to determine and influence the factors affecting the professional staff organization affiliation decision.

INTEGRATED MARKETING ORGANIZATION

4. Is there a vice president or director of marketing responsible for planning, executing, and coordinating the marketing functions?
   A. No such individual exists.
   B. Yes, but there is little integration of this individual within the planning/decision-making process. This individual primarily provides marketing services.
   C. Yes, and the individual participates in HSO/HS policy making as well as providing marketing services.
5. To what extent are marketing-oriented functions (e.g., planning, public relations, marketing research, advertising, promotion, and fund-raising) coordinated in the HSO/HS?
   A. Not very well. There is sometimes unproductive conflict among these functions.
   B. Somewhat. There is some formal integration, but less than satisfactory coordination and control.
   C. Very well. There is effective coordination and control of these functions.

6. Is there a formal systematic procedure for evaluating potential new services and technologies?
   A. There is no formal procedure.
   B. A procedure exists, but it does not include major input from marketing.
   C. The procedure is well developed and includes major input from marketing.

MARKETING INFORMATION SYSTEM

7. Does the HSO/HS conduct patient exit interviews and other surveys of patient satisfaction and suggestions?
   A. Rarely or never
   B. Occasionally, but not on a formal basis.
   C. Yes, systematically, on a formal basis.

8. Does the HSO/HS collect information regarding trends in demand for various types of treatments and the availability in the market of competitive services?
   A. Rarely or never
   B. Occasionally
   C. Yes, on a systematic, continuous basis.

9. Does the HSO/HS have an information system containing relevant and up-to-date marketing data?
   A. Such information is limited, and is not maintained on an ongoing basis.
   B. Adequate records are maintained and updated on a routine basis, essentially in hardcopy form.
   C. An extensive, computer-based information system is provided for systematic storage, maintenance, update, and analysis of marketing data.

STRATEGIC ORIENTATION

10. Does the HSO/HS regularly monitor and evaluate patient services to identify potential new services to offer and current services to curtail or drop?
    A. The HSO/HS does not evaluate the marketing viability of its various services.
    B. The HSO/HS occasionally evaluates its current services and studies potential new services.
    C. The HSO/HS regularly evaluates its current services and systematically studies potential new services.

11. Does the HSO/HS carry out strategic market planning as well as annual marketing planning?
    A. Strategic market planning is only initiated under special circumstances, such as when considering facility expansion or debt financing
    B. Strategic market planning is carried out regularly but is not done very well.
    C. Strategic market planning is carried out regularly and is done very well.

12. Does the HSO/HS prepare contingency plans?
    A. No
    B. Contingency plans are occasionally developed to meet a major threat.
    C. Contingency plans are routinely developed as part of the normal planning process.

13. Does HSO/HS management know the costs and profitability of its various services?
    A. Such information is not available.
    B. Limited information is available.
    C. HSO/HS management knows the costs and profitability of its various services.

14. Are marketing resources used effectively on a day-to-day basis?
    A. Such resources are either not available or are inadequately used.
    B. The resources are adequate and used to a significant extent, but not in an optimal manner.
    C. Yes. Such resources are employed adequately and effectively.
15. Does management examine the results of its marketing expenditures to know what it is accomplishing for its money?
    A. No
    B. To a limited extent
    C. Yes

SCORING

For all of the 15 questions, indicate the number of

A responses _____ × 0 = _____
B responses _____ × 1 =
C responses _____ × 2 = _____
Total score _____

The following scale shows the HSO's/HS's level of marketing effectiveness:

0–5 = None
6–10 = Poor
11–15 = Fair
16–20 = Good
21–25 = Very good
26–30 = Superior

QUESTION

1. How does the HSO/HS that you evaluated score on the marketing effectiveness rating instrument? If it was low, explain why.

CASE STUDY 2: HSO STRATEGIC ASSESSMENT

Assume that you are the chief executive officer of a single HSO such as a hospital, nursing facility, or HMO. It may be one in your present locale or elsewhere, if details about it are known. Using the strategic planning model as a guide (see Figure 8.5), conduct a strategic assessment including: 1) external environmental analysis, 2) marketing audit, and 3) internal capability analysis.

QUESTIONS

1. Compile a detailed list of "strategic assessment" considerations (e.g., factors, items) that are relevant to the HSO selected.
2. Using Porter's five forces model of competition, what is the HSO's competitive position?
3. List the "yields" (risks, issues, deficiencies, and gaps) confronting the HSO.
4. Attempt to identify and describe past and present organizational strategies the HSO has implemented or is implementing.
5. Are you aware whether any of the "context of strategy choice" variables are present in the situation? If so, describe them and discuss the reasons why they are applicable.

CASE STUDY 3: CLOSING PEDIATRICS

City Hospital has a pediatrics department with 35 beds. For the past several years the occupancy has varied between 40% and 60%. There is a definite downward trend, but it appears to be stabilizing at about 45% occupancy. The low occupancy has caused a financial strain. Other area hospitals are experiencing a similar situation. As a result, several hospitals have proposed forming a community task force to study the situation and determine whether one or more pediatric departments should be closed, thereby increasing occupancy for those remaining. It is hoped that this will reduce costs and increase quality.

Although this proposal may benefit the community as a whole, it raises questions for City Hospital. Among them is the effect on two objectives: to provide a full range of quality services and to offer a full range of graduate medical education, including residencies in pediatrics.

QUESTIONS

1. What effect would the retrenchment strategy have on City Hospital's objectives?
2. Identify the stakeholders that influence the decision.
3. Are there other strategies that can be considered by City Hospital?
4. Argue against the closure. What reasons support your position?

CASE STUDY 4: NATIONAL HEALTH INSURANCE

Yesterday, the president signed a bill passed by Congress establishing universal-comprehensive health insurance. It will cover all U.S. residents for medically necessary hospital inpatient and outpatient services, physician and other licensed independent practitioner services, and nursing facility care. The National Health Insurance (NHI) program becomes effective 12 months from yesterday. Funding for the NHI program will be through a national value-added tax. All residents, whether employed or unemployed, from birth to death ("womb to tomb") are covered by the NHI program, and there are no beneficiary deductibles or copayments. State government State Health Insurance Boards (SHIBs) will be the fiscal intermediaries. Private health insurance for covered services will be barred when the NHI program takes effect.

Delivery of services will be private, as before, and will be done through existing providers (e.g., hospitals, nursing facilities, private practitioners). Institutional providers' services and capacities will be frozen in place the day the NHI program begins. They may only be changed (added to or deleted) subject to SHIB approval based on the SHIB's assessment of area needs. Start-up and facility expenditures for approved expansions in services and capabilities will be fully funded by the federal NHI board through the SHIB.

Amounts paid to all independent providers, such as physicians for care rendered to beneficiaries, will be fee-for-service. National rates for all services will be determined by the federal NHI board and will vary in amount only by geographic area based on a market-basket consumer price index. Institutional providers will not be reimbursed on fee-for-service but will receive annual global budgets that are fixed. These budgets will be determined by each SHIB and will be largely based on capacity, such as type and number of beds. Providers will not be allowed to balance bill patients. Because uninhibited access is an objective of the NHI program, all providers will be required to serve all people who present themselves.

QUESTIONS

1. Is the NHI program a threat or an opportunity for providers? Why?
2. If you were a hospital CEO, what organizational strategies would you recommend for implementation before the start of the NHI program? What strategies after it begins?
3. Once NHI becomes effective, what changes in stakeholder relations would you predict?

CASE STUDY 5: VIOLATION

Bill Richardson, purchasing department storeroom clerk at Parks Manor, a 200-bed nursing facility, spotted a fire in a difficult-to-reach air shaft. He ran to the nearest call box, turned in the alarm, and asked a nearby employee to stay at the box and direct the fire department to the fire location in shaft No. 2 when they arrived. After grabbing a soda-acid fire extinguisher, he crawled into the air shaft and, at considerable risk to himself because the fire was near electrical wiring, put out the fire. When the fire department arrived, 3 minutes after the alarm was sounded, a smoke-befuddled Richardson was crawling out of the shaft.

Richardson was congratulated and his department head said he would write a commendation report to be attached to his personnel record. Their conversation had scarcely ended when another fire broke out in the vicinity of the air shaft. Acidulated water from the extinguisher had seeped down into a high-voltage junction box, and within moments a severe electrical fire, worse than the one Richardson had put out, was raging. The fire department, with some difficulty, brought the fire under control.

Richardson was censured by the director of maintenance for using the wrong type of fire extinguisher. On the top rim band the soda-acid extinguisher was a large, commercial placard stating that the extinguisher was not to be used on electrical fires. A carbon dioxide extinguisher, approved for electrical fires, was located near the one Richardson used. "You should leave things to trained personnel!" yelled the maintenance director. "There is a policy that, in case of fire, employees are to activate the nearest alarm, notify their supervisor, see to the safety of patients, and not attempt to extinguish the fire themselves unless specifically trained to do so. Now you have created a real mess!"

QUESTIONS

1. Did Richardson violate a policy or a procedure? What is the difference between them?
2. Is something wrong with this policy/procedure? If so, what is it and how can it be corrected?
3. When is it appropriate to deviate from policy/procedure? Can one be ignored with less potential damage to the organization than the other?
4. Should Richardson have been reprimanded? Why or why not?

CASE STUDY 6: TRENDS FOR THE FUTURE—
INDUSTRY STRUCTURE AND COMPETITIVE POSITION

The health services environment is changing. "The future healthcare environment shows no signs of being 'kinder and gentler' to providers. A number of trends on the horizon will affect providers and their decisions about the future."[128] The following trends were identified by Zuckerman[129]:

1. **Providers will assume increasing risk for underutilization and overutilization of services.** Economic risk is shifting from insurance companies and employers to providers. Comprehensive systems will assume risk for a defined population group, and will be paid a fixed fee per covered life. By keeping the group covered lives healthy, and providing and controlling a full continuum of services for their patients, providers will reduce utilization and, ultimately, costs. The philosophical shift from building volume by increasing admissions, tests, and procedures, to keeping a population healthy and reducing utilization will not come easily.
2. **Only unique or geographically isolated providers will remain independent.** Providers in the healthcare system of the future will be closely aligned. Partnerships, alliances,

mergers, and consolidations are the watchwords for healthcare providers of the future. Adversarial relationships will lead to failure.

3. **Healthcare reform is occurring parallel to, and in spite of, state and federal healthcare reform initiatives.** Universal insurance coverage, healthcare purchasing groups, and other reform measures may eventually develop. In the meantime, many providers are reforming themselves. Legislation may simply formalize changes already occurring.

4. **Technological advances will enhance and challenge healthcare delivery.** Existing and developing technology has enormous potential to improve efficiency and productivity, but often at a high price. Use of technology may increase operational costs and drain resources if the value of the technology is not proven to reduce staffing or resource utilization.

5. **Providers must manage excess capacity.** As inpatient and specialist utilization continues to drop and many services move beyond the traditional institutional setting, providers must cope with the burden of excess capacity. Consolidating or closing down services and reallocating resources to provide services that maintain or improve economic viability are imperatives facing providers.

6. **Limitations on reimbursement for high-cost services will stimulate continued growth of ambulatory care services and increase demand for post-acute options.** With continued emphasis on cost containment, providing services on an outpatient basis will be a viable, cost-saving option for providers. Home healthcare, skilled nursing centers, and rehabilitation facilities will help healthcare organizations downstage patients out of costly acute care settings. Primary care, including dramatically increased use of physician extenders, will continue as a substitute for specialty medical services.

7. **As healthcare moves toward an all managed care system, the number of physicians needed will drop dramatically resulting in an oversupply of physicians, particularly specialists.** The oversupply of physicians may have lasting effects on the quality, availability, and costs of healthcare. Options for physicians include planning early retirement, practicing in underserved communities, and seeking retraining as primary care physicians.

QUESTIONS

1. For each of the above predictions, indicate whether you "agree" or "disagree" and list several reasons to support your position.
2. For each of the above predictions, indicate how it will affect a HSO's/HS's competitive position by applying the Porter competitive model (i.e., rivalry, threat of new entrants, threat of substitutes, bargaining power of buyer, bargaining power of supplier).
3. For the predictions that suggest that a provider should follow a particular organizational strategy, identify the strategies that are suggested.
4. Drawing on the information in Chapter 2 and the information in this chapter concerning strategic issues management, relative to Prediction 3:
   A. At the national level, in what stage of the issue's life cycle is reform of health care (i.e., national health insurance)?
   B. What path has the issue followed through the years?
   C. If, as stated, "many providers are reforming themselves," what issue strategies (i.e., tactics) are providers pursuing, and how will those strategies make the environment more favorable for them?

NOTES

1. Carroll, Lewis. *Alice's Adventures in Wonderland,* 57. New York: Delacorte Press/Seymour Lawrence, 1978.
2. Donnelly, James H., Jr., James L. Gibson, and John M. Ivancevich. *Fundamentals of Management,* 10th ed., 140. Boston: Irwin/McGraw-Hill, 1998.

3. Pearce, John A., II, and Richard B. Robinson, Jr. *Management,* 12. New York: Random House, 1989; see also Ivancevich, John M., James H. Donnelly, Jr., and James L. Gibson. *Management Principles and Functions,* 4th ed., 68. Homewood, IL: BPI/Irwin, 1989.
4. Donnelly, James H., James L. Gibson, and John M. Ivancevich. *Fundamentals of Management,* 139.
5. Kaluzny, Arnold D., D. Michael Warner, David G. Warren, and William N. Zelman. *Management of Health Services,* 8. Englewood Cliffs, NJ: Prentice-Hall, 1982.
6. Higgins, James M. *The Management Challenge: An Introduction to Management,* 141. New York: Macmillan, 1991.
7. Zuckerman, Alan M. "Hospital and Medical Staff Strategic Planning: Developing an Integrated Approach." *Physician Executive* 20 (August 1994): 16.
8. Orlikoff, James E., and Mary Totten. "Strategic Planning by the Board." *Trustee* 48 (July/August 1995): 2.
9. McManis, Gerald L. "The Board's Role in Strategic Planning." *Healthcare Executive* 5 (September/October 1990): 22.
10. Gibson, C. Kendrick, David J. Newton, and Daniel S. Cochran. "An Empirical Investigation of Hospital Mission Statements." *Health Care Management Review* 15 (Summer 1990): 35.
11. Zuckerman, Alan M. *Healthcare Strategic Planning: Approaches for the 21st Century,* 37. Chicago: Health Administration Press, 1998.
12. Pearce, John A., II, and Richard B. Robinson, Jr. *Strategic Management: Formulation, Implementation, and Control,* 5th ed., 33. Burr Ridge, IL: Irwin, 1994.
13. Thompson, Arthur A., Jr., and A. J. Strickland, III. *Strategic Management: Concepts and Cases,* 10th ed., 24. Boston: Irwin/McGraw-Hill, 1998.
14. Zuckerman, *Healthcare Strategic Planning,* 41.
15. Whyte, E. Gordon, and John D. Blair. "Strategic Planning for Health Care Providers." In *Health Care Administration: Principles, Practices, Structure, and Delivery,* 2nd ed., edited by Lawrence F. Wolper, 293. Gaithersburg, MD: Aspen Publishers, 1995.
16. Zuckerman, *Healthcare Strategic Planning,* 8.
17. American Diabetes Association. "Association Approves Future Plans and Core Values Statement." *Diabetes Forecast* (November 1998): 123.
18. Georgopoulos, Basil S., and Floyd C. Mann. *The Community General Hospital,* 5. New York: Macmillan, 1962.
19. http://www.henryfordhealth.org/, February 2, 1999.
20. Sahney, Vinrod K., and Gail L. Warden. "The Role of CQI in the Strategic Planning Process." *Quality Management in Health Care* 1 (Summer 1993): 6.
21. American Hospital Association. *Evaluating Diversification Strategies: Management Advisory,* 3. Chicago: American Hospital Association, 1990.
22. Donnelly, Gibson, and Ivancevich, *Fundamentals of Management,* 154–155.
23. Labovitz, George H. "Customer Expectations in the New Millenium." *Healthcare Executive* 13 (January/February 1998): 47.
24. Brown, Montague. "Commentary: Competition, Managed Care, and Trusteeship—Can Voluntary Hospital Governance Survive? Will Not-for-Profit Hospitals Survive?" *Health Care Management Review* 20 (Winter 1995): 84.
25. MacStravic, Robin E. "The End of Health Care Marketing." *Health Marketing Quarterly* 7 (1990): 3.
26. See Sturm, Arthur C., Jr. *The New Rules of Healthcare Marketing: 23 Strategies for Success.* Chicago: Health Administration Press, 1998.
27. For myths about marketing in HSOs, see Kotler, Philip, and Roberta N. Clarke. *Marketing for Health Care Organizations,* 2nd ed., 22–25. Englewood Cliffs, NJ: Prentice-Hall, 1987.
28. Cooper, Philip D. "Managed Care Positives and Negatives for Health Care Marketing." *Health Marketing Quarterly* 12 (1995): 59.
29. Cooper, Philip D. "Marketing from Inside Out." In *Health Care Marketing: Issues and Trends,* 2nd ed., edited by Philip D. Cooper, 109. Rockville, MD: Aspen Publishers, 1985.
30. Proenca, E. Jose. "Market Orientation and Organizational Culture in Hospitals." *Journal of Hospital Marketing* 11 (1996): 6.
31. Kotler and Clarke, *Marketing for Health,* 4.
32. Seidel, Lee F., John W. Seavey, and Richard J.A. Lewis. *Strategic Management for Healthcare Organizations,* 36. Owings Mills, MD: National Health Publishing/AUPHA Press, 1989.

33. Fisk, Trevor A. "Strategic Planning and Marketing." In *The AUPHA Manual of Health Services Management,* edited by Robert J. Taylor and Susan B. Taylor, 311. Gaithersburg, MD: Aspen Publishers, 1994.

34. Kotler and Clarke, *Marketing for Health,* 90.

35. Kotler, Philip, and Gary Armstrong. *Marketing: An Introduction,* 4th ed., 10. Upper Saddle River, NJ: Prentice-Hall, 1997.

36. Cooper, Philip D., Ed. "What Is Health Care Marketing?" In *Health Care Marketing: Issues and Trends,* 2nd ed., edited by Philip D. Cooper, 6. Rockville, MD: Aspen Publishers, 1985.

37. Kotler and Clarke, *Marketing for Health,* 5. For similar definitions of the marketing concept, see Cooper, Philip D. "What Is Health Care Marketing?" In *Health Care Marketing: Issues and Trends,* 2nd ed., edited by Philip D. Cooper, 3. Rockville, MD: Aspen Publishers, 1985; Keith, Jon G. "Marketing Health Care: What the Recent Literature Is Telling Us." In *Health Care Marketing: Issues and Trends,* 2nd ed., edited by Philip D. Cooper, 15–16. Rockville, MD: Aspen Publishers, 1985; MacStravic, Robin E. *Marketing Religious Health Care,* 1. St. Louis: The Catholic Health Association of the United States, 1987; and Winston, William J. *How To Write a Marketing Plan for Health Care Organizations,* 3. New York: Haworth, 1985.

38. Zelman, William N., and Deborah L. Parham. "Strategic, Operational, and Marketing Concerns of Product-Line Management in Health Care." *Health Care Management Review* 15 (Winter 1990): 29.

39. Costello, Michael M., and Daniel J. West. "A New Way of Thinking: How Managed Care Networks Will Affect Physician and Hospital Marketing Efforts." *Journal of Hospital Marketing* 10 (1996): 4; Paul, David P., III and Earl D. Honeycutt. "An Analysis of the Hospital-Patient Marketing Relationship in the Health Care Industry." *Journal of Hospital Marketing* 10 (1995): 36.

40. Bigelow, Barbara, and John F. Mahon. "Strategic Behavior of Hospitals: A Framework for Analysis." *Medical Care Review* 46 (Fall 1989): 298.

41. A good review of methods to measure customer satisfaction can be found in Ford, Robert C., Susan A. Bach, and Myron D. Fottler. "Methods of Measuring Patient Satisfaction in Health Care Organizations." *Health Care Management Review* 22 (Spring 1997): 74–89.

42. Kotler and Armstrong, *Marketing,* 51–53; Mobley, Mary F., and Ralph E. Elkins. "Megamarketing Strategies for Health Care Services." *Health Marketing Quarterly* 7 (1990): 13.

43. Keith, "Marketing Health Care," 17.

44. MacStravic, Robin E. "Price of Services." In *Health Care Marketing: Issues and Trends,* 2nd ed., edited by Philip D. Cooper, 232–234. Rockville, MD: Aspen Publishers, 1985.

45. Kotler and Clarke, *Marketing for Health,* 25.

46. Bruton, Garry D., Benjamin M. Oviatt, and Luanne Kallas-Bruton. "Strategic Planning in Hospitals: A Review and Proposal." *Health Care Management Review* 20 (Summer 1995): 17.

47. Pointer, Dennis D. "Offering-Level Strategy Formulation in Health Services Organizations." *Health Care Management Review* 15 (Summer 1990): 18; Rakich, Jonathon S., and Kurt Darr. "Outcomes of Hospital Strategic Planning. *Hospital Topics* 66 (May/June 1988): 23–24.

48. Whyte and Blair, "Strategic Planning," 293.

49. Savage, Grant T., Rosemary L. Taylor, Timothy M. Rotarius, and John A. Buesseler. "Governance of Integrated Delivery Systems/Networks: A Stakeholder Approach." *Health Care Management Review* 22 (Winter 1997): 7.

50. For an extensive treatment of stakeholder analysis, see Blair, John D., and Myron D. Fottler. *Challenges in Health Care Management: Strategic Perspectives for Managing Key Stakeholders.* San Francisco: Jossey-Bass, 1990. For a model suggesting ways to assess stakeholders' potential for threat, potential for cooperation, and relevance to the HSO as well as negotiation approaches to use, see Blair, John D., Grant T. Savage, and Carlton J. Whitehead. "A Strategic Approach for Negotiating with Hospital Stakeholders." *Health Care Management Review* 14 (Winter 1989): 13–23; Savage, Grant T., and John D. Blair. "The Importance of Relationships in Hospital Negotiation Strategies." *Hospital & Health Services Administration* 34 (Summer 1989): 231–253. A good presentation of stakeholder relationships for medical groups can be found in Blair, John D., Terence T. Rock, Timothy M. Rotarius, Myron D. Fottler, Gena C. Bosse, and J. Matthew Driskill. "The Problematic Fit of Diagnosis and Strategy for Medical Group Stakeholders—Including IDS/Ns." *Health Care Management Review* 21 (Winter 1996): 7–28; Savage, Grant T., Rosemary L. Taylor, Timothy M. Rotarius, and John A. Buesseler. "Governance of

Integrated Delivery Systems/Networks: A Stakeholder Approach." *Health Care Management Review* 22 (Winter 1997): 7–20.

51. Bower, Joseph L., Christopher A. Bartlett, C. Roland Christensen, Andrall E. Pearson, and Kenneth R. Andrews. *Business Policy: Text and Cases,* 7th ed., 109. Homewood, IL: Irwin, 1991.
52. Adapted from Whyte and Blair, "Strategic Planning," 295; reprinted with permission.
53. Porter, Michael E. *Competitive Strategy: Techniques for Analyzing Industries and Competitors,* 4. New York: The Free Press, 1980.
54. Thompson and Strickland, *Strategic Management,* 74.
55. Porter, *Competitive Strategy,* 17–23.
56. Porter, *Competitive Strategy,* 23–24.
57. Thompson and Strickland, *Strategic Management,* 81.
58. Porter, *Competitive Strategy,* 7–17.
59. Porter, *Competitive Strategy,* 24–27.
60. Brown, Montague. "Mergers, Networking, and Vertical Integration: Managed Care and Investor-Owned Hospitals." *Health Care Management Review* 21 (Winter 1996): 30.
61. Ernst & Young, LLP. *Mapping Your Competitive Position: Medicare PSOs and Health Plans* (Score Retrieval File No. 000168), 12. Washington, DC: Ernst & Young, 1997.
62. Brown, "Mergers, Networking," 30.
63. Porter, *Competitive Strategy,* 27–29.
64. Walston, Stephen L., John R. Kimberly, and Lawton R. Burns. "Owned Vertical Integration and Health Care: Promise and Performance." *Health Care Management Review* 21 (Winter 1996): 84.
65. See Burns, Lawton R., and Darrell P. Thorpe. "Trends and Models in Physician-Hospital Organization." *Health Care Management Review* 18 (Fall 1993): 7–20.
66. Kongstvedt, Peter R. *Essentials of Managed Care,* 2nd ed., 42. Gaithersburg, MD: Aspen Publishers, 1997.
67. Kongstvedt, *Essentials,* 42–43.
68. Reeves, Philip N. "Organizational Competence Analysis for Strategic Planning." In *Strategic Management in the Health Care Sector: Toward the Year 2000,* edited by Farhad Simyar and Joseph Lloyd-Jones, 65–84. Englewood Cliffs, NJ: Prentice-Hall, 1988.
69. Adapted from Whyte and Blair, "Strategic Planning," 296–297; reprinted by permission.
70. Reeves, Philip N. "Strategic Planning for Every Manager." *Clinical Laboratory Management Review* 4 (July/August 1990): 272.
71. Porter, *Competitive Strategy,* 35.
72. McIlwain, Thomas F., and Melody J. McCracken. "Essential Dimensions of a Marketing Strategy in the Hospital Industry." *Journal of Hospital Marketing* 11 (1997): 42.
73. Clement, Jan P. "Vertical Integration and Diversification of Acute Care Hospitals: Conceptual Definitions." *Hospital & Health Services Administration* 33 (Spring 1988): 99; Luke, Royce D., and James W. Begun. "The Management of Strategy." In *Health Care Management: A Text in Organization Theory and Behavior,* 2nd ed., edited by Stephen M. Shortell and Arnold Kaluzny, 481. New York: John Wiley & Sons, 1988.
74. Conrad, Douglas A., and William L. Dowling. "Vertical Integration in Health Services: Theory and Managerial Implications." *Health Care Management Review* 15 (Fall 1990): 9–10.
75. Brown, Montague, and Barbara P. McCool. "Vertical Integration: Exploration of a Popular Strategic Concept." *Health Care Management Review* 11 (Fall 1986): 7.
76. Satinsky, Marjorie A. *The Foundations of Integrated Care: Facing the Challenges of Change,* 10. Chicago: American Hospital Publishing, 1998.
77. Haglund, Claudia L., and William L. Dowling. "The Hospital." In *Introduction to Health Services,* 3rd ed., edited by Stephen J. Williams and Paul R. Torrens, 194. Albany, NY: Delmar Publishers, 1988.
78. Smith, Tyler. "Hospitals Are Using Fitness Centers To Improve Health Status and Lower Costs." *Health Care Strategic Management* 14 (July 1996): 16.
79. Campbell, Sandy. "Using Wellness and Prevention as a Strategic Platform for a Hospital System." *Health Care Strategic Management* 16 (May 1998): 15.
80. Health Care Advisory Board. *The Great Product Enterprise: Future State for the American Health System,* 3. Washington, DC: The Advisory Board Company, 1997.

81. Conrad and Dowling, "Vertical Integration," 10; Harrigan, Kathryn Rudie. "Vertical Integration and Corporate Strategy." *Academy of Management Journal* 28 (June 1985): 397.

82. Flexner, William A., Eric N. Berkowitz, and Montague Brown. *Strategic Planning in Health Care Management,* 15. Rockville, MD: Aspen Publishers, 1981.

83. Satinsky, *Foundations,* 5.

84. "Beverly Enterprises." *Value Line* 4 (June 2, 1998): 652.

85. Shortell, Stephen M., Ellen M. Morrison, and Susan Hughes. "The Keys to Successful Diversification: Lessons from Leading Hospital Systems." *Hospital & Health Services Administration* 43 (Winter 1989): 472.

86. Ginter, Peter M., Linda M. Swayne, and W. Jack Duncan. *Strategic Management of Health Care Organizations,* 3rd ed., 177–178. Malden, MA: Blackwell, 1998.

87. Sabatino, Frank. "Home Health, Diagnostic Centers Were Financial Winners in 1990." *Hospitals* 65 (January 20, 1991): 27.

88. For a good discussion of hospital diversification into long-term care, see Giardina, Carole W., Myron D. Fottler, Richard M. Shewchuk, and Daniel B. Hill. "The Case for Diversification into Long Term Care." *Health Care Management Review* 15 (Winter 1990): 71–82.

89. Ginter, Swayne, and Duncan, *Strategic Management,"* 180.

90. Zuckerman, Howard S., Arnold D. Kaluzny, and Thomas C. Ricketts, III. "Alliances in Health Care: What We Know, What We Think We Know, and What We Should Know." *Health Care Management Review* 20 (Winter 1995): 54.

91. Zuckerman, Kaluzny, and Ricketts, "Alliances in Health Care," 56.

92. Campbell, Sandy. "Columbia/HCA Has a Vision and a Mission for Its Future, but No Strategic Plan." *Health Care Strategic Management* 15 (December 1997): 15.

93. "Columbia/HCA." *Value Line* 4 (April 3, 1998): 653. For an interesting critique of Columbia/HCA and its strategies, see Goldsmith, Jeff. "Columbia/HCA: A Failure of Leadership." *Health Affairs* 17 (March/April 1998): 27–29.

94. Ginn, Gregory O., and Gary J. Young. "Organizational and Environmental Determinants of Hospital Strategy." *Hospital & Health Services Administration* 37 (Fall 1992): 293.

95. Scotti, Dennis J. "Cultural Factors in Choosing a Strategic Posture: A Bridge Between Formulation and Implementation." In *Strategic Management of the Health Care Sector: Toward the Year 2000,* edited by Farhad Simyar and Joseph Lloyd-Jones, 156. Englewood Cliffs, NJ: Prentice-Hall, 1988.

96. Others use the terms *planning, entrepreneurial,* and *adaptive mode*—see Hunger, J. David, and Thomas L. Wheelen. *Essentials of Strategic Management,* 12. Reading, MA: Addison-Wesley, 1997.

97. Whyte and Blair, "Strategic Planning," 293.

98. Craig, Tim T. "Formulating Patterns of Strategic Behavior." In *Strategic Management in the Health Care Sector: Toward the Year 2000,* edited by Farhad Simyar and Joseph Lloyd-Jones, 193. Englewood Cliffs, NJ: Prentice-Hall, 1988.

99. Bower, Bartlett, Christensen, Pearson, and Andrews, *Business Policy,* 341.

100. Digman, Lester A. *Strategic Management: Concepts, Decisions, Cases,* 2nd ed., 335. Homewood, IL: BPI/Irwin, 1990.

101. Hunger and Wheelen, *Essentials of Strategic Management,"* 90–91.

102. Rutsohn, Phil, and Nabil A. Ibrahim. "Strategically Positioning Tomorrow's Hospital Today: Current Indications for Strategic Marketing." *Journal of Hospital Marketing* 9 (1995): 15.

103. Sheldon, Alan, and Susan Windham. *Competitive Strategy for Health Care Organizations,* 118. Homewood, IL: Dow Jones–Irwin, 1984.

104. Harrell, Gilbert D., and Matthew F. Fors. "Planning Evolution in Hospital Management." *Health Care Management Review* 12 (Winter 1987): 12; Malhotra, Naresh K. "Hospital Marketing in the Changing Health Care Environment." *Journal of Health Care Marketing* 6 (September 1986): 38. For application of strategic business unit analysis by diagnosis-related group, see Reynolds, James X. "Using DRGs for Competitive Positioning and Practical Business Planning." *Health Care Management Review* 11 (Summer 1986): 39.

105. Pegels, C. Carl, and Kenneth A. Rogers. *Strategic Management of Hospitals and Health Care Facilities,* 98. Rockville, MD: Aspen Publishers, 1988.

106. Pegels and Rogers, *Strategic Management,* 98.

107. A matrix using financial strength and profit/price of service is found in Cleverley, William O. "Promotion and Pricing in Competitive Markets." *Hospital & Health Services Administration* 32 (August 1987): 329–333. An interesting growth and nongrowth opportunity matrix is presented by Breindel, Charles L. "Nongrowth Strategies and Options for Health Care." *Hospital & Health Services Administration* 33 (Spring 1988): 37–45.

108. Whyte and Blair, "Strategic Planning," 289.

109. Blair, Savage, and Whitehead, "A Strategic Approach," 17–20.

110. Reeves, Phillip N. "Issues Management: The Other Side of Strategic Planning." *Hospital & Health Services Administration* 38 (Summer 1993): 233.

111. Bigelow, Barbara, Margarete Arndt, and Melissa Middleton Stone. "Corporate Political Strategy: Incorporating the Management of Public Policy Issues into Hospital Strategy." *Health Care Management Review* 22 (Summer 1997): 54.

112. Bigelow, Arndt, and Stone, "Corporate Political Strategy," 53.

113. Reeves, Phillip N. "Strategic Planning Revisited." *Clinical Laboratory Management Review* 20 (November/December 1994): 550–551.

114. Bigelow, Arndt, and Stone, "Corporate Political Strategy," 56–57.

115. Bigelow, Arndt, and Stone, "Corporate Political Strategy," 54.

116. Bigelow, Arndt, and Stone, "Corporate Political Strategy," 55.

117. Although the term *strategy* is used by Bigelow and colleagues in Table 8.5, it is not equivalent to the term's use in the Porter or general strategy classifications. A more appropriate term would be *tactic*. However, for the sake of this presentation, the term *strategy* is retained.

118. Bigelow, Arndt, and Stone, "Corporate Political Strategy," 61.

119. Bigelow, Arndt, and Stone, "Corporate Political Strategy," 54.

120. Bigelow, Arndt, and Stone, "Corporate Political Strategy," 61.

121. Bigelow, Barbara, Liam Fahey, and John Mahon. "A Typology of Issue Evolution." *Business and Society* 32 (April 1993): 23–26.

122. Bigelow, Fahey, and Mahon, "A Typology," 22.

123. Bigelow, Fahey, and Mahon, "A Typology," 22.

124. Bigelow, Fahey, and Mahon, "A Typology," 23.

125. Reeves, "Strategic Planning Revisited," 552.

126. Reeves, "Strategic Planning Revisited," 551.

127. Adapted from Kotler, Philip, and Roberta N. Clarke. *Marketing for Health Care Organizations,* 2nd ed., 32–35. Englewood Cliffs, NJ: Prentice-Hall, 1987; reprinted by permission. This instrument was prepared by Rick Heidtman under the supervision of Professor Philip Kotler.

128. Zuckerman, *Healthcare Strategic Planning,* 7.

129. From Zuckerman, Alan M. *Healthcare Strategic Planning: Approaches for the 21st Century,* 7–9. Chicago: Health Administration Press, 1998; reprinted by permission.

SELECTED BIBLIOGRAPHY

Bigelow, Barbara, Margarete Arndt, and Melissa Middleton Stone. "Corporate Political Strategy: Incorporating the Management of Public Policy Issues into Hospital Strategy." *Health Care Management Review* 22 (Summer 1997): 53–63.

Bigelow, Barbara, Liam Fahey, and John Mahon. "A Typology of Issue Evolution." *Business and Society* 32 (April 1993): 18–29.

Bigelow, Barbara, and John F. Mahon. "Strategic Behavior of Hospitals: A Framework for Analysis." *Medical Care Review* 46 (Fall 1989): 295–311.

Blair, John D., and Myron D. Fottler. *Challenges in Health Care Management: Strategic Perspectives for Managing Key Stakeholders.* San Francisco: Jossey-Bass, 1990.

Blair, John D., Terence T. Rock, Timothy M. Rotarius, Myron D. Fottler, Gena C. Bosse, and J. Matthew Driskill. "The Problematic Fit of Diagnosis and Strategy for Medical Group Stakeholders—Including IDS/Ns." *Health Care Management Review* 21 (Winter 1996): 7–28.

Blair, John D., Grant T. Savage, and Carlton J. Whitehead. "A Strategic Approach for Negotiating with Hospital Stakeholders." *Health Care Management Review* 14 (Winter 1989): 13–23.

Bower, Joseph L., Christopher A. Bartlett, C. Roland Christensen, Andrall E. Pearson, and Kenneth R. Andrews. *Business Policy: Text and Cases,* 7th ed. Homewood, IL: Irwin, 1991.

Breindel, Charles L. "Nongrowth Strategies and Options for Health Care. *Hospital & Health Services Administration* 33 (Spring 1988): 37–45.

Brown, Montague. "Commentary: Competition, Managed Care, and Trusteeship—Can Voluntary Hospital Governance Survive? Will Not-For-Profit Hospitals Survive?" *Health Care Management Review* 20 (Winter 1995): 84–89.

Brown, Montague. "Mergers, Networking, and Vertical Integration: Managed Care and Investor-Owned Hospitals." *Health Care Management Review* 21 (Winter 1996): 29–37.

Brown, Montague, and Barbara P. McCool. "Vertical Integration: Exploration of a Popular Strategic Concept." *Health Care Management Review* 11 (Fall 1986): 7–19.

Bruton, Garry D., Benjamin M. Oviatt, and Luanne Kallas-Burton. "Strategic Planning in Hospitals: A Review and Proposal." *Health Care Management Review* 20 (Summer 1995): 16–25.

Burns, Lawton R., and Darrell P. Thorpe. "Trends and Models in Physician-Hospital Organization." *Health Care Management Review* 18 (Fall 1993): 7–20.

Campbell, Sandy. "Columbia/HCA Has a Vision and a Mission for Its Future, but No Strategic Plan." *Health Care Strategic Management* 15 (December 1997): 15.

Clement, Jan P. "Vertical Integration and Diversification of Acute Care Hospitals: Conceptual Definitions." *Hospital & Health Services Administration* 33 (Spring 1988): 99–110.

Cleverley, William O. "Promotion and Pricing in Competitive Markets." *Hospital & Health Services Administration* 32 (August 1987): 329–339.

Conrad, Douglas A., and William L. Dowling. "Vertical Integration in Health Services: Theory and Managerial Implications." *Health Care Management Review* 15 (Fall 1990): 9–22.

Cooper, Philip D. "Marketing from Inside Out." In *Health Care Marketing: Issues and Trends,* 2nd ed., edited by Philip D. Cooper, 109–111. Rockville, MD: Aspen Publishers, 1985.

Cooper, Philip D. "What Is Health Care Marketing?" In *Health Care Marketing: Issues and Trends,* 2nd ed., edited by Philip D. Cooper, 1–8. Rockville, MD: Aspen Publishers, 1985.

Cooper, Philip D. "Managed Care Positives and Negatives for Health Care Marketing." *Health Marketing Quarterly* 12 (1995): 55–61.

Costello, Michael M., and Daniel J. West. "A New Way of Thinking: How Managed Care Networks Will Affect Physician and Hospital Marketing Efforts." *Journal of Hospital Marketing* 10 (1996): 3–10.

Craig, Tim T. "Formulating Patterns of Strategic Behavior." In *Strategic Management in the Health Care Sector: Toward the Year 2000,* edited by Farhad Simyar and Joseph Lloyd-Jones, 179–202. Englewood Cliffs, NJ: Prentice-Hall, 1988.

Donnelly, James H., Jr., James L. Gibson, and John M. Ivancevich. *Fundamentals of Management,* 10th ed. Boston: Irwin/McGraw-Hill, 1998.

Fisk, Trevor A. "Strategic Planning and Marketing." In *The AUPHA Manual of Health Services Management,* edited by Robert J. Taylor and Susan B. Taylor, 311–331. Gaithersburg, MD: Aspen Publishers, 1994.

Ford, Robert C., Susan A. Bach, and Myron D. Fottler. "Methods of Measuring Patient Satisfaction in Health Care Organizations." *Health Care Management Review* 22 (Spring 1997): 74–89.

Georgopoulos, Basil S., and Floyd C. Mann. *The Community General Hospital.* New York: Macmillan, 1962.

Giardina, Carole W., Myron D. Fottler, Richard M. Shewchuk, and Daniel B. Hill. "The Case for Diversification into Long-Term Care." *Health Care Management Review* 15 (Winter 1990): 71–82.

Gibson, C. Kendrick, David J. Newton, and Daniel S. Cochran. "An Empirical Investigation of Hospital Mission Statements." *HealthCare Management Review* 15 (Summer 1990): 35–45.

Ginn, Gregory O., and Gary J. Young. "Organizational and Environmental Determinants of Hospital Strategy." *Hospital & Health Services Administration* 37 (Fall 1992): 291–302.

Ginter, Peter M., Linda M. Swayne, and W. Jack Duncan. *Strategic Management of Health Care Organizations,* 3rd ed. Malden, MA: Blackwell, 1998.

Goldsmith, Jeff. "Columbia/HCA: A Failure of Leadership." *Health Affairs* 17 (1998): 27–29.

Haglund, Claudia L., and William L. Dowling. "The Hospital." In *Introduction to Health Services,* 3rd ed., edited by Stephen J. Williams and Paul R Torrens, 160–211. Albany, NY: Delmar Publishers, 1988.

Health Care Advisory Board. *The Great Product Enterprise: Future State for the American Health System.* Washington, DC: The Advisory Board Company, 1997.

Horowitz, Judith L. "Using Strategic Planning To Address Managed Care Growth." *Healthcare Financial Management* 49 (April 1994): 22–24.

Hunger, J. David, and Thomas L. Wheelen. *Essentials of Strategic Management.* Reading, MA: Addison-Wesley, 1997.

Kaluzny, Arnold D., D. Michael Warner, David G. Warren, and William N. Zelman. *Management of Health Services.* Englewood Cliffs, NJ: Prentice-Hall, 1982.

Kongstvedt, Peter R. *Essentials of Managed Care,* 2nd ed. Gaithersburg MD: Aspen Publishers, 1997.

Kotler, Philip, and Gary Armstrong. *Marketing: An Introduction,* 4th ed. Upper Saddle River, NJ: Prentice-Hall, 1997.

Kotler, Philip, and Roberta N. Clarke. *Marketing for Health Care Organizations,* 2nd ed. Englewood Cliffs, NJ: Prentice-Hall, 1987.

Labovitz, George H. "Customer Expectations in the New Millennium." *Healthcare Executive* 13 (January/February 1998): 47.

MacStravic, Robin E. *Marketing Religious Health Care.* St. Louis: Catholic Health Association of the United States, 1987.

McIlwain, Thomas F., and Melody J. McCracken. "Essential Dimensions of a Marketing Strategy in the Hospital Industry." *Journal of Hospital Marketing* 11 (1997): 39–59.

Orlikoff, James E., and Mary Totten. "Strategic Planning by the Board." *Trustee* 48 (July/August, 1995): SS1–SS4.

Paul, David P., III, and Earl D. Honeycutt, Jr. "An Analysis of the Hospital-Patient Marketing Relationship in the Health Care Industry." *Journal of Hospital Marketing* 10 (1995): 35–49.

Pearce, John A., II, and Richard B. Robinson, Jr. *Strategic Management: Formulation, Implementation, and Control,* 5th ed. Burr Ridge, IL: Irwin, 1994.

Pegels, C. Carl, and Kenneth A. Rogers. *Strategic Management of Hospitals and Health Care Facilities.* Rockville, MD: Aspen Publishers, 1988.

Pointer, Dennis D. "Offering-Level Strategy Formulation in Health Services Organizations." *Health Care Management Review* 15 (Summer 1990): 15–23.

Porter, Michael E. *Competitive Strategy: Techniques for Analyzing Industries and Competitors.* New York: The Free Press, 1980.

Proenca, E. Jose. "Market Orientation and Organizational Culture in Hospitals." *Journal of Hospital Marketing* 11 (1996): 3–18.

Rakich, Jonathon S., and Kurt Darr. "Outcomes of Hospital Strategic Planning." *Hospital Topics* 66 (May/June 1988): 23–27.

Reeves, Phillip, N. "Issues Management: The Other Side of Strategic Planning." *Hospital & Health Services Administration* 38 (Summer 1993): 229–241.

Reeves, Phillip, N. "Strategic Planning Revisited." *Clinical Laboratory Management Review* 20 (November/December 1994): 549–554.

Rutsohn, Phil, and Nabil A. Ibrahim. "Strategically Positioning Tomorrow's Hospital Today: Current Indications for Strategic Marketing." *Journal of Hospital Marketing* 9 (1995): 13–23.

Sahney, Vinrod K., and Gail L. Warden. "The Role of CQI in the Strategic Planning Process." *Quality Management in Health Care* 1 (Summer 1993): 1–11.

Satinsky, Marjorie, A. *The Foundations of Integrated Care: Facing the Challenges of Change.* Chicago: American Hospital Publishing, 1998.

Savage, Grant T., and John D. Blair. "The Importance of Relationships in Hospital Negotiation Strategies." *Hospital & Health Services Administration* 34 (Summer 1989): 231–253.

Savage, Grant T., Rosemary L. Taylor, Timothy M. Rotarius, and John A. Buesseler. "Governance of Integrated Delivery Systems/Networks: A Stakeholder Approach." *Health Care Management Review* 22 (Winter 1997): 7–20.

Seidel, Lee F., John W. Seavey, and Richard J.A. Lewis. *Strategic Management for Healthcare Organizations.* Owings Mills, MD: National Health Publishing/AUPHA Press, 1989.

Shortell, Stephen M., Ellen M. Morrison, and Susan Hughes. "The Keys to Successful Diversification: Lessons from Leading Hospital Systems." *Hospital & Health Services Administration* 43 (Winter 1989): 471–492.

Sturm, Arthur C., Jr. *The New Rules of Healthcare Marketing: 23 Strategies for Success.* Chicago: Health Administration Press, 1998.

Thompson, Arthur A., Jr., and A. J. Strickland, III. *Strategic Management: Concepts and Cases,* 10th ed. Boston: Irwin/McGraw-Hill, 1998.

Walston, Stephen L., John R. Kimberly, and Lawton R. Burns. "Owned Vertical Integration and Health Care: Promise and Performance." *Health Care Management Review* 21 (Winter 1996): 83–92.

Whyte, E. Gordon, and John D. Blair. "Strategic Planning for Health Care Providers." In *Health Care Administration: Principles, Practices, Structure, and Delivery,* 2nd ed., edited by Lawrence F. Wolper, 289–326. Gaithersburg, MD: Aspen Publishers,1995.

Williams, Stephen J., and Paul R. Torrens. *Introduction to Health Services.* Albany, NY: Delmar Publishers, 1988.

Zelman, William N., and Deborah L. Parham. "Strategic, Operational, and Marketing Concerns of Product-Line Management in Health Care." *Health Care Management Review* 15 (Winter 1990): 29–35.

Zuckerman, Alan, M. "Hospital and Medical Staff Strategic Planning: Developing an Integrated Approach." *Physician Executive* 20 (August 1994): 15–17.

Zuckerman, Alan M. *Healthcare Strategic Planning: Approaches for the 21st Century.* Chicago: Health Administration Press, 1998.

Zuckerman, Howard S., Arnold D. Kaluzny, and Thomas C. Ricketts, III. "Alliances in Health Care: What We Know, What We Think We Know, and What We Should Know." *Health Care Management Review* 20 (Winter 1995): 54–64.

9 Quality and Competitive Position

Continuous Quality Improvement in health care comes in a variety of "shapes, colors, and sizes" and is referred to by many names. Don't be confused. . . . [It] is a structured organizational process for involving personnel in planning and executing a continuous stream of improvements in order to provide quality health care that meets or exceeds customer expectations.[1]

The management model in Figure 1.7 shows how health services organizations (HSOs) and health systems (HSs) convert input resources into outputs. Individual and organizational work results (i.e., outputs) are achieved only when structure, tasks/technology, and people elements are integrated. The quality of output is affected by this conversion process and by the types and nature of inputs.

This chapter presents two dimensions of the quality of output. The philosophy of continuous quality improvement (CQI) is described, and the importance of improving the processes that are used to generate output is discussed. The relationships among CQI, productivity, cost-effectiveness, and HSO/HS competitive position are analyzed. Included are benchmarking and ISO 9000. The work of quality experts W. Edwards Deming, Joseph M. Juran, and Philip B. Crosby is profiled. The chapter develops a CQI model based on doing the right things and doing the right things right. It also introduces a CQI process improvement model, and the relationship between problem solving and the team approach to process improvement is discussed. Productivity improvement is defined, and various productivity improvement methods to improve work systems and job design, capacity and facilities layout, and production control, scheduling, and materials handling are presented.

The subject of reengineering is explored as another approach to quality. Reengineering is customer focused and involves the radical redesign of end-to-end processes. It seeks to give HSOs/HSs a competitive advantage. Facilitators and barriers to reengineering are presented. A discussion of strategic quality planning follows. Strategic quality planning is a top-down process linking quality improvement (QI) to the strategic plans of the HSO/HS. Steps include choosing the HSO's/HS's focus of what it wants to become and prioritizing the key critical processes that are necessary to achieve success and to maintain or attain competitive position. Sections on organizational align-ment and implementation follow. The chapter concludes with an examination of two subjects: physician involvement in QI, including proactive steps that management can take to gain the com-mitment and involvement of clinicians; and the next iteration of the quality movement, interorga-nizational communitywide initiatives.

There has been a shift in the health services paradigm with respect to quality[2]: "[I]t represents a 'new order of things' in the provision of health care."[3] This shift has occurred at two levels: the definition of quality output and the means of achieving it. First, the traditional definition of quality of care and service (i.e., output) has been expanded beyond meeting specifications or standards to incorporate conformance to requirements and fitness for use, both of which include meeting or ex-ceeding patient/customer expectations. Second, there is recognition of the importance of focusing on improving the inputs and processes that generate outputs (product and service outcomes).[4] This expanded definition of quality output and the focus on improving inputs and processes are the twin pillars of CQI. Adopting the philosophy and methods of CQI will positively affect HSO/HS man-agement and organizational arrangements; resource allocation, utilization, cost-effectiveness, and productivity improvement; the quality of services provided (i.e., conformance and customer satis-faction); and the HSO's/HS's competitive position in the marketplace.

Intense international competition and increased consumer demands and expectations for qual-ity products and services profoundly affected the American industrial sector in the 1980s, and in-dustry was found wanting. There was an awakening in the 1990s with an increased awareness by business of the importance of quality and satisfying customers; the implementation of initiatives to improve the quality of outputs to be more effective in the face of global competition; and, as de-scribed by Deming, the beginning of the transformation of American business[5] that is ongoing.

Like industry, the health services system in the United States is undergoing profound change. The 1980s and 1990s were years of turmoil for HSOs/HSs, especially hospitals. Environmental forces and required changes that occurred then will continue in the 21st century. Some of the changes are revenue and cost pressures; increased competition from alternate forms of delivery, such as man-aged care organizations; and health services system restructuring, with some closures, mergers, and consolidations resulting from the formation of many more HSs.[6] The environment for HSOs/HSs is turbulent, and they are at risk with increasingly greater demands from and accountability to cus-tomers for lower-cost care with improved quality. These customers include patients as well as major payers such as government and self-insured businesses.[7] HSOs/HSs must respond to all of these cus-tomer expectations and other stakeholder expectations.

QUALITY—TWO DIMENSIONS

Traditionally, quality in HSOs/HSs focused on product or service content[8] and meeting specifica-tions or standards. The evaluation of quality tended to be retrospective and assessed the product or service using predetermined criteria. Examples are accuracy of diagnosis, physiological change and improvement in patients at discharge, mortality and morbidity rates, and the efficacy of medical procedures and drugs. Methods of quality evaluation include inspection, peer review, and quality assurance, as well as tracking indicators such as infection rates, unanticipated readmissions after discharge, and accuracy and timeliness of diagnostic tests.

The contemporary view of quality in HSOs/HSs includes two dimensions: conformance to re-quirements and fitness for use—both of which incorporate satisfying customer needs and meeting or exceeding customer expectations. The American Society for Quality defines quality as "the totality of features and characteristics of a product or service that bear on its ability to satisfy [customer] stated or implied needs."[9] The American Production and Inventory Control Society indicated that

Quality can be defined through five principal approaches: (1) Transcendent quality is an ideal, a condition of excellence. (2) Product-based quality is based on a product attribute. (3) User-based quality is fitness for use. (4) Manufacturing based quality is the conformance to requirements. (5) Value-based quality is the degree of excellence at an acceptable price. Also, quality has two major components: (1) quality of conformance—quality is defined by the absence of defects, and (2) quality of design—quality is measured by the degree of customer satisfaction with a product's characteristics and features.[10]

Quality judgments occur when the HSO/HS or individuals within it generate outputs.[11] Quality considerations include questions such as: Are there defects? Does the product work? Was the service appropriate? Is treatment reliable? Was the service on time? Was it delivered in a friendly manner? Was it the right service? Did it meet the customer's needs? Was the customer delighted—did the product or service attributes exceed the customer's expectations?[12] The answers to such questions about expectations by customers are influenced by their experiences, perceptions, and values. The Hospital Research and Educational Trust (HRET) Quality Measurement and Management Project (QMMP) calls this "delivery quality," and it refers to all aspects of the HSO's/HS's interaction with the customer.[11] In a general way, delivery quality describes customers' satisfaction with their experiences based on interacting with the HSO/HS.

In HSOs/HSs conformance and expectation quality monitoring and improvement must be directed at every level and at every process.[14] Customers are not just patients and external stakeholders[15]; they also are physicians, internal customers, payers, the community,[16] and any internal downstream user of a unit's output.[17] For example, the nursing service is a customer of the pharmacy with regard to medications and a customer of dietary services with regard to food service for patients; physicians are customers of diagnostic testing; the intensive care unit is a customer of the emergency department with respect to trauma patients being admitted; third-party payers are customers of patient billing; and all HSO departments and units to some degree are customers of administration. Depending on the transaction, any HSO process, department, unit, or person may switch from supplier to processor to customer.[18] In HSs, such as those vertically integrated along the continuum of care, the HS's skilled nursing facility may be the customer of the acute care hospital. Figure 9.1 shows how a hospital's functional departments have internal and external customers.

CQI PHILOSOPHY

CQI, the pervasive philosophy about quality in health care that gained acceptance in the 1990s, is based largely on the work of the industrial quality experts W. Edwards Deming,[19] Joseph M. Juran,[20] and Philip B. Crosby.[21] CQI philosophy has four attributes. First, output quality includes meeting or exceeding customer expectations. Second, monitoring and evaluating the quality of outputs is both retrospective (after the fact) and prospective (before the fact); poor quality can be prevented. Third, "quality is not the responsibility of just one department or individual"[22]; it is organizationwide and involves all HSO/HS staff. Fourth, quality and QI focus on both process (and inputs) and outcomes, not just outcomes.[23] The Joint Commission on Accreditation of Healthcare Organizations' (Joint Commission's) *Agenda for Change* recognized the need for outcome and process quality.[24] The philosophical context of the *Agenda for Change* is based on QI that emphasizes the following:

> Quality as a central priority: organizationwide devotion to quality, leadership involvement in promoting and improving quality
>
> Customers: attention to customer needs, feedback from internal and external customers, customer–supplier dialogue

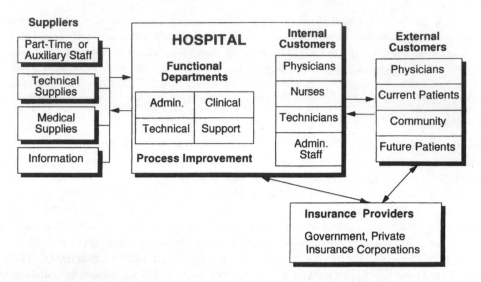

Figure 9.1.　Internal and external customers of hospital functional departments. (From Carol Greebler, TQM Plus, San Diego, CA, 1989; reprinted by permission.)

Work processes: describing key clinical and managerial processes, systems approach, and
　　cross-disciplinary teams
Measurement: use of data, understanding of variation, search for underlying causes
Improvement: never-ending commitment to improving performance[25]

As observed in the chapter's opening quote, CQI comes in a variety of shapes, colors, and sizes and has many different names. It is sometimes called quality management,[26] total quality management (TQM),[27] total quality care,[28] or QI.[29] CQI is used here rather than TQM. CQI suggests the major break with previous efforts to achieve quality, it is the most positive way to state the concept, and it eliminates the suggestion that quality is the job only of managers.

CQI is defined as an ongoing, organizationwide framework in which HSOs/HSs and their employees and clinical staff are committed to and involved in monitoring and evaluating all aspects of the HSO's/HS's activities (inputs and processes) and outputs in order to continuously improve them.[30] The essential elements of this definition are

- CQI is organizationwide. CQI can be successful only if the organization is transformed to seek quality in all that it does. It requires a total commitment to quality—a philosophical transformation—by the governing body and senior-level management; it involves all HSO/HS employees, including clinical staff[31]; and it is rooted in a cultural setting that supports quality initiatives, teamwork, adaptability, and flexibility.[32]
- CQI is process focused. CQI seeks to understand processes, identify process characteristics that should be measured, and monitor processes as changes are made to determine the effect of changes. The result is more efficient and effective processes that improve productivity through better use of resources. In sum, CQI improves conversion processes, thereby generating higher-quality products and service (outputs).
- CQI empowers employees. Process understanding and improvement requires a team-based approach in which employees are involved and empowered to effect change.

- CQI uses output or inspection measures. Outcomes of care (indicators) provide macro-level measures to determine how well groups of processes and the HSO/HS as a whole are performing. Indicators allow a HSO/HS to perform time-series comparisons and do inter-HSO/HS comparisons, for example. They are crude arrows that point the HSO/HS toward needs for process analysis and improvement.
- CQI is customer driven. The goal is to meet or exceed customer expectations. "Customer" is defined in its broadest possible sense, both internally and externally.

The literature is replete with CQI applications in HSOs.[33] Selected examples are individual hospitals,[34] integrated health systems,[35] and medical specialty clinics.[36] Success stories in specific departments abound—clinical medicine,[37] laboratory,[38] diagnostic radiology,[39] medical records,[40] and pharmacy.[41] In a survey of U.S. and Canadian hospitals, it was found that, among those responding, approximately 90% had implemented CQI and 65% had conducted over six CQI projects. There was a significant relationship between CQI and hospital size and teaching status. Larger teaching hospitals were more likely to be involved in CQI initiatives than smaller nonteaching hospitals.[42]

CQI MODEL

The HRET QMMP presented the CQI challenge as follows: "Continuous Quality Improvement demands that health care providers answer three questions. Are we doing the right things? Are we doing things right? How can we be certain that we do things right the first time, every time?"[43] Figure 9.2 answers these questions in the context of a CQI model. The discussion in this section references components of the model by number.

Are We Doing the Right Things?

Output quality [3] is the first pillar of CQI and determines whether the HSO/HS is doing the right things. Products and services that are in conformance and that meet or exceed customer expectations result in the organization doing the right things. From the CQI perspective, customers are not only patients and external stakeholders but also internal users of a department, unit, or individual's outputs. Customers are the next downstream process that relies on another process for inputs.[44] Output that is in conformance/meets customers' expectations is a quality product or service and means that the HSO/HS is doing the right things.

Are We Doing Things Right?

Process improvement [2] is the second pillar of CQI for three reasons. First, output quality can be improved only by improving the processes that produce it (or the inputs used in the process, or both). Second, all processes can be improved. As observed by the president of the Joint Commission, "patient care systems, particularly because of their high degree of human dependency, can always be improved."[45] He states further, "Quality improvement turns us 180 degrees from where we have been. It means if it ain't broke, it can still be improved."[46] Others have conveyed the message as follows: "If it isn't perfect, make it better."[47]

Third, monitoring, evaluating, and intervening to improve processes are continuous. A prerequisite is systematic understanding and documentation of processes. In addition, all employees must seek opportunities to improve work results and the way in which they produce them. The outcome is not only improved output quality [3] but also productivity improvement, in which there is more effective resource use [4] and enhanced competitive position [5]. The goal of process improvement, as expressed by Crosby, is to do it right the first time.[48] Although this goal may never be attained, if a HSO/HS continuously improves processes, it is moving in the direction of "do it right the first time."

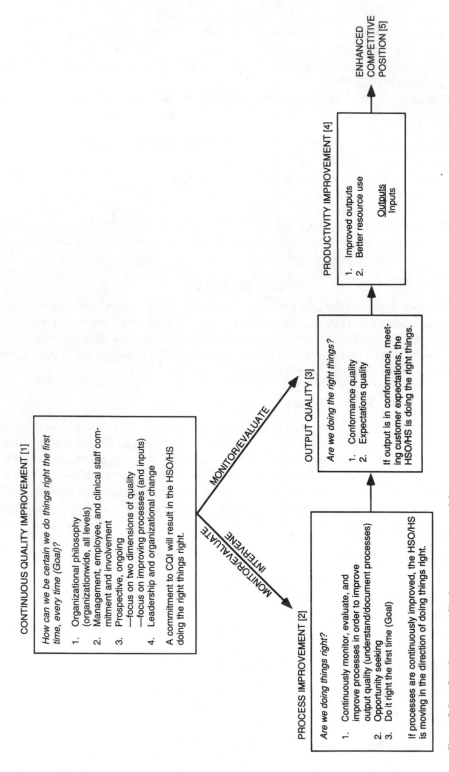

CONTINUOUS QUALITY IMPROVEMENT [1]

How can we be certain we do things right the first time, every time (Goal)?

1. Organizational philosophy (organizationwide, all levels)
2. Management, employee, and clinical staff commitment and involvement
3. Prospective, ongoing
   —focus on two dimensions of quality
   —focus on improving processes (and inputs)
4. Leadership and organizational change

A commitment to CQI will result in the HSO/HS doing the right things right.

MONITOR/EVALUATE

MONITOR/EVALUATE
INTERVENE

OUTPUT QUALITY [3]

Are we doing the right things?

1. Conformance quality
2. Expectations quality

If output is in conformance, meeting customer expectations, the HSO/HS is doing the right things.

PROCESS IMPROVEMENT [2]

Are we doing things right?

1. Continuously monitor, evaluate, and improve processes in order to improve output quality (understand/document processes)
2. Opportunity seeking
3. Do it right the first time (Goal)

If processes are continuously improved, the HSO/HS is moving in the direction of doing things right.

PRODUCTIVITY IMPROVEMENT [4]

1. Improved outputs
2. Better resource use

   <u>Outputs</u>
   Inputs

ENHANCED COMPETITIVE POSITION [5]

Figure 9.2.   Continuous quality improvement model.

How Can We Be Certain We Do Things Right the First Time, Every Time?

The goal of CQI is to do things right the first time, every time. If there is quality output (the right things) and process improvement (doing things right) with CQI, the HSO/HS will move in the direction of doing things right the first time, every time (goal).[49] The essential attributes of CQI [1] are as follows (see Figure 9.2):

- CQI is an organizational philosophy that becomes part of the culture—the ingrained beliefs and values of the HSO/HS. It is pervasive throughout the organization. CQI is customer driven and requires the transformation of the existing beliefs and values regarding quality.
- CQI requires the total commitment and involvement of everyone in the HSO/HS. Management must commit resources and create an atmosphere that is conducive to continuous improvement in which quality is integral to the work of all employees and clinical staff.[50] They must participate and be committed to continuously improving their work results and the way in which those results are achieved. This requires extensive collaboration and cross-functional coordination among work units and departments.[51] Employees must be involved in problem solving, particularly as it relates to seeking and identifying opportunities for improvement.
- CQI is prospective and ongoing. The focus on output quality must be prospective, not just retrospective; it must be continuous, not intermittent.[52] The aim is to prevent poor quality before it happens and to seek opportunities to improve processes in an organized fashion.
- CQI requires management to meet its leadership responsibility to train employees; to encourage innovation, worker participation and empowerment, and team building so that employees can contribute to process improvement problem solving; and to facilitate organizational change that leads to improvement.

QI, PRODUCTIVITY IMPROVEMENT, AND COMPETITIVE POSITION

The result of the CQI paradigm is the reciprocal of the traditional cost-containment initiatives that were prevalent during the 1970s and 1980s. At that time, in the context of the management model in Figure 1.7, HSOs/HSs primarily focused on increasing the ratios of outputs to inputs. Such initiatives were narrowly applied, episodic, and short term. They often had low worker involvement and commitment and primarily focused on reducing input costs rather than enhancing output quality. In the CQI model, improvement initiatives are broad based, long term, and ongoing; have extensive management and employee involvement and commitment; are customer driven; and focus on improving both process and output quality versus simply reducing costs.

Figure 9.2 depicts the ways in which CQI improves quality and productivity improvement [4] leading to enhanced competitive position [5]. Deming asserted that productivity improvement does not result in improved output quality but that improved quality does result in productivity improvement. As presented in Figure 9.3, Deming's chain reaction denotes that improved quality results in improved productivity, which leads to decreased prices and increased market share; thus the organization stays in business, provides jobs, and yields greater returns. Consequently, the HSO's/HS's competitive position is enhanced. According to Deming's philosophy, improved quality results in better resource use (lower costs) because improved processes result in less rework (readmissions), fewer mistakes (repeats of tests), fewer delays (waiting for service), and better use of resources. These results occur because the prospective and continuous assessment of, and changes made to, work processes and inputs yield both improved quality and improved productivity.[53]

In its review of quality initiatives by 20 high-scoring applicants for the Malcolm Baldrige National Quality Award (MBNQA), the U.S. General Accounting Office (GAO) developed the quality

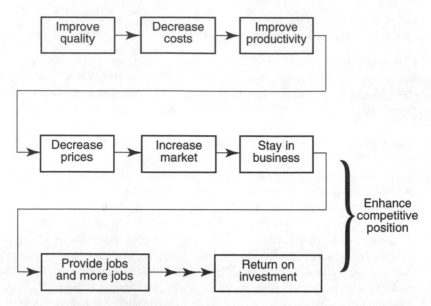

Figure 9.3. Deming chain reaction. (Adapted from Joiner, Brian L. *Fourth Generation Management: The New Business Consciousness,* 23. New York: McGraw-Hill, 1994; reprinted by permission.)

management model that appears in Figure 9.4. It presents the essential attributes of CQI: management leadership for continuous improvement; quality systems (i.e., programs) and employee involvement; enhancing product and service quality (increased reliability, decreased errors or defects); and customer satisfaction. The GAO found that increased quality resulted in greater customer satisfaction (increased customer retention and decreased customer complaints); organization benefits such as increased productivity, reduced employee turnover, and decreased costs; and enhanced competitive position (market share and profits).[54]

The MBNQA was created in 1987 and named for a former Secretary of Commerce. Since 1988 it has been awarded to companies that excel in quality achievement and quality management. The application process is rigorous; the award is prestigious. Its purpose is to promote quality excellence; recognize U.S. organizations that have made significant improvements in products, services, and competitive position; and foster information sharing among U.S. organizations. The MBNQA criteria are based on the concept of customer-driven quality, a de facto definition of TQM, and, together with scoring criteria, represent an assessment device.[55] Criteria are based on seven categories; among them are leadership, strategic quality planning, management of process quality and results, and customer focus and satisfaction.[56]

APPROACHES TO QI

Three recognized leaders on achieving quality—W. Edwards Deming, Joseph M. Juran, and Philip B. Crosby—have greatly influenced the philosophy and practice of QI, and their principles are being adopted in HSOs/HSs.[57] These experts provide philosophies and methodologies for organizations seeking to establish a quality culture. They are not of like mind on many of the specifics of how to achieve QI: Deming is the philosopher and statistician, Juran uses a more managerial approach, and Crosby is the organizational behavioralist and motivator. Although the routes differ somewhat, their destination is the same. They are three different preachers with the same religion—quality.[58]

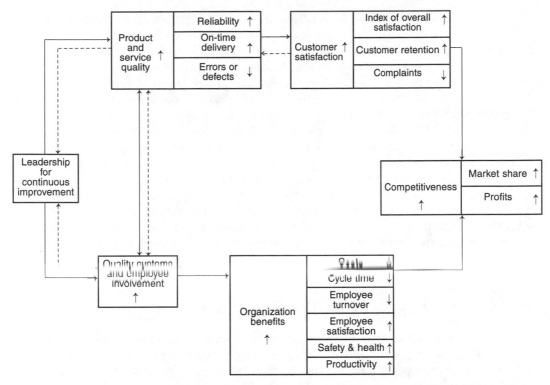

Figure 9.4. Quality management model. *Note:* The solid line shows the direction of the total quality processes to improve competitiveness. The dotted line shows the information feedback that is necessary for continuous improvement. The arrows in the boxes show the expected direction of the performance indicators. (From National Security and International Affairs Division, General Accounting Office. *Management Practices: U.S. Companies Improve Performance* [GA Report NSIAD-91-190], 15. Washington, DC: General Accounting Office, February 14, 1994.)

W. Edwards Deming

Deming was most influential in assisting post–World War II Japan in transforming its industry into the economic power it became. His underlying premise, like that of Juran, is that poor quality is the result of badly designed or malfunctioning processes—not worker behavior—and that poor quality can be prevented. Therefore, his approach emphasizes monitoring and evaluating processes through statistical quality control and searching for ways to improve processes. It was not until the 1980s that his work was recognized in the United States, yet his theories and principles about quality are much older.[59] His most significant book, *Out of the Crisis,* was published in 1986.

Like Crosby and Juran, Deming incorporates the essential characteristics of CQI: total organization commitment and worker involvement and education in the improvement of processes. The following profile of Deming is insightful:

> *Quality must become a central focus of the corporation. The emphasis must shift from inspection to prevention. Preventing defects before they occur and improving the process so that defects do not occur are goals for which a company should strive.*
>
> *Training and retraining of employees is critical to the success of the corporation. Deming believes that it is management's job to coach employees. Education and training are investments in people. They help to avoid employee burnout, reenergizing employees, and give a clear message to*

employees that management considers employees to be a valuable resource. Finally, Deming also believes that management must pay attention to variability within processes. He advocates systematic understanding of variation and reduction of variations as a strategy to improve processes.

   Deming believes that the road to enhanced productivity is through continuous quality improvement called the Deming Chain Reaction. Improving quality through improving processes leads to a reduction of waste, rework, delays, and scrap. This reduction causes productivity as well as quality to improve.[60]

The Deming chain reaction is presented in Figure 9.3. It indicates that improving quality and eliminating variability in processes decrease costs, increase productivity, and enhance the organization's competitive position. This sequence is incorporated in the CQI model in Figure 9.2.

   The Deming method has two distinct components. The first step is critical: Managers must establish and perpetuate an environment in which QI is integral to the work of all employees. For most HSOs/HSs this means a transformation—a major philosophical shift and commitment to quality. The second, concurrent component is that efforts to improve quality are supported by the statistical analysis of activities—management must understand what the organization is doing and how well it is being done. These data and their analyses allow managers to identify and correct problems.

   Deming's 14 points for quality[61] have been discussed extensively by other writers.[62] The 14 points have been applied to HSOs by Batalden and Vorlicky, as cited in Deming[63] and Darr.[64]

1. *Create constancy of purpose toward improvement of product and service with the aim to become competitive, to stay in business, and to provide jobs.*[65] This means identifying customers, giving good-quality service to them, and ensuring organization survival through innovation and constant improvement.

2. *Adopt the new philosophy.* Commonly accepted levels of nonquality are unacceptable.

3. *Cease dependence on inspection to achieve quality.* Health services should

     require statistical evidence of quality of incoming materials, such as pharmaceuticals, serums, and equipment. Inspection is not the answer. Inspection is too late and is unreliable. Inspection does not produce quality. . . . Require corrective action, where needed, for all tasks that are performed in the hospital or other facility, ranging all the way from bills that are produced to processes of registration. Institute a rigid program of feedback from patients in regard to their satisfaction with services.[66]

4. *End the practice of awarding business on the basis of price tag.* The intent is to develop long-term relations with suppliers so that they can improve the quality of the products (and services) they provide as an input to the HSO/HS.

5. *Improve constantly and forever the system of production and service, to improve quality and productivity, and thus constantly decrease costs.* Improvement is not a one-time effort. Management is obligated to continually look for ways to reduce waste and improve quality.

6. *Institute training on the job.* Too often, workers learn their jobs from other workers who were never trained properly. They cannot do their jobs well because no one tells them how.

7. *Institute leadership.* A supervisor's job is not to tell people what to do or to punish them, but to lead.

     Supervisors need time to help people on the job. Supervisors need to find ways to translate the constancy of purpose to the individual employee. Supervisors must be trained in simple statistical methods for aid to employees, with the aim to detect and eliminate special causes of mistakes and rework.[67]

8. *Drive out fear, so that everyone may work effectively for the company.* Many workers are afraid to take a position or ask questions even when they do not understand the job or what is right or wrong.

     We must break down the class distinctions between types of workers within the organization—physicians, nonphysicians, clinical providers versus nonclinical providers, physician to physician. . . . Cease to blame employees for problems of the system. Management should be held responsible for faults of the system. People need to feel secure to make suggestions.[68]

9. *Break down barriers between departments.* Often, areas compete with one another or have conflicting goals. They do not work as a team to solve or foresee problems. Worse, one department's goals may cause trouble for another department.

10. *Eliminate slogans, exhortations, and targets for the workforce asking for zero defects and new levels of productivity.* "Instead, display accomplishments of the management in respect to assistance to employees to improve their performance."[69]

11. *Eliminate work standards (quotas) on the factory floor.* Quotas that represent measured day work or output alone without regard to quality should be eliminated. "It is better to take aim at rework, error, and defects [all measures of quality], and to focus on help to [sic] people to do a better job."[70]

12. *Remove barriers that rob the hourly worker of the right to pride of workmanship.* People are eager to do a good job and distressed when they cannot. Too often, misguided supervisors, faulty equipment, and defective materials stand in the way. These barriers must be removed.

13. *Institute a vigorous program of education and self-improvement.* "Institute a massive training program in statistical techniques. Bring statistical techniques down to the level of the individual employee's job, and help him to gather information in a systematic way about the nature of his job."[71] Also, the training "program should keep up with changes in model, style, materials, methods, and if advantageous, new machinery."[72]

14. *Put everyone in the company to work to accomplish the transformation.* As observed by Darr, "taking action to accomplish the transformation . . . will take a special top management team with a plan of action to carry out the quality mission. Workers can't do it on their own, nor can managers."[73]

Joseph M. Juran

Joseph M. Juran, a consultant and the founder and chairman emeritus of the Juran Institute, is a leading advocate of TQM. He pursued a varied career in management as engineer, industrial executive, government administrator, university professor, corporate director, and management consultant.[74] Juran defines quality as fitness for use, which includes being free from deficiencies and meeting customer needs.[75] Juran's quality trilogy is a universal way of thinking about quality. It is applicable to all functions, levels, and product lines.[76] The quality trilogy involves three activities: quality planning, quality control, and quality improvement.

> *Quality Planning.* This is the activity of developing the products and services required to meet customers' needs. It involves a series of universal steps essentially as follows:

1. Determine who the customers are.
2. Determine the needs of customers.
3. Develop product features that respond to customers' needs.
4. Develop the processes that are able to produce those product features.
5. Transfer the resulting plans to the operating forces.

> *Quality Control.* This process consists of the following steps:

1. Evaluate actual quality performance.
2. Compare actual performance to quality goals.
3. Act on the differences.

> *Quality Improvement.* This process is a means of raising quality performance to unprecedented levels ("breakthrough"). The methodology consists of a series of universal steps:

1. Establish the infrastructure that is needed to secure annual quality improvement.

2. Identify the specific needs for improvement—the improvement projects.
3. For each project, establish a project team with clear responsibility for bringing the project to a successful conclusion.
4. Provide the resources, motivation, and training that are needed by teams to diagnose the causes, stimulate the establishment of a remedy, [and] establish controls to hold the gains.[77]

Juran, like Crosby, argues that there is a cost to nonquality, including reworking defective products, scrap, liability from lawsuits, and lost sales from previously dissatisfied customers or customers who purchase competitors' products or services because of their better quality.[78]

The relationship of the parts of the trilogy is presented in Figure 9.5. Juran described it as follows:

The Juran Trilogy diagram is a graph with time on the horizontal axis and cost of poor quality (quality deficiencies) on the vertical axis. The initial activity is quality planning. The planners determine who are the customers and what are their needs. The planners then develop product and process designs that are able to respond to those needs. Finally, the planners turn the plans over to the operating forces.

The job of the operating forces is to run the processes and produce the products. As operations proceed it soon emerges that the process is unable to produce 100 percent good work. [Figure 9.5] shows that 20 percent of the work must be redone as a result of quality deficiencies. This waste then becomes chronic because the operating process was designed that way.

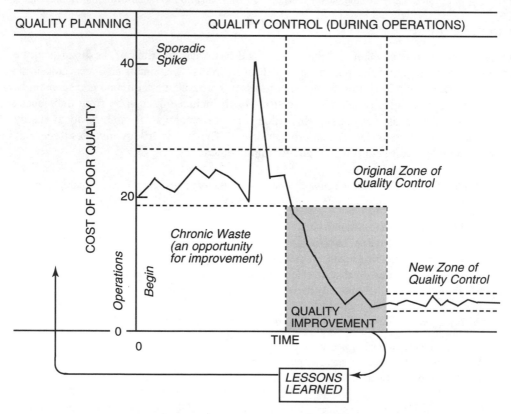

Figure 9.5.   Juran quality trilogy. (From Juran, Joseph M. "The Quality Trilogy." *Quality Progress* 19 [August 1986]: 20; reprinted by permission.)

Under conventional responsibility patterns, operating forces are unable to get rid of that planned chronic waste. What they do instead is carry out quality control—to prevent things from getting worse. Control includes putting out the fires, such as that sporadic spike.

The chart also shows that in due course the chronic waste is driven down to a level far below the level that was planned originally. That gain is achieved by the third process of the trilogy: quality improvement. In effect, it is realized that chronic waste is also an opportunity for improvement, and steps are taken to seize that opportunity.[79]

Juran advocates QI, the third step in the trilogy, as a way to improve an existing process (redesigned, if necessary) so that the "original zone" of quality control and the chronic waste associated with it can be reduced below the (original) existing level. This is represented in Figure 9.5 by the "new zone" of quality control. Juran views QI as seeking and finding opportunities for improvement that result in achieving the new zone. In his earlier writings, Juran called this the "breakthrough" zone consisting of a new and better level of performance and quality. A breakthrough necessitates accepting the premise that current performance is not good enough and can be improved, as well as making an attitudinal change about quality that becomes part of the organization's culture.[80] In Crosby's terms it involves attaining and surpassing the enlightenment stage of organization maturity and moving to the certainty stage.

Philip B. Crosby

Crosby, a former vice president of quality at ITT and a consultant to many industrial organizations, published his significant work, *Quality is Free,* in 1979. He stated that "Quality is free. It's not a gift, but it is free. What costs money are the nonquality things—all the actions that involve not doing jobs right the first time."[81] Crosby viewed quality as "conformance to requirements," and he stated that the goal of an organization should be to "satisfy the customer first, last, and always."[82] Sahney and Warden profiled Crosby and his basic principles as follows:

> *Crosby strongly advocates a system of quality improvement that focuses on prevention rather than appraisal. Prevention involves careful understanding of the process and identification of problem areas, followed by improvement of the process.*
>
> *Crosby strongly advocates the ultimate goal of quality as "Zero Defects" and that a company should constantly strive to achieve this goal. He believes that the best measure of quality is "cost of quality" and that this cost can be divided into two components: the price of nonconformance, and the price of conformance. The price of nonconformance includes the cost of internal failures (i.e., the cost of reinspection, retesting, scrap, rework, repairs, and lost production) and external failures (i.e., legal services, liability, damage claims, replacement, and lost customers). Crosby estimates that an organization's cost of nonconformance can be as high as 25 to 30 percent of operating costs. The price of conformance, on the other hand, includes the cost of education, training, and prevention as well as costs of inspection and testing. An organization must minimize the sum of both costs. The focus on process improvement, error-cause removal, employee training, management leadership, and worker awareness of quality problems are all important tenets.*[83]

Crosby also emphasized that organizations should recognize the hidden costs of poor quality. In health services, malpractice is one such cost. Figure 9.6 uses an iceberg model to present examples of the visible and hidden costs of poor quality for a HSO/HS. Crosby's ultimate goal of "do it right the first time" and the derivative concept of "zero defects"[84] are just that—ultimate goals that may never be attained but that give direction for the organization with regard to quality.[85] To move in this direction, the HSO/HS must go through a maturing process with respect to a philosophy about quality and then use Crosby's 14 steps of QI.

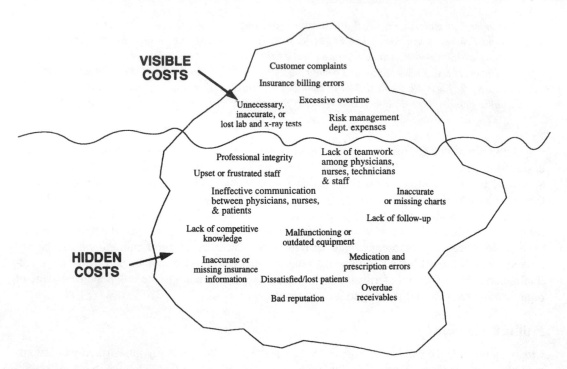

Figure 9.6. The iceberg of visible and hidden costs of poor quality. (From Carol Greebler, TQM Plus, San Diego, CA, 1989; reprinted by permission.)

Crosby's organizational maturity model includes the stages of uncertainty, awakening, enlightenment, wisdom, and certainty.[86] Enlightenment is the stage in which management's understanding and attitude about QI are heightened and management is supportive of and accepts QI; problems are faced openly and resolved in an orderly manner; and there is implementation of the 14-step approach to quality. Crosby states that in the last stage, certainty, CQI is ingrained in the organization's culture.

Crosby's 14 steps of QI are not necessarily consecutive; in fact, many are parallel:

1. Management commitment to and involvement in quality
2. Use of QI teams composed of people with process knowledge and a commitment to action
3. Quality measurement so that areas for improvement can be identified and action can be taken
4. Measuring the cost of quality—meaning the cost of nonquality
5. Quality awareness by all organization members
6. Corrective actions—seek opportunities for improvement
7. Zero defects planning—striving to "do it right the first time"
8. Employee education with formal orientation at all levels of management (and employees) about the 14 steps
9. Zero Defect Day, which is management's demonstration of its commitment to quality
10. Goal setting—the ultimate is zero defects, but "intermediate goals move in that direction"
11. Error-causal removal, in which people describe problems that prevent error-free work
12. Recognition of those who meet their goals
13. Quality councils composed of quality professionals assisting others in QI
14. Do it all (Steps 1–13) over again[87]

Crosby stated that his 14-step program is "a systematic way of guaranteeing that organized activities happen the way they are planned."[88] It results in doing the right things the right way and doing them right the first time.

Table 9.1 presents differences and similarities among Deming's, Juran's, and Crosby's philosophies. Included are their definitions of quality, the objectives they envision for QI, their general approaches to quality, their methods for QI, and their views of management responsibilities.

Statistical Control

Deming and Juran believed that poor quality is overwhelmingly caused by processes rather than by workers. They emphasized the use of statistical methods for quality control and to identify process variation.[89] Deming was especially vocal in support of his contention that most poor quality results from variation. He defined variation in statistical control as "performance within three standard deviations of the mean—a generous amount of variation, although management can set more stringent limits."[90] Typically HSOs/HSs use two standard deviations. Variation within these limits is known as common cause variation and results from the process itself. Variation beyond these limits is called special cause variation. Such variation can be either positive or negative. Reasons for negative special cause variation must be identified and corrected.[91] Examples are a sudden malfunction or broken equipment, or delays in service resulting from an unanticipated surge in arrivals in the emergency department, which may indicate a capacity problem. Special cause variation for Juran is the "sporadic spike," in which a process is not "in control." Deming and Juran believed that, once processes are in control, they can be improved. In Juran's terminology this is moving to the "new zone of quality control." In Deming's terminology it is improving the process by decreasing common cause variation around the mean. For Crosby it is moving through the organizational maturity stages toward certainty and striving for the goal of "do it right the first time."

Deming used control charts to determine whether a process is in control. The applications of such charts are numerous and can range from analyzing customer waiting time in the admitting office or units of output from a laboratory to monitoring equipment and capacity utilization. Figure 9.7 is a control chart of average (i.e., mean) patient waiting time from arrival to the start of service in the admitting office. The mean waiting time is 4 minutes, with an upper control limit (UCL) of 8 minutes. The lower control limit (LCL) is zero—on a given day no patient waited for service. Common cause variation is variation between the UCL and the LCL; special cause variation occurs outside this range. The average patient waiting time for this set of observations exceeded the UCL on Days 5 and 10. Deming advocates finding the reason for this special cause variation. Perhaps a computer was down or a new, untrained employee was on duty. Once found, the negative special cause variation is eliminated, if possible.

The more important focus must be reducing common cause variation in a process that is in statistical control because it will do the most to improve quality. Deming avers that all processes can be improved and that initiatives to lower the UCL to UCL' (see Figure 9.7) will result in higher quality (greater customer satisfaction) as well as productivity improvement. In Juran's terminology this is moving to the new zone of quality control. In Crosby's terminology this is moving toward the goal of zero defects.

PROCESS IMPROVEMENT MODELS

CQI uses statistical techniques such as control charts to understand a process. As monitoring continues, changes are made to proactively improve the process. The Find-Organize-Clarify-Understand-Select–Plan-Do-Check-Act (FOCUS–PDCA) model is the most widely known. It is based on the work of Walter Shewhart, an early pioneer of quality who developed the PDCA cycle, and was ex-

TABLE 9.1. DIFFERENCES AND SIMILARITIES IN THE APPROACHES TO QUALITY OF DEMING, JURAN, AND CROSBY

Dimension	Deming	Juran	Crosby
Definition of quality	A product or service that helps someone and has a good, sustainable market	Fitness for use—free of deficiencies and meeting customer needs	Conformance to requirements, including "satisfy the customer"
Poor quality	Overwhelmingly caused by process, not workers; common cause variation	Caused by poor planning/design (chronic) and sporadic spike (see Figure 9.5)	Nonconformance; there are (hidden) costs of nonquality (see Figure 9.6)—quality is free
Quality objective	Error-free (reduce common cause variation); hit target every time	Reduce chronic poor quality and sporadic spike; move to "new zone" of quality control	Zero defects (objective): "do it right the first time"
Customer orientation	Yes, transformation—improve quality (so customers buy products) to improve competitive position (see Figure 9.3)	Yes, meet customer needs	Yes, satisfy the customer
General approach to quality	Prospective prevention in all processes, not retrospective inspection; understand and reduce variation through statistical quality control; transform organization (change culture)	General management approach; find opportunities for improvement; "breakthrough"; change culture regarding quality	Managerial approach: QI teams, project basis for improvements, move to "certainty" stage, prevention and error-cause removal
Method for quality improvement	14 points for QI	Trilogy (quality planning, quality control, QI)	14 steps to QI
Management responsibility	Commitment to quality control (central focus); cause transformation; establish and perpetuate environment in which quality is integral to work of all employees; don't blame employees; drive out fear; break down barriers; and train, coach, and teach statistical methods to employees	Commitment to quality, especially design; instill quality culture; support operating forces and QI project teams	Commitment, leadership, and involvement in QI; worker training; promote quality awareness by all employees and management

420

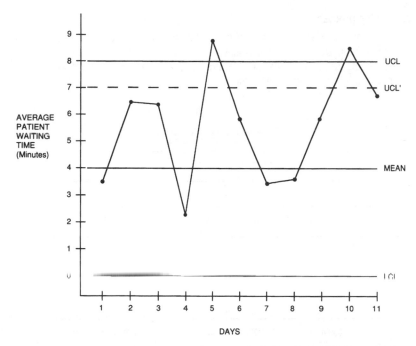

Figure 9.7.   Control chart for average patient waiting time prior to service in an admitting department. UCL and LCL are ±3 standard deviations from the mean. UCL' is improved process—reducing the range of common cause variation.

panded by Columbia/HCA (formerly the Hospital Corporation of America). The FOCUS–PDCA process improvement model is shown in Figure 9.8. Table 9.2 is a detailed description of the FOCUS–PDCA cycle. Data collection is important throughout to monitor and evaluate, to determine whether an opportunity for improvement is present, to clarify the current understanding of and knowledge about the process under investigation, and to uncover causes of variation.

In 1989 HRET published the results of the QMMP, a 3-year research project supported by 15 hospital systems and alliances. QMMP is a QI model that is similar to the FOCUS–PDCA model.[92] Although the QMMP model made a major contribution to the health services field in that it is still useful and incorporates the essential elements of CQI, HRET did not continue its development. Instead, in the late 1990s HRET research projects focused on areas such as the impact of health maintenance organizations (HMOs) on integrated networks and services, the organizational typology of health systems and networks, and the effects of hospital mergers on market power and effectiveness.[93]

The HRET QMMP model includes the following steps[94]:

1. Find a process that needs improvement.
2. Assemble a team that knows the process. In general, those who understand it best are the employees involved in it. "Through its members, the team must also have an understanding of continuous quality improvement principles, statistical quality control, the use of data management systems, and access to management so that organizational roadblocks to improvement can be overcome."
3. Identify customers and process outputs and measure customer expectations regarding outputs. Different processes have different outputs, and "the team's first task is therefore to list the outputs of the process, identify its customers, and measure expectations of outputs." Customers may be patients, external stakeholders, or an internal downstream process.

4. Document the process.

    A process consists of a series of steps that convert inputs to outputs. They are usually hierarchical; that is, the main process may be broken down into subprocesses, each with subinputs and suboutputs. The hierarchical chain may be followed to that level of detail necessary to understand the process.

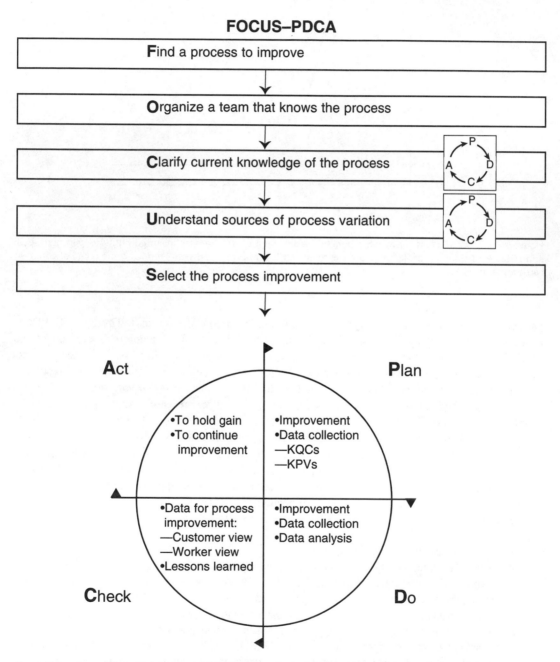

Figure 9.8.   Process improvement model. (KQCs, key quality characteristics; KPVs, key process variables.) (From Columbia/HCA [formerly Hospital Corporation of America], Nashville, TN; reprinted by permission. FOCUS–PDCA is a registered servicemark of Columbia/HCA.)

5. Generate output and process specifications. "A specification is an explicit, measurable, statement regarding an important attribute of an output (a customer expectation) or the (sub)process that produces it."
6. Eliminate inappropriate variation (implement).
7. Document continuous improvement (innovate).

> The team can select those ideas that seem most promising and then apply them on a test basis within their process. . . . The proposed change can then be discarded, implemented, or modified and tried again, based on the results of the test.

TABLE 9.2. WHAT TO LOOK FOR ON A FOCUS–PDCA STORYBOARD

F(ind)
- Who is the customer?
- What is the name of the process?
- What are the process boundaries?
- Is the opportunity statement there? Is it clear?
- Who will benefit from the improvement?
- How is the process tied to the hospital as a sys-
  ꞏꞏꞏꞏꞏ ꞏꞏꞏꞏ ꞏꞏ ꞏꞏꞏꞏꞏꞏꞏꞏ ꞏ

O(rganize)
- How big is the team?
- Do the members represent people who work in the process or did the "organizational chart" show up?
- Does the team's knowledge of the process align with the boundaries in the opportunity statement?

C(larify)
- Is the process presented at a level of detail that identifies possible causes of variation?
- Is there evidence of agreement on a best method as represented by a single flow diagram?
- Do the boundaries of the flow diagram align with the opportunity statement and the team?
- Were there quick and easy improvements made in the "C" phase using PDCA? Did the team defer any improvements to the "S" phase?
- Is there evidence that the "actual" flow of the process was documented rather than some perceived flow?

U(nderstand)
- How did the team identify the key quality characteristic (KQC) and potential key process variables (KPVs)?
- Is there an operational definition for the KQC and the potential KPVs?
- Is there a data collection plan? Is it clear how the data will be collected? Who will collect them?
- Does the team understand how long it will take to collect enough data to make a decision?
- How does the performance of the process vary over time?
- Can the team show a relationship between the KQC and the KPVs?

S(elect)
- How did the team select the opportunity for improvement?
- Are there any data or other evidence to support the selection?
- What were the criteria for making the decision?

Roadmap
- Does the roadmap indicate key actions that the team is likely to take?
- What is the time frame?
- Is the team on track?
- Is there evidence of updating or reviewing the roadmap?
- Where is the team on the roadmap?

P(lan)
- Does the team have a plan for piloting the improvement and collecting data?
- Does the pilot plan indicate dates, communications, and ownership of specific steps?
- What training was necessary?

D(o)
- How was the plan executed?
- Did any contingencies arise?
- Were dates on the data collection plan met?

C(heck)
- Do the data on the run chart suggest that the process changed?
- How did the data change?
- Does the team know anything that helps explain any evident change?
- Is the team comfortable that enough data are present to support an action?
- If the team is not comfortable with the amount of data or the knowledge provided by the data, what is the plan for obtaining more?

A(ct)
- Did the team act to implement the process gain beyond the pilot?
- Did the team act to generalize the lessons learned from the pilot? Or did the team act to discard the planned improvement?
- Can the team find another opportunity for improvement within this process?
- What did the team learn from the effort?

From Columbia/HCA (formerly Hospital Corporation of America), Nashville TN: reprinted by permission. FOCUS–PDCA is a registered servicemark of Columbia/HCA.

Understanding and Measuring a Process

The first step in any process improvement is to select a process to improve. People with process knowledge are critical to understanding and documenting the process. Flowcharts are used to describe it. It is only after the process is understood that data about process variables can be collected to determine whether the process is in control. If the process is not in control, it must be brought into control, which means eliminating special cause variation. Once in control, process variables can be measured and decisions can be made as to where changes should be implemented. Data collection is continued so that the effects of changes can be measured.

Figure 9.2 shows that monitoring and evaluation are crucial elements of process improvement. There are many formal sources, such as reports, data from control charts, and customer questionnaires, as well as informal sources (i.e., complaints), from which information can be obtained. These data must be organized so they become information that is usable for decision making. Two examples of such organization are helpful.

Pareto analysis is a way to prioritize—to separate the "important few" from the "trivial many."[95] The principle is that 80% of defects, errors, volume, or whatever is being measured are caused by 20% of the variables or process factors. The 80/20 rule in marketing is an application of the Pareto principle. That is, 80% of sales are derived from 20% of a firm's products. In a hospital Pareto analysis could indicate that 80% of operative case delays are caused by 20% of surgeons.[96] The 80/20 ratio is not fixed or magical; instead, it is the notion of understanding relationships that is important. A Pareto diagram is a useful tool in understanding what is happening in a process and for prioritizing because it shows the relative importance of elements in a process that contribute to a result. Figure 9.9 is an example of a Pareto diagram. It shows that physicians' untimed routine orders and discharge orders are the two areas in which the greatest improvement can occur, and attention should be focused there.

Figure 9.10 is a second way to display data. Scatter diagrams depict the relationship between two variables. Here, the relationship is that between number of operations per year (x axis) and percentage mortality (quality) for coronary artery bypass graft operations (y axis). The data suggest a decline in mortality as the number of operations increases, perhaps as a result of a learning or experience curve.

The statistical technique of least squares linear regression can be applied to scatter diagram plots to show a "best fit line" as well as UCLs and LCLs, which are set by some number of positive and negative standard deviations, respectively, from the best fit line. If three standard deviations are used, there is 99.74% confidence that an outlying plot is not due to chance. Figure 9.10 indicates that the single outlying plot above the UCL and the two below the LCL would be, in Deming's terms, special cause variation, and in Juran's terms, a sporadic spike. All three outliers are of interest. The one above the UCL would be investigated to determine why the undesirable result occurred so it might be prevented in the future. Those below the LCL would be investigated to understand the reasons for the good results and to learn, for example, whether a surgical team was doing something that could be replicated by other teams. Outliers may result from input differences such as the skill and training of surgical teams, how acutely ill the patient is, or from the process—the way in which the surgery was performed and techniques that were used.

Benchmarking

At a macro level, systematic data collection provides information that allows priorities to be set about which processes to improve. At a process improvement level—a more micro level—data enable the quality improvement team (QIT) to understand variables in a process, a requisite to improvement. For both, benchmarking is important. Benchmarking can be internal to the HSO/HS, in which case it involves comparing similar activities or processes to "best practices." It can also be

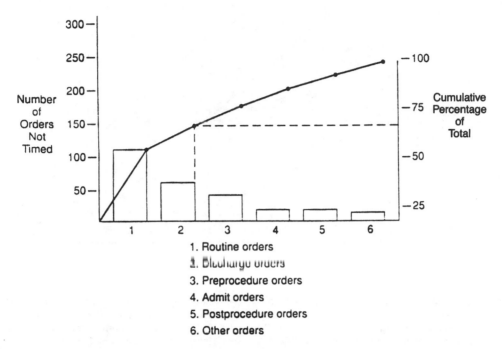

Figure 9.9.   Pareto diagram showing the rank order of untimed physicians' orders in a major hospital. This diagram ranks classes of orders that failed to be timed with a plot line showing that the correction of the first two classes of orders would lead to a greater than 50% improvement in all untimed orders. (From Re, Richard N., and Marie A. Krousel-Wood. "How to Use Continuous Quality Improvement Theory and Statistical Quality Control Tools in a Multispecialty Clinic." *Quality Review Bulletin* 16 [November 1990]: 394; reprinted by permission. Copyright 1990 by the Joint Commission on Accreditation of Healthcare Organizations, Oakbrook Terrace, IL.)

external, in which case comparison is made to identical or similar activities and processes in the same or similar industries. Benchmarking provides norms, standards, and comparative measures for any attribute chosen, such as for a particular process (i.e., patient admitting), customer service and satisfaction, quality outcomes, or financial performance.

Competitive benchmarking involves comparison to competitors that are providing the same service in similar markets. On an advanced level, it may include identifying the "best patient outcomes for each service measured by such factors as mortality rates, nosocomial infections, [and] patient mobility" as well as practice patterns and resource consumption profiles relative to competitors.[97] World-class benchmarking can be applied by comparing the HSO/HS to organizations within or outside the health services industry that excel and have similar processes. Common examples would be order fulfillment and supplier relations and billing and collections.[98]

The steps that are involved in benchmarking include identifying what to benchmark, collecting data internally and externally, and applying conclusions to improving existing processes. Processes in HSOs/HSs that can be benchmarked are admitting, billing, transportation, and surgical scheduling, to name a few. Information obtained about other organizations also is used for control. For example, in Chapter 10 databases are described that present information about peer organizations in the areas of performance and financial outcomes as well as resource consumption. These data are benchmarks against which a HSO/HS can compare itself to other peer or "best in class" organizations. The process of benchmarking enables the HSO/HS to improve results. It provides standards for use in QI and control and, ultimately, to improve competitive position.

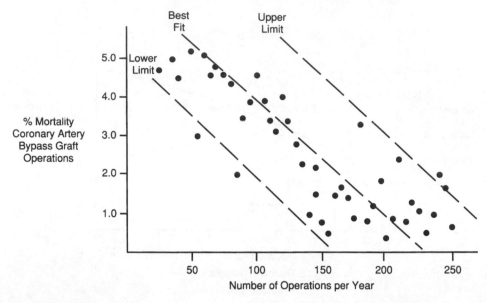

Figure 9.10.   Scatter diagram used to determine a possible relationship between two variables: the mortality rate for a surgical procedure and the number of times the procedure is performed during a 12-month period. Each dot represents one surgical team. (From Merry, Martin D. "Total Quality Management for Physicians: Translating the New Paradigm." *Quality Review Bulletin* 16 [March 1990]: 103; reprinted by permission. Copyright 1990 by the Joint Commission on Accreditation of Healthcare Organizations, Oakbrook Terrace, IL.)

In Chapter 8 external environmental analysis is emphasized. To attain and sustain competitive position, a HSO/HS must have knowledge about its competitors and how it performs relative to them. Table 9.3 presents a summary of differences among approaches for competitive analysis and benchmarking.

ISO 9000

ISO 9000 is an "international protocol for organizing and documenting the process and procedures used to establish a quality system."[99] Sponsored by the International Organization for Standardization, located in Switzerland, these standards provide for an organization establishing, documenting, and maintaining a quality system "that once implemented, is certifiable by independent auditors and is recognized throughout the world."[100] Like Joint Commission or academic accreditation, the ISO 9000–compliant organization can present itself as one that meets minimum standards with regard to a quality system and that "it does what it says it will do." ISO 9000 is basically a CQI approach in

TABLE 9.3.   SUMMARY OF DIFFERENCES AMONG APPROACHES FOR COMPETITIVE ANALYSIS AND BENCHMARKING

Item	Competitive analysis	Benchmarking
Generic purpose	Analyze competitive strategies	Analyze what, why, and how well competition or leading companies are doing
Usual focus	Competitive strategies	Business practices that satisfy customer needs
Application	Marketplace and products	Business practices as well as products
Usually limited to	Marketplace activities	Not limited; competitive, functional, and internal benchmarking are used
Information sources	Industry analysts, etc.	Industry leaders as well as competitors

From Camp, R.C. *Benchmarking: The Search for Industry Best Practices that Lead to Superior Performance.* Milwaukee, WI: ASCQ Quality Press, 1989; reprinted by permission.

which the organization is committed to quality coupled with documentation in order to ensure consistency. Originating in Europe and the Common Market, the International Organization for Standardization was founded in 1946 and adopted a series of quality standards in 1987, which were revised in 1994. Organizations certified (technically they are registered) under ISO 9000 standards are ensured to have a quality system in place that is equal to that of their peers. The standards are recognized by more than 100 countries, and they apply to all types of businesses, including health care.[101]

ISO 9000 standards do not define quality—the applicant organization does. However, the 150 guidelines in the standards provide the structure for developing and maintaining a quality system. Certified organizations must follow procedures in more than 20 areas, among them management responsibility, quality system, process control, inspection and testing, corrective and preventive action, control of quality records, training, and statistical techniques. The value of ISO 9000 certification is that the organization must have a quality commitment in order to attain this distinction, including self-examination and improvement and documentation of processes. Customers are aware that the organization is structured to produce consistent results, and that its suppliers may be required to be ISO 9000 certified. A trend since the late 1990s has been that of certain industries developing industry-specific standards using ISO 9000 as a base.[102] For example, U.S. automotive and truck manufacturers have imposed QS 9000 on their suppliers.[103] The purpose is to extend quality system requirements backward to their suppliers to ensure conformance to requirements. Other industries have developed similar standards: AS 9000 in the aerospace industry and TL 9000 in the telecommunications industry.[104] As HSOs/HSs embrace ISO 9000, it is likely that they too will extend quality system certification to their suppliers.

The five objectives of the ISO 9000 standards are to

1. Achieve, maintain, and seek continuously to improve product quality (including services).
2. Improve the quality of operations to continually meet customers' and stakeholders' stated and implied needs.
3. Provide confidence to internal management and other employees that quality requirements are being fulfilled and that improvement is taking place.
4. Provide confidence to customers and other stakeholders that quality requirements are being achieved in the delivered product (including services).
5. Provide confidence that quality system requirements are fulfilled.[105]

Although both MBNQA and ISO 9000 certification (i.e., registration) are prestigious designations, there are differences. A comparison is presented in Table 9.4. Both address improvement and results; however, ISO 9000 is narrower. MBNQA deals with continuous improvement and customer satisfaction. ISO 9000 standards mostly fall within the process management dimension of MBNQA.[106] MBNQA focuses on competitiveness and customer values, the definition of quality is customer driven, and there is heavy dependence on output results and improvement. ISO 9000, in contrast, focuses on conformity to practices that are specified by the organization's own quality system, and the definition of quality is conformity to specific operations and to the documented requirements. It does not assess outcome-oriented results but the documentation of the processes to achieve the results.

IMPROVEMENT AND PROBLEM SOLVING

Process improvement requires problem solving[107] and uses the steps in the problem-solving model presented in Figure 7.4. Conditions that initiate problem solving are deviation (actual results are inconsistent with desired results), crisis, opportunity or threat, and improvement (see Figure 7.3). Problem solving under the condition of improvement, like other conditions, involves 1) problem

TABLE 9.4. CONTRASTS BETWEEN THE BALDRIGE AWARD AND ISO 9000 REGISTRATION

	Baldrige award program	ISO 9000 registration
Focus	Competitiveness; customer value and operational performance	Conformity to practices specified in the registrant's own quality system
Purpose	Educational; shares competitiveness learning	To provide a common basis for assuring buyers that specific practices conform with the provider's stated quality systems
Quality definition	Customer-driven	Conformity of specified operations to documented requirements
Improvement/results	Heavy dependence on results and improvement	Does not assess outcome-oriented results or improvement trends
Role in the marketplace	A form of recognition, but not intended to be a product endorsement or certification	Provides customers with assurances that a registered supplier has a documented quality system and follows it
Nature of assessment	Four-stage review process	Evaluation of quality manual and working documents and site audits to ensure conformance to stated practices
Feedback	Diagnostic feedback on approach, deployment, and results	Audit feedback on discrepancies and findings related to practices and documentation
Criteria improvement	Annual revision of criteria	Revisions of 1987 document issued in 1994, focusing on clarification
Responsibility for information sharing	Winners required to share quality strategies	No obligation to share information
Service quality	Service excellence a principal concern	Standards focused on repetitive processes without a focus on critical service quality issues, such as customer relationship management and human resource development
Scope of coverage	All operations and processes of all work units; includes all ISO 9001 requirements	Covers only design/development, production, installation, and servicing; addresses less than 10% of Baldrige criteria
Documentation requirements	Not spelled out in criteria	A central audit requirement
Self-assessment	Principal use of criteria in the area of improvement practices	Standards primarily for "contractual situations" or other external audits

From Reimann, Curt W., and Harry S. Hertz. "The Malcolm Baldrige National Quality Award and ISO 9000 Registration." *ASTM Standardization News* (November 1993): 42–53.

analysis, 2) developing assumptions, 3) identifying tentative alternative solutions, 4) developing and applying decision criteria, 5) selecting the alternative that best fits the criteria, 6) implementation, and 7) evaluating the solution. Results of the change in performance are compared with desired results.

The steps of process improvement in Figure 9.8 and the FOCUS–PDCA cycle are similar to those of problem solving. CQI also involves problem solving under the condition of deviation when outliers are investigated, for example. However, CQI is primarily concerned with improving processes—proactively seeking opportunities for improvement. In applying the problem-solving model to seeking opportunities for improvement, the situation analysis step is different. It involves collecting and evaluating information not in terms of recognizing or defining a problem (as under the condition of deviation), but in terms of recognizing and defining opportunities to improve a process that is in control—that is, to make the acceptable better. Improvement problem solving for Deming is reducing common cause variation; for Juran, it is moving a process to the new zone of quality control; and for Crosby, it is moving toward the goal of doing it right the first time.

The discussion of the "assumptions step" in problem solving in Chapter 7 states that narrow, restrictive structural, personal, and problem-centered assumptions result in lower-quality solutions. This occurs because assumptions narrow the range of alternatives that is considered. The same issue arises in process improvement. Organizing for improvement means assembling a team of people with process knowledge. This necessitates large-scale worker involvement because they have the most process knowledge.[108] The advantages of group problem solving presented in Chapter 7 apply to process improvement. Beyond these advantages, a QIT's members will learn new tasks and become aware of one another's problems. They will be more eager to assist one another in solving problems, team spirit will develop, and motivation and sense of worth will be enhanced.[109]

Commitment by management to provide resources, a participative philosophy, and employee team building[110] are essential. Deming, Juran, and Crosby advocated giving employees the authority to act. Others call it empowerment.[111] QITs, sometimes called process improvement teams permit a systematic discussion of the problem being investigated and greater understanding of it. A QIT's development of a cause-and-effect diagram such as the one presented in Figure 9.11 results from team brainstorming and identifies the problems in a process, as well as ways to solve them.

Walton indicated that the cause-and-effect diagram is "also known as the 'fishbone' diagram because of its shape, or the Ishikawa diagram, after its originator Kaoru Ishikawa." These diagrams "are used in brainstorming sessions to examine factors that may influence a situation. An 'effect' is a desirable or undesirable situation, condition, or event produced by a system of 'causes'."[112] The cause-and-effect diagram in Figure 9.11 shows reasons for laboratory test delays for patients in an emergency department. Primary process variables are represented by the long arrows, and minor process variables relate to each of the primary variables.

A cause-and-effect diagram is a systematic way to identify key process variables—in this case, the process by which a CQI team can improve a work process. The QMMP step of "document the process" requires that "fundamental knowledge about it" be gathered. This knowledge "usually re-

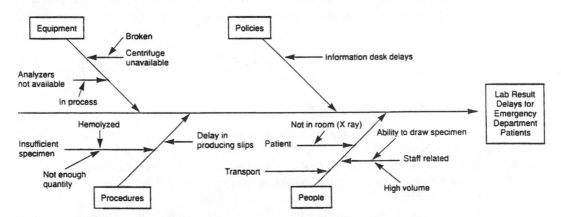

Figure 9.11.   A fishbone, or cause-and-effect, diagram examining reasons for delays in laboratory test results for emergency department patients. The fishbone diagram is drawn after a brainstorming session. The central problem is visualized as the head of the fish, with the skeleton divided into branches showing contributing causes of different parts of the problem. (From Merry, Martin D. "Total Quality Management for Physicians: Translating the New Paradigm." *Quality Review Bulletin* 16 [March 1990]: 102; reprinted by permission. Copyright 1990 by the Joint Commission on Accreditation of Healthcare Organizations, Oakbrook Terrace, IL.)

sides in front-line workers who deal with the process in a detailed manner on a daily basis."[113] Understanding the process leads to ideas about how it can be improved.

PRODUCTIVITY IMPROVEMENT

Cost- (resource use) effectiveness and productivity improvement result from CQI. Figure 9.2 indicates that process improvement [2] leads to higher-quality outputs [3], which leads to productivity improvement and better resource use [4] and, thus, enhanced competitive position [5]. The Deming chain reaction in Figure 9.3 shows that improved quality decreases costs, and this results in productivity improvement and an enhanced competitive position. CQI and productivity improvement are integral. They cannot be separated, nor can input resource costs be separated from output quality. They must be evaluated simultaneously.

Productivity and Productivity Improvement

Productivity is the index of outputs relative to inputs.[114] Alternately, productivity is results that are achieved relative to resources consumed[115]:

$$\text{Productivity} = \frac{\text{Outputs}}{\text{Inputs}} = \frac{\text{Results achieved}}{\text{Resources consumed}}$$

Productivity is increased by any change that increases the ratio of outputs to inputs, which is achieved by altering either the conversion process (structure, tasks/technology, people; see Figure 1.7) or the inputs. For example, fewer nurses caring for the same number of patients increases productivity: same output, fewer inputs. More radiographic procedures per day with the same staff and equipment has the same result. However, increasing productivity (output) without maintaining or enhancing the level of quality—conformance and satisfaction—does not lead to productivity improvement. Producing poor-quality radiographs or performing unnecessary radiographic procedures (nonconformance output) is not productivity improvement. Decreasing the number of surgical assistants and increasing patient and physician waiting time (lower customer satisfaction) is not productivity improvement. Productivity improvement occurs only when the index ratio of outputs to inputs increases and conformance/expectation quality is maintained or enhanced. This is denoted in the following formula[116]:

$$\text{Productivity improvement} = \frac{\text{Outputs}}{\text{Inputs}} = \frac{\text{Quantity}}{\text{Inputs}} + \text{Quality} = \frac{\text{Results achieved}}{\text{Resources consumed}}$$

CQI and Productivity Improvement

Figure 9.12 shows the relationship of the productivity improvement triangle to CQI. Productivity improvement occurs only when lowest reasonable costs (inputs) are consistent with highest possible quality (outputs). QMMP called this the "value of health care."[117] Because productivity improvement focuses on the relationship of outputs and quality to inputs and costs, both inputs and processes are investigated in productivity improvement, as they are in CQI.

HSOs/HSs are service organizations with high levels of customer interaction. Most HSOs/HSs, but especially hospitals, must have flexible capacity to meet surges in demand.[118] For others, such as nursing facilities, there is little need for flexible capacity, particularly when occupancy is 100%.

CQI focuses on improving processes (see Figure 9.8), which commonly necessitates evaluating inputs. For example, a QIT may determine that a process will be more efficient if better-skilled

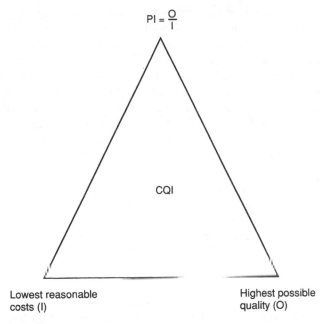

Figure 9.12.   Productivity improvement (PI) triangle.

employees are recruited or if employees are cross-trained so reassignment is more flexible when workloads change. Enhancing technology inputs can improve work systems and substitute equipment for people. Magnetic resonance imaging improves clinical diagnosis, and microcomputers enhance accuracy and productivity in billing and admitting. Other techniques may be used to add efficiency to inputs: increasing the quality of materials and supplies by working closely with suppliers (Deming advocates sole-source suppliers); using a just-in-time inventory system to eliminate inventory beyond that needed for safety stock; and using ABC inventory analysis[119] (similar to Pareto analysis) to indicate which supplies are the most expensive or critical and require special attention. Management information systems provide data for control and utilization evaluation, and forecasting enables managers to anticipate demand and alter capacity. Use of work measurement to monitor employee utilization and workloads and information from a patient acuity classification system permits efficient nurse staffing patterns.

Productivity may be improved in numerous ways other than by analyzing inputs. Examination of a process or work system in a CQI framework should ask questions such as: Is what we do really necessary? Are we doing the right things? Can the work be done in another way with the same or improved quality? How are the work results of one job interdependent with other jobs, materials, or processes? Can we improve the process with a different mix of resources that will improve quality, decrease costs, or both? The following sections describe methods to answer these questions: 1) analysis and improvement of work systems and job design; 2) capacity planning and facilities layout; and 3) production control, scheduling, and materials handling. Inputs are integral to each.

Analysis and Improvement of Work Systems and Job Design

Analysis and improvement of work systems and job design is integral to CQI process improvement and leads to productivity improvement. The basic objectives are to find better ways to work in general, improve specific jobs in particular, and increase the ratio of quality relative to costs—with the same, fewer, or a different, less costly mix of inputs.

Work systems (i.e., processes) are interrelated jobs that form an integrated whole. Hospitals, for example, have many systems and subsystems: nonpatient care systems, such as admitting, discharge, accounts payable, transportation, central services, material distribution, patient food delivery, and medication order fulfillment; direct patient care, including nursing service; ancillary services such as laboratory, radiology, and respiratory therapy; and administration. Analysis of a system can be exclusive (how it functions) or inclusive (how it interrelates with other systems); the purpose is to identify ways to improve systems so that output quality and productivity are enhanced. Process and methods analysis are techniques that are used to evaluate systems.[120] In health services, processes are the series of operations, steps, or activities through which patients, material, or information flows. Documenting flow permits the evaluation of the sequence of events[121] and whether altering the flow, combining or eliminating operations, or methods redesign will result in higher-quality outputs and productivity improvement.[122] One of the first activities of a QIT is to flow diagram the process.

Figure 9.13 is an example of a flow diagram of the process of implementing physicians' orders. Understanding the sequence of events in a physician's order will show how the process can be improved—the bottlenecks, delays, or steps that can be eliminated. In processes with high customer interaction, flow analysis will indicate where interactions may be enhanced or lessened, if either results in higher patient satisfaction.

Because HSO work systems are interdependent, multisystem process flow analysis is necessary to identify areas for improvement. For example, timely reading and reporting of test results (radiology, electrocardiography, electroencephalography, and laboratory) positively affects patient care and shortens length of stay; delayed reading or reporting negatively affects patient care and increases length of stay. Knowledge about and improvement of system or process output that becomes input elsewhere positively affects productivity.

Methods analysis involves evaluating how work is done—the specific operations, steps, or activities that are performed. Such analyses include evaluating the appropriateness of the operations, steps, or activities; considering alternative inputs, such as personnel and equipment substitution or redesigning jobs; or evaluating information flow and the media used.

At a micro level, job design improvement evaluates the tasks in a job or a cluster of jobs that constitute an operation or activity in a process. Included are the sequence of job tasks, design of physical layout, and employee–machine relationships, including equipment, material, and supplies used. Job design improvement or a variant, work simplification, is used to eliminate unnecessary tasks, reduce time between tasks, reallocate tasks among different jobs, combine jobs, or centralize common tasks in one job (i.e., specialization).

Finally, work simplification, which involves dividing work into specific tasks and making it easier, is a way to evaluate and improve jobs and enhance work results. User-friendly, menu-driven microcomputers in the admissions department enable employees to admit patients faster with greater accuracy, both of which improve quality as well as productivity.

Capacity Planning and Facilities Layout

Facilities analysis is an important dimension of process improvement. It focuses on the physical aspects of a process, the need for flexibility in meeting variable demand, and balancing timeliness of service and idle resources. Facility layout is the arrangement of equipment and work areas. Facilities, process flow, equipment, and workstations may be rearranged to improve sequence and flow, decrease unnecessary worker movement and material transportation, eliminate bottlenecks and congestion, and yield faster patient throughput. Layout analysis can be accomplished by using drawings, proximity charts, templates, or three-dimensional models. Computer simulation can be used to design the physical layout of a facility within predetermined constraints and assumptions.

The analysis of traffic patterns and material flows consists of observing and recording movement to decrease travel, eliminate or reduce delays, or substitute alternate material handling or de-

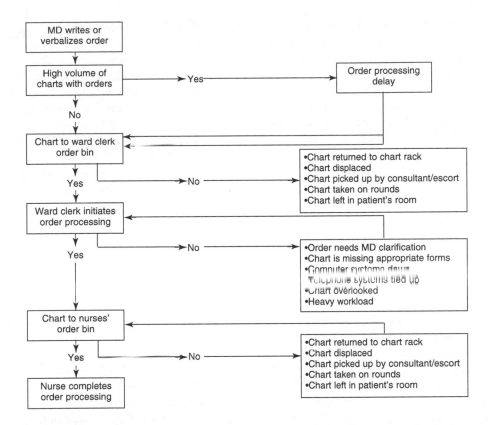

Figure 9.13. Flowchart outlining the initial steps in implementing physicians' orders, clearly identifying points of consumer–producer interchange (e.g., the interaction of physician and ward clerk) and sites of possible system failure or delay. (From Re, Richard N., and Marie A. Krousel-Wood. "How to Use Continuous Quality Improvement Theory and Statistical Quality Control Tools in a Multispecialty Clinic." *Quality Review Bulletin* 16 [November 1990]: 393; reprinted by permission. Copyright 1990 by the Joint Commission on Accreditation of Healthcare Organizations, Oakbrook Terrace, IL.)

livery methods. For example, the analysis of traffic patterns may reveal that restricting the use of certain elevators to patients and employees reduces delays in transporting patients and equipment. Similarly, materials and supplies flow analyses may justify an exchange cart system to improve logistical movement, decrease inventory and staffing, and ensure that patient care supplies and medications are on units when needed.

Production Control, Scheduling, and Materials Distribution

Production control in HSOs involves matching workload with capacity through work scheduling and is applicable to areas such as admitting, operating rooms, diagnostic testing, clinics, physician offices, and outpatient services. Often, production-smoothing techniques are used to spread the workload throughout a shift. For example, if all patients were brought to radiology or all outpatients arrived at 9:00 A.M., waiting lines would build, staff would be overworked, and quality such as patient satisfaction would be reduced because of increased waiting time. In the afternoon, staff would be underutilized. If workload can be spread throughout the day, then patient waiting time is minimized and staff are productive during the entire shift. If demand cannot be controlled through scheduling, then part-time staff may be used or other adjustments made to meet peak load demands.

Workload balancing through scheduling of demand or capacity ensures that staff, equipment, and facilities are used efficiently and customer waiting time is lessened. Many manual and computerized scheduling techniques are available, including short-interval scheduling, multiple activity charts, and work distribution analysis. Another is simulation, which is discussed in Chapter 10.

The timely distribution of materials and supplies is important to downstream processes. Improvement techniques are as simple as using general stores exchange carts to deliver supplies to nursing units. Each day one cart is filled and the other is used. Once a day the carts are exchanged. In the operating room a case cart system may be used. Each surgeon has a list of supplies and equipment that are needed for each procedure, and before surgery starts the case cart for that procedure is packed and delivered to the operating room. The unit dose system is used to distribute drugs. Medications are purchased individually prepackaged or are packaged in the pharmacy and distributed to nursing units. Each medication dose is available as needed by the patient, and the risk of error is reduced.

REENGINEERING

CQI represents a fundamental shift in thinking. It focuses on the customer, whether internal or external, and is customer driven. It is systematic and organizationwide, with top management commitment to improving processes (and inputs) through employee empowerment in order to improve quality as perceived by the customer. The result is improved quality and customer satisfaction, productivity improvement (i.e., effectiveness), and enhanced competitive position.

Reengineering is another approach to quality. Relative to CQI, Michael Hammer, an ardent advocate of reengineering, stated, "Reengineering and TQM [i.e., CQI] are merely different pews in the church of process improvement. The two share an orientation toward process, a dedication to improvement, and dogma that one begins with the customer."[123] Deming, Juran, and Crosby were three preachers with the same religion of quality, but each took different approaches. Hammer's reengineering is another approach in the continuum of improvement that builds on the principles and tools of CQI.[124] It includes additional features—radical change and process redesign. Some have called it "beyond CQI" or "Phase II CQI."[125]

Outward-In, Right to Left

In order to create quality and enhance competitive position, an outward-in orientation is required. Enhanced competitive position is accomplished by HSOs/HSs that achieve high-quality service with productivity improvement. To obtain this position, HSOs/HSs must work backward, thinking right to left, to improve the processes that generate quality and enhanced competitive position. The CQI model in Figure 9.2 focuses on market changes and customer needs and results in attaining and maintaining competitive advantage (see [5]). This is done through quality outcomes that are in conformance and meet or exceed customer expectations (see [4]). Hammer contended that CQI focuses on incrementally improving existing processes to achieve higher quality.[126] That is, CQI seeks to modify processes (and inputs) to achieve higher levels of quality. For Deming this is reducing common cause variation; for Juran it is quality improvement. However, periodically there is a change in customers' needs or in competition resulting in a performance gap. "[I]f the world has changed dramatically since the process was (or most recently [was]) redesigned, the current design may be fundamentally flawed and incapable of delivering the required performance. Reengineering is then called for. Reengineering does not merely enhance the individual steps of the process but entirely reconsiders how they are put together."[127] Movement from inpatient care to outpatient care in HSOs/HSs,[128] including support mechanisms, apparatus, facilities, and staffing, is one example of a radical change to the process of patient care delivery. The formation of HSs is another case in which management has had to redesign how care is integrated and delivered among entities. Prospective pricing and managed care requires rethinking how HSOs/HSs do business because of a fundamental shift that increased the bargaining power of one of their stakeholders, the payer.

Reengineering Defined

Hammer and Champy defined reengineering as "the fundamental rethinking and radical redesign of business processes to achieve dramatic improvements in critical, contemporary measures of performance, such as costs, quality, service, and speed."[129] Sometimes termed *process innovation* or *core process redesign,*[130] reengineering as applied to health services seeks to make fundamental and radical changes in processes and how health care is arranged and delivered, including time and place.[131]

Attributes

The attributes of reengineering are as follows:

- It is *outward-in,* focusing on the customer's needs to attain and maintain competitive advantage.
- It involves *fundamental* change by identifying first what HSOs/HSs must do (vision) and then how to do it.
- It is *radical.* Radical design means disregarding existing structures and procedures and developing new ones to accomplish work.[132] "It is about throwing it away and starting over; beginning with the proverbial clean slate and reinventing how you do your work."[133] It is analogous to "breaking the china," challenging the purpose and assumptions of a process and putting it back together (redesigned) in a new way.[134]
- It is *dramatic,* resulting in breakthrough leaps in performance versus marginal or incremental improvements.
- It involves *processes,* "the collection of activities that takes one or more kinds of input and creates an output that is of value to the customer."[135] The focus is on end-to-end, interlinked processes.

What Reengineering Is Not (Reengineering and CQI)

A major criticism of reengineering is that it is considered equivalent to *downsizing,* a term encompassing several cost reduction strategies: reducing labor costs, outsource contracting of work that was previously done in-house, replacement of permanent employees with temporary employees,[136] or discontinuing programs or services. Hammer and Champy differentiated reengineering by what it is not. They asserted that it is not automation, restructuring or downsizing, or reorganization, delayering, or flattening the organization. However, these results often occur with use of the "clean sheet of paper" radical, cross-functional redesign with a customer focus. Furthermore, they contend that reengineering is not the same as QI, TQM, or CQI. They stated: "Quality improvement seeks steady incremental improvement to process performance. Reengineering . . . seeks breakthroughs, not by enhancing existing processes, but by discarding and replacing them with entirely new ones."[137] The disciples of reengineering assert that it is macro in scope; it is the next quality iteration beyond CQI.

> *TQM [i.e., CQI] stresses incremental improvement through structured problem solving, whereas reengineering is about radical improvement through total process redesign. TQM assumes the underlying process is sound and looks to improve it. Reengineering is best seen as the next step after TQM. Success with TQM can position an organization to take that next step.*[138]

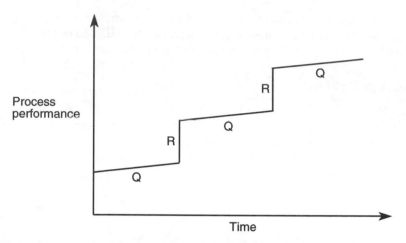

Figure 9.14. Relationship between CQI and reengineering. (Q, quality programs: continued and continuous; R, reengineering: episodic and discontinuous.) (From Hammer, Michael. *Beyond Reengineering: How the Process-Centered Organization Is Changing Our Work and Our Lives,* 83. New York: HarperBusiness, 1996; reprinted by permission.)

Others reinforce this point that reengineering pushes the CQI philosophy and mindset upstream to the customer and a more macro level—to more quality consciousness that is external to the HSO/HS.[139] The differences also can be distinguished as scale and pace. Reengineering involves improvements that are discontinuous or cause quantum leaps in performance.[140] Figure 9.14 illustrates the conceptual relationship between CQI and reengineering. CQI improves processes and performance. At some point, however, because of performance gaps such as diminished or weakened competitive position and changed customer needs and demands, the replacement of some processes must occur through reengineering. Once that occurs, CQI—improvement in the new, radically designed process—continues until such time as external forces require another breakthrough change.

The triggers or drivers of reengineering efforts may include a strategy of retrenchment because the HSO/HS no longer has a competitive advantage or market strength for a program or service (see Chapter 8); because of limited resources that can more effectively be allocated to other existing or new services; or because of changing needs of patients/customers, including shifts in market demand or composition. However, negative connotations may arise from the implementation step of a HSO/HS strategy. Examples would include a decision to exit a product or service line based on external assessment of threats and opportunities and internal strengths and weaknesses, or a situation in which the HSO/HS cannot maintain or cannot attain a comparative advantage; or a decision to reallocate limited resources to other more promising products or services by discontinuing a hospital-based trauma center or obstetrical services. Because reengineering is about the organization's response to a changing marketplace, including competition, and what customers want, it can be viewed as strategic in nature, whereas CQI is tactical.[141]

Elements

The critical elements of reengineering are as follows:

1. An outside-in, customer focus, putting the organization in the shoes of the customer to understand and meet customer needs

2. A focus on cross-functional end-to-end processes, versus intradepartmental processes
3. An understanding of processes and customer requirements to recognize weaknesses of the existing process and the performance requirements of the new one[142]
4. An articulated vision of where the HSO/HS wants to be in the future, with that vision communicated and understood by all organization members
5. Top-down rather than bottom-up leadership initiated with committed senior-level management who elicit and obtain acceptance by process owners
6. Identification and questioning of the underlying assumptions about processes
7. The design of new processes, including piloting (small-scale use), to see whether they work, and redesigning, and rolling out the new process in rapid fashion
8. An organizational environment that supports reengineering, including communication throughout the organization, supportive leader personal behavior, measurements, rewards, and "selling the new way of working and living to the organization as a whole"[143]

Implementation of additional elements are senior-level management's commitment to and participation in the reengineering effort; identification of process owners—those who have a direct interest in and responsibility for a process—and empowering them to initiate change; formation of reengineering teams—groups that diagnose existing processes, oversee their redesign, and implement new processes; and use of a steering committee—"a policy-making body of senior managers who develop the organization's overall reengineering strategy and monitor its progress."[144]

Handling Resistance to Change

Inevitably CQI and reengineering initiatives will encounter resistance. As discussed in Chapter 12, resistance to change is a natural phenomenon; it may be visible, overt, and explicit, or it may be indirect. Resistance may be political in nature, or it may stem from individuals who will be adversely affected, those who have low tolerance for change and prefer the status quo, or those who are in denial that change is needed. Complete and open communication is one way to lessen fear and to dispel uncertainty; employee involvement can lead to them accepting ownership. Hammer and Champy urged managers to uncover resistance, understand the motivations, provide incentives for accepting and disincentives for not accepting change, and deal with people's concerns.[145] Hammer contended that HSOs/HSs must be oriented toward change as a way of life in order to improve: "Do it or be done to; change or be changed."[146]

Applications

Various reengineering applications in HSOs/HSs are described in the literature. Among them are service decentralization, clinical resource management, patient aggregation, skill-mix changes, and alterations to noncore processes. In their research based on interviews with 255 senior managers, physicians, and staff at 14 hospitals, Walston and Kimberly found that service decentralization occurred in 13 of the HSOs examined. They reported that ancillary services such as respiratory therapy, physical therapy, and dietary, laboratory, and radiology services were segmented departments in hospitals. To decrease multiple patient hand-offs and "throwing services over the wall" to another department, which resulted in scheduling complications and increased waiting time, a redesign was undertaken that resulted in initiating responsibility for some support services, such as phlebotomy and respiratory services, on the nursing unit. "[H]ousekeeping, dietary, and EKGs were often combined into new patient services positions titled patient care associates, patient care partners, or support partners."[147] Clinical resource management initiatives involved the creation of clinical protocols to lessen treatment variation and to provide a day-to-day schedule for different types of patients by diagnosis using physician "best practices." Only modest success was reported.[148]

Patient aggregation and redesign involves combining patients who require similar skills and resources. By examining historical admitting locations of patients, reallocation of beds by specialty and aggregation of patients with common resource needs result in better care. Homogeneous patient populations requiring similar clinical resources enable dedicated delivery teams to enhance their skills, provide for coordination and continuity of care, decrease unnecessary clinical variation, and enhance outcomes of quality and customer satisfaction.[149] Skill-mix changes reported were use of nursing assistants versus licensed practical nurses and abandoning primary care nursing. Nonpatient care reengineering examples were increasing charge capturing, improving materials contracts, and modifying employee benefits.[150]

Finally, although the preachers of reengineering indicate that downsizing and delayering are not the focus of reengineering, Walston and Kimberly report "it was our experience that downsizing through layoffs was specifically a focus of many executives,"[151] in part because of situations of decreased inpatient census and diminished competitive position. Others also are critical of reengineering, citing that it may be used as a cover to absolve the HSO from blame if layoffs are negatively perceived by stakeholders.[152]

Facilitators and Barriers

Based on their interviews, Watson and Kimberly identified the facilitators and barriers to reengineering shown in Table 9.5, which are similar to CQI initiatives. It is clear that vision, organizational philosophy, senior-level management commitment, physician participation, process design and implementation, and performance measures are critical to QI initiatives.

TABLE 9.5.   REENGINEERING FACILITATORS AND BARRIERS

Facilitators	Barriers
Establish and maintain a constant, consistent vision	Lack of continuity of vision/purpose Disconnection of vision with environment
Prepare smooth transitions for the reengineering effort	Poor transition between project phases Planning to implementation Implementation to a continued process
Prepare and train for reengineering changes	Inadequate administrative skills Inadequate clinical/technical skills
Establish continual, multiple communication methods	Historical practices Lack of continuity of communication Little or inadequate feedback Perceived dishonest communication
Establish strong support and involvement	Inconsistent support and involvement Lack of consistent and even administrative support Lack of equitable departmental participation
Establish mechanisms to measure reengineering's progress and outcomes	Inability to measure progress Complexity of changes without understanding causal mechanisms
Effectively establish both new authority and responsibility relationships	Inadequate authority/responsibilities assigned
Find methods to involve physicians	Lack of time and interest

From Walston, Stephen L., and John R. Kimberly. "Reengineering Hospitals: Evidence from the Field." *Hospital & Health Services Administration* 42 (Summer 1997): 153; reprinted by permission.

STRATEGIC QUALITY PLANNING: HOSHIN PLANNING[153]

Reengineering is a customer-focused, top-down, outside-in, radical change to HSO/HS end-to-end processes that seeks to maintain or attain competitive advantage. A strategic approach to quality is referred to in the literature as *hoshin* planning. *Hoshin* is Japanese for "shining metal compass" or "pointing direction."[154] It is also known as focused planning, policy deployment, or strategic quality planning.[155] It, too, is customer oriented, is primarily externally focused, and seeks to achieve breakthroughs in performance, quality, and competitive position. It is a way of linking quality planning such as that in CQI and reengineering to the overall HSO's/HS's strategic planning process discussed in Chapter 8. It identifies and focuses improvement activities on a few key areas that are strategic priorities to meet customer needs and enhance competitive position.[156]

Hoshin planning has various definitions, but its attributes are similar. AT&T uses the definition of "an organizationwide and customer-focused management approach aimed at planning and executing breakthrough improvements in business performance."[157] The Juran Institute defines it as "the systematic process by which an entire organization sets and achieves specific long-term goals with respect to quality."[158] Another definition is that hoshin planning is "a systems approach to management planning. It is a step-by-step process for building consensus on the vital few strategic areas within which breakthroughs must occur if an organization is to meet and exceed the needs of its customers."[159]

There are six key and consistent attributes of hoshin planning:

1. A *focus for the organization,* in the form of a few breakthrough goals that are vital to the organization's success.
2. A *commitment to customers,* including targets and means at every level of the organization that are based on meeting the needs and expectations that customers rank as most important.
3. *Deployment of the organization's focus* so that employees understand their specific contributions to it. This is referred to as the "golden thread" that links employees to what is important to customers and to one another.
4. *Collective wisdom to develop the plan* through a top-down, bottom-up communication process called "catchball."
5. *Tools and techniques* that make the hoshin planning process and the plan helpful, clear, and easy to use.
6. *Ongoing evaluation of progress* to facilitate learning and continuous improvement. The evaluation system emphasizes both results and the processes that are used to achieve results.[160]

Hoshin planning is vertical, as opposed to the horizontal planning that is done in CQI; is based on the strategic vision of the organization in conjunction with its mission; and is a systematic way of prioritizing and integrating key success factor (KSF) process improvement initiatives.[161] It also allocates resources and aligns or restructures the organization so that "all units attempt to achieve or contribute to the same few key organizational goals or objectives."[162] Hoshin planning is a step beyond CQI and reengineering that is strategic in nature.

As health services shift focus from predominantly illness to wellness and from independent HSOs to HSs, managers need to address critical questions for their organizations:

- How do we *plan* a successful integrated system?
- What are the right things for people to *focus* on to ensure long-term success of the system?
- How do we *align* many different people, departments, and organizations to work together toward the success of the whole system?
- How can we increase employee *understanding* of the system's priorities and plans?
- How can we *balance* the need for organizational direction with opportunities for employee initiative and creativity?
- How can we promote *breakthrough thinking and results*?[163]

Strategic quality planning (i.e., hoshin planning) is one method to answer these questions and for a HSO/HS to achieve the suggested results. An overview of the hoshin planning process is shown in Figure 9.15. The main activities are 1) choose the focus, 2) align the organization, 3) implement the plan, and 4) review and improve.

Choose the Focus

Choosing the focus includes some of the tasks that are inherent in strategic planning as presented in Chapter 8, such as understanding the mission and vision; analyzing the external environment opportunities and threats, including customers, markets, and competitive position; and assessing the HSO's/HS's internal environment to identify strengths and weaknesses. In hoshin planning the focus relates to strategic vision—identifying and articulating what the HSO/HS wants to be in the future. Examples are 1) be the highest value health care provider in the area, 2) promote the development of integrated delivery networks to enhance community health, 3) expand delivery capacity and capability to serve patients in the service area, and 4) provide information on demand for all customers.[164]

Figure 9.16 presents a sample vision statement for a HSO to be "a catalyst to continuously improve the region's health status" that is derived from its mission to "provide tertiary hospital services." The focus is developed by incorporating the values of the HSO (e.g., compassion, excellence, respect) and understanding the trends in its performance (such as 2% decrease in market share and 6% decrease in admissions) as presented in Step 1 of Figure 9.16. The vision of what the HSO wants to become is articulated in Step 2. The third step identifies the HSO's focus if it is to achieve its vision, including KSF and gap analysis. The focus component of hoshin planning provides a methodology by which senior-level management can identify what is most important to customers and a structure to ensure that the focus drives behavior and work at all levels of the HSO/HS.

Align the Organization

The alignment component of Figure 9.15 identifies the performance targets for the key success factors that are part of the strategies to meet customers' needs.[165] An iterative process involving substantial communication throughout the HSO/HS is intended to ensure that all employees understand the vision and accept ownership of the performance targets.

By polling customers and management, gap analysis will reveal discrepancies between expectations and actual performance in the quality of services delivered.[166] Through an iterative organization-wide process, targets for key process performance are developed, negotiated, and communicated.[167] The "golden thread" is interconnected targets at all levels that tie the organization together. *Catchball* is the term that is used to describe the iterative process by which implementation plans and targets are developed. As plans and targets are developed, they are communicated to those involved in implementation, modified, and thrown back for redevelopment.

> *In the catchball process, one level of management throws the ball—the tasks to be accomplished—to the next level of management or another planning team. [There is] . . . input to the development of means to achieve the targets. Dialogue about targets and means proceeds within and across departments, down to the next level of the people closest to the relevant customers and work processes, until the plan is developed in sufficient detail. Then, the process reverses itself. As the plan is finalized, it is rolled back up the organization and checked for gaps, overlaps, and feasibility.*[168]

The collective wisdom of staff within the HSO/HS emerges from the iterative process to develop specific targets at all organizational levels and the plans to achieve them. This collective, it-

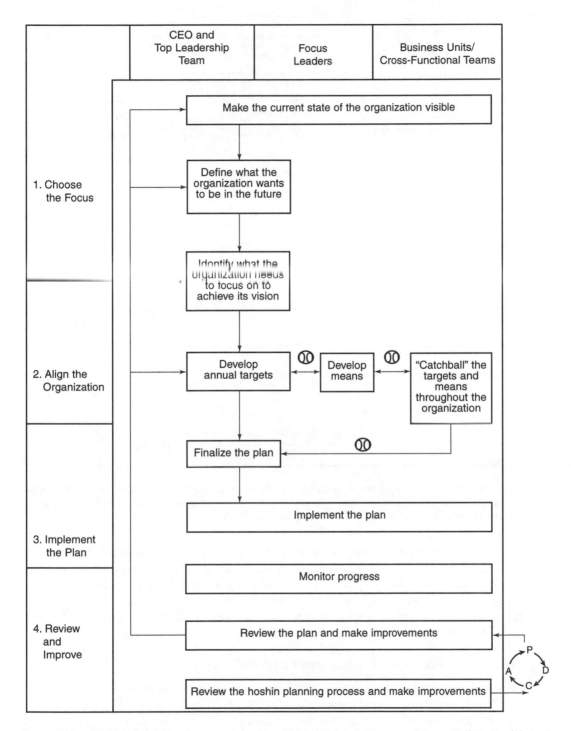

Figure 9.15.   Hoshin planning system overview. (From Melum, Mara Minerva, and Casey Collett. *Breakthrough Leadership: Achieving Organizational Alignment Through Hoshin Planning*, 127. Chicago: American Hospital Publishing, 1995; reprinted by permission.)

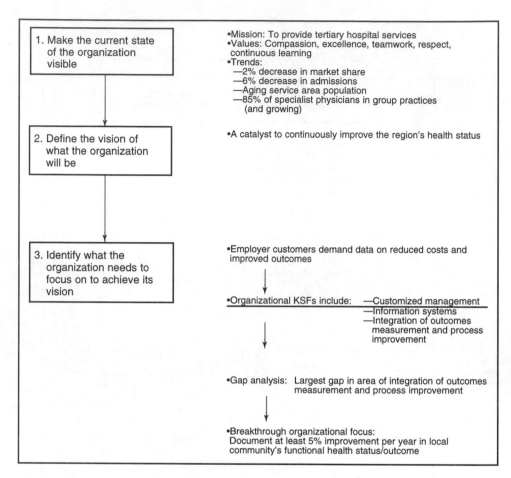

Figure 9.16. Choosing the focus: a health care example. KSF = key success factors. (From Melum, Mara Minerva, and Casey Collett. *Breakthrough Leadership: Achieving Organizational Alignment Through Hoshin Planning, 29.* Chicago: American Hospital Publishing, 1995; reprinted by permission.)

erative procedure is composed of top-down, horizontal, and bottom-up cascades throughout the HSO/HS. Important outcomes are an understanding of how the targets and plans relate to other organizational processes and how they are interconnected. It is evident that empowering employees in the planning and implementation process enhances acceptance of the strategic plan, as well as the commitment and motivation to achieve the results. Furthermore, catchball and the resulting understanding of interrelationships facilitate teamwork.

Implement the Plan and Review and Improve

Examination of Figure 9.15 (Steps 3 and 4) shows that implementation of the plan, reviewing, and improving involve the same steps as those in the FOCUS–PDCA cycle. Based on identified targets at all organizational levels for the processes that are critical to organizational success and resulting plan(s), implementation occurs. Performance relative to each target is tracked using collected data. Reviewing and improving the plan are concurrent and interactive with implementation. It is essentially a problem-solving and control type of activity. If desired results are not attained in key processes, then assessment will determine whether the deviation can be corrected and how to do it. Assessment also may indicate no deviation but that further improvement can be made. As in the

PDCA cycle, lessons learned can be communicated. This can be done with reviews by process improvement teams, the next level of management, and senior-level management. All will facilitate achieving the vision that was developed in the focus stage.

PHYSICIAN INVOLVEMENT IN QI

HSOs/HSs are unique because they are a structural blend of administrative and patient care activities in which clinicians are accorded significant autonomy. Historically, the blended structure created conflict between the two. However, the quality philosophy is changing this relationship. There is now greater collective managerial and clinical accountability for quality, more collaborative participation in quality initiatives, and a mutual interest in both retrospective and concurrent process performance.[169] Both HSO/HS managers and physicians realize they must respect each other's competencies and collaborate to succeed in providing quality services and introducing organizational change, such as improved processes, reengineering, or strategic quality planning. One such change has been the greater use of practice parameters.

Practice Parameters

Practice parameters, also known as practice guidelines, clinical guidelines, protocols, or clinical pathways,[170] are methods for patient management that assist physicians in clinical decision making. To elicit physician support in clinical QI, physicians must be involved and have ownership,[171] there must be physician champions, and physicians must be convinced that such initiatives will enhance quality without inappropriately jeopardizing their professional autonomy or individual patients' needs.[172]

In the provider-at-risk environment, with capitated and per case revenues as well as managed care initiatives,[173] clinical QI initiatives can positively reduce costs. Clinical pathways are an analytical tool to identify optimal timing for clinical interventions by diagnosis and to obtain more effective resource use and better outcomes.[174] Another QI technique is practice guidelines to promote more consistent clinical decision making. As a result, improving clinical processes can have a significant effect on costs and quality for the simple reason that physicians control clinical resource allocation and utilization.[175] Better and wiser physician decisions and less unnecessary variability in diagnosis and treatment from physician "best practices" can leverage quality initiatives regarding inputs consumed and outcomes attained. For example, the practice guideline in Figure 9.17 suggests hospital-based emergency department treatment responses for acute exacerbations of asthma in adults. This protocol can guide physicians in their decision-making process in initial assessment, initial treatment, continued assessment and continued treatment, as well as present alternatives ranging from discharge to admission. In the case of a HS with multiple units providing services along the same continuum of care, practice parameters such as practice guidelines, clinical guidelines, protocols, and clinical pathways should be monitored for "best practices" consistency.[176]

Involving Physicians

James, a physician, identified three general categories of work in most HSOs/HSs: 1) support services, including admission/discharge, billing, medical records, and scheduling; 2) medical infrastructure, including services directly involved in patient care, such as blood bank, laboratory, radiology, and other ancillary services; and 3) medical products, which are "the diagnostic and treatment processes that hospitals provide to patients. For example, normal obstetrical delivery, medical treatment of acute myocardial infarction (heart attack), and surgical treatments of appendicitis are all clinical products."[177] James suggested ways to increase physician involvement in CQI initiatives, which apply by extension to reengineering and strategic quality planning.[178]

Acute Exacerbations of Asthma in Adults: Emergency Department Management

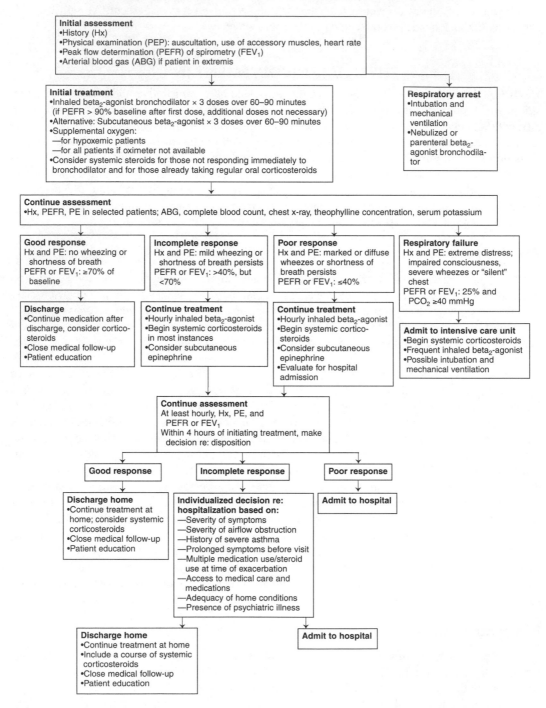

Figure 9.17.   Flowchart illustrating the steps of a treatment protocol for hospital-based emergency department management of acute asthma attack. (From Kibbe, David C., Arnold J. Kaluzny, and Curtis P. McLaughlin. "Integrating Guidelines with Continuous Quality Improvement: Doing the Right Thing the Right Way to Achieve the Right Goals." *Joint Commission Journal on Quality Improvement* 20,4 [1994]: 181–191; reprinted by permission.)

First, QI is not new to physicians. They are trained in scientific, numbers-oriented investigation and reasoning. Management must train physicians to use QI techniques, and "quality improvement theory should be presented as a direct extension of the principles that the medical profession has always espoused."[179] Because clinical quality initiatives seek to improve medical outcomes,[180] physicians should be comfortable with their data-driven scientific approaches and process orientation. These initiatives will result in better mobilization and utilization of resources to meet the needs of physicians and patients.[181]

Second, physicians often distrust clinical measurement efforts that are unilaterally initiated by management.[182] Management efforts should dispel distrust and the possible perception that quality projects are "thinly disguised efforts to reduce health care resource utilization, seemingly without regard for the potential impact of such actions on patients' health."[183] When trust exists, physicians and managers will work toward common goals in the delivery of high-quality and cost-effective services.[184]

Third, quality teams already exist for clinical products, and they should be involved in other quality initiatives. Quality assurance (see Chapter 10) includes peer review "typically organized through sub-specialty medical staff groups and reports through an independent medical staff organization."[185] QI techniques can be incorporated in this process. Because of physicians' independent self-interest in husbanding their time, James recommends structuring clinical improvement projects within staff meetings and allocating salaried physicians' use of work time.[186] Management "should consider physician's self-perceived role as customers or providers as they plan physician involvement on quality improvement teams."[187]

Fourth, physicians should be encouraged to become involved in clinical product quality initiatives with other organization members and provided with administrative support.[188] This may also include assigning staff to collect and analyze data and to support clinical QI teams, along with investing in real-time clinical/management information systems.[189]

Fifth, clinical QI requires stable diagnostic and treatment processes. Because physicians control these processes, management must ensure that they participate in the initiative and regard themselves as owners of the process used to improve it. As James observed, "It is more important how you [managers] implement than what you implement. The aim is to manage clinical processes, not to manage the physicians."[190]

Sixth, a 2-year study to identify and assess attributes of successful CQI initiatives in acute care hospitals concluded that physician involvement on clinical process improvement teams early in the CQI program is essential for success.[191] Management must train a nucleus of physicians at the outset of a QI initiative so that there is a sense of physician ownership.[192]

Seventh, the focus should be on strategically important clinical issues and procedures, such as those that are high cost and high volume, in which data are readily available and improvement opportunities are present.[193] It is suggested that management identification of these conditions will serve as an important motivating factor and reinforce the HSO's/HS's commitment to improving areas of concern to physicians.[194] Those involved should be physician leaders who may have administrative appointments as well as independent clinicians who are highly respected by their peers.[195]

Eighth, management must be both patient and opportunistic[196] and be prepared to respond to the "neutral" majority of physicians who identify a clinical problem or concern.[197] When they do, management should be ready to show them how QI relates to them or their practices, orient them to QI methods, and arrange for them to interact with physician champions who are committed to QI.[198]

Results

The rise of managed care has given impetus to improving the consistency of clinical practice and the development of evidence-based "best practice" guidelines. A research study surveyed approaches used to implement clinical guidelines and improve clinical performance in 25 integrated delivery systems and managed health care plans. Together they provided health care to 40 million people. The organizations surveyed were 13 HMOs, 8 multispecialty group practices, 2 indemnity insurance companies, and 2 Blue Cross Blue Shield plans. The most frequently cited method for improving clinical practice was feedback or clinical profiles of individual clinicians through audits of medical records and comparing their practice with peers or other benchmarks. The second most frequently cited method was clinician feedback from clinical department or administrative heads though regular department meetings. The third most frequent method was involvement of local physicians in developing practice parameters; the same number of organizations also reported using or considering the use of financial incentives by "tying a small percentage of income to factors such as patient satisfaction, rates of preventative services, and efforts to improve quality."[199]

Failed approaches to achieving improvement in clinical performance reported were simply sending information to physicians or increasing their knowledge alone; feedback with group data alone; and development of practice guidelines outside of the managed care plan or practice unit without local physician involvement.[200] The success of clinical improvement was based on HSO/HS leadership promoting a QI culture, respect for physicians, involvement of physicians and other workers, a customer perspective, organizational support, and "viewing physicians as important participants but not necessarily the focus of a system whose performance is to be improved."[201] The latter point paraphrases Deming—blame the process for poor quality, not the workers.

QI—THE NEXT ITERATION

What lies in the future of QI? The next iteration of QI, beyond that practiced within a single HSO within a HS, will be a quantum leap to involve multiple independent HSOs/HSs within a community. The acceptance of QI by community organizations will be more difficult to achieve, and the complexity of arrangements will be great.[202] Three essential features will be 1) data sharing among participating HSOs/HSs, which may represent a threat to them and a possible barrier to cooperation; 2) accommodating different organizational cultures and dealing with the issue of control; and 3) the shift in quality activities from independent HSOs/HSs to a collection within the community that represents "a transformation from hierarchies to markets."[203] QI initiatives beyond the single HSO or HS will likely use a public health model that relies on health status indicators, community satisfaction, and overall community benefit.[204] The PRECEDE–PROCEED model in Figure 2.2 reflects these factors.

QI within the context of a communitywide model will require the application of QI principles, perhaps reengineering, and certainly strategic quality planning. However, it will be necessary to manage the changed leadership patterns among participating HSOs/HSs, lessen threats to them, and gain the cooperation of HSOs/HSs that have traditionally competed with one another. Whether this can be achieved is problematic. However, the following steps will facilitate this transformation from traditional HSO/HS–based quality initiatives to those that are community oriented[205]:

1. *Be cautious in implementing a conventional quality improvement infrastructure that may have worked in intraorganizational initiatives.* All organizations may not have the same experience with quality initiatives; they may have different agendas and different priorities.
2. *Achieve the commitment of top management to community-based needs assessment.* Community-based indicators of need and quality must be developed, with HSO/HS leaders focusing on the needs of the community versus those of their own organization.
3. *Develop long-run objectives, but also set short-term measurable objectives.* Because there is likely to be variability in commitment among different organizations, short-run objectives, perhaps involving modest initiatives, are necessary to demonstrate that communitywide quality initiatives can work.

4. *Select topics to utilize network participants who are ready for a common quality improvement approach to specific objectives, capitalizing on small wins.* To build consensus, "select issues and areas for cooperation where the majority of key participants appear to be ready to implement quality improvement on a communitywide basis, capitalizing on emergent interest and activities."

5. *Emphasize data feedback and improved insight.* Use feedback to lessen the concerns of HSOs/HSs as well as autonomous professionals who will, to some degree, be conceding their sovereignty.

6. *Avoid "religious" wars.* One organization should not preach its own approach to quality as the one true approach.

7. *Build the network of organizations carefully.* Elicit the cooperation of community stakeholders who are critical to success.

8. *Recognize initial efforts as a coalition arrangement.* Indicate to potential participants how the community quality initiatives will benefit them and help to achieve their organization's objectives. Also, permit them to participate or not participate in initiatives; in a confederation, it is necessary to allow some degree of freedom.

SUMMARY

This chapter examines the health services paradigm shift with respect to quality. Quality must incorporate not only conformance to requirements but also the dimension of meeting or exceeding patient/customer expectations. The philosophy of CQI is described and modeled. CQI is defined as an ongoing, organizationwide framework that commits managers, employees, and clinical staff to improving quality and involves them in monitoring and evaluating all HSO/HS activities (inputs and processes) and outputs to improve them.

The CQI model presented in Figure 9.2 rests on two pillars: improving output quality and improving processes. Through both, productivity improvement occurs and the HSO's/HS's competitive position is enhanced.

Profiles of three quality experts—W. Edwards Deming, Joseph M. Juran, and Philip B. Crosby—are presented. Included are Deming's 14 points for improved quality and organization transformation, Juran's quality trilogy, and Crosby's 14 steps for QI. The role of statistical quality control is emphasized.

Two process improvement models are presented: FOCUS–PDCA and QMMP. Both are similar and suggest steps to improve processes. MBNQA, benchmarking, and ISO 9000 standards provide methods or measures for achievement in quality. CQI and problem solving, the role of QITs, and methods that can assist QITs in analyzing processes are discussed. For CQI to be effective, there must be commitment to it by all HSO/HS members.

The subjects of productivity and productivity improvement are presented. Productivity is the index of outputs to inputs. Productivity improvement is a function of the index of results achieved, which includes quantity and quality, relative to resources consumed. The productivity improvement triangle (Figure 9.12) presents the relationship between CQI and productivity improvement, and indicates that productivity improvement occurs only when the highest quality possible (outputs) is attained for the lowest reasonable costs (inputs). Various approaches to productivity improvement are presented: analysis and improvement of work systems and job design; capacity planning and facilities layout; and production control, scheduling, and materials distribution.

Reengineering is defined as the fundamental rethinking and radical redesign of business processes to achieve dramatic improvements in critical, contemporary measures of performance, such as costs, quality, service, and speed. Through the radical redesign of processes, it seeks to meet customer needs and enhance HSO/HS competitive position. Reengineering is differentiated from CQI. Resistance to reengineering, examples of applications in HSs, and facilitators and barriers to reengineering are discussed.

Strategic quality planning, referred to as hoshin planning, is a method by which the HSO/HS links QI initiatives to strategic planning. Hoshin planning focuses on the key critical processes that are requisite for satisfying customers and achieving an enhanced competitive position. Its attributes include choosing the focus (i.e., vision), aligning the organization, implementation, and review.

Clearly, physician involvement in QI is necessary for success, particularly in clinical areas. Practice parameters are one method to improve clinical decision making. Recommendations to enhance physician participation and commitment to QI are presented. Finally, the next iteration of QI will involve communitywide initiatives among multiple HSOs and HSs. The leap will be quantum, involving many pitfalls. A communitywide public health model is suggested by some. Recommendations are made to facilitate this iteration of QI.

DISCUSSION QUESTIONS

1. What are some of the important changes that occurred in health services delivery in the 1980s and 1990s that induced HSOs/HSs to adopt the philosophy of CQI?
2. Define CQI. Why is it an organizational philosophy? What are its attributes? How can CQI lead to an enhanced HSO/HS competitive position?
3. Think about the nursing service in a hospital. Who or what are its customers? If the nursing service is the customer, who or what provides inputs (is the supplier)?
4. Identify several difficulties and several benefits of working with licensed independent practitioners to improve quality. What considerations should managers keep in mind when working with them?
5. Based on the profiles of Deming, Juran, and Crosby, identify the similarities and differences in their approaches to quality.
6. How does the FOCUS–PDCA process improvement model relate to the problem-solving model in Figure 7.4?
7. Define reengineering. What are its attributes? How are CQI and reengineering related?
8. What are the four steps in strategic quality planning? How is it related to strategic planning as described in Chapter 8?
9. Why is it necessary for physicians to be involved in QI? What steps are recommended to increase their involvement?

CASE STUDY 1: FED UP IN DALLAS [206]

Dear Ann Landers:

I've done at least $20,000 worth of business with a local printer. I've always paid my bills in installments, some as large as $1,000 a month.

My printer told me my payments were too small and she had to have all her money in one lump from then on. I paid her off and took my printing elsewhere.

I've patronized the same dry cleaner for 5 years. They know me on sight and have never asked for identification when they cash my checks. Suddenly, they are losing and damaging my clothes and acting as if it's not their fault.

This morning I drove into the service station where I've been a customer for 3 years. I asked the man to please check the pressure in a low tire. I was told that I'd have to buy gas in order to get full service. When I said, "OK," the attendant continued to gripe and then the owner got into the act. I told them to forget it, that I'd go elsewhere. The attendant replied, "You want me to take the air back out of your tire?" Needless to say, they won't see me again.

I've even had a run-in with a doctor I've been seeing for 6 years. I walked out of his office after being kept waiting for an hour and a half.

Ann, what's wrong with these people? Why don't they value those of us who keep them in business? In these times of economic hardship, you'd think they would do everything possible to please their customers. Am I wrong to expect a little service and courtesy in exchange for my business?

—Fed Up in Dallas

QUESTIONS

1. CQI focuses on improving processes and quality. It is customer oriented. In the letter to Ann Landers, it is evident that "Fed Up in Dallas" is not a satisfied customer. In our society in general, why do you think there is indifference to customers by organizations (and their employees) that provide products and services?
2. Describe instances in which you or acquaintances encountered a negative customer orientation by a HSO. What was your (their) reaction?

CASE STUDY 2: THE CARBONDALE CLINIC [207]

The Carbondale Clinic, located in Carbondale, Illinois, is a large group practice of about 30 physicians. The clinic employs about 100 people and serves a regional population of about 100,000. Specialties ranging from pediatrics to psychiatry are offered by the clinic, which also operates its own lab, x-ray room, and outpatient surgical center.

For some years, the clinic has been receiving complaints from its patients that appointment times are not being met. For instance, a patient with an appointment for two o'clock might not get in to see the physician until four o'clock. However, the clinic has felt that such delays are unavoidable due to the uncertainty involved in the time it takes to adequately examine each patient and the possibility of emergency cases that must be inserted into the schedule.

Several criteria are used for scheduling. For instance, many patients are scheduled for annual physical exams. These are usually scheduled at least several weeks in advance because they require coordination of lab facilities and the physician's time. However, some physicians will begin examining a patient and decide that the patient needs a physical immediately. The physicians feel this does not really cause problems because they can send the patient down to the lab while they continue to see other patients.

Some patients also phone the clinic for an appointment when they have nonemergency, routine problems such as a mild fever or sore throat. Such patients are scheduled into available time slots as soon as possible—usually a day or two from the time they call. The objective here is to fit such patients in as quickly as possible without overloading the schedule with more patients than can reasonably be examined in a time period. Usually the plan is to schedule four patients per hour.

However, each day various emergencies occur. These can range from a splinter in the eye to a heart attack, and these cases cannot wait. For an emergency that is not life threatening, the approach is to try to squeeze the person into a time slot that is not too heavily scheduled. However, a case of life or death—such as a heart attack—means that the schedule must be disrupted and the patient treated immediately.

Currently, all scheduling of appointments is done centrally. However, this frequently causes problems because the people making appointments often do not know how long it should take to examine a patient with a particular complaint. On the other hand, the nurses in each department are usually too busy to do the scheduling themselves. Generally, if there is a doubt about whether a patient can be fitted into a time slot, the preference is to go ahead and schedule the patient. This is because the physicians prefer not to have any empty times in their schedules. At times, if it looks as if there might be an available opening, the clinic even calls patients who were originally scheduled for a later time and asks them to come in early.

QUESTIONS

1. "For some years, the clinic has received complaints from its patients that appointment times are not being met." Why has no action to correct the situation been taken?
2. As a member of a QIT, you are charged with evaluating the appointment/scheduling process. Are there some "assumptions" in the narrative that you question? If there were sufficient data to prepare a Pareto diagram, what do you think the items would be? Please list them.
3. Draw a cause-and-effect diagram (fishbone chart) of the causes for patient complaints.
4. What recommendations would you make to improve the situation and decrease patient waiting time?

CASE STUDY 3: TOTAL QUALITY MANAGEMENT (TQM) INVENTORY[208]

Continuous quality improvement (CQI) and total quality management (TQM) are frequently used interchangeably in the literature. This TQM inventory is an instrument to measure an organization's TQM (or CQI) orientation. It contains three parts, eight criteria questions, a scoring sheet, and an interpretation sheet.

PART 1: TQM INVENTORY

Instructions: For each of the eight TQM criteria listed below, circle the statement that best describes the present situation in your organization.

Criterion 1: Top Management Leadership and Support

A. Top managers are directly and actively involved in activities that foster quality.
B. Top managers participate in quality leadership activities.
C. Most top managers support activities that foster quality.
D. Many top managers are supportive of and interested in quality improvement.
E. Some top managers are beginning to tentatively support activities that foster quality.
F. No top management support exists for activities involving quality.

Criterion 2: Strategic Planning

A. Long-term goals for quality improvement have been established across the organization as part of the overall strategic planning process.
B. Long-term goals for quality improvement have been established across most of the organization.
C. Long-term goals for quality improvement have been established in key parts of the organization.
D. Short-term goals for quality improvement have been established in parts of the organization.
E. The general goals of the organization contain elements of quality improvement.
F. No quality improvement goals have been established anywhere in the organization.

Criterion 3: Focus on the Customer

A. A variety of effective and innovative methods are used to obtain customer feedback on all organizational functions.
B. Effective systems are used to obtain feedback from all customers of major functions.

C. Systems are in place to solicit customer feedback on a regular basis.
D. Customer needs are determined through random processes rather than by using systematic methods.
E. Complaints are the major methods used to obtain customer feedback.
F. No customer focus is evident.

Criterion 4: Employee Training and Recognition

A. The organization is implementing a systematic employee training and recognition plan that is fully integrated into the overall strategic quality planning process.
B. The organization is assessing the employee training and recognition that are needed, and the results of that assessment are being evaluated periodically.
C. An employee training and recognition plan is beginning to be implemented.
D. An employee training and recognition plan is under active development.
E. The organization has plans to increase employee training and recognition.
F. There is no employee training, and there are no systems for recognizing employees.

Criterion 5: Employee Empowerment and Teamwork

A. Innovative, effective employee empowerment and teamwork approaches are used.
B. Many natural workgroups are empowered to constitute quality improvement teams.
C. A majority of managers support employee empowerment and teamwork.
D. Many managers support employee empowerment and teamwork.
E. Some managers support employee empowerment and teamwork.
F. There is no support for employee empowerment and teamwork.

Criterion 6: Quality Measurement and Analysis

A. Information about quality and timeliness of all products and services is collected from internal and external customers and from suppliers.
B. Information about quality and timeliness is collected from most internal and external customers and from most suppliers.
C. Information about quality and timeliness is collected from major internal and external customers and from major suppliers.
D. Information about quality and timeliness is collected from some internal and external customers.
E. Information about quality and timeliness is collected from one or two external customers.
F. There is no system for measuring and analyzing quality.

Criterion 7: Quality Assurance

A. All products, services, and processes are designed, reviewed, verified, and controlled to meet the needs and expectations of internal and external customers.
B. A majority of products, services, and processes are designed, reviewed, verified, and controlled to meet the needs and expectations of internal and external customers.
C. Key products, services, and processes are designed, reviewed, verified, and controlled to meet the needs and expectations of internal and external customers.
D. A few products and services are designed, reviewed, and controlled to meet the needs of internal and external customers.
E. Products and services are controlled to meet internally developed specifications that may or may not include customer input.
F. There is no quality assurance in this organization.

Criterion 8: Quality and Productivity Improvement Results

A. Most significant performance indicators demonstrate exceptional improvement in quality and productivity over the past 5 years.
B. Most significant performance indicators demonstrate excellent improvement in quality and productivity over the past 5 years.
C. Most significant performance indicators demonstrate good improvement in quality and productivity.
D. Most significant performance indicators demonstrate improving quality and productivity in several areas.
E. There is evidence of some quality and productivity improvement in one or more areas.
F. There is no evidence of quality and productivity improvement in any area.

PART 2: TOTAL QUALITY MANAGEMENT (TQM) INVENTORY SCORING SHEET

To determine your scores on the inventory, complete the following three steps:

1. For each of the *Total Quality Management Criteria* listed in the left column [see following table], find the letter under the heading labeled *Response Categories/Points* that corresponds to the one you chose on the questionnaire.
2. Circle the one- or two-digit *Point* number that corresponds to the letter you chose.
3. Add up the points circled for all eight criteria to determine your *Overall Score*.

Note: The numbers you are about to circle correspond to the relative weights attached to individual Quality/Productivity Criteria in the President's Award. Therefore in addition to helping score your responses, the points also identify the categories that are more significant than others. For example, scores on Criterion 8 (Quality and Productivity Improvement Results) are better indicators of an organization's orientation toward quality and productivity than are its scores on Criterion 4 (Employee Training and Recognition).

TQM CRITERIA	RESPONSE CATEGORIES/POINTS					
	A	B	C	D	E	F
1. Top Management Leadership and Support	20	16	12	8	4	0
2. Strategic Planning	15	12	9	6	3	0
3. Focus on the Customer	40	32	24	16	8	0
4. Employee Training and Recognition	15	12	9	6	3	0
5. Employee Empowerment and Teamwork	15	12	9	6	3	0
6. Quality Measurement and Analysis	15	12	9	6	3	0
7. Quality Assurance	30	24	18	12	6	0
8. Quality and Productivity Improvement Results	50	40	30	20	10	0
Scores for Choice Categories:	——	——	——	——	——	——
Overall Score:	—— (Range: 0–200)					

PART 3: TOTAL QUALITY MANAGEMENT (TQM) INVENTORY INTERPRETATION SHEET

160–200 points: An overall score in this range indicates a "world-class" organization with a deep long-term and active commitment to improving quality and productivity. At this level, goals should focus on the challenge of maintaining gains as well as seeking ways to attain even higher levels of quality and productivity.

120–159 points: An overall score in this range indicates that an organization with a sound, well-organized philosophy of quality and productivity improvement is beginning to emerge. At this level, goals should focus on fully implementing a sound TQM effort while continuing to build on current levels of excellence.

80–119 points: An overall score in this range indicates an organization that is starting to learn about and plan quality and productivity improvements. At this level, goals should focus on moving from the planning stages to actually implementing a TQM effort in order to gain the necessary hands-on experience.

40–79 points: An overall score in this range indicates an organization that is vaguely aware of quality and productivity improvement but has no plans to learn about or implement such activity. Scores at this level approach the danger point; if long-term organizational viability is sought, progress must be made quickly. Goals should focus on strongly encouraging top managers to learn more about TQM while re-examining their assumptions about possible contributions that the process can make to the health of their organization.

0–39 points. An overall score in this range indicates an organization that currently has neither an awareness of nor an involvement with quality- and productivity-improvement programs. Unless an organization has an absolute, invulnerable monopoly on extremely valuable products or services, this level represents a de facto decision to go out of business. Goals should focus on an emergency turnaround. Learning about TQM must occur at an accelerated rate, and plans to bring quality and productivity consciousness to the organization must be implemented immediately.

CASE STUDY 4: NONINVASIVE CARDIOVASCULAR LABORATORY

The associate vice president for operations at Barbarosa Hospital had a problem concerning the noninvasive cardiovascular laboratory (NCVL). First, patients complained to their physicians about long waits and interruptions during tests. Second, the NCVL technician complained about being overworked. After observing the technician and talking with him and his supervisor, the following information was obtained.

The NCVL is located on the third floor of the hospital. It is adjacent to the stress test laboratory, which has twice the space of the noninvasive laboratory but uses only half of it. Also, the stress test technician is productive only 60% of the time. Loren Findley is the only technician assigned to the NCVL. Findley's workspace is cramped and crowded with two patient beds, a very large desk, and supplies in stacked boxes. The equipment layout in the room does not permit easy movement, and some of the equipment must be placed in the hall. Consequently, Findley spends an average of 10 minutes moving equipment in or out of the room when setting up for a test that differs from the preceding one.

Findley is qualified to administer the following three tests:

1. Echocardiogram (ECHO): A graphic recording generated by ultrasound that is used to study the structures and motions of the heart.
2. Ocular plethysmograph (OPG): A test to measure changes in size and volume of the eye.
3. Pulse volume recording (PVR) plethysmograph: A test to measure changes in volume of a cross-section of a blood vessel over several heartbeats.

Findley schedules the inpatient and outpatient tests ordered by house staff and attending physicians. Frequent phone calls to schedule tests are received throughout the day. On average, three of four tests Findley administers are interrupted by phone calls. It takes 10 minutes to return to the point before the interruption (2 minutes talking on the phone and 8 minutes to restart the test).

From extensive observation, the following standard times for each test were determined (assume there is no standard time difference for inpatients and outpatients):

Test	Standard time
ECHO	1 hour
OPG	1/2 hour
PVR	1/2 hour

With the expansion of the professional staff organization at the beginning of the year, the number of tests ordered increased.

Findley complained to his supervisor about being overworked and unable to keep up with the workload. He stated that he wanted a full-time assistant or he might quit. The hospital has no other employees who could perform the tests, even though they are not difficult to learn. Findley could train someone to perform the tests in about 2 months.

Hospital records were used to compare the number of tests performed last year with the number performed in the first 3 months of this year:

		No. performed	
		This year	
Test	Previous year	First 3 months	Annualized
ECHO	800	300	1,200
OPG	200	75	300
PVR	200	75	300

The typical pattern for scheduled tests on any given day is ECHO, ECHO, OPG, ECHO, ECHO, PVR, ECHO, ECHO, OPG, and so forth.

QUESTIONS

1. Is Findley overworked? Why or why not? Should another technician be hired?
2. Assume that the addition of a new technician is not a viable alternative. How can the present NCVL process be changed to improve quality and productivity?

CASE STUDY 5: TRYING HARD MEMORIAL HOSPITAL AND DO IT RIGHT MEDICAL CENTER[209]

Trying Hard Memorial Hospital

At Trying Hard Memorial, the chief executive officer (CEO) frequently reminds the staff of her commitment: "Keep up all of your good work on TQM! It's an important project for this organization and one that should bring impressive results quickly." The CEO stops by the major TQM training sessions to give the opening remarks and visits quality council meetings when her schedule permits. She also tries periodically to observe [quality] improvement team meetings.

The hospital holds special quarterly meetings to discuss the progress of TQM. When time permits, TQM also is discussed under "other business" at regular management meetings.

TQM is ostensibly a major goal in the organization's strategic plan. However, because of severe financial constraints, the TQM budget includes only a half-time coordinator, four facilitators, and $10,000 for TQM training.

Trying Hard Memorial made sure that it provided TQM training for most of the vice-presidents and for facilitators in the first year of TQM implementation. The director of human resources designed the curriculum and training workbook. Courses included an awareness session, 4 days of training for facilitators, and a 1-day training session for vice presidents. The hospital focused its training on TQM analytical tools so that people could see that TQM really differs from quality assurance (QA)—that total quality incorporates, advances, and extends beyond the traditional QA process. The first TQM team started work 2 months after the training session.

A few physicians at the hospital have expressed interest in TQM, and the chief of staff is a standing member of the quality council. Unfortunately, however, most physicians at the hospital do not really understand TQM, and they cannot afford to take time away from their practices to attend the training sessions. Thus, Trying Hard Memorial plans to hold one TQM informational meeting that would be open to all members of the medical staff. The hospital also hopes to generate more physician interest in TQM when the results of the pilot improvement team on turnaround time in the OR are announced.

Because of the financial constraints mentioned previously and because of an upcoming Joint Commission site visit, Trying Hard Memorial had decided to delay until next year the development of new TQM information systems, a new TQM planning and budgeting process, and other new management systems.

Do It Right Medical Center

Meanwhile, at Do It Right Medical Center, the CEO is continually reminding employees by her actions that she is committed to TQM. The management committee has been designated as the quality council, chaired by the CEO, to guide the organizationwide effort. The CEO has gone through 15 days of TQM training from internal TQM staff, working with an outside consultant, to become a facilitator and team leader. She also teaches one TQM course every month. She is currently serving as team leader of an improvement team that is applying TQM to the cost management process. The CEO has restructured her job to delegate more operational responsibilities so that she can spend at least 50% of her time directly with internal and external customers. "What could be a more important use of my time?" she asks those who question her schedule.

At Do It Right Medical Center, quality is the first item on the agenda at all management and board meetings. Every month a quality report is presented. This report monitors agreed-on quality performance measures, much as the financial report monitors financial performance measures.

At Do It Right Medical Center, the quality vision statement and the quality goal that is specified in the strategic plan have been integrated into operational plans at every level of the organization. The result is specific, directed action. To accomplish this integration, the quality council first developed performance measures for the vision and goals, in consultation with employees, physicians, patients, and purchasers. Then each department was asked to develop a plan to contribute to the achievement of the organization's vision and goal. Each departmental plan was then translated into employee work plans and budgets.

The medical center's education budget has doubled over the past 2 years. An annual training plan directs allocation of these resources. The training plan is developed by the quality council based on input from customers and results from the annual leadership profile completed by all managers. Current courses, which were tailored for the organization, include Managing by TQM, TQM for Team Leaders, TQM for Facilitators, TQM for Teams, Empowerment, Customer Expectations, and TQM Planning. In addition, the first half hour of every improvement team meeting is devoted to just-in-time training, which prepares teams for the specific project at hand, and continuing education about TQM in general. The training curriculum is balanced between analytical techniques, such as statistical process control, and behavioral modules, such as team building.

Physicians are an integral part of TQM at Do It Right Medical Center. Led by three physician champions, physicians serve on the quality council, help identify operational and clinical processes that would benefit from improvement teams, serve on quality improvement teams, and discuss the hospital's quality report at the beginning of their department and executive committee meetings. The medical center is assisting the three largest physician practices to implement TQM in their offices.

TQM seems to be everywhere at the medical center. For example, all budget requests must document how they contribute to TQM. Customer satisfaction ratings are a major factor in performance evaluations. And the CEO always seems to be asking, "What root cause did your team discover for our problem? What data led you to that conclusion?"

QUESTIONS:

1. Relative to CQI, what is "Trying Hard Memorial Hospital" doing wrong?
2. Relative to CQI, what is "Do It Right Medical Center" doing right?

NOTES

1. McLaughlin, Curtis P., and Arnold D. Kaluzny. *Continuous Quality Improvement in Health Care: Theory, Implementation and Applications,* 3. Gaithersburg, MD: Aspen Publishers, 1994.
2. Laffel, Glenn, and David Blumenthal. "The Case for Using Industrial Management Science in Health Care Organizations." *Journal of the American Medical Association* 262 (November 24, 1989): 2870; Merry, Martin D. "Total Quality Management for Physicians: Translating the New Paradigm." *Quality Review Bulletin* 16 (March 1990): 104; McLaughlin, Curtis P., and Arnold D. Kaluzny. "Total Quality Management in Health: Making It Work." *Health Care Management Review* 15 (Summer 1990): 7.
3. Kaluzny, Arnold D., and Curtis P. McLaughlin. "Managing Transitions: Assuring the Adoption and Impact of TQM." *Quality Review Bulletin* 37,4 (November 1992): 380.
4. American Hospital Association. *Quality Management: A Management Advisory,* 1. Chicago: American Hospital Association, 1990; James, Brent C. *Quality Management for Health Care Delivery—Quality Measurement and Management Project,* 10. Chicago: Hospital Research and Educational Trust, 1989; Laffel and Blumenthal, "The Case for Using," 2870; O'Connor, Stephen J. "Service Quality: Understanding and Implementing the Concept in the Clinical Laboratory." *Clinical Laboratory Management Review* 3 (November/December 1989): 330; Schumacher, Dale N. "Organizing for Quality Competition: The Coming Paradigm Shift." *Frontiers of Health Services Management* 5 (Summer 1989): 113. For a useful model of quality, see Lanning, Joyce A., and Stephen J. O'Connor. "The Health Care Quality Quagmire: Some Signposts." *Hospital & Health Services Administration* 35 (Spring 1990): 42.
5. Deming, W. Edwards. *Out of the Crisis,* 18. Boston: Massachusetts Institute of Technology, 1986.
6. Milakovich, Michael E. "Creating a Total Quality Health Care Environment." *Health Care Management Review* 16 (Spring 1991): 9.
7. Casurella, Joe. "Managing a 'Total Quality' Program." *Federation of American Health Systems Review* 22 (July/August 1989): 31.
8. James, *Quality Management,* 11.
9. American Production and Inventory Control Society. *APICS Dictionary,* 9th ed., 78. Falls Church, VA: American Production and Inventory Control Society, 1998. For ease of reading, these two components of quality are referred to as conformance and expectation quality. For further discussion of quality, see Casalou, Robert F. "Total Quality Management in Health Care." *Hospital & Health Services Administration* 36 (Spring 1991): 135; James, Brent C. "Implementing Continuous Quality Improvement." *Trustee* 43 (April 1990): 16; Juran, Joseph M. *Juran on Planning for Quality,* 4. New York: The Free

Press, 1988; Re, Richard N., and Marie A. Krousel-Wood. "How to Use Continuous Quality Improvement Theory and Statistical Quality Control Tools in a Multispecialty Clinic." *Quality Review Bulletin* 16 (November 1990): 392.

10. Heizer, Jay, and Barry Render. *Production and Operations Management: Strategic and Tactical Decisions,* 4th ed., 74. Upper Saddle River, NJ: Prentice-Hall, 1996.

11. James, *Quality Management,* 10.

12. McLaughlin and Kaluzny, *Continuous Quality Improvement,* 12.

13. James, *Quality Management,* 11.

14. Re and Krousel-Wood, "How to Use," 392.

15. Milakovich, "Creating a Total," 11.

16. Arndt, Margarete, and Barbara Bigelow. "The Implementation of Total Quality Management in Hospitals: How Good Is the Fit?" *Health Care Management Review* 20 (Fall 1995): 9.

17. McLaughlin and Kaluzny, "Total Quality Management," 8.

18. Marszalek-Gaucher, Ellen, and Richard J. Coffey. *Transforming Healthcare Organizations: How to Achieve and Sustain Organizational Excellence,* 85. San Francisco: Jossey-Bass, 1990; Arndt and Bigelow, "The Implementation of," 9.

19. Deming, W. Edwards. "Improvement of Quality and Productivity Through Action by Management." *National Productivity Review* 1 (Winter 1981–1982): 12–22; Deming, W. Edwards. *Quality, Productivity, and Competitive Position.* Boston: The MIT Press, 1982; Deming, W. Edwards. "Transformation of Western Style Management." *Interfaces* 15 (May/June 1985): 6–11; Deming, *Out of the Crisis.*

20. Juran, Joseph M. *Managerial Breakthrough: A New Concept of the Manager's Job.* New York: McGraw-Hill, 1964; Juran, Joseph M. "The Quality Trilogy." *Quality Progress* 19 (August 1986): 19–24; Juran, Joseph M. *Juran on Leadership for Quality.* New York: The Free Press, 1989; Juran, *Juran on Planning.*

21. Crosby, Philip B. *Quality Is Free.* New York: McGraw-Hill, 1979; Crosby, Philip B. *Let's Talk Quality.* New York: McGraw-Hill, 1989; Crosby, Philip B. *Quality Without Tears.* New York: McGraw-Hill, 1984.

22. American Hospital Association, *Quality Management,* 2.

23. For ease of reading, when reference is made in this chapter to process improvement, it also includes input improvement.

24. Joint Commission on Accreditation of Healthcare Organizations. *The Joint Commission's Agenda for Change: Stimulating Continual Improvement in the Quality of Care,* 1–4. Oakbrook Terrace, IL: Joint Commission on Accreditation of Healthcare Organizations, 1990; Joint Commission on Accreditation of Healthcare Organizations. *Transitions: From QA to CQI—Using CQI Approaches to Monitor, Evaluate, and Improve Quality,* 6–7. Oakbrook Terrace, IL: Joint Commission on Accreditation of Healthcare Organizations, 1991.

25. Joint Commission on Accreditation of Healthcare Organizations. *Brief Overview of Joint Commission's Agenda for Change* (internal working document), 1. Oakbrook Terrace, IL: Joint Commission on Accreditation of Healthcare Organizations, 1990; see also Joint Commission, *Transitions,* 21.

26. James, *Quality Management,* 1.

27. Anderson, Craig A., and Robin D. Daigh. "Quality Mind-Set Overcomes Barriers to Success." *Healthcare Financial Management* 45 (February 1991): 21; Kroenberg, Philip S., and Renee G. Loeffler. "Quality Management Theory: Historical Context and Future Prospect." *Journal of Management Science & Policy Analysis* 8 (Spring/Summer 1991): 204; McLaughlin and Kaluzny, "Total Quality Management," 7; Sahney, Vinod K., and Gail L. Warden. "The Quest for Quality and Productivity in Health Services." *Frontiers of Health Services Management* 7 (Summer 1991): 2.

28. Milakovich, "Creating a Total," 9.

29. McEachern, J. Edward, and Duncan Neuhauser. "The Continuous Improvement of Quality at the Hospital Corporation of America." *Health Matrix* 7 (Fall 1989): 7; Postal, Susan Nelson. "Using the Deming Quality Improvement Method to Manage Medical Records Department Product Lines." *Topics in Health Records Management* 10 (June 1990): 34.

30. American Hospital Association, *Quality Management,* 2; James, *Quality Management,* 1; Lynn, Monty L., and David P. Osborn. "Deming's Quality Principles: A Health Care Application." *Hospital & Health Services Administration* 36 (Spring 1991): 113.

31. Berwick, Donald M. "Managing Quality: The Next Five Years." *Quality Letter for Healthcare Leaders* 6,6 (July–August 1994): 3.
32. Boerstler, Heidi, Richard W. Foster, Edward J. O'Connor, James L. O'Brien, Stephen M. Shortell, James M. Carman, and Edward F.X. Hughes. "Implementation of Total Quality Management: Conventional Wisdom Versus Reality." *Hospital & Health Services Administration* 41 (Summer 1996): 143.
33. A good review, including barriers to CQI, can be found in Bigelow, Barbara, and Margarete Arndt. "Total Quality Management: Field of Dreams?" *Health Care Management Review* 20 (Fall 1995): 15–25; and Gustafson, David H., and Ann Schoofs Hundt. "Findings of Innovation Research Applied to Quality Management Principles for Health Care." *Health Care Management Review* 20 (Spring 1995): 16–33.
34. Lynn and Osborn, "Deming's Quality Principles."
35. Green, Deborah K. "Implementing a Corporate Quality Management Program: The AMI Experience." *Topics in Health Records Management* 10 (March 1990): 23–31; Postal, "Using the Deming"; McEachern and Neuhauser, "The Continuous Improvement"; Sahney and Warden, "The Quest for Quality"; Walton, Mary. *Deming Management at Work.* New York: Putnam, 1990.
36. Re and Krousel-Wood, "How to Use."
37. James, Brent C. "TQM and Clinical Medicine." *Frontiers of Health Services Management* 7 (Summer 1991): 42–46.
38. Laffel and Blumenthal, "The Case for Using."
39. Cascade, Philip N. "Quality Improvement in Diagnostic Radiology." *American Journal of Radiology* 154 (May 1990): 1117–1120.
40. Postal, "Using the Deming."
41. Peterson, Charles D. "Quality Improvement in Pharmacy: A Prescription for Change." *Quality Review Bulletin* 16 (March 1990): 106–108.
42. Chan, Yee-Ching Lilian, and Shih-Jen Kathy Ho. "Continuous Quality Improvement: A Survey of American and Canadian Healthcare Executives." *Hospital & Health Services Administration* 42 (Winter 1997): 529–534.
43. James, *Quality Management.*
44. Casalou, "Total Quality Management," 138.
45. O'Leary, Dennis S. "CQI—A Step Beyond QA." *Joint Commission Perspectives* 10 (March/April 1990): 2.
46. President of the Joint Commission, cited in Patterson, Pat. "JCAHO Shifts Its Emphasis to QI—Quality Improvement." *OR Manager* 6 (May 1990): 1.
47. Everett, Michael, and Brent C. James. "Continuous Quality Improvement in Healthcare: A Natural Fit." *Journal for Quality and Participation* (January/February 1991): 10.
48. Crosby, *Let's Talk Quality,* 63.
49. See also Berwick, Donald M., A. Blanton Godfrey, and Jane Roessner. *Curing Health Care: New Strategies for Quality Improvement,* 32–43. San Francisco: Jossey-Bass, 1990.
50. Darr, Kurt. "Applying the Deming Method in Hospitals: Part 1." *Hospital Topics* 67 (November/December 1989): 4.
51. Milakovich, "Creating a Total," 12.
52. Kaluzny, Arnold D., Curtis P. McLaughlin, and B. Jon Jaeger. "TQM as a Managerial Innovation: Research Issues and Implications." *Health Services Management Research* 6 (May 1993): 79.
53. Deming, *Out of the Crisis,* 3; Walton, Mary. *The Deming Management Method,* 25. New York: Perigee Books, 1986.
54. National Security and International Affairs Division, General Accounting Office. *Management Practices: U.S. Companies Improve Performance* (GA Report NSIAD-91-190), 15. Washington, DC: General Accounting Office, February 14, 1994.
55. Reimann, Curt W. "Malcolm Baldrige National Quality Award Criteria." In *Total Quality Management,* edited by Mara Minerva Melum and Marie Kuchuris Sinioris, 282. Chicago: American Hospital Publishing, 1992.
56. National Security and International Affairs Division, General Accounting Office, *Management Practices,* 8–9; Jennings, Kenneth, and Fred Westfall. "A Survey-Based Benchmarking Approach for Health

Care Using the Baldrige Quality Criteria." *Joint Commission Journal on Quality Improvement* 20 (September 1994): 502.

57. Lowe, Ted A., and Joseph M. Mazzeo. "Crosby, Deming, Juran: Three Preachers, One Religion." *Quality* 25 (September 1986): 22–25; Sahney and Warden, "The Quest for Quality," 4–7.
58. Lowe and Mazzeo, "Crosby, Deming, Juran," 22.
59. Darr, Kurt. "Eulogy to the Master: W. Edwards Deming." *Hospital Topics* 72 (Winter 1994): 4.
60. Sahney and Warden, "The Quest for Quality," 4–5.
61. Deming, "Improvement of Quality"; Deming, *Quality, Productivity*; Deming, "Transformation of Western"; Deming, *Out of the Crisis.*
62. Darr, "Applying the Deming Method (Part 1)"; Darr, Kurt. "Applying the Deming Method in Hospitals: Part 2." *Hospital Topics* 68 (Winter 1990): 4–6; Gabor, Andrea. *The Man Who Discovered Quality: How W. Edwards Deming Brought the Quality Revolution to America—The Stories of Ford, Xerox, and GM.* New York: Random House, 1990; Gitlow, Howard S., and Shelly J. Gitlow. *The Deming Guide to Quality and Competitive Position.* Englewood Cliffs, NJ: Prentice-Hall, 1987; Neuhauser, Duncan. "The Quality of Medical Care and the 14 Points of Edwards Deming." *Health Matrix* 6 (Summer 1986): 7–10; Scherkenbach, William W. *The Deming Route to Quality and Productivity.* Washington, DC: CEEP Press, 1986; Walton, *The Deming Management Method*
63. Deming, *Out of the Crisis,* 199–203.
64. Darr, "Applying the Deming Method (Part 1)," 4.
65. Deming's 14 points (in italics) are drawn from Deming, *Out of the Crisis,* 22–24.
66. Deming, *Out of the Crisis,* 200.
67. Deming, *Out of the Crisis,* 201.
68. Deming, *Out of the Crisis,* 202.
69. Deming, *Out of the Crisis,* 202.
70. Deming, *Out of the Crisis,* 202.
71. Deming, *Out of the Crisis,* 203.
72. Deming, "Improvement of Quality," 22.
73. Darr, "Applying the Deming Method (Part 1)," 5.
74. Juran Institute, personal communication, January 1999.
75. Juran, *Managerial Breakthrough*; Juran, "Quality Trilogy"; Juran, *Juran on Planning*; Juran, *Juran on Leadership,* 361.
76. Sahney and Warden, "The Quest for Quality," 6–7.
77. From Juran, Joseph M. *Juran on Leadership for Quality,* 20–21. New York: The Free Press, 1989; reprinted by permission.
78. Juran, *Juran on Planning,* 1.
79. From Juran, Joseph M. *Juran on Leadership for Quality,* 21–22. New York: The Free Press, 1989; reprinted by permission.
80. Juran, *Managerial Breakthrough,* 7.
81. Crosby, *Quality Is Free,* 1.
82. Crosby, *Let's Talk Quality,* 104.
83. Sahney and Warden, "The Quest for Quality," 6.
84. The industrial concept of zero defects means conformance to standards or specifications. For example, size is allowed to vary by ±3 millimeters. "Zero defects" does not mean that the product is perfect, although "zero defects" has been used in industry as a slogan—an exhortation directed at workers. Deming opposes setting specifications except as general guides. He argues that efforts to seek perfection are thwarted if the goal is only to meet specifications. Point 10 expresses Deming's opposition to slogans. In his judgment, management has been unwilling to accept blame for poor processes and, instead, blamed the workers, an attitude that caused management to substitute slogans for process improvement. Deming believes slogans alone only cause worker anger and frustration.
85. Crosby, *Let's Talk Quality,* 9.
86. Crosby, *Quality Is Free,* 38–39.
87. Crosby, *Quality Is Free,* 132–138; Crosby, *Quality Without Tears,* 101–124; Crosby, *Let's Talk Quality,* 106–107. The quotation in Point 10 is from Crosby, *Quality Without Tears,* 117.

88. Crosby, *Quality Is Free,* 22.
89. Lowe and Mazzeo, "Crosby, Deming, Juran," 23.
90. Darr, "Applying the Deming Method (Part 2)," 4.
91. Darr, "Applying the Deming Method (Part 2)," 4.
92. James, *Quality Management,* iii.
93. Readers interested in HRET research projects can find information on the American Hospital Association website at *http://www.aha.org/hret/R_ehm.html.*
94. James, *Quality Management,* 26–28, 32.
95. Vonderembse, Mark A., and Gregory P. White. *Operations Management: Concepts, Methods, and Strategies,* 2nd ed., 723. St. Paul, MN: West Publishing, 1991.
96. Werner, John P. "Productivity and Quality Management." In *Productivity and Performance Management in Health Care Institutions,* edited by Mark D. McDougall, Richard P. Covert, and V. Brandon Melton, 110. Chicago: American Hospital Publishing, 1989.
97. Anderson, Craig, and Peggy A. Rivenburgh. "Benchmarking." In *Total Quality Management: The Health Care Pioneers,* edited by Mara Minerva Melum and Marie Kuchuris Sinioris, 326. Chicago: American Hospital Publishing, 1992.
98. Anderson and Rivenburgh, "Benchmarking," 226.
99. Schuler, Charles, Jesse Dunlap, and Katharine Schuler. *ISO 9000: Manufacturing, Software, and Service,* 6. Albany, NY: Delmar Publishers, 1996.
100. Tambolas, Stephen F. "ISO 9000: A Guide to World-Class Quality Standards." *Hospital Material Management Quarterly* 18 (February 1997): 63.
101. Evans, James R., and William M. Lindsay. *The Management and Control of Quality,* 4th ed., 528. Cincinnati, OH: South-Western Publishing, 1999.
102. Litsikas, Mary. "QS-9000 Scores High Among Suppliers." *Quality* 36 (October 1997): 24.
103. Keenan, Tim. "Cashing in on QS-9000." *Ward's Auto World* 33 (February 1997): 45.
104. Gupta, Praveen, and Dan Pongetti. "Are ISO/QS-9000 Certifications Worth the Time and Money?" *Quality Progress* 31 (October 1998): 19.
105. Evans and Lindsay, *The Management and Control,* 528.
106. Evans and Lindsay, *The Management and Control,* 533–534.
107. Mosard, Gil R. "A TQM Technical Skills Framework." *Journal of Management Science & Policy Analysis* 8 (Spring/Summer 1991): 242–244.
108. James, "Implementing Continuous Quality," 16.
109. Goldense, Robert A. "Attaining TQM Through Employee Involvement: Imperatives for Implementation." *Journal of Management Science & Policy Analysis* 8 (Spring/Summer 1991): 268.
110. Schermerhorn, John R., Jr. "Improving Health Care Productivity Through High-Performance Managerial Development." *Health Care Management Review* 12 (Fall 1987): 51.
111. Kazemek, Edward A., and Rosemary M. Charny. "Quality Enhancement Means Total Organizational Involvement." *Healthcare Financial Management* 45 (February 1991): 15; Kronenberg and Loeffler, "Quality Management Theory," 211–212.
112. Walton, *The Deming Management Method,* 99.
113. James, *Quality Management,* 27.
114. Eastaugh, Steven R. *Financing Health Care: Economics, Efficiency, and Equity,* 258. Dover, MA: Auburn House, 1987.
115. Fogarty, Donald W., Thomas R. Hoffmann, and Peter W. Stonebraker. *Production and Operations Management,* 18. Cincinnati, OH: South-Western Publishing, 1989.
116. Selbst, Paul L. "A More Total Approach to Productivity Improvement." *Hospital & Health Services Administration* 30 (July/August 1985): 86.
117. James, *Quality Management,* 7.
118. Shukla, Ramesh K. "Effect of an Admission Monitoring and Scheduling System on Productivity and Employee Satisfaction." *Hospital & Health Services Administration* 35 (Fall 1990): 430.
119. In ABC inventory analysis, items are classified into A, B, or C groups based on volume, criticalness, or dollar value. A is high; C is low. The A group should have highest priority.
120. Laliberty, Rene, and W.I. Christopher. *Enhancing Productivity in Health Care Facilities,* chap. 5. Owings Mills, MD: National Health Publishing, 1984.

121. Mosard, "A TQM Technical Skills," 237.

122. Anderson and Daigh, "Quality Mind-Set," 26.

123. Hammer, Michael. *Beyond Reengineering: How the Process-Centered Organization Is Changing Our Work and Our Lives,* 81–82. New York: HarperBusiness, 1996.

124. Kennedy, Maggie. "Reengineering in Healthcare." *Quality Letter for Healthcare Leaders* 6 (September 1994): 2–3.

125. Griffith, John R., Vinod K. Sahney, and Ruth A. Mohr. *Reengineering Health Care: Building on CQI,* 14. Ann Arbor, MI: Health Administration Press, 1995; Kaluzny, Arnold D., Thomas R. Konrad, and Curtis P. McLaughlin. "Organizational Strategies for Implementing Clinical Guidelines." *Journal on Quality Improvement* 21 (July 1995): 349.

126. Hammer, *Beyond Reengineering,* 80.

127. Hammer, *Beyond Reengineering,* 82.

128. Leatt, Peggy G., Ross Baker, Paul K. Halverson, and Catherine Aird. "Downsizing, Reengineering, and Restructuring: Long-Term Implications for Healthcare Organizations." *Frontiers of Health Services Management* 13 (June 1997): 17.

129. Hammer, Michael, and James Champy. *Reengineering the Corporation: A Manifesto for Business Revolution,* 32. New York: HarperBusiness, 1993.

130. Hammer, Michael. "Reengineering: The Hot New Management Tool." *Fortune* 130 (August 1993), 11.

131. Bergman, Rhonda. "Reengineering Health Care." *Hospitals & Health Networks* 68 (February 5, 1994): 30.

132. Hammer and Champy, *Reengineering the Corporation,* 33.

133. Hammer, Michael, and Steven A. Stanton. *The Reengineering Revolution: A Handbook,* 4. New York: HarperBusiness, 1995.

134. Johansson, Henry J., Patrick McHugh, A. John Pendlebury, and William A. Wheeler, III. *Business Process Reengineering: Breakpoint Strategies for Market Dominance,* 6. New York: John Wiley & Sons, 1993.

135. Hammer and Champy, *Reengineering the Corporation,* 35.

136. Leatt, Baker, Halverson, and Aird, "Downsizing, Reengineering," 5–6.

137. Hammer and Champy, *Reengineering the Corporation,* 49.

138. Hammer and Stanton, *The Reengineering Revolution,* 97.

139. Johansson, McHugh, Pendlebury, and Wheeler, *Business Process Reengineering,* 6.

140. Kaluzny, Konrad, and McLaughlin, "Organizing Strategies," 349; Leatt, Baker, Halverson, and Aird, "Downsizing, Reengineering," 17.

141. Johansson, McHugh, Pendlebury, and Wheeler, *Business Process Reengineering,* 15; Griffith, Sahney, and Mohr, *Reengineering Health Care,* 14.

142. Hammer and Stanton, *The Reengineering Revolution,* 56.

143. Hammer and Stanton, *The Reengineering Revolution,* 57.

144. Hammer and Champy, *Reengineering the Corporation,* 102.

145. Hammer and Champy, *Reengineering the Corporation,* 128–133.

146. Grayson, Mary. "Stuck on a Strategy: Interview with Michael Hammer." *Hospitals & Health Networks* 17 (October 5, 1997): 76.

147. Walston, Stephen L., and John R. Kimberly. "Reengineering Hospitals: Evidence from the Field." *Hospital & Health Services Administration* 42 (Summer 1997): 150.

148. Walston and Kimberly, "Reengineering Hospitals," 151.

149. Schweikhart, Sharon Bergman, and Vicki Smith-Daniels. "Reengineering the Work of Caregivers: Role Redefinition, Team Structures, and Organizational Redesign." *Hospital & Health Services Administration* 41 (Spring 1996): 22.

150. Walston and Kimberly, "Reengineering Hospitals," 151–152.

151. Walston and Kimberly, "Reengineering Hospitals," 151–152.

152. Arndt, Margarete, and Barbara Bigelow. "Reengineering: Déjà Vu All Over Again." *Health Care Management Review* 23 (Summer 1998): 63.

153. This section adapted from Rakich, Jonathon S. "Strategic Quality Planning." *Hospital Topics* 78(2) (Winter 2000).

154. Melum, Mara Minerva, and Casey Collett. *Breakthrough Leadership: Achieving Organizational Alignment Through Hoshin Planning,* 15. Chicago: American Hospital Publishing, 1995; Campbell, S. "Fo-

cusing and Aligning Hospitals Through Hoshin Planning." *Health Care Strategic Management* 15 (February 1997): 1.

155. Stonestreet, Jana S., and Suzanne S. Prevost. "A Focused Strategic Plan for Outcomes Evaluation." *Nursing Clinics of North America* 32 (September 1997): 616.

156. See O'Brien, James L., Stephen M. Shortell, Edward F.X. Hughes, Richard W. Foster, James M. Carman, Heidi Boerstler, and Edward J. O'Connor. "An Integrative Model for Organization-wide Quality Improvement: Lessons from the Field." *Quality Management in Health Care* 3,4 (1995), 21; Hyde, Rebecca S., and Joan M. Vermillion. "Driving Quality Through Hoshin Planning." *Joint Commission Journal on Quality Improvement* 22 (January 1996): 28; Horak, Bernard J. *Strategic Planning in Healthcare: Building a Quality-Based Plan Step by Step,* 2–4. New York: Quality Resources, 1997.

157. Melum and Collett, *Breakthrough Leadership,* 16.

158. Melum and Collett, *Breakthrough Leadership,* 16.

159. Demers, David M. "Tutorial: Implementing Hoshin Planning at the Vermont Academic Medical Center." *Quality Management in Health Care* 1 (Summer 1993): 64.

160. Melum and Collett, *Breakthrough Leadership,* 16.

161. Shortell, Stephen M., Daniel Z. Levin, James L. O'Brien, and Edward F.X. Hughes. "Assessing the Evidence on CQI: Is the Glass Half Empty or Half Full?" *Hospital & Health Services Administration* 40 (Spring 1995): 6.

162. Kennedy, Maggie. "Using Hoshin Planning in Total Quality Management: An Interview with Gerry Kaminski and Casey Collett." *Journal on Quality Improvement* 20 (October 1994): 577.

163. Melum and Collett, *Breakthrough Leadership,* 4.

164. Melum and Collett, *Breakthrough Leadership,* 17.

165. Griffith, John R. "Reengineering Health Care: Management Systems for Survivors." *Hospital & Health Services Administration* 39 (Winter 1994): 451.

166. Hyde and Vermillion, "Driving Quality," 30.

167. Plsek, Paul E. "Techniques for Managing Quality." *Hospital & Health Services Administration* 40 (Special CQI Issue, Spring 1995): 68–69.

168. Melum and Collett, *Breakthrough Leadership,* 21.

169. McLaughlin and Kaluzny, "Total Quality Management," 8.

170. Kibbe, David C., Arnold D. Kaluzny, and Curtis P. McLaughlin. "Integrating Guidelines with Continuous Quality Improvement: Doing the Right Thing the Right Way to Achieve the Right Goals." *Journal on Quality Improvement* 20 (April 1994): 181.

171. Bigelow and Arndt, "Total Quality Management," 21.

172. Weiner, Bryan J., Stephen M. Shortell, and Jeffrey Alexander. "Promoting Clinical Involvement in Hospital Quality Improvement Efforts: The Effects of Top Management, Board, and Physician Leadership." *Health Services Research* 32 (October 1997): 492.

173. James, Brent C. "Implementing Practice Guidelines Through Clinical Quality Improvement." *Frontiers of Health Services Management* 10 (November 1993): 4.

174. Coffey, Richard J., Janet S. Richards, Carl S. Remmert, Sarah S. LeRoy, Rhonda R. Schoville, and Phyllis J. Baldwin. "An Introduction to Critical Paths." *Quality Management in Health Care* 1 (Fall 1992): 46.

175. Weiner, Shortell, and Alexander, "Promoting Clinical Involvement," 492.

176. Gillies, Robin P., Stephen M. Shortell, and Gary J. Young. "Best Practices in Managing Organized Delivery Systems." *Hospital & Health Services Administration* 42 (Fall 1997): 303.

177. James, Brent C. "How Do You Involve Physicians in TQM?" *Journal for Quality and Participation* (January/February 1991): 43.

178. See also Kaluzny, Arnold D., Curtis P. McLaughlin, and David C. Kibbe. "Continuous Quality Improvement in the Clinical Setting: Enhancing Adoption." *Quality Management in Health Care* 1 (Fall 1992): 37–44; and Berwick, Donald M. "The Clinical Process and Quality Process." *Quality Management in Health Care* 1 (Fall 1992): 1–8, for ways to enhance physician involvement in QI.

179. James, "Implementing Practice Guidelines," 44.

180. Schumacher, "Organizing for Quality," 11.

181. Laffel and Blumenthal, "The Case for Using," 2870.

182. Lagoe, Ronald J., and Deborah L. Aspling. "Enlisting Physician Support for Practice Guidelines in Hospitals." *Health Care Management Review* 21 (Fall 1996): 61–67.

183. James, "How Do You Involve," 44.
184. Succi, Melissa J., Shou-Yih Lee, and Jeffrey A. Alexander. "Trust Between Managers and Physicians in Community Hospitals: The Effects of Power Over Hospital Decisions." *Journal of Healthcare Management* 43 (September/October 1998): 398.
185. James, "How Do You Involve," 44.
186. James, "How Do You Involve," 44.
187. James, "How Do You Involve," 47.
188. James, "How Do You Involve," 47.
189. Shortell, Stephen M., James L. O'Brien, Edward F.X. Hughes, James M. Carman, Richard W. Foster, Heidi Boerstler, and Edward J. O'Connor. "Assessing the Progress of TQM in U.S. Hospitals: Findings from Two Studies." *Quality Letter for Healthcare Leaders* 6 (April 1994): 15–16.
190. James, "Implementing Practice Guidelines," 7.
191. Carman, James M., Stephen M. Shortell, Richard W. Foster, Edward F.X. Hughes, Heidi Boerstler, James L. O'Brien, and Edward J. O'Connor. "Keys for Successful Implementation of Total Quality Management in Hospitals." *Health Care Management Review* 21 (Winter 1996): 58.
192. Shortell, O'Brien, Hughes, Carman, Foster, Boerstler, and O'Connor, "Assessing the Progress," 15.
193. Lagoe and Aspling, "Enlisting Physician Support," 61.
194. Shortell, O'Brien, Hughes, Carman, Foster, Boerstler, and O'Connor, "Assessing the Progress," 15.
195. Berwick, "The Clinical Process," 3.
196. Kaluzny, McLaughlin, and Kibbe, "Continuous Quality Improvement," 40.
197. Shortell, O'Brien, Hughes, Carman, Foster, Boerstler, and O'Connor, "Assessing the Progress," 16.
198. Shortell, O'Brien, Hughes, Carman, Foster, Boerstler, and O'Connor, "Assessing the Progress," 16; Carman, Shortell, Foster, Hughes, Boerstler, O'Brien, and O'Connor, "Keys for Successful," 50.
199. Sisk, Jane. "How Are Health Care Organizations Using Clinical Guidelines?" *Health Affairs* 17 (September/October 1998): 97.
200. Sisk, "How Are Health Care," 99–100.
201. Sisk, "How Are Health Care," 106.
202. Kaluzny, Arnold D., Curtis P. McLaughlin, and David C. Kibbe. "Quality Improvement: Beyond the Institution." *Hospital & Health Services Administration* 40 (Special CQI Issue, Spring 1995): 176.
203. Kaluzny, McLaughlin, and Kibbe, "Quality Improvement," 175.
204. Kaluzny, McLaughlin, and Kibbe, "Quality Improvement," 178–180.
205. Adapted from Kaluzny, McLaughlin, and Kibbe, "Quality Improvement," 181–185.
206. From the *Akron Beacon Journal,* July 12, 1991, C14; reprinted by permission of Ann Landers and Creators Syndicate, *The Chicago Tribune,* Chicago, IL.
207. From Vonderembse, Mark A., and Gregory P. White. *Operations Management: Concepts, Methods, and Strategies,* 2nd ed., 549–550. St. Paul, MN: West Publishing, 1991; reprinted by permission. Copyright © 1991 by West Publishing Company. All rights reserved.
208. From Reagan, Gaylord. "Total Quality Management (TQM) Inventory." In *The 1992 Annual: Developing Human Resources,* edited by J. William Pfeiffer, 149–162. San Diego, CA: Pfeiffer & Company, 1992; reprinted by permission. This instrument is based on information in Federal Quality Institute. *Federal Total Quality Management Handbook 2: Criteria and Scoring Guidelines for the President's Award for Quality and Productivity Improvement.* Washington, DC: Office of Personnel Management, 1990.
209. From Melum, Mara Minerva, and Marie Kuchuris Sinioris, Eds. *Total Quality Management: The Health Care Pioneers,* 5–6. Chicago: American Hospital Publishing, 1992; reprinted by permission. The term *continuous quality improvement (CQI)* may be substituted for total quality management (TQM).

SELECTED BIBLIOGRAPHY

American Hospital Association. *Quality Management: A Management Advisory,* 1–3. Chicago: American Hospital Association, 1990.

American Production and Inventory Control Society. *APICS Dictionary,* 9th ed. Falls Church, VA: American Production and Inventory Control Society, 1998.

Arndt, Margarete, and Barbara Bigelow. "The Implementation of Total Quality Management in Hospitals: How Good Is the Fit?" *Health Care Management Review* 20 (Fall 1995): 7–14.

Arndt, Margarete, and Barbara Bigelow. "Reengineering: Déjà Vu All Over Again." *Health Care Management Review* 23 (Summer 1998): 58–66.

Bergman, Rhonda. "Reengineering Health Care." *Hospitals & Health Networks* 68 (February 5, 1994): 28–36.

Berwick Donald M. "The Clinical Process and Quality Process." *Quality Management in Health Care* 1 (Fall 1992): 1–8.

Berwick, Donald M. "Managing Quality: The Next Five Years." *Quality Letter for Healthcare Leaders* 6,6 (July–August 1994): 1–7.

Berwick, Donald M., A. Blanton Godfrey, and Jane Roessner. *Curing Health Care: New Strategies for Quality Improvement.* San Francisco: Jossey-Bass, 1990.

Bigelow, Barbara, and Margarete Arndt. "Total Quality Management: Field of Dreams?" *Health Care Management Review* 20 (Fall 1995): 15–25.

Boerstler, Heidi, Richard W. Foster, Edward J. O'Connor, James L. O'Brien, Stephen M. Shortell, James M. Carman, and Edward F.X. Hughes. "Implementation of Total Quality Management: Conventional Wisdom Versus Reality." *Hospital & Health Services Administration* 41 (Summer 1996): 143–159.

Campbell, S. "Focusing and Aligning Hospitals Through Hoshin Planning." *Health Care Strategic Management* 15 (February 1997): 1, 18–23.

Carman, James M., Stephen M. Shortell, Richard W. Foster, Edward F.X. Hughes, Heidi Boerstler, James L. O'Brien, and Edward J. O'Connor. "Keys for Successful Implementation of Total Quality Management in Hospitals." *Health Care Management Review* 21 (Winter 1996): 48–60.

Chan, Yee-Ching Lilian, and Shih-Jen Kathy Ho. "Continuous Quality Improvement: A Survey of American and Canadian Healthcare Executives." *Hospital & Health Services Administration* 42 (Winter 1997): 525–544.

Crosby, Philip B. *Quality Is Free.* New York: McGraw-Hill, 1979.

Crosby, Philip B. *Quality without Tears.* New York: McGraw-Hill, 1984.

Crosby, Philip B. *Let's Talk Quality.* New York: McGraw-Hill, 1989.

Darr, Kurt. "Eulogy to the Master: W. Edwards Deming." *Hospital Topics* 72 (Winter 1994): 4–5.

Darr, Kurt, and Anjna Vij. "The Malcolm Baldrige National Quality Awards for Healthcare Organizations." *Hospital Topics* 73 (Summer 1995): 4–7.

Demers, David M. "Tutorial: Implementing Hoshin Planning at the Vermont Academic Medical Center." *Quality Management in Health Care* 1 (1993): 64–72.

Deming, W. Edwards. "Improvement of Quality and Productivity Through Action by Management." *National Productivity Review* 1 (Winter 1981–1982): 12–22.

Deming, W. Edwards. *Quality, Productivity, and Competitive Position.* Boston: Massachusetts Institute of Technology, 1982.

Deming, W. Edwards. "Transformation of Western Style Management." *Interfaces* 15 (May/June 1985): 6–11.

Deming, W. Edwards. *Out of the Crisis.* Boston: Massachusetts Institute of Technology, 1986.

Evans, James, and William M. Lindsay. *The Management and Control of Quality,* 4th ed. Cincinnati, OH: South-Western Publishing, 1999.

Everett, Michael, and Brent C. James. "Continuous Quality Improvement in Healthcare: A Natural Fit." *Journal for Quality and Participation* (January/February 1991): 10–14.

Gabor, Andrea. *The Man Who Discovered Quality: How W. Edwards Deming Brought the Quality Revolution to America—The Stories of Ford, Xerox, and GM.* New York: Random House, 1990.

Gillies, Robin P., Stephen M. Shortell, and Gary J. Young. "Best Practices in Managing Organized Delivery Systems." *Hospital & Health Services Administration* 42 (Fall 1997): 299–321.

Gitlow, Howard S., and Shelly J. Gitlow. *The Deming Guide to Quality and Competitive Position.* Englewood Cliffs, NJ: Prentice-Hall, 1987.

Goodman, Davis. "Earning the ISO 9000 Seal of Approval—Part II: Balancing the Costs and Benefits of Certification." *World Trade* 11 (September 1998): 46–49.

Grayson, Mary. "Stuck on a Strategy: Interview with Michael Hammer." *Hospitals & Health Networks* 17 (October 5, 1997): 74–76.

Griffith, John R. "Reengineering Health Care: Management Systems for Survivors." *Hospital & Health Services Administration* 39 (Winter 1994): 451–470.

Griffith, John R., Vinod K. Sahney, and Ruth A. Mohr. *Reengineering Health Care: Building on CQI.* Ann Arbor, MI.: Health Administration Press, 1995.

Gupta, Praveen, and Dan Pongetti. "Are ISO/QS-9000 Certifications Worth the Time and Money?" *Quality Progress* 31 (October 1998): 19–24.

Gustafson, David H., and Ann Schoofs Hundt. "Findings of Innovation Research Applied to Quality Management Principles for Health Care." *Health Care Management Review* 20 (Spring 1995): 16–33.

Hammer, Michael. *Beyond Reengineering: How the Process-Centered Organization Is Changing Our Work and Our Lives.* New York: HarperBusiness, 1996.

Hammer, Michael, and James Champy. *Reengineering the Corporation: A Manifesto for Business Revolution.* New York: HarperBusiness, 1993.

Hammer, Michael, and Steven A. Stanton. *The Reengineering Revolution: A Handbook.* New York: Harper-Business, 1995.

Horak, Bernard J. *Strategic Planning in Healthcare: Building a Quality-Based Plan Step by Step.* New York: Quality Resources, 1997.

Hyde, Rebecca S., and Joan M. Vermillion. "Driving Quality Through Hoshin Planning." *Joint Commission Journal on Quality Improvement* 22 (January 1996): 27–35.

James, Brent C. *Quality Management for Health Care Delivery—Quality Measurement and Management Project.* Chicago: Hospital Research and Educational Trust, 1989.

James, Brent C. "How Do You Involve Physicians in TQM?" *Journal for Quality and Participation* (January/February 1991): 42–47.

James, Brent C. "TQM and Clinical Medicine." *Frontiers of Health Services Management* 7 (Summer 1991): 42–46.

James, Brent C. "Implementing Practice Guidelines Through Clinical Quality Improvement." *Frontiers of Health Services Management* 10 (November 1993): 3–37.

Jennings, Kenneth, and Fred Westfall. "A Survey-Based Benchmarking Approach for Health Care Using the Baldrige Quality Criteria." *Joint Commission Journal on Quality Improvement* 20 (September 1994): 500–509.

Joiner, Brian L. *Fourth Generation Management: The New Business Consciousness.* New York: McGraw-Hill, 1994.

Juran, Joseph M. *Managerial Breakthrough: A New Concept of the Manager's Job.* New York: McGraw-Hill, 1964.

Juran, Joseph M. "The Quality Trilogy." *Quality Progress* 19 (August 1986): 19–24.

Juran, Joseph M. *Juran on Planning for Quality.* New York: The Free Press, 1988.

Juran, Joseph M. *Juran on Leadership for Quality.* New York: The Free Press, 1989.

Kaluzny, Arnold D., Thomas R. Konrad, and Curtis P. McLaughlin. "Organizational Strategies for Implementing Clinical Guidelines." *Journal on Quality Improvement* 21 (July 1995): 347–351.

Kaluzny, Arnold D., and Curtis P. McLaughlin. "Managing Transitions: Assuring the Adoption and Impact of TQM." *Quality Review Bulletin* 18,11 (November 1992): 380–384.

Kaluzny, Arnold D., Curtis P. McLaughlin, and B. Jon Jaeger. "TQM as a Managerial Innovation: Research Issues and Implications." *Health Services Management Research* 6 (May 1993): 78–88.

Kaluzny, Arnold D., Curtis P. McLaughlin, and David C. Kibbe. "Continuous Quality Improvement in the Clinical Setting: Enhancing Adoption." *Quality Management in Health Care* 1 (Fall 1992): 37–44.

Kaluzny, Arnold D., Curtis P. McLaughlin, and David C. Kibbe. "Quality Improvement: Beyond the Institution." *Hospital & Health Services Administration* 40 (Special CQI Issue, Spring 1995): 172–188.

Keenan, Tim. "Cashing in on QS-9000." *Ward's Auto World* 33 (February 1997): 45.

Kennedy, Maggie. "Reengineering in Healthcare." *Quality Letter for Healthcare Leaders* 6 (September 1994): 2–10.

Kennedy, Maggie. "Using Hoshin Planning in Total Quality Management: An Interview with Gerry Kaminski and Casey Collett." *Journal on Quality Improvement* 20 (October 1994): 577–581.

Kibbe, David C., Arnold D. Kaluzny, and Curtis P. McLaughlin. "Integrating Guidelines with Continuous Quality Improvement: Doing the Right Thing the Right Way to Achieve the Right Goals." *Journal on Quality Improvement* 20 (April 1994): 181–191.

Lagoe, Ronald J., and Deborah L. Aspling. "Enlisting Physician Support for Practice Guidelines in Hospitals." *Health Care Management Review* 21 (Fall 1996): 61–67.

Leatt, Peggy G., Ross Baker, Paul K. Halverson, and Catherine Aird. "Downsizing, Reengineering, and Restructuring: Long-Term Implications for Healthcare Organizations." *Frontiers of Health Services Management* 13 (June 1997): 3–37.

Litsikas, Mary. "QS-9000 Scores High Among Suppliers." *Quality* 36 (October 1997): 24–30.

Lowe, Ted A., and Joseph M. Mazzeo. "Crosby, Deming, Juran: Three Preachers, One Religion." *Quality* 25 (September 1986): 22–25.

Lynn, Monty L., and David P. Osborn. "Deming's Quality Principles: A Health Care Application." *Hospital & Health Care Administration* 36 (Spring 1991): 111–120.

McLaughlin, Curtis P., and Arnold D. Kaluzny. *Continuous Quality Improvement in Health Care: Theory, Implementation, and Applications.* Gaithersburg, MD: Aspen Publishers, 1994.

Melum, Mara Minerva, and Casey Collett. *Breakthrough Leadership: Achieving Organizational Alignment Through Hoshin Planning.* Chicago: American Hospital Publishing, 1995.

Melum, Mara Minerva, and Marie Kuchuris Sinioris, Eds. *Total Quality Management: The Health Care Pioneers.* Chicago: American Hospital Publishing, 1992.

Milakovich, Michael E. "Creating a Total Quality Health Care Environment." *Health Care Management Review* 16 (Spring 1991): 9–20.

National Security and International Affairs Division, General Accounting Office. *Management Practices: U.S. Companies Improve Performance* (GA Report NSIAD-91-190), 1–42. Washington, DC: General Accounting Office, February 14, 1994.

Neuhauser, Duncan. "The Quality of Medical Care and the 14 Points of Edwards Deming." *Health Matrix* 6 (Summer 1988): 7–10.

O'Brien, James L., Stephen M. Shortell, Edward F.X. Hughes, Richard W. Foster, James M. Carman, Heidi Boerstler, and Edward J. O'Connor. "An Integrative Model for Organization-wide Quality Improvement: Lessons from the Field." *Quality Management in Health Care* 3,4 (1995), 21.

Plsek, Paul E. "Techniques for Managing Quality." *Hospital & Health Services Administration* 40 (Special CQI Issue, Spring 1995): 50–79.

Re, Richard N., and Marie A. Krousel-Wood. "How to Use Continuous Quality Improvement Theory and Statistical Quality Control Tools in a Multispecialty Clinic." *Quality Review Bulletin* 16 (November 1990): 391–397.

Scherkenbach, William W. *The Deming Route to Quality and Productivity.* Washington, DC: Ceep Press, 1986.

Schuler, Charles, Jesse Dunlap, and Katharine Schuler. *ISO 9000: Manufacturing, Software and Service.* Albany, NY: Delmar Publishers, 1996.

Schweikhart, Sharon Bergman, and Vicki Smith-Daniels. "Reengineering the Work of Caregivers: Role Redefinition, Team Structures, and Organizational Redesign." *Hospital & Health Services Administration* 41 (Spring 1996): 19–35.

Shortell, Stephen M., James L. O'Brien, Edward F.X. Hughes, James M. Carman, Richard W. Foster, Heidi Boerstler, and Edward J. O'Connor. "Assessing the Progress of TQM in U.S. Hospitals: Findings from Two Studies." *Quality Letter for Healthcare Leaders* 6,3 (April 1994): 14–17.

Shortell, Stephen M., Daniel Z. Levin, James L. O'Brien, and Edward F.X. Hughes. "Assessing the Evidence on CQI: Is the Glass Half Empty or Half Full?" *Hospital & Health Services Administration* 40 (Spring 1995): 4–24.

Sisk, Jane. "How Are Health Care Organizations Using Clinical Guidelines?" *Health Affairs* 17 (September/October 1998): 91–109.

Stewart, Thomas A. "Reengineering: The Hot New Managing Tool." *Fortune* 128 (August 1993): 41–43, 48.

Stonestreet, Jana S., and Suzanne S. Prevost. "A Focused Strategic Plan for Outcomes Evaluation." *Nursing Clinics of North America* 32 (September 1997): 615–631.

Succi, Melissa J., Shou-Yih Lee, and Jeffrey A. Alexander. "Trust Between Managers and Physicians in Community Hospitals: The Effects of Power Over Hospital Decisions." *Journal of Healthcare Management* 43 (September/October 1998): 397–415.

Tambolas, Stephen F. "ISO 9000: A Guide to World-Class Quality Standards." *Hospital Material Management Quarterly* 18 (February 1997): 62–68.

Walston, Stephen L., and John R. Kimberly. "Reengineering Hospitals: Evidence from the Field." *Hospital & Health Services Administration* 42 (2) (Summer 1997): 143–163.

Walton, Mary. *Deming Management at Work.* New York: Putnam, 1990.

Weiner, Bryan J., Stephen M. Shortell, and Jeffrey Alexander. "Promoting Clinical Involvement in Hospital Quality Improvement Efforts: The Effects of Top Management, Board, and Physician Leadership." *Health Services Research* 32 (October 1997): 491–510.

10

Control and Resource Allocation

Management control . . . continuously gathers data on the quantity of services rendered, the quality and other characteristics of these services, and the resources consumed in their provision. Data from the sensor (management reports) are monitored against preestablished standards of quantity (production and service goals), quality of care, efficiency of the service process, and patient outcomes. When standards are not met, a control process is activated to initiate necessary changes and improvements.[1]

Chapter 9 focuses on quality—doing the right things right—and productivity improvement—providing the highest quality products and services at the lowest reasonable cost. This chapter focuses on control and resource allocation. How do we know whether a health services organization's (HSO's) or health system's (HS's) products and services are high quality? How do we determine whether processes that generate output are functioning effectively? How do we know whether input resources are of high quality, whether they are properly allocated, and whether the amount used is appropriate? How do we know whether organization objectives are being achieved? One word answers these questions—control. Those who understand HSOs/HSs know about quality control, infection control, performance improvement (PI), risk management (RM), cost control, utilization review, narcotics control, and credentials review. All are control or control-like activities.

In this chapter a control model that integrates continuous quality improvement (CQI) is presented. It compares actual results to standards and expectations and suggests appropriate action when deviation occurs. Because control is information dependent, management information systems (MIS) and clinical information systems (CIS) and their applications are discussed.

A special section addresses RM and PI, which are critical to control in HSOs/HSs. Other methods of control examined are budgeting, activity-based costing (ABC), and ratio analysis. The final section discusses analytical techniques relevant to resource allocation and use, such as volume analysis, capital budgeting, cost–benefit analysis, and simulation.

CONTROL AND PLANNING

Managers control to ensure that what is planned and expected actually occurs.[2] Organization results occur when HSO/HS managers integrate structure-tasks/technology-people components and allocate and use input resources. As the opening quote suggests, control is information dependent; that information is conveyed to a sensor unit—managers, who continuously monitor inputs, process, and outputs to ensure that individual work results are desirable and organization objectives are accomplished. As indicated by the management process model in Figure 1.7, managers use control to ensure that actual and desired outputs are consistent, work and conversion processes are effective, and resource consumption is appropriate.

Chapter 1 describes the controlling function of management as gathering information about and monitoring activities and performance, comparing actual results with expected results, and, when appropriate, intervening to take corrective action by changing inputs or processes. Control is also the means "by which managers assure that the organization is reaching its objectives and carrying out associated plans in an effective and efficient manner."[3] Control and planning are closely linked; the standards and desired results used in control are derived from the HSO's/HS's strategic and operational plans.

MONITORING (CONTROL) AND INTERVENTION POINTS

Control systems are information based. Figure 10.1 shows a generic control system that identifies monitoring (control) and intervention points. In the process of control, information is collected at three monitoring points: input utilization, functioning of conversion processes, and outputs. If results at these three monitoring points are inconsistent with expectations or standards, then intervention and change can occur at the input [A] or process [B] points or both.

Output Control

The best known type of control is that exercised over output. It is often called feedback control[4] and is retrospective—after the fact. Feedback in HSOs/HSs focuses on all levels of quantitative and qualitative output and ranges from individual and departmental to overall organizational results. Throughout, standards and expectations denote desired results, which usually are expressed numerically. Examples at the individual and departmental levels include individual job performance

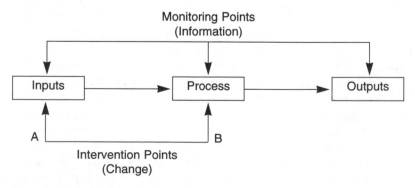

Figure 10.1.   Generic control system.

and departmental measures such as number or units of output (e.g., laboratory tests, radiography, surgical procedures, meals served, patients admitted, drug orders filled, pounds of laundry processed), as well as quality dimensions of outputs such as accuracy, timeliness, and customer satisfaction. At the organizational level, examples are average length of stay, occupancy rate, quality of care, range of services, stakeholder satisfaction, financial integrity, and market share. Output standards and expectations are derived from and reflect unit/departmental subobjectives and overall organization objectives.

Process Control

Converting inputs to outputs requires processes. The quality of outputs is determined by the efficacy and efficiency of process, the amount and appropriateness of inputs, or both. In controlling, attention usually is directed at outputs (quantity and quality of service), but it is equally important to monitor the myriad integrative conversion processes whose total effort generates outputs. The foundation principle of CQI is that processes can be improved. For this to occur there must be a monitoring system to identify how well they are functioning. Examples of integrative conversion processes in HSOs/HSs include

- Work systems such as patient admitting and discharge, transportation, materials handling and distribution, direct patient care, and ancillary services
- Specific job design and staff, and machine, technology, and facility interrelationships
- Financial record keeping and information collection, storage, retrieval, and dissemination systems
- Decision and resource allocation and planning processes
- Managerial methods, practices, and styles along with organizational structuring, coordination, and communication methods and flows

Because process (in combination with inputs) yields outputs, concurrent process control is important. Also referred to as screening control,[5] it "focuses on activities that occur as inputs are being transformed to outputs."[6] Furthermore, process is one of two points at which intervention can occur if outputs are inconsistent with expectations (see Point B in Figure 10.1). Standards and expectations are easier to develop for processes that deal with tangibles, are consistent, and are simple to document and understand. It is more difficult when a process is less tangible. For example, what are the effects on conversion (and, ultimately, on output) of different managerial methods of problem solving and decision making, leadership and supervisory styles, approach to motivation, or methods of communication? Perhaps this is one reason why control historically has focused more on outputs generated and inputs consumed and less on process. One inherent element of CQI is that control is directed at process.

Input Control

As stated in the opening quotation, control must focus on "resources consumed" in creating outputs. Virtually all HSOs/HSs exercise control over inputs by developing standards and expectations about resource consumption. Examples include nursing hours per patient day, materials and supplies consumed, and the ratio of personnel to beds. Often called feedforward control, "it is an approach to control that uses inputs to a system of organizational activities as a means of controlling the accomplishment of organizational objectives [outputs]."[7] The philosophy of CQI suggests choosing the best inputs before conversion to avoid problems. In HSOs/HSs one way to control the quality of human resources inputs is credentialing and licensure, which help ensure that clinical and other staff possess certain levels of training and skills. Input control alone, however, is no substitute for process and output control.

CONTROL MODEL

Thus far, control has been described as a process by which information is gathered about results and performance at the monitoring (control) points of inputs, process, and outputs. Comparing actual results with preestablished standards and expectations, appraising comparisons, and making interventions and changes at the inputs, the process points, or both as needed are the remaining components of control. Figure 10.2 incorporates these components in an expanded control process model and shows that actual results are measured and compared with standards and expectations. Depending on results, the control process follows one of four loops, each of which indicates whether intervention and change are necessary.

In Control Loop

In Figure 10.2 the "in control loop" is the simplest. When an appraisal of results, based on information at the three monitoring points—inputs, process, and outputs, indicates that they meet standards and expectations, no intervention or change is required. Whatever is being monitored is judged to be in control; activity continues.

Acceptance Control Loop

When appraisal based on information at the three monitoring points indicates that actual results and performance do not meet standards and expectations, managers investigate to determine the cause

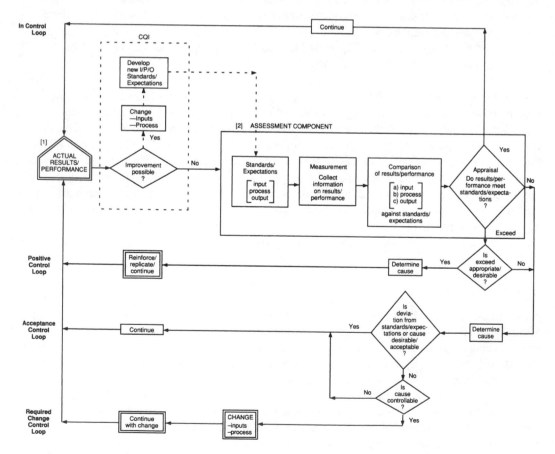

Figure 10.2.   Expanded control model.

of the deviation. If the deviation is desirable or acceptable, or its cause is uncontrollable, then activities continue with no intervention or change. For example, actual overtime, which is higher-than-budgeted overtime (standard), may be acceptable if the census is higher than expected.

If the deviation is undesirable and the cause is uncontrollable, then actual results and performance must be accepted. For example, a decrease in the ratio of registered nurse hours per patient to below the desired standard but above the minimum needed for good patient care may result from a shortage of registered nurses—an inadequate pool of this resource in the service area.

Required Change Control Loop

When information indicates that deviation is unacceptable and the cause is controllable, intervention should occur. For example, if average length of stay is substantially above standard, intervention and change are required. This may occur if physicians (input point) do not discharge patients in a timely manner or if work systems (process point) are ineffective and there are delays in administering and reporting tests. Another example is higher-than-normal personnel turnover, which may result from a poor organizational climate, inadequacy of the compensation system, or poor supervision. Here, too, intervention and change at the input or process points are required.

Positive Control Loop

There is a general perception that control has a negative focus; however, this is not always the case. For example, if performance is better than standards, then the cause should be identified, reinforced, frozen in place, and, if possible, replicated elsewhere. A department consistently under budget with superior individual work results and high quality and customer satisfaction may be the result of factors such as effective managerial style, positive employee attitude and commitment, and well-designed processes. Necessarily control is concerned with maintaining performance at a certain level—identifying negative deviation; however, improvement control also recognizes and emphasizes the positive.

There are instances in which actual performance exceeds (is better than) standards, but this is undesirable. For example, it may seem desirable that nursing service hours per patient are below budget (i.e., standard), but evaluation may show this to be unacceptable if quality of care is diminished. Physical plant maintenance expenditures may be below budget, yet this may be undesirable if preventive maintenance is postponed. If actual results and performance are better than standards and expectations but are not desirable or appropriate, then the cause should be determined and either the "acceptance" or "required change" control loops should be used in the control process.

LEVELS OF CONTROL

There are three basic levels of control: strategic, operational, and functional. Strategic control focuses on attaining overall organization objectives, including financial performance of the HSO/HS. Senior-level managers monitor to determine whether implemented strategies are successfully accomplishing objectives and whether the organization's external environment requires a reevaluation of those strategies. Part V of the strategic planning model in Figure 8.5 depicts strategic control. Operational control focuses on monitoring operational plans and day-to-day unit or department activities. Control at this level is largely the responsibility of middle- and first-level managers who are concerned with their unit or department work schedules, budgets, and use of associated resources. Finally, functional control focuses on specific logically grouped functional areas such as clinical services, finance, IS, and marketing. Senior functional-area managers, as well as middle- and first-level managers, have responsibility for control in these areas.[8]

CONTROL AND CQI

In HSOs/HSs meeting standards is never the end of the control process. The philosophy of CQI uses continuous inquiry to improve processes and inputs so that outputs can be improved. The control model in Figure 10.2 shows use of CQI in the box outlined by dashes. If no improvement of process or inputs is possible, the control loop flows from actual results/performance [1] through to the assessment component [2]. If improvement is possible, change is made to inputs, process, or both and new standards and expectations are developed to replace those used previously in the assessment component [2].

CONTROL AND PROBLEM SOLVING

As presented in Chapter 7 problem solving depends on information that is generated by control. The four conditions that initiate problem solving are deviation, opportunity/threat, crisis, and improvement. The most common is deviation, which occurs when individual and organizational work results are found to be inconsistent with those that are desired. Comparison of actual results with prospective standards for inputs, processes, or outputs shows deviation. Problem solving under the condition of deviation is triggered by monitoring and evaluation during control. Problem solving under the condition of improvement improves processes or inputs to affect outputs positively. Information that is obtained from control is requisite to process investigation and improvement activities.

CONTROL CONSIDERATIONS

Several managerial and design considerations are important when control systems are established and maintained.

Managerial Considerations

Managerial questions to be answered when a control system is established or modified are

- *Where is control focused?* Control may focus on input (review of resource use), process or conversion (review of efficiency of work systems in converting inputs to outputs), or output (concern for overall organizational results).
- *What types of measures are used for standards and monitoring results?* Measures used in control depend on focus, quantifiability of results, and the extent to which measures convey accurate, usable, and meaningful information.
- *Who has the authority to establish standards?* A principle of control is that those whose activities are monitored have input but not sole authority to establish standards and monitor results. Checks and balances are universal in accounting systems; for example, cashiers who handle cash do no final audits or reconciliations. Similarly, utilization review is not performed by those providing the services.
- *How flexible should standards be?* Blind and inflexible use of numerical measures for control purposes can cause distortions. Changes and unforeseen circumstances require that judgment, common sense, and flexibility be used in control systems.
- *Who has access to control system information?* Controlling requires dissemination of information, but certain information is appropriately restricted to certain levels of management or specific managers.
- *Who is responsible for intervention?* Just as organizations have a defined authority-responsibility hierarchy, managerial consideration of control includes who is responsible and who intervenes when appropriate.

Design Considerations

There are situations in which control systems cause unintended and undesirable consequences, cost more than they are worth, measure the wrong things, or focus on the wrong points. Design of control systems should include the following considerations to decrease the occurrence of such dysfunctional outcomes:

- *When possible, control should be prospective.* Control cannot always be forward looking or predictive. Usually, information flows or organizational constraints limit it to being concurrent or retrospective. If available, however, feedforward control provides information to managers that enables them to anticipate deviation and makes them more effective.
- *Control should be organizationally realistic and understandable to users.* Control systems need to be in harmony with the organization, realistically fit, and be understandable. A system that creates barriers or artificial constraints is dysfunctional. For example, control of inventories and supplies is best centralized in materials management. Centralizing access to and control of photocopiers in one office may be unrealistic.
- *Control should be accurate, timely, and reliable.* In addition, control systems, standards and measurements need to be accurate and reliable. Making corrections based on inaccurate or unreliable information defeats the purpose of control, as does using obsolete data that do not reflect the current situation.
- *Control should be significant, should have economic benefit, or both.* "Significant" refers to the importance of what is controlled. "Economic benefit" refers to the cost of control relative to the value of what is controlled. There is little economic benefit to disposal (destruction) control of used syringes. It is beneficial, however, for such reasons as preventing use by drug addicts and protecting those who handle medical waste. Narcotics control has significant clinical and economic benefits and is required by law. Conversely, an elaborate control system for the use of disposable surgical clothing may have low economic benefit; the cost of control exceeds the benefit. Because it is nearly impossible to control every input, process, or output, managers need to focus on what is important.
- *Control should be information appropriate.* Too much or too little information is undesirable. Important indicators are lost in the avalanche of paper that is caused by excessive information. Too little information denies managers the ability to focus on critical elements. Control systems should be designed to give managers sufficient and discriminating information at the right time and in a usable format.

INFORMATION SYSTEMS AND CONTROL

HSO/HS managers depend on information. Effective planning, problem solving, and control occur only when managers receive appropriate, accurate, and timely information in the proper format. As observed by Enthoven and Vorhaus, "the organization that can successfully and efficiently manage information will produce better-quality health care because it will be able to measure, monitor, and improve the care it delivers."[9] In addition to improved access to information, IS can facilitate communication among providers and team members, contribute to reduced costs, and enhance the HSO's/HS's competitive position.[10]

Management information systems is a generic term that refers to computer IS that gather, format, process, store, and report data to managers and make them retrievable by managers so that they can plan, execute, and control the organization's activities. Most traditional IS are applications driven; information is retrieved from discrete files that are created for specific purposes by organization units. In their design, users specify the type and extent of information desired. Historically,

MIS design was performed by in-house systems analysts and programmers. However, there has been an increasing trend to purchase application programs from commercial vendors.[11]

IS in HSOs/HSs generally fall into two broad categories. First, administrative and financial systems provide information supporting administrative operations and managerial planning, resource allocation, and control activities. Second, clinical and medical systems provide information to support patient care activities.[12] A survey of 2,400 senior-level hospital managers rated these as the two most important categories. Others are cost accounting, resource utilization and productivity analysis, and market intelligence.[13] Table 10.1 presents associated IS applications by core functions for a managed care organization.

The person responsible for managing a HSO's/HS's IS is the chief information officer (CIO), who is a senior-level manager. The qualities that are important in a CIO include 1) technical competence, including managing the internal system and awareness of technology used by competitors and new developments; 2) compatibility with organization objectives, stage of evolution of information technology, and clientele; 3) business perspective, to realize information's importance in a competitive market and the technology's high cost; and 4) leadership, especially as a change agent, team builder, and communicator.[14]

Information Systems: LANs, WANs, and CHINs

The sophistication of information systems ranges from applications reporting systems to database management systems to decision support systems. Applications reporting is the most familiar to HSO/HS managers and consists of tailored reports about organizational operations or areas of activity such as payroll, inventory, budgets, admission, census, and scheduling.

Rapid technological advances in computer hardware and software have made database IS increasingly common in HSOs/HSs. Data from throughout the organization are integrated and consolidated in a single database or multiple databases that are accessible by authorized users rather than segregated for specific applications reporting. These systems are often inquiry based.

Local-area networks (LANs) permit communication and information transmission between computers as well as peripheral equipment within an organization.[15] Wide-area networks (WANs) allow long-distance input and inquiry information access. WANs enable far-flung operating units to "interchange information, create computer-based patient records, and develop integrated outcome measures and statistics."[16] Chapter 6 examines a further evolution of IS in community health information networks (CHINs), which link together multiple parties such as the HSO/HS provider, payers, physicians at remote sites, and pharmacies. It is reported that there are more than 500 CHINs in operation nationwide.[17] Figure 6.7 depicts health care data links.

An extension of IS applications is management decision support systems (MDSS), sometimes called expert systems, which are model based and have statistical and simulation capabilities. They are interactive, which permits managers to use online terminals to ask "what if" questions.[18] A financial example is "What would be the effect on profit margin of a 20% increase in Medicare patients?" Another is implications for resource allocation and utilization through a bed assignment model.[19] The applications of decision support systems are not restricted to administration; clinical applications are evolving in the form of clinical decision support systems (CDSS).[20]

Clinical–Patient Care IS and Electronic Medical Records

Clinical, patient care–type IS are widely used in areas such as the laboratory and the pharmacy and in department management in radiology, physical therapy, respiratory therapy, nursing service, critical care units, and emergency medicine.[21] Clinical IS can improve quality and achieve control by comparing clinical outcomes with historical results[22] and can be used to profile physician practices. In addition, electronic medical records (EMRs) that can be accessed within the HSO/HS or by

TABLE 10.1.   MANAGED CARE ORGANIZATION FUNCTIONS AND ASSOCIATED INFORMATION REQUIREMENTS

Core functions	Examples of applications
Financial monitoring	Balance sheets Income statements Financial statements General accounting Cost accounting Premium billing and accounts receivable Payment tracking for contracts, subcontracts
Preparation of standard analytical reports and decision models	Performance statistics Utilization management Provider reporting: inpatient and outpatient Referral patterns Inpatient and outpatient out-of-network use Case-mix analysis Provider profiling Actuarial analysis
Management control and reporting	Membership analysis Eligibility/verifications tracking Utilization rates by groups, age, gender Quality indicators Financial reporting Regulatory reporting Budgeting models Forecasting models Contract modeling and projections
Claims payment and prospective/ capitation payment processing	Capitation payments Claims payment, network and out-of-network Claims adjudication Encounter statistics Claims grouping by episodes of care
Management of multiple lines of business	Government accounts (Medicare, Medicaid, etc.) Individual coverage Group billing, benefits management, eligibility
Marketing and sales support	Enrollment and disenrollment trends Geographic distribution of members and providers Contract negotiation and management Rate management/actuarial services Account management and analysis Forecasting models Provider databases and credentials
Profitability	Per member per month costs and premiums Medical loss ratios
Member/customer services	Customer service inquiry Internet access to MCO Member health/wellness education and promotion Epidemiological analysis
Employer information needs	HEDIS reporting Outcomes measurement Employer group enrollment tracking and reporting Utilization history and claims experience of covered population

From Austin, Charles J., and Stuart B. Boxerman. *Information Systems for Health Services Administration*, 5th ed., pp. 350–351. Chicago: AUPHA/Health Administration Press, 1998; reprinted by permission.

physicians from off-site locations represent a major technological advance. (Chapter 6 provides additional information concerning the advantages and disadvantages of EMRs.)

With EMRs, patients' medical records can be accessed to obtain chart abstracting reports, pharmacy orders, nursing progress reports, and laboratory reports.[23] CDSS, similar to MDSS, represent a leap in technology application. CDSS "generally consist of static and dynamic modeling routines, driven by normative data bases and vast stores of 'automated' clinical knowledge; their outputs consist of quantitative comparisons of clinical outcomes associated with alternative medical decisions."[24]

A contemporary extension of the information explosion is *medical informatics,* a generic term that is used to describe the application of computing and communication technology in health services delivery. One definition of medical informatics is "the science of storage, retrieval, and optimal use of biomedical information for problem solving and medical decision making."[25] It also incorporates management and health network applications such as WANs and CHINs.

IS Issues

The advances in IS technology during the 1990s were profound, making major contributions to enhanced resource utilization through better managerial control and improved-quality patient care outcomes through better clinical decision making. However, the advances have not occurred without cost. Hardware and software are expensive, as are IS support staff. Relative to patient care and clinical IS use, many issues have been raised. For example, applications such as CDSS typically build on IS originally designed for administrative and claims/transactions processing,[26] and thus may be working from contaminated databases or may lack standardization when different databases are accessed. Incompatible system architectures create problems relative to compatibility. As observed by Austin and colleagues, "Patient and financial tracking across the network requires integrated information systems that operate on multiple vendor hardware and software. Standardization of databases and coding mechanisms are imperative."[27]

Additional issues for CHINs are that some community HSOs/HSs may not want to share information with competitors,[28] and there can be encounter and episode information fragmentation among organizations. That is, "patient information over time and geographical space as patients move through a fragmented treatment system"[29] is likely to be incomplete. Telemedicine, the delivery of patient care in remote areas through IS and telecommunications technology, raises potential issues of regulation and licensure. For example, there are legal/licensure implications if a multistate managed care organization had a physician network in which consultation and coordination of care were provided by a physician in one state to a patient in another state. EMRs, whether or not linked to CHINs, raise issues of unauthorized access, patient privacy (e.g., relative to genetic testing results), backup, and compliance with licensure and regulatory requirements.[30] Uses and issues regarding IS are discussed in Chapter 6; legal issues are covered in Chapter 14.

IS Uses

Given that quality and control in HSOs/HSs depend on information, Austin delineates a number of areas in which IS can support managers and clinicians:

> *Medical Quality Assurance.* Clinical information abstracted from patient medical records provides the basic material utilized by health professionals in peer review systems to assess diagnostic and treatment practices. . . . One goal of a computerized information system is to make such data readily accessible and retrievable from a central patient data file for purposes of quality assessment and initiation of necessary corrective action.
>
> *Cost Control and Productivity Enhancement.* Health services organizations are under increasing pressure to contain increases in the cost of services. Computerized information systems offer

the potential for providing cost analyses and productivity reports for use by management and board members in improving the efficiency of operation. Such systems require the ability to integrate clinical and financial information systems.

Utilization Analysis and Demand Estimation. A complete information system should provide current and historical data on utilization of health services. Such data systems serve to assist in current analysis of the efficiency of utilization of resources and also provide a basis for predicting future demand for services.

Program Planning and Evaluation. Information obtained for the above purposes—quality assurance [performance improvement, PI], cost control, utilization analysis, and demand estimation—serves as the basic input for management decisions related to evaluation of present programs and services. When combined with projections about future changes in the demographic characteristics of the service population, the information system can provide an important resource for planning future programs and services.[31]

From a control perspective, IS should provide information that meets the specific needs of managers so that they can monitor activities at the input, process, and/or output points; provide each level of management with specific reports it before in its area of responsibility that contain accurate, relevant, and timely information to improve decisions on control (intervention or change); and extract and pinpoint critical and high-priority items requiring management's analysis and, perhaps, intervention.

RM AND QUALITY IMPROVEMENT

Historically, safety programs and efforts to measure the quality of clinical services were separate control activities that usually were limited to acute care hospitals. In the early 1970s safety programs began evolving into the broader concept of RM and included proactively managing risk.

> *[R]isk management functions encompass activities in health [services] organizations that are intended to conserve financial resources from loss. Those functions include a broad range of administrative activities intended to reduce losses associated with patient, employee, or visitor injuries; property loss or damages; and other sources of potential organizational liability.[32]*

A comprehensive RM program includes identifying, controlling, and financing risks of all types. Inherent in RM is preventing risk and minimizing the effect of untoward events, should they occur. RM programs are common in HSOs/HSs and are required in a number of states.[33]

Both internal and external factors caused these changes. Internally, HSO/HS managers increasingly recognized their ethical duty to provide a safe environment for patients, staff, and visitors, and to provide high-quality clinical services. External stimuli included 1) an increasingly litigious society and court decisions that put greater legal liability on the HSO/HS; 2) state laws mandating RM programs, as indicated above; 3) federal laws such as the Occupational Safety and Health Act of 1970 (PL 91-596),[34] which mandated the study of hazards in acute care hospitals so that national standards could be set; and 4) the requirements of private organizations such as the Joint Commission on Accreditation of Healthcare Organizations (Joint Commission) and public bodies such as the Department of Health and Human Services and their state counterparts, which increasingly emphasized the quality of services and managing risk. Better programs followed as it became apparent that HSOs/HSs had to effectively manage the economic costs of all types of risk.

In the 1990s improving clinical quality (quality assessment and improvement, QA/I) for patients was an important part of this expanded concept of RM. In 1992 the Joint Commission moved away from the terms and methodology of quality assurance and mandated QA/I as a better, more proactive and effective focus to evaluate and improve quality. Those standards linked but did not integrate QA/I and RM activities. The 1998 Joint Commission *Comprehensive Accreditation Man-*

ual for Hospitals, Refreshed Core, continued this evolution, and RM and quality improvement (QI) are now integrated. Performance improvement (PI) standard PI.3.3 includes the following: "Data on important process and outcomes are also collected from . . . risk management activities; and quality control activities." The Joint Commission's intent is that

> *When integrated with other performance-improvement data, autopsies, risk-management activities, and quality control activities can provide important information for systematic, hospital wide improvement—but only if data collection is guided by clear assessment criteria, and data is [sic] shared with those responsible for improvement of hospital performance. . . . Cooperation [of other departments, disciplines, and individuals] is especially important for risk-management functions, which have operational links to the clinical aspects of patient care, patient safety, and performance improvement.[35]*

Integrating QI and RM is prudent and enhances the effectiveness of both. HSOs/HSs must be certain, however, not to suggest that they are more concerned with reducing economic risk than with providing high-quality clinical services.

RM and efforts to improve clinical quality have similar but not identical activities. The Venn diagram in Figure 10.3 shows the overlap between RM and QI, most of which is found in PI. Risk financing, employee benefits, and general liability issues have been unique to RM and are likely to remain so. Patient satisfaction, employee empowerment, and process improvement are largely unique to QI, even though they may affect risk. The evolution of quality assurance to PI expands the historical focus of quality assurance beyond clinical activities to include the processes that support them. This change further diminishes the distinctions between RM and clinical activities and increases their linkages and the need for integration. Certainly, opportunities to benefit from cooperation will increase. In the meantime,

> *[F]or some professionals on both sides, integration means that one function envelops and subsumes the other—a circumstance that would not be in the best interests of either function. . . . Operational linkages is a term that is vague enough to allow for a variety of organizational models, reporting relationships, and data flow.[36]*

Risk Management

As late as the 1970s, even larger HSOs often assigned the director of maintenance collateral duties in facility safety. These managers were unlikely to have any formal preparation in RM and issues regarding patient safety. RM was underdeveloped, and various risks facing the HSO were neither

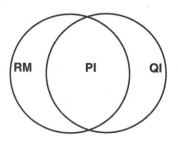
•Patient/customer focus
•Data-driven, complementary databases
•Includes clinical *and* administrative areas
•Process improvement orientation
•Staff involvement at all levels
•Loss(es) viewed as process failure
•Leadership from the top
•Ongoing education of staff
•QI viewed as step to managing risk
•Problem identification
•Culturally embedded

Figure 10.3.   Relationship and integration of RM and QI.

integrated nor handled comprehensively. Insurance was the typical means of protecting HSOs against monetary loss; proactive efforts or programs to reduce risk likely came from insurance companies seeking to decrease their exposure. Figure 10.4 shows a risk control (management) system with the quadrants of bodily injury, liability losses, property losses, and consequential losses. It illustrates the relationships that arise among governance, senior-level management, and the HSO's/HS's organization, actors, and activities.

Link to Senior-Level Management

Regardless of the extent of integration between RM and QI, encouragement and commitment at the HSO's/HS's senior levels are necessary if an RM program is to be successful. Governing body sup-

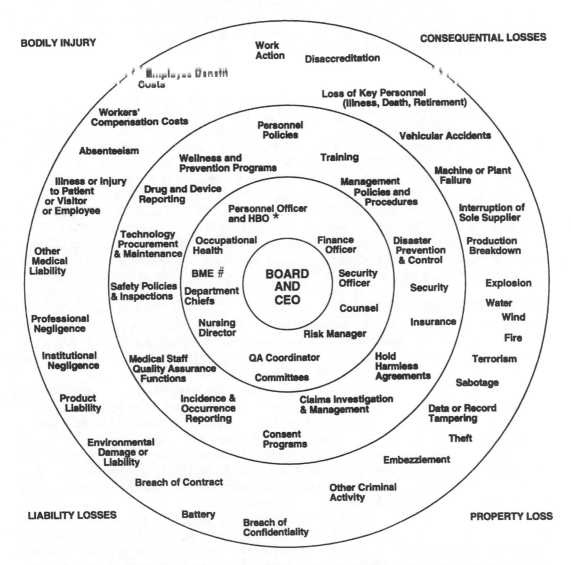

Figure 10.4.   Risk control (management) system (*HBO, health benefits officer; #BME, biomedical equipment). (From Kavaler, Florence, and Allen D. Spiegel. *Risk Management in Health Care Institutions: A Strategic Approach,* 6. Sudbury, MA: Jones & Bartlett, 1997; reprinted by permission.)

port is evidenced by allocating adequate resources to the chief executive officer (CEO) for RM activities, support that should be readily available once the economics of prevention are known. RM has a staff rather than a line relationship to the CEO.

The RM committee develops policy and provides general oversight. To the extent that RM and QI are integrated, this committee includes members of professional staff organization committees and has a greater clinical orientation.

Risk Manager

Common preparation for health services risk managers includes an understanding of RM, nursing, health care and hospital administration, insurance, and law.[37] Larger HSOs and HSs need a full-time risk manager. Integrating RM and QI suggests the need for more academic preparation, perhaps as an adjunct to a clinical background. Managing the RM program in a HS is likely to be the responsibility of someone with significant operational experience, perhaps supplemented by training in the law and clinical preparation. A master of Health Services Administration degree is useful preparation for either the HSO or HS risk manager.

Risk managers have become increasingly important in HSOs/HSs. As the risk managers' role matured, their duties came to include identifying and evaluating risks, loss prevention/reduction, managing the insurance program, safety and security administration, litigation management and claims handling, assisting in adjusting losses, RM consultation, and QI and related activities.[38] A review of business relationships (including contracts) is an appropriate and important activity for risk managers. Examples include clinical and educational affiliations, vendor relationships, interorganizational relationships (in a HS and among HSOs), contracts with clinicians, management services, employment contracts, equipment purchase and lease agreements, and joint ventures.[39]

Risk managers depend on the efforts of various HSO/HS units and constituent departments. Working effectively with people over whom the risk manager has no line authority requires good interpersonal skills and an ability to coordinate and integrate various resources and sources of information. The risk manager may have the effect of exerting line authority by presenting information that is the basis for senior-level management decision making, as well as by persuading senior management to take action. The risk manager's influence is, nevertheless, indirect.

Principles of Managing Risk

The steps in managing risk include identifying, evaluating, eliminating, reducing, and transferring risk. Risk is identified in several ways. The most common is to collect and aggregate data about problems so that patterns become foci for action. However, managing risk must be more than reactive. It should concentrate on eliminating, reducing, and transferring risk.

Evaluating risk means reviewing and categorizing information about problems over time, which allows the RM to concentrate efforts where problems are greatest. Evaluating risk should be prospective, too, because it can be predicted actuarially that certain types of problems will occur or have a probability of occurring. Prospective, retrospective, and concurrent efforts can use evaluative techniques such as cost–benefit and cost-effectiveness analyses to select the best course of action. Evaluative efforts also aid in identifying strategies to eliminate, reduce, or transfer risk. Safety inspections and audits of various activities and functions (ranging from financial [e.g., contracts] to fire protection) are ways to prospectively identify problem areas.

Eliminating or reducing risk (or both) can be achieved in many ways. Examples include sponsoring education and awareness programs for staff, modifying physical plant and structure, enhancing the credentialing process and review of clinical staff activities, improving processes and procedures, initiating material management systems, improving patient and staff relations, and hiring qualified personnel in appropriate categories. It is preferable to eliminate risk, but this may be impossible for many types of risk. Here, the emphasis must be on minimizing risk.

Corporate reorganization (restructuring) can eliminate certain economic risks. For example, assets of a separately incorporated operating HSO may be leased from the HS, which makes them immune from attachment by successful plaintiffs. Establishing trusts and foundations in the corporate reorganization that is common when HSs are established or when restructuring occurs has the same effect. Putting HSO assets beyond the legal reach of successful plaintiffs has its place and is a legitimate business strategy. Failing to provide a means of fairly compensating people who have been clinically or financially injured because of interacting with a HSO or HS, however, is socially irresponsible and unethical.

Some risks can be transferred to others. A common example is the "hold harmless" agreement. It requires that a party doing business with a HSO/HS indemnify it for any liability incurred because of that party's negligence. Equipment purchase contracts commonly include such clauses. As the law permits, risk transfer clauses should be used in all agreements with subcontractors.

Financing Risk

Some risks, such as casualty (e.g., fire, water damage, wind storm), general liability (e.g., injury to visitors or tradespeople), business interruption (e.g., equipment failure, strike, vandalism), theft (e.g., embezzlement), and medical malpractice, cannot be eliminated or transferred. The financial viability of the HSO/HS must be protected from them; insurance is the most common way of doing so. Commercial insurance requires the insured to pay a premium. Coverage under the contract of insurance provides specified protection against certain losses for a fixed period. This contract between the HSO/HS (the insured) and the insurer (carrier) puts obligations on the insured as well. Examples include prompt reporting of problems with potential liability and cooperating in the carrier's investigation and defense of claims. In addition to commercial insurance, HSOs/HSs may participate in insurance programs through captive insurance companies that have been established by the state, a trade association, a consortium of HSOs/HSs, or a large HSO/HS. "Off-shore" insurance companies are an example. After the malpractice crises in the late 1960s and early 1970s and in the 1980s, which are discussed in Chapter 14, rapid increases in malpractice insurance premiums made these variations popular. Some commercial insurance carriers stopped writing medical malpractice liability insurance, and this made availability a factor as well.

Prior to the 1980s, medical malpractice liability insurance usually was written on an occurrence basis, which means that the insured has coverage if a policy is in effect at the time of the event (occurrence). Occurrence coverage protects the insured from a claim regardless of how long after the occurrence it is filed. This resulted in a "long tail"; in other words, claims could be brought months and even years after the event that caused a claim to be filed. In addition, the statute of limitations begins to run only after the event is discovered, and this adds more length to the "tail." For example, a newborn infant could bring suit for 21 years plus the statute of limitations for negligent medical treatment. Insurance carriers argued that this made it difficult or impossible to predict their risk (exposure) actuarially, which made it impossible to determine what the premiums should be. To avoid this problem, they began to write policies with claims-made coverage, which "eliminates the long tail of occurrence coverage because the insurer knows at the expiration of a given policy all of the claims that will be reported against that policy. The insurer need not be concerned with unknown claims that may be made in future years at inflated costs."[40] This change meant that the insured must have a policy in effect when the claim is brought rather than when the insured event occurs, as in occurrence coverage. The effect of this shift on HSOs/HSs seems to have reduced the rate of increase of medical malpractice liability insurance premiums.

Larger HSOs/HSs are more able to self-insure. Self-insurance programs usually are broader than medical malpractice liability and may include financial protection against risks such as business interruption, fire and other casualty losses, and bonding for employees with financial responsibilities. Establishing a self-insurance program involves much more than simply stating that the

HSO/HS is self-insured. Actuarial studies must be done to determine the potential for various types of losses, including special attention to the specific risk from clinical services offered or contemplated. Based on these data, the HSO/HS must establish dedicated reserves to meet expected claims. Usually several years are needed to accumulate the reserves for a self-insurance program to be financially viable. In the interim, commercial coverage is necessary. In addition, after the program is fully established, vigilance is necessary so that the fund both is adequate to meet expected claims and is not raided for other purposes. Underfunding or stripping reserves for self-insurance protection can have disastrous consequences for the economic viability of the organization.

Even when the self-insurance program is mature, most HSOs/HSs carry excess liability and casualty coverage against large claims. For example, a HSO/HS might self-insure for all losses up to $3 million; beyond that it may have a policy with a commercial carrier to a total coverage of $20 million. It is important to note that, even if a HSO/HS has only commercial insurance, the policy is likely have a deductible, which is a form of self-insurance. Deductibles must be met from reserves.

Good business practice demands that HSOs/HSs protect themselves against a range of financial risks. In addition, it is socially responsible and ethical that they do so. "Going bare" in terms of medical malpractice claims means that the HSO/HS neither self-insures nor carries commercial insurance. This practice is not uncommon among licensed independent practitioners (LIPs) with a poor medical malpractice liability record. Their assets are in a spouse's name or otherwise beyond the reach of plaintiffs. This, too, is socially irresponsible. It is prudent that HSOs/HSs require that LIPs on their professional staffs provide evidence of insurance coverage that meets minimum requirements as a condition of having clinical privileges. This is standard practice in acute care hospitals.

Non–LIP caregivers and managers should carry personal liability insurance to protect themselves as individuals from legal actions for alleged negligence. Individual malpractice policies have become common among registered nurses, for example, and their professional association recommends it. Managers should not forget that they, too, are liable for errors and omissions (malpractice) committed in their professional activities. The HSO's/HS's umbrella liability policy covers employees. Nonetheless, the effects of litigation have many nuances for employers and employees. Soon after litigation begins, it becomes apparent that the various parties have substantially different interests. Umbrella policies of the type commonly found in HSOs/HSs do not include employees as named insureds. This means, for example, that, legally, an individual employee has no voice in a decision to settle a lawsuit. Although not a legal determination, settling suggests an admission of fault. This may be adverse to the employees' interests from the standpoints of professional reputation, licensure, certification, and references. Conversely, a personal policy gives one a much more powerful position. The Health Care Quality Improvement Act of 1986,[41] described in Chapter 14, requires that payments made for the benefit of physicians and LIPs be reported to a national data bank. This greatly increases the effects of settling a malpractice claim and makes it important for affected parties to have maximum control.

Members of the HSO's/HS's governing body are not employees. They should be protected against legal actions for errors and omissions under a directors' and officers' liability policy, a policy that should be provided by the HSO/HS. They, too, should consider a personal errors and omissions liability insurance policy.

Process of RM

It is crucial that a RM program systematically report circumstances that put HSOs/HSs at risk. These can be fire and safety problems, accidents, or any type of negligence. Data collection for analysis of actual and potential loss may be a sophisticated RM software program or a simple manual entry system. "Establishing data bases for incident reports, claims, insurance coverages, hazardous materials, and other sources of information may be accomplished through the use of both internal and external sources. One of the richest internal sources is quality data . . . ."[42]

Common to internal control systems is a written statement, usually called an incident or occurrence report. Incident or occurrence reports alert risk managers to specific problems, and aggregating the data will show problem areas and patterns. Figure 10.5 is a sample occurrence report form. Because incidence reporting and associated activities are used to improve the quality of care as part of peer review, laws in most states prevent plaintiffs' attorneys from obtaining (discovering) them. Such laws were passed in the belief that access to such information would have a chilling effect on physicians' willingness to engage in peer review. A collateral result of limiting access to documents is that the plaintiff (injured party) is less likely to prevail. On balance, however, society's interests are served by promoting activities that seek to improve quality of care.

Analysis of data from reporting systems is used in the feedback loop—it informs the risk manager about problems and suggests steps to correct them. For example, data about falls resulting from patients' excessive waits for assisted toileting could be used to support a nursing service request for more staff. Data about postsurgical wound infections could be used to improve the training of staff in central sterile supply, or it could be used to teach correct handwashing techniques to clinical staff. Data about back injuries to staff who move patients could stimulate development of a training program about proper lifting techniques.

Legal counsel review of the RM program is indispensable. If counsel are available on site (in-house counsel), then it is likely they will be more involved in a RM program than would be retainer counsel. Some HSOs/HSs use in-house counsel as risk managers. Regardless, legal counsel must participate in the program.

The risk manager can minimize loss after injury to patients has occurred by immediately taking four steps. First, if the patient has been discharged, then the medical record (including radiographs) should be obtained and absolute custody of it retained by the risk manager. Second, if the patient continues under treatment and the record is active, then it should be photocopied (new entries are photocopied on a regular basis) and the copies retained by the risk manager. This standard operating procedure should be known throughout the HSO/HS. Third, meetings should be held with the patient, the family, or both to determine their interest in settling any potential claim. Once legal counsel is retained by the patient, the case is almost certain to become more complex and costly. Fourth, the HSO/HS should do whatever it can to retain the patient's goodwill; above all, insult should not be added to injury. An injured patient who needs additional treatment should never be sent a bill for the extra services. Angry patients are much more likely to sue than are those who believe the HSO/HS did the best it could under the circumstances and acted responsibly.

Efforts at early settlement raise a potential conflict of interest. Patients and their relatives should clearly understand that the risk manager is an employee of the HSO/HS. Risk managers must never allow patients or family members to believe that they are advocates for the patient or acting as legal counsel on the patient's behalf. Honesty and forthrightness succeed far better than other tactics. Fraud or misrepresentation by the risk manager not only is unethical but will cause a court to set aside any agreement and may result in criminal charges or punitive damages being levied against the HSO/HS.

Improving Quality and Performance

Early concerns about the quality of clinical practice in HSOs focused on hospitals and were addressed through peer review, which is defined as physician review of the care that is provided by physicians and other types of caregivers. The American College of Surgeons began developing the concept of peer review in 1912. In 1918 it published the "Minimum Standard," part of which addressed peer review of medical practice: "The [medical] staff [shall] review and analyze at regular intervals their clinical experience in the various departments of the hospital."[43] As noted in Chapter 2, the work of the American College of Surgeons was continued by the Joint Commission when it was formed in 1951.

Occurrence Report

The George Washington University WASHINGTON DC MEDICAL CENTER

This form is to report the facts of any unusual, unexpected or unplanned events. It is not to document opinions or conclusions concerning potential causes of or solutions to those events. Staff may verbally communicate any such opinion and / or conclusion directly to the Risk Management Office at 994-2849.

Patient ID Plate

☐ Patient ☐ Staff ☐ Other	Name:		SEX ☐ Male ☐ Female	Age	Date of Birth

Diagnosis		Location of Occurrence: ☐ BR ☐ Hall ☐ Patient Room Unit:	☐ Other	Date	Time	☐ AM ☐ PM

Person completing Report (include title and phone number):

Complete all sections which pertain to the type of occurrence being reported - Check all boxes that apply. Please see the reverse side of this form for specific instructions / definitions.

FALLS
- ☐ Found On Floor
- ☐ From Bed
- ☐ From Bedside Commode
- ☐ From Chair/Wheelchair
- ☐ From Stretcher/Table
- ☐ From Toilet
- ☐ While Ambulating: w/Assistance
- ☐ While Ambulating: w/o Assistance
- ☐ While Ambulating: w/Device
- ☐ Repeat or Multiple Falls
- ☐ On Fall Prevention Program
- ☐ Other (Please Comment)

MEDICATION
- ☐ Adverse Drug Reaction
- ☐ Extra Dose
- ☐ IV Related
- ☐ Missed Dose
- ☐ Narcotic Count
- ☐ Pharmacy Related
- ☐ Transcription Related
- ☐ Transfusion Related
- ☐ Dosage Related
- ☐ Wrong Medication
- ☐ Wrong Patient
- ☐ Wrong Route
- ☐ Wrong Time
- ☐ Other(Please Comment)

MISCELLANEOUS Please Comment
- ☐ AMA/Walkout
- ☐ Behavior
- ☐ Complaint
- ☐ Discharge Delayed
- ☐ Employee Injury
- ☐ Exposure to Infection
- ☐ Equipment Related
- ☐ Patient ID Related
- ☐ Property Damaged/Lost
- ☐ Results Delayed
- ☐ Self Injury
- ☐ Service Delayed
- ☐ Support Service Related
- ☐ Transfer Delayed
- ☐ Transcription Related
- ☐ Other (Please Comment)

MD Notified?- YES☐ NO☐   MD Responded?- YES☐ NO☐

Name of Attending Physician:

TYPE OF INJURY
- ☐ None Apparent
- ☐ Abrasion
- ☐ Burn
- ☐ Damaged Teeth
- ☐ Dislocation
- ☐ Fracture
- ☐ Hematoma
- ☐ IV Infiltration
- ☐ Laceration
- ☐ Rash/Hives
- ☐ Sprain/Strain
- ☐ Other(Please Comment)

TREATMENT
- ☐ Additional Procedure
- ☐ Break In Sterile Technique
- ☐ Cancelled After Induction
- ☐ Consent Variation
- ☐ Count Variation
- ☐ Foreign Body Retained
- ☐ Incorrect Procedure
- ☐ Injury to Organ
- ☐ Prep Omitted/Wrong
- ☐ Returned to OR
- ☐ Other (Please Comment)

Name of Responding Physician:

Studies Ordered:

Narrative/Comments
Use this section for details related to any "OTHER" box checked or to provide necessary details regarding the event being reported.

ADDITIONAL INFORMATION

Condition Before Event:
- ☐ Oriented
- ☐ Confused
- ☐ Other (Please Comment)

Activity Level:
- ☐ Ad Lib
- ☐ OOB With Assistance
- ☐ Bathroom Privileges
- ☐ Bedside Commode
- ☐ Complete Bedrest

Bed Position:
- ☐ Low   ☐ High

Bed Side Rails Up:
- ☐ Upper L ☐ Upper R
- ☐ Lower L ☐ Lower R

Call Bell w/in Patient's Reach
- ☐ Yes   ☐ No

LABORATORY SPECIMEN
- ☐ Damaged
- ☐ Destroyed
- ☐ Improperly Collected
- ☐ Lost
- ☐ Mislabeled
- ☐ Misplaced
- ☐ Wrong Patient
- ☐ Other (Please Comment)

Restraints:
- ☐ None
- ☐ Soft Wrist
- ☐ Posey Vest
- ☐ Leather
- ☐ Other (Please Comment)

Supervisor's Signature: Date:

Figure 10.5. Sample occurrence report form. (From The George Washington University Medical Center; reprinted by permission.)

The process of peer review was called medical audit, terminology that was used into the 1960s. Enactment of Medicare codified utilization review (UR), which focused on the use of services by beneficiaries. UR did not directly affect the quality of care in hospitals, except that judging the appropriateness of admission, use of ancillary services, and length of stay minimized nosocomial (institution-caused) and iatrogenic (physician-caused) problems. The focus of UR in Medicare is discussed in Chapter 2. Medical audit and UR placed little emphasis on solving the problems that were identified.

Efforts to measure quality continued to evolve. In the early 1970s the Joint Commission required quality assessment activities, a variation on medical audit. In the middle 1970s the words were changed to "medical care evaluation," but it remained essentially medical audit. By 1980 the concept of quality assurance had become a Joint Commission standard. Quality assurance meant that Joint Commission standards had evolved from problem finding (medical audit) to a more proactive and dynamic concept. Quality assurance went beyond identifying and describing problems and stressed problem solving to improve clinical quality. As noted earlier, in 1991 the Joint Commission changed quality assurance to QA/I, and by 1998 the standards had fully integrated RM and QI into PI.

Historically, quality has been defined as the degree of adherence to standards or criteria. As applied in health services, ensuring quality meant using prospectively determined criteria to measure performance, with the measurement being done retrospectively. Newer definitions of quality are discussed in Chapter 9 in the context of CQI. These include conformance to requirements and fitness for use or fitness for need and are customer driven because they focus on customer expectations and do not exclusively reflect criteria or standards that are developed through professional expertise. It is suggested that quality should be defined as meeting latent needs—identifying "needs" customers may not even know they have but may be pleased to have identified and met by the provider. CQI defines "customer" broadly to include all who receive goods or services.

Measuring quality using the concepts of quality assurance required that the HSO/HS establish standards (criteria), typically through peer judgment. Developing criteria was only the first step, however. Two other elements were necessary: a means of surveillance to identify deviations that required action, and stopping the deviation or minimizing its recurrence—the corrective action. These steps were simple in theory and may have been in practice as well, depending on what was being measured. Much of the conceptual framework buttressing efforts to measure quality was developed by Avedis Donabedian, a physician, whose nomenclature of structure, process, and outcome is standard in the health services field. Structure and process were the major foci of the Joint Commission's quality assurance standards in the 1980s.

Donabedian noted the difficulty of developing a definition of quality medical care and measuring the quality of the interpersonal relationship between physician and patient—a relationship that is essential to the process of care as well as reflected in the outcome of care. Technical aspects of care are more definable and measurable than are interpersonal relationships.[44] Regardless, however, measuring quality under traditional quality assurance began with criteria that were developed internally, were externally imposed, or were a combination of the two.

Structure, Process, and Outcome in Quality Assessment

Donabedian defined structure as the tools and resources that providers of care have at their disposal and the physical and organizational settings where they work.[45] Process is the set of activities that occur within HSOs/HSs and between practitioners and patients. Here, judgments of quality may be made either by direct observation or by reviewing recorded information. Donabedian considered this means of measuring quality to be largely normative in that the norms come either from the science of medicine or from the ethics and values of society.[46] Outcome is a change in a patient's current and future health status that can be attributed to antecedent health care.[47] Donabedian defined outcome broadly to include improvement of social and psychological function in addition to physical and physiological aspects. Also included are patient attitudes, health-related knowledge acquired by the patient, and health-related behavioral change.[48]

Donabedian concluded that "good structure, that is, a sufficiency of resources and proper system design, is probably the most important means of protecting and promoting the quality of care."[49] He added that assessing structure is a good deal less important than assessing process and outcome. Comparing process and outcome, Donabedian concluded that neither is clearly preferable. Either may be superior, depending on the situation and what is being measured. He emphasized that it is critical, however, to know the link between the content of the process and the resulting outcome. Only by knowing this link (preferably at the level of a causal relationship) can what is done or not done in the process be modified to improve the outcome. A desirable outcome without knowing how it was achieved means that replication is impossible. Table 10.2 shows the advantages and disadvantages of focusing on process and outcome to measure quality. Outcome indicators in Donabedian's taxonomy focus on the overall outcomes of medical care, such as health status and disability.

Developments for Beyond 2000: Practice Parameters

Development and application of quality assurance reached a peak in the late 1980s with development of a 10-step quality assurance process. At that point the Joint Commission began a long-term effort to emphasize outcome indicators; in 1988 its "Agenda for Change"[50] initiated a major shift to adopting CQI, a process that is detailed in Chapter 9. It is generally conceded that quality assurance as implemented in the 1980s was less than effective in improving the quality of care. "On the whole, to the extent that quality measurement tools have been developed at all, they tend to unveil the fact of flaw, not its cause."[51]

The Joint Commission's shift to a focus on outcome in 1988 followed by about 1 year the much-criticized release of hospital mortality data by the Health Care Financing Administration. The first clinical indicators to be developed were hospitalwide care and obstetrical and anesthesia care.[52] In early 1989, 12 key principles of organizational and management effectiveness were announced by the Joint Commission, and pilot testing was undertaken. The purpose was to characterize an acute care hospital's commitment to continuously improve its quality of care. A central tenet was that identifying and monitoring outcome indicators were necessary for a hospital to focus its QI activities. By 1991 indicators had been developed for anesthesia, obstetrics, cardiovascular medicine, oncology, and trauma care.[53] These indicators were focused on high-risk, high-volume, and problem-prone aspects of care. By the mid-1990s the Joint Commission's Indicator Monitoring System (IMSystem) included 31 measures for five patient populations, including those receiving perioperative, obstetrical, trauma, oncologic, or cardiovascular care, together addressing well over half of all inpatient admissions. Eleven additional measures focused on clinical functions of medication use and infection control.[54] The effort to develop and implement outcome indicators proved too difficult, however, and by the late 1990s the Joint Commission began to implement the ORYX program, which is described in Chapter 2.

The practice parameters (guidelines) developed by various physician organizations are separate from and complement the Joint Commission's efforts to develop outcome indicators and its ORYX program. "Practice parameters are a generic term for acceptable approaches to the prevention, diagnosis, treatment, or management of a disease or condition, as determined by the medical profession based on the best medical evidence currently available."[55] Various names are used to express the concept of practice parameters: critical paths, practice guidelines, clinical guidelines, clinical protocols or algorithms, care or target tracks, case management, and clinical pathways. (An example of a clinical protocol appears in Figure 9.17.) A 1996 survey of hospitals found that 81% used critical paths, and many of the remainder were planning to use them in the near future.[56] HSOs/HSs may define these terms differently and with various levels of precision. Regardless,

TABLE 10.2. ADVANTAGES AND DISADVANTAGES OF PROCESS AND OUTCOME MEASURES OF QUALITY

Process		Outcome	
Advantages	Disadvantages	Advantages	Disadvantages
Practitioners have no great difficulty specifying technical criteria for standards of care. Even not fully validated standards and criteria can serve as interim measures of acceptable practice. Information about technical aspects of care is documented in the medical record and usually is accessible as well as timely—it can be used for prevention and intervention. Use of this information permits specific attribution of responsibility so that credit or blame can be more easily ascertained and specific corrective action can be taken.	Great weakness in the scientific basis for much of accepted practice and use of prevalent norms as the basis for judging quality may encourage dogmatism and perpetuate error. Because practitioners prefer to err on the side of doing more than is necessary, there is a tendency toward overly elaborate and costly care; this is reflected in the norms. Although technical aspects are overemphasized, the management of the interpersonal process tends to be ignored, partly because the usual sources of data give little information about the physician–patient relationship.	When the scientific basis for accepted practice is in doubt, emphasis on outcome tends to discourage dogmatism and helps maintain a more open and flexible approach to management. An open and flexible approach may help in the development of less costly but no less effective strategies of care. Outcomes reflect all of the contributions of all of the practitioners to the care of the patient and thus provide an inclusive, integrative measure of the quality of care. Also reflected in the outcome is the patient's contribution to the care that may have been influenced by the relationship between patient and practitioners; a more direct assessment of the patient–physician relationship can be obtained by including aspects of patient satisfaction among measures of care.	Even expert practitioners are unable to specify the outcomes of optimal care, as to their magnitude, timing, and duration. When indicators of health status are obtained, it is difficult to know how much of the observed effect can be attributed to medical care. Choosing outcomes that have marginal relevance to the objectives of prior care is an ever-present pitfall; even when relevant outcomes are selected, information about many outcomes often is not available in time to make it useful for certain types of monitoring. Waiting for a pattern of adverse outcomes can be questioned on ethical grounds. Examining outcomes without examining means of attaining them may result in a lack of attention to the presence of redundant or overly costly care.

Adapted from Donabedian, Avedis. *Explorations in Quality Assessment and Monitoring. Vol. 1, The Definition of Quality and Approaches to its Assessment*, 119–122. Ann Arbor, MI: Health Administration Press, 1980.

there is evidence that the efforts that integrated delivery systems and managed care organizations are making to implement clinical guidelines and improve performance and quality will profoundly affect health services delivery.[57]

Practice parameters are not the same as indicators, but they lead to measurable indicators. Practice parameters are a means for describing what should be done; indicators are a means for measuring. "Once one moves from determining what ought to be done to seeing if or how often it is done, one moves from guidelines [parameters] to indicators."[58]

The American Academy of Pediatrics was the first organization to develop practice parameters in 1938. It was not until the late 1970s that such efforts gained momentum. By 1990, 26 physician organizations had developed practice parameters for their specialties[59]; by 1995 approximately 1,800 medical practice guidelines had been catalogued.[60] The use of clinical guidelines for congestive heart failure developed by the Agency for Health Care Policy and Research has meant fewer readmissions and decreased cost and length of stay by boosting the use of recommended posthospital medications.[61] Table 10.3 shows the preferred practice pattern guideline for a comprehensive adult eye evaluation that was developed by the American Academy of Ophthalmology.

In addition to setting guidelines for physicians, practice parameters will be another source in establishing the legal standard of care, which is described in Chapter 14. During litigation, physicians will be entitled to explain variations from practice guidelines. Deviations are likely because practice guidelines are meant to assist providers but not to replace individualized patient treatment plans.[62] It is possible, however, that practice guidelines will become presumptive reflections of the standard of care and that this will place the burden on the practitioner to prove that the deviations were justified.

Work by the American Society of Anesthesiologists in setting practice parameters for intraoperative monitoring (monitoring during surgery) has been credited with virtually eliminating hypoxic (insufficient oxygen) injury lawsuits and causing a significant reduction in medical malpractice insurance premiums.[63] Another important potential benefit of guidelines is major reductions in losses per malpractice claim in high-risk areas such as the emergency department, maternity ward, and operating rooms, with one study reporting a 96% reduction when guidelines were used in all three areas.[64]

Importance of QI

The importance of evaluating quality was suggested in Chapter 2. Several reasons should be reiterated, however. HSOs/HSs that seek Joint Commission accreditation must have organized, effective QI activities. Unaccredited HSOs/HSs are not in "deemed status" for purposes of Medicare reimbursement and must meet the conditions of participation that were established by the Department of Health and Human Services. Accreditors of medical education programs in HSOs/HSs usually demand Joint Commission accreditation. Insurance carriers that write coverage for HSOs/HSs expect them to be accredited, and lending institutions and organizations that rate bond offerings consider accreditation to be important in their decisions. Chapter 4 details the importance of credentialing the clinical staff, an activity that is indispensable to QI. In addition, failing to effectively assess and improve quality increases the probability of adverse medical malpractice judgments because the HSO has not met the legal standard of care.

QI is considered important by managerial, clinical, and support staff who want to do their best. They strive to do so because they are professionals who have internalized the motivation to provide high-quality care and be part of an excellent HSO/HS. This includes and necessitates the need to learn what is being done correctly and what is not, as well as how to improve performance.

Figure 10.6 shows the flow of QI activities. Data sources (many of which will be outcome indicators) focus the attention of the coordinating body, which may be called the quality improvement council. The coordinating body sanctions the establishment of cross-functional quality improvement teams (QITs) to analyze processes and recommend changes to improve them. Intradepartmental QITs are established by departments and monitored by them and by the quality improvement council. In addition, departments may assign individual workers who are process owners to monitor and improve a process. The coordinating body may have authority to approve major changes and expenditures resulting from QIT recommendations, or CEO or governing body approval may be required.

QI and Quality Assurance Compared

As HSOs/HSs fully adopt the philosophy and techniques of CQI, it is useful to understand how it differs from traditional approaches to quality. As described in Chapter 9, QI necessitates a paradigm shift because it uses powerful tools that are supported by a radically different philosophy about re-

TABLE **10.3.** EXCERPTS FROM A PREFERRED PRACTICE GUIDELINE FOR A COMPREHENSIVE ADULT EYE EVALUATION

Brief Summary

TITLE:
Comprehensive Adult Eye Evaluation

RELEASE DATE:
1996 September

MAJOR RECOMMENDATIONS:
Evaluation Process

A comprehensive eye evaluation includes history, examination, diagnosis and initiation of management. Included within each are a series of items particularly relevant to the detection, diagnosis, and choice of appropriate therapy for ocular, visual and systemic disease. The items listed are basic areas of evaluation or investigation and are not meant to exclude additional elements when appropriate. For example, because history taking is an interactive process, additional questions and evaluation may be suggested by the patient's responses.

History

In general, a thorough history includes the following items, although the exact composition varies with the patient's particular problem and needs.

- Demographic data: includes name, date of birth, gender and race
- The identity of the patient's other pertinent health care providers
- Chief complaint and history of present illness (including a review of systems relevant to eye conditions)
- Present status of visual function: includes a review of the patient's assessment of his/her visual status, visual needs, any recent or current ocular symptoms, and use of eyeglasses or contact lenses (type, wearing habits)
- Past history (ocular): prior eye disease (e.g., amblyopia), injuries, diagnoses, and surgery or other treatments and medications
- Past history (systemic): allergies or adverse reactions to medications, medication use, pertinent medical conditions, and previous surgeries
- Family history: poor vision (and cause, if known) and other pertinent familial ocular and systemic disease
- Medications: ophthalmic and systemic medications currently used
- Social history: occupation, smoking history, alcohol use, for example

Examination

The comprehensive examination consists of an evaluation of the physiologic function and the anatomic status of the eye, visual system and its related structures. In general, this will include, but not necessarily be limited to, the following elements:

- Visual acuity with present correction (the power of the present correction recorded) at a distance and close
- Measurement of best corrected visual acuity (with refraction when indicated)
- Ocular alignment and motility
- Pupillary function
- Intraocular pressure measurement
- Visual fields by confrontation when indicated
- External examination: lids, lashes and lacrimal apparatus, orbit, and pertinent facial features
- Slit-lamp examination: eyelid margins and lashes, tear film, conjunctive, sclera, cornea, anterior chamber and assessment of peripheral anterior chamber depth, iris, lens and anterior vitreous
- Examination of the fundus: vitreous, retina (including posterior pole and periphery), vasculature, and optic nerve

Examination of anterior segment structures routinely involves gross and biomicroscopic evaluation prior to and after dilation. Evaluation of structures situated posterior to the iris may require a dilated pupil. Optimal examination of the peripheral retina requires the use of an indirect ophthalmoscope and sometimes a Goldmann three-mirror lens.

(continued)

TABLE **10.3.** (*continued*)

Based on the patient's history and findings, additional tests or evaluations might be indicated to evaluate further a particular structure or function. Components that are not routinely part of the comprehensive eye evaluation include:

- Gonioscopy
- Visual fields by perimetry
- Color-vision testing
- Microbiology and cytology
- Amsler grid
- Functional evaluation of the lacrimal system
- Fluorescein angiography
- Radiologic testing
- Electrophysiological testing
- Stereophotography and/or analysis of the optic disc

Diagnosis and Management

The ophthalmologist evaluates and integrates the findings of the comprehensive ophthalmologic examination with all aspects of the patient's health status and social situation in determining an appropriate course of action. The evaluation results may be considered in one of three general categories: patients with no risk factors, patients with risk factors, and patients with conditions requiring intervention.

Developed by the American Academy of Ophthalmology. Used by permission of the Academy. From the National Guideline Clearinghouse. *http://www.ngc.gov/VEWS/summary.as . . . =comprehensive+adult+eye+evaluation,* March 26, 1999.

lationships between managers and staff. Table 10.4 suggests the differences, but several deserve additional attention.

Despite some anecdotes or case experience to the contrary, quality assurance was seen as a negative process. It focused on the "who," and this meant risk for anyone who worked in a process from which problems arose. QI seeks the "why" of a problem or inefficiency; those who are part of a process are not the focus. In this regard, QI adopts the view of W. Edwards Deming, whose theories are described in Chapter 9, that 85%–94% of problems result from the process; few, if any, are caused by those who work in it.

Typically, quality assurance exclusively measured the quality of clinical practice, which until the 1990s was the Joint Commission's focus. QI measures clinical practice but is equally concerned with myriad processes and systems that support the delivery of clinical services, as well as those that are administrative, such as admitting and patient accounts. Clinical and administrative aspects of many processes cannot be easily separated, and QI seeks to improve integrated or cross-functional processes as well as those that are intradepartmental. Improved quality in a HSO's/HS's support and administrative areas positively affects clinical areas because there is greater organizationwide quality consciousness and because, without exception, these areas affect clinical services. Admitting is an example. Inefficient intradepartmental or interdepartmental admitting processes directly and indirectly affect patient care.

Another important difference is that QI focuses on improving processes, whereas quality assurance focuses on solving problems. Traditionally, quality assurance meant dealing with the unusual or unique—what Deming called special causes—and investigated indicators that exceeded thresholds. Similarly, under this philosophy managers spend much of their time "fighting fires." At times, "putting out fires" is necessary, but it does not improve processes and does not increase efficiency or effectiveness. Putting out a fire only returns the process, more or less, to the state it was in before the fire started. QI asserts that unique and unusual results or outcomes should be ignored unless they pose a significant risk or danger; attention should focus on improving the process. HSO/HS managers cannot ignore unusual or unique events that affect patients, but the effort spent on them should be minimized because the real gain comes from improving processes to reduce variation, error rates, and other inefficiencies.

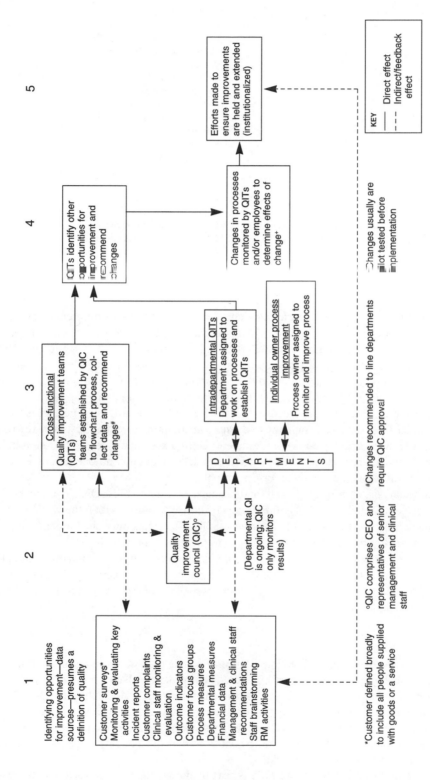

Figure 10.6.   Steps in the process of QI.

TABLE 10.4.   CHARACTERISTICS OF QI VERSUS QA

QI	QA
"Why" focused (positive)	"Who" focused (negative)
Prospective	Retrospective
Internally directed	Externally directed
Follows patients	Follows organizational structure
Involves the many	Delegated to the few
Integrated analysis	Divided analysis
Bottom up	Top down
Proactive	Reactive
Employee focused	Management focused (directing)
Full staff involvement	Limited staff involvement
Process based	Event based
Process approach	Inspection approach
Quality is integral activity	Quality is separate activity
Focus on all processes to improve fitness for use	Focus on meeting clinical criteria
Focus on improving processes	Focus on solving problems
Makes no assumption about irreducibility of problems	Assumes problems/numbers of problems reach irreducible number

Finally, assumptions that have been made about the irreducibility of problems were the most insidious dimension of the philosophy of quality assurance and have probably been responsible for delaying improvement in the quality of care. Psychologically, it is crucial that "good enough" is no longer acceptable; the QI philosophy rejects it. An element of "good enough" is suggested when HSOs/HSs compare outcome indicators or other performance measures with their own criteria or with external criteria. Criteria and indicators are an important starting point and provide a macro-level understanding of outcomes produced by a HSO/HS or from a process. The fact is that organizations in which CQI has been implemented improve quality by reducing waste, rework, and redundancy, not by accepting a place within the herd. Until a systematic search for the root causes of medication errors has been done using the tools of QI, for example, no one knows what the irreducible level of medication errors in an organization is.

In the final analysis, improving clinical (and managerial) quality in HSOs/HSs requires change. If Deming is correct that only 6%–15% of problems result from causes within the worker's control, then management must work with staff to improve quality. Managers must shed the traditional view that poor quality occurs because employees choose to perform suboptimally.

What must be remembered, especially with the increased emphasis on outcome indicators, is that it is crucial to understand the link between process and outcome. Unless it is known how the outcome was produced, desired outcomes cannot be purposefully replicated, nor can a process be changed to prevent undesired outcomes.

Summary

Readers should have a clear sense of the importance of managing risk and assessing and improving the quality of clinical and managerial performance. These processes have an important place in the control function of managers in HSOs/HSs. Making changes is often difficult in HSOs/HSs, where much that is done is a personal service that is rendered by clinical staff who are, in many cases, independent contractors. For the manager, this requires attention to interpersonal skills and an ability to work with and through people. Maintaining quality of care for patients and protecting employees and visitors depend largely on these skills.

Improving quality (and minimizing risk) is part of the manager's control function described previously and shown in the control model in Figure 10.2. In terms of clinical practice, the purpose is to improve the quality of care. Size, organizational complexity, severity of patient illness, and intensity of service necessitate that acute care hospitals have sophisticated RM programs and make extensive efforts to improve quality. Increasingly, similar programs are found in all HSOs/HSs. Pragmatically, there are no differences between the type of statistical quality control used in industry and that which can be applied to many HSO/HS activities. Even the methodologies used in clinical areas are remarkably similar to those that are used in industrial settings.

It is platitudinous, but true nevertheless, to say that managers must be part of the solution or they will remain part of the problem. Managers should be unwilling to accept an attitude anywhere in the HSO/HS that what is being done is "good enough."

CONTROL METHODS

Managers use numerous methods and techniques to monitor and control inputs, processes, and/or outputs. RM and PI are examples of structured, programmatic control methods. Others are budgeting, ABC, and operational-activity and financial ratio analysis.

Budgeting

One of the most common methods for control is the use of budgets. They serve a dual purpose. First, they are numerical expressions of plans,[65] and second, they become control standards against which results are compared.[66] Types of budgets and time frames vary. Most, such as operating expense and revenue budgets, are made for 1 year; capital expenditure budgets, however, may be multiyear.

Budgeting depends on planning and forecasting. Individual cost centers or departments forecast the volume of service that they expect to deliver, the workload demand, and the resources that are needed in the next budget period. Cost centers are organizational units in which there is a well-defined relationship between inputs and outputs. Examples are surgery, nursing service, clinics, laboratories, pharmacy, diagnostic testing, dietary, patient billing, medical records, and maintenance. Based on expected workloads, revenue budgets can be derived for those units with which revenues can be associated; examples are the emergency department, clinics, diagnostic testing, pharmacy, and surgery. For all departments, including those in which revenues typically cannot be directly associated, such as nursing service, social services, maintenance, and administration, operating expense budgets are derived that reflect the amount and types of resources that are necessary to perform the projected workload.

Operating expense budgets include two types: direct and indirect. Direct expenses are those that are incurred by a cost center or a department and can be specifically attributed to it. They include labor and nonlabor components. Human resources requirements must be converted to dollars paid for salary, wages, and fringe benefits. Nonlabor expenses are supplies and equipment. From a cost perspective, indirect expenses can be allocated, including overhead costs, such as general facility maintenance, building depreciation, utilities, and management staff not identified with specific cost centers. These indirect costs usually are allocated among cost centers on some basis such as space occupied, number of employees, or volume of output.[67] Usually, cost centers have control over only their direct expenses.

Operating budgets can be fixed, variable, or fixed-variable. Fixed budgets represent a resource commitment to a cost center or department for the budget period. They are based on planned workload. Variable budgets recognize that, as volume, workload, or service demands change, so will resource needs.[68] Often, hybrid fixed-variable operating budgets are developed. They separate costs into fixed and variable components, with the latter changing as workload increases or decreases.

Budgets force managers to be aware of how input resources are used and the associated costs for staff, materials, equipment, or supplies. Preparing a budget requires managers to think about the cost and amount of resources that will be consumed and used in conversion. Also, budgets are standards against which results can be compared. Typically, budget reports are prepared monthly to compare actual expenditures for the month and the year-to-date with the amount budgeted. Variances that indicate deviations of actual from budgeted amounts can be identified and used for control purposes.

A sample hospital emergency services department budget for a 100-bed acute care hospital is presented in Table 10.5. It reports inpatient and outpatient revenues and direct operating expenses (but not allocated indirect costs such as overhead). It shows total net operating revenues (OR) of $267,363 and total operating expenses (OE) of $82,563 for the current period (i.e., month) [Column A] to the budget for the current period (OR = $230,739; OE = $71,458) [Column B], and the variance (OR = $36,624; OE = $11,105) [Column C]; year-to-date actual net operating revenues ($2,336,096) and operating expenses ($689,714) [Column D] to the year-to-date budget (OR = $2,367,046; OE = $682,766) [Column E], as well as the year-to-date variance [Column F]; and year-to-date for last year [Column G]. Budget reports such as these enable managers to exercise greater control over resource use and determine whether department activities such as revenue generation or costs incurred are below, meet, or exceed expectations.

Cost Allocation

HSOs/HSs typically control resource consumption and conversion through the budget process at cost center or department level. This form of budgeting, in which direct and indirect costs are identified and monitored, has limitations, however. Prior to implementing prospective pricing, the Health Care Financing Administration required providers to use step-down costing for Medicare payments. Subsequently, this costing system was used by HSOs to develop base rates that became the basis for diagnosis-related group (DRG) reimbursement. Step-down cost allocation allocates direct costs and pools of indirect costs to specific services and or departments. For example, pooled indirect costs such as those for maintenance, housekeeping, utilities, administration, information services, and marketing would be allocated to cost centers on some logical basis such as labor hours, space occupied, number of employees, or units of service, and the direct and indirect costs of a department would be stepped down to specific services. The goal of step-down cost allocation is to present a more complete financial picture of the costs of treating individual patients and providing specific services. By analyzing input—labor, materials, and equipment—and indirect and overhead costs throughout the organization and associating them with different products or services, standard costs by type of output can be determined. Control is exercised by comparing actual costs of final output with prospectively determined standard costs. Analysis of variance allows inferences to be drawn about the appropriateness of input consumption and efficiency of conversion.

Before cost allocation procedures were widely adopted by HSOs/HSs, managers had difficulty defining end products (services) and the costs associated with producing them and had few incentives to do so. A unit of service such as patient day is a poor output measure because it fails to reflect variations in resource use resulting from factors such as admission type or severity of medical problems (e.g., acuity level). For example, providing care for a high-risk premature infant requires very different resources from various cost centers than does care for a full-term infant not at risk. Also, the nursing service resources that are necessary to care for severely ill rather than convalescing patients differ, although the intermediate output measure, patient day, is the same.

Activity-Based Costing

ABC differs from conventional approaches to cost allocation.[69] It is a bottom-up method of allocating costs, in contrast to the top-down method of step-down allocation, which begins with all costs and allocates them downward to various services.[70] This is depicted in Figure 10.7. ABC is a bottom-up method "because it finds the costs of each service at the lowest level, the point where resources are used, and aggregates them upward into products. ABC is based on the paradigm that

TABLE 10.5. COMMUNITY HOSPITAL EMERGENCY DEPARTMENT REVENUES AND EXPENSES[a]

	A Current month this year	B Current month budget	C[b] Current month variance	D Year-to-date this year	E Year-to-date budget	F[b] Year-to-date variance	G Year-to-date last year
Operating revenue							
Inpatient	76,858	49,072	27,786	65,580	629,564	25,016	593,286
Outpatient	190,505	181,667	8,838	1,681,516	1,737,482	-55,966	1,675,505
Total net revenue	267,363	230,739	36,624	2,336,096	2,367,046	-30,950	2,268,791
Operating expenses							
Salaries & wages	72,044	61,319	10,725	598,818	586,746	12,072	547,616
Purchased services	0	116	-116	5,797	1,044	4,753	925
Repair, maintenance, rent, lease	987	2,115	-1,128	31,806	19,035	-12,229	18,819
Supplies, pharmacy, food	9,336	7,626	1,710	75,524	73,402	2,122	69,932
Other	196	282	-86	2,769	2,538	231	3,041
Total operating expenses	82,563	71,458	11,105	589,714	682,766	6,948	640,333
Department profit (loss)	184,800	159,281	25,519	1,545,382	1,684,280	-37,898	1,628,458

[a]All amounts in U.S. dollars.

[b]Minus denotes the revenue and/or expenses were under the budget amount for the period.

Traditional Costing

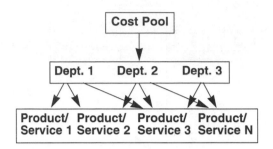

- •Costs (labor, supplies, facilities) of various kinds of functions (purchasing, setup, monitoring, service delivery)

- •Organizational units that deliver or support the delivery of service

- •Various services (lab tests, CBC, physical exam)

Activity-Based Costing

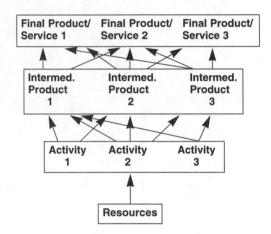

- •Normal delivery, bypass surgery, etc.

- •Physical, well-baby visits, meals, lab tests, radiology procedures, etc.

- •Patient history, writing orders, chest X-ray, urinalysis, test setups, purchasing, billing, 15-min outpatient visits, echocardiogram, telemetry, etc.

- •Labor, supplies, materials

Figure 10.7.   Comparison of traditional and activity-based costing. (From Zelman, William N., Michael J. McCue, and Alan R. Millikan. *Financial Management of Health Care Organizations: An Introduction to Fundamental Tools, Concepts, and Applications,* 465. Malden, MA: Blackwell, 1998; reprinted by permission.)

activities consume resources and processes consume activities."[71] It is a more precise way of allocating all direct and indirect costs to the many activities that result in patient services; provides managers with more precise measures of the cost of services, or residuals in the case of revenue centers (revenues minus costs); and is useful in identifying non–value-added activities.

There are two dimensions to ABC. They are, first, process assessment and, second, identification of activities involved in patient service, called cost drivers, and cost assignment for resources used in each activity. Thus, ABC focuses not only on expenses but also on the process that generates the expenses. It enhances control over resource consumption and is a logical adjunct to CQI by facilitating an understanding of processes and activities that do or do not add value.[72] By focusing on process, Peter Drucker observed that "activity-based costing asks, 'Does it have to be done?' "[73]

By evaluating the flow, for example, of a patient who receives services, it is possible to identify all activities (i.e., elements) of work. These activities are called cost drivers because they result in resource use. ABC allocates both indirect and direct costs to each individual activity. By tracing costs across cost centers and departments to the final product/service, a more accurate understanding of work process and the costs to provide service is achieved.[74] For example, for a given service such as a surgical procedure, ABC will "develop cost information on all different activities along the critical path from preadmission to discharge."[75] The cost of admission, billing, and accounts receivables can be assigned to the final product (surgery), as can other costs such as nursing service, operating suite, and recovery costs that are associated with the particular surgical procedure. To identify costs, the specific resources consumed for any patient encounter must be identified. To do so, there must be process analysis of required activities. The implications for management control are that ABC is a more precise way of matching costs of resources consumed to services provided[76] and a way of evaluating processes to identify activities that can be improved, substituted, or eliminated. Furthermore, by understanding the true cost of a service, HSOs/HSs and individual practitioners, such as physicians, can make better strategic and tactical pricing decisions, determine whether a service is really profitable, and know more precisely what resources are needed to provide it.[77] In addition, providers are better able to evaluate services, programs, and managed care contracts. Data can contribute to CQI evaluation because the process input costs are more easily recognized.

Financial Statements

All HSO/HS activity is eventually translated into its financial statements. The two most important are the income statement and the balance sheet. Both are indispensable for management control. Table 10.6 presents income statements and balance sheets for the years 1993 and 1997 for the U.S. hospital industry. They are composite averages prepared by the Center for Healthcare Industry Performance Studies (CHIPS) based on data from a sample of 1,500 voluntary not-for-profit hospitals (excluding investor-owned and specialty hospitals).[78] The income statement presents revenues and expenditures for a 1-year period, including the excess of revenues over expenditures (i.e., profit). Gross revenues usually are presented in categories such as inpatient, outpatient, premium, and other revenues, such as those from grants, investments, and auxiliary operations. Premium revenues are those earned from capitated contracts. Gross revenues are those that the HSO/HS would have received if everyone paid full price (i.e., charges). However, most third-party payers negotiate prices as a percentage of charges. The difference between charges and negotiated price as well as the value of charity care are discounts and contractual allowances that are deducted from gross revenue. Thus net patient revenue is what the HSO/HS actually received for the services it provided.[79]

The balance sheet presents the assets, both current and fixed, and the liabilities and equity of the organization. From these statements, management can identify for control purposes profitability (such as profit margin, return on investment, and return on equity), capital structure risk (such as debt to assets), and asset utilization efficiency (e.g., fixed and total asset turnover, accounts receivable collection period, inventory turnover). (A discussion of these measures can be found in "Financial Analysis.")

Ratio Analysis

The language that is common to all organizations is numerically expressed data. For example, HSOs/HSs are described by number and type of beds, by number and type of employees, and by size and specialty mix of members of the professional staff organization; they are evaluated, in part, by number of patients admitted, procedures performed, and expenditures.

Managers use similar data to control (monitor) the HSO's/HS's functioning and how well it is accomplished. This may be done by comparing any activity to predetermined standards or by ratio analysis. The latter involves evaluating the relationship between two pieces of data that may be expressed as an index or a percentage. They are simple measures and typically occur in two modes: point specific and longitudinal. In general, the analysis is applied to two areas, operational-activity and financial status.[80]

TABLE 10.6. COMPOSITE AVERAGE INCOME STATEMENT AND BALANCE SHEET, U.S. HOSPITAL INDUSTRY, 1993, 1997[a]

	1993	1997	Annual growth rate
Income Statement			
Revenues			
Net patient revenue	$62,595	$77,361	5.4%
Premium revenue	0	1,153	Inf.
Other revenue	4,293	6,715	11.8%
Total revenues	$66,888	$85,229	6.1%
Expenses			
Interest expense	1,407	1,529	2.1%
Depreciation & amortization	3,481	4,641	7.5%
Bad debt expense	3,107	3,982	6.4%
Other expense	56,076	69,687	5.6%
Total expenses	$64,071	$79,839	5.7%
Excess of revenues over expenses (profit)	2,817	5,390	17.6%
+ Other equity changes	(112)	1,180	Inf.
Increase in equity	$2,705	$6,570	24.8%
Balance Sheet			
Assets			
Cash & short-term investments	$6,009	$9,462	12.0%
Accounts receivable	11,189	13,103	4.0%
Inventory	934	1,136	5.0%
Other current assets	1,772	2,733	11.4%
Total current assets	$19,904	$26,434	7.4%
Net fixed assets	32,634	41,416	6.1%
Replacement funds	12,936	22,166	14.4%
Other assets	7,047	10,694	11.0%
Total assets	$72,521	$100,710	8.6%
Liabilities & equity			
Current liabilities	$10,594	$14,230	7.7%
Long-term debt	23,235	26,991	3.8%
Other liabilities	3,303	4,999	10.9%
Equity	35,389	54,490	11.4%
Total liabilities & equity	$72,521	$100,710	8.6%

From Center for Healthcare Industry Performance Studies. *The 1998–1999 Almanac of Hospital Financial and Operating Indicators*, 4–5. Columbus, OH: Center for Healthcare Industry Performance Studies, 1998; reprinted by permission.

[a] Data in thousands.

Operational-Activity Analysis

Operational-activity analysis is a control method that involves the evaluation of any activity—input, process, or output variable—that is of interest to the manager and that can be expressed numerically. Control charts are one form of operational-activity analysis. Control charts have predetermined standards—upper and lower control limits—that can be developed for any form of unit volume or measurable product or service attribute. Data tracking will identify both common cause variation and special cause variation. Figure 9.7 includes a control chart for patient waiting time in the admitting department. Other types of control charts could include portion size of meals, age of blood in the blood bank, or time to answer incoming telephone calls.

Another method for operational-activity analysis is through the use and evaluation of nonfinancial indices expressed as ratios or percentages. Managers can design any type of operational-activity ratio (or percentage index) to meet specific control needs as long as it can be expressed in numerical terms. Such ratios are valuable in controlling because they can be used as point-specific input, conversion, and output standards and as indicators of improvement, and they can be tracked and compared longitudinally to show trends. The variety and derivations of such ratios are endless. Three broad categories are performance-utilization ratios, input-to-output ratios, and key indicator ratios.

Performance-utilization ratios provide index information about specific activities such as inventory turnover by area (dietary services, pharmacy, general stores, laboratory), inventory dollar value per occupied bed, percentage of readmissions, and personnel turnover and absenteeism by area or type of employee. These ratios also yield information about capacity utilization, such as average length of stay, percentage occupancy, and efficient use of space and time (surgical suites, clinics, emergency department, radiology). Finally, they can provide indices of specific process outputs usually expressed in patient days or some other common denominator—for example, radiographs per admission, laboratory tests per patient day, clinic visits per day, pounds of laundry processed per occupied bed, and full-time employee equivalents (FTEs) per occupied bed.

Input-to-output ratios are indicators of resource consumption. They relate specific measures of resource use to units of output. Examples include the whole range of labor hours per unit of service, such as nursing hours per patient day, radiographs per radiology technician hour, and square feet cleaned per housekeeping hour. Others are total revenue to FTE, cost per discharge, and cost per patient day.

Key indicator ratios fall outside the previous two groups but are important to control. Incident ratios yield inferences about quality. Examples are patient incidents and injuries per 100 patient days, percentage of incomplete medical records 30 days after discharge, gross and net death rates, anesthesia deaths per 10,000 surgical procedures, infection rates, and percentage of normal tissue removed in operative procedures. Other key indicator ratios include patient mix by type of payer, average age of clinical staff or mix by specialty, and patient origin by service area segment.

This discussion of performance-utilization, input-to-output, and key indicator ratio groupings is not exhaustive, but it does illustrate that ratios can be derived by comparing any two sets of numbers. When used in control, ratio analysis should address two issues. First, does the ratio make sense? Many do, some do not—the ratio of maintenance expenditures per Medicare patient day is meaningless. Managers must evaluate the underlying derivation of the ratio, what it measures, and its meaning. Second, judgment must be used in interpreting results. Particularly important is assessing the many causes of single-point deviation (that occurring at one point) or longitudinal deviation (change over time). Ratios are only one of many indicators that show how actual results deviate from desired results at the input, process, or output points. The cause of the deviation must be investigated, understood, and corrected, if necessary. Blindly using ratios without evaluation may result in inappropriate conclusions and intervention and, perhaps, undesirable consequences.

Data Analysis Services

Data analysis services that provide comparative performance-utilization, input-to-output, key indicator, financial, and productivity and efficiency analyses for hospitals are available from vendors. CHIPS has already been mentioned; another is HCIA.[81] Both sources provide industry data for a large number of performance indicators. Reports for a specific hospital can be generated to show its change in indicators longitudinally over time, be tailored to benchmark against similar hospitals, and even present specific hospital and comparative results for virtually all departments. Furthermore, both CHIPS and HCIA provide industry indicators by various classifications such as bed size, urban-rural, region, state, teaching-nonteaching, system affiliation, and national averages. The combinations are almost endless.

Table 10.7 presents a summary of 57 performance measures for all U.S. hospitals in the HCIA database by percentile (top [75th], middle [50th], and lower [25th]) groups for 1992–1996.[82] The 50th percentile group is the median. The categories of indicators are capacity and utilization, patient and payer mix, capital structure, liquidity, revenues and expenses, productivity and efficiency, and pricing strategies. Table 10.7 reveals that a median-sized U.S. nongovernmental hospital in 1996 had 114 acute care beds in service, 4,243 discharges, an average occupancy rate of 44.17%, and an average length of stay of 4.18 days, with Medicare discharges representing 43.54% of all discharges. Such a hospital had an average age of plant of 9.26 years, a current ratio of 2.05, gross revenue per adjusted discharge of $7,695, and 5.28 FTEs per adjusted average daily census.

Benchmarking

Benchmarking involves comparative analysis to determine performance in areas such as operational and clinical outcomes relative to reference standards and industry "best practices."[83] Most often the comparison of performance or outcome measures is to HSOs/HSs with similar characteristics. Both HCIA and CHIPS provide benchmark data such as those presented in Table 10.7; they also provide "best practices" reference information. In addition, benchmarking can occur internally, as in the case of a horizontally integrated HS that compares system hospitals' performance with one another. For control purposes, benchmarking provides standards against which comparisons can be made. Further information about benchmarking appears in Chapter 9.

Information from data services is valuable because reports are very extensive, and the HSO/HS can choose the other institutions to be used for comparison. Furthermore, point-specific as well as longitudinal information that is useful for controlling the HSO's/HS's activities is available to managers.

Financial Analysis

If data expressed in numerical terms represent the common language of organizations, their lifeblood is finance as it relates to the value of resources. Financial ratio analysis is the process of calculating and evaluating various indices that measure the HSO's/HS's financial status: its risk exposure, activity, and profitability. The accepted conventions for these measures typically are grouped into four categories, as summarized in Table 10.8[84]:

1. Liquidity ratios are risk measures that refer to the organization's ability to meet short-term obligations. Included are current ratio, acid test (also called quick ratio), and accounts receivables collection period.
2. Capital structure ratios are also risk measures. They reflect the ratio of debt (borrowed funds) to total capital structure and, in the case of investor-owned HSOs/HSs, the proportion of debt to owners' investment (equity). In general, higher debt ratio(s) mean greater leverage and higher risk. Other risk-measuring ratios include cash flow to debt and times interest earned.
3. Activity ratios are turnover measures that reflect asset utilization. In a sense, this is the degree to which various categories of assets generate revenues. Those presented in Table 10.8 compare operating revenues to total, net fixed, and current assets as well as to inventory.
4. Profitability ratios are indicators of the HSO's/HS's performance expressed in financial terms. Particularly critical measures are deductions (allowances for contractual adjustments and uncollectible accounts), operating margin, nonoperating revenue contribution, and return on assets. A measure that is important to investor-owned organizations is return on equity (operating income plus interest divided by stockholders' equity).

Financial and other data analysis services for comparison purposes are available from vendors. Table 10.9 presents an executive summary report of a number of financial control measures for a sample

CHIPS hospital. The hospital's results are presented for 1993–1997 and compared with the median value for all not-for-profit, nongovernmental hospitals in Ohio.[85] Included are profitability, liquidity, capital structure, asset efficiency, and other financial ratios. Just as with the national hospital industry indicators presented in Table 10.7, such data can be obtained by various classifications for comparison purposes, such as by hospital bed size, urban-rural, region, state, teaching-nonteaching, system affiliation, and national averages.

Viewing the hospital financial ratios in Table 10.9, in 1997 the sample hospital had a total margin of –1.1% (as compared with the median for Ohio hospitals of 6.4%); earnings before interest, depreciation, and amortization to assets of 7.2% (versus 11.8%); current ratio of 2.03 (versus 1.96); equity financing of 46.6% (versus 60.6%); and total asset turnover of 0.97 (versus 0.90).

USE OF ANALYTICAL TECHNIQUES IN RESOURCE ALLOCATION

Converting inputs to outputs requires allocation and use of resources. One dimension of control is determining whether such allocation and use are appropriate and meet expectations. One dimension of control is improving processes to more efficiently use resources. It is imperative that managers understand the wide range of analytical techniques that is available as they make decisions about allocating resources, using resources, and improving processes.

Analytical techniques are methods or procedures that systematically arrange and permit the evaluation of information in a specific fashion. They help managers focus on important considerations and judge them against criteria. Results are expressed in objective terms. The problem-solving model in Figure 7.4 shows that analytical techniques are useful in evaluating and selecting alternatives, especially those concerning resource allocation. It should be remembered that nonquantitative considerations are important when evaluating alternatives and that only when both nonquantitative and quantitative measures are included do effective problem solving and decision making occur. Analytical techniques are the predominant means for deriving objective information.

Analytical techniques can be used to evaluate the allocation and utilization of resources for new projects and the improvement of existing processes. Those techniques described in the following sections are volume analysis (with and without revenue as a variable), capital budgeting, cost–benefit analysis, and simulation. Volume analysis with revenue as a variable is used to evaluate the economic viability of an alternative, such as adding a service or buying equipment. When revenue is not a variable, volume analysis can be used to evaluate alternatives with different fixed and variable cost characteristics and to evaluate the resource implications of improving an existing process. Capital budgeting is a ranking method that is used to compare several proposed alternatives. Cost–benefit analysis identifies and compares the resource consequences of two or more proposed alternatives, one of which can be an existing situation. Finally, simulation yields "what if" information about the resource consequences of changes in existing situations—such as adding staff to decrease patient waiting time or modifying the flow of a process—without actually making a change. Analytical techniques not included here but that are also used are decision matrix analysis, inventory analysis, linear programming, queuing, network analysis, and statistical techniques such as regression, forecasting, and hypothesis testing.[86] Table 10.10 provides brief descriptions of some of these techniques.

Volume Analysis with Revenue

Volume analysis with revenue as a variable is often called breakeven analysis. It is one of the simplest analytical techniques available to evaluate the economic viability of a proposed alternative

TABLE 10.7. PERCENTILE VALUES FOR THE 57 PERFORMANCE MEASURES, ALL HOSPITALS

Percentile	1996 75th	1996 50th	1996 25th	1995 75th	1995 50th	1995 25th	1994 25th	1994 50th	1994 75th	1993 50th	1992 50th
CAPACITY & UTILIZATION											
Beds in Service, Acute Care	222	114	55	227	116	56	57	119	235	121	122
Total Discharges, Acute Care	9,586	4,243	1,707	9,618	4,280	1,743	1,742	4,234	9,515	4,244	4,359
Occupancy Rate (%)	58.68	44.17	28.84	59.89	45.33	29.62	30.75	47.14	61.73	48.08	50.00
Average Length of Stay	4.97	4.18	3.51	5.17	4.33	3.62	3.80	4.58	5.49	4.79	4.95
ALOS, Case Mix-Adjusted	3.79	3.20	2.75	3.96	3.37	2.88	3.06	3.61	4.25	3.80	3.95
ALOS, Medicare	6.47	5.52	4.64	6.87	5.84	4.86	5.14	6.28	7.40	6.63	6.95
ALOS, Non-Medicare	3.89	3.15	2.62	3.98	3.23	2.66	2.81	3.40	4.19	3.55	3.67
PATIENT & PAYER MIX											
% Medicare Discharges	52.30	43.54	34.51	51.86	42.58	33.72	33.36	41.81	51.03	40.55	39.47
% Medicaid Discharges	20.31	13.01	7.65	20.83	13.56	8.09	8.00	13.70	21.46	13.99	13.88
% Medicare Acute Care Days	65.20	57.48	47.59	65.41	57.77	47.66	47.87	57.55	64.72	56.23	55.42
% Medicaid Acute Care Days	15.52	9.80	5.92	15.99	10.12	6.12	6.07	10.13	15.94	10.13	10.08
% Special Care Days	12.96	9.38	6.17	12.77	9.02	5.99	5.79	8.68	12.28	8.42	8.16
Medicare Case Mix Index	1.4304	1.2722	1.1389	1.4166	1.2603	1.1296	1.1191	1.2480	1.4006	1.2384	1.2277
% Outpatient Revenue	48.06	39.15	30.37	45.98	37.24	28.90	27.16	34.85	42.90	33.00	31.15
CAPITAL STRUCTURE											
Average Age of Plant	11.64	9.26	7.34	11.37	9.04	7.14	6.83	8.78	11.28	8.58	8.40
Net PP&E per Bed ($)	176,755	111,416	61,473	164,609	105,038	57,095	54,259	99,697	156,359	93,854	88,124
Debt per Bed ($)	194,879	103,962	42,252	185,538	100,761	41,478	40,441	99,480	179,547	94,333	88,197
% Capital Costs	9.13	7.19	5.44	9.46	7.24	5.49	5.61	7.43	9.76	7.43	7.42
Capital Costs per Adj Disch ($)	501	346	233	506	342	219	223	347	523	342	325
LT Debt to Total Assets	0.42	0.29	0.14	0.44	0.30	0.16	0.16	0.32	0.47	0.32	0.33
LT Debt to Net Fixed Assets	0.99	0.63	0.33	1.00	0.65	0.34	0.35	0.69	1.04	0.70	0.69
LT Debt to Capitalization	0.50	0.34	0.17	0.53	0.36	0.18	0.20	0.38	0.56	0.39	0.40
Cash Flow to Total Debt	0.47	0.26	0.15	0.47	0.26	0.16	0.15	0.24	0.42	0.25	0.25
Debt Service Coverage Ratio	10.20	4.70	2.38	8.54	4.20	2.25	2.07	3.77	7.36	3.55	3.46
LIQUIDITY											
Current Ratio	3.05	2.05	1.44	3.01	2.04	1.44	1.45	2.07	3.00	2.06	2.09
Acid Test Ratio	0.91	0.38	0.10	0.91	0.36	0.09	0.09	0.33	0.84	0.32	0.30
Days in Net Accounts Receivable	80.56	66.89	55.18	80.65	67.14	55.30	56.75	68.66	83.14	68.58	71.80
Average Payment Period	75.97	57.16	42.32	75.26	55.69	42.36	41.37	55.06	74.00	54.59	54.24
Days Cash on Hand	n/a	n/a	n/a	119.25	54.56	14.18	12.17	48.69	108.78	46.20	44.17

REVENUES & EXPENSES

Gross Rev per Adj Disch ($)	11,101	7,695	5,655	10,767	7,425	5,343	0,469	7,227	5,157	6,886	6,357
Gross Rev per Adj Disch* ($)	8,160	6,555	5,359	7,968	6,308	5,143	7,792	6,205	4,996	5,981	5,574
Operating Rev per Adj Disch ($)	6,467	4,972	3,960	6,311	4,812	3,763	6,201	4,741	3,692	4,600	4,356
Expense per Adj Disch ($)	6,124	4,736	3,762	6,000	4,600	3,608	5,951	4,539	3,551	4,424	4,228
Expense per Adj Disch* ($)	4,684	4,033	3,494	4,578	3,915	3,388	4,566	3,915	3,386	3,864	3,673
Lab Cost per Adj Disch** ($)	322	258	205	320	258	209	326	263	214	268	262
Radiology Cost per Adj Disch** ($)	303	234	181	299	231	176	300	232	181	230	226
Pharmacy Cost per Adj Disch** ($)	257	202	157	253	200	156	258	205	161	202	193
Admin Cost per Adj Disch ($)	798	569	416	788	555	404	764	546	399	526	496
% Deductions from Gross Rev	45.64	36.87	28.95	45.18	36.61	28.69	44.26	35.82	27.73	34.33	32.58
Operating Profit Margin (%)	7.95	3.84	0.29	7.78	3.89	0.66	7.04	3.37	0.30	3.12	3.03
Total Profit Margin (%)	9.67	5.37	1.63	9.27	5.31	1.87	8.25	4.44	1.30	4.32	4.46
Cash Flow Margin (%)	16.74	12.24	7.76	16.69	12.36	8.29	15.71	11.66	7.78	11.65	12.02
Return on Assets (%)	9.11	5.34	1.66	9.09	5.34	2.09	8.18	4.50	1.45	4.46	4.53
Cash Flow per Bed ($)	52,742	30,304	13,932	49,172	29,580	13,606	2,856	25,579	12,666	23,719	23,205

PRODUCTIVITY & EFFICIENCY

FTEs per Adj Avg Daily Census	6.22	5.28	4.48	6.07	5.20	4.41	5.94	5.07	4.34	4.98	4.81
FTEs per 100 Adj Disch	7.31	6.02	4.98	7.38	6.04	5.04	7.59	6.26	5.25	6.43	6.48
FTEs per 100 Adj Disch**	5.57	4.70	4.01	5.61	4.79	4.08	5.86	5.02	4.27	5.16	5.21
Salary & Benefits Exp per FTEs ($)	45,606	39,883	34,696	44,255	38,410	33,441	2,441	36,825	32,057	35,230	33,363
% Salary and Benefits Expense	55.49	50.47	45.12	55.70	50.70	45.55	56.07	51.01	45.88	51.29	51.67
% Overhead Expense	36.42	32.71	29.26	37.00	33.22	29.87	37.60	33.88	30.60	34.15	34.49
Discharges per Bed	46.77	37.02	26.60	46.18	36.98	26.54	14.41	36.13	26.04	35.44	35.26
Total Assets Turnover Ratio	1.25	0.96	0.75	1.28	0.98	0.77	1.28	0.99	0.79	1.00	1.00

PRICING STRATEGIES

Markup, All Ancillary Services	2.91	2.39	2.02	2.84	2.36	2.00	2.75	2.29	1.96	2.23	2.16
Markup Ratio, Medical Supplies	3.95	2.73	1.99	3.99	2.73	1.97	3.89	2.69	1.95	2.63	2.54
Markup Ratio, Drugs Sold	4.03	2.99	2.25	3.97	3.01	2.27	3.88	2.97	2.24	2.90	2.82
Markup Ratio, Laboratory	3.30	2.54	1.96	3.22	2.50	1.96	3.09	2.44	1.91	2.35	2.28
Markup Ratio, Diagnostic Radiology	2.85	2.28	1.83	2.73	2.20	1.78	2.55	2.08	1.70	1.99	1.94

From HCIA. *The Comparative Performance of U.S. Hospitals: The Sourcebook,* 12. Baltimore: HCIA, Inc., ▨ reprinted by permission. © 1998 by HCIA Inc. and Deloitte & Touche LLP.

*Case mix– and wage-adjusted; **Case mix-adjusted.

TABLE 10.8. COMMON FINANCIAL RATIOS USED FOR CONTROL

LIQUIDITY

1. Current $= \dfrac{\text{Current Assets}}{\text{Current Liabilities}}$

2. Acid Test $= \dfrac{\text{Cash + Marketable Securities}}{\text{Current Liabilities}}$

3. Collection Period $= \dfrac{\text{Net Accounts Receivable}}{\text{Average Daily Operating Revenue}}$

4. Average Payment Period $= \dfrac{\text{Current Liabilities}}{(\text{Total Operating Expenses} - \text{Depreciation}) \div 365}$

CAPITAL STRUCTURE

5. Long-Term Debt to Fixed Assets $= \dfrac{\text{Long-Term Debt}}{\text{Net Fixed Assets}}$

6. Long-Term Debt to Equity $= \dfrac{\text{Long-Term Debt}}{\text{Unrestricted Fund Balance}}$

7. Times Interest Earned $= \dfrac{\text{Net Income + Interest}}{\text{Interest}}$

8. Debt Service Coverage $= \dfrac{\text{Net Income + Depreciation + Interest}}{\text{Principal Payment + Interest}}$

9. Cash Flow to Debt $= \dfrac{\text{Net Income + Depreciation}}{\text{Total Liabilities}}$

ACTIVITY

10. Total Asset Turnover $= \dfrac{\text{Total Operating Revenue}}{\text{Total Assets}}$

11. Fixed Asset Turnover $= \dfrac{\text{Total Operating Revenue}}{\text{Net Fixed Assets}}$

12. Current Asset Turnover $= \dfrac{\text{Total Operating Revenue}}{\text{Current Assets}}$

13. Inventory Turnover $= \dfrac{\text{Total Operating Revenue}}{\text{Inventory}}$

PROFITABILITY

14. Mark-up $= \dfrac{\text{Gross Patient Revenue}}{\text{Operating Expenses}}$

15. Deductible $= \dfrac{\text{Allowances for Contractual Adjustments and Uncollectible Accounts}}{\text{Gross Patient Revenue}}$

16. Operating Margin $= \dfrac{\text{Operating Income}}{\text{Operating Revenue}}$

17. Nonoperating Revenue Contribution $= \dfrac{\text{Nonoperating Revenue}}{\text{Net Income}}$

18. Return on Assets $= \dfrac{\text{Operating Income + Interest}}{\text{Total Assets}}$

COMPOSITE

19. Viability Index $= \dfrac{[\text{Total Liabilities}]}{[\text{Total Assets}]} \times \dfrac{[\text{Operating Expense}]}{[\text{Operating Revenue}]} \times \dfrac{1}{\text{Current Ratio}} \times 4.0$

From Cleverley, William O. "Financial Ratios: Summary Indicators for Management Decision-Making." *Hospital & Health Services Administration* 26 (Special Issue, 1981): 30–31; reprinted by permission. © 1981, Foundation of the American College of Healthcare Executives, Ann Arbor, MI: Health Administration Press.

TABLE 10.9. HOSPITAL FINANCIAL RATIOS, EXECUTIVE SUMMARY—CHIPS SAMPLE HOSPITAL (COMPARED WITH OHIO)

	1993	1994	1995	1996	1997	1997 median (Ohio)
Profitability ratios						
Total margin	3.6	2.2	−2.4	0.4	−1.1	6.4
EBIDA to revenues	14.9	12.7	7.4	8.9	7.4	13.6
EBIDA to assets	13.1	11.8	6.8	8.6	7.2	11.8
Oper. cash flow to revenue	−3.6	−1.1	−2.6	−2.6	−2.0	3.9
Oper. cash flow to assets	−3.2	−1.0	−2.4	−2.5	−1.9	3.6
Bad debt expense	5.9	6.4	6.5	7.4	7.8	4.4
Reported income index	0.705	0.661	1.108	0.563	−0.531	0.897
Return on investment (PLA)[a]	11.2	10.0	5.7	7.2	6.0	10.0
Return on equity	7.6	4.6	−5.0	0.8	−2.3	9.9
Growth rate in equity	10.8	6.9	−4.5	1.5	4.3	11.5
Economic value added (EVA)	1,534,194	−998,398	−2,871,994	−1,676,301	−1,649,021	540,104
EVA to capital	4.3	−2.7	−8.0	−4.6	4.3	1.0
Liquidity ratios						
Current ratio	1.38	1.67	1.59	1.57	2.03	1.96
Days in accounts receivable	53.5	58.7	63.8	64.3	65.4	66.0
Days in A/R w/3rd party	N/A	N/A	58.4	50.1	61.3	58.4
Average payment period	64.5	54.5	56.5	54.9	42.5	59.0
Days cash on hand, ST sources	24.5	20.2	17.7	9.2	10.1	26.0
Days cash on hand, all sources	137.1	123.2	123.2	112.7	124.0	128.7
Capital structure ratios						
Equity financing	42.1	45.4	43.3	43.1	46.6	60.6
Long-term debt to capitalization	50.8	47.7	49.4	49.4	46.0	26.8
Fixed asset financing	92.4	89.8	90.2	90.8	93.4	53.5
Cash flow to total debt	14.9	13.8	6.0	10.2	8.6	29.7
Capital expense	11.7	10.7	9.7	8.6	8.4	7.5
Times interest earned	1.70	1.48	0.38	1.12	0.62	4.93
Debt service coverage	1.83	1.63	1.23	2.35	2.15	4.26
Cushion ratio	4.17	3.98	5.29	7.66	9.46	10.70
Asset efficiency ratios						
Total asset turnover	0.88	0.93	0.92	0.97	0.97	0.90
Fixed asset turnover	1.88	2.01	1.96	2.09	2.29	2.17
Fixed asset turnover (PLA)[a]	1.38	1.45	1.40	1.45	1.55	1.59
Other asset turnover	2.62	2.83	2.92	3.00	2.74	2.92
Current asset turnover	4.55	4.37	4.32	4.51	4.43	3.68
Inventory ratio	124.06	103.62	105.69	92.50	69.78	77.84
Other financial ratios						
Average age of plant	8.30	9.17	9.80	10.80	11.07	9.86
Depreciation rate	5.9	5.7	5.5	5.1	5.3	5.7
Capital expend. growth rate	57.3	4.4	6.3	5.4	4.1	6.4
Working capital absorption	−0.4	50.5	−1.8	32.7	76.9	11.3
Restricted equity	0.1	0.1	0.1	0.1	0.1	0.4
Replacement viability	40.9	35.0	33.1	31.0	32.7	22.9
Financial flexibility index	1.470	0.323	−1.928	−1.707	−2.044	3.697

From Center for Healthcare Industry Performance Studies. *Financial Performance Report*, 8. Columbus, OH: Center for Healthcare Industry Performance Studies, 1988; reprinted by permission. Copyright © 1998 by the Center for Healthcare Industry Performance Studies.

[a]Price-level adjusted.

TABLE 10.10. QUANTITATIVE TECHNIQUES FOR DECISION ANALYSIS

Technique	Linear programming	Queuing theory	Network analysis	Regression analysis
Description	This technique attempts to optimize the distribution of scarce resources among competing activities. This is accomplished by the maximization or minimization of a dependent variable, which is a function of several independent variables that are subject to a set of restraints, i.e., limited resources. This method is capable of being executed manually, but is very adaptable to solution by a computer.	Queuing theory is the study of the probabilities associated with the length of a waiting line and the time an individual must wait in the queuing system. This information is used to achieve a balance between the cost of waiting for a service and the cost associated with providing this service. "Cost in a medical setting invariably includes elements defined by 'good medical care' which are, at best, difficult to quantify but must be included with monetary cost to obtain the proper solution." In queuing theory, the waiting line may be organized on a first-in–first-out basis, a random basis, or by some other priority technique. The waiting line can have a finite or infinite calling population, and it is assumed that the average service rate is greater than the average arrival rate for a single-channel–single-server queuing model.	Network analysis is characterized by a network of events and activities. Activities are defined as the actual performance of tasks, whereas events represent the start of completion of an activity. Events do not consume time. This technique allows the determination of probabilities of meeting specified deadlines; identifies bottlenecks in the project; evaluates the effect of shifting resources from a noncritical activity to a critical activity and vice versa and enables the manager to evaluate the effect of a deviation of the actual time requirement for an activity from what had been predicted. Specific network analysis models include critical path methods (CPM), program evaluation and review techniques (PERT), and graphical evaluation and review techniques (GERT). The difference between these systems lies in their different abilities to analyze complex network systems.	This is a technique that derives a mathematical equation to describe or express the relationship between the data of two or more variables over a period of time. The variable to predict in this equation is referred to as the dependent variable. The other variables in the equation are called independent variables or predicting variables. The basic measure of the relationship between the dependent variable and the independent variable(s) is depicted by a regression line, which is computed by the method of least squares. This will result in an equation, based on historical data, that will predict the future behavior of the dependent variable. This technique is used primarily for the purpose of forecasting and control.
Hospital applications	Physician, nurse, and patient scheduling problems; purchasing problems associated with hospital supplies and equipment; hospital transportation problems and assignment problems	Determination of the most effective serving system for food service operations, outpatient clinic operations, admission operations, telephone switchboard operations, etc. In each of these situations, queuing theory balances the cost of an individual waiting with the cost of additional facilities that would be incurred to prevent the individual from waiting.	Hospital planning and control efforts associated with building or research and development projects or the determination of flow allocations through a health care system, such as a mass screening facility	Used to forecast dependent variables such as a number of hospital admissions, inpatient days, outpatient days, outpatient visits, average daily census, cost per patient day, etc., and to control deviations from the planned costs associated with each of these variables

508

				Historical data compiled daily, monthly, quarterly, or annually with respect to the dependent and independent variables of the problem
Data required	Manager must express desires in a unidimensional objective function; data that pertain to an objective function expressed in terms of maximization of benefits or minimization of costs, set of constraints, variables, and alternative courses of action	Average number of arrivals per a unit of time; specified unit of time; average service time per arrival; number of waiting lines, number of waiting line phases, and number of people in the waiting line	Data that pertain to the determination of project activities and events; determination of optimistic, pessimistic, and most likely time estimates with associated mean activity times and time required for an activity in terms of probability distribution and associated parameters	
Advantages	Optimum use of productive factors; potential to increase decision quality; highlights problem bottlenecks; forces objectivity and quantification	Description of probabilities that a waiting line will contain a certain number of individuals; expected length of the waiting line and the expected waiting time for the individual	Determination of longest time paths through a network; identification of the relative frequency of occurrence of different paths; evaluation of program changes	Provides accurate forecasts of dependent variables in a three-month to two-year time frame. Allows management to analyze deviations from the planned cost of an activity or event.
Disadvantages	Inability to represent several goals/objectives in a unidimensional objective function; costs associated with data upkeep; homogeneous values in constraints; assumption of linearity	Assumption that both arrival and service completion lines follow a Poisson distribution; upkeep of data	Accurate time forecasts for activities	Cost of data upkeep; assumption of linearity; the assumption that no causal relationship exists between the variables

Excerpted from Helmer, F. Theodore, William H. Kucheman, Edward B. Oppermann, and James D. Suver. "Basic Management Science Techniques for Decision Analysis." *Hospital & Health Service Administration* 27 (March/April 1982): 68–69; reprinted by permission. © 1982, Foundation of the American College of Healthcare Executives, Ann Arbor, MI: Health Administration Press.

involving resource allocation. To use such analysis, identifiable costs and identifiable revenue must be available. Important components of volume analysis with revenue as a variable are

- Identifiable revenues measured by price or charge (P) per unit of output or service (x) (e.g., charge per emergency department, outpatient, or office visit; per laboratory test, electrocardiogram, or radiograph; or per day of hospital or nursing facility stay)
- Identifiable fixed costs (FC)—costs that do not vary with output or volume (e.g., associated capital costs for facility and equipment lease or depreciation, minimum staffing levels)
- Identifiable variable costs (VC)—costs that vary with output or volume (supplies, materials, medications, additional staff beyond minimum levels, overtime)

Three variants of volume analysis yield different results depending on which variables are known. The breakeven model determines the economic viability of an alternative. If fixed and variable costs and price/charge per unit of output/service are known, the breakeven model determines the volume of output/service (x) needed to break even. It should be noted that type of provider reimbursement (fixed, such as DRG; capitated; cost-based; or charges) and payer mix significantly complicate the use of volume analysis.[87] Breaking even occurs when total revenue (price per unit of service times volume) equals total costs (fixed plus variable). The general formula is (solve for x)

$$\text{Breakeven point} = \frac{FC + VC(x)}{P(x)}$$

or

$$(P)(x) - VC(x) = FC$$

$$(P - VC)x = FC$$

$$x = \frac{FC}{P - VC}$$

A second variant of volume analysis is determining the net (positive or negative) contribution (NC) that results from an alternative when price or charge, total volume, and fixed and variable costs are known. Positive net contribution occurs when total revenue (volume times price) exceeds total costs (fixed plus variable); net contribution is negative when total costs exceed total revenue. The general formula is (solve for NC)

$$P(x) = FC + VC(x) + NC$$

or

$$NC = P(x) - [FC + VC(x)]$$

The third variant of volume analysis is to use it as a price- or charge-setting model. If fixed and variable costs and volume are known, the technique yields the price or charge per unit of output/service required to meet end-result criteria ranging from breaking even (where total revenue equals total costs) to attaining a specific net positive contribution. When NC is set at the value desired—which may be zero—the general formula is (solve for P)

$$P(x) = FC + VC(x) + NC$$

or

$$P = \frac{FC + VC(x) + NC}{x}$$

HSOs/HSs encounter many situations with identifiable cost and revenue attributes in which volume analysis can be applied. Examples are acquiring new equipment (magnetic resonance imager, laboratory diagnostic equipment), expanding facilities (new beds, parking deck), adding new services (neonatology, open heart surgery), and embarking on new ventures (emergency care center, ambulatory surgery center, physicians' office building). Depending on known variables or assumptions made about them, volume analysis can determine economic viability. Will the project break even? Will it have a net positive or negative contribution? Volume analysis also can be used as a price-setting model to meet specific criteria (i.e., break even or yield a net positive contribution). Figure 10.8 provides an example: A freestanding satellite urgent care center is proposed by a hospital. Fixed costs (building and equipment depreciation, minimum staffing levels) are $600,000/year. Variable costs (supplies and materials) per patient visit are assumed to be $20. The average price/charge per patient visit is $80. Volume analysis can be used to determine what number of pa-

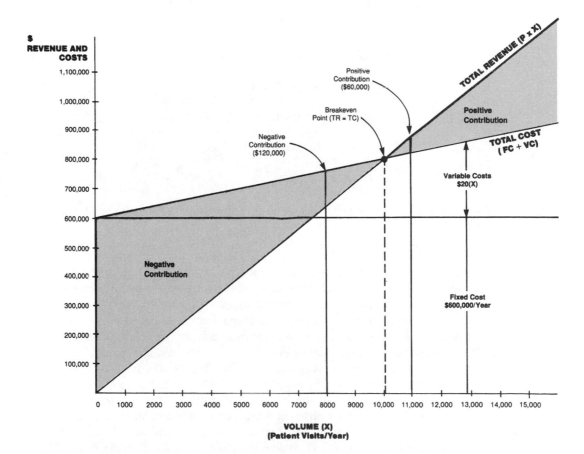

Figure 10.8.   Urgent care center volume analysis.

tient visits per year (or per day) will be necessary to break even. This is determined as follows (solve for x):

$$P(x) = FC + VC(x)$$

$$\$80(x) = \$600,000 + \$20(x)$$

$$\$60(x) = \$600,000$$

$$x = \frac{\$600,000}{\$60}$$

$$x = 10,000$$

Thus, to break even, 10,000 patient visits per year (28/day) will be necessary.

If other information (knowledge about competition, population in the service area) is available, the decision maker can judge whether it is reasonable to expect 10,000 patient visits per year (28/day) and determine the economic viability of the project. If only 8,000 patient visits can be expected each year, the net (negative) contribution would be –$120,000 as indicated in Figure 10.8. Algebraically, this is determined as follows (solve for NC):

$$P(x) = FC + VC(x) + NC$$

$$\$80\,(8,000) = \$600,000 + \$20\,(8,000) + NC$$

$$\$60\,(8,000) = \$600,000 + NC$$

$$\$480,000 = \$600,000 + NC$$

$$NC = \$480,000 + (-\$600,000)$$

$$NC = -\$120,000$$

Similarly, if volume were 11,000 patient visits per year, net (positive) revenue would be $60,000.

Volume Analysis without Revenue

Often, HSOs/HSs have alternative situations that do not have an identifiable revenue attribute but do have volume and fixed and variable cost attributes. Volume analysis without revenue is useful to evaluate and compare cost consequences of alternatives with one another. It may be used in situations in which there is no revenue or when revenue is indeterminate. Because revenue is not a variable, the analysis focuses on fixed and variable cost trade-offs among volume alternatives.

Figure 10.9 illustrates the concept. Renting one of two copying machines is under consideration. Machine A is slow (10 copies per minute) and leases for $200/month (fixed cost). Machine B is faster (30 copies per minute) and leases for $600/month. Machine A has a lower fixed cost than Machine B ($FC_a < FC_b$); however, the variable cost of staff waiting at the machine while photocopying is higher ($VC_a > VC_b$). Given the different fixed and variable cost attributes, the preferred alternative is different at various volume levels. If volume is x_1, then Machine A is preferred because total costs are lower ($TC_{a1} < TC_{b1}$). If volume is x_2, then Machine B is preferred ($TC_{b2} < TC_{a2}$). Alternative preference is thus dependent on the extent to which there are fixed and variable cost trade-offs relative to volume.

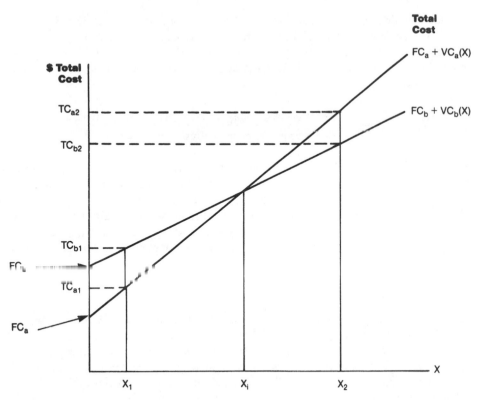

Figure 10.9.   Volume analysis without revenue.

Volume analysis without revenue is powerful because it focuses on the relationship of cost components to volume alternatives. Applications include equipment replacement and machine/technology-people substitution. As larger portions of HSO/HS revenues are prospectively determined by case (i.e., DRGs) or capitated, alternative evaluation from a cost trade-off perspective becomes important.

Capital Budgeting

Capital budgeting commonly refers to several techniques to evaluate, compare, and rank multiple capital investment alternatives or to compare single alternatives to a given criterion such as rate of return. The degree of sophistication ranges from simply determining payback period to complex evaluations of revenue and cost streams that are discounted to net present value.[88]

Payback is an uncomplicated capital budgeting technique because it does not consider the net present value of revenue and cost streams for investment alternatives under consideration. It simply determines the number of years that are needed to recoup an initial investment and yields a gross index of the desirability of investment alternatives. In any comparison of multiple investment alternatives, the one with the shortest payback period (lowest index) is preferred. Results, however, are distorted if revenue and cost streams are dissimilar and the useful life of alternatives differs appreciably. Type of provider payment and payer mix also affect the analysis. A more precise ranking index is the net present value of alternatives.

In payback analysis, necessary components for each alternative are

Identifiable annual revenue generated
Identifiable annual costs
Identifiable investment and salvage value

The payback technique has two basic elements. The first is net investment; initial cost minus salvage value. The second is annual net benefit from the investment, if selected. Net benefit is determined by revenues generated minus operating expenses. Dividing net investment by net benefit determines the number of years to return the cost of the investment. The general formula for the payback period is

$$\text{Payback period} = \frac{(\text{Cost of the proposed investment}) - (\text{Salvage value})}{(\text{Revenue generated from investment}) - (\text{Operating expenses})}$$

It should be noted that payback is used predominantly to rank and compare multiple capital investment alternatives—whether to acquire personal computers for managers or fetal monitoring equipment—or alternatives for the same use—which vendor's personal computers to acquire. If investment, cost, and revenue streams are discounted to present value (and assuming a given rate of interest), then a new present value index that is similar to the payback index can be used to rank alternatives. Applications in general involve equipment or facility expansion alternatives such as adding or replacing equipment, building a parking deck or an office building, or expanding facilities.

Cost–Benefit Analysis

Conceptually, cost–benefit analysis, which is "an evaluation of the relationship between benefits and costs of a particular project or program,"[89] is similar to payback analysis. However, unlike payback analysis, a capital budgeting technique, cost–benefit analysis may be used whether or not there is an identifiable revenue stream. Used widely to evaluate government programs, such as the cost–benefit of infant immunization or federally supported prenatal care, cost–benefit analysis also can be applied to HSOs/HSs.

Cost–benefit analysis has wide applicability in almost all areas of a HSO's/HS's operations and can readily be used in making process improvement decisions. It involves comparing two or more alternatives to each other, one of which may be an existing situation. Cost components are required; a revenue component can be incorporated if present, although revenues are not required to perform the analysis.

Important components in analysis are

- Identifiable imputed or actual costs that are associated with the proposed alternatives (one of which may be an existing situation)
- Identifiable changes in productivity (and imputed value of the productivity) that represent cost savings that are associated with the proposed alternatives (one of which may be an existing situation)
- Identifiable changes in revenue that are associated with the proposed alternatives (this variable is not required to perform the analysis)
- Other considerations that may not be quantifiable

Costs that are associated with an alternative, which may be actual or imputed, can include capital expenditures for equipment, space, employees, and materials and supplies. Net benefit is the marginal difference between the components listed previously for each of the proposed alternatives. That is, net benefit equals Alternative A minus Alternative B for the previous components. If the net benefit is positive, this suggests that the proposed alternative is preferred. However, other nonquantifiable considerations, such as the impact on customer satisfaction or organizational control, may suggest acceptance of a particular alternative even though it may have higher costs, fewer benefits, or both. In this instance the decision maker must evaluate the importance of the nonquantifiable considerations and whether they outweigh the quantifiable results.

Applications of cost–benefit analysis exist in virtually every area and operational activity of HSOs/HSs. Examples include evaluating the cost/benefit of using disposable versus nondisposable tableware in the cafeteria, computer system upgrading, owning or leasing a phone system, or contract outsourcing to vendors for present in-house services such as IS, housekeeping, or food service. Applications can occur in any situation with identified or imputed costs and benefits (which may be revenue based but more often are cost-savings based) associated with different alternatives, one of which may be the existing situation.

Table 10.11 shows an application of cost–benefit analysis. Community Memorial Medical Center, a 211-bed facility, is considering two alternatives. Alternative A involves upgrading its existing computer information system to include more sophisticated cost accounting and decision support capability. Alternative B is to outsource this application to a vendor. Table 10.11 indicates that Alternative A would require Community Memorial Medical Center to make a one-time expenditure for additional hardware of $4,000; pay software purchasing/licensing fees of $75,865 in the first year and $15,173/year thereafter; incur annual costs of standards maintenance of $15,628 starting in the second year and inflated thereafter; and add one new FTE at an annual cost of $56,250, which is inflated in subsequent years. Alternative B, outsourcing, would require an initial monthly fee of $5,055, (composed of a base of $4,000 plus a volume charge of $5 per adjusted occupied bed) during the first year, which totals $60,660, and is inflated in subsequent years.

TABLE 10.11. COMMUNITY MEMORIAL MEDICAL CENTER, ANYTOWN, USA (211 ADJUSTED OCCUPIED BEDS)[a]

	Year 1	Year 2	Year 3	Year 4	Year 5	Year 6	Year 7
Alternative A: medical center–related costs							
Annual costs							
Computer hardware	4,000						
Software license	75,865	15,173	15,173	15,173	15,173	15,173	15,173
Annual cost standards maintenance (starts in second year)		15,628	16,097	16,580	17,077	17,590	18,117
Added client staff costs (1 FTE)	56,250	57,938	59,676	61,466	63,310	65,209	67,165
Total package cost per year	136,115	88,739	90,946	93,219	95,560	97,972	100,456
Discounted annual cost— medical center related	136,115	82,165	77,971	74,000	70,240	66,678	63,304
Alternative B: outsourcing costs [b]							
Service fee for 12 months	60,660	62,480	64,354	66,285	68,273	70,322	72,431
Discounted annual cost—outsourcing	60,660	57,852	55,173	52,619	50,183	47,860	45,644

	Alternative A: medical center	Alternative B: outsourcing	Cost–benefit A–B	Savings (%) (A–B) ÷ A
Summary of life cycle costs				
5-Year sum of discounted costs	440,491	276,487	164,004	37.2%
7-Year sum of discounted costs	570,474	369,991	200,483	35.1%

[a]All amounts in U.S. dollars. Assumptions:
1. Annual increase in CPI — 3.0%
2. Discount rate — 8.0%
3. Annual cost of 1 FTE with benefits — $56,250
4. Annual software maintenance percent — 20.0%

[b]Outsourcing pricing formula:
1. Number of adjusted occupied beds (AOB) — 211
2. Volume charge per bed (VOL) — $5
3. Monthly service fee = $4,000 + (VOL*AOB) — $5,055

Table 10.11 presents the stream of costs—discounted to present value—for both alternatives with the assumptions that annual inflation measured by the Consumer Price Index will be 3.0%; the discount rate will be 8%; and the annual cost standards maintenance will increase 3%/year, starting with the second year. Evaluation of the 5- and 7-year sums of discounted costs for both alternatives indicates that outsourcing (Alternative B) is more cost-effective for both time periods. Over a 5-year time period, outsourcing, compared to the in-house alternative, would save $164,004; it would save $200,483 for the 7-year time period. Given this information, a logical decision would be to outsource the cost accounting and decision support applications. However, a nonquantitative consideration should be whether the HSO wants to be dependent on an outside vendor for such critical information.

Simulation

Simulation is one of the most powerful analytical tools available to health services managers in making resource allocation decisions and in determining whether and how processes can be improved. It enables managers to ask "what if" questions and review the implications and consequences of alternatives without altering the present situation.

Simulation involves constructing a detailed, computer-based mathematical model representing situations and variables. The model has detailed rules that each variable follows as it interacts with the "system," which may be a work process such as diagnostic testing or surgery and recovery. (The simulation literature uses the term *system* to denote such a process, and that term is used here.) The simulation model replicates and reflects variables in the system, and it is constructed using mathematical expressions of relationships, attributes, and probability distributions of events derived from empirical observations of the system. The model is activated by use of a random number generator to represent events, such as admission, arrival for service, a particular type of surgical case, and length of stay.

Simulation models are dynamic. When variables, rules, or assumptions are changed, the model produces the consequences of that change. When no change is made in the relationships of variables in the model (static state), simulation can forecast the effect of increased demand on the system and suggest what resource allocation and capacity changes are needed to meet the desired level of quality. In a dynamic state, variable relationships can be changed, "what if" questions can be asked, and the results will indicate whether and how systems can be improved to enhance the quality of a product or service.

Simulation is applicable to any activity that involves scheduling and service rates and capacity constraints, for both physical plant and staffing.[90] Examples are admissions, operating room,[91] emergency department, diagnostic testing, clinics, ancillary services, bed planning, and nurse staffing.[92]

To solve a capacity problem and to increase patient satisfaction, a simulation model for diagnostic testing was designed for a 500-bed acute care hospital. Management was concerned about the quality of patient service, specifically complaints about waiting times in radiology.[93] The simulation model depicted arrival, processing, and waiting times for eight types of inpatients and outpatients. Procedures tracked included fluoroscopy, radioisotope scanning, computed tomography (CT) scan, and ultrasound. Distributions of arrival rates by type of patient and service times by type of procedure were constructed by observing the actual system. The simulation determined the effects of various capacity changes on queues and patient waiting time. Figure 10.10 shows the results of simulating changes in capacity—increasing the number of radiologists (note the scale is reversed and the *x* axis should be read right to left). Patient waiting time before the start of service decreased substantially (approximately 22 minutes for all four procedures) when capacity was increased from five to six radiologists. Increasing the number of radiologists provided the largest marginal gain for all capacity configurations. Only a modest decrease in waiting time (about 6 minutes) occurred when a seventh radiologist was added.[94] This simulation provided "what if" information

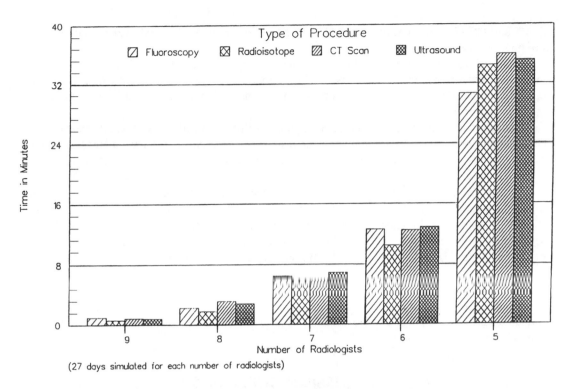

Figure 10.10.   Patient wait time by procedure (excludes processing time); average wait time for greater than zero. (Based on data from Klafehn, Keith A., Paul J. Kuzdrall, Jonathon S. Rakich, and Alan G. Krigline. "Application of Simulation in Hospital Resource Allocation and Utilization." *Journal of Management Science & Policy Analysis* 8 [Spring/Summer 1991]: 346–356.)

useful in deciding whether and how to alter a capacity-bound process. Such information enables managers to make more informed resource allocation and utilization decisions.

The power of simulation as an analytical technique in resource allocation and utilization and in process improvement is evident. To the extent that health services managers are generally familiar with it and the other techniques presented here, they can positively affect the quality of output, improve the processes that generate it, make more informed resource allocation decisions, and control to ensure that actual results meet or exceed expected results.

SUMMARY

The management function of control involves gathering information about and monitoring HSO/HS activities, comparing actual and expected results, and intervening with corrective action as appropriate by introducing change in inputs or process. Control depends on planning. Preestablished standards and expectations of performance and results are based on organizational plans and objectives. The three control monitoring points are outputs, in which control is retrospective; processes, in which it may be concurrent; and inputs, in which control may be prospective. The control model in Figure 10.2 integrates CQI and uses a systematic approach to control in HSOs/HSs. The positive control loop, in which desirable organizational work results/performance exceed standards/expectations, suggests the CQI philosophy—determine why good results occur, replicate them elsewhere, and encourage continued improvement.

Control depends on information. Cost allocation methods such as ABC, MIS, and CIS are critical if managers are to plan, solve problems, control, and appropriately allocate and utilize resources.

MDSS and CDSS permit managers and clinicians to exercise greater control over the HSO's/HS's activities and the quality of care.

RM is a structured, programmatic control method important in HSOs. PI has elements of control and is partially or fully integrated with RM. The methodology and philosophy of PI, however, focuses on improving processes and thereby avoids the inspection approach that is inherent in most traditional control activities.

Control is not happenstance. Budgeting is the most prevalent of the traditional control methods. Budgets are numerical plans that show the resources that are available for the HSO's/HS's activities and plans. Other important control methods presented are operational-activity analysis and financial ratio analysis.

Converting inputs to outputs requires that resources be allocated and their utilization be controlled. The final section of this chapter presents analytical techniques used in resource allocation: volume analysis, capital budgeting, cost–benefit analysis, and simulation. Cost–benefit analysis is especially useful in many areas of the HSO/HS without assignable revenue. Simulation is a powerful tool for investigating how systems (i.e., processes) can be improved. The ability to ask "what if" questions without having to actually change the system allows managers to understand theoretically the effects of changes in activities such as traffic and materials flow, capacity design, staffing patterns, patient service and waiting times, and reallocation of beds among services. Based on the simulated results, resources can be allocated or reallocated, thereby ensuring greater control over their effective use.

DISCUSSION QUESTIONS

1. Define control. What are the major elements of control?
2. What are the three monitoring and two intervention points for control? Why is MIS important to control?
3. Review the control model in Figure 10.2 and give examples of situations for each of the control loops. What are the similarities between the control model (Figure 10.2) and the problem-solving model presented in Figure 7.4?
4. How does CQI relate to control? Specifically, what control point is its focus and how does this affect the control model (see Figure 10.2)?
5. Describe the purpose, structure, and process of RM and QI. Why are both important to HSOs/HSs from a control perspective?
6. What are the duties of risk managers? How do they fit into the organization of HSOs? HSs?
7. Discuss the concept of insurance and its applicability in RM.
8. Contrast traditional quality assurance with QI as formulated by W. Edwards Deming (see Chapter 9). How are they complementary? Contradictory?
9. Distinguish Donabedian's conceptualization of quality as a function of and measurable by process and outcome. Provide and discuss a clinical or nonclinical example that shows the application of this conceptualization.
10. Identify control methods presented in this chapter. Why are budgets and ratio analysis so important? How does each relate to the control model in Figure 10.2?
11. Identify the analytical techniques for resource allocation that were presented in this chapter. Explain how and why they are useful.

CASE STUDY 1: ADMITTING DEPARTMENT

Shelley York is supervisor of the admitting department at Newhealth, a health maintenance organization. Three clerks—Shemenski, Turner, and Underwood—report to her. All are responsible for processing patients. Using a sampling method for monitoring productivity, York obtained the following data for a 2-hour period:

Clerk	Patients processed
Shemenski	14
Turner	16
Underwood	11

Each clerk is expected to process seven patients per hour.

QUESTIONS

1. What should York do?
2. What is the control point (input, process, or output)?
3. What kind of information should York obtain relative to Turner and Underwood? What might be some of the "causes" for the deviations?

CASE STUDY 2: CENTRALIZED PHOTOCOPYING

Carey Snook saw Ted Rath drinking coffee in the cafeteria. "I thought you guys in management services were up to your eyeballs in productivity improvement projects," Snook said as he walked over to sit down with Rath.

"We are," Rath said. "In fact, we have so much work and so many project deadlines coming up, we've had to work Saturdays."

Snook responded, "Then how come you're goofing off by wasting time and drinking coffee?"

"I'm not wasting time," said Rath, "I'm waiting."

"For what?" said Snook.

"For some layout prints to be reproduced. We're in the middle of a systems analysis project. We're redesigning the outpatient department layout and work process flow. I can't continue with the project until I get the template layout drawings copied in central photocopying. Our secretary took them over there 20 minutes ago and they won't be ready for another 20 minutes. So, I'm waiting. This happens about three times a week to each of the three of us in my department."

Rath continued, "We used to have a photocopier in our department. Well, some people were caught copying personal documents. This probably cost the hospital about $10 a week, so they centralized all photocopying equipment to save money on use and have fewer machines. Now we have to walk our materials way over there to the central building and wait until it's our turn to have them reproduced."

"I guess the biggest gripe I have is with Smith, head of centralized photocopying. Sometimes it takes 10 minutes to convince Smith that the reproduction job is hospital business and is important. Smith really seems to like the authority. Anyway, take this isometric drawing I have here; I bet Smith will think it's my 6-year-old daughter's homework assignment. I wonder how long it will take me to convince Smith it is job related."

"Want some more coffee?" asked Snook.

QUESTIONS

1. What is the focus of control in this situation?
2. What dysfunctional results have occurred from centralizing photocopying?

CASE STUDY 3: BARRIERS TO AN EFFECTIVE QI EFFORT

District Hospital is a 260-bed, public, general acute care hospital owned by a special tax district. Its service area includes five communities with a total population of 180,000 in a southeastern coastal state in one of the nation's fastest growing counties. It is one of three hospitals owned by the special tax district. The seven other hospitals in District Hospital's general service area make the environment highly competitive.

District Hospital has a wide range of services and a medical staff of 527 from most specialties. The emergency department (ED) is a major source of admissions. Last year, 26,153 patients visited the ED and 3,745, or 14.3%, were admitted. This was 42% of total hospital admissions. Some admissions were sent to the ED by private physicians and some came by ambulance, but most were self-referred.

The hospital chief executive officer, W.G. Lester, noted that the number of visits to the ED was decreasing. Over a 3-year period they had declined from a high of 29,345 to the current low of 26,153. Only part of this reduction seemed attributable to competition. Lester also was concerned about an increasing number of complaints about the quality of emergency services. These complaints related to excessive waiting time, poor attitudes of physicians, and questions about the quality of care. Investigation found that many complaints were justified, but the causes of these problems were difficult to discern.

Registered nurses (RNs) employed in the ED want a larger role in triaging and treating patients, but the overwhelming dominance of ED physicians limits the RNs' duties and frustrates other staff as well. This is manifested among the RN staff by high turnover, low morale, and difficulty in recruitment and retention.

Another factor is the emergency medical technician (EMT) program started in the county a few years ago. The EMTs are an important community medical resource and are very influential in deciding to which hospital ED patients will be transported. It will be necessary for District Hospital, through the ED physicians, to participate actively in training and managing the EMT program if District Hospital is to receive its share of emergency patients. ED physicians have refused to participate in teaching or directing the program, however. In fact, they often alienate the EMTs.

Lester is concerned, too, that the position of full-time director of emergency medicine at District Hospital has been vacant for 4 years. Residency programs in emergency medicine are producing physicians who are seeking positions with higher salaries and better working conditions than those that were available at District Hospital.

There has been little turnover among the six physicians who staff the ED: one retired general surgeon, two internists, and three foreign medical graduates trained in family practice. The ED physicians lack a clear commitment to District Hospital. All of them contract separately with the hospital to provide ED services. District Hospital bills ED patients and collects the physicians' fees: moneys above the guaranteed minimum are paid to them pro rata. They participate in District Hospital's fringe benefits and are covered by its professional liability insurance.

One ED physician, Dr. Balck (the retired surgeon), recognizes the progress being made nationally in emergency medicine. She made several unsuccessful attempts to move District Hospital in the same direction. With great effort she instituted programs on intradepartmental education and mandatory attendance at approved courses in emergency medicine. Quality-related activities are done perfunctorily. Also, she had tried to obtain full recognition of the ED and its work by other members of the professional staff organization (PSO).

The members of the PSO seem satisfied with the situation. Its executive committee did not understand the changing status of emergency medicine. As evidence of its unwillingness to grant full recognition to the department, the PSO has consistently denied its requests for full departmental status.

QUESTIONS

1. Use the problem-solving methodology described in Chapter 7 to define the problem facing Lester. Which alternative solution do you prefer? Why?
2. Describe the relationship between inpatient census and ED admissions. Outline a strategy to educate the members of the ED physician staff as to the relationship and importance of the ED to the financial good health of District Hospital.
3. Use the principles of CQI from Chapter 9 to outline a basic effort to improve quality in the ED.
4. Analyze the role of the EMTs and their relationship with District Hospital. What should be the role of ED physicians and staff at District Hospital in terms of educating the EMTs? What are the negative aspects of this educational activity? Is there a potential conflict of interest?
5. Identify some control measures that could be used by Lester.

CASE STUDY 4: DON'S RISK MANAGEMENT

Don Phelps is the director of engineering at Sunrise Village, a large life-care community located in a semirural area on the West Coast. Phelps has a staff of 19, including those who maintain and repair heating, ventilation, and air conditioning (HVAC) and electrical wiring and plumbing. There are several utility repairmen who do carpentry, locksmithing, and general maintenance. The grounds are maintained by two full-time employees, supplemented by high school students in the summer.

Senior management at Sunrise feels lucky to have Phelps on its staff. Phelps is a baccalaureate mechanical engineer and has done graduate work in electrical engineering. He is dedicated, hardworking, and genuinely concerned that his department perform efficiently.

Sunrise self-insures for all risks, including malpractice liability, up to $1 million. It has an excess liability insurance policy to $5 million. Last year the excess liability carrier recommended that Sunrise develop a risk management program, but provided little specific information on how to do it. Phelps thinks such a program is a good idea.

Phelps has some data on visitor and resident accidents, but has had no time to do anything with them. He has no data on the quality of care provided in the skilled nursing unit at Sunrise, but he knows there have been several "incidents" in the past few years. He knows, too, that one of the reasons that Sunrise began to self-insure was that there had been dramatic premium increases in its liability coverage because of three large settlements paid by its previous insurance carrier.

Senior management asked Phelps to organize a risk management program, but he isn't sure where to start.

QUESTIONS

1. Should Sunrise have a risk management program? Why?
2. Outline the steps that Phelps should take in establishing a risk management program. Which types of people should help him?
3. Identify and describe the types of links, including data collection, that should be present among risk management and quality improvement.
4. Incident or occurrence reporting is considered an important part of a risk management program. Why do staff often regard it as negative? What can be done to change this perception?

CASE STUDY 5: THE ARRAY MACHINE

An equipment acquisition proposal was being considered by a large hospital laboratory. An array machine would enable the hospital to perform autoimmunity tests (for immunoglobulins G, M, and A and complements C3 and C4) in-house rather than sending them to a reference laboratory. As a result, test turnaround time would be decreased by 2 days. The array machine costs $50,000, with a useful life of 5 years. The depreciation schedule would be $10,000/year.

The hospital's volume for the five autoimmunity tests is one of each test per day. Having the tests done by the reference laboratory costs the hospital an average of $10/test. The hospital's average charge to patients is $20/test. If the array machine were acquired and the autoimmunity tests done in-house, the costs of reagents used would average $2/test.

The array machine can run a maximum of 40 patient samples and perform 20 different tests on each sample every 2 hours. Except in extraordinary circumstances, tests would be run Monday through Saturday.

The machine requires approximately 1 hour of technician time (valued at $15/hour) each day to calibrate it, to conduct a test run for control purposes, and to perform general maintenance. This is a fixed cost because it does not vary by volume. Technician set-up time to run tests is negligible. Beyond the five autoimmunity tests the laboratory wants to perform in-house, the machine can also perform apolipoprotein cardiac profiles that are currently done on equipment in the clinical chemistry department. The array machine can provide a quantitative measure and not just the positive or negative indicator that the clinical chemistry department's current equipment gives.

QUESTIONS

1. How many autoimmunity tests per year will have to be performed on the array machine to break even?
2. Given the present volume of tests, would there be an annual net contribution and, if so, how much?
3. If half of the patients have Medicare coverage (DRG reimbursement includes all tests), would the laboratory break even on the equipment? If not, should the equipment be acquired anyway?

CASE STUDY 6: FINANCIAL RATIOS

General Hospital (GH) is a freestanding 265-bed nongovernmental, not-for-profit HSO. Review the income statement and balance sheet provided here.

GENERAL HOSPITAL INCOME STATEMENT (YEAR ENDING DECEMBER 31, 2000)

Revenues	
Operating revenue	
Inpatient	$38,800,000
Outpatient	49,000,000
Gross patient revenue	$87,800,000
Less contractual allowances & deductions	($23,500,000)
Net patient operating revenue (operating revenue)	$64,300,000
Other income	
contributions	$ 2,000,000
misc. income	5,400,000
Total other income	7,400,000
Total operating revenue and income	$71,700,000
Expenses	
Salaries and benefits	$27,000,000
Depreciation and amortization	3,400,000
Interest	300,000
Other expenses	30,000,000
Total operating expenses	$60,700,000
Net income	$11,000,000
Net operating income[a]	$ 3,600,000

[a]Net operating revenue/income = 11,000,000 less $7,400,000 = $3,600,000.

GENERAL HOSPITAL BALANCE SHEET (YEAR ENDING DECEMBER 31, 2000)

Assets

Current assets

Cash	$ 4,000,000
Temporary investments	2,700,000
Accounts receivables	11,000,000
(less allowance for uncollectable accounts receivables)	(2,800,000)
Other receivables	1,400,000
Inventory	1,100,000
Prepaid expenses	20,000
Total current assets	$17,420,000

Fixed assets

Land and improvements	$ 3,000,000
(less accumulated depreciation)	(1,500,000)
Buildings	24,000,000
(less accumulated depreciation)	(10,000,000)
Equipment	45,000,000
(less accumulated depreciation)	(25,000,000)
Total fixed assets	$35,500,000
Other assets (investments long term)	$25,400,000
Total assets	**$78,320,000**

Liabilities

Current liabilities

Accounts payable	$ 3,000,000
Wages and salaries payable	4,200,000
Short-term loans	4,000,000
Total current liabilities	$11,000,000

Long-term liabilities

Mortgage payable	$12,000,000
Other long-term debt	4,200,000
Total long-term liabilities	$16,200,000
Total liabilities	**$27,200,000**

Equity

General fund balance	$51,120,000
Total liabilities and equity	**$78,320,000**

Use the financial ratio formulas provided in Table 10.8 to calculate the values listed in the following table.

Item	Calculated value	Benchmark value
1. Current ratio		1.95
2. Acid test		0.31
3. Average payment period		60 days
4. Long-term debt to fixed assets		0.70
5. Operating profit margin		4.3%
6. Return on total assets		5.7%
7. Collection period		46.4 days
8. Total asset turnover		0.92
9. Contractual allowances and discounts as percentage of operating patient revenue[a]		41.3%

[a]Contractual allowances and discounts divided by gross patient revenue.

QUESTION

1. What do you conclude when comparing the calculated values for GH to the benchmark values that are supplied by HCIA for hospitals of similar size and type in the same state?

NOTES

1. Austin, Charles J., and Stuart B. Boxerman. *Information Systems for Health Services Administration,* 5th ed., 32. Chicago: AUPHA/Health Administration Press, 1998.

2. Donnelly, James H., Jr., James L. Gibson, and John M. Ivancevich. *Fundamentals of Management,* 241. Boston: Irwin/McGraw-Hill, 1998.

3. Higgins, James M. *The Management Challenge: An Introduction to Management,* 568. New York: Macmillan, 1991.

4. Bartol, Kathryn M., and David C. Martin. *Management,* 3rd ed., 523. Boston: Irwin/McGraw-Hill, 1998.

5. Bartol and Martin, *Management,* 523.

6. Van Fleet, David D. *Contemporary Management,* 444. Boston: Houghton Mifflin, 1991.

7. Pearce, John A., II, and Richard B. Robinson, Jr. *Management,* 584. New York: Random House, 1989.

8. Bartol and Martin, *Management,* 515.

9. Enthoven, Alain C., and Carol B. Vorhaus. "A Vision of Quality in Health Care Delivery." *Health Affairs* 16 (May/June 1997): 48.

10. Brown, Michael S. "Industry Information: Technology Trends." *CARING Magazine* 16 (December 1997): 69.

11. Austin, Charles J. "Information Technology and the Future of Health Services Delivery." *Hospital & Health Services Administration* 34 (Summer 1989): 159.

12. Austin, Charles J., and Richard C. Howe. "Information Systems Management." In *The AUPHA Manual of Health Services Management,* edited by Robert J. Taylor and Susan B. Taylor, 237–238. Gaithersburg, MD: Aspen Publishers, 1994.

13. Jones, V. Brewster, and L. Clark Taylor. "Expectations and Outcome Skills of a Generalist Health Care Administrator." *Journal of Health Administration Education* 8 (Winter 1990): 46.

14. Nilson, Julie T. "How To Hire the Right CIO." *Healthcare Executive* 13 (May/June 1998): 8–13.

15. Austin and Boxerman, *Information Systems,* 436.

16. Shaffer, Michael D., and Michael J. Shaffer. "Business Reengineering, Information Technology, and the Healthcare Connection." *Hospital Topics* 74 (Spring 1996): 12.

17. Stipe, Suzanne. "Health Information Networks: A Connection to an Efficient Future?" *Best's Review: Life/Health Insurance Edition* 96 (February 1996): 28.

18. Stamen, Jeffrey P. "Decision Support Systems Help Planners Hit Their Targets." *Journal of Business Strategy* 11 (March/April 1990): 30.

19. Clerkin, Daniel, and Peter J. Fos. "A Decision Support System for Hospital Bed Assignment." *Hospital & Health Services Administration* 40 (Fall 1995): 386.

20. Martin, James B. "The Environment and Future of Health Information Systems." *Journal of Health Administration Education* 8 (Winter 1990): 19.

21. Austin and Boxerman, *Information Systems,* 273.

22. Jelinek, Richard C., and Matthew M. Person, III. "Clinical Data Systems: Management Imperative for Tomorrow." *Journal of Health Administration Education* 6 (Spring 1988): 341.

23. Guiney, Mary Ann. "Community Hospital Computer Links Distant Physicians." *Health Systems Review* 27 (May/June 1994): 34.

24. Kleinke, J.D. "Release 0.0: Clinical Information Technology in the Real World." *Health Affairs* 17 (November/December 1998): 27.

25. Austin and Boxerman, *Information Systems,* 18.

26. Kleinke, "Release 0.0," 2: 27.

27. Austin, Charles J., Jerry M. Trimm, and Patrick M. Sobczak. "Information Systems and Strategic Management." *Health Care Management Review* 20 (Summer 1995): 31.

28. Muldoon, Jeannine D., and Joseph L. Sardinas, Jr. "Confidentiality, Privacy, and Restrictions for Computer-Based Patient Records." *Hospital Topics* 74 (Summer 1996): 32.

29. Kleinke, "Release 0.0," 29.

30. Wager, Karen A., Shyam Heda, and Charles J. Austin. "Developing a Health Information Network within an Integrated Delivery System: A Case Study." *Topics in Health Information Management* 17 (May 1997): 26.

31. Austin, Charles J. *Information Systems for Hospital Administration,* 11. Ann Arbor, MI: Health Administration Press, 1988.

32. Harpster, Linda Marie, and Margaret S. Veach, Eds. *Risk Management Handbook for Health Care Facilities,* 378. Chicago: American Hospital Association, 1990.

33. Kavaler, Florence, and Allen D. Spiegel. "Risk Management Dynamics." In *Risk Management in Health Care Institutions: A Strategic Approach,* edited by Florence Kavaler and Allen D. Spiegel, 18–19. Sudbury, MA: Jones & Bartlett, 1997. ("At least 10 states [Arkansas, Colorado, Florida, Kansas, Maryland, Massachusetts, New York, North Carolina, Rhode Island, and Washington] have legislative mandates for risk management programs. These state regulations relate to the administration of a risk management program, investigation and analysis of identified risks, education programs, patient grievance procedures, and confidentiality of risk management data." [p. 18])

34. [illegible]

35. Joint Commission on Accreditation of Healthcare Organizations. *Comprehensive Accreditation Manual for Hospitals, Refreshed Core,* PI-21. Oakbrook Terrace, IL: Joint Commission on Accreditation of Healthcare Organizations, January 1998.

36. Harpster and Veach, *Risk Management Handbook,* 107.

37. Sedwick, Jeannie. "The Risk Manager Role." In *Risk Management Handbook for Health Care Organizations,* 2nd ed., edited by Roberta Carroll, 4. Chicago: American Hospital Publishing, 1997.

38. Sedwick, "The Risk Manager Role," 17.

39. Nakamura, Peggy L.B. "The Risk Manager's Role in Contract Review." In *Risk Management Handbook for Health Care Organizations,* 2nd ed., edited by Roberta Carroll, 499 513. Chicago: American Hospital Publishing, 1997.

40. Mahaffey, Paul F. "Lawyers Professional Liability Insurance." *Lawyers' Liability Review Quarterly Journal* (April 1989): 1–3.

41. Health Care Quality Improvement Act of 1986, PL 99-660, 100 Stat. 3784 (1986).

42. Sedwick, "The Risk Manager Role," 19.

43. American College of Surgeons. *The Minimum Standard.* Chicago: American College of Surgeons, 1918.

44. Donabedian, Avedis. *Explorations in Quality Assessment and Monitoring. Vol. II, The Criteria and Standards of Quality.* Ann Arbor, MI: Health Administration Press, 1982.

45. Donabedian, Avedis. *Explorations in Quality Assessment and Monitoring. Vol. I, The Definition of Quality and Approaches to Its Assessment,* 81. Ann Arbor, MI: Health Administration Press, 1980.

46. Donabedian, *Explorations, Vol. I,* 79–89.

47. Donabedian, *Explorations, Vol. I,* 8.

48. Donabedian, *Explorations, Vol. I,* 83.

49. Donabedian, *Explorations, Vol. I,* 82.

50. Joint Commission on Accreditation of Healthcare Organizations. *Agenda for Change* 2 (June 1988).

51. Berwick, Donald M., A. Blanton Godfrey, and Jane Roessner. *Curing Health: New Strategies for Quality Improvement,* 11. San Francisco: Jossey-Bass, 1990.

52. Joint Commission. *Agenda for Change,* 3, 4.

53. Joint Commission on Accreditation of Healthcare Organizations. *Accreditation Manual for Hospitals,* Appendix D, 225–232. Oakbrook Terrace, IL: Joint Commission on Accreditation of Healthcare Organizations, 1992.

54. Nadzam, Deborah M., and Mary Nelson. "The Benefits of Continuous Performance Measurement." *Nursing Clinics of North America* 32 (September 1997): 548.

55. Kelly, John T., and James E. Swartwout. "Development of Practice Parameters by Physician Organizations." *QRB* 16 (February 1990): 54. (Use of the term "practice parameters" is preferred by the American Medical Association, the American Academy of Neurology Quality Standards Subcommittee, and the American Academy of Pediatrics; Merritt, T. Allen, Donald Palmer, David A. Bergman, and Patricia

H. Shiono. "Clinical Practice Guidelines in Pediatric and Newborn Medicine: Implications for Their Use in Practice." *Pediatrics* 99,1 [January 1997]: 100–114.)

56. Larsen-Denning, Lorie, Catherine Rommal, and Annie Stoekmann. "Clinical Practice Guidelines." In *Risk Management Handbook for Health Care Organizations,* 2nd ed., edited by Roberta Carroll, 575. Chicago: American Hospital Publishing, 1997.

57. Sisk, Jane E. "How Are Health Care Organizations Using Clinical Guidelines?" *Health Affairs* 17 (September/October 1998): 91–109.

58. Marder, Robert J. "Relationship of Clinical Indicators and Practice Guidelines." *QRB* 16 (February 1990): 60. (This article defines practice parameters and indicators and discusses their uses and relationships.)

59. Kelly, John T., and James E. Swartwout. "Development of Practice Parameters by Physician Organizations. *QRB* 16 (February 1990): 55.

60. Citrome, Leslie. "Practice Protocols, Parameters, Pathways, and Guidelines: A Review." *Administration and Policy in Mental Health* 25 (January 1998): 258.

61. "Good News on Guidelines." *Hospitals & Health Networks* 72 (January 5, 1998): 13.

62. Larsen-Denning, Rommal, and Stoekmann, "Clinical Practice Guidelines," 579.

63. Kelly and Swartwout, "Development of Practice," 55.

64. "Risk Management: Guideline Payoff." *Trustee* 51 (October 1998): 7.

65. Esmond, Truman H., Jr. *Budgeting for Effective Hospital Resource Management,* 26. Chicago: American Hospital Association, 1990.

66. Neumann, Bruce R., James D. Suver, and William N. Zelman. *Financial Management: Concepts and Applications for Health Care Providers,* 2nd ed., 269. Owings Mills, MD: National Health Publishing/AUPHA Press, 1988.

67. Meeting, David T., and Robert O. Harvey. "Strategic Cost Accounting Helps Create a New Competitive Edge." *Healthcare Financial Management* 20 (December 1998): 43.

68. Finkler, Steven A. "Flexible Budgeting Allows for Better Management of Resources as Needs Change." *Hospital Cost Management and Accounting* 8 (June 1996): 1.

69. Stiles, Renee A., and Stephen S. Mick. "What Is the Cost of Controlling Quality? Activity-Based Cost Accounting Offers the Answer." *Hospital & Health Services Administration* 42 (Summer 1997): 199.

70. Zelman, William N., Michael J. McCue, and Alan R. Millikan. *Financial Management of Health Care Organizations: An Introduction to Fundamental Tools, Concepts, and Applications,* 365. Malden, MA: Blackwell, 1998.

71. Zelman, McCue, and Millikan, *Financial Management,* 365–366.

72. Finkler, Steven A. "Responsibility Accounting in a Dynamic Environment: Activity-Based Cost Management." *Hospital Cost Management and Accounting* 8 (October 1996): 3.

73. Drucker, Peter F. "The Information Executives Truly Need." *Harvard Business Review* 73 (January-February 1995): 14.

74. Baker, Judith J., and Georgia F. Boyd. "Activity-Based Costing in the Operating Room at Valley View Hospital." *Journal of Health Care Finance* 24 (Fall 1997): 2.

75. Upda, Suneel. "Activity-Based Costing for Hospitals." *Hospital & Health Services Administration* 21 (Summer 1996): 84.

76. Meeting and Harvey, "Strategic Cost Accounting," 47.

77. Zelman, McCue, and Millikan, *Financial Management,* 365.

78. Center for Healthcare Industry Performance Studies. *The 1998–99 Almanac of Hospital Financial and Operating Indicators,* 3. Columbus, OH: Center for Healthcare Industry Performance Studies, 1998.

79. Zelman, McCue, and Millikan, *Financial Management,* 32.

80. Those interested in more information about this subject may refer to Zelman, McCue, and Millikan, *Financial Management,* Chapter 4.

81. The Center for Healthcare Industry Performance Studies is located at 1550 Old Henderson Road, Suite S-277, Columbus, OH 43220 (telephone 1-800-859-2447; website *www.chipsonline.com*); HCIA is located at 300 East Lombard Street, Baltimore, MD 21202 (telephone 1-800-324-1746; website address: *www.hcia.com*).

82. HCIA. *The Comparative Performance of U.S. Hospitals: The Sourcebook,* 12. Baltimore: HCIA, 1988.

83. "What Is Benchmarking?" *Hospital Cost Management and Accounting* 7 (January 1996): 8; Freeman, James M. "Benchmarking for Success." *Healthcare Executive* 13 (March/April 1998): 51.

84. Cleverley, William O. "Financial Ratios: Summary Indicators for Management Decision Making." *Hospital & Health Services Administration* 26 (Special Issue, 1981): 30–31. See also Berman, Howard J., Lewis E. Weeks, and Steven F. Kukla. *The Financial Management of Hospitals,* 6th ed., 664–665; Zeller, Thomas L., Brian B. Stanko, and William O. Cleverley. "New Perspectives on Hospital Financial Ratio Analysis." *Healthcare Financial Management* 51 (November 1997): 62–66.

85. Center for Healthcare Industry Performance Studies. *Financial Performance Report,* 8. Columbus, OH: Center for Healthcare Industry Performance Studies, 1998.

86. Smith-Daniels, Vicki L., Sharon B. Schweikhart, and Dwight E. Smith-Daniels. "Capacity Management in Health Care Services: Review and Future Directions." *Decision Sciences* 19 (Fall 1988): 889–919.

87. Breakeven analysis with formulas incorporating revenues from three types of payers—cost, fixed price, and charge—is presented in Cleverley, William O. "Break-Even Analysis in the New Payor Environment." *Hospital Topics* 20 (March/April 1988): 36–37.

88. Further reading about capital budgeting analytical technique in HSOs can be found in Berman, Weeks, and Kukla, *Financial Management,* chap. 18; Broyles, Robert W., and Michael D. Rosko. *Fiscal Management of Healthcare Institutions,* chap. 13. Owings Mills, MD: National Health Publishing, 1990; Cleverley, William O. *Handbook of Health Care Accounting and Finance,* chap. 8. Rockville, MD: Aspen Publishers, 1982; Cleverley, William O. *Essentials of Health Care Finance,* chap. 13. Rockville, MD: Aspen Publishers, 1986; Neumann, Suver, and Zelman, *Financial Management,* chap. 12; and Zelman, McCue, and Millikan, *Financial Management.* chap. 7.

89. Ziebell, Mary T., and Don T. DeCoster. *Management Control Systems in Nonprofit Organizations,* 913. San Diego: Harcourt Brace Jovanovich, 1991.

90. An excellent review of the literature concerning the application of simulation and other operations research techniques to health care is found in Smith-Daniels, Schweikhart, and Smith-Daniels, "Capacity Management." For classic reviews of applications, see Stimpson, David H., and Ruth H. Stimpson. *Operations Research in Hospitals: Diagnosis & Prognosis,* chap. 2. Chicago: Hospital Research and Educational Trust, 1972; and Valinsky, David. "Simulation." In *Operations Research in Health Care: A Critical Analysis,* edited by Larry J. Shuman, R. Dixon Speas, Jr., and John P. Young, 114–176. Baltimore: The Johns Hopkins University Press, 1975.

91. Kwak, N.K., Paul J. Kuzdrall, and Homer H. Schmitz. "The GPSS Simulation of Scheduling Policies for Surgical Patients." *Management Science* 22 (May 1976): 982–989.

92. Hashimoto, Fred, Staughton Bell, and Sally Marshment. "A Computer Simulation Program To Facilitate Budgeting and Staffing Decisions in an Intensive Care Unit." *Critical Care Medicine* 15 (March 1987): 256–259.

93. Klafehn, Keith A., Paul J. Kuzdrall, Jonathon S. Rakich, and Alan G. Krigline. "Application of Simulation in Hospital Resource Allocation and Utilization." *Journal of Management Science & Policy Analysis* 8 (Spring/Summer 1991): 346–356.

94. Klafehn, Kuzdrall, Rakich, and Krigline, "Application of Simulation," 351.

SELECTED BIBLIOGRAPHY

Austin, Charles J., and Stuart B. Boxerman. *Information Systems for Health Services Administration,* 5th ed. Chicago: AUPHA/Health Administration Press, 1998.

Austin, Charles J., and Richard C. Howe. "Information Systems Management." In *The AUPHA Manual of Health Services Management,* edited by Robert J. Taylor and Susan B. Taylor, 229–251. Gaithersburg, MD: Aspen Publishers, 1994.

Austin, Charles J., Jerry M. Trimm, and Patrick M. Sobczak. "Information Systems and Strategic Management." *Health Care Management Review* 20 (Summer 1995): 26–33.

Baker, Judith J., and Georgia F. Boyd. "Activity-Based Costing in the Operating Room at Valley View Hospital." *Journal of Health Care Finance* 24 (Fall 1997): 1–9.

Bartol, Kathryn M., and David C. Martin. *Management,* 3rd ed. Boston: Irwin/McGraw-Hill, 1998.

Brown, Michael S. "Industry Information: Technology Trends." *CARING Magazine* 16 (December 1997): 68–70, 72.

Carroll, Roberta, Ed. *Risk Management Handbook for Health Care Organizations,* 2nd ed. Chicago: American Hospital Publishing, 1997.

Center for Healthcare Industry Performance Studies. *Financial Performance Report.* Columbus, OH: Center for Healthcare Industry Performance Studies, 1998.

Center for Healthcare Industry Performance Studies. *The 1998–99 Almanac of Hospital Financial and Operating Indicators.* Columbus, OH: Center for Healthcare Industry Performance Studies, 1998.

Citrome, Leslie. "Practice Protocols, Parameters, Pathways, and Guidelines: A Review." *Administration and Policy in Mental Health* 25 (January 1998): 257–269.

Clerkin, Daniel, and Peter J. Fos. "A Decision Support System for Hospital Bed Assignment." *Hospital & Health Services Administration* 40 (Fall 1995): 386–400.

Cleverley, William O. "Break-Even Analysis in the New Payor Environment." *Hospital Topics* 20 (March/April 1988): 36–37.

Darr, Kurt. "Quality Improvement and Quality Assurance Compared." *Hospital Topics* 69 (Summer 1991): 4–5.

Donabedian, Avedis. *Explorations in Quality Assessment and Monitoring. Vol. I, The Definition of Quality and Approaches to Its Assessment.* Ann Arbor, MI: Health Administration Press, 1980.

Donabedian, Avedis. *Explorations in Quality Assessment and Monitoring. Vol. II, The Criteria and Standards of Quality.* Ann Arbor, MI: Health Administration Press, 1982.

Donnelly, James H., Jr., James L. Gibson, and John M. Ivancevich. *Fundamentals of Management.* Boston: Irwin/McGraw-Hill, 1998.

Drucker, Peter F. "The Information Executives Truly Need." *Harvard Business Review* 73 (January–February 1995): 12–21.

Enthoven, Alain C., and Carol B. Vorhaus. "A Vision of Quality in Health Care Delivery." *Health Affairs* 16 (May/June 1997): 44–57.

Finkler, Steven A. "Flexible Budgeting Allows for Better Management of Resources as Needs Change." *Hospital Cost Management and Accounting* 8 (June 1996): 1–5.

Finkler, Steven A. "Responsibility Accounting in a Dynamic Environment: Activity-Based Cost Management." *Hospital Cost Management and Accounting* 8 (October 1996): 1–5.

Freeman, James M. "Benchmarking for Success." *Healthcare Executive* 13 (March/April 1998): 51.

Guiney, Mary Ann. "Community Hospital Computer Links Distant Physicians." *Health Systems Review* 27 (May/June 1994): 34–37.

Harpster, Linda Marie, and Margaret S. Veach. *Risk Management Handbook for Health Care Facilities.* Chicago: American Hospital Association, 1990.

HCIA. *The Comparative Performance of U.S. Hospitals: The Sourcebook.* Baltimore: HCIA, 1998.

Kavaler, Florence, and Allen D. Spiegel. *Risk Management in Health Care Institutions: A Strategic Approach.* Sudbury, MA: Jones & Bartlett, 1997.

Klafehn, Keith A., Paul J. Kuzdrall, Jonathon S. Rakich, and Alan G. Krigline. "Application of Simulation in Hospital Resource Allocation and Utilization." *Journal of Management Science & Policy Analysis* 8 (Spring/Summer 1991): 346–356.

Kleinke, J.D. "Release 0.0: Clinical Information Technology in the Real World." *Health Affairs* 17 (November/December 1998): 23–38.

Marder, Robert J. "Relationship of Clinical Indicators and Practice Guidelines." *QRB* 16 (February 1990): 60.

Meeting, David T., and Robert O. Harvey. "Strategic Cost Accounting Helps Create a New Competitive Edge." *Healthcare Financial Management* 20 (December 1998): 42–51.

Muldoon, Jeannine D., and Joseph L. Sardinas, Jr. "Confidentiality, Privacy, and Restrictions for Computer-Based Patient Records." *Hospital Topics* 74 (Summer 1996): 32–37.

Nilson, Julie T. "How to Hire the Right CIO." *Healthcare Executive* 13 (May/June 1998): 8–13.

Palmer, R. Heather, Avedis Donabedian, and Gail J. Povar. *Striving for Quality in Health Care: An Inquiry into Policy and Practice.* Ann Arbor, MI: Health Administration Press, 1991.

Shaffer, Michael D., and Michael J. Shaffer. "Business Reengineering, Information Technology, and the Healthcare Connection." *Hospital Topics* 74 (Spring 1996): 10–15.

Stiles, Renee A., and Stephen S. Mick. "What Is the Cost of Controlling Quality? Activity-Based Cost Accounting Offers the Answer." *Hospital & Health Services Administration* 42 (Summer 1997): 193–204.

Stipe, Suzanne. "Health Information Networks: A Connection to an Efficient Future?" *Best's Review: Life/ Health Insurance Edition* 96 (February 1996): 28–31.

Udpa, Suneel. "Activity-Based Costing for Hospitals." *Hospital & Health Services Administration* 21 (Summer 1996): 83–96.

Wager, Karen A., Shyam Hoda, and Charles J. Austin. "Developing a Health Information Network Within an Integrated Delivery System: A Case Study." *Topics in Health Information Management* 17 (May 1997): 20–31.

"What is Benchmarking?" *Hospital Cost Management and Accounting* 7 (January 1996): 8.

Zeller, Thomas L., Brian B. Stanko, and William O. Cleverley. "New Perspective on Hospital Financial Ratio Analysis." *Healthcare Financial Management* 51 (November 1997): 62–66.

Zelman, William N., Michael J. McCue, and Alan R. Millikan. *Financial Management of Health Care Organizations: An Introduction to Fundamental Tools, Concepts, and Applications.* Malden, MA: Blackwell, 1998.

11

Human Resources and Labor Relations

A hospital needs an appropriate number of qualified people to fulfill its mission and meet the needs of the patients it serves. The goal of this function [human resources management] is to identify and provide the right number of competent staff to meet the needs of patients served . . .[1]

In 1999 there were 10 million individuals employed in all sectors of the health services delivery system representing 7.1% of the U.S. workforce.[2] Because employee costs represent approximately two thirds of expenditures in most health services organizations (HSOs) and health systems (HSs), staff is one of the most important input components in the provision of health services.

To implement strategies, accomplish objectives, and fulfill their mission, HSOs/HSs must be staffed with adequate numbers of properly trained personnel. When managers integrate technology and people into formal structures (organizational arrangements), meaningful work occurs. The human element is the catalyst in the organizational equation that causes other inputs (material, supplies, technology, information, and capital) to be converted into outputs in the form of individual and organizational work results (see the management model for HSOs/HSs, Figure 1.7). It is through people that work gets done, patient care is delivered, organizational objectives are accomplished, mission is fulfilled, and competitive position is maintained or enhanced.[3]

A HSO's/HS's human resources (employees) are its most important asset.[4] Without people, organizations are inert. If employees are insufficient in number, inadequately qualified, or improperly matched to the organization's needs, less-than-optimal work results will occur—quality and productivity improvement will be adversely affected. As indicated by the opening quote and Figure 11.1, the Joint Commission on Accreditation of Healthcare Organizations (Joint Commission) standards pertinent to the human resources function focus on management defining the qualifications, competencies, and level of staff to achieve the hospital's mission; acquiring and maintaining the right number of competent people to meet the needs of patients served; and continuously as-

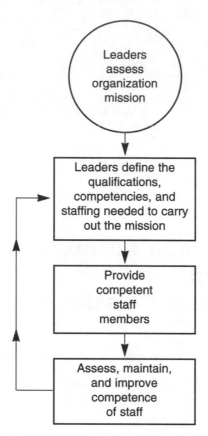

Figure 11.1.　Management of human resources function. (From Joint Commission on Accreditation of Healthcare Organizations. *1996 Accreditation Manual for Hospitals: Volume II, Scoring Guidelines,* 310. Oakbrook Terrace, IL: Joint Commission on Accreditation of Healthcare Organizations, 1995; reprinted by permission.)

sessing and improving the competencies of employees. Although the Joint Commission standard references hospitals, the same focus is applicable to HSOs and HSs as well. It is senior-level management's responsibility to implement and coordinate a total human resource system—composed of workforce acquisition, retention/maintenance, separation—to ensure that the HSO/HS is properly staffed; and to develop a labor-relations environment so that the mutual needs of the organization and staff are met to the benefit of patients/customers.

ROLE OF HUMAN RESOURCES MANAGEMENT

Personnel administration is the historical term that is used to describe a wide range of centralized staffing activities, programs, and policies related to acquisition, retention and maintenance, and separation of human resources. All managers play a part in and have some degree of responsibility for staffing activities such as selection, performance appraisal, promotion, training and development, discipline and corrective counseling, and compensation of their employees. However, most staffing activities are centralized in and coordinated by a single department—or, in the case of a HS, a corporate office[5]—that establishes organizationwide/systemwide policies and procedures and provides human resources acquisition, retention, and separation services for other departments/units.

The contemporary designation for the centralized staffing activities in HSOs/HSs is *human resources management* (HRM); this term is used here when referring to the set of centralized staffing activities, programs, and policies concerned with the acquisition, retention and maintenance, and separation of employees, as well as labor relations (i.e., union–management relationships); *human resources department* refers to the organizational component responsible for staffing and labor relations activities, programs, and policies; and *human resources manager* refers to managers of that department or unit.

The human resources department is responsible for bringing employees into the HSO/HS and placing them in the existing structure (acquisition); enhancing the competencies of existing employees and keeping those who are effective in the organization (retention and maintenance); facilitating the exit of those who leave (separation); and developing policies for employees in the organization (coordinating). It is a staff versus line department that assists other departments and managers with special expertise and programs.[6] Because of the centralized role of the human resources department and because employees are the organization's most important resource, the human resources manager is typically a member of senior-level management who influences the formulation and implementation of human resources policies for the whole organization. This manager integrates all HRM activities with the HSO's/HS's strategic plans.[7]

Even though staffing activities are centralized in the human resources department, other managers must be familiar with them. First, HRM policies provide structure and define the interactions among managers, who are ultimately accountable for the quality and productivity of their operations, and employees. Second, HRM policies reflect societal norms that are expressed in legislative enactments and judicial decisions in areas such as nondiscriminatory hiring, discipline, promotion, and compensation. Better-informed managers will be more effective in using human resources and less likely to act unethically or illegally.

STAFFING ACTIVITIES

HRM staffing activities can be viewed as a time flow of distinct phases (Figure 11.2). *Acquisition* includes human resources planning, recruitment, selection, and orientation. *Retention and maintenance* include performance appraisal, placement, training and development, discipline and corrective counseling, compensation and benefits administration, employee assistance and career counseling, and safety and health. *Separation* is the third phase. These phases, along with the legislation affecting them, are described later in this chapter. Another activity that is generally centralized in the human resources department—labor relations or, more specifically, union–management relations and collective bargaining—is presented in the final sections of this chapter.

ACQUIRING HUMAN RESOURCES

Human Resources Planning

Acquisition, the first activity in the time flow model in Figure 11.2, highlights the fact that human resources planning precedes the recruitment, selection, and orientation of new employees. A HSO/HS determines staffing needs through human resources planning. Because organizations are dynamic, these needs change. The workforce must be considered in the context of a changing environment: Present staff must be retained and new employees recruited to meet changing needs.[8] In the context of changing social values, it may be necessary to develop and tap new labor markets.

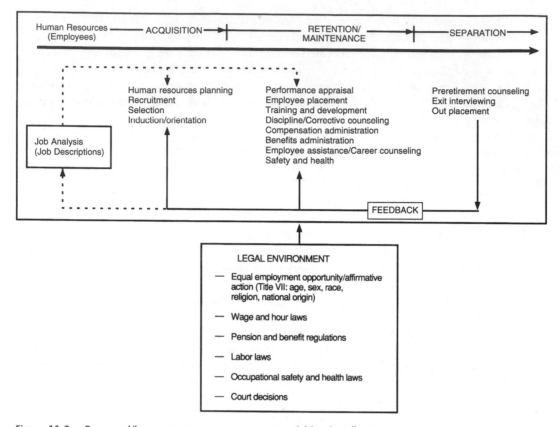

Figure 11.2.   Personnel/human resource management activities time flow.

Staff needs in HSOs/HSs are driven by organizational growth and employee turnover. Growth occurs through increased demand for services, facility expansion, the addition of new services, or intensifying services. Furthermore, staffing needs differ when services are eliminated or point of delivery changes. Each necessitates a different level of employees and mix of skills. Employee turnover through resignation, discharge, and retirement is the normal process of employee separation (exit). In addition to employee turnover and organizational growth, changes in technology drive the need for staff with different skills. The HSO/HS must constantly monitor the need for new employees. The human resources manager ensures that current and future needs for adequate numbers of qualified employees are met. This makes human resources planning integral to HRM, and the latter must be supportive of the organization's strategic plans.

Human resources planning ensures that the HSO/HS has the right number of people, with the appropriate qualifications and skills, to deliver appropriate levels and quality of service.[9] It involves five steps: profiling, estimating, inventorying, forecasting, and planning.

Step 1: Profiling

Whether the human resources plan is short term (less than 2 years) or long term (2 years or more), the initial step is to profile the HSO/HS at some future point and estimate numbers and types of jobs (skills). This often is subjective, but factors such as anticipated demand for services, changes in professional practice or labor supply, and staffing for new technologies can be taken into account in the projections.

Step 2: Estimating

Once a profile is developed, human resources estimates are made. Unless drastic changes are expected, such as major new services, reengineering initiatives, or strategic organizational changes, this step is straightforward because the health services industry has established staffing ratios for most major functions. If the determining variables can be identified and quantified, then a projection of needed staff can be made. For example, knowing the number of square feet in a new facility allows accurate projections of the number of additional housekeepers that are needed. Similarly, if inpatient beds are added, accepted nurse staffing ratios can be used. Outpatient expansion for which the volume of services can be projected allows a determination of staff needed.

Step 3: Inventorying

Present employees and their skills must be inventoried. Sometimes called talent inventory, the assessment of human resources skills, abilities, and potential and how they are being used is vital.[10] Human resources audit (skills and use inventory) involves compiling facts about each employee's job title, experience, length of service, performance, education, special skills, and placement. Modified, this technique can be used to inventory all employees, including managers and clinical staff, whether salaried or independent contractors.

Step 4: Forecasting

Having obtained an assessment of present employees, the planner can forecast changes in the present workforce in terms of entries and exits, as well as transfers within the HSO/HS. All organizations experience turnover through retirement, death, voluntary separation, and discharge, and historical data are used to forecast future patterns.

Also related to these losses is movement within the organization. One factor that distinguishes HSOs/HSs from other organizations is that much of the workforce is credentialed and/or licensed for specific jobs and delivers clinical services (examples are provided in Chapter 2). This means that there is less upward or lateral movement to unrelated positions as compared with other types of organizations. Nevertheless, some upward movement does occur because of promotion, particularly into managerial positions, and lateral movement occurs as a result of transfer, such as nurses from inpatient to outpatient services or to satellite facilities. Succession planning is performed for managerial positions,[11] but all such movement must be taken into account when forecasting changes in the present workforce.

It is likely that the skills inventory of experience and education will have to be adjusted upward over time. An older, mature organization will have stabilized in this sense (reached a norm), whereas a new organization will have wider statistical variation. As noted in Chapter 2, many states have continuing education requirements for certain health services occupations. Particular emphasis is placed on managers of nursing facilities, physicians, and nurses. Professional associations that certify their members are likely to have similar requirements.

Step 5: Planning

Assumptions that are made and information that is acquired in Steps 1 through 4 are the basis for an action plan that ensures the appropriate number of employees with requisite skills are available. Human resources needs that are identified through an organizationwide or systemwide continuous quality improvement (CQI) program are factored into the human resources plan.

Summary

Human resources planning deals with a dynamic situation in which the human resources department interacts with other managers to forecast staffing needs on the basis of changes that will occur in the present workforce and develops an action plan to fill those needs through recruiting and hiring, transferring, or enhancing the skills of existing employees through training and development. The human resources plan determines how the HSO's/HS's future staffing needs will be met.

Human Resources Sources

Sources of human resources are categorized as internal and external.[12] Using internal sources means the HSO/HS fills a vacancy by transferring or promoting from within. Using internal sources is cost effective, usually is quicker, reduces recruiting and relocation costs, and enhances employee morale. To use present employees effectively, it is important that the skills inventory include career path planning, when appropriate, and that necessary training be provided to upgrade employees with the potential for promotion or transfer.

In addition to internal sources, new employees may be recruited from outside the organization. Advertising vacancies or relying on present employees to "pass the word" to potential employees often generates applications. Visits to schools and colleges, contacts with public and private employment agencies, and recruitment through professional organizations also may be useful.

Other sources of workers include those who inquire about employment and temporary help agencies and contract employees.[13] Selecting the source depends on the qualifications required, labor market supply, geographic area, employer's reputation, and perhaps teaching affiliations. The significant recruiting problems in many areas are exacerbated by job fragmentation and specialization, uneven workforce distribution, increasing demand for health services, career alternatives for women, and differences in public educational support.

Approximately 200 different types of positions are required to staff a general acute care community hospital and more than 300 for a large metropolitan teaching facility, and the numbers are growing. Acquiring and retaining a suitably qualified workforce is one of the major tasks facing management.

Job Analysis and Job Descriptions

A fundamental responsibility of the human resources department is developing and maintaining job descriptions for all positions. HRM staffing activities such as workforce planning, recruitment, selection, performance appraisal, and compensation administration depend on job descriptions.[14] In addition, much of equal employment opportunity law uses the job description as a basic document. Thus efforts to develop and maintain job descriptions are a good investment.

Job Analysis

New employees cannot be recruited until it is known what types of training, skills, and experience are required. In general, this information is obtained from job analysis.[15] The human resources department is responsible for this analysis, which consists of observing and studying a job to determine its content (duties and responsibilities), the conditions under which it is performed, and its relationships to other jobs. Furthermore, the analysis results in identifying the skills, training, and abilities that are necessary to perform the required work.[16] There are three primary ways to conduct job analysis: observation, questionnaires, and interviews.[17] The information that is obtained is the source for developing a job description.

Job Descriptions

The content and format of job descriptions vary among organizations. The general practice is to include job title, location, job summary, from five to nine general duties and responsibilities, supervision given or received, special working conditions (including equipment or systems used), hazards, and qualifications. A statement of qualifications should include the minimum education, training, experience, and demonstrated skills required. Sometimes the statement of qualifications is in a "job specifications" document; however, it is more common for essential qualifications to be incorporated into the job description document.[18] Job descriptions should be concise for ease of understanding and, where possible, worded to permit maximum flexibility in work design. Tables 11.1 and 11.2 are sample job descriptions for a senior-level management and a service position, respectively.

Job descriptions for each job should be updated whenever job content, performance requirements, or qualifications change. This basic document is used for virtually all other HRM functions—recruitment, selection, training, performance appraisal, career counseling, and compensation[19]—and is a fundamental document in legal disputes. With this information, communication among managers, employees, applicants, and the human resources department is greatly simplified. For example, when a vacancy occurs, the human resources department is notified by means of a requisition to fill the position, and recruitment for someone who meets the requirements stated in the document begins.

Recruitment

Recruitment involves searching for and attracting prospective employees either from outside or within the HSO/HS.[20] There are many ways to recruit potential employees, and selecting among them is related largely to the labor market. If no special skills or training is required for the job and labor supply is ample, recruitment may mean reviewing applications from those who simply inquire. For other jobs, shortages may have existed for years. Here, HSOs/HSs must compete for available supply. Internal job posting, promotion, and transfer of existing employees are sources for recruitment. External sources can consist of recruiting at schools, job fairs, employment agencies, and professional associations.[21]

Selection

When recruitment is effective, the organization or system will have applicants. The next step in the acquisition process is to select from among them using job qualifications as a guide. The essence of selection is determining whether an applicant is suited for the job in terms of training, experience, and ability.[22] Three basic sources of information are used in selection: application forms, preemployment interviews, and testing.

As indicated in Figure 11.2, all HSO/HS managers must function within a complex legal environment relative to equal employment opportunity and nondiscriminatory practices. Human resources managers, in particular, are responsible for ensuring that the organizationwide staffing function and HRM policies comply with federal, state, and local laws. All other managers also must have a basic understanding of the legal environment. The following presentation is not meant to be definitive as to legal or illegal employment practices, but it is meant to alert operating managers to the complexity of the employment legal environment. The main point is, when in doubt, check with the human resources manager, legal counsel, or both.

Application Forms and Preemployment Interviews

Background information about the applicant, such as education, training, and previous employment, can be obtained from the application form. Figure 11.3 shows a portion of a sample form. References, letters of recommendation, previous employment verification, and background checks are used to confirm application data. Also, properly conducted interviews can yield useful information about an applicant.

Two types of interviews are used widely. The directed or structured interview is planned and led by the interviewer. It is confined to verifiable facts that the interviewer expects to hear by ask-

TABLE 11.1. SAMPLE JOB DESCRIPTION FOR A SENIOR-LEVEL MANAGEMENT POSITION

Job Title: President
(Administrator)
(Chief executive officer)

Brief Summary:

Provide leadership, direction, and administration of all aspects of hospital/multiorganizational activities and other corporate entities to [e]nsure compliance with established objectives and the realization of quality, economical health care services, and other related lines of business.

Principal Duties and Responsibilities:

Participate with the governing board in charting the course the hospital is to take in response to the developing needs of the community and carrying it out accordingly.

Recommend and update long-range plans which support the institution's philosophy and general objectives.

Recommend hospital policy positions regarding administrative policy, legislation, government, and other matters of public policy.

Inform and advise trustees regarding current trends, problems, and activities in health care to facilitate policy making.

Participate in and coordinate selection process of new board members.

In coordination with the board, the [clinical] staff and other hospital personnel, respond to the community's needs for quality health care services by monitoring the adequacy of the hospital's medical activities.

Consult with relevant personnel and departments prior to recommending/establishing new policies and the availability of resources to implement same.

Coordinate efforts of [clinical] staff, board, and administrative staff in the recruitment and retention of medical personnel.

[E]nsure the provision of affordable health care services by the acquisition, utilization, and organization of available resources (human, financial, and physical) and the development of improved techniques and practices. Coordinate the long-range fund raising efforts of the institution.

[E]nsure compliance with all regulatory agencies governing health care delivery and the rules of accrediting bodies by continually monitoring the operations and its programs and physical properties, and initiating changes where required.

Encourage the integration of the hospital with the community through effective communication and public relations programs.

Direct and supervise all hospital activities through administrator and/or competent administrative support staff and department heads. Provide assistance to supervisory personnel in establishing department philosophy and objectives; determining staffing needs and standards of productivity; establishing policies and procedures and job classifications; complying with federal, state, and local codes, regulations, and ordinances. Consult with and advise department heads on a regular basis; evaluate competence of work force and make changes as necessary; keep lines of communication open; seek to maintain high employee morale and a professional, healthful atmosphere and environment in the hospital.

Serve as liaison and channel of communication between the board and any of its committees and [clinical] staff and assist with organizational and medicoadministrative problems and responsibilities.

Represent hospital in its relationships with other health agencies, organizations, groups; in dealings with government agencies and third party payers; at top level meetings (national, state, local). May assign administrative support personnel, department heads, others to this task.

Maintain professional affiliations and enhance professional growth and development to keep abreast of latest trends in hospital administration.

Perform other related administrative/managerial duties as directed/required.

Working Conditions:

Subject to long and irregular hours; many interruptions. Generally sedentary position.

Knowledge, Skills, Experience Required:

MHA/MBA/MS in hospital administration, health care administration, or equivalent educational experience. Sufficient previous management experience in hospital administration.

From American Society for Health Care Human Resources Administration. *Health Care Occupations: A Comprehensive Job Description Manual,* 19–20. Chicago: American Society for Health Care Human Resources Administration, 1985; reprinted by permission.

TABLE 11.2. SAMPLE JOB DESCRIPTION FOR A SERVICE POSITION

Title: Cook I   Position #:   00006968
Department: 4146-PUH Nutr/Fs Kitchen Allo
Age of patient population: NON

Basic Functions:
Under the supervision of the Food Production Manager is responsible for the preparation of all cold food items and the mixing, arranging and garnishing of all patient and cafeteria salads according to standards.

Qualifications:
A high school diploma or equivalent is desired. At least six months prior food production experience is required.

Responsibilities:
1. Carries out job responsibilities in a manner that is consistent with the service management vision of Presbyterian University Hospital which includes the demonstration of appropriate behavior toward patients, visitors, staff, peers and physicians.
2. Accurately perform the duties of the assigned positions as outlined in the performance standards.
3. Product is prepared following standard recipes.
4. Following daily production sheets, complete all salad/cold production within designated time period.
5. Utilizing proper serviceware appropriately, plates and garnishes all salads in an appetizing manner.
6. Retrieve, handle and store all products properly.
7. Break down leftover food items and store properly.
8. Observe sanitary regulations in handling and preparing foods and keep work area clean.
9. Notify Food Production Manager/Team Leader of any food item shortages in sufficient time to make necessary adjustments to menu.
10. Assist in the training of new employees.
11. Other duties as assigned in order for the Nutrition and Food Service Department to fulfill its responsibilities.

Problem Solving:
The ability to accurately follow documented production forecasts and recipes by applying knowledge of both traditional and metric measurement scales.

Physical Demands and Hazards:
Potential exists for fatigue and stress due to physical requirements of the position's constant standing, heavy lifting and meeting mealtime deadlines. The potential exists for physical injury if safety precautions are ignored when using kitchen utensils and equipment.

From University of Pittsburgh Medical Center Health System; reprinted by permission.

ing specific questions. This type of interview is most often used when employees are being selected, when job descriptions are being prepared, and when an employee is exiting (exit interview). The second type is a nondirected interview that has the more ambitious purpose of achieving understanding beyond specific facts.[23] In practice the two often merge, and effective interviewers change interview types as the situation warrants.

The primary purpose of the application form and preemployment interview is to provide the organization with information about the applicant. However, federal and state laws, as well as judicial decisions concerning fair employment practices and equal employment opportunity, identify certain application form and preemployment interview practices as discriminatory and, therefore, illegal. Questions asked must have a job-related business purpose. Many employers collect information such as race, marital status, number of dependent children, and date of birth on a separate form that is not given to those who make the employment decision. These data can then be used for Equal Employment Opportunity Commission (EEOC) reporting requirements.[24] If such a separate reporting system is not in place, "once an employer tells an applicant that he or she is hired [the 'point of hire'], inquiries that were prohibited earlier can be made."[25] Table 11.3 presents guidelines to lawful and unlawful preemployment inquiries based on court and regulatory decisions.[26]

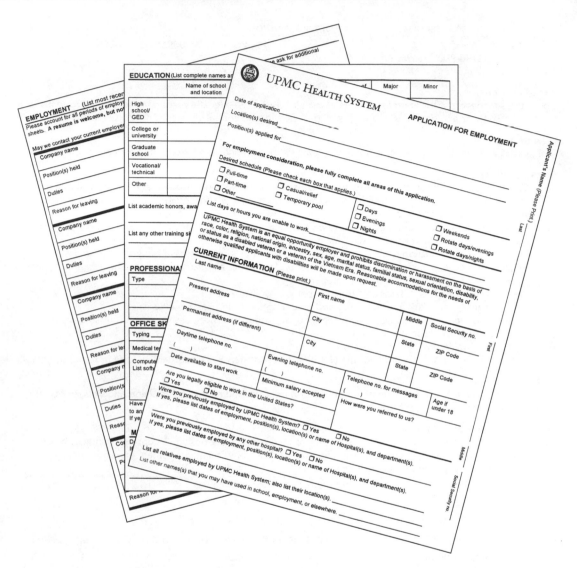

Figure 11.3. Sample application for employment. (From University of Pittsburgh Medical Center Health System; reprinted by permission.)

Testing

Given the importance of a decision to hire, it is understandable that human resources and first-level managers have sought more refined methods to evaluate and screen applicants. A wide variety of preemployment tests are used to determine which candidate is best suited for a position.

Preemployment testing has been closely scrutinized by several federal agencies, including the EEOC and the Department of Labor. Basic regulations have been compiled in the "Uniform Guidelines on Employee Selection Procedures" and are aimed at the issues of adverse impact.[27] In *Griggs v. Duke Power Co.,*[28] the Supreme Court stated that if a test has an adverse impact on the selection of women or minorities, which occurs when they fail the test in significantly greater percentages than the overall failure rate, the employer using the test must prove that it is a valid indicator of the abilities that are needed to perform the job. This showing must be made even if there is proof that the employer did not intend to discriminate.

TABLE 11.3. GUIDELINES TO LAWFUL AND UNLAWFUL PREEMPLOYMENT INQUIRIES

Subject of inquiry	It may not be discriminatory to inquire about:	It may be discriminatory to inquire about:
1. Name	a. Whether applicant has ever worked under a different name	a. The original name of an applicant whose name has been legally changed b. The ethnic association of applicant's name
2. Age	a. If applicant is over the age of 18 b. If applicant is under the age of 18 or 21 if job related (i.e., selling liquor in retail store)	a. Date of birth b. Date of high school graduation
3. Residence	a. Applicant's place of residence; length of applicant's residence in state and/or city where employer is located	a. Previous addresses b. Birthplace of applicant or applicant's parents
4. Race or color		a. Applicant's race or color of ⁂⁂⁂⁂
5. National origin and ancestry		a. Applicant's lineage, ancestry, national origin, parentage, or nationality b. Nationality of applicant's parents or spouse
6. Sex and family composition		a. Sex of applicant b. Dependents of applicant c. Marital status d. Child-care arrangements
7. Creed or religion		a. Applicant's religious affiliation b. Church, parish, or holidays observed
8. Citizenship	a. Whether the applicant is a citizen of the United States b. Whether the applicant is in the country on a visa that permits him or her to work or is a citizen	a. Whether applicant is a citizen of a country other than the United States
9. Language	a. Language applicant speaks and/or writes fluently, if job related	a. Applicant's native language; language commonly used at home
10. References	a. Names of people willing to provide professional and/or character references for applicant	a. Name of applicant's pastor or religious leader
11. Relatives	a. Names of relatives already employed by the employer	a. Name and/or address of any relative of applicant b. Whom to contact in case of emergency
12. Organizations	a. Applicant's membership in any professional, service, or trade organization	a. All clubs or social organizations to which applicant belongs
13. Arrest record and convictions	a. Convictions, if related to job performance (disclaimer should accompany)	a. Number and kinds of arrests b. Convictions unless related to job performance

(continued)

TABLE 11.3. *(continued)*

Subject of inquiry	It may not be discriminatory to inquire about:		It may be discriminatory to inquire about:	
14. Photographs			a.	Photographs with application, with resume, or before hiring
15. Height and weight			a.	Any inquiry into height and weight of applicant except where a bona fide occupational qualification
16. Physical limitations	a.	Whether applicant has the ability to perform job-related functions with or without accommodation	a.	The nature or severity of an illness or the individual's physical condition
			b.	Whether applicant has ever filed a workers' compensation claim
			c.	Any recent or past operations or surgery and dates
17. Education	a.	Training applicant has received if related to the job under consideration		
	b.	Highest level of education attained, if validated that having certain educational background (e.g., high school diploma or college degree) is necessary to perform the specific job		
18. Military	a.	What branch of the military applicant served in	a.	Type of military discharge
	b.	Type of education or training received in military		
	c.	Rank at discharge		
19. Financial status			a.	Applicant's debts or assets
			b.	Garnishments

From Mathis, Robert L., and John H. Jackson. *Human Resources Management: Essential Perspectives*, 187–189. Cincinnati, OH: South-Western, 1999; reprinted by permission from Mathis & Associates. Developed by Robert L. Mathis, Mathis & Associates, L.L.C., 1429 North 31st Avenue Circle, Omaha, NE 68153. All rights reserved.

There are three forms of validity in testing[29]:

> *Content validity:* The test recreates or represents significant sample parts of the job, such as typing tests.
>
> *Construct validity:* The test identifies a psychological or personality trait [that is] important to successful performance, such as leadership or problem solving abilities.
>
> *Criterion-related validity:* The test contains elements on which anyone who would do well on the job will perform well, or anyone who would do poorly on the job will perform poorly.

The strict and complex guidelines for preemployment testing suggest it should be used only for specialized or high-level positions or when incorrect selection will have significant cost and patient care consequences. Experts should be consulted to develop the test instruments. Content-valid tests are the simplest and legally safest.

Selection—A Shared Responsibility

The question of who makes the final employment selection from among screened candidates is critical. Selection remains an inexact science despite all of the techniques that have been developed and used. Ideally, the decision is made by the manager to whom the new employee will report, with the advice and counsel of the human resources department. This approach has the advantages that stipulated and necessary credential requirements are met, organizational policies and employment laws are followed, and individuals selected meet the HSO's/HS's quality standards and conform to its values and culture.

Orientation

After selection, induction and orientation occur. Induction activities are typically carried out by the human resources department and include enrolling new employees in benefit plans, issuing an identification badge, and creating a database for the individual. Most HSOs/HSs require a physical before new employees' start dates to screen for communicable diseases, to ensure that individuals can perform the job without danger to themselves or others, to determine workers' compensation risk, and to detect and document preexisting health conditions.

The orientation program should include information about the physical facility, organizational structure, universal precautions, fire and safety programs, employee health service, employee assistance program (EAP), and other human resources department methods. Organization policies and benefits should be explained in detail. In some departments, orientation may include an extended period of training and orienting the employee to department-specific work methods. This is done through such techniques as on-the-job training, using preceptors, and formal classroom training.

An important part of inducting new employees into the HSO/HS is informing them about its mission, vision, and values. Successful orientation builds employees' sense of identification with the organization, helps them gain acceptance by fellow workers, and gives them a clear understanding of what they need to know. Ideally, the orientation program enables new employees to become familiar with the entire organization as well as their own work area and department. This can be accomplished via a group or personal tour, a pictorial description such as a slide program, or a combination of these.

Equal Employment Opportunity

In recruiting and selecting new employees, and throughout their employment, one responsibility of the human resources department is to establish and implement nondiscriminatory HRM policies that comply with state and federal law.[30] Such legislation and regulations affect the employment relationship from recruitment and selection to retention activities such as promotion, transfer, and compensation, as well as layoffs. Table 11.4 presents major federal legislation that is relevant to the employment relationship.[31]

The legal concept of equal employment opportunity was articulated in Title VII of the Civil Rights Act of 1964.[32] This law, as amended, and its regulations dominate the field and prohibit discriminatory practices based on "race, color, national origin, religion or sex," but it is not the only noteworthy relevant legislation. In 1963 Congress passed the Equal Pay Act, which amended the Fair Labor Standards Act by requiring "equal pay" for substantially equal work, without regard to sex.[33]

Age discrimination legislation also is rooted in the 1960s. The Age Discrimination in Employment Act of 1967 prohibited discrimination against employees between the ages of 40 and 65.[34] Similar to the Equal Pay Amendment, its full effect was felt in 1979 when the minimum mandatory retirement age was raised from 65 to 70, and in 1986 when mandatory retirement was barred.[35] In 1978 Congress enacted the Pregnancy Discrimination Act protecting women from discrimination based on the ability to become or actually being pregnant. Employers must treat pregnant employees in the same way as any other employee with a medical condition.[36]

Other legislation that affects HRM selection and retention activities is the Americans with Disabilities Act (ADA) of 1990.[37] It prohibits discrimination against Americans who have disabilities

TABLE 11.4. HUMAN RESOURCES LEGISLATION

Law	Year	Description
Workers' compensation laws	Various	State-by-state laws that establish insurance plans to compensate employees injured on the job
Social Security Act	1935	Payroll tax to fund retirement benefits, disability and unemployment insurance
Fair Labor Standards Act	1938	Established minimum wage and overtime pay
Equal Pay Act	1963	Prohibits unequal pay for same job
Title VII of Civil Rights Act	1964	Prohibits employment decisions based on race, color, religion, sex, and national origin
Executive Order 11246	1965	Same as Title VII; also requires affirmative action
Age Discrimination in Employment Act	1967	Prohibits employment decisions based on age when person is 40 or older
Occupational Safety and Health Act (OSHA)	1970	Establishes safety and health standards for organizations to protect employees
Employee Retirement Income Security Act (ERISA)	1974	Regulates the financial stability of employee benefit and pension plans
Vietnam-Era Veterans Readjustment Act	1974	Prohibits federal contractors from discriminating against Vietnam-era veterans and encourages affirmative action plans to hire Vietnam veterans
Pregnancy Discrimination Act	1978	Prohibits employers from discriminating against pregnant women
Job Training Partnership Act	1982	Provides block money grants to states, which pass them on to local governments and private entities that provide on-the-job training
Consolidated Omnibus Budget Reconciliation Act (COBRA)	1985	Requires continued health insurance coverage (paid by employee) following termination
Immigration Reform and Control Act	1986	Prohibits discrimination based on citizenship status; employers required to document employees' legal work status
Worker Adjustment and Retraining Act (WARN)	1988	Employers required to notify workers of impending layoffs
Drug-Free Workplace Act	1988	Covered employers must implement certain policies to restrict employee drug use
Americans with Disabilities Act (ADA)	1990	Prohibits discrimination based on disability
Civil Rights Act	1991	Amends Title VII; prohibits quotas, allows for monetary punitive damages
Family and Medical Leave Act	1993	Employers must provide unpaid leave for childbirth, adoption, illness
Uniformed Services Employment and Reemployment Rights Act	1994	Employers must not discriminate against individuals who take leave from work to fulfill military service obligations

From Gómez-Mejía, Luis R., David B. Balkin, and Robert L. Cardy. *Managing Human Resources*, 3rd ed., 113–114. Upper Saddle River, NJ: Prentice-Hall, 1998; reprinted by permission.

and, as of 1997, applies to employers with more than 15 employees.[38] Part of Congress's findings with passage of ADA in 1990 was that more than 43 million people had one or more physical or mental disabilities.[39] ADA's wording is almost identical to that of the Rehabilitation Act of 1973 and prohibits discrimination in virtually all areas of employment on the basis of handicap or disability. During the selection process, employers may not make inquiries or conduct medical examinations that are designed to identify applicants with disabilities.[40] Private employers must make "reasonable accommodation" for qualified workers unless it can be shown that such accommodation would cause "undue hardship" for the employer. Examples of reasonable accommodation are modifying facilities, job restructuring, part-time and modified work schedules, and reassignment.

Individuals are covered by ADA if they have[41]

> *a physical or mental impairment that substantially limits a major life activity. The ADA also protects individuals who have a record of a substantially limiting impairment, and people who are regarded as having a substantial limiting impairment.*
>
> *A substantial impairment is one that significantly limits or restricts a major life activity such as hearing, seeing, speaking, breathing, performing manual tasks, walking, caring for oneself, learning or working.*

The broad range of disabilities includes blindness, paralysis, heart disease, cancer, acquired immunodeficiency syndrome (AIDS) or a human immunodeficiency virus (HIV)–positive condition,[42] emotional illness, low IQ, and learning disabilities.[43] People who use illegal drugs are not covered by ADA, and they as well as those who abuse alcohol "may be denied employment or fired on the basis of such use,"[44] Employers can administer drug tests to applicants because such tests are not considered to be part of medical examinations under ADA, and are not prohibited. Employers do not have to show that the test is job related. However, alcohol and drug abusers who rehabilitate themselves are covered by ADA.[45]

ADA does not preclude the employer from hiring the best-qualified individual, nor does it impose affirmative action obligations. It does, however, prohibit discrimination because of disability. Employers can ask applicants questions about their ability to perform job-related functions as long as the questions are not phrased in terms of a disability.[46]

What Is Equal Opportunity and Discrimination?

The Civil Rights Act of 1964 defines unlawful employment practices in broad terms.[47] Title VII, section 703, of the act specifically forbids employers from

> *Failing or refusing to hire; or*
>
> *to discharge or otherwise discriminate against any individual with respect to terms, conditions, or privileges of employment; or*
>
> *to limit, segregate, or classify employees in any way that would deprive or tend to deprive any individual of employment opportunity or otherwise adversely affect the individual's status as an employee due to race, color, religion, sex, or national origin.*[48]

These provisions broadly prohibit employers from using the specified categories to adversely affect employees or candidates for employment. The 1991 amendments to the Civil Rights Act of 1964 overturned U.S. Supreme Court decisions and now place the burden of proof of nondiscrimination on the employer, prohibit quotas, and allow plaintiffs to collect punitive damages.[49]

Passage of the Civil Rights Act of 1964 and its subsequent interpretation by the courts caused HSOs/HSs to realize that some of their HRM practices were discriminatory. The criteria for determining whether a practice was illegal was based primarily on whether it had an adverse effect on a class of people protected by the act or whether the practice was a bona fide occupational qualification.

Adverse Impact

In a case of adverse impact, the question is whether a certain practice in recruitment, selection, compensation, transfer, or discharge has been shown to adversely affect a protected class. This can be determined with the aid of sophisticated statistical measures that show the variance between the percentage of a class of minorities in the local population and its percentage in the employer's workforce. If the employer's workforce has fewer employees of that class than one would expect on the basis of population, then courts may assume that discrimination, either intentional or unintentional, has taken place.

Bona Fide Occupational Qualifications

Title VII, section 703, of the Civil Rights Act

> *defines what employment practices are unlawful. This same section, however, exempts several key practices from the scope of Title VII. The most important are the bona fide occupational qualification exemption, the testing and educational requirements section, and the seniority system exemption.*[50]

Bona fide occupational qualifications provide an opportunity for employers to justify or explain a suspect practice by giving nondiscriminatory business reasons for it. However, the burden of proof is on the employer.[51] The following are examples of applying these concepts:

- *Testing*—Preemployment tests are not illegal per se, but they are closely scrutinized. Often, they are found to be culturally biased because they cause more minority applicants to be rejected. Bona fide occupational qualifications determine that what is being tested is related to the job or serves as a valid predictor of success.
- *Physical requirements*—A formerly common but now illegal practice was a requirement that applicants be a certain size or be able to lift certain weight. Such requirements must be justified as necessary to the job (bona fide occupational qualifications) or they risk being found discriminatory based on sex.
- *Educational background*—In an earnest but misguided effort to upgrade their labor force, many managers specified educational requirements for a job that adversely affected a protected class. For example, the job description for a housekeeper may require that the employee be a high school graduate. This requirement has been shown to adversely affect minorities because fewer of them graduate from high school. Coupled with the fact that it is not a bona fide occupational qualification (only basic reading and math skills are needed), the requirement often has been set aside as discriminatory.

Where a bona fide seniority system exists, such as in union contracts, differences in employment conditions are allowed if they are not caused by an intent to discriminate. That is, employees with longer continuous service have a "priority claim to a job over others with fewer years of experience."[52]

Affirmative Action

Another factor to be considered in recruitment and selection is affirmative action planning. "Affirmative action focuses on the hiring, training, and promotion of protected groups where there are deficiencies."[53] Contrary to common belief, affirmative action is neither defined nor required under Title VII of the federal Civil Rights Act of 1964, as amended. However when the EEOC, the administrative and enforcement agency for Title VII of the Civil Rights Act, finds that an employer has discriminated, it may request that the employer adopt a voluntary affirmative action plan. If the employer refuses, then the EEOC may appeal to the courts, which can order affirmative action to correct the deficiencies.

An affirmative action plan is an organization's positive remedy for activities that created inequality or lack of equal opportunity in its employment program. It is a results-oriented program that is designed to materially affect the status quo by increasing the number of employees from a target group, such as African Americans, women, or Hispanic Americans. An example would be an employer who did not hire Hispanics in an area where the population and workforce is 13% Hispanic. An affirmative action plan might require the employer to hire only Hispanics until they represented 13% of the workforce.

A voluntarily adopted affirmative action plan simply formalizes the development and implementation of an employer's nondiscrimination policy by establishing goals to be achieved in a specific time frame. A comprehensive affirmative action plan defines all aspects of the employer–employee relationship: employment, promotion, demotion, layoff, termination, recruitment, rates of pay, employee benefits, and selection for training. The plan may include provisions that the organization will not purchase from or contract with firms that discriminate. A business providing services or products under contract to the federal government must meet special provisions that strictly delineate affirmative action requirements.

Sexual Harassment

Title VII of the 1964 Civil Rights Act does not specifically address sexual harassment in the workplace; however, subsequent court rulings recognized it as a form of discrimination.[54] Managers should have a working knowledge of what sexual harassment is and how to prevent it.

EEOC guidelines define sexual harassment as follows:

> *Unwelcome sexual advances, requests for sexual favors, and other verbal or physical conduct of a sexual nature constitute sexual harassment when (1) submission to such conduct is made either explicitly or implicitly a term or condition of an individual's employment, (2) submission to or rejection of such conduct by an individual is used as the basis for employment decisions affecting such individual, or (3) such conduct has the purpose or effect of unreasonably interfering with an individual's work performance or creating an intimidating, hostile, or offensive working environment.*[55]

The first two forms are categorized as *quid pro quo* because specific outcomes are linked to the granting of sexual favors. The third is hostile environment harassment.[56] The sexual advances need not have been made by the subject's supervisor to be defined as sexual harassment. Co-workers and customers can cause the employer to be liable if the employer "knows or should have known of the conduct and fails to take immediate and appropriate corrective action."[57] Victims do not have to be of the opposite sex and do not have to be the person harassed, but they could be anyone affected by the offensive conduct; also, unlawful harassment need not result in economic injury or discharge of the victim.[58]

Figure 11.4 presents the American College of Healthcare Executives' policy statement on harassment of all types, including articulation, employee training relative to it, procedure for reporting, procedure for investigation, and standards for corrective action.[59] It is management's ethical and legal responsibility to provide a work environment that is free from all forms of harassment. In doing so, costs of litigation are avoided, morale and productivity are increased, absenteeism and turnover are reduced, and the psychological and physical consequences to victims are eliminated.[60]

Table 11.5 presents the number of (and percentage of total) discrimination charges filed, by type, with the EEOC for fiscal years (FYs) 1991–1997. In FY 1997 the three highest categories of charges were race (36.2%), sex (30.7%), and disability (22.4%).

RETAINING EMPLOYEES

After human resources needs have been determined and people are recruited and selected, HRM maintenance and retention activities occur throughout the term of employment. These HRM activ-

PREVENTING AND ADDRESSING HARASSMENT IN THE WORKPLACE

Statement of the Issue

Healthcare executives have a professional responsibility to provide a work environment that protects staff from unwanted and inappropriate behavior. To this end, healthcare executives have a responsibility to their staffs, their organizations, and themselves to create a culture that clearly conveys zero tolerance for harassment and to implement and enforce policies prohibiting harassment. Furthermore, healthcare executives must provide the necessary resources and mechanisms to safeguard against such behavior.

Harassment in the workplace may cause profound damage to both individuals and organizations. Besides the potential legal consequences of such activity, harassment can be linked to loss of productivity, absenteeism, turnover, low morale, lack of trust, communication breakdowns, and long-term career and psychological damage.

Policy Position

The American College of Healthcare Executives believes that all healthcare executives have a professional and ethical responsibility to promote a workplace that is free from harassment on the basis of sex, sexual orientation, age, race, color, religion, national origin, disability, or any other protected characteristic, and to demonstrate zero tolerance for harassment. On behalf of their employing organizations, healthcare executives must further realize that they are responsible for policy implementation and monitoring compliance among their managers. To this end, healthcare executives should promote multifaceted programs in their organizations to prevent harassment and employees should be encouraged to avoid or limit the harm from harassment. Sample program components include, but are not limited to, the following:

Clearly articulated policy against harassment. The policy should define "harassment" (preferably as defined by the Equal Employment Opportunity Commission), explicitly state that harassment is not tolerated in the organization, include examples of prohibited conduct, delineate methods for making and investigating complaints, and provide that appropriate corrective action will be taken. The policy should be incorporated into the employee handbook as well as discussed in new employee orientation.

Employee training on harassment and its prevention. Training should be conducted by human resources staff or other individuals who have a technical and legal understanding of the issue in addition to a demonstrated ability to stimulate discussion about this sensitive topic. Training should be conducted with the goal of raising awareness of harassment, clarifying misconceptions about what constitutes harassment, explaining managers' role and responsibility in providing a harassment-free work environment, and finally, the specifics of the organization's policy prohibiting harassment.

Procedure for reporting allegations of harassment. The procedure should provide as much confidentiality as possible, for both the complaining employee and the employee accused of harassment. Employees should be protected from retaliation for filing a complaint of harassment or appearing as a witness in a harassment investigation. Further, if the procedure requires employees to make initial complaints to their supervisors, an alternate person should be designated to handle complaints when the supervisor is the alleged harasser.

Procedure for expeditiously investigating complaints of harassment. According to EEOC guidelines, once an employee complains of harassment, employers should take "immediate and appropriate corrective action." The organization should, therefore, have a process in place for investigating complaints quickly, discreetly, and completely. Investigations should be conducted by an objective party, and the results of the investigation should be reported to both the complaining employee and the employee accused of harassment. Other staff should be informed only on a "need to know" basis.

Standards for corrective action. Standards for corrective action are an essential part of any plan to prevent sexual harassment. Disciplinary action should be proportionate to the severity of any harassment found; however, avoid providing specific punishments for specific actions. The policy, as it relates to corrective action, should be broad enough to give the freedom to exercise appropriate action. For example, the policy might state that harassing behavior may result in discipline, up to and including discharge.

Legal counsel should review policies and procedures related to harassment because of the potential exposure to liability.

Figure 11.4.   American College of Healthcare Executives public policy statement on harassment in the workplace. (From American College of Healthcare Executives. "Preventing and Addressing Harassment in the Workplace: Public Policy Statement." *Healthcare Executive* 15 [May/June 2000]: 67–68; reprinted by permission.)

ities include appraising each employee's job performance; moving employees within the organization through promotion, demotion, and transfer; disciplinary counseling and separation, when necessary; administering compensation and benefits; providing employee assistance and career counseling; and ensuring a healthful workplace and personal safety (see Figure 11.2). These activities are critical to providing competent staff to meet patient needs.

TABLE 11.5. DISCRIMINATION CHARGES FILED WITH EEOC, BY TYPE OF DISCRIMINATION, FY 1991–1997

	FY 1991	FY 1992	FY 1993	FY 1994	FY 1995	FY 1996	FY 1997
Total charges[a]	63,898	72,302	87,942	91,189	87,529	77,990	80,680
Race	27,981	29,548	31,695	31,656	29,986	26,287	29,199
	43.8%	40.9%	36.0%	34.8%	34.3%	33.8%	36.2%
Sex	17,672	21,796	23,919	25,860	26,181	23,813	24,728
	27.7%	30.1%	27.2%	28.4%	29.9%	30.6%	30.7%
Nation origin	6,692	7,434	7,454	7,414	7,035	6,687	6,712
	10.5%	10.3%	8.5%	8.1%	8.0%	8.6%	8.3%
Religion	1,192	1,388	1,449	1,546	1,581	1,564	1,709
	1.9%	1.9%	1.6%	1.7%	1.8%	2.0%	2.1%
Retaliation	7,906	10,932	12,644	14,415	15,342	14,412	18,113
	12.4%	15.1%	14.4%	15.8%	17.5%	18.5%	22.5%
Age	17,550	19,573	19,809	19,618	17,416	15,719	15,785
	27.5%	27.1%	22.5%	21.5%	19.9%	20.2%	19.6%
Disability	NA	1,048	15,274	18,859	19,798	18,046	18,108
		1.4%	17.4%	20.7%	22.6%	23.1%	22.4%
Equal pay act	1,197	1,291	1,360	1,101	1,171	969	1,140
	1.9%	1.0%	1.5%	1.3%	1.3%	1.2%	1.4%

From Equal Employment Opportunity Commission. *http://www.eeoc.gov/stats/charges.html*, October 9, 1998. The data are compiled by the Office of Research, Information, and Planning from EEOC's Charge Data System—quarterly reconciled Data Summary Reports, and the national database.

[a] The number for total charges reflects the number of individual charge filings. Because individuals often file charges claiming multiple types of discrimination, the number of total charges for any given fiscal year will be less than the total of the eight types of discrimination listed.

Performance Appraisal

The human resources department establishes and maintains an organizationwide employee performance appraisal system to be used by all managers.[61] Appraisal systems evaluate an employee's work by comparing actual with expected performance.

Uses of Performance Appraisal

The results of performance appraisal have many uses. Among them are

- Determining whether individual work results are consistent with expectations. As managers integrate the structure, tasks/technology, and people components of the organization, work results occur (see the management model in Figure 1.7). Performance appraisal is a systematic way of collecting information to assess whether results are those expected and, if not, to determine why not.
- Providing feedback to both employee and supervisor. The performance appraisal interview is a formal opportunity for two-way communication. Positive performance can be reinforced. Less-than-satisfactory performance can be discussed, reasons for it identified, interventions formulated, and future expectations established.
- Identifying high, marginal, and unsatisfactory performers. Depending on the assessment of employee performance levels and their causes, various interventions can be used. Less-than-satisfactory performance often results from employee variables such as a lack of technical job skills or experience, or poor process or job design. Based on this information, interventions such as developmental education, skills training, or job redesign may be warranted. If performance is unsatisfactory for reasons of attitude and behavior, then counseling, discipline, or separation may be warranted. The purpose of performance appraisal is to monitor and, when possible, to constructively improve each employee's ability to do the job well.
- Identifying potential and desirable employee movement within the organization. The results of performance appraisal can influence an employee's candidacy for promotion as well as trans-

fer and demotion. High performers may be promoted with or without further skill building; low performers may be transferred or demoted to a more suitable job.

- Providing information for compensation. If organizations have a wage and salary system that incorporates merit compensation, performance appraisal provides data for determining wage adjustments that are based on performance.
- Providing information for employee assistance and counseling. If an employee's performance is unsatisfactory because of substance abuse or off-the-job personal problems, then the performance appraisal process may reveal that external assistance is recommended.

Virtually all HRM retention activities are linked to performance appraisal. As a result, it is a control and information-gathering system of great importance to managers and the HSO/HS. Joint Commission accreditation standard HR3 requires that processes be "designed to ensure competence of all staff members is assessed, maintained, demonstrated, and improved on an ongoing basis,"[62] including an objective, measurable system that is used to evaluate employee job performance, unmet competencies, and skills.[63]

Appraisal Methods

There are many approaches to employee performance appraisal. Among them are the rating scale, person-to-person comparison, checklist, and critical incident methods.[64] The most commonly used appraisal system is the rating scale method completed by the employee's supervisor. The scales typically specify: 1) personal traits and behaviors such as cooperativeness, dependability, initiative, judgment, and attitude; and 2) job dimension attributes such as quantity of work, quality of work, and job knowledge. For each scale there is usually a scoring mechanism using descriptive adjectives such as "poor" to "excellent," key descriptive phrases, or some other method of differentiation, such as numerical values that often range from 1 (poor) to 10 (excellent). Figure 11.5 presents a sample rating scale employee evaluation (appraisal) form consisting of both personal/behavioral and job dimension scales, with a key phrase scoring system. There also are other approaches to job performance appraisal. Input from peers and subordinates (in the case of a manager), self-appraisal, and customers can provide information that is helpful in assessing job performance. Multirater or 360-degree feedback is a systematic method by which the above-mentioned sources can provide information about an individual's job performance.[65]

Benefits of Systematic Appraisal

A formal performance evaluation system provides a standard format by which managers throughout the organization assess their employees' performance. It also forces managers to observe how well employees are performing and to consider what can be done to improve performance. A formal appraisal system serves another important purpose. Employees have a right to know how well they are performing and what can be done to improve their performance. Most employees want to know what supervisors think of their work out of concern for self-worth and a need for reassurance.

Formal written appraisals of all employees are normally required on an annual basis; however, good management practice and maintenance of high productivity require more frequent feedback on an informal basis. If an employee has just started a new or more responsible position, then an appraisal within 3 months is advisable. In some organizations, appraisals are made according to hire dates; in others, all appraisals are made once or twice a year on fixed dates. As an employee achieves longevity, periodic appraisals have an important influence on morale. They reaffirm the manager's interest in the employee's continuous development and improvement.

Appraisal Problems

Despite the apparent simplicity of performance appraisal forms, a manager often is faced with a number of problems when completing them.[66] First, raters sometimes do not agree on the definitions

EMPLOYEE PERFORMANCE EVALUATION

Date: _____

Employee Name: _____

Job Title: _____

Department: _____

Check ($\checkmark$) one of the following as the reason for this particular performance evaluation.

( ) Prior to the end of the three (3) month probationary period for all new employees or when it is sufficiently clear that new employee is not likely to be satisfactory for the job.

( ) Termination of employment.

( ) Annual: 12 months from last evaluation.

( ) Other, specify: _____

PERFORMANCE REVIEW

APPRAISER: Consider the following five columns as a scale: The extreme right as outstanding, the extreme left as unusually poor. Based on your opinions, place an "X" in the box under the groups of words that best describe each quality of the individual. On the lines below each grouping, make a brief statement showing why certain conclusions were made. Evaluate only the qualities you have observed. Use additional blank sheets for opinion if necessary.

QUALITY: Freedom from errors and mistakes; accuracy; Quality of work in general.	Excessive errors and mistakes. Very poor quality.	Acceptable by minimum standards. Improvement needed.	No more mistakes than should be expected. Quality definitely acceptable.	Quality above average. Few errors & mistakes.	Highest possible quality. Final job virtually perfect.
	☐	☐	☐	☐	☐

COMMENTS: _____
_____

QUANTITY: The actual work output of the employee relative to other employees.	Extremely low output. Definitely not acceptable.	Acceptable but low output. Below average.	Average output. Definitely acceptable.	Produces more than most. Above average.	Definitely a top producer.
	☐	☐	☐	☐	☐

COMMENTS: _____
_____

JOB KNOWLEDGE: Knowledge of the techniques, skills, processes, equipment, and procedures.	Lacks knowledge to perform work properly.	Minimum knowledge for doing job.	Has adequate knowledge of duties.	Good knowledge of duties.	Excellent understanding of job assignments.
	☐	☐	☐	☐	☐

COMMENTS: _____
_____

LEARNING ABILITY: Alertness & ability to advance and grow with the department.	Seems unable to learn new tasks. Cannot adjust from one job to another. Resists change.	Learns new tasks slowly. Has difficulty understanding and going from one assignment to another.	Neither slow nor fast. Can perform several related tasks. Handles new assignments with some difficulty.	Catches on fast. Learns new tasks easily. Handles new assignments with minimum amount of difficulty.	Very adaptable and flexible. Masters new tasks easily. Handles various assignments without difficulty.
	☐	☐	☐	☐	☐

COMMENTS: _____
_____

Figure 11.5. Sample employee evaluation form.   (continued)

INITIATIVE: Degree to which employee can be relied upon to do job without close supervision.	Never volunteers to undertake work. Requires constant prodding to do work. Has no drive or ambition. ☐	Needs some prodding to do work. Dislikes responsibilities. Has very little drive. Believes in just getting by. ☐	Seldom seeks new tasks. Will accept responsibilities when necessary but does not go out of way. Routine worker. ☐	Occasionally seeks new tasks. Works well when given responsibility. Makes occasional suggestion. ☐	Definitely a self-starter. Goes out of way to accept responsibility. Very alert and often constructive. ☐

COMMENTS: _____
_____

COOPERA-TIVENESS: Willingness to work harmoniously with others in getting a job done. Readiness to observe and conform to the policies of management.	Extremely negative and hard to get along with. ☐	Indifferent. Makes no effort to cooperate. ☐	Cooperative. Gets along well with others; has a good attitude. ☐	Goes out of his way to cooperate and get along. ☐	Extremely cooperative. Stimulates teamwork and good attitude in others. ☐

COMMENTS: _____
_____

ATTENDANCE: Faithfulness in coming to work daily and conforming to work hours.	Often absent without good excuse and/or frequently reports for work late. ☐	Lax in attendance and reporting for work on time. ☐	Usually present and on time. ☐	Very prompt. Regular in attendance. ☐	Always regular and prompt. ☐

COMMENTS: _____
_____

PERSONAL APPEARANCE:

This quality refers to the employee's personal grooming, attire, and overall appearance. Does the employee's personal appearance meet the standards for the job? An employee's attire is usually dictated by the nature of the work, which should be considered in evaluating this quality.

Needs Improvement _____   Satisfactory _____

Specific action to be taken by supervisor and/or employee to improve weaknesses.	BY WHOM	BY WHEN

ADDITIONAL RATER'S COMMENTS: _____
_____

_____   _____
Rater's Signature   Date:

EMPLOYEE COMMENTS: _____
_____
_____

_____   _____
Employee's Signature: Date:

COMMENTS RESULTING FROM INTERVIEW: _____
_____
_____
_____

COMMENTS AND RECOMMENDATIONS: (Reviewed by Rater's Supervisor) _____
_____
_____

_____   _____
Reviewer's Signature: Date:

Figure 11.5.   *(continued)*

of terms such as *excellent, good, average,* or *poor.* Descriptive phrases or sentences added to each of these adjectives are helpful in choosing the level that most adequately describes the employee.

Another problem is that one manager's appraisal of employees may be more critical than another's. Some managers do not give low ratings because they are afraid of antagonizing subordinates, whom they believe will then be less cooperative. In addition, low ratings may be perceived as reflecting negatively on the manager's performance and suggesting that employees have not been motivated to improve themselves. Finally, rater perceptual biases can emerge, as exemplified by the appraiser who assumes that no one is "excellent."

The manager also should recognize that one factor may influence others. When employees are very capable in one area, such as quantity of work, the manager may tend to rate them high on most scales without critically analyzing them. One way to avoid this "halo" effect is to rate all employees on one area before starting on the next.

Finally, it is important to show employees their ratings (note the space for the employee's signature on the sample form in Figure 11.5) and to allow them to discuss their rating with their supervisor and to make comments in writing if they wish. Performance evaluations are one of the most important tools an employer has to build a high-quality and competent workforce. Employee involvement is central to a successful appraisal system.

Continuous Quality Improvement

Drucker noted that "quantity without quality is the worst thing and will result in total failure."[67] Performance appraisals are critical to monitoring quality; they provide data to measure the success of current job design and work flow (processes), progress toward achieving objectives, and individual performance. Real-time performance feedback is required to achieve continuous improvement of affected processes. Cascio identified criteria for evaluation, including having customer expectations drive quality improvement team or individual performance expectations, or both; preidentification of results-expectations and whether they are met or exceeded; and identification and measurement of behavioral skills that make a difference in improving quality results and customer satisfaction (see the discussion of CQI in Chapter 9).[68]

Training and Development

Another basic HRM activity of maintaining and retaining human resources is training, which involves changing behavior and expanding employee knowledge and skills through an organized process by which employees learn skills, abilities, and attitudes that are needed for successful job performance.[69] When not performed by a separate department, this function often is assigned to the human resources department. In most HSOs/HSs training is organized into staff or line training or both. Training departments are found in most large HSOs, and they educate staff on organization-wide issues such as CQI, they develop managers and supervisors, and they facilitate departmental (line) training. Another method is cooperative: several independent HSOs may share staff training, specialists, and cost; or, in the case of HSs a centralized training unit can provide services to system members.

Line training is department specific and usually is the responsibility of department managers. Examples include a nursing service department that provides in-service training for nursing assistants or recently graduated registered nurses (RNs) and a housekeeping department that trains employees in proper cleaning or infection control.

Special mention should be made of supervisory and management development as a type of training. HSOs/HSs have special needs in preparing supervisors and managers because so many are drawn from technically trained staff. Management development is a way to increase the capabilities of managers beyond their technical base.[70] Development focuses on general managerial skills such as leadership, motivation, communication, and problem solving. Specific skills training in report writing and budgeting may be included.

Management development may be internal or external. Internally, job rotation or vendor-delivered on-site programs that are structured or simulation based can be used to develop middle-level and senior-level managers.[71] Externally, periodically attending off-site seminars or professional association programs can be beneficial. Other approaches include senior-level managers coaching lower level managers (mentoring) and inclusion of managers on important committees.

The training and development of employees, whether by skills enhancement or cross-training in more than one job function, is an investment.[72] Clearly, it is a value-added activity that is an important part of quality and productivity improvement and ensures that the HSO/HS has competent staff.

Discipline (Corrective Counseling)

Discipline may be the least-understood aspect of the HSO's/HS's relationship with employees. Most people associate discipline with punishment—a negative concept. Accurately understood, however, discipline is positive and means corrective counseling, which involves creating a climate and an attitude among employees that encourages them to accept policies and practices because they understand that doing so contributes to their success and to the organization's success. If discipline is to be seen as positive, then policies and practices must be reasonable and employees must understand what is expected of them. In addition, it must be understood that the employer has a right to a well-disciplined, cooperative workforce and has the authority to take action if rules are violated.

To be effective, discipline/corrective counseling should be formalized and include established procedures. Although there is no one best process, certain provisions should be included[73]:

> Disciplinary/corrective counseling actions should be based on facts with clear and demonstrable justification.
>
> Employees should be treated consistently, with the background and circumstances of each case considered separately.
>
> Disciplinary actions should be progressive and related to behavior; in order of severity, typical actions are: 1) unrecorded oral warning, 2) oral warning noted in the employment record, 3) written warning noted in the employment record, 4) suspension from the job, and 5) discharge.

Including these provisions does not guarantee that a disciplinary program will meet its objectives, but they go far toward ensuring a positive approach to discipline in HSOs/HSs.

Compensation Administration

One of the most important aspects of maintaining and retaining a suitable workforce is effective compensation administration. Compensation is a generic term for wages, salaries, and fringe benefits and directly affects the organization's ability to attract and retain qualified employees. In HSOs/HSs the human resources department has responsibility for developing, implementing, and administering an organizationwide compensation program.[74]

Equity is the primary objective of compensation programs. Depending on its size and programs, a single HSO might have more than 200 different types of jobs. Determining what each job should be paid involves consideration of three factors: internal and external equity and philosophy.

- *Internal equity*—How does the pay of various jobs compare? What should a nurse earn compared to a social worker or dietitian? There are various ways to achieve internal equity; at a minimum, job requirements must be identified and their complexity evaluated. Evaluation usually is reduced to a numerical factor (rating) so that jobs can be more easily compared.

- *External equity*—How does the HSO's/HS's pay for jobs compare with that at competing organizations? External equity became more important as the supply and demand of market forces began to affect HSOs/HSs. Shortages of certain types of staff such as medical technologists and pharmacists caused wage wars, and union pressures prompted HSOs/HSs to analyze the market for pay competitiveness.
- *Philosophy*—How does the HSO/HS pay relative to the market? A mature pay philosophy succinctly describes how the HSO/HS uses data that are obtained by answering the first two questions to compete for staff in the labor market. For example, the philosophy might be "Our pay range midpoints will be 10% above the projected median of our market for professional (higher level) jobs, and equal to the projected median of our market for service (lower level, entry) jobs." There is no "right" pay philosophy because factors such as labor supply, market definition, projected human resources needs, type of organization, and fiscal constraints must be considered.

Establishing and Administering a Compensation System

Job evaluation is a formal system to determine the relative value of jobs in an organization and is the heart of a wage and salary administration program.[75] Jobs are analyzed using job descriptions. Each job is rated according to an evaluation plan with the purpose of establishing specific rates of pay or specific wage ranges (salary grades).

There are four major methods of job evaluation. The two that are the least complex are ranking and job classification; the point and factor comparison systems are quite complex.[76] Regardless of method, the expected outcome is a system of hourly rates, wage ranges, or both that relate logically to one another, a procedure that permits changes in compensation within grades using criteria such as performance and experience, a means to move employees to new grades or classifications based on changes such as job expansion, and a way to maintain internal equity.

There are several advantages for employees and managers in a well-structured and well-administered wage program. For example,

- Inequities tend to be reduced because employees are objectively paid according to job requirements.
- Managers can explain the wage program's basis because it results from a systematic analysis of job and wage data.
- Favoritism in assigning wage rates is minimized.
- Employee morale and motivation are increased because the wage program is easily explained, is based on fact, and shows employees where they stand.
- Managers can systematically plan and control labor costs.
- The program attracts qualified employees by paying fair and competitive wages.

One of the most important pieces of legislation affecting compensation administration is the federal Fair Labor Standards Act (FLSA) of 1938, amended in 1967 to include many HSOs/HSs. The FLSA requires HSOs/HSs to pay overtime for hours worked beyond 40 in a 7-day period, just as a non–HSO must. An option for hospitals recognizes their 24-hour, 7-days-a-week operation and permits them to pay overtime differently: Hours beyond 8/day and 80/14-consecutive-day period require overtime pay.[77]

The FLSA prohibits employers whose workers are subject to minimum wage requirements from discriminating based on gender in paying wages for equal work. It also sets a minimum age of 17 for general employment and 18 for work found hazardous by the U.S. Secretary of Labor. Minors ages 14 and 15 may be employed outside school hours in certain occupations and under specified conditions. Evaluations, judgments, determinations, and decisions relating to wage and salary administration may be reviewed by the Wage and Hour Division of the Department of Labor. Inquiries and follow-up investigations can be made randomly or based on employee complaint.

Executive and Incentive Compensation

The need to recruit and retain senior-level managers has prompted HSOs/HSs to evaluate executive incentive compensation plans, such as bonuses. HSOs/HSs joined industry in using this feature, in which compensation incentives are linked to organization performance.[78] According to data from a survey of 1,200 hospitals that was co-sponsored by the American Hospital Association, 78% of health care management companies and 49% of hospitals have an incentive component in their senior-level management compensation programs.[79] Incentive compensation can achieve substantial savings by attracting talented leaders, encouraging development of multiple skills, increasing tolerance for risk taking, motivating innovative behavior, and rewarding cost reductions.

Benefits Administration

Fringe benefits account for an increasingly large proportion of total employee compensation. Benefits commonly provided include health insurance (hospital, professional service, and sometimes dental and vision), pension, life insurance, short- and long-term disability insurance, vacation, holidays, and sick leave. Some benefits are legally mandated federal and state insurance programs. Examples include Social Security, no-fault workers' compensation for on-the-job injuries, and unemployment insurance. Benefits typically average one fourth to one third of payroll costs, and prudent management of employer contributions is essential. HSOs/HSs and industry have sought to control benefits costs through concepts such as self-insuring. Self-insuring is ordinarily done through an employer-established trust fund to pay claims directly without using an insurance carrier. Dollars that the employer would have paid in premiums fund the trust and cover claims. Excess liability coverage ("stop loss" insurance) with a high deductible is used to limit employer risk and losses.

Another way to effectively curb benefits costs while maximizing employee satisfaction is the cafeteria or full flexible benefit plan.[80] In this arrangement the employer allocates a dollar allowance to employees and each designs a benefits package from a menu of items. Because employees choose benefits to suit their needs, their satisfaction is enhanced and employer costs are more predictable.

Flexible spending accounts for health and child care expenses are key parts of cafeteria plans and frequently are offered as freestanding benefits. Employees place pretax dollars in accounts reserved for use during the year. Unused dollars are lost. Employers do not pay Social Security or income taxes on reserved dollars, and this further reduces cost and increases employee take-home pay.

With a high percentage of female and single-parent employees, HSOs/HSs have become increasingly involved in providing on-site child care services. The value of such services to employers is in reduced absenteeism, enhanced recruitment, increased morale and retention, and reduced parental stress.

The Consolidated Omnibus Budget Reconciliation Act of 1985 (COBRA) requires employers to allow former employees to participate in group health insurance for as long as 18 months.[81] A full premium must be paid (with a small surcharge for employer administration), but former employees pay considerably less than they would for nongroup coverage. The Health Insurance Portability and Accountability Act of 1996 had the intended purpose of lessening employee lock-in to a job because of health insurance benefits. The act, under certain conditions, enables employees to change jobs and be exempt from preexisting conditions restrictions when joining the health plan of the new employer.[82]

The Family and Medical Leave Act of 1993 is a noncompensation benefit that covers employers with more than 50 employees.[83] It permits employees to take employment leaves for the "birth, adoption or foster-care placement of a child, caring for a spouse, child or parent with a serious health condition, or serious health condition of the employee."[84] It requires employers to grant up to 12 weeks of unpaid leave per year.[85]

Pension Programs

Although pension programs are only one of several benefits programs provided for HSO/HS employees, they are particularly significant because they show increased involvement of the federal government in employer–employee relations. Pension programs can be contributory, in which both employer and employee contribute, or noncontributing, in which only the employer contributes.[86] They may also be defined contribution or defined benefit pension programs. Defined benefit programs obligate the employer to a specific pension amount when the employee retires based on years of service and age versus amount contributed. This carries some unknown risk. Defined contribution plans are those in which an employer makes specific contributions, such as to an employee's tax-deferred 401(k) plan, for which the employee can choose various individual contribution levels and various investment options. The employee's retirement benefit is based on the appreciated value of the contributions at retirement and does not obligate the employer to an annuity stream based on age and years of service as in a defined benefit plan.[87]

The Employee Retirement Income Security Act (ERISA) was enacted in 1974 and reflects a basic philosophical change about pension plans.[88] The old theory was that a pension rewarded long and faithful service and that it was an incentive for employees to remain with the employer. The new theory is that a pension is a contractual right—a form of wages deferred as part of employment similar to workers' and unemployment compensation. The law sought to prevent loss of pension benefits when plans were terminated because of plant closings, bankruptcies, sales and mergers of businesses, or voluntary termination.

To carry out ERISA's purpose of protecting employees and their heirs in pension and welfare plans, Congress established requirements for preparing and filing reports, making plan documents available, and providing statements of benefits. Reports must be written in simple language and must highlight benefit design, complaint procedures, vesting, financial integrity, and employee rights. The net effect has been to shift the information-sharing burden from employees, who previously often had to ask for information, to employers, who now must provide it, and to protect the rights of employees. Effectively managing the act's legal requirements provides further opportunities for employee communications that help HSOs/HSs maintain and retain employees. The legal aspects of health benefits and ERISA are discussed further in Chapter 14.

Employee Assistance Programs

Employees are an asset, and many organizations have established EAPs to help employees with a problem that adversely affects their work. Early programs dealt only with alcoholic employees, but the focus has broadened and includes help for substance abuse as well as legal, financial, and emotional problems. The first EAPs were developed by a few progressive industrial corporations and were justified by claims of reduced absenteeism and work-related accidents. It is now clear that their value is much greater given estimates that 15%–20% of the workforce either use illicit drugs or abuse alcohol. These employees are three to four times more likely to be injured at work than nonusers, have 47% of serious workplace accidents, file close to 50% of workers' compensation claims, and are 33% less productive.[89] There is value in reducing employee chemical dependency problems and behavioral illnesses. Health services environments have ready access to drugs and are emotionally difficult settings. EAPs have the potential for significant savings through decreased turnover rates, lower insurance costs, decreased use of sick time, improved employee job performance, enhanced quality and productivity,[90] and salvaged human resources.

HSOs/HSs have become active in providing comprehensive EAP services to industry as an extension of outpatient activities. They are ideal sources for two reasons. First, an effective EAP incorporates confidentiality. The employee must receive help without fear of retribution or any record of counseling that might affect future employment. Services provided by a separate HS entity enhance confidentiality.

Career counseling is a second area in which human resources departments effectively provide employee assistance. Shortages have led to development of current employees to meet future human resources needs. Expenditures for direct skills training, subsidized professional education, and management development have become a large part of the organization's investment in its staff. Career counseling and needs assessment are ways in which the human resources department can reduce costs of mismatching people and jobs and enhance an organization's return on its employee investment.

Health education and promotion is a third and increasingly vital area of employee assistance. By educating the workforce to better manage their own health and supporting efforts in areas such as stress management and weight and smoking reduction, employers can improve productivity, reduce health insurance expense, and contribute significantly to the positive climate required for longer employee retention. These initiatives are an investment in the HSO's/HS's human resources.

Workplace Health and Safety

A final aspect of retaining a workforce is ensuring workplace health and safety. HSOs/HSs, like other types of organizations, have long been concerned with employee health and safety. Significant impetus for formal health and safety programs was provided by the enactment of most state workers' compensation laws between 1910 and 1925. These laws hold employers financially responsible for work injuries regardless of fault.

Enactment of the Occupational Safety and Health Act of 1970, also known as the Williams-Steiger Act, had far-reaching effects on organizations of all types.[91] The law was designed to solve safety and health problems associated with complex and dangerous machinery, chemicals, pollutants, and environmental threats found in the workplace. The act focused on the traditional industrial workplace, but the law was broad enough to include nongovernmental HSOs. The Occupational Safety and Health Administration (OSHA) implements the law and requires organizations to perform three major activities: 1) promulgation and enforcement of safety standards to eliminate or lessen hazards, 2) record keeping, and 3) training and education.

HSOs/HSs are dangerous places. Caustic and toxic chemicals in the laboratory and pharmacy, slicing equipment in food services, radiation in radiology, ethylene oxide in supply processing, and infections in patient care areas are a few of the many hazards. The health services industry has recognized this danger, and the Joint Commission has formulated standards for safety in HSOs/HSs, including requirements for multidisciplinary committees to identify and correct safety problems and educate employees on the importance of safety. Finally, increasing attention is being given to reducing workplace violence.[92] Employers have a responsibility to provide a secure and safe workplace for their employees and customers.

AIDS poses a unique problem for HSOs/HSs: Protecting health care workers from patients is compounded by the need to protect patients from health care workers. Universal precautions protect workers (and other patients by reducing the risk of cross-infection) by assuming that every patient is HIV positive. A focus of the public debate about protecting patients has been testing of health care workers, especially physicians and dentists. This debate tends to be emotional and is complicated by concerns that employees who test positive for the virus will be discriminated against or suffer emotionally. Chapter 13 discusses the ethical issues surrounding AIDS, and Chapter 14 discusses the legal issues.

SEPARATION FROM EMPLOYMENT (EXIT)

Employees leave HSOs/HSs for various reasons—better job opportunities, discharge, retirement, or death. Most human resources departments engage in activities to assist and monitor exit. Traditional activities include easing the individual's departure; collecting employer-provided equipment, keys, and records; completing personnel records; processing final pay; and collecting information through an exit interview. Other activities include preretirement planning and outplacement.

Preretirement Planning

Preretirement counseling is an important function of the human resources department. The purpose is to prepare employees for the psychological, emotional, and financial changes at retirement. Such programs typically use experts to help employees understand lifestyle changes, emotional and physical needs, financial planning, Social Security benefits, pensions, and legal affairs such as estate planning. A preretirement planning program is effective in building employee relations.

Outplacement

HSOs/HSs now face "industrial" problems of changing demand, downsizing, consolidation, and mergers. Outplacement occurs most often when jobs are eliminated because services are retrenched or abandoned or facilities close or merge. Outplacement recognizes a social and financial commitment by the employer to assist employees in securing employment because their services have been valued. Contacts with other employers, advertising on employees' behalf, counseling, and retraining are typical, as is arranging for the services of professional outplacement firms. Increasing competitiveness in health care has made outplacement a key element in managing the separation of managers, too. Here, counseling usually means exploring alternate careers.

Exit Interviews

It is hoped that employees who leave a HSO/HS will provide candid feedback, and many organizations use exit interviews to learn about employee relations. Usually, this means an interview with someone in the human resources department. Employees are asked about job likes and dislikes and their opinions of supervisors, the facility, the benefits package, and compensation. The reason for separation is confirmed. An attempt is made to resolve problems so that the employee leaves on a positive note. If the process is to be credible, information from exit interviews must be confidential. It is combined with other data to provide a profile of programmatic strengths and weaknesses and, possibly, the need for intervention.[93] The technique has limitations—it usually deals with problems after the fact—but is important in providing feedback to management.

HUMAN RESOURCES DEPARTMENT AND CLINICAL STAFF

It is noteworthy that, although the functions and scope of the human resources department have grown significantly, professional staff organization (PSO) relations are the exclusive domain of the HSO/HS governing body and chief executive officer. When private practice clinical staff are involved this is understandable, because licensed independent practitioners (LIPs) typically are not employees and are controlled by the HSO/HS only as required by the PSO bylaws and the clinical privileges granted. However, when LIPs are salaried (clinical managers or facility-based specialists such as pathologists and radiologists), they have many characteristics of employees and may be included in the HSO's/HS's employee benefit program as well. Even here, however, the human resources department is rarely involved in wage administration or personnel file maintenance. The HSO/HS does not view these individuals as typical employees.

HUMAN RESOURCES IN HSs

To this point, HRM activities relative to acquiring and retaining as well as maintaining employees have been discussed primarily from the perspective of a freestanding HSO; they also apply to HSs but in a more centralized way. The human resources role in HSs includes setting overall policy, co-ordinating all HRM activities among system component organizations, and supporting their programs rather than always administering staffing activities. Corporate efforts may range from establishing overall systemwide policy guidelines on compensation and benefits, regional training and development, and recruitment and selection, to intraorganizational behaviors such as workplace romances and sexual harassment. Corporate assistance also can be provided to components relative to specific programs, such as succession planning and regional training. Corporate support can range from informal consultation on compensation plan design to benefit plan administration. Well-directed corporate human resources functions save time and money for individual component facilities as well as expand their human resources services.

LABOR RELATIONS

Staffing the HSO/HS with qualified people to fulfill its mission entails all of the acquisition and re-tention and maintenance HRM activities presented previously, including that of complying with state and federal laws. In addition, for those HSOs/HSs in which some employees are members of an employee organization (i.e., union) or seek to be represented by an employee organization, the human resources department has centralized responsibility for union–management relations and collective bargaining. Even though union–management relations are centralized, all managers need to be aware of the legislation affecting this relationship, including the rights of employees as well as those of the employer, reasons why employees may seek to join a union, and permissible management behavior in a union-organizing election.

Labor relations is a generic term that is used to describe the employer–employee relationship. Collective bargaining "is the process by which union leaders representing groups of employees negotiate terms of employment with representatives designated by management."[94] That relationship and the process of bargaining are important because employee unions and management negotiate about wages, conditions of work, promotion policies, discipline procedures, and sometimes job design and work assignments. Consequently, the employer–employee relationship and the collective bargaining agreement between the two ultimately affect the HSO's/HS's costs and allocation and utilization of human resources, and can influence managerial decision-making, planning, directing, and controlling functions. The remaining sections of this chapter describe the evolution of labor law, including that in health services, its current status, and issues pertinent to labor relations in HSOs/HSs.

LABOR MOVEMENT

It was not until the passage of federal labor legislation, beginning in the 1930s, that the labor movement picked up momentum in the United States. In 1935 the number of unionized workers (and their percentage of the workforce) was 3.7 million (6.7%). It peaked in 1975 at 20.7 million (22.6%) and was 16.2 million (13.9%) in 1998.[95]

Subsequent to the unionization of basic manufacturing industries such as automobiles, steel, chemicals, and rubber from the 1930s through the 1950s, increased attention was given by union organizers to service industries, including health care. During the 10-year period from 1985 to 1994, there were 886 union elections in nongovernment, not-for-profit acute care hospitals involving 147,600 employees. Unions were successful in 51.4% of the elections. Similarly, during the same time period, there were 33,833 union elections in all economic sectors, involving 2.1 million individuals. Unions were successful in 48.7% of the elections—a rate similar to that in health services.[96]

FEDERAL LABOR LEGISLATION

In general, the federal government was anti-union before the 1930s. However, during the Great Depression a shift occurred. The Protestant work ethic, factory systems, and common law employer property rights were challenged by a social ethic. Although some states had progressive labor legislation, the Depression contributed to an awareness that the federal government had responsibilities to blue-collar workers. The legal setting changed in 1932 with passage of the Norris-LaGuardia Act. Other subsequent federal labor legislation examined in this chapter includes the Wagner Act of 1935, the Taft-Hartley Act of 1947, and the 1974 Nonprofit Hospital Amendments to the Taft-Hartley Act.

Norris-LaGuardia Act (Anti-Injunction Act, 1932)

The Norris-LaGuardia Act of 1932, officially called the Anti-Injunction Act,[97] was landmark legislation. It represented a major change in Congress's attitude toward labor–management relations. The law's basic philosophy was that individuals were at a disadvantage when bargaining with employers. As a consequence, to enable the individual employee "to protect his freedom of labor," it prohibited employer use of "yellow dog" contracts, which required employees not to join a union. If they did join a union, it was a breach of the contract and cause for termination.[98] The Norris-LaGuardia Act also focused on federal court injunctions in labor disputes. Prior to 1932, preliminary injunctions were frequently issued to forestall union activity (e.g., a recognition strike) that could cause "irreparable" harm while the court examined the merits of the case. Employers were able to obtain injunctions enjoining union activity from sympathetic courts. Although activities such as strikes or picketing were not illegal, failure to comply with an injunction was. Norris-LaGuardia stripped employers of nonmeritorious use of injunctions.

Wagner Act (National Labor Relations Act, 1935)

The second major labor–management relations law enacted in the 1930s was the Wagner Act, officially known as the National Labor Relations Act (NLRA) of 1935.[99] The primary purpose of NLRA was to ensure that private-sector employees had the right to organize and bargain collectively, free from employer influence or coercion, and to establish a balance of bargaining power between employers and employees. To achieve this purpose, NLRA specified employer unfair labor practices and established the National Labor Relations Board (NLRB) to oversee issues involving union recognition and collective bargaining.[100]

Employer Unfair Labor Practices

Section 8 of NLRA specified five employer unfair labor practices. These are summarized in Table 11.6 to reflect subsequent amendments, and examples are given. Unfair labor practices define what employers may not do when employees want to unionize. In addition, they specify how employers must deal with the certified representative (union) of the employees once recognition occurs. In sum, the employer must bargain in good faith.

National Labor Relations Board

The second major provision of NLRA established the NLRB, defined union recognition, and provided the means to resolve allegations of unfair labor practices. The thrust of NLRA is that the duly elected representative of a majority of employees for an appropriate bargaining unit shall be the exclusive agent for the purpose of collective bargaining. Basically, if a majority of employees want to form a union, they can impose their will on the minority. NLRB conducts elections for representation and certifies the exclusive agent for a particular bargaining unit.

TABLE 11.6.   EMPLOYER UNFAIR LABOR PRACTICES AND EXAMPLES

1. *To interfere with, restrain, or coerce employees in the exercise of their rights to organize* [Section 8(a)(1)].
   —Threaten employees with loss of job or benefits if they vote for a union
   —Grant wage increases deliberately timed to discourage employees from joining a union

2. *To dominate or interfere with the affairs of a union* [Section 8(a)(2)].
   —Take an active part in the affairs of a union, such as a nurse supervisor actively participating in a nurses' association representing RNs
   —Show favoritism to one union over another in an organizing attempt

3. *To discriminate in regard to hiring, tenure, or any employment condition for the purpose of encouraging or discouraging membership in any union organization* [Section 8(a)(3)].
   —Discharge employees who urge others to join a union
   —Demote an employee for union activity

4. *To discriminate against or discharge an employee because he has filed charges or given testimony under this act* [Section 8(a)(4)].
   —Discriminate against, fire, or demote employees because they gave testimony to NLRB officials or filed charges against the employer with the NLRB

5. *To refuse to bargain collectively with representatives of the employees; that is, "bargain in good faith"* [Section 8(a)(5)].
   —Refuse to provide information, if requested, by the union, that is relevant and necessary to allow employees' representative to bargain intelligently and effectively with respect to wages, hours, and other conditions of employment
   —Refuse to bargain about a "mandatory" subject such as hours and wages
   —Refuse to meet with union representatives duly appointed by a certified bargaining unit
   —Take unilateral action in current conditions of employment without notifying the union, such as subcontracting x-ray or food service activities if those employees are currently unionized

From Office of the General Counsel, National Labor Relations Board. *A Guide to Basic Law and Procedures Under the National Labor Relations Act*, 22–23. Washington, DC: National Labor Relations Board, 1990.

Prior to passage of NLRA, unions often had to strike to force employers to recognize them as the employees' bargaining agent. NLRA changed that. At the request of at least 30% of employees, NLRB holds an election and, if a majority of voting employees in the defined bargaining unit vote for a particular union to represent them, then that union becomes their exclusive bargaining agent. Furthermore, the employer must bargain in good faith with that agent.

The second function of NLRB concerns unfair labor practices. If it is found, for example, that an employer committed an unfair labor practice, then NLRB can provide remedies through cease-and-desist orders and take corrective action, "including reinstatement of employees with or without back pay"[101] who were discharged in violation of the act. NLRB's objective is to eliminate unfair labor practices and to undo the effects of the violation.

Taft-Hartley Act (Labor–Management Relations Act, 1947)

The employer unfair labor practices listed in Table 11.6 indicate that, as of 1935, unprecedented constraints were applied against employers while restrictions on the behavior of labor were minimal. Clearly, the intent of NLRA was to create a legal environment promoting the rights of workers to unionize.[102] However, by the late 1940s, the balance of power had swung so far in favor of labor that Congress passed, over President Truman's veto, the Taft-Hartley Act in 1947.[103]

The Taft-Hartley Act, officially titled the Labor–Management Relations Act (LMRA) of 1947,[104] amended the Wagner Act (NLRA) of 1935. Its purpose was "to define and protect the rights of employees and employer, to encourage collective bargaining, and to eliminate certain practices on the part of labor and management that are harmful to the general welfare."[105] The major provisions of the Taft-Hartley Act changed the structure of NLRB, protected employee rights not to join a union, enumerated union unfair labor practices, provided legislative prescriptions for certain bargaining procedures, and established procedures for handling national emergencies.

The act restructured NLRB around two functions: to conduct representation elections and certify the results, and to prevent employers and unions from engaging in unfair labor practices. When requested, NLRB intervenes in both of these areas. A five-member board hears cases. The NLRB general counsel investigates and prosecutes cases.[106] This structural change separated prosecution of cases from judging them by separating quasi-executive from quasi-judicial functions.

Employee Protection

Another major change was that Taft-Hartley protected both workers who wanted to organize and those who did not. When a "substantial" number of employees (defined by NLRB as a "showing of interest" by at least 30% of the bargaining unit) petition to hold a recognition election, NLRB conducts one. If a majority of employees vote against the union, Section 9(c)(3) prohibits any union from petitioning for an election for 1 year.[107] Therefore, the right of employees not to join a union is preserved and employers are not harassed with endless elections. Similarly, by majority vote employees can exercise their right to decertify a union that is currently representing them.

Union Unfair Labor Practices

Employer unfair labor practices were specified in the 1935 Wagner Act. A major provision of the 1947 Taft-Hartley Act is enumeration of union unfair labor practices. These are contained in Section 8(b) of the Taft-Hartley Act, as amended, and are summarized with examples in Table 11.7.

Bargaining Procedures

Other Taft-Hartley provisions specify that 1) nonthreatening handbilling is not an unfair labor practice; 2) a 60-day notice of contract termination or modification must be given to the other party; 3) supervisors cannot be part of a bargaining unit; and 4) guards and professional employees cannot be mixed with other employees in a bargaining unit, except in the case of professional employees who have concurred. Taft-Hartley also has an 80-day cooling off period that begins when the president declares a national emergency. During this time there can be no strike.[108]

The Wagner (NLRA) and Taft-Hartley (LMRA) acts were amended by the 1959 Landrum-Griffin Act, officially known as the Labor–Management Reporting and Disclosure Act of 1959.[109] Landrum-Griffin primarily addresses internal union affairs such as election of officers and provides safeguards for union members, but Title VII adds a seventh union unfair practice (8[b][7]): picketing an employer for recognition of a second union when one union is already certified.[110] Examples include engaging in picketing to obtain recognition by the employer (recognition picketing) or acceptance by employers of the employees' representative (organizational picketing) when the employer has lawfully recognized another union, when a valid NLRB election has been held within the previous 12 months, or when no representation petition has been filed with NLRB within 30 days of the commencement of such picketing.[111]

Nonprofit Hospital Amendments to the Taft-Hartley Act (1974)

Pre-1974 Environment

Prior to 1974, the collective bargaining legal framework covering HSOs/HSs varied by type of ownership. Taft-Hartley specifically excluded from its definition of employer "any corporation or association operating a hospital, if no part of the net earnings inures to the benefit of any private share holder or individual" (Section 2[2]). This meant that not-for-profit hospitals were excluded from federal labor law. Federal and nonfederal (state, local) government hospitals continued to be excluded.

Investor-owned HSOs/HSs (for-profit hospitals, nursing facilities, or systems of them) continued to be covered by provisions of NLRA, as amended, although NLRB exerted no jurisdiction until 1967.[112] NLRB developed revenue standards that trigger a presumption that an investor-

TABLE 11.7. UNION UNFAIR LABOR PRACTICES AND EXAMPLES

1. *To restrain or coerce employees in the exercise of their right to join or not to join a union except when an agreement is made by the employer and union that a condition of employment will be joining the union (called a union security clause authorizing a "union shop")* [Section 8(b)(1)(A)].
    —Picket as a mass and physically bar other employees from entering a health care facility
    —Act violently toward nonunion employees
    —Threaten employees for not supporting union activities

2. *To cause an employer to discriminate against an employee other than for nonpayment of dues or initiation fees* [Section 8(b)(2)].
    —Cause an employer to discriminate against an employee for antiunion activity
    —Force the employer to hire only workers "satisfactory" to the union

3. *To refuse to bargain with an employer in "good faith" about wages, hours, and conditions of employment* [Section 8(b)(3)].
    —Insist on negotiating illegal provisions such as management's prerogative to appoint supervisors
    —Refuse to meet with the employer's representative
    —Terminate an existing contract or strike without the appropriate notice

4. *To engage, induce, encourage, threaten, or coerce any individual to engage in strikes, refusal to work, or boycott when the objective is to* [Section 8(b)(4)]:
    (a) *Force or require any employer or self-employed person to recognize or join any labor organization or employer organization.*
    (b) *Force or require any employer or self-employed person to cease using the products of or doing business with another person, or force any other employer to recognize or bargain with the union unless it has been certified by the NLRB.*
    (c) *Force an employer to apply pressure to another employer to recognize a union.*

    —Picketing a hospital so that it will apply pressure on a subcontractor (food service, maintenance, emergency department) to recognize a union, or forcing an employer to do business only with others, such as suppliers, who have a union, or picketing by another union for recognition when a different one is already certified

5. *To charge excessive or discriminatory membership fees* [Section 8(b)(5)].
    —Charge a higher initiation fee to employees who did not join the union until after a union-security agreement (union shop) is in force

6. *To cause an employer to give payment for services not performed (featherbedding)* [Section 8(b)(6)].
    —Force an employer to add people to the payroll when they are not needed
    —Force payment to employees who provide no services

From Office of the General Counsel, National Labor Relations Board. *A Guide to Basic Law and Procedures Under the National Labor Relations Act*, 27–40. Washington, DC: National Labor Relations Board, 1990.

owned HSO/HS affects interstate commerce and is subject to NLRA jurisdiction.[113] President Kennedy's Executive Order 10988, which was modified in 1970 by President Nixon's Executive Order 11491,[114] established recognition and bargaining procedures and unfair labor practices for federal employees (and management), including those in federal hospitals.[115] These provisions were incorporated into Title VII of the 1978 Civil Service Reform Act. Neither the executive orders nor the 1978 act ended the prohibition on strikes by federal employees.[116]

1974—A Changed Environment

PL 93-360, the Nonprofit Hospital Amendments to the Taft-Hartley Act, was passed on July 26, 1974, and ended the nongovernmental, not-for-profit hospital exclusion in the 1947 act.[117] For-profit HSOs/HSs were already covered by Taft-Hartley, if they met the revenue test. By 1973, 16.8% of not-for-profit hospitals had at least one collective bargaining agreement that had been obtained without federal labor law protection and procedural benefits.[118] Excluding not-for-profit hospitals from federal labor law coverage and the absence or inadequacy of state legislation often caused highly publicized work stoppages (strikes) initiated for purposes of union recognition.

Thus, since 1974 not-for-profit and investor-owned (nongovernmental) HSOs/HSs, as well as unions, have complied with recognition, election, and unfair labor practice provisions of the Wagner and Taft-Hartley acts. The 1974 amendments define a health care organization as "any hospital, convalescence hospital, health maintenance organization, health clinic, nursing home, extended care facility, or any other institution devoted to the care of sick, infirm, or aged persons" (Section 2[2][b][14]). NLRB defines health care delivery to include hospitals, health maintenance organizations (HMOs), and long-term care facilities that provide inpatient or outpatient care, including private institutions providing for the care of people with mental retardation,[119] as well as other noninstitutional providers such as medical associations, laboratories, group practices, and home health agencies.

Unique Provisions

The 1974 amendments included provisions that are unique to HSOs/HSs: contract notices, notification preceding a strike, conciliation of disputes, and payment of union dues by individuals with religious convictions.[120]

Contract Notices

Because HSOs/HSs provide unique and essential services, the amendments require a 90-day (compared to 60-day for other sectors) notification to the other party to modify an existing contract and a 60-day notice to the Federal Mediation and Conciliation Service (FMCS) and the applicable state agency.[121] If a breakdown occurs during bargaining for an initial contract following recognition and NLRB certification of a labor organization, a 30-day notice must be given to the FMCS and the appropriate state agency before a strike can be called. These provisions provide a longer time for the parties to reach agreement or plan for a work stoppage and to enable the FMCS to provide assistance.

Strike Notice

If there is an existing collective bargaining agreement, then the union must give at least 10 days' notice to the employer preceding a work stoppage, which cannot occur before the end of the 90-day notice of a desire to change an existing contract. Striking, picketing, or a concerted refusal to work without properly notifying the HSO/HS or the FMCS is a union unfair labor practice.[122] In bargaining for an initial contract after recognition, the strike notice cannot be given until the end of the 30-day notice of an impasse. The strike notice allows the HSO/HS to discharge or transfer patients, or otherwise plan for continuity of care.

Conciliation of Labor Disputes

The amendments provide that if the director of the FMCS believes "a threatened strike or lockout affecting a health care institution will . . . substantially interrupt the delivery of health care in the locality concerned" (Section 213[a]) the director can appoint an impartial board of inquiry to help resolve the issues. The act specifies a time for appointing the board and investigating and reporting, during which the employer and union must maintain the status quo, unless they agree to a change. This allows the FMCS to begin discussions and help resolve issues before negotiations break down.

Individuals With Religious Convictions

PL 93-360 exempted HSO/HS employees from paying union dues, even in a union shop, when the individual "is a member of and adheres to established and traditional tenets or teachings of a bona fide religion, body, or sect which has historically held religious conscientious objections to joining or financially supporting labor organizations." The individual must, however, donate an equivalent amount to a charitable fund approved by the institution and labor organization. In 1980 this provision was extended to all employees covered by NLRA.[123]

LABOR ORGANIZATIONS IN HEALTH SERVICES

The labor organizations most active in health services are the American Federation of State, County, & Municipal Employees (AFSCME) union, the American Nurses Association, the Service Employees International Union (SEIU), the Teamsters, and the National Health and Human Services Employees Union (often referred to as District 1199),[124] as well as many independent local unions not affiliated with a national labor organization. District 1199 in New York State represents 117,000 members in more than 200 hospitals and nursing facilities.[125] AFSCME has 1.3 million members. It represents 360,000 workers in HSOs/HSs of all types and is particularly active in government-owned hospitals[126] as well as nursing facilities. More than 45,000 RNs and licensed practical nurses are represented by the United Nurses of America.[127] SEIU, part of the AFL-CIO, represents about 500,000 health care workers.[128] It is especially active in investor-owned chain settings and nursing facilities.[129] It was reported to account for one fourth of all health care organizing activity in 1998, with RNs the most frequently targeted group.[130]

Physicians who may be full-time salaried employees of HSOs/HSs, such as a closed panel HMO, are a professional group that may be interested in unionizing, especially as managed care policies restrict their practice autonomy. It is estimated that 40% of physicians are employed in some form of managed care setting and that 6% of U.S. physicians are members of a union.[131] Among the unions representing physicians are the United Salaried Physicians and Dentists union (affiliated with SEIU),[132] the Union of American Physicians and Dentists (affiliated with AFSCME), and the Federation of Physicians and Dentists (affiliated with the AFL-CIO).[133]

Historically, NLRB considered residents to be students and thus ineligible to join a union under NLRA, as amended. On November 29, 1999, however, NLRB ruled in the case *Boston Medical Center Corporation and House Officers' Association/Committee of Interns and Residents* that residents and fellows were "employees" and therefore eligible to join a labor organization under section 2(3) of NLRA, as amended. A similar sea change occurred in July 1999 when the American Medical Association's (AMA) House of Delegates voted to form a national labor organization that would represent the interests of physicians who are employed by HSOs/HSs; those who are self-employed are barred from collective bargaining by federal antitrust laws. The AMA resolution contained the guiding principles that the physicians' labor organization would not affiliate with traditional labor unions nor would it strike.[134]

WHY EMPLOYEES UNIONIZE

Employees unionize when they are dissatisfied with conditions of employment and elements of and democracy in the work setting, and when they perceive that collective bargaining will yield positive outcomes. Simply put, unions are a vehicle for redress when employee needs are not met by the HSO/HS. The union's primary role is to improve the job security and economic interests,[135] and at times the professional interests, of employees. In addition, the collective bargaining process allows unions to address other terms and conditions of employment, organizational policies and procedures affecting the employer–employee relationship and, in some instances, the occupational status of members.

Conditions of employment are concerned primarily with economic and security issues, as well as elements of the work setting. Economic concerns relate to compensation, such as wages and salaries and fringe benefits. Wages and salaries include absolute pay rates, relative pay among similar organizations, pay differentials among job classifications, and shift differentials. Fringe benefits typically include health and life insurance, retirement programs, holidays and vacation time, and EAPs.

Elements of the work setting include hours of employment, scheduling patterns, breaktimes, the physical work environment, and personal security. Finally, job security as affected by a changing mix of part-time and full-time employees, the outside contracting (i.e., outsourcing) of work previously performed in-house, and employee reductions during organization mergers, acquisitions, and downsizing will continue to legitimately concern employees. Collective bargaining subjects all of these elements to negotiation.

Democracy in the work setting describes the organization's prevailing attitude toward employees and the application of policies and procedures. Policies and criteria for promotion, transfer, discipline, termination, job reassignment, performance appraisal, grievances, and compensation changes are important, along with consistent application and fairness in treatment among individuals or groups of employees.[136] Lack of clearly stated policies or inconsistency in application leads to dissatisfaction, which is an important cause of unionization.

The HSO's/HS's philosophy about human resources greatly influences the context of the employment relationship. Employees want to be treated as individuals, not just another resource, and they want to know that the HSO/HS is sincerely concerned about them and their well-being. Employees' perceptions of the organization and its policies and attitudes toward workers are largely derived from their immediate supervisor—the organization's representative with whom employees most frequently interact.[137] The supervisor's management practices affect this perception. If supervision is fair, consistent, and concerned, then employee dissatisfaction will be lower than if the reverse is true, particularly it conditions of employment and democracy in the work setting are positive. An organizational philosophy and management practices that recognize the importance of employees and their individuality are progressive. Chapter 16 amplifies this point.

Such an atmosphere of employment necessarily incorporates meaningfulness of work in job design and involves, when possible, shaping jobs to individual strengths, skills, and interests. It is dependent on two-way communications, which lessen information vacuums and encourage two-way listening. Risk-free upward communication and downward communication to be informed are important employee needs (see Chapter 17). Perceptive, well-qualified first-level managers contribute greatly to fostering this positive atmosphere.

Job autonomy and empowerment are important to many HSO/HS employees, especially to professionals such as RNs and technicians. They are concerned with their work roles and the way in which they relate to the task-structure elements of the organization and patient care delivery. Their ability to fulfill professional and autonomy needs is important. They seek to expand their job responsibilities and be involved in decision making within their areas of competence. Assertiveness among professionals who increasingly seek recognition and greater participation in managing patient care is a powerful force, particularly for RNs. For them, job dissatisfaction stems from unclear roles, conflict with physicians, and inadequately performing or insufficient numbers of staff. These employees may view unionization as an alternative to what they perceive to be the HSO's/HS's indifference or unwillingness to deal with professional issues.

Symptoms of an Organizing Campaign

HSOs/HSs and managers must be sensitive to employees' needs relative to conditions of employment, democracy in the work setting, and the content of employment, including professional autonomy. As Fennell notes, "In many cases an insensitive employer is a union's best organizer."[138] If HSOs/HSs and managers are sensitive and are proactive to address deficiencies, it is less likely that employees will seek to join a union. In general, the climate of labor–management relations is sufficiently clear that an attempt to organize employees is evident. Some of the symptoms are[139]

> A sudden lack of communication between supervisors and normally friendly or conversant employees
>
> New informal leaders within the employee group
>
> Employees asking unusual questions or seeking information about the HSO's/HS's policies and procedures

Unusual group activity among employees before and after working hours as well as employees congregating in small groups during work hours

Increased contact among employees in off-site locations

A greater-than-usual number of rumors and expressions of insecurity

Changing tardiness and absentee patterns

Abnormal attention given to a recently discharged or disciplined employee

Attempts by employees to provoke confrontations with supervisors

Distribution of union literature

Off-site union meetings held by organizers

Bargaining Units

After a petition for an initial recognition election in which there is a "showing of interest" by at least 30% of the proposed bargaining unit, NLRB determines whether it has jurisdiction and determines the appropriate bargaining unit. In 1989 NLRB administratively ruled on the bargaining unit composition in acute care hospitals. The board was frustrated by inconsistent court rulings on NLRB bargaining unit determination between 1974 and 1989 in which NLRB sought to follow the congressional admonition in the legislation's conference report to "give due consideration" to avoid bargaining unit proliferation. Consequently, in 1989 NLRB administratively ruled on the classification of bargaining units for acute care hospitals. Affirmed by the U.S. Supreme Court in 1991, the approved bargaining units are

1. All registered nurses
2. All physicians
3. All professional employees except registered nurses and physicians
4. All technical employees
5. All skilled maintenance employees
6. All business office clerical employees
7. All guards
8. All other nonprofessional employees except for those classified above[140]

There are certain exemptions and exceptions. First, existing noncomforming bargaining units may continue. Second, in extraordinary circumstances, such as when a defined unit would have five or fewer employees, NLRB will determine the appropriate unit. The rule applies to acute care hospitals in which more than 50% of patients have an average length of stay that is less than 30 days, even if the facility provides long-term, psychiatric, or rehabilitative care. All other HSOs are excluded.

Solicitation and Distribution

It is in the interest of HSOs/HSs to have policies in place that restrict union solicitation and distribution prior to a union-organizing campaign. Solicitation is defined as one person talking with another about joining a union and includes handing out the authorization cards that document a showing of interest. Distribution is defined as handing out union literature. A HSO/HS may restrict distribution if the policy began before a union campaign and if it is not overly broad. Overly broad and all-encompassing policies such as "absolutely no solicitation or distribution by anyone on the HSO's/HS's premises at any time" are presumed by NLRB to be invalid. For example, employees cannot be prohibited from soliciting or distributing, although times and specific locations can be restricted. "It is an unfair labor practice under section 8(a)(1) [of NLRA] for an employer to impose an unlawfully broad rule against solicitation or distribution interfering with the employee's statutory rights to engage in concerted activity" to organize.[141]

NLRB has baseline rules about solicitation and distribution. If the organization has an exclusion rule, outside union organizers (i.e., nonemployees) can be denied access to the premises for the purposes of solicitation and distribution, if the rule is enforced consistently and in a nondiscriminatory manner.[142] If outsiders such as charitable (except for United Way)[143] and volunteer organizations may come on the premises for non–HSO/HS business, NLRB may require that the same privilege be granted to outside union organizers.[144]

The second baseline is that internal organizers (i.e., employees) may legally engage in soliciting and distributing union literature on HSO/HS property, but only during nonworking time and in nonworking areas.[145] Working hours are from the beginning to the end of a shift. Working time is time spent working, excluding meal and breaktime, which is considered nonworking time. Employees can be prohibited from soliciting and distributing union material in any working area during the solicitor's or the recipient's working time.[146]

Guidelines on solicitation and distribution for HSOs/HSs issued by the NLRB general counsel subsequent to the 1974 amendments recognized that HSOs are unique. As a consequence, there may be additional restrictions on where solicitation and distribution may occur. To "protect patients from disturbance," employees may not solicit for union membership or distribute union literature during nonworking time[147] if patient care will be disrupted. Patient care areas include patient rooms, operating rooms, treatment rooms, patient area corridors and sitting rooms, and elevators and stairways frequently used in transporting patients.[148] A ban cannot be enforced in nonpatient areas to which only employees have access, including kitchens; laundry supply rooms; the housekeeping, bookkeeping, and medical records departments; and employee lounges, locker rooms, and restrooms.[149] Policies regarding areas of public access, such as cafeterias, lobbies, gift shops, grounds, and walkways, are examined by NLRB on a case-by-case basis.[150]

HSOs/HSs must be concerned that, absent a preexisting policy, prohibiting solicitation and distribution may be an unfair labor practice like that of enforcing an overly broad policy or one that has not been enforced in a consistent, nondiscriminatory manner. Gilmore recommends the following guidelines in formulating a policy: HSOs/HSs must avoid promulgating a solicitation and distribution policy that is overly broad, must predicate the policy on the need to prevent or minimize disruption of patient care, and must time the introduction of the policy so that NLRB will not conclude that its sole purpose is to deprive employees of their right to union solicitation.[151]

Employer Conduct During an Election Campaign

When NLRB finds a "showing of interest" by employees, an election is held. During an election campaign there are permissible and prohibited activities on the part of the employer and its representatives—managers and supervisors. Section 1(11) of NLRA defines a supervisor (manager) as

> *any individual having authority, in the interest of the employer, to hire, transfer, suspend, lay off, recall, promote, discharge, assign, reward, or discipline other employees, or responsibility to direct them, or to adjust their grievances, or effectively to recommend such action, if in connection with the foregoing the exercise of such authority is not of a merely routine clerical nature, but requires the use of independent judgment.*

Employers or managers and supervisors cannot interfere, restrain, or coerce employees in exercising their right under Section 7 of NLRA to organize.[152] It is an unfair labor practice to interfere with employees' right to organize, such as lawful solicitation and distribution, or to act coercively, such as inappropriately interrogating or conducting surveillance of employees. Other activities defined by the NLRB as interfering with employee free choice are[153]

> Threats of loss of jobs or benefits by an employer to influence the votes or union activities of employees

A grant of benefits or promise to grant benefits to influence the votes or union activities of employees

Firing employees to discourage or encourage their union activities

Making campaign speeches to assembled groups of employees on HSO/HS time within the 24-hour period before an election

Incitement of racial or religious prejudice by inflammatory campaign appeals

Employers and their agents have the right of free speech during an organizing campaign. However, their statements must not contain the threat of reprisal or force or promise benefits. Feldacker indicates that

> *Section 8(c) of the Labor Management Relations Act [Taft-Hartley] states that the "expressing of any views, arguments or opinions or the dissemination thereof, whether in written, printed, graphic or visual form, shall not constitute or be evidence of an unfair labor practice under any provision of this Act, if such expression contains no threat of reprisal or force or promises of benefits."*[154]

The employer may respond to union organizing charges and communicate its general views about unionism and predictions of the economic realities of unionization as long as the predictions are based on objective facts.[155] An example would be the experience the employer or other employers have had with unions, such as the union not successfully negotiating higher wages.

Readers should be aware that NLRB and court rulings on permissible and prohibited employer activities are evolutionary, complex, and dependent on the facts of each situation. In the event of an organization campaign, legal counsel should provide advice to management about permissible and prohibited activities.

MANAGERIAL RESPONSIBILITIES IN LABOR RELATIONS

Managers must use resources effectively to meet customer and other stakeholder needs and to accomplish the HSO's/HS's objectives. This is easier to achieve with greater managerial freedom for resource interchange. By definition, a union lessens management's prerogatives because the collective bargaining agreement restricts management decisions about allocating and utilizing personnel and other resources. HSOs/HSs are labor intensive. Union constraints on utilizing employees could have a major impact on personnel costs, productivity, and possibly quality. Retaining administrative flexibility is a powerful incentive to remain union free. Unions have an impact on compensation costs; may demand restrictive work rules; generally dissipate management energy and time; may cause strife and conflict, particularly when the relationship is adversarial; and ultimately have the potential for a work stoppage.

Metzger observes that a HSO/HS with a positive labor relations atmosphere, "an organization that provides all the benefits and protection afforded by a union contract—such as competitive wages, a seniority system, a grievance and arbitration procedure—need not be unionized."[156] He also observes that, in a nonunion environment[157]

> The employer has greater latitude in running of the operation and directing employees.
>
> It is easier to change work processes, task–technology relationships, and schedules.
>
> There is freedom to introduce new technologies and productivity programs and quality improvement.

It is easier to introduce new and varying programs directed at increasing the motivation of employees, such as gain sharing, and, through employee involvement and participation, achieve greater employee commitment to organization initiatives such as CQI.

Setting the Tone and Environment

It is clear that human resources are the HSO's/HS's most important asset. As a consequence, managers must be concerned with the way in which employees view the organization, as well as their needs and aspirations. Metzger reinforces this point in his statement that "we must start to think of our employees not as adversaries but as partners."[158] Human resources managers, as well as all other managers, need to collectively establish sound relationships with employees and to develop HRM and other programs to maximize employees' commitment to their jobs and the HSO/HS. All managers are responsible for facilitating this partnership. Process and work systems design and technology are important, but people are everything. Providing employees the opportunity for participation, involvement, and empowerment is more likely to lead to success and enhanced competitive position.[159] A contentious and adversarial labor-management relationship will likely preclude these goals. A positive work atmosphere and a well-developed organizational culture and philosophy about employees are absolutely critical.

Proactive Steps

There are three steps that management can take to strengthen its partnership with employees and their commitment to the organization. They are effective first-level supervision, increased two-way communication, and, in union-free organizations, the establishment of a formal grievance procedure.

Immediate supervisors are the representatives of management with whom employees most frequently interact. Supervisors set the tone and climate and confirm or disaffirm the organization's philosophy toward employees. Adequately trained and technically competent supervisors who, by their practices and behavior, affirm the organization's philosophy will be much more effective in managing subordinates and achieving higher performance. The supervisor's awareness of employee feelings, treatment of subordinates as individuals, and sincere concern for job-related problems foster a positive environment and eliminate many of the reasons why employees unionize.

Communication also is critical to a smoothly functioning organization. Managers must keep employees informed and listen to them.[160] Effective two-way communication contributes greatly to a positive organizational environment and is especially important during times of organizational change. It is very difficult to bond a partnership when only one party speaks.

Promoting upward communication simply makes good sense. This can be accomplished by listening sessions, employee opinion or attitude surveys, or formal interviews conducted by consultants. A mechanism that is especially useful is a formal grievance procedure.[161] The American Hospital Association advocates establishing a grievance procedure, especially in nonunion hospitals, so that employee complaints or disagreements arising "out of disagreements over rule infractions, misunderstandings, and involuntary terminations or temporary suspensions from work" can be resolved.[162]

Grievance procedures provide employees with an easily accessible and fair means to be heard, to alert management to causes of employee dissatisfaction, and "to contribute to the improvement of morale and productivity and the development of mutual respect, trust, and rapport between supervisors and employees."[163] When employees perceive that management is interested in legitimate complaints, dissatisfaction is decreased. A formal grievance procedure is a vehicle to vent frustration. It also makes senior-level management more aware of employee concerns. Whether these concerns are legitimate is not the point—it is employee perception, whether right or wrong, that will remain if not addressed. Designing a formal grievance procedure should involve some employee participation, which will promote its legitimacy and instill a sense of commitment to making it work.

COLLECTIVE BARGAINING

Thus far, federal labor law prescribing how the employer and union interact, extent of unionization in health services, reasons why employees join unions, and managerial responsibilities in labor relations have been discussed. However, even if a sound employer–employee relationship is developed, it is still possible that employees will unionize. If so, or if the HSO/HS is already unionized, then management and union representatives engage in collective bargaining (i.e., contract negotiation and subsequent administration of the contract).

The provisions of an employer-union contract establish parameters for conduct of management and the employees' representative (union), and such contracts are legally enforceable.[164] Federal laws do not specify contract provisions. They do, however, set limits on accomplishing recognition, indicate the range of behavior and bargaining issues that are legal, and mandate that both parties bargain fairly and in good faith.

Negotiation

Collective bargaining begins after a union has been recognized. During an organizing campaign, neither employer nor union may commit unfair labor practices (see Tables 11.6 and 11.7). Contract negotiations begin after NLRB certifies the employees' representative.[165] Both parties spend a great deal of time preparing: warm-up meetings are held and proposals and counterproposals are made.

Federal labor law restricts how the parties act toward one another and what can and cannot be part of the contract. They must meet with each other's representatives and cannot interfere with each other's rights.[166] The union can demand that the employer negotiate about NLRA–specified mandatory subjects, which include wages and hours, conditions of employment, and, as specified in subsequent rulings, pensions, bonuses, grievance procedures, safety practices, seniority, procedures for layoff and recall, discipline and discharge, and union security.[167] Unions may seek to bargain about nonmandatory subjects such as scope of management of the HSO's/HS's operations, decisions about allocating and utilizing resources, and management rights regarding employee overtime, scheduling, determining job content, and transferring employees. The employer may choose not to negotiate about these subjects.

Neither negotiations nor the contract can include unlawful issues such as operating a closed shop (which requires new employees to be union members before they can be hired), including supervisors in a bargaining unit, or the HSO/HS pressuring a subcontractor to recognize a union.

Unions usually seek to negotiate provisions about union security and the grievance process. Union security relates to the union's desire to secure and strengthen its position. The employer may accept a union shop provision that requires all new employees in a bargaining unit to join the union after a brief period, generally 30 days. At a minimum the union may seek an agency shop, in which an employee who does not join must pay the equivalent of dues to it or a charity.[168] Finally, there may be a checkoff provision that requires the employer to deduct union dues from each member's pay and remit it to the union or other mutually approved organization.

Contracts may specify the disciplinary procedure for workplace infractions such as absenteeism, insubordination, and theft. The procedure may include a sequence such as oral warning for the first infraction, written warning for the second, then disciplinary layoff (perhaps a week without pay), and finally termination. Furthermore, it may identify infractions that skip the initial steps. For example, assaulting a supervisor or any other employee may carry a penalty of "up to and including discharge" without progressing through the other steps. An employee who thinks the procedure has not been followed or disagrees with the result may file a grievance.

A formal grievance procedure to resolve employee disputes about the contract may be negotiated. The first step of the grievance procedure is a meeting between the supervisor and the union steward, the second involves the human resources manager, and finally a more senior manager meets with a union official. If the grievance is not resolved, then an arbitrator (a neutral third party) may hear the facts and render a decision, which may be advisory or binding, depending on the collective bargaining agreement.[169]

Impasses

Failure of the parties to agree about mandatory bargaining subjects during negotiations results in an impasse. There are several options when an impasse occurs. The union may call a strike after appropriate notification. Strikes are an economic burden that may induce the employer to modify its position. Strikes in HSOs/HSs are costly in terms of monetary impact and patient welfare.

Organizations that are struck may hire replacements, provided that the strike was for economic reasons and the employer did not commit an unfair labor practice.[170] Health team members, however, are highly interdependent, and striking employees are not easily replaced. Furthermore, if employees are striking legitimately because the employer committed an unfair labor practice, then NLRB can force the employer to reinstate striking workers even if this means discharging replacements. However, if the strike was not called because the employer has committed an unfair labor practice or if the union struck illegally (an unfair labor practice), striking employees need not be reinstated.

Another option available during an impasse is mediation. Such assistance can be requested from the state or FMCS. Mediators are third-party neutrals who meet with the parties, stimulate the negotiating process, and try to persuade the two sides to agree to a solution. A mediator's only power is persuasion, and the impasse may not be resolved. Binding arbitration is a final option. Here the parties agree to accept the arbitrator's findings and decision. During contract negotiations, however, neither party wants to give a third party such authority. As a result, binding arbitration is most commonly used to settle grievances during an existing contract rather than to resolve impasses.

Agreement is eventually reached through some method. The resulting contract is a private law that binds the parties. The contract and the manner of reaching agreement—whether by mutual respect or adversary power dominance—greatly influences future labor–management relations and the organizational climate.

THE HUMAN RESOURCES PERSPECTIVE

Contemporary human resources management in HSOs/HSs is appreciably different from what it was in the early 1980s, not only in its role and process but also, more important, in terms of perspective and philosophy. The new environment has placed HSOs/HSs at risk; accountability for resource use has increased; new delivery arrangements have affected staffing levels; and consumer and payer stakeholders and Joint Commission accreditation standards have called for improved performance and quality outcomes. All of these forces have significantly affected the employer–employee relationship. The major current outcome—the HSO's/HS's view of employees—can be labeled the "human resources perspective."[171]

Progressive HSOs/HSs and managers who embrace the human resources perspective in general subscribe to the following:

- Employees are the catalyst for individual and organizational work results; they are the principal components in converting inputs to outputs. Human resources are the HSO's/HS's most important asset.

- Employees are crucial to the organization because of the cost of employing them, the investment in their training and development, and their knowledge and on-the-job experience.
- Organizations and employees have reciprocal obligations to and interests in each other, and both gain from these relationships.
- Management views all employees, including those represented by a labor organization, as partners, not adversaries.
- Management and employee values and attitudes are congruent; both seek to change organizational arrangements and work processes to 1) accommodate and capitalize on interests, needs, abilities, and skills of employees; and 2) improve output quality on the dimensions of conformance and customer expectations.
- There is a permeating climate of mutual respect, positive interaction, shared problem solving, and involvement to improve quality outcomes along with employee work life quality.

The human resources perspective is a management and organizational philosophy describing how HSO/HS managers view and interact with employees as they carry out managerial functions and engage in managerial roles. The human resources department is responsible for the HRM programs and systems of acquiring and retaining and maintaining employees in the organization, as well as labor relations with those who are members of a union. It facilitates implementation of this management philosophy as it administers the programs and systems, which, in turn, are integrated into the HSO's/HS's strategic plans.

Contemporary human resources management is interventionist and proactive because it integrates human resources acquisition and retention activities with the organization's operational components and strategic plans. The human resources department is a catalyst for organizational changes such as CQI.

The human resources department has a major role in monitoring and improving the employment climate through employee needs assessments and attitude surveys and by identifying employee satisfiers and dissatisfiers. Interventions to change structure and work processes are included so that all resources are used more effectively; employer and employee seek to accomplish objectives as partners.

Performance appraisal systems not only yield information for compensation changes but also are integrated with programs of positive behavior modification and corrective counseling to improve performance. Training and development focus on skills enhancement and technological upgrading, both of which increase employee competencies—they are critical to successful implementation of CQI initiatives. In addition, training and development can address social skills such as coping with work, reducing stress, and fostering interpersonal relationships.

Career counseling based on aptitude and interest assessment is performed to enable people to achieve their fullest potential. Although the HSO's/HS's payback may not seem tangible, this activity serves long-range human resources planning by upgrading employee skills in areas in which supply is short, by building loyalty to the organization, and by demonstrating that employees are respected as individuals with unique needs.

EAPs that preserve and salvage human resources are integrated with other retention activities. The direct and indirect costs of alcoholism and drug abuse in lost time, low productivity, poor quality, and human wreckage are staggering. Providing treatment without recrimination to the employee who seeks help makes sense from the human resources perspective. Corollary programs include marital and financial counseling and health awareness and fitness. They are good investments in the organization's human resources.

Accomplishing the HSO's/HS's objectives, especially quality care and improved efficiency, fulfilling its mission, and achieving an enhanced competitive position depends on people. Embracing the human resources perspective reflects a commitment by the HSO/HS to people as its most important resource.

SUMMARY

Human resources management is composed of the wide range of centralized staffing activities, programs, and policies related to acquisition, retention and maintenance, and separation of a HSO's/ HS's human resources (see Figure 11.2), as well as union–management relations. Management is responsible for defining the qualifications, competencies, and level of staffing to achieve the HSO's/HS's mission; acquiring and maintaining the right number of competent people to meet the needs of patients served; and continuously assessing and improving the competencies of employees. Acquiring human resources involves workforce planning, recruitment, selection, and, ultimately, induction into the HSO/HS and orientation. All depend on an effective job analysis program and well-developed job descriptions. In recruitment and selection, as well as throughout employees' tenure, one role of the human resources department is to establish and implement nondiscriminatory personnel policies that comply with state and federal law. Other department activities are preemployment applications and interviews and testing; monitoring of equal employment opportunity, adverse impact, and affirmative action; and administering compensation.

In addition to centralized acquisition, the human resources department is also responsible for activities related to retaining human resources. These include performance appraisal (methods, uses, and benefits), training and development, and discipline. The discussion of compensation administration includes job analysis methods, pay philosophies, and the inherent activities involved in developing and administering a compensation system. Benefits administration, including pension programs and EAPs, follow. Promotion of safety and health of employees within the HSO/HS and separation activities such as preretirement planning and outplacement are discussed.

Because HSOs/HSs are labor intensive, effectively utilizing personnel and retaining management's prerogatives are extremely important. Management's responsibilities regarding unionization focus on providing a positive environment in which employees see no advantage to bargaining collectively. Federal legislation relative to labor relations is presented, including the 1974 amendments to the Taft-Hartley Act, which brought not-for-profit acute care hospitals under the umbrella of federal labor law. Employer and union unfair labor practices, reasons employees unionize, the collective bargaining process, and managerial responsibilities are presented.

HSO/HS management must be concerned with its prerogative to manage—to allocate and utilize resources. There is, however, a reciprocal responsibility of meeting employees' legitimate concerns and interests. Management is responsible for nurturing a workplace environment that enables the organization to accomplish objectives, fulfill its mission, and maintain its competitive advantage. These all require that there be an appropriate number of qualified and competent employees who share the organization's goals and are empowered to meet the needs of the patients served. The organizational perspective about its human resources must be one in which employees are viewed as partners rather than adversaries.

DISCUSSION QUESTIONS

1. The human resources department is responsible for centralized staffing activities related to acquisition, retention and maintenance, and separation of employees. Describe those activities presented in the chapter using a time flow perspective.
2. Job descriptions are used for many HRM purposes. How is the job description document derived and what does it contain?
3. What is equal employment opportunity? How does it affect HRM activities?
4. All health services managers appraise the work performance of subordinates. How are appraisals used? What are the benefits and potential problems of performance appraisal?
5. Discuss equity and job evaluation relative to compensation administration. What benefits result from a well-designed and implemented compensation program? What results can occur

from an ill-designed or a poorly implemented program? What employee benefits are there beyond wages and salaries?

6. What economic and noneconomic justification is there for employee assistance, preretirement planning, and outplacement programs? Be specific.

7. Discuss the reasons why HSOs/HSs must be concerned about unionization. What impact does a union have on managing the organization? Discuss the impact relative to the management model for HSOs/HSs presented in Figure 1.7.

8. Discuss the meaning and give general examples of employer and union unfair labor practices. How do they restrain behavior for both parties?

9. From the point of view of the employee, what are the advantages and disadvantages of joining a union? Should health services professionals such as physicians, RNs, and pharmacists unionize? Discuss and support your position.

10. This chapter gives several reasons why employees join unions. Which are the most important? Do they vary for different occupational groups, such as nonprofessional and professional employees? Are there reasons other than those presented?

11. What is the human resources perspective? Describe it. Is it consistent with the opening quote to the chapter? Why?

CASE STUDY 1: PERSONNEL POLICIES AT ROBBINS MEMORIAL HOSPITAL

Lindsey King is vice president of human resources at a 127-bed facility located in a small farming town. She has been at Robbins Memorial Hospital for only 2 weeks, but has already concluded that the human resources department is not well developed and there are no policies for many situations.

SITUATION A

One morning King had a meeting with Nicholas Jens, director of the clinical laboratory, who told King she has a problem with an employee who is chronically late and frequently absent. King reviewed the employee's records for the past 6 months, the extent of record keeping. They show the employee has been tardy 70 times and absent 15 times. King learned from Jens that the employee is a Hispanic medical technician who has been employed in the lab for 18 months. The technician is working on a degree at a local college and is frequently late because of her class schedule or sorority activities.

King checked the personnel policy manual. The policy regarding absenteeism or tardiness states "the facility requires employees to be at their work stations on a timely and regular basis. Failure to adhere to regular attendance and punctuality standards may cause the facility to take disciplinary action." King then consulted the personnel manual for a policy on discipline and found no guidelines other than a general statement that "failure to adhere to facility policies and procedures may cause the facility to take necessary measures." King reviewed other files and found no documentation of what had been done in similar cases. Jens is pressing King to know what action she can take to correct this problem or to terminate the employee.

SITUATION B

King was informed by the director of the intensive care unit that a female night employee has told other staff that, when she comes to work, she carries a small-caliber handgun for personal protection. The handgun has been shown to other employees and allegedly waved carelessly about in the unit. King responded by stating that the facility has a clear policy that prohibits employees from bringing firearms onto the premises. The director of security, however, reminded King that recently a night shift employee was assaulted in the parking lot and that many female employees are concerned for their safety. The director of security is worried that there might be other ramifications if this employee is disciplined. For example, other night shift employees might say that the facility is not concerned about their safety and that carrying a firearm is both a Second Amendment (constitutional) guarantee and necessary because of poor facility security. King agreed that this might become an issue and was also concerned that the facility has had difficulty getting nurses for the night shift.

SITUATION C

The following situation was described to King by the food service manager:

> A cook at Robbins Memorial Hospital was observed taking a chicken and other food from a storage area and putting the items in a bag under his coat. As the employee entered his car to go home, he was stopped by security officers and told that they were making a package check of the contents of the bag he was carrying. The employee objected, but the security officers insisted, stating that there was a policy allowing inspection of all packages removed from the facility. The employee relented and the food items were found in the bag.
>
> The employee was terminated by the food service manager for theft. He filed a complaint with the EEOC alleging that his dismissal resulted from discrimination based on the fact that he is the only food service employee who is an ethnic Italian and that other employees regularly take food from the department. Therefore, his termination was based solely on the fact that he is Italian and he was "singled out." King and the security director have no knowledge that other employees are stealing.

QUESTIONS

1. What should King do about the attendance problems described in Situation A? Why?
2. What should King do about the firearms possession and personnel security issues described in Situation B? Why?
3. Regarding Situation C, what position should the facility take when contacted by EEOC?

CASE STUDY 2: COMPLAINT OF LPN PAY INEQUALITY

You are the vice president of human resources at a large HMO. A representative of the licensed practical nurses (LPNs) has complained to you about pay inequity. The HMO employs both RNs and LPNs, whose training and state licensure differ significantly. Because of a shortage of RNs and an abundance of LPNs, LPNs have been performing many RN duties. However, the difference in pay is more than 30%. Because this practice has occurred for some time, the LPNs want a wage increase. They argue they should be paid the same as a RN if they perform the same work. Neither the LPNs nor the RNs are represented by a union.

QUESTIONS

1. Should the pay for the LPNs be increased to equal that of RNs? Why or why not?
2. What are the implications throughout the organization if LPN pay is increased to that of RNs?
3. What should be done to solve the problem of the two groups performing similar duties?
4. Are there quality-of-patient-care considerations?

CASE STUDY 3: SUBSTANCE ABUSE AND EAP

Alex has been a clerk in the Fairfax Clinic's medical records department for 15 years. He is a good employee and is liked by all. In the last 9 months, however, his performance has deteriorated and relationships with co-workers have been strained. As vice president of human resources, several years ago Brittany Kim set up an EAP for staff with personal problems or who are involved with drug or alcohol abuse. Unknown to Kim (and consistent with EAP policy), Alex contacted the EAP and has been receiving counseling for alcohol abuse for the past month. His supervisor is not aware of the source of the problem and has been disciplining Alex through the steps of progressive discipline (oral warning, formal warning, and a 2-day suspension) for poor performance.

Again this morning Alex came to work with the smell of alcohol on his breath. His speech was slurred and he had poor coordination. The supervisor called Kim and requested that Alex be fired immediately. Kim called Alex to her office and found that his condition had improved. She informed Alex of his supervisor's decision to terminate him and discussed his alcohol abuse and poor performance. Alex became irate and cited EAP policy stating that the clinic seeks to help employees with such problems. All information was to have been kept confidential and no one was to have been at risk or terminated as a result of voluntarily using EAP. Because Kim set up the EAP, she is concerned about its credibility and success.

QUESTIONS

1. Should Alex be discharged? Why or why not?
2. Develop a policy for supervisors on confidentiality and EAPs.
3. What are the pros and cons of a HSO's/HS's use of outside counseling versus in-house counseling?

CASE STUDY 4: MISSING NARCOTICS

You are the vice president of human resources in a community hospital that is the largest employer in town. The vice president of nursing services, Michelle Gates, calls at 5:00 P.M. on Friday. She asks you to come to her office and witness a confrontation with Helen Jones, a RN who works in the inpatient postanesthesia care unit "caught red-handed stealing drugs."

Gates tells you that two staff members saw Jones put five containers of Demerol in her pocket as she prepared to give medications and reported it to the charge nurse, Nancy Gray. Gray checked the drug count and verified the shortage. At the end of Jones's rounds, Gray asked her to empty her pockets. This produced five containers of Demerol.

In Gates's office a few minutes later, you listen while she repeats the incident and asks Jones whether she is stealing drugs. Jones calmly says, "Yes." Gates tells Jones there is no choice but to fire her for theft. Without emotion, Jones asks that someone clean out her locker and bring its contents to her. Gates says, "Yes, I'm sure we're all very anxious to go home."

Left alone with Jones while the two nurse managers arrange for a security guard to clean out her locker, you quietly begin talking with Jones and ask why she stole the drugs. "You can't stop me," she replies. "If I can't take an overdose, I'll just leave here and drive my car into a wall. I'm not going home." After several more minutes of revealing conversation, Gates and Gray return with Jones's belongings.

Jones has been an employee for 14 years. She started as a nursing student after her children were placed in school. Her eldest daughter is now a student nurse here as well. Your proposal to start an EAP has not yet been accepted.

QUESTIONS

1. Is this a clear case of theft? What actions should be taken?
2. What are the implications for the hospital of the actions taken in Question 1? What responsibility (obligation) does the organization have to Jones? To patients?
3. What should be done about Jones's threat to harm herself?
4. Does Jones's threat raise legal or ethical duties for you?

CASE STUDY 5: PHYSICIAN HARASSMENT

After participating in a management development workshop on employee counseling in which a sexual harassment example was used, the operating room (OR) supervisor, Leslie McClung, asked for an appointment with Brynna Euston, the OR manager. One of McClung's nurses, Amy Kelly, complained to her last month that Dr. Ray "had made several passes at her," including asking her for a date. She refused and told him she didn't appreciate his unprofessional behavior in surgery.

When the next OR schedule was posted, Kelly noticed that her name had been crossed off Dr. Ray's cases. When asked why, McClung told her that Dr. Ray asked that Kelly be removed from his cases until she has more experience.

McClung told Euston that she had smoothed over the incident, but now wonders if that was the right thing to do.

QUESTIONS

1. Was Kelly sexually harassed? Give reasons for your answer.
2. Was smoothing over the incident appropriate? Why?
3. Is there an obligation to confront the issue of sexual harassment since the physician is not a hospital employee?
4. What are the political implications of disciplining or not disciplining the physician?

CASE STUDY 6: UNION MEMBERSHIP SOLICITATION AND DISTRIBUTION OF UNION MATERIAL AT DUNLAP MEMORIAL HOSPITAL

Ambrose Catan is a housekeeping supervisor on the 7:00 A.M.–3:00 P.M. shift at Dunlap Memorial Hospital. The hospital has a clear and concise no solicitation or distribution policy that is as restrictive as the law permits. It has existed for many years and has always been enforced in a nondiscriminatory manner. Walking down the hallway by the employee's lounge at 12:45 P.M., Catan saw one of his subordinates, Mary, talking with Bill, an X-ray technician who had just handed her a pamphlet. Mary's job assignment is to clean the hallway and lounge area. She was on duty and Bill was on break. Because the X-ray technicians recently filed a petition with NLRB for a recognition election of their unit, Bill was trying to get Mary to support them.

QUESTIONS

1. What should Catan do?
2. Would the situation and Catan's action be different if Mary were on break in the lounge and Bill were a 3:00 P.M.–11:00 P.M. shift employee who had come to the hospital before his shift started for the purpose of talking about the union with other employees?
3. Would the situation and Catan's action be different if Mary and Bill were both same-shift employees on break and Catan saw Bill (pro-union) and Mary (anti-union) arguing and scuffling with each other? What should Catan do: Initiate discipline against Bill? Initiate

discipline against Mary? Initiate discipline against both? What are the implications of each option?

CASE STUDY 7: PROMOTION AT VISITING NURSE SERVICE

Butler County Visiting Nurse Service (VNS) is a not-for-profit home health agency with 150 full-time and part-time employees, most of whom are RNs and home health aides. There are, however, three secretarial and five information systems (IS) nonsupervisory employees who have similar clerical responsibilities. The job classification and pay grade for those employees in IS is one level higher than that for the secretaries.

VNS has a union contract that specifies that "For the purpose of promotion, the most senior person with sufficient ability shall be promoted." Tracy Alexander and Barbara Lucas are both secretaries at VNS. Alexander has 4 years of service and Lucas has 3 years of service. Both have equal abilities and skills. When an opening occurred in IS, both Alexander and Lucas bid for it. Lucas was promoted. Previously, both had been temporarily assigned to IS. Alexander's performance when assigned to IS was mediocre at best, whereas Lucas's performance was very good to excellent. Alexander filed a grievance stating that she should have been promoted under the terms of the contract because she has seniority.

QUESTIONS

1. If you were an arbitrator and this case came before you, what would you decide? What would be the basis for your decision?
2. How would you rewrite the "promotion policy" in the contract to avoid a similar grievance from being filed in the future?

NOTES

1. Joint Commission on Accreditation of Healthcare Organizations. *1996 Accreditation Manual for Hospitals: Volume II, Scoring Guidelines,* 309. Oakbrook Terrace, IL: Joint Commission on Accreditation of Healthcare Organizations, 1995.
2. Bureau of Labor Statistics. *http://stats.bls.gov/newsrel.htm,* March 15, 1999.
3. Kleiman, Lawrence S. *Human Resource Management: A Tool for Competitive Advantage,* 12. Minneapolis-St. Paul, MN: West Publishing, 1997.
4. American Hospital Association. *Human Resources: Management Advisory,* 1. Chicago: American Hospital Association, 1990.
5. Joint Commission, *1996 Accreditation Manual,* 313.
6. For a good overview of HRM, see Metzger, Norman. "Human Resources Management." In *Health Care Administration: Principles, Practices, Structure, and Delivery,* edited by Lawrence F. Wolper, 327–362. Gaithersburg, MD: Aspen Publishers, 1995.
7. Hernandez, S. Robert, Myron D. Fottler, and Charles L. Joiner. "Integrating Strategic Management and Human Resources." In *Essentials of Human Resources Management in Health Services Organizations,* edited by Myron D. Fottler, S. Robert Hernandez, and Charles L. Joiner, 2. Albany, NY: Delmar Publishers, 1998.
8. Fottler, Myron D., Robert L. Phillips, John D. Blair, and Catherine A. Duran. "Achieving Competitive Advantage Through Strategic Human Resource Management." *Hospital & Health Services Administration* 35 (Fall 1990): 348.
9. Gómez-Mejía, Luis R., David B. Balkin, and Robert L. Cardy. *Managing Human Resources,* 3rd ed., 147. Upper Saddle River, NJ: Prentice-Hall, 1998.
10. Cascio, Wayne F. *Managing Human Resources: Productivity, Quality of Work Life, Profits,* 5th ed., 148. Boston: Irwin/McGraw-Hill, 1998.

11. Hernandez, S. Robert, Cynthia Carter Haddock, William M. Behrendt, and Walter F. Klein, Jr. "Management Development and Succession Planning: Lessons for Health Services Organizations." *Journal of Management Development* 10 (Special Issue on Health Care Management Development, 1991): 19–22.

12. Mathis, Robert L., and John H. Jackson. *Human Resource Management: Essential Perspectives,* 72. Cincinnati, OH: South-Western Publishing, 1999.

13. Gómez-Mejía, Balkin, and Cardy, *Managing Human Resources,* 153–154.

14. Cascio, *Managing Human Resources,* 134–136.

15. Fottler, Myron D. "Job Analysis." In *Essentials of Human Resources Management in Health Services Organizations,* edited by Myron D. Fottler, S. Robert Hernandez, and Charles L. Joiner, 118. Albany, NY: Delmar Publishers, 1998.

16. Harris, Michael. *Human Resource Management: A Practical Approach,* 120. Fort Worth, TX: Dryden Press/Harcourt Brace, 1997.

17. Cascio, *Managing Human Resources,* 140–141.

18. Mathis and Jackson, *Human Resource Management,* 58.

19. Harris, *Human Resource Management,* 121.

20. Friedman, Tamara T. "Recruitment Strategies." In *Human Resource Management in the Health Care Sector,* edited by Amarjit S. Sethi and Randall S. Schuler, 74–89. New York: Quorum Books, 1989.

21. Landau, Jacqueline, and Michael Abelson. "Recruitment and Selection." In *Essentials of Human Resources Management in Health Services Organizations,* edited by Myron D. Fottler, S. Robert Hernandez, and Charles L. Joiner, 134–165. Albany, NY: Delmar Publishers, 1998.

22. See Fottler, "Job Analysis," 117–133.

23. Foster, Charles, and Lynn Godkin. "Employment Selection in Health Care: The Case for Structured Interviewing." *Health Care Management Review* 23 (Winter 1998): 46.

24. Dessler, Gary. *Personnel/Human Resource Management,* 4th ed., 214. Englewood Cliffs, NJ: Prentice-Hall, 1991.

25. Mathis, Robert L., and John H. Jackson. *Personnel/Human Resource Management,* 6th ed., 139. St. Paul, MN: West Publishing, 1991.

26. Mathis and Jackson, *Human Resource Management,* 187–189. Readers interested in more information about permissible and nonpermissible preemployment questions and activities are referred to the following sources: Equal Employment Opportunity Commission. *Laws Administered by the EEOC,* 1–48. Washington, DC: Equal Employment Opportunity Commission, 1981; Equal Employment Opportunity Commission. *Uniform Employee Selection Guidelines—Interpretation and Clarification—Questions and Answers, Sect. 4175.01–4175.08.* Chicago: Commerce Clearing House, Inc., 1985; Equal Employment Opportunity Commission. "Uniform Guidelines on Employee Selection Procedures." *Code of Federal Regulations,* sect. 29, pt. 1607, 206–233. Washington, DC: Office of the Federal Register, 1988; Office of Public Affairs, Equal Employment Opportunity Commission. *Pre-employment Inquiries and Equal Employment Opportunity Law,* 1–8. Washington, DC: Equal Employment Opportunity Commission, 1981.

27. Equal Employment Opportunity Commission. "Uniform Guidelines on Employee Selection Procedures," 29 C.F.R. 1607. July 1, 1998.

28. Griggs v. Duke Power Co., 401 U.S. 424 (1971).

29. Garbin, Margery. "Validity of EAS Tests." *Quality Assessment Quarterly* 1 (Spring, 1991): 2; Mathis and Jackson, *Personnel/Human,* 120–123. For guidelines on testing see Dessler, *Personnel/Human,* 174–191.

30. For further information, see the following government publication: Equal Employment Opportunity Commission, *Laws Administered,* 1–48 (covers Title VII of the Civil Rights Act of 1964; as amended; the Age Discrimination in Employment Act of 1967, as amended; the Equal Pay Act of 1963; and Section 501 of the Rehabilitation Act of 1973); see also the Americans with Disabilities Act of 1990, PL 101-336, 42 U.S.C. § 12101 *et seq.*

31. Gómez-Mejía, Balkin, and Cardy, *Managing Human Resources,* 113–114; see also Lehr, Richard I., Robert A. McLean, and Gregg L. Smith. "The Legal and Economic Environment." In *Essentials of Human Resources Management in Health Services Organizations,* edited by Myron D. Fottler, S. Robert Hernandez, and Charles L. Joiner, 21–43. Albany, NY: Delmar Publishers, 1998.

32. Civil Rights Act of 1964, PL 88-352, 42 U.S.C. § 2000(a) *et seq.*
33. Fair Labor Standards Act of 1963, PL 106-73, 29 U.S.C. § 201 *et seq.*
34. Age Discrimination in Employment Act of 1967, PL 90-202, 29 U.S.C. § 621 *et seq.*; see also Older Workers Benefit Protection Act of 1991, PL 101-433, 104 Stat. 978.
35. The Age Discrimination Act does not apply when age is a job-related occupational qualification, such as for airline pilots. The 1986 amendments eliminated the age 70 ceiling.
36. Pregnancy Discrimination Act of 1978, PL 95-555, 92 Stat. 2076; Gómez-Mejía, Balkin, and Cardy, *Managing Human Resources,* 93.
37. Americans with Disabilities Act of 1990, PL 101-336, 42 U.S.C. § 12101 *et seq.*
38. Equal Employment Opportunity Commission. "The ADA: Your Responsibilities as Employer," 3. *http://www.eeoc.gov/facts/ada17.html,* January 15, 1997; Gillman, Steven L., and Davi L. Hirsch. "The Americans with Disabilities Act: Civil Rights for Handicapped Workers." *The Brief* 20 (Summer 1991): 16.
39. Equal Employment Opportunity Commission. "The Americans with Disabilities Act of 1990: Titles I and V," 1. *http://www.eeoc.gov/laws/ada.html,* January 15, 1997.
40. Equal Employment Opportunity Commission, "The ADA," 4.
41. Equal Employment Opportunity Commission, "The ADA," 2.
42. Equal Employment Opportunity Commission, "The Americans with Disabilities Act," 17.
43. Equal Employment Opportunity Commission, "The ADA," 7.
44. Equal Employment Opportunity Commission, "The ADA," 4.
45. Coil, James H., III, and Lori J. Shapiro. "The ADA at Three Years: A Statute in Flux." *Employee Relations Law Journal* 21 (Spring 1996): 9–10.
46. Equal Employment Opportunity Commission, "The ADA," 4.
47. Civil Rights Act of 1964, PL 88-352, 42 U.S.C. § 2000 *et seq.*
48. Twomey, David P. *A Concise Guide to Employment Law, EEO & OSHA,* 1–2. Cincinnati, OH: South-Western Publishing, 1986.
49. Gómez-Mejía, Balkin, and Cardy, *Managing Human Resources,* 93–96.
50. Twomey, *A Concise Guide,* 25.
51. Cascio, *Managing Human Resources,* 45.
52. Twomey, *A Concise Guide,* 28.
53. Mathis and Jackson, *Personnel/Human,* 134.
54. Gómez-Mejía, Balkin, and Cardy, *Managing Human Resources,* 94.
55. Equal Employment Opportunity Commission. "Guidelines on Discrimination Because of Sex." *Code of Federal Regulations,* sect. 29, pt. 1604.11. Washington, DC: Office of the Federal Register, 1990.
56. Kinard, Jerry L., J. Reagan McLaurin, and Beverly Little. "Sexual Harassment in the Hospital Industry: An Empirical Inquiry." *Health Care Management Review* 20 (Winter 1995): 48.
57. Equal Employment Opportunity Commission, "Guidelines on Discrimination."
58. Equal Employment Opportunity Commission. "Facts About Sexual Harassment," 1. *http://www.eeoc.gov/stats/charges.html,* August 11, 1998.
59. American College of Healthcare Executives. "Preventing and Addressing Sexual Harassment in the Workplace: Public Policy Statement." *Healthcare Executive* 11 (November/December 1996): 43.
60. Decker, Phillip J. "Sexual Harassment in Health Care: A Major Productivity Problem." *Health Care Supervisor* 16 (September 1997): 1–2.
61. See Joiner, Charles L., and John C. Hyde. "Performance Appraisal." In *Essentials of Human Resources Management in Health Services Organizations,* edited by Myron D. Fottler, S. Robert Hernandez, and Charles L. Joiner, 223–247. Albany, NY: Delmar Publishing, 1998.
62. Joint Commission on Accreditation of Healthcare Organizations, *1996 Accreditation Manual,* 295.
63. For a discussion of competency-based evaluation models, see Decker, Phillip J., Marlene K. Strader, and Rebecca J. Wise. "Beyond JCAHO: Using Competency Models to Improve Healthcare Organizations: Part 1." *Hospital Topics* 75 (Winter 1997): 23–27; Decker, Phillip J., Marlene K. Strader, and Rebecca J. Wise. "Beyond JCAHO: Using Competency Models to Improve Healthcare Organizations: Part 2." *Hospital Topics* 75 (Spring 1997): 10–17.
64. Cascio, *Managing Human Resources,* 310–313.

65. Cascio, *Managing Human Resources,* 318.
66. Kleiman, *Human Resource Management,* 224–226.
67. Drucker, Peter F. *Managing the Non-Profit Organization,* 62. New York: HarperCollins, 1990.
68. Cascio, *Managing Human Resources,* 321.
69. Noe, Raymond A. *Employee Training and Development,* 4. Boston: Irwin/McGraw-Hill, 1999.
70. Smith, Howard L., and Myron D. Fottler. "Training and Development." In *Essentials of Human Resources Management in Health Services Organizations,* edited by Myron D. Fottler, S. Robert Hernandez, and Charles L. Joiner, 197–222. Albany, NY: Delmar Publishers, 1998.
71. Rakich, Jonathon S., Paul J. Kuzdrall, Keith A. Klafehn, and Alan G. Krigline. "Simulation in the Hospital Setting: Implications for Managerial Decision Making and Management Development." *Journal of Management Development* 10 (Special Issue on Health Care Management Development, 1991): 36.
72. Fottler, Myron D. "The Role and Impact of Multiskilled Health Practitioners in the Health Services Industry." *Hospital & Health Services Administration* 41 (Spring 1996): 56.
73. Dessler, *Personnel/Human,* 463–469.
74. See Joiner, Charles L., Kerma N. Jones, and Carson F. Dye. "Compensation Management." In *Essentials of Human Resources Management in Health Services Organizations,* edited by Myron D. Fottler, S. Robert Hernandez, and Charles L. Joiner, 248–270. Albany, NY: Delmar Publishers, 1998.
75. Noe, Raymond A., John R. Hollenbeck, Barry Gerhart, and Patrick M. Wright. *Human Resource Management: Gaining a Competitive Advantage,* 2nd ed., 463. Boston: Irwin/McGraw-Hill, 1997.
76. Friss, Lois. "Designing a Compensation System in the Strategic Human Resource Management Model." In *Human Resource Management in the Health Care Sector,* edited by Amarjit S. Sethi and Randall S. Schuler, 151–158. New York: Quorum Books, 1989.
77. Bernat, John. "Employee Rights Strategies." In *Human Resource Management in the Health Care Sector,* edited by Amarjit S. Sethi and Randall S. Schuler, 255–256. New York: Quorum Books, 1989.
78. Hofrichter, David A., and Gordon W. Hawthorne. "Governing Performance: Examining the Board's Role in Executive Compensation." *Trustee* 50 (June 1997): 7; Keefe, Thomas J., George R. French, and James L. Altman. "Incentive Plans Can Link Employee and Company Goals." *Journal of Compensation and Benefits* 9,4 (January/February 1994): 27.
79. Williams, James B., and R. Scott Coolidge. "Annual Survey: Incentive Plans on the Rise in Hospitals." *Hospitals* 65 (September 5, 1991): 26.
80. Kleiman, *Human Resource Management,* 272.
81. Consolidated Omnibus Budget Reconciliation Act of 1985, PL 99-272, 7 U.S.C. § 1314(g) *et seq.*
82. Health Insurance Portability and Accountability Act of 1996, PL 104-191, 29 U.S.C. § 1181 *et seq.*
83. Family and Medical Leave Act of 1993, PL 103-3, 29 U.S.C. § 2601 *et seq.*
84. Mathis and Jackson, *Human Resource Management,* 135.
85. Kleiman, *Human Resource Management,* 335.
86. Mathis and Jackson, *Human Resource Management,* 137.
87. Harris, *Human Resource Management,* 282.
88. Employee Retirement Income Security Act of 1974, PL 93-406, 29 U.S.C. § 1001 *et seq.*
89. Fernberg, Patricia. "Substance Abuse Is Risky Business." *Occupational Hazards* 60 (October 1998): 67.
90. Howard, John C., and David Szcerbacki. "Employee Assistance Programs in the Hospital Industry." *Health Care Management Review* 13 (Spring 1988): 74.
91. Occupational Safety and Health Act of 1970, PL 91-596, 29 U.S.C. § 651 *et seq.*; Twomey, *A Concise Guide,* 109.
92. Kleiman, *Human Resource Management,* 412.
93. Kennedy, Marilyn Moats. "What Managers Can Find Out from Exit Interviews." *Physician Executive* 22 (October 1996): 45.
94. Carrell, Michael R., and Christina Heavrin. *Collective Bargaining and Labor Relations: Cases, Practice, and Law,* 3. New York: Merrill, 1991.
95. Sloane, Arthur A., and Fred Witney. *Labor Relations,* 9th ed., 24. Upper Saddle River, NJ: Prentice-Hall, 1997; Bureau of Labor Statistics. *http://stats.bls.gov/news.release/union2.nws.htm,* March 29, 1999.
96. Data compiled by the authors from National Labor Relations Board monthly election reports, 1985–1994.

97. Anti-Injunction Act of 1932, PL 106-73, 62 Stat. 968.
98. Anti-Injunction Act of 1932.
99. National Labor Relations Act of 1935, PL 106-73, 29 U.S.C. § 151 *et seq.*
100. Office of the General Counsel, National Labor Relations Board. *A Guide to Basic Law and Procedures Under the National Labor Relations Act,* 1. Washington, DC: National Labor Relations Board, 1990; Sloane, Arthur A., and Fred Witney. *Labor Relations,* 7th ed., 93. Englewood Cliffs, NJ: Prentice-Hall, 1991.
101. Office of the General Counsel, National Labor Relations Board, *A Guide to Basic Law,* 47.
102. Office of the General Counsel, National Labor Relations Board, *A Guide to Basic Law,* 1.
103. Sloane and Witney, *Labor Relations,* 9th ed., 112.
104. Labor–Management Relations Act of 1947, PL 106-73, 29 U.S.C. § 151 *et seq.*
105. Office of the General Counsel, National Labor Relations Board, *A Guide to Basic Law,* 1.
106. Office of the General Counsel, National Labor Relations Board, *A Guide to Basic Law,* 41–42; National Labor Relations Board. "Fact Sheet on the National Labor Relations Board," 2. *http://www.nlrb.gov/ facts.html,* December 11, 1998; Byars, Lloyd L., and Leslie W. Rue. *Human Resources Management,* 428. Boston: Irwin/McGraw-Hill, 1997.
107. Office of the General Counsel, National Labor Relations Board, *A Guide to Basic Law,* 15.
108. Office of the General Counsel, National Labor Relations Board, *A Guide to Basic Law,* 7–13.
109. Labor–Management Reporting and Disclosure Act of 1959, PL 86-257, 29 U.S.C. § 401 *et seq.*
110. Leap, Terry L. *Collective Bargaining and Labor Relations,* 79–80, 87–88. New York: Macmillan, 1991; Office of the General Counsel, National Labor Relations Board, *A Guide to Basic Law,* 27.
111. Office of the General Counsel, National Labor Relations Board, *A Guide to Basic Law,* 23.
112. Becker, Edmund R., Frank A. Sloan, and Bruce Steinwald. "Union Activity in Hospitals: Past, Present, and Future." *Health Care Financing Review* 3 (June 1982): 2; Scott, Clyde, and Jim Simpson. "Union Election Activity in the Hospital Industry." *Health Care Management Review* 14 (Fall 1989): 21.
113. Office of the General Counsel, National Labor Relations Board, *A Guide to Basic Law,* 44.
114. Carrell and Heavrin, *Collective Bargaining,* 22.
115. Byars and Rue, *Human Resources Management,* 430–431.
116. Civil Service Reform Act of 1978, PL 95-454, 92 Stat. 1111; Byars and Rue, *Human Resources Management,* 431.
117. Nonprofit Hospital Amendments to the Taft-Hartley Act, of 1974, PL 93-360.
118. Miller, Richard U. "Hospitals." In *Collective Bargaining: Contemporary American Experience,* edited by Gerald G. Somers, 391. Madison, WI: Industrial Relations Research Association, 1980.
119. Office of the General Counsel, National Labor Relations Board. "Guidelines Issued by the General Counsel of the National Labor Relations Board for Use of Board Regional Offices in Unfair Labor Practice Cases Arising Under the 1974 Nonprofit Hospital Amendments to the Taft-Hartley Act" (Memorandum 74-79, August 20, 1974). *Labor Relations Reporter* 86 (No. 33, 1974): 369–393; see also Appropriate Bargaining in the Health Care Industry, 29 C.F.R. 103.30.
120. Office of Legal and Regulatory Affairs, American Hospital Association. *The New NLRB Bargaining Unit Rules: Hospitals Prepare Yourselves,* 89–90. Chicago: American Hospital Association, 1989; Becker, Edmund R., and Jonathon S. Rakich. "Hospital Union Election Activity, 1974–1985." *Health Care Financing Review* 9 (Summer 1988): 59–60.
121. Office of the General Counsel, National Labor Relations Board, *A Guide to Basic Law,* 8.
122. Office of the General Counsel, National Labor Relations Board, *A Guide to Basic Law,* 22.
123. Feldacker, Bruce. *Labor Guide to Labor Law,* 5. Englewood Cliffs, NJ: Prentice-Hall, 1990.
124. Richman, Dan. "Struggle of a Lifetime." *Modern Healthcare* 17 (August 14, 1987): 110.
125. District 1199. *http://www.1199.org/intro.html,* March 29, 1999.
126. Kilgour, John G. "Union Organization Activity in the Hospital Industry." *Hospital & Health Services Administration* 29 (November/December 1984): 87.
127. American Federation of State, County, and Municipal Workers. *http://www.afscme.org/una/content. htm,* 1, March 16, 1999.
128. Robinson, Michele L. "Labor Pains." *Health Systems Review* 29 (July/August 1996): 18.

129. Carrell, Michael R., and Christina Heavrin. *Labor Relations and Collective Bargaining: Cases, Practices, and Law,* 5th ed., 29. Upper Saddle River, NJ: Prentice-Hall, 1998.

130. Weinstock, Matthew. "Labor Organizing on Upswing Among Health Care Workers." *AHA News* 34 (November 16, 1998): 6.

131. Havighurst, Craig. "A Union Answer." *American Medical News* (January 11, 1999): 1. (*http://www. ama-assn.org/sci-pubs/amanews/feat_99/feat0111.htm*)

132. *http://www.cirdocs.org/,* March 29, 1999.

133. Jaklevic, Mary Chris. "Physicians Find Power in Unions." *Modern Healthcare* 27 (October 6, 1997): 104.

134. See [330 NLRB No. 30] Boston Medical Center Corporation and House Officers' Association/Committee of Interns and Residents, Petitioner. (*http://frwebgate4.access.gpo.gov/cgi-bin/...ocID=6685319725+ 0+0+0&WAISaction=retrieve*); "AMA to Establish National Collective Bargaining Unit." *American Medical News* (July 5, 1999): 2

135. Byars and Rue, *Human Resources Management,* 442.

136. Joiner, Charles L. "Preventive Labor-Management Relations." In *Handbook of Health Care Human Resources Management,* edited by Norman Metzger, 511. Rockville, MD: Aspen Publishers, 1990.

137. Eubanks, Paula. "Avoiding Unions: Supervisors Are the First Line of Defense." *Hospitals* 64 (November 20, 1990): 40.

138. Fottler, Karen S. "The Unionization of the Health Care Industry: General Trends and Emerging Issues." *Journal of Health and Human Resources Administration* 10 (Summer 1987): 73

139. Office of Legal and Regulatory Affairs, American Hospital Association, *New NLRB Bargaining,* 13–16.

140. National Labor Relations Board. "Collective-Bargaining Units in the Health Care Industry: Final Rule." *Federal Register* (April 21, 1989): 16347–16348.

141. Feldacker, *Labor Guide,* 74.

142. Office of Legal and Regulatory Affairs, American Hospital Association, *New NLRB Bargaining,* 30.

143. Holley, William H., Jr., and Kenneth M. Jennings. *The Labor Relations Process,* 6th ed., 191. Ft. Worth, TX: Dryden Press, 1997.

144. Hopson, Edwin S. "NLRB Cracks Down on Hospital No-Solicitation/Right of Access Rules." *Kentucky Hospitals* 6 (No. 4, 1989): 28.

145. See Office of Legal and Regulatory Affairs, American Hospital Association, *New NLRB Bargaining,* 30–31; Fossum, John A. *Labor Relations,* 162–163. Boston: Irwin/McGraw-Hill, 1999.

146. Harty, James Q. "Union Organizing Drive: An Introduction." In *American Law Institute–American Bar Association Continuing Legal Education (ALI-ABA Course of Study SB36),* 1706. Chicago: American Law Institute–American Bar Association, 1997.

147. Office of the General Counsel, National Labor Relations Board. "Guidelines for Handling No-Solicitation, No-Distribution Rules in Health-Care Facilities" (Memorandum 79-76), 1–15. Washington, DC: National Labor Relations Board, 1979.

148. Feldacker, *Labor Guide,* 76.

149. Rhodes, Rhonda. "Employee Solicitation: What Should Your Policy Include?" *Trustee* 2 (March 1989): 25.

150. See Feldacker, *Labor Guide,* 76; Gilmore, Carol B. "When Hospitals Limit Organizing Activity." *Employee Relations Law Journal* 14 (Summer 1988): 100; Rhodes, "Employee Solicitation," 25.

151. Gilmore, "When Hospitals Limit," 103.

152. Office of the General Counsel, National Labor Relations Board, *A Guide to Basic Law,* 2.

153. Office of the General Counsel, National Labor Relations Board, *A Guide to Basic Law,* 17.

154. Feldacker, *Labor Guide,* 82.

155. Feldacker, *Labor Guide,* 83.

156. Metzger, Norman. "The Union Movement: Dead or Alive?" In *Handbook of Health Care Human Resources Management,* edited by Norman Metzger, 385. Rockville, MD: Aspen Publishers, 1990.

157. Metzger, "The Union Movement," 384–385.

158. Metzger, "The Union Movement," 389–390.

159. McLaurin, James R., Arthur Berkely, and Robert R. Taylor. "Perspectives on Unionization in Hospitals." *Journal of Health and Human Resources Administration* 14 (Winter 1992): 269.

160. Bolon, Douglas S. "Health Care Supervisors and Employee Relations Success: Three C's a Day Keeps the Union Away." *Health Care Supervisor* 14 (September 1995): 33–36.

161. Eubanks, Paula. "Employee Grievance Policy: Don't Discourage Complaints." *Hospitals* 64 (December 20, 1990): 36.

162. American Hospital Association. *Establishing an Employee Grievance Procedure: Management Advisory,* 1. Chicago: American Hospital Association, 1990.

163. American Hospital Association, *Establishing an Employee,* 1.

164. Byars and Rue, *Human Resources Management,* 451.

165. An overview of negotiating and administering labor contracts can be found in Metzger, Norman, and Donna M. Malvey. "Negotiating and Administering the Labor Relations Contract." In *Strategic Management of Human Resources in Health Services Organizations,* 2nd ed., edited by Myron D. Fottler, S. Robert Hernandez, and Charles L. Joiner, 436–479. Albany, NY: Delmar Publishers, 1994; Holley and Jennings, *The Labor Relations Process,* 221–257 and 302–331.

166. Office of the General Counsel, National Labor Relations Board, *A Guide to Basic Law,* 32–33.

167. Office of the General Counsel, National Labor Relations Board, *A Guide to Basic Law,* 24–25.

168. Byars and Rue, *Human Resources Management,,* 453.

169. Carrell and Heavrin, *Labor Relations,* 5th ed., 384–386.

170. Carrell and Heavrin, *Labor Relations,* 5th ed., 218–219.

171. Robbins, Stephen A., and Jonathon S. Rakich. "Hospital Personnel Management in the Early 1990s: A Follow-Up Analysis." *Hospital & Health Services Administration* 34 (Fall 1989): 385–396.

SELECTED BIBLIOGRAPHY

American College of Healthcare Executives. "Preventing and Addressing Sexual Harassment in the Workplace: Public Policy Statement." *Healthcare Executive* 11 (November/December 1996): 43.

Bolon, Douglas S. "Health Care Supervisors and Employee Relations Success: Three C's a Day Keep the Union Away." *Health Care Supervisor* 14 (September 1995): 32–41.

Carrell, Michael R., and Christina Heavrin. *Collective Bargaining and Labor Relations: Cases, Practice, and Law.* New York: Merrill, 1991.

Carrell, Michael R., and Christina Heavrin. *Labor Relations and Collective Bargaining: Cases, Practices, and Law,* 5th ed. Upper Saddle River, NJ: Prentice-Hall, 1998.

Cascio, Wayne, F. *Managing Human Resources: Productivity, Quality of Work Life, Profits,* 5th ed. Boston: Irwin/McGraw-Hill, 1998.

Coil, James H., III, and Lori J. Shapiro. "The ADA at Three Years: A Statute in Flux." *Employee Relations Law Journal* 21 (Spring 1996): 5–38.

Decker, Phillip J. "Sexual Harassment in Health Care: A Major Productivity Problem." *Health Care Supervisor* 16 (September 1997): 1–14.

Decker, Phillip J., Marlene K. Strader, and Rebecca J. Wise. "Beyond JCAHO: Using Competency Models to Improve Healthcare Organizations: Part 1." *Hospital Topics* 75 (Winter 1997): 23–27.

Decker, Phillip J., Marlene K. Strader, and Rebecca J. Wise. "Beyond JCAHO: Using Competency Models to Improve Healthcare Organizations: Part 2." *Hospital Topics* 75 (Spring 1997): 10–17.

Drucker, Peter F. *Managing the Non-Profit Organization.* New York: HarperCollins, 1990.

Equal Employment Opportunity Commission. *Laws Administered by the EEOC,* 1–48. Washington, DC: Equal Employment Opportunity Commission, 1981.

Equal Employment Opportunity Commission. *Uniform Employee Selection Guidelines—Interpretation and Clarification—Questions and Answers, Sect. 4175.01–4175.08.* Chicago: Commerce Clearing House, 1985.

Equal Employment Opportunity Commission. "The ADA: Your Responsibilities as an Employer," 1–9. *http:2//www.eeoc.gov/facts/ada17.html,* January 15, 1997.

Equal Employment Opportunity Commission. "The Americans with Disabilities Act of 1990, Titles I and V," 1–18. *http://www.eeoc.gov/laws/ada.html,* January 15, 1997.

Equal Employment Opportunity Commission. "Facts About the Americans with Disabilities Act," 1–2. *http://www.eeoc.gov/facts/fs-ada.html,* January 15, 1997.

Equal Employment Opportunity Commission. "Facts About Sexual Harassment." 1–2. *http://www.eeoc.gov/stats/charges.html,* August 11, 1998.

Fernberg, Patricia. "Substance Abuse Is Risky Business." *Occupational Hazards* 60 (October 1998): 67.

Fossum, John A. *Labor Relations.* Boston: Irwin/McGraw-Hill, 1999.

Foster, Charles, and Lynn Godkin. "Employment Selection in Health Care: The Case for Structured Interviewing." *Health Care Management Review* 23 (Winter 1998): 46–51.

Fottler, Myron D. "Job Analysis." In *Essentials of Human Resources Management in Health Services Organizations,* 2nd ed., edited by Myron D. Fottler, S. Robert Hernandez, and Charles L. Joiner, 117–133. Albany, NY: Delmar Publishers, 1994.

Fottler, Myron D. "The Role and Impact of Multiskilled Health Practitioners in the Health Services Industry." *Hospital & Health Services Administration* 41 (Spring 1996): 55–75.

Gillman, Steven L., and Davi L. Hirsch. "The Americans with Disabilities Act: Civil Rights for Handicapped Workers." *The Brief* 20 (Summer 1991): 16–21, 43.

Gómez Mejía, Luis R., David B. Balkin, and Robert L. Cardy. *Managing Human Resources,* 3rd ed. Upper Saddle River, NJ: Prentice-Hall, 1998.

Harris, Michael. *Human Resource Management: A Practical Approach.* Fort Worth, TX: Dryden Press/Harcourt Brace, 1997.

Harty, James Q. "Union Organizing Drive: An Introduction." In *American Law Institute–Amercan Bar Association Continuing Legal Education* (ALI-ABA Course of Study SB36), 1699. Chicago: American Law Institute–American Bar Association, 1997.

Hernandez, S. Robert, Myron D. Fottler, and Charles L. Joiner. "Integrating Management and Human Resources." In *Essentials of Human Resources Management in Health Services Organizations,* edited by Myron D. Fottler, S. Robert Hernandez, and Charles L. Joiner, 1–20. Albany, NY: Delmar Publishers, 1998.

Hernandez, S. Robert, Cynthia Carter Haddock, William M. Behrendt, and Walter F. Klein, Jr. "Management Development and Succession Planning: Lessons for Health Services Organizations." *Journal of Management Development* 10 (Special Issue on Health Care Management Development, 1991): 19–30.

Holley, William H., Jr., and Kenneth M. Jennings. *The Labor Relations Process,* 6th ed. Fort Worth, TX: Dryden Press, 1997.

Jaklevic, Mary Chris. "Physicians Find Power in Unions." *Modern Healthcare* 20 (October 6, 1997): 99–106.

Joiner, Charles L., and John C. Hyde. "Performance Appraisal." In *Essentials of Human Resources Management in Health Services Organizations,* edited by Myron D. Fottler, S. Robert Hernandez, and Charles L. Joiner, 223–247. Albany, NY: Delmar Publishers, 1998.

Joiner, Charles L., Kerma N. Jones, and Carson F. Dye. "Compensation Management." In *Essentials of Human Resources Management in Health Services Organizations,* edited by Myron D. Fottler, S. Robert Hernandez, and Charles L. Joiner, 248–270. Albany, NY: Delmar Publishers, 1998.

Joiner, Charles L., Norman Metzger, John C. Hyde, and Donna M. Malvey. "Labor Relations." In *Essentials of Human Resources Management in Health Services Organizations,* edited by Myron D. Fottler, S. Robert Hernandez, and Charles L. Joiner, 271–313. Albany, NY: Delmar Publishers, 1998.

Kennedy, Marilyn Moats. "What Managers Can Find Out from Exit Interviews." *The Physician Executive* 22 (October 1996): 45–47.

Kinard, Jerry L., J. Reagan McLaurin, and Beverly Little. "Sexual Harassment in the Hospital Industry: An Empirical Inquiry." *Health Care Management Review* 20 (Winter 1995): 47–53.

Kleiman, Lawrence S. *Human Resource Management: A Tool for Competitive Advantage.* Minneapolis/St. Paul: West Publishing, 1997.

Landau, Jacqueline, and Michael Abelson. "Recruitment and Selection." In *Essentials of Human Resources Management in Health Services Organizations,* edited by Myron D. Fottler, S. Robert Hernandez, and Charles L. Joiner, 134–165. Albany, NY: Delmar Publishers, 1998.

Landau, Jacqueline, and Daniel S. Fogel. "Selection and Placement." In *Essentials of Human Resources Management in Health Services Organizations,* 2nd ed., edited by Myron D. Fottler, S. Robert Hernandez, and Charles L. Joiner, 166–196. Albany, NY: Delmar Publishers, 1998.

Lehr, Richard I., Robert A. Mclean, and Gregg L. Smith. "The Legal and Economic Environment." In *Essentials of Human Resources Management in Health Services Organizations,* edited by Myron D. Fottler, S. Robert Hernandez, and Charles L. Joiner, 21–43. Albany, NY: Delmar Publishers, 1998.

Mathis, Robert L., and John H. Jackson. *Human Resource Management: Essential Perspectives.* Cincinnati, OH: South-Western Publishing, 1999.

Metzger, Norman. "Human Resources Management." In *Health Care Administration: Principles, Practices, Structure, and Delivery,* 2nd ed., edited by Lawrence F. Wolper, 327–362. Gaithersburg, MD: Aspen Publishers, 1995.

National Labor Relations Board. "Collective-Bargaining Units in the Health Care Industry: Final Rule." *Federal Register* (April 21, 1989): 16336–16348.

National Labor Relations Board. "Fact Sheet on the National Labor Relations Board," 1–3. *http://www.nlrb. gov/facts.html,* December 11, 1998.

Noe, Raymond A., John R. Hollenbeck, Barry Gerhart, and Patrick M. Wright. *Human Resource Management: Gaining a Competitive Advantage,* 2nd ed. Boston: Irwin/McGraw-Hill, 1997.

Noe, Raymond A. *Employee Training and Development.* Boston: Irwin/McGraw-Hill, 1999.

Office of the General Counsel, National Labor Relations Board. "Guidelines Issued by the General Counsel of the National Labor Relations Board for Use by Board Regional Offices in Unfair Labor Practice Cases Arising Under the 1974 Nonprofit Hospital Amendments to the Taft-Hartley Act," (Memorandum 74-79, August 20, 1974). *Labor Relations Reporter* 86 (No. 33, 1974): 369–393.

Office of the General Counsel, National Labor Relations Board. *A Guide to Basic Law and Procedures Under the National Labor Relations Act.* Washington, DC: National Labor Relations Board, 1990.

Office of Public Affairs, Equal Employment Opportunity Commission. *Pre-employment Inquiries and Equal Employment Opportunity Law,* 1–8. Washington, DC: Equal Employment Opportunity Commission, 1981.

Rakich, Jonathon S., Paul J. Kuzdrall, Keith A. Klafehn, and Alan G. Krigline. "Simulation in the Hospital Setting: Implications for Managerial Decision Making and Management Development." *Journal of Management Development* 10 (Special Issue on Health Care Management Development, 1991): 31–37.

Robbins, Stephen A., and Jonathon S. Rakich. "Hospital Personnel Management in the Early 1990s: A Follow-Up Analysis." *Hospital & Health Services Administration* 34 (Fall 1989): 385–396.

Robinson, Michele L. "Labor Pains." *Health Systems Review* 29 (July/August 1996): 18–20.

Sloane, Arthur A., and Fred Witney. *Labor Relations,* 9th ed. Upper Saddle River, NJ: Prentice-Hall, 1997.

Smith, Howard L., and Myron D. Fottler. "Training and Development." In *Essentials of Human Resources Management in Health Services Organizations,* edited by Myron D. Fottler, S. Robert Hernandez, and Charles L. Joiner, 197–222. Albany, NY: Delmar Publishers, 1998.

12 Organizational Change

Change is inevitable and the future is uncertain.[1]

One of the most important contributions that managers make to their health services organization's/ health system's (HSO's/HS's) ability to attain its organizational objectives and desired levels of overall organizational performance is to know when organizational change is needed and how to smoothly and effectively implement it. How organizations and systems manage change affects the commitment that people feel toward their organizational homes.[2]

Organizational changes are made because managers perceive a performance gap—a discrepancy between a desired and actual state—in their areas of responsibility and take action to address the gap. In effect, managers must know how to act as change agents. This chapter is about managers as agents of change in HSOs/HSs. In particular, the chapter provides a model of the complex process of organizational change that provides a framework for what managers do while carrying out their change agent responsibilities.

Change in any organization or system of organizations takes place whenever a measurable modification in "form, quality, or state over time"[3] is made in the organization's or system's purpose or objectives, culture, strategies, tasks, technologies, people, or structures.[4] These possible foci of organizational change in HSOs/HSs are shown in Table 12.1. Such modifications occur in HSOs/HSs so ubiquitously that organizational change can be considered a constant.

Another way to envision the enormous variety of organizational changes that managers in HSOs/HSs make is to review the management model in Figure 1.7, which illustrates that managers have numerous options. For example, inputs can be changed and managers can increase, decrease, or modify the HSO's/HS's human resources, obtain additional information, employ new technologies, or obtain better supplies. They might employ new staff with specific education or experience in an effort to achieve a desired output. If such people are not available or if the HSO/HS cannot compete effectively for them with other employers, then the change may involve more or different training for current staff. It might also involve the introduction of technology that permits other in-

TABLE 12.1.   FOCI FOR ORGANIZATIONAL CHANGES IN HSOs/HSs, WITH EXAMPLES

Points of focus	Examples of organizational changes
Purpose and objectives	Changes in a HSO's/HS's mission statement; addition or deletion of organizational objectives; modification of existing objectives
Cultures	Changes in value that drive HSO/HS; new emphasis on entrepreneurial behaviors
Strategies	Changes in strategic plans or in means to operationalize their accomplishment
Tasks	Changes in job designs; use of cross-functional teams
Technologies	Adoption of new technologies
People	Training of personnel in new techniques; changes in hiring criteria in use; clarification of roles
Structures	Redesign of reporting relationships; downsizing of HSO/HS; addition of new units

Adapted from Longest, Beaufort B., Jr. "Organizational Change and Innovation." In *Handbook of Health Care Management,* edited by W. Jack Duncan, Peter M. Ginter, and Linda E. Swayne, 371. Malden, MA: Blackwell, 1998.

puts to be used more effectively. Computerizing much of the information exchanged within a HSO/HS is a good example of such a change.

Managers also can change the organizational structure or design, the relationships among people, and the conditions of work. They might change the mix of technologies used in converting inputs to outputs, reassign tasks, or change the assignment of people. Such changes can be modest: changing job design or work schedules or adding rules and procedures to increase standardization. Or the changes can be extensive, such as increasing centralization to speed decision making in a HS or combining departments or units to remove vertical layers of a HSO. Sometimes structural changes are more extensive, as would be the case if the structure of a HSO were transformed into a matrix design (see Chapter 3). As discussed in Chapter 9, changes in structure and design often arise through continuous quality improvement (CQI) programs, reengineering activities, and strategic quality planning.

Managers also can change or redefine outputs. It is senseless to produce an output with no market. A well-managed HSO/HS seeks to identify and respond to unmet needs in its service area, thus ensuring a continuous reconsideration of the mix of desired outputs. Marketing studies can guide a HSO/HS to reduce inpatient services and increase ambulatory services or provide industrial medicine services for employers.

Because HSOs/HSs do not exist in a vacuum, another option for change is that management alters the HSO's/HS's relationships with its external environment and stakeholders. The most important task facing any organization or system is to fit its external environment.[5] Changes in inputs, organizational structure, tasks/technology, and outputs (e.g., those described previously) can help fit the organization or system to the opportunities and threats in its external environment. A HSO's/HS's managers also can try to change the external environment to make it more closely fit the organization's input requirements and output capabilities. This can be done through marketing a HSO's/HS's services (outputs) or lobbying for more resources for production of an input. Seeking to increase federal funding for nursing education is an example of the latter type of activity.

Managers can change the HSO's/HS's culture, although this usually occurs over a long period of time. Finally, as can be seen in Figure 1.7, managers can even change their own functions, skills, roles, or competencies.

PRESSURES FOR CHANGE IN HSOs/HSs

Managers must be able to make changes continuously in HSOs/HSs because the pressures for change are pervasive, constant, diverse, and numerous. Pressures to change come from internal and external sources. Internally, a new strategic plan that includes diversifying into new services is a potent force for change. It may stimulate recruiting staff or retraining current personnel. It may stimulate changes in accounting systems or marketing programs. The arrival of a new chief executive officer (CEO) often portends significant organizational changes, sometimes bordering on upheaval. Leadership changes often are followed by significant shifts in strategic direction and the structure of HSOs/HSs. They are powerful internal forces for change.

The dynamic external environments of HSOs/HSs are another set of forces for change. For example, growing, declining, or aging populations in their market areas or the plans and actions of competitors have significant implications for HSOs/HSs, usually requiring them to change in a variety of ways in response. Public policies and regulations also exert strong and direct external pressures for change.[6] Changes in reimbursement policy for the Medicare and Medicaid programs routinely drive changes in HSOs/HSs. Similarly, National Labor Relations Board (NLRB) rulings can instantly change how HSOs/HSs relate to unionized employees. Because HSOs/HSs are so dependent on technologies, technological advances exert a strong force for change on them. The dramatic shift from inpatient to outpatient surgery that began in the early 1980s was largely attributable to better anesthesia, surgical techniques, and postoperative care technologies.

A HSO's/HS's senior-level managers are primarily responsible for assessing the external environment and determining what changes are needed and when. Care must be exercised by CEOs and other senior-level managers in environmental assessment and in interpreting and predicting the effects of environmental conditions on their organizations or systems. This is no easy task, the key steps of strategic planning and environmental assessment are covered in Chapter 8. A reason that this task is difficult is that perceptions of the environment are influenced by the characteristics of those who observe it. As has been noted

> *A top management team with a primarily marketing background may be more sensitive to changes in market structure and performance data related to market share than a team with financial or production backgrounds, who may be more sensitive to changes in traditional financial performance indicators or tax and legal changes. Individuals pay selective attention to the environment according to interests and selectively interpret the information they receive.*[7]

The continuing internal and external pressures for change, coupled with managers' responsibilities to maximize organizational performance—including implementing changes when necessary—means that the capability to implement organizational changes is among the most important that managers can possess. In the next section organizational change is defined and clarified. Then, a four-stage model of the complex process of managing organizational change is presented and discussed, with actual applications to managerial practice in HSOs/HSs.

ORGANIZATIONAL CHANGE DEFINED

To build on the concept of organizational change discussed earlier, organizational change can be defined as a discernible, measurable modification in form, quality, or state over time in a HSO's/HS's purpose or objectives, culture, strategies, tasks, technologies, people, or structures. Stated slightly differently, organizational change is "any modification in operations, structure, or ends."[8] This means that organizational changes span a spectrum from a fundamental shift in a HSO's/HS's purpose to a small refinement in a single job description.

Not all organizational change is alike. It is especially important to distinguish among organizational changes on the dimension of creativity. As discussed in Chapter 8, creativity involves imagination and ingenuity.[9] A creative change occurs when a HSO/HS (or a part of it) develops and is the first user of a concept, practice, or thing. Most organizational changes, however, occur through the adoption of concepts or ideas, practices, or things that have been developed in other organizations or systems. The distinction among organizational changes in terms of their creativity leads to the identification of three types of change based on the source of the particular concepts or ideas, practices, or things involved in a change.[10] In this conceptualization, concepts or ideas, practices, or things involved in organizational changes can be borrowed directly and without modification; they can be borrowed but adapted to fit; or they can originate in the HSO/HS that is making the change.

Origination involves more creativity, which is not to say, however, that it is necessarily better to originate than to borrow or to adapt when organizational changes are being made. In general, borrowing or adapting means easier implementation (another's experience can be very informative) and lower cost than an originated concept, practice, or thing because someone else has borne the development costs.

Adapting and borrowing are the most common sources of organizational changes in HSOs/HSs and reflect the ready diffusion of innovations. In fact, widespread diffusion of clinical and administrative innovations characterizes the health care industry. The diffusion of medical technologies such as those involved in imaging, surgery, and diagnostic laboratory procedures has received a great deal of attention, but administrative changes also are routinely diffused by adaptation or borrowing. For example, concepts of strategic alliance formation were widely adapted and borrowed by HSOs/HSs in the 1990s,[11] as were concepts of CQI.[12]

The fact that adaptation and borrowing in HSOs'/HSs' organizational changes is so commonplace does not mean that originated changes are unimportant. After all, there must always be someone who creates and initially uses a new concept, practice, or thing before others can borrow or adapt it. One way to increase creativity in a HSO/HS and enhance the likelihood that it will originate innovations is to hire and sustain creative people. Another is to create an organizational climate in which creativity and innovation are stimulated. The following items characterize such a climate:

- People are encouraged to experiment without fear of the consequences should they fail.
- Mistakes are treated as learning opportunities.
- Rules, regulations, policies, and similar controls are kept to a minimum.
- Jobs are defined broadly. Narrowly defined jobs create myopia, but diverse job activities give people a broader perspective.
- Ambiguity is accepted because too much emphasis on objectivity and specificity constrains creativity.
- Conflict is tolerated and differences of opinion are encouraged. Harmony and agreement between and among individuals and/or units are not assumed to be evidence of high performance.
- The impractical is tolerated. Individuals who offer impractical, even foolish, answers to "what if" questions are not stifled. There is recognition that what seems impractical at first might lead to creative solutions.
- There is a focus on ends rather than means: Objectives are made clear, and individuals are encouraged to consider alternative routes to attain them. Focusing on ends suggests that there might be several right answers to a problem.
- Communication is open and flows in all directions in the HSO/HS because this facilitates cross-fertilization of ideas.[13]

The best way to understand the complex process of organizational change is to consider what managers in HSOs/HSs actually do when they manage change. The next section presents a four-stage model, with each stage incorporating specific tasks that must be successfully accomplished if organizational change is to be well managed.

PROCESS OF MANAGING ORGANIZATIONAL CHANGE[14]

To effectively manage organizational change, managers must accomplish an extensive series of interrelated tasks.[15] As managers make organizational changes, these tasks are accomplished in four stages, as illustrated in Figure 12.1. In the first stage, they 1) recognize situations and circumstances that require an organizational change; and 2) identify and specify the nature of the change needed. These two tasks are closely related and are triggered by the internal and external pressures for change discussed earlier.

The second stage of managing organizational change is implementation planning, which involves 1) developing alternative changes to be considered, 2) choosing the change from among the alternatives, 3) shaping a general approach to making the change, and 4) developing and selecting the techniques to build support and minimize resistance to the change. Only after effective implementation planning has been done can managers be certain they are prepared for actually implementing a change.

Implementation is accomplished in the third stage of the process through three additional tasks, descriptively labeled as 1) unfreezing, 2) changing, and 3) refreezing.[16] Unfreezing disrupts the status quo and convinces those involved of the necessity for and appropriateness of the change. If they cannot be convinced, then managers must at least apprise them of the impending change and prepare them as much as possible. The unfreezing task is followed by actually making the

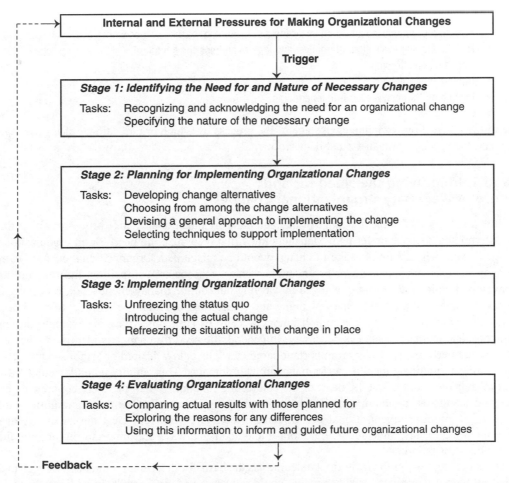

Figure 12.1. A model of the process of managing organizational changes. (From Longest, Beaufort B., Jr. "Organizational Change and Innovation." In *Handbook of Health Care Management,* edited by W. Jack Duncan, Peter M. Ginter, and Linda E. Swayne, 375. Malden, MA: Blackwell, 1998; reprinted by permission.)

change. Some concept or idea, practice, or thing, or some combination of them, is used to modify the HSO's/HS's purpose or objectives, culture, strategies, tasks, technologies, people, or structure. The change is followed by refreezing to stabilize the context and circumstances surrounding the change. This is necessary if the newly implemented change is to have any chance of stability and durability.

The effective and systematic management of organizational change does not end with implementation. Managers who have the most success with the complex process of managing organizational change evaluate the results of the changes they make and use the information as feedback for future iterations of the change process. Tasks in this fourth stage include 1) comparing actual results with those that were planned, 2) exploring the reasons for differences, and 3) using this information to guide future changes.

The similarities between the process of managing an organizational change as illustrated in Figure 12.1 and the process by which managers solve problems that is presented in Chapter 7 are striking. In fact, it is useful to think of managing organizational change as an exercise in problem solving. Recall that problem solving was described in Chapter 7 as a process by which managers cause change so that actual HSO/HS results or outputs more closely align with those that are desired. The process by which managers solve problems, as presented in Chapter 7, includes

- Selecting or identifying and then analyzing a situation that requires a decision
- Developing and evaluating alternative solutions to address the situation
- Choosing an alternative
- Implementing the alternative
- Evaluating the results after implementation

The following sections examine each stage of the process by which organizational change is managed and the specific tasks that must be performed.

Stage 1: Identifying the Need for and Nature of Necessary Organizational Changes

As shown in Figure 12.1, the first stage of managing the organizational change process requires that two interrelated tasks be performed. Managers must first recognize the need for an organizational change because change for the sake of change would be misguided. Organizational changes carry a variety of costs and should never be undertaken unless reasons are compelling. Information that is developed while managers are engaged in carrying out routine management work, especially in their performance of the functions of planning and controlling, often helps them identify real need for change. Deviations from the accomplishment of a HSO's/HS's objectives, for example, are important indicators that a change is necessary. In general, the need for change is identified when organizational performance along an important parameter falls below desired or established targets.

Managers routinely monitor performance in their domains. This activity is fundamental to the work of managers and lies at the heart of the controlling function. When there are concrete objectives and standards, monitoring outcomes and comparing them to standards is straightforward. However, to monitor organizational performance effectively, managers must observe more than mere operating results, although such bottom-line outcomes always are important in judging ultimate success or failure.

One problem with relying on final outcomes as the basis for determining the need for a change is that by then it is too late for changes that could prevent a bad final result. In addition, final results may not identify why deviations occurred and thus give little information about the nature of the changes needed. To overcome such problems, managers must design their monitoring systems and techniques carefully. For example, management information systems (MISs) can be designed so that information that is useful in identifying when organizational change is needed can be collected, formatted, stored, and retrieved in a timely way. This means that they must focus on interim measures and not rely solely on final results.

If MISs (see the discussion about MISs in Chapter 10) are to be useful in identifying the need for change, and especially if they are to contribute to determining the nature of changes needed, then several factors should be considered, including the following:

- HSO/HS managers should match the elements of information covered by their MISs to organizational purposes or objectives, cultures, strategies, tasks, technologies, people, and structures that may need to be changed to improve organizational performance.
- The elements of information in a MIS should point out exceptions at critical points. Effectively managing change requires that managers concentrate on issues and activities that are the most critical to organizational performance.
- The MIS should report deviations promptly. The ideal MIS helps managers identify when change is needed by detecting deviations soon after they occur. Only timely information allows managers to make changes when they are needed.
- The MIS should be forward-looking. When relying on MISs to help them determine when a change is needed, managers usually prefer a forecast of what will probably happen next week or next month—even though this projection contains a margin of error—in contrast to a report, accurate to several decimal points, on the past, about which nothing can be done.

When a change is indicated, the next step in the first stage of managing organizational change is to identify the nature of the change that is needed. Again, this depends on information, although, typically, the information that is necessary to determine the nature of the change is more detailed than the information that signals only that a change is needed. An example that occurred at Butterworth Hospital's respiratory therapy department will clarify how information is used both in recognizing a need for change and in the more extensive task of identifying the needed change.[17]

When Butterworth Hospital's MIS indicated that the department was not able to meet the demand for respiratory services, a change was needed. Information on the number of missed respiratory therapy sessions was sufficient to reveal the need for change. Determining the nature of the change, however, required more information.

To obtain this information, a quality improvement team (see Chapter 9) that included members from respiratory therapy and other departments that interacted with it was formed to determine why the department could not meet demands for services. The team first held a brainstorming session to identify reasons why the respiratory therapy department could not meet demand. They organized the possible explanations into eight categories and developed the cause-and-effect, or fishbone, diagram shown in Figure 12.2.

To move their analysis beyond speculation, the team surveyed respiratory therapy department staff, who were asked to rank order the reasons the team had identified in its brainstorming session. The results were displayed in a Pareto diagram (see Figure 12.3), which shows the six most frequently mentioned reasons why members of the department missed service appointments.

On examining their Pareto diagram, the team realized that three of the top six reasons for missed services related to equipment: equipment availability, equipment misstocked, and equipment out of order. The team decided to look more specifically into the equipment

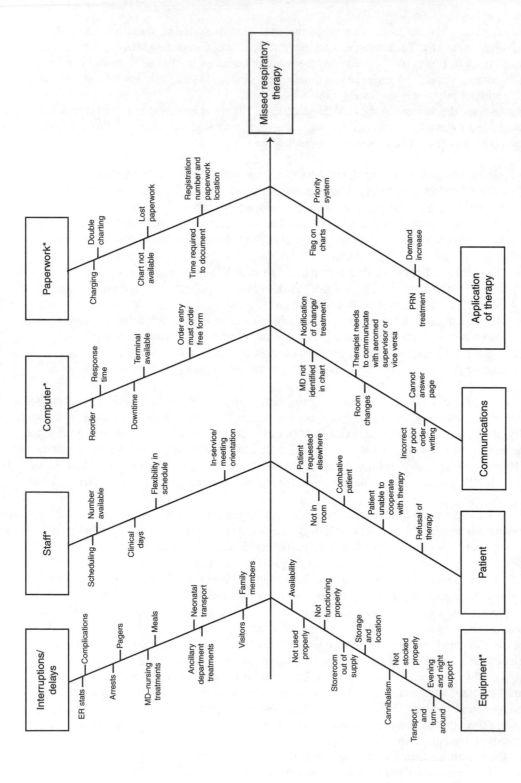

Figure 12.2. Reasons for missed respiratory therapy: a cause-and-effect diagram. *Most important in group ratings. (From Berwick, Donald M., A. Blanton Godfrey, and Jane Roessner. *Curing Health Care: New Strategies for Quality Improvement*, 95. San Francisco: Jossey-Bass, 1990; reprinted by permission.)

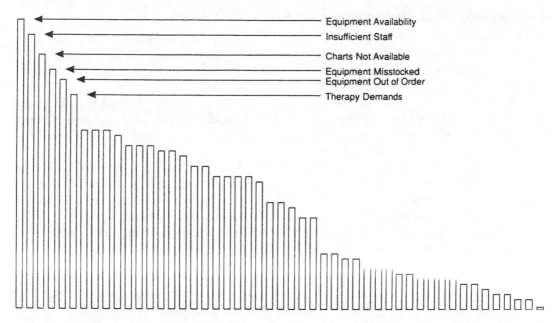

Figure 12.3.   Reasons for missed respiratory therapy: a Pareto diagram of survey results. (From Berwick, Donald M., A. Blanton Godfrey, and Jane Roessner. *Curing Health Care: New Strategies for Quality Improvement,* 96. San Francisco: Jossey-Bass, 1990; reprinted by permission.)

problem. By surveying members of the respiratory therapy department again, the team learned that the specific problems were flowmeter and oximeter unavailability and oxygen analyzer downtime. Armed with this information, the specific organizational changes that needed to be made in this situation were easily identified.

This example illustrates both steps in the change identification stage of the process of managing organizational change. At first, managers knew only that an organizational change was needed. This conclusion was based simply on the information that the respiratory therapy department was not meeting demand for its services. However, additional, more detailed information showed the specific nature of the changes needed to address the problem. In other words, the managers involved accomplished the task of identifying the need for organizational change and the task of determining the nature of the change needed. They had successfully completed the first stage, but their work had only begun in terms of completely managing this organizational change situation.

Stage 2: Planning for Implementing Organizational Change

As Figure 12.1 shows, the second stage in the overall process of managing organizational change contains four interrelated tasks. The first is to develop viable alternative changes for consideration. Usually, when there is an indication that something in a HSO/HS needs to be changed, a variety of possibilities for change exist. Even when much is known about the nature of the change needed, there may be multiple possibilities. Developing a set of alternatives for consideration is the first task in planning for implementation of an organizational change. The second task is selecting from among the alternatives. Then, a general approach to implementing the change can be devised or determined. The final task in this stage is the selection of techniques to support implementation of the change being planned and to reduce resistance to it. The planning stage is a crucial precursor to successful implementation. Each of the four tasks within this stage must receive attention.

Developing a Set of Viable Alternative Changes for Consideration

When carrying out the task of developing a set of viable alternative changes, it is important to remember that organizational changes can be borrowed, adapted, or originated. The essence of this task is that, once the need for a change is clear and the nature of the change that is needed has been identified, managers must develop alternatives that might work.

When considering alternative changes, managers should not necessarily think in terms of one best alternative. More realistic, several options with both positive and negative features are possible responses to the need for an organizational change. The challenge in this task is to develop as many potentially satisfactory choices as possible.

Managers who wish to increase the likelihood that their organizations or systems will be able to originate the concepts and ideas, practices, and things necessary for creative changes must establish an organizational climate in which creativity and innovation are valued, stimulated, and facilitated.[18] The characteristics of such an organizational climate were listed earlier.

Just as there are organizational characteristics that encourage creativity in HSOs/HSs, there are behaviors that stifle it. More important, for example, the isolation of senior-level managers from their organization or system "fosters misunderstandings about conditions and people in the organization and contributes to a risk-averse climate."[19] A myopic focus on short time horizons and short-term organizational performance can reduce the chances of developing creative solutions to problems, as can incentive and reward systems that do not effectively support creativity. Kanter cautions, only slightly tongue-in-cheek, that managers who want to foster creativity should avoid the temptation to "regard any new idea from below with suspicion—because it's new, and because it's from below."[20]

Through combinations of borrowing, adapting, and originating, managers can successfully carry out the task of developing sets of possible alternatives to consider. The existence of various alternatives permits their comparison as managers perform the second task in planning for implementing organizational change.

Choosing from Among the Change Alternatives

The purpose of choosing from among the change alternatives is straightforward: to select the alternative that has the most desired, and the fewest undesired, consequences (see the section on "Developing and Applying Decision Criteria" in Chapter 7). Selecting among the alternatives is easy if one alternative is clearly superior. Most often, however, the choice is not easy. Change situations in HSOs/HSs tend to be gray rather than black or white. In addition, they tend to be dynamic. The most appropriate alternative may become less desirable as circumstances change. Complicating matters further is that, although there are several bases on which to choose an alternative (i.e., experience, intuition, advice from others, experimentation, scientific or analytical decision making), no basis is always best. Choosing from among available alternatives usually is challenging, and there is no way to ensure that managers will select the best, or even an adequate, alternative. However, if three factors regarding the choice of alternatives are compared, then the quality of the choices often can be improved.

First, the manager should assess how each alternative contributes to the attainment of organizational objectives. This implies that the alternatives in organizational change are a means to an end that has been clearly stated as an organizational performance or outcome objective. For example, a change is being undertaken to increase patient demand by 10%, or to decrease costs by 5%, or to increase the level of employee satisfaction. An alternative that does not support the achievement of stated performance or outcome objectives better than other alternatives should be scrutinized carefully. To be selected, such an alternative must have other positive features. Perhaps it will enhance subsequent performance by facilitating other changes.

Second, the manager should assess the relative degree of economic effectiveness of the alternatives. Which alternative makes the maximum use of available resources? There are times when economic considerations should not be used as a criterion for making these choices. This is especially the case in HSOs/HSs, where quality considerations are paramount and could suffer if only economic considerations are taken into account in choosing among alternatives. Usually, however, the economic consideration is a useful guideline in choosing among alternatives for change.

Finally, the manager should compare alternatives as to their inherent feasibility and the HSO's/HS's ability to implement them effectively. In making these comparisons, managers must think about how alternatives will be implemented in view of the resources available and the circumstances of the organizational change. Consideration of these three factors does not guarantee that the best alternative—or even a good one—will be chosen. It does, however, increase the chances that managers will make their selections wisely.

Devising a General Approach to Implementing Organizational Change

The third task in the implementation planning stage of managing organizational change is devising an overall approach to making the change. Managers must consider the range of general change approaches in their implementation planning, all of which fit into one of two broad categories. One set is based on the use of power, in which managers use coercion or sanctions to bring about change. Such approaches are also called force-coercion approaches and are top-down in nature.[21] Alternatively, the general approach to change can rely on reason and rational persuasion. In these approaches, managers make organizational changes by convincing those involved of the need for change and explaining the rationale.

In the power (force-coercion) approaches, managers determine and announce the changes that they wish to make; other participants in the HSO/HS are expected to accept them. Usually, there is a penalty for not accepting top-down directives to make organizational changes.

Changes in the strategic direction of HSOs/HSs often require top-down power approaches, as do quick responses to important environmental changes. For example, a change in the reimbursement policy of a major insurance carrier may require an immediate change that leaves little time for anything but a top-down edict. Top-down approaches offer the advantage of speed by "requiring only a few people to make timely, comprehensive decisions that can be communicated quickly to lower levels. A top-down change (approach) carries great weight and usually reaches deeply into the organization."[22]

Approaches that rely on reason and persuasion to implement organizational change come in many forms, although they share the common element of being participative. In these approaches, managers and staff participate in implementing organizational change, although the degree of participation can vary widely. In general, increasing the level of participation or involvement of employees in decisions about the design and management of HSOs/HSs—including decisions about organizational change—can reap substantial rewards, including "higher quality products and services, less absenteeism, less turnover, better decision making, and better problem solving—in short, greater organizational effectiveness."[23] Approaches that rely on participation are very different from top-down approaches. Participation suggests the opposite of top-down edicts from senior-level managers who direct what and how change will be made.

Lawler has identified three approaches to increasing employee participation or involvement in organizations: parallel suggestion involvement, job involvement, and what he terms high-involvement approaches.[24] These approaches vary in the degree to which the following four features are moved downward: 1) information about organizational performance, 2) rewards based on organizational performance, 3) knowledge that enables employees to understand and contribute to organizational performance, and 4) power to make decisions that influence organizational performance.[25]

When information, rewards, knowledge, and power are concentrated at the top of a HSO/HS, little opportunity exists elsewhere for meaningful involvement or participation in change. In contrast, when these factors are moved downward, opportunities to participate actively in managing change are greatly increased throughout the HSO/HS.

Parallel suggestion involvement encourages staff to make suggestions about changes that are needed as well as about how to implement and manage the changes. Participation is encouraged, although staff only recommend or suggest changes. Decisions are reserved for managers.

Job involvement enriches work so that people have more influence over it. In effect, staff are empowered to make changes in their own work, although not elsewhere in the HSO/HS. This approach does not give staff the power to change the structures or operations of the organizations or systems within which they work or to change their strategic directions. However, staff are permitted a much greater degree of involvement than in the parallel suggestion approach.

In high involvement, staff not only decide about changes in their work but also have meaningful input into changes in the HSO's/HS's purpose or objectives, culture, strategies, tasks, technologies, people, and structures. In some instances of high involvement in implementing change, staff working in quality improvement teams actually devise the means of implementing organizational change. Such high involvement, which is sometimes called a bottom-up approach, works best when senior-level managers encourage and facilitate its use. The primary advantage of a high-participation, bottom-up approach to organizational change is that it stimulates creativity in the HSO/HS.[26] It also fosters commitment to implementing changes for those who have roles in deciding how to make changes. HSOs/HSs frequently use high-involvement, bottom-up approaches to organizational changes that involve small parts of the organization or system, such as single departments, or when changes are modest and operational.

The circumstances of each change situation determine which approach to increased involvement is best.

> *Because they position power, information, knowledge, and rewards differently, these approaches tend to fit different situations and to produce different results. It is not that one is always better than another, but that they are different and, to some degree, competing.*[27]

Managers must exercise care when determining how much responsibility to delegate to implement organizational change. For example, parallel suggestion involvement is often appropriate in organizations with a traditional hierarchy, well-developed and entrenched management systems, and independent, relatively simple, and repetitive work. However, in new HSOs/HSs or in new units where there is complex and highly interdependent work and managers who value employee involvement, a high-involvement approach may be better.

Whether the approach to implementing change is based on power or persuasion, managers facing organizational change must determine how best to convince others that change is needed and that a suitable alternative has been chosen. Beyond this, as change agents managers must influence others to make the decisions and take the actions that are required to implement the change. In thinking about how to exert this influence, managers can use five different bases or sources.[28]

One base from which managers can exert influence in change situations is the formal power and authority derived from their organizational position in a HSO/HS, as was discussed in Chapter 3. This formal source of influence or authority exists because organizations assign certain powers to individuals so that they can do their jobs. All managers have a degree of formal power or authority that flows from their position. Of course, managers at different levels of HSOs/HSs possess different amounts of this kind of influence.

Another source of managers' ability to exert influence over organizational change is their ability to reward desirable behavior. This source stems partly from the positional source; in other words, because of their positions, managers are granted authority to use certain rewards to buttress their positional power and authority. Rewards include pay increases, promotions, work schedules, recognition of accomplishments, and status symbols such as office size and location. These rewards and many others are a source of influence for managers in change situations. Conversely, managers have the authority to punish or prevent others from obtaining rewards. This, too, is a source of influence as managers implement change.

Another important source of managers' ability to influence change is their knowledge or expertise, which is valued by the HSO/HS and which enhances their ability to influence the thinking of others. This source of influence is personal to the individual, in contrast to the positional sources of authority, which are granted to managers by virtue of position. A related source of influence is that some managers engender admiration, loyalty, and emulation that enable them to influence others. At the senior level of management, this quality is sometimes called charisma. Charismatic managers typically have a vision for their HSO/HS, possess strong convictions about the correctness of the vision, exude great self-confidence about their ability to realize the vision, and are perceived by others in their organizations or systems as legitimate agents of change in pursuit of the vision.[29]

After accomplishing the tasks of identifying alternatives in a change situation, choosing from them, and devising a general approach to implementing change, managers can turn to the final task in this stage of managing the change process. They must determine how to build support for the change and minimize resistance so as to maximize the likelihood of success.

Selecting Techniques to Support Implementation

Selecting techniques to support implementation, the fourth and final task in the implementation planning stage, involves selecting the techniques that will be used to develop support for or reduce resistance to the change.[30] Managers cannot ensure that an organizational change will be successfully implemented, although certain actions increase the likelihood of success. Perhaps the most important action is that those involved in or affected by a change understand the necessity for it. Managers should provide information as far in advance as possible—including details concerning reasons for the change, its nature and timing, and the expected impact on the HSO/HS and the people who work in it.

It may be useful for a change to be introduced on a trial basis. Familiarity gained through experience with a change, as well as assurances that it is not irrevocable, can reduce initial insecurity and increase the likelihood of acceptance. Allowing time for a change to be digested by those involved almost always will increase their acceptance of it.

Another useful action for managers when implementing organizational change is to minimize the disruption of customs and informal relationships. The culture developed in a HSO/HS has value because it helps people adjust to the workplace and to their roles in it. Change almost invariably disrupts the culture of a HSO/HS, but such disturbances can be reduced by facilitating widespread participation in planning and implementing the change. People feel less stress from the changes that they help plan because they understand them. They also are likely to be more committed to the success of a change if they are involved in planning and implementation.

In considering what support techniques they might use, managers must remember that people respond to change in predictable, often negative, ways. Managers who view change as the logical response to problems or opportunities may be surprised to learn that others have a different view. Sometimes other managers may not support changes that a manager thinks are important. Whereas a manager contemplating a change may view resistance as irrational, it may seem perfectly rational to affected people, especially if their past experiences with change were negative. Each change is judged by attitudes and feelings, which in turn determine how people respond to it. These attitudes and feelings are caused by numerous factors.

Roots of Resistance to Change

People may view change negatively and resist it because of their background and experience. They also may react negatively to change because of the work environment. For example, when a HSO/HS has been very stable for a long time, it may be especially difficult to introduce organizational change. When people become part of the status quo and believe it is permanent, even minor changes can be disruptive. Conversely, in HSOs/HSs where change is part of the culture, people expect change and accept it more readily.

Reasons for the often-encountered resistance to change include insecurity, possible social and economic losses, inconvenience, resentment of control, union opposition, and threats to the influence that people have in their HSOs/HSs.[31] Each of these bases for resistance to change is explored briefly here.

Insecurity is a major source of resistance to change. For many people, there is great comfort in the status quo; any change introduces uncertainty. Even a seemingly simple change such as moving the photocopying machine can have far-reaching repercussions. To some, such a move symbolizes management's lack of concern for inconvenienced employees. To others, it means more traffic, noise, and interference around their work area. A third group may see it as further evidence of managerial autocracy. Change, then, can reduce the level of satisfaction. People affected by change may not know what will actually happen, but past experience may have taught them to expect the worst. In addition, change suggests that performance may have been unsatisfactory.

Social losses of various kinds may result from change, and even the fear of such losses can cause people to resist change. Complex informal relationships may be affected by organizational change. Following a change, close friends may have to work in separate rooms or not be able to interact during work. Status symbols such as office size or location may be lost when a HSO/HS is reorganized. Social acceptance by co-workers may be jeopardized if some people cooperate in a change inaugurated by management and others reject it. In such circumstances people must choose between cooperating with management and retaining the friendship of co-workers. Thus what may seem a desirable and logical change can meet heavy resistance because the price in disrupted social relationships is too great.

In addition to social losses, economic losses can accompany organizational changes. In many cases new technology allows more work to be done by fewer staff. Resistance by those affected is understandable. Even if employees do not lose their jobs, a change may require them to work faster or contribute in other ways without additional compensation. Such economic losses frequently concern people who face workplace changes.

Inconvenience is part of many organizational changes, even when they do not involve significant economic or social losses. Any change usually causes some inconvenience, and extra effort is required to adjust to it. Old habits and ways of doing things often must be replaced with new practices. Inconvenience alone stimulates resistance. However, if inconvenience is the only factor, then resistance may be minor.

Resentment is a normal human reaction to close control of actions and behaviors. Management's control is never more apparent than during change. In such situations people are made keenly aware that they do not fully control their own destinies in the HSOs/HSs within which they work.

Unions are a source of resistance to some organizational change. HSOs/HSs with unions often encounter opposition to changes that managers want to make. Unions, after all, do not exist to cooperate with management; their role is to protect the interests of their members.

Threats to an individual's position and influence within a HSO/HS are another reason that some people fear and resist change. In fact, change that threatens the power base or influence of individuals, groups, departments, or even entire HSOs in HSs goes to the heart of their organizational existence and role and thus stimulates some of the strongest resistance to change. For example, physicians in HSOs/HSs routinely and vigorously resist changes that threaten their power and influence.

All of these factors can cause people to resist change in HSOs/HSs. Furthermore, they often occur in combination, thus strengthening the resolve of the people affected. An important aspect of effective implementation planning in this respect is for managers to consider how to address resistance effectively. Several of the most important options for dealing with resistance to change are outlined in Table 12.2 and discussed in the following section.

Techniques to Reduce Resistance

Education and communication are among the most common and useful ways for managers to overcome resistance to organizational change. These techniques involve communicating so that those affected are educated about the nature of the change and informed about its implications before it is implemented. Effective communication about a change and education regarding its implementation and implications can turn resistance into support.

Similarly, participation or involvement in planning for and implementing change can help overcome resistance, especially when the people who are most likely to resist it are involved. Such involvement reduces uncertainty and misunderstanding about a change and its implications. Participation in decisions about a change gives people a clearer picture of the change and enhances their commitment to its success.

Managers can help people accept change by facilitating and supporting their adaptation to it. This can be accomplished through training programs, granting requests for leave during a painful transition period, or even special counseling.

TABLE 12.2. TECHNIQUES FOR REDUCING RESISTANCE TO ORGANIZATIONAL CHANGE

Approach	Situational use	Advantages	Drawbacks
Education and communication	Where there is a lack of information or inaccurate information and analysis	Once persuaded, people often will help with the implementation of the change.	Can be very time-consuming if many people are involved
Participation and involvement	Where the initiators do not have all of the information they need to design the change, and where others have considerable power to resist	People who participate will be committed to implementing change, and any relevant information they have will be integrated into the change plan.	Can be very time-consuming if participants design an inappropriate change
Facilitation and support	Where people are resisting because of adjustment problems	No other approach works as well with adjustment problems.	Can be time-consuming, expensive, and still fail
Negotiation and agreement	Where someone or some group clearly will lose out in a change, and where that group has considerable power to resist	Sometimes it is a relatively easy way to avoid major resistance.	Can be too expensive in many cases if it alerts others to negotiate for compliance
Manipulation and co-optation	Where other tactics will not work or are too expensive	It can be a relatively quick and inexpensive solution to resistance problems.	Can lead to future problems if people feel manipulated
Explicit and implicit coercion	Where speed is essential, and the change initiators possess considerable power	It is speedy and can overcome any kind of resistance.	Can be risky if it leaves people feeling angry at the initiators

From Kotter, John P., and Leonard A. Schlesinger. "Choosing Strategies for Change." *Harvard Business Review* 57 (March/April 1979): 111; reprinted by permission. Copyright 1979 by the President and Fellows of Harvard College; all rights reserved.

Negotiating agreement among those affected by a change is a technique for reducing resistance to change. When using this technique, managers negotiate with opponents of the change and exchange something of value for reduced resistance. If resistance is centered in a few people or a department, then it may be possible to negotiate reduced resistance by allocating additional resources or promising to make another desired change later. Collective bargaining agreements often require that changes in how work is performed must be negotiated with the union. If agreement is reached, then the HSO/HS may implement a change but grant union members added compensation or other concessions.

Some managers use manipulation and co-optation techniques to reduce resistance to organizational change. These techniques raise serious ethical concerns if taken to an extreme. Devious manipulative techniques include withholding information about changes from people who might resist, releasing false or misleading information, and playing the interests of one person or group off others. Co-optation is a form of manipulation, but it is usually less devious than other forms. It may be as simple as bringing a person who is resisting change, or one who might resist it, into planning for the change so that this individual becomes a proponent. However, co-optation may also involve deceit, which clearly is unethical.

The bottom of the continuum of techniques for overcoming resistance to change as shown in Table 12.2 is the use of explicit or implicit coercion. Because of managers' positional power, such techniques are available to them as a way of getting people to accept changes. For example, people can be threatened with firing or reduced promotion opportunities in an effort to stop them from resisting change. Acceptance of significant change can be forced on people by the threat of even more drastic measures, up to and including closing or selling the HSO/HS. Coercion techniques, like manipulation techniques, can easily lead to unethical behavior. The potential for unethical behavior, added to the inevitable anger of people forced into accepting change, makes coercive techniques inappropriate in overcoming resistance to change.

The necessary support-building and resistance-reducing techniques that managers use to overcome resistance typically form a "package" of techniques aimed at different people. Selecting appropriate and effective support techniques, as well as selecting a suitable general or overall approach to implementing organizational change, bears directly on the success of implementing any change in a HSO/HS.

Stage 3: Implementing Organizational Change

The implementation stage of managing the process of organizational change as presented in Figure 12.1 involves the introduction of a new concept or idea, practice, or thing—or some combination of them—to a HSO/HS. Whether using a general approach to implementing change that is based on power or one that relies on persuasion, and no matter which supportive techniques they plan to employ, managers must accomplish three actions in sequence to implement any organizational change. They must first disrupt or "unfreeze" the status quo, then introduce the actual change, and finally stabilize or "refreeze" the modified organizational situation.[32] The three steps involved in the implementation stage of an organizational change are illustrated in Figure 12.4.

In the unfreezing step, managers prepare those who will participate in or be affected by the change by making them aware of the impending change and reducing or minimizing their resistance. Using a power approach may involve little more than announcing the change and directing those involved as to their roles in the change. When a persuasion approach is being taken, preparing people for change involves providing adequate information about the need for it and may also require soliciting their participation in its implementation. As noted in the discussion of Stage 2 in the process, people are far more likely to be receptive to change and to help implement it when they understand the advantages of a change and their part in it, especially when they are allowed to par-

Figure 12.4. Lewin's three steps to implementing organizational changes. (Adapted from Lewin, Kurt. "Group Decision and Social Change." In *Readings in Social Psychology,* 2nd ed., edited by Guy E. Swanson, Theodore M. Newcomb, and Eugene L. Hartley, 459–473. New York: Holt, Rinehart, 1952; reprinted by permission.)

ticipate in its planning and implementation. They also are more likely to fulfill their responsibilities in the change.

Once the status quo of an organizational situation is broken, whether through a simple, top-down announcement of an impending change or a much more elaborate participatory approach, the change actually can occur. This second step in implementation is the actual application or insertion of different concepts or ideas, practices, or things in the HSO/HS. As shown in Table 12.1, organizational changes can be directed to modify any aspect of a HSO/HS—including its purpose or objectives, culture, strategies, tasks, technologies, people, or structures. In this step some aspect of the organizational situation is changed. If the change involves the use of a thing that is different, such as a piece of equipment, then it is put in place and people begin using it. If the change involves the introduction of a different concept or practice, such as new reporting relationships, a revised marketing strategy, or a modified accounting system, then use of the concept or practice is initiated.

During the changing step, people affected by a change typically go through four distinct periods in the experience.[33] First, there is an awareness period in which they recognize that things are not—or will not be—the same. A disorientation period follows immediately after awareness that a change has been introduced. In this difficult period people begin to see a difference in the workplace and perhaps in their jobs. They may wonder whether anyone is in charge or what the priorities are of those in charge. They may be confused about what is expected of them. Disorientation can lead to people's losing confidence in the change or their enthusiasm for it, even though they supported the change initially. Opponents of change during this period typically believe that their worst fears about the change are coming true.

With most changes, the people affected begin to reestablish a sense of normalcy. This is the reorientation period in the implementation stage, and it is vital to successful changes. People may still feel some discomfort about a change but are less concerned and more confident. Their fear of the unknown is replaced with growing acquaintance with the new circumstances.

Finally, when changes are being implemented, the people involved typically experience an integration period. People accept the change as part of the new equilibrium in the workplace. This important period occurs in Lewin's third step of implementing an organizational change (see Figure 12.4). The change is incorporated into the routines of those responsible for and otherwise involved in its implementation. Ideally, a new equilibrium is established as people adapt to the change and accept it as the norm. The manager's efforts in this step are to restabilize the situation and establish conditions that will make the change permanent. The most important action that a manager can take to ensure the long-term stability of an organizational change is to overcome the resistance to the change before implementation. Postimplementation, a manager can offer appropriate rewards to those who have successfully implemented the change, positive reinforcement intended to maintain the change, and adequate resources to ensure its continuation. If a change is to be permanent, then it is also important for the responsible managers to maintain continuing oversight of the change and its results.

In effect, again using Lewin's[34] word for this step, the organizational situation is "refrozen" with the modification in place. Refreezing the HSO/HS after a change makes the change permanent, at least until a future circumstance leads to a decision that the change is inadequate or flawed and should be modified or abandoned. Such determinations are made through managers' systematic efforts to evaluate the organizational changes they have implemented, as is discussed in the following description of the fourth and final stage of managing organizational change.

Stage 4: Evaluating Organizational Change

Evaluation, the final stage in the process of managing organizational change, often is given inadequate attention by managers and may be overlooked altogether. However, evaluating changes is a vitally important stage in any manager's efforts to manage organizational change effectively. In fact, managers should evaluate all of their decisions and actions, including those that are related to organizational change, because they have a responsibility to use optimally the resources that are entrusted to them. All organizational change involves expending organizational resources such as money and time, which have alternative uses. Systematic evaluation permits managers to determine whether the resources that are used in implementing change have yielded the intended benefits.

Evaluating change involves collecting data and information that are sufficient to determine whether a change has been implemented effectively, whether the objectives established for the change were achieved, and what other related changes or modifications may be needed. Information that a change led to the desired or undesired outcomes provides important input to the overall process of managing organizational change.

When the evaluation stage shows that the results of a change are as desired, managers can turn to other matters. When it does not, the change must be modified. As shown in Figure 12.1, the feedback loop goes all the way back to Stage 1. When changes do not accomplish their purposes, the process begins again, although this time the manager has more information, new insights into what may or may not work, and more experience with the challenge of managing change.

HUMAN RESOURCES CHANGES

Pervasive in HSOs/HSs is changing the attitudes, values, skills, and behaviors of people. Human resources changes frequently result from a manager's observation or perception that the organizational climate does not facilitate optimum performance. An additional impetus for human resources changes, however, arises when managers think that other changes being implemented should be supported by human resources changes.[35] Examples of changes that may benefit from simultaneous human resources changes include downsizing, mergers, or the introduction of new services.

TABLE 12.3. FREQUENTLY USED TECHNIQUES IN HUMAN RESOURCES CHANGES

Technique	Examples
Organizational diagnoses	Interviews, surveys, group meetings
Team building	Improvement of existing groups; creation of teams for problem solving and quality improvement
Survey feedback	Provision of survey results to members; interpretation of results by members
Education	Classroom training for "sensitivity" skills and interpersonal skills
Intergroup activities	Communication development; conflict reduction
Third-party peacemaking	Negotiation, mediation by "outsider" for interpersonal and intergroup conflict
Technostructural/ sociotechnical activities	Joint examination of technology, structure, and people systems
Process consultation	Observation of groups in action with immediate feedback on processes observed
Life/career planning	Future oriented—development of personal goals and acquisition of skills to help individuals fit into the HSO/HS and the HSO/HS match individual needs
Coaching	Nonevaluative feedback to individuals describing how others see them
Planning and goal setting	Training of individuals to improve personal planning and goal-setting

Adapted from French, Wendell L., and Cecil H. Bell, Jr. *Organization Development*, 6th ed., pp. 151–152. Upper Saddle River, NJ: Prentice-Hall, 1998.

Table 12.3 contains a list of standard techniques to facilitate human resources changes. Surveys to gather information about the social and psychological conditions in the HSO/HS are even more useful when the information gathered is made available to those surveyed. Information from surveys stimulates consideration of potential problems and their causes and may provide clues to solutions.[36]

Another especially important category of human resources change techniques is team building or team development efforts, which "remove barriers to group effectiveness, develop self-sufficiency in managing group process, and facilitate the change process."[37] These techniques help in the changing and refreezing steps and often feature the use of outside consultants to help the group in its development.

A widely used team-building or development technique in HSOs/HSs is the quality improvement team, which undertakes CQI activities (CQI is discussed in Chapter 9). For example, the University of Illinois at Chicago Medical Center (UICMC) has adopted CQI as "the central operating strategy used at UICMC to achieve our mission," and uses CQI tools and techniques in its efforts to improve "both operational and clinical processes that impact delivery of every service offered."[38] A central element in its approach is a diverse and comprehensive set of quality improvement teams, as described in the following[39]:

> A **quality lead team** is in place composed of clinical and administrative leaders. This team is accountable to the CEO/medical staff executive committee. Reporting to the quality lead team are three **functional lead teams—clinical practice, clinical operations, and administrative operations.** Each lead team has a 1-year plan that details their purpose, strategies, and an integration plan for coordinating their efforts with other initiatives, such as clinical resource management and customer service. These three teams guide the formation of **individual quality improvement teams** that will address key organizational priorities. Priorities are identified both from the top down (surveys and focus group research regarding satisfaction) and the bottom up (from staff on teams that are closest to the processes).

The director of continuous quality improvement oversees the development of this program at all levels. This includes providing training to all UICMC employees, facilitator support for teams, tracking, and communicating results. In addition, individual departments have established quality performance indicators that they monitor regularly, which in turn may support or identify the need for a cross-functional CQI initiative.

CONSTANCY OF THE CHANGE AGENT'S RESPONSIBILITY IN MANAGEMENT WORK IN HSOs/HSs

Organizational change in HSOs/HSs does not occur absent certain conditions. Key are the people who are catalysts for change and who can manage the organizational change process. Such people are called change agents. Anyone can be a change agent, although this role usually is played by managers. Scientists and clinicians also can be change agents in HSOs/HSs, especially regarding technology. On occasion, change agents are outside consultants who specialize in change. Managers who are effective change agents are more likely to successfully perform management work in the dynamic context of HSOs/HSs.

Health care professionals in the United States, including managers of HSOs/HSs, have achieved some marvelous successes. Among them are world-class diagnostic and therapeutic capabilities, biomedical research that has begun to understand disease at the molecular level and to intervene in diseases at the genetic level, the widespread availability of the latest technology and most sophisticated clinical facilities, and the widespread provision of excellent health care services and insurance coverage. Coexisting with a justifiable sense of pride and accomplishment about these achievements is a growing awareness that the nation faces fundamental problems regarding health care. The most serious is the cost of health care, which threatens the capacity of the nation to keep pace and which exacerbates the health problems of those who lack adequate financial resources to gain access to the health care system. In addition to and contributing to the central cost problem, the health care system simultaneously creates excesses and shortages of various capabilities and facilities. Primary care and preventive services are underused by many, whereas high-technology services are overused.[40] Some Americans lack access to basic health care services, whereas others are overtreated. One of the consequences of these problems is an inexorable pressure for change. This pressure falls directly on HSOs/HSs and on their managers, requiring that they be effective change agents.

Indeed, if the problems of cost and access are to be addressed successfully, then managers as change agents will be key to the solution. Beyond their desire to solve access and cost problems, many managers envision an improved health care system. Such visions create their own positive pressure for change. Thus knowledge of how best to manage the complex process of change—how to be effective change agents—is vital for the managers of HSOs/HSs now and will be even more so in the future. In acting as change agents, managers should remember that

- Something always precipitates organizational change—an event, trend, development, signal of dissatisfaction with the status quo from internal or external stakeholders, or the preferences of a change agent position the HSO/HS for change; without a stimulus, there is no change.
- The HSO/HS must be ready to change, or the change agent must convince others that old, comfortable ways should be replaced by different, perhaps unfamiliar concepts or ideas, practices, or things.
- The change agent must recognize that any organizational change involves changing individuals; they must not only learn something new but also must unlearn something that may be well integrated into their personalities and social relationships.
- Individuals will not change without *motivation;* inducing that motivation is often the most difficult part of change in HSOs/HSs and the greatest challenge for the change agent.
- The change agent, perhaps in concert with others, must select the approach or combination of approaches that are necessary to convince others of the need for change (for example, by plant-

ing seeds for change through a governing body—management—professional staff organization educational process and/or by using task forces or quality improvement teams).

- The change agent must create a body of shared values and attitudes, a new consensus in which key individuals within a HSO/HS reinforce one another in selling the new way and in defending it against inertia, reluctance, or outright opposition.[41]

Being a change agent in HSOs/HSs is never easy. It is most difficult when it involves major or complex changes. As Figure 12.5 shows, the successful management of a complex change requires that the change agent have a purpose for the change, the skills that are necessary to make the change, incentives and resources to make the change possible, and a plan for making the change. If any of the necessary ingredients are missing, then the change will not succeed. Two examples of complex changes in HSOs/HSs can be seen in retrenchment or significant downsizing or in combining HSOs into HSs. These special cases are treated separately.

Special Case of Being a Change Agent in Retrenchment

Retrenchment means reducing a HSO's/HS's size or scope of activities. An entire HSO/HS may be downsized, although more frequently only a part is involved. There are several approaches to retrenchment: internal consolidation, wherein parts of the HSO/HS are melded into a simpler organizational design; divestiture, wherein parts of the HSO/HS or its subsidiary organizations or both are sold; and liquidation, wherein business ceases through bankruptcy or sale.

Downsizing in HSOs/HSs often involves activities in one or more of the following broad classifications[42]:

- *Staff reductions* through layoffs, attrition, or transfers. Downsizing-related staff reductions differ from other staff reductions in three important ways. First, downsizing-related staff reductions usually affect all levels of the HSO/HS, whereas non–downsizing-related layoffs often are confined to a particular department or service. Second, downsizing-related staff reductions usually are accompanied by organizational restructuring (combining of departments or units) and a reduction in capacity (fewer beds); non–downsizing-related layoffs often are implemented unilaterally, without corresponding changes in organizational structure. Third, downsizing-related staff reductions tend to be permanent, whereas traditional layoffs tend to be temporary, in response to a "short-term downturn" in patient volume.
- *Organizational restructuring,* which usually consists of departmental consolidation or elimination. It should be noted that organizational changes such as department consolidations often occur on an interim basis. These short-term actions should not be confused with downsizing-related organizational changes, which usually are permanent.
- *Plant capacity reduction* through reduction of beds or operating rooms, closing a wing or floor, or sale of excess equipment and supplies
- *Conversion of use of the facilities,* such as changing a hospital inpatient operating room to outpatient use or changing acute care beds into a skilled nursing unit or a palliative care unit

A number of problems are associated with downsizing: 1) loss of credibility for senior-level managers; 2) increased infighting and politicking for position in the retrenched HSO/HS, which increases conflict among first- and middle-level managers; and 3) decaying motivation and increased voluntary turnover in affected parts of the HSO/HS.

Effective management of these problems is an added burden of managing organizational change caused by retrenchment. There are no easy answers, but managers can take two actions that are especially useful in minimizing these problems in HSOs/HSs. First, they can address the ambi-

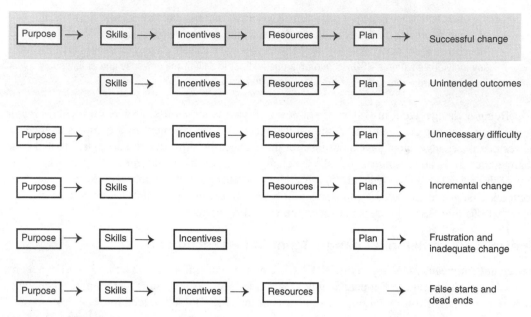

Figure 12.5. Managing complex change.

guity that organizational retrenchment invariably creates among stakeholders. This is best done by clarifying or restating the HSO's/HS's purpose and organizational objectives: Where is it going? What is its future and potential? By addressing these questions, management demonstrates that it understands the problem and has a vision of what the new, smaller organization will look like. Stakeholders in a retrenching HSO/HS want to believe that management is not content to conduct a going-out-of-business sale or a fire sale.

Second, organizational retrenchment demands that management communicate openly and frequently with stakeholders (see Chapter 17). The primary focus should be to explain the rationale for needed changes, but there also should be two-way communication so that stakeholders can vent their fears and frustrations and have important questions answered. In cases of retrenchment, managers' credibility is likely to be diminished, and rumors will be rampant. This puts a premium on making every effort to explain the reasons for, and implications of, all significant changes.[43]

Special Case of Being a Change Agent in Health Systems (HSs)

As noted earlier, being a change agent is most difficult in situations involving major organizational change. Just as downsizing or retrenchment makes the change agent role difficult, building HSs requires managers to be change agents in challenging circumstances. The challenges for the change agents in HSs are shaped by unique aspects of managerial work in these complex settings.

The work of managers in HSs—whether at the level of the HS or in its component HSOs— differs from that of managers in independent organizations in several fundamental ways.[44] In highly integrated HSs managers are involved in managing a spectrum of services spanning the life cycles of the people in the populations that they serve rather than simply meeting the episodic needs of individuals for specific services. The fact that HSs provide coordinated continua of health care services (see Chapter 4) significantly alters the work of managers. In independent HSOs, managers focus on the organization's particular service domain, whether acute care, ambulatory services, long-term care, rehabilitation services, palliative care, hospice care, or some other type of health care service. In HSs, however, managers must be knowledgeable in many or all of these domains. Linking primary care, ambulatory care, acute care, home care, rehabilitation, long-term care, palliative care, and hospice care into coordinated continua, especially when these are then integrated with financing arrangements, greatly expands the work of managers and requires them to make numerous and complex changes.

Another difference in management work in HSs is that managers, especially at senior levels, are accountable for the health status of the populations they serve. Managers in independent HSOs typically are accountable for the outcomes that are achieved in the provision of their organizations' specific services, but not for the overall health status of those whom they serve. This accountability changes in HSs, however, where a range of different types of services are linked and provided to populations. When managers bear responsibility for the health status of defined populations, they must move past the traditional focus on care and cure to broader, more positive perspectives on health, including prevention and health promotion. Furthermore, if they are to be accountable for health status, then managers must be able to measure and document changes in health status. These new responsibilities and capabilities impose substantial demands for change.

When HSs assume fiscal accountability, as they do increasingly under capitated arrangements, the work of their managers is changed. Payment on the basis of a prospectively determined rate, or capitation payment for a comprehensive package of services provided to defined populations, generates complex new work requirements and necessitates many changes. For example, to respond to the risks that are imposed by capitation, managers must know how to evaluate physicians' practice patterns for efficiency and how to prevent or minimize malpractice litigation across a much broader range of clinical activities.

Finally, the fact that HSs are, by definition, composed of multiple HSOs changes much about the work of managers within them. Whether the links are based on ownership, contracts, or alliances, the resulting networks of organizations exhibit significant organizational complexity. Quite aside from the implications of working in a context in which a coordinated continuum of diverse services is provided, the structural complexity that is imposed by working in a context made up of multiple HSOs of different types linked in a variety of ways expands the work of managers. They must be adept at forging a variety of organizational relationships and links. Frequently, these relationships and links are not based on the traditional models of ownership but on trust, commitment to shared objectives and purposes, and mutual recognition of interdependence. All of these aspects of organization design and organization building represent expanded demands for effective management of change.

The change agent role in HSs is widely agreed to be a key factor in the success of these systems.[45] As with all organizational change, the ability of managers in HSs to manage change involves a composite of skills, including[46]

- Creatively disrupting those participants in the HS who cling to the status quo
- Communicating a vision for the HS in terms that can be understood and realized by all
- Developing comprehensive and focused implementation plans for changes
- Providing ongoing support during the process of change and in follow-up to changes

SUMMARY

Significant external and internal pressures drive organizational change in HSOs/HSs. When change is needed, managers have several options. Inputs can be changed, as can the organizational structure, relationships among people, and conditions of work. In short, managers can change the processes that convert inputs into outputs. Outputs, too, can be changed. Finally, the HSO/HS can try to change its external environment.

In this chapter organizational change is defined as a discernible modification in any aspect of an organization's purpose or objectives, culture, strategies, tasks, technologies, people, or structures. It is noted that most organizational change occurs by adopting borrowed or modified concepts or ideas, practices, or things. However, change also can involve creativity, which is presented as a special kind of change in a HSO/HS when someone invents or develops a new concept or idea, practice, or thing.

The complex process of managing organizational change is presented in this chapter as a four-stage model (see Figure 12.1) including identification, planning, implementation, and evaluation/feedback stages. Each stage incorporates several tasks that must be successfully accomplished if organizational change is to be well managed. The first task is for managers to recognize situations and circumstances that require an organizational change. Then they must identify the nature of the change needed in a particular situation. These two tasks are related and can be triggered by various pressures for change.

Identifying the need for and nature of the change needed in a particular situation is followed by other tasks that ensure effective planning for implementation. The tasks involved in implementation planning are developing alternative changes to be considered, choosing the alternative to be implemented, shaping a general approach to making the change, and developing the techniques to build support for the change and minimize resistance to it.

Actual implementation of an organizational change is accomplished through three additional tasks: unfreezing the status quo, introducing the change, and refreezing the organizational situation with the change in place. Unfreezing occurs when managers disrupt the status quo and prepare those involved for change. Unfreezing is followed by making the change. Some concept or idea, practice, or thing, or a combination of them, is inserted into a situation to modify the organization's purpose or objectives, culture, strategies, tasks, technologies, people, or structure. The change is followed by refreezing the organizational situation to give the change stability and durability.

The management of organizational change does not end with implementation, however. Managers who have the most success evaluate the results of change and use the information obtained to provide feedback to future iterations of the change process. The task essentially is comparing actual results with those planned, exploring the reasons for differences, and using this information to inform and guide future changes.

The model of the process of managing organizational change emphasizes that the stages in the process—and the steps within each stage—are sequential. If any are done poorly, then managers are not adequately playing their important role as change agents and the entire process is jeopardized.

DISCUSSION QUESTIONS

1. Discuss the pressures for change confronting managers in HSOs/HSs.
2. Discuss the possible foci for organizational change in HSOs/HSs and give an example of each.
3. What are the three sources of change that are available to managers? Discuss the differences among them.
4. Discuss creativity in the change process.
5. Briefly describe the four stages in the process of managing organizational change, including the steps in each stage.
6. Discuss the similarities between the process of managing an organizational change and the process by which managers solve problems.
7. Discuss the role of information in the change identification stage of managing organizational change.

8. Describe and compare the two broad categories of approaches to organizational change that are presented in this chapter.
9. What are the three steps in the implementation stage of managing an organizational change?
10. Why is resistance so often the human response to change? What can managers do to overcome resistance?
11. Discuss the manager's role as change agent.

CASE STUDY 1: LABOR, DELIVERY, RECOVERY, POSTPARTUM (LDRP) STAFFING SITUATION

Traditionally, Community Hospital has staffed LDRP with obstetricians, registered nurses (RNs), and nursing assistants. Recently, senior management learned that, in addition to routine cleanup tasks, nursing assistants were being assigned a number of nonpatient duties by RNs. Because delegating nonpatient duties did not reduce or hinder patient care in the LDRP and it appeared to be acceptable to the obstetricians, management permitted the pattern to continue and remain under the control of those in the LDRP.

However, as pressures for cost containment mounted, efficiency became the watchword at Community Hospital, and staffing patterns in the LDRP were reviewed by the unit manager. The manager's study revealed that significant savings could be realized by eliminating the nursing assistants. The manager decided that some of the nonpatient duties being performed by the nursing assistants could be reassigned to the RNs and some others to clerks in the LDRP and that housekeeping could assign staff to the LDRP for cleanup tasks. The projected savings resulted primarily from the fact that both clerks and housekeeping personnel were paid about 20% less per hour in wages and benefits than were the nursing assistants.

The new staffing pattern was implemented in January by directive from the CEO, but by June it was clear that there were problems. Nurses were complaining to the unit manager about the lack of support staff (nursing assistants), which they believed caused them to be overworked. In turn, this turmoil upset the obstetricians who used the rooms for their patients. They, too, complained about the situation. In July a majority of obstetricians informed the CEO in writing of their displeasure. By October, no action had been taken.

QUESTIONS

1. Identify and discuss the problem(s).
2. How could it/they have been prevented?
3. What should be management's plan at this point? How should it be implemented?

CASE STUDY 2: A RESPONSE TO CHANGE

As business office manager of Group HMO, Inc., Dana Smith was responsible for the work of approximately 45 employees, of whom 26 were classified as secretarial or clerical. At the direction of the plan president, a team of outside systems analysis consultants was contracted to make a time study and work-method analysis of Smith's area to improve the efficiency and output of the business office.

The consultants began by observing and recording each detail of the work of the secretarial and clerical staff. After 2 days of preliminary observation, they indicated that they were prepared to begin their time study on the following day.

The next morning five of the business office employees participating in the study were absent. On the following day 10 employees were absent. Concerned, Smith sought to find reasons for the absenteeism by calling her absent employees. Each related basically the same story. Each was nervous, tense, and physically tired after being a "guinea pig" during the 2 days of preliminary observation. One told Smith that his physician had advised him to ask for a leave of absence if working conditions were not improved.

Shortly after the telephone calls, the head of the study team told Smith that, if there were as many absences on the next day, then his team would have to delay the study. He stated that a scientific analysis would be impossible with 10 employees absent. Realizing that she would be held responsible for the failure of the study, Smith was very concerned.

QUESTIONS

1. What caused the reactions to the study?
2. Could these reactions have been predicted? How?
3. What steps should Smith take to get the study back on track?

CASE STUDY 3: HOW READY ARE YOU FOR MANAGING IN A TURBULENT WORLD?[47]

Instructions: Listed below are some statements a 37-year-old manager made about his job at a large, successful HSO. After each statement are five letters, A–E. Circle the letter that best describes how you think you would react to these characteristics according to the following scale:

A *I would enjoy this very much; it's completely acceptable.*

B *This would be enjoyable and acceptable most of the time.*

C *I'd have no reaction to this feature one way or another, or it would be about equally enjoyable and unpleasant.*

D *This feature would be somewhat unpleasant for me.*

E *This feature would be very unpleasant for me.*

1. I regularly spend 30%–40% of my time in meetings. A B C D E
2. A year and a half ago, my job did not exist, and I have been essentially inventing it as I go along. A B C D E
3. The responsibilities I either assume or am assigned consistently exceed the authority I have for discharging them. A B C D E
4. At any given moment in my job, I have an average of a dozen telephone calls to return. A B C D E
5. There seems to be very little relationship in my job between the quality of my performance and my actual pay and fringe benefits. A B C D E
6. About 2 weeks a year of formal management training is needed in my job just to stay current. A B C D E
7. Because we have very effective equal employment opportunity (EEO) regulations in my HSO and because it is located in a major urban area, my job consistently brings me into close contact at a professional level with staff of many races, ethnic groups, nationalities, and both sexes. A B C D E
8. There is no objective way to measure my effectiveness. A B C D E
9. I report to three different bosses for different aspects of my job, and each has an equal say in my performance appraisal. A B C D E
10. On average, about one third of my time is spent dealing with unexpected emergencies that force all scheduled work to be postponed. A B C D E

11. When I schedule a meeting of the staff who report to me, it takes my secretary most of a day to find a time when all are available, and, even then, I have yet to have a meeting in which everyone was present the entire time. A   B   C   D   E

12. The college degree I earned in preparation for this type of work is obsolete, and I probably should go back for another degree. A   B   C   D   E

13. My job requires that I absorb 100–200 pages per week of technical materials.
    A   B   C   D   E

14. I am out of town overnight at least 1 night per week. A   B   C   D   E

15. My department is so interdependent with several other departments in the HSO that all distinctions about which departments are responsible for which tasks are quite arbitrary.
    A   B   C   D   E

16. I probably will get a promotion in a year to a job in another division that has most of these same characteristics. A   B   C   D   E

17. During the period of my employment here, either the entire HSO or the division that I worked in has been reorganized every year or so. A   B   C   D   E

18. I am offered several possible promotions, but in my estimation neither I have no real career path. A   B   C   D   E

19. I can foresee several possible promotions, but I think I have no realistic chance of getting to the top levels of the HSO. A   B   C   D   E

20. I have many ideas about how to make things work better, but I have no direct influence on either the business policies or the personnel policies that govern my division.
    A   B   C   D   E

21. My HSO recently created an "assessment center"; all of the other managers and I will be required to take an extensive battery of psychological tests to assess our potential.
    A   B   C   D   E

22. My HSO is a defendant in an antitrust suit, and if the case goes to trial, I probably will have to testify about some decisions that were made a few years ago.
    A   B   C   D   E

23. Advanced computer and other electronic office technology is continually being introduced to my division, necessitating constant learning on my part. A   B   C   D   E

24. The computer terminal and screen in my office can be monitored in my bosses' offices without my knowledge. A   B   C   D   E

Scoring: Score four points for each A, three for each B, two for each C, one for each D, and zero for each E. Compute the total, divide by 24, and round to one decimal place.

Although the results are not intended to be more than suggestive, the higher your score, the more comfortable you seem to be with change. The test's author suggests analyzing scores as if they were grade point averages. In this way, a 4.0 average is an A, a 2.0 is a C, and scores below 1.0 flunk.

Using replies from nearly 500 MBA students and young managers, the range of scores was found to be narrow—between 1.0 and 2.2. The average score was between 1.5 and 1.6, which is equivalent to a D+/C−.

CASE STUDY 4: A HUMAN RESOURCES CHANGE AT SUN COAST HEALTH SYSTEM

A large vertically integrated HS, with HSOs located in several western states, undertook a human resources change in response to problems stemming from dissatisfaction with their work among the system's 250 medical technologists. The HS's senior management initiated the program when the vice president for human resources reported the results of an employee satisfaction study of the system's central laboratory and the satellite laboratories located in a number of HSOs in the Sun Coast Health System. The study had been conducted with focus groups of medical technologists and through an extensive written survey that had been administered to the technologists and to which they responded anonymously. Results from the focus groups and the written survey indicated widespread job dissatisfaction among medical technologists who worked in the HS's laboratories.

The data gathered in the study revealed several sources of the dissatisfaction. Some of it arose from a small fraction of the surveyed staff who felt that their skills were underused. Others expressed dissatisfaction with communications within the laboratories, although this problem varied widely from one laboratory to another in the system. The problem did not appear to be significant in the central system laboratory where about 100 of the technologists worked. However, in the central laboratory there was significant concern expressed about how unevenly the workloads were distributed. The survey of medical technologists at Sun Coast also revealed that more than half (52%) did not think that the pathologists with whom they worked gave them the level of respect their professional status deserved. By far the most consistent concern that was expressed in the focus groups and by the surveyed technologists was over the pressure they felt from the constant requirements that they adjust to the introduction of new and very complex technology in the laboratories as the HS sought to remain at the forefront of medical technology.

Sun Coast's human resources department discussed the implications of the data gathered in the employee satisfaction study with the vice president for professional affairs, with the manager of the laboratory division, and with the heads of each of the system's laboratories. All agreed that an effort should be undertaken to help the medical technologists become more comfortable adapting to the changing technology that they faced. They all agreed that this could improve the effectiveness of the HS's laboratories and enhance the technologists' work satisfaction. Their challenge was to develop a human resources change program that could increase the technologists' capability to adjust to the constant pressure that they faced from new technology.

QUESTIONS

1. Assume that you are the project manager with responsibility for managing this change. Outline the steps that you would take in carrying out the change.
2. What specific human resources change techniques (see Table 12.3) would you employ? Explain your choice.

CASE STUDY 5: "YOU DIDN'T TELL ME!"

Metropolitan Hospital has 500 beds with 1,500 full-time employees and a professional staff organization of 400. As part of a comprehensive analysis of communication at Metropolitan, a consulting firm called Management Strategies, Inc., surveyed all of the employees. The results of one question troubled the CEO. The question was: "Does your immediate superior tell you about changes well in advance of their implementation so that you are prepared for them?"

The responses (in percentages) were as follows:

	Always	Often	Sometimes	Seldom	Never
Senior-level managers	90	8	2		
Middle-level managers (department heads)	78	12	10		
First-level managers	65	25	10		
Nonmanagers	40	20	18	12	10

QUESTIONS

1. What do these results show? Why?
2. What reasons could explain these results?
3. What steps should the CEO take based on these results?

NOTES

1. Kaluzny, Arnold D. "Patients, Populations, and Caregivers: Opportunities and Challenges at the Intersection." *Frontiers of Health Services Management* 15 (Fall 1998): 46.

2. Aon Consulting. *America@Work.* Chicago: Aon Consulting Worldwide, Inc., 1998.

3. Van de Ven, Andrew H., and Marshall S. Poole. "Explaining Development and Change in Organizations." *Academy of Management Review* 20 (July 1995): 512.

4. Schermerhorn, John R., Jr., James G. Hunt, and Richard N. Osborn. *Organizational Behavior,* 6th ed. New York: John Wiley & Sons, 1998.

5. Ginter, Peter M., Linda M. Swayne, and W. Jack Duncan. *Strategic Management of Health Care Organizations,* 3rd ed., chap. 1. Malden, MA: Blackwell, 1998.

6. Longest, Beaufort B., Jr. *Seeking Strategic Advantage Through Health Policy Analysis.* Chicago: Health Administration Press, 1997; Longest, Beaufort B., Jr. *Health Policymaking in the United States,* 2nd ed. Chicago: Health Administration Press, 1998.

7. Shortell, Stephen M., Ellen M. Morrison, and Bernard Friedman. *Strategic Choices for America's Hospitals: Managing Change in Turbulent Times,* 34. San Francisco: Jossey-Bass, 1990.

8. Hernandez, S. Robert, and Arnold D. Kaluzny. "Organizational Change and Innovation." In *Health Care Management: Organization Design and Behavior,* 3rd ed., edited by Stephen M. Shortell and Arnold D. Kaluzny, 296. Albany, NY: Delmar Publishers, 1994.

9. Couger, Daniel J. *Creative Problem Solving and Opportunity Finding,* 18. Danvers, MA: Boyd & Fraser, 1995.

10. Pelz, David C., and Fred C. Munson. "A Framework for Organizational Innovating." Paper presented at the Academy of Management Annual Meeting, 1980.

11. Zuckerman, Howard S., Arnold D. Kaluzny, and Thomas C. Ricketts, III. "Strategic Alliances: A Worldwide Phenomenon Comes to Health Care." In *Partners for the Dance: Forming Strategic Alliances in Health Care,* edited by Arnold D. Kaluzny, Howard S. Zuckerman, and Thomas C. Ricketts, III, 1–18. Chicago: Health Administration Press, 1995.

12. Berwick, Donald M. "Blazing the Trail of Quality: The HFHS Quality Management Process." *Frontiers of Health Services Management* 7 (Summer 1991): 47–50; Berwick, Donald M., A. Blanton Godfrey, and Jane Roessner, Eds. *Curing Health Care: New Strategies for Quality Improvement.* San Francisco: Jossey-Bass, 1990; Rakich, Jonathon S., Kurt Darr, and Beaufort B. Longest, Jr. "An Integrated Model for Continuous Quality Improvement and Productivity Improvement in Health Services Organizations." *Clinical Laboratory Management Review* 7 (1993): 292–303.

13. Robbins, Stephen P., and Mary K. Coulter. *Management,* 6th ed., 539. Upper Saddle River, NJ: Prentice-Hall, 1998.

14. This section is adapted from Longest, Beaufort B., Jr. "Organizational Change and Innovation." In *Handbook of Health Care Management,* edited by W. Jack Duncan, Peter M. Ginter, and Linda E. Swayne, 369–398. Malden, MA: Blackwell, 1998.

15. Dunham, Randall B., and Jon L. Pierce. *Management.* Reading, MA: Addison-Wesley, 1989.

16. Lewin, Kurt. "Group Decision and Social Change." In *Readings in Social Psychology,* 2nd ed., edited by Guy E. Swanson, Theodore M. Newcomb, and Eugene L. Hartley, 459–473. New York: Holt, Rinehart, 1952.

17. Berwick, Donald M., A. Blanton Godfrey, and Jane Roessner. *Curing Health Care: New Strategies for Quality Improvement,* 94–97. San Francisco: Jossey-Bass, 1990.

18. Schermerhorn, John R., Jr. *Management for Productivity,* 4th ed. 664–672. New York: John Wiley & Sons, 1993.

19. Schermerhorn, *Management for Productivity,* 663.
20. Kanter, Rosabeth M. *The Change Masters: Innovation for Productivity in the American Corporation,* 101. New York: Simon & Schuster, 1985.
21. Chinn, Robert, and Kenneth D. Benne. "General Strategies for Effecting Changes in Human Systems." In *The Planning of Change,* 4th ed., edited by Warren G. Bennis, Kenneth D. Benne, and Robert Chinn, 22–45. New York: Harcourt Brace, 1985.
22. Holt, David H. *Management: Principles and Practices,* 2nd ed., 618. Englewood Cliffs, NJ: Prentice-Hall, 1990.
23. Lawler, Edward E., III. "Choosing an Involvement Strategy." *The Executive* 2 (August 1988): 197.
24. Lawler, "Choosing an Involvement Strategy," 197.
25. Lawler, "Choosing an Involvement Strategy," 197.
26. Lawler, Edward E., III, and Susan A. Mohrman. "Quality Circles After the Fad." *Harvard Business Review* 63 (January-February 1985): 65–71.
27. Lawler, "Choosing an Involvement Strategy," 197.
28. French, John R.P., and Bertram H. Raven. "The Basis for Social Power." In *Studies of Social Power,* edited by Dorwin Cartwright, 150–167. Ann Arbor, MI: Institute for Social Research, 1959.
29. Conger, Jay A., and Rabindra N. Kanungo. *Charismatic Leadership in Organizations.* Thousand Oaks, CA: Sage Publications, 1998.
30. Dunham and Pierce, *Management.*
31. Mondy, R. Wayne, Robert M. Noe, and Shane R. Premeaux. *Human Resource Management,* 7th ed., 637–640. Upper Saddle River, NJ: Prentice-Hall, 1998.
32. Lewin, "Group Decision and Social Change."
33. Adapted from Aon Consulting. "Managing the Stages of Change." *Forum* (October 1998): 6–7.
34. Lewin, "Group Decision and Social Change."
35. Hernandez and Kaluzny, "Organizational Innovation," 375–378.
36. Schneider, Benjamin. *Organizational Climate and Culture.* San Francisco: Jossey-Bass, 1990.
37. Hernandez and Kaluzny, "Organizational Innovation," 375.
38. University of Illinois at Chicago Medical Center. *http://www.uic.edu/hsc/,* January 1999.
39. Adapted from the website of the University of Illinois at Chicago Medical Center. *http://www.uic.edu/hsc/,* January 1999.
40. Bodenheimer, Thomas S., and Kevin Grumbach. *Understanding Health Policy: A Clinical Approach,* chap. 1. Stamford, CT: Appleton & Lange, 1995.; Wallace, Robert B. "Public Health and Preventive Medicine: Trends and Guideposts." In *Public Health & Preventive Medicine,* 14th ed., edited by Robert B. Wallace and Bradley N. Doebbeling, chap. 1. Stamford, CT: Appleton & Lange, 1998.
41. Peters, Joseph P., and Simone Tseng. "Managing Strategic Change." *Hospitals* 57 (June 1, 1983): 65; Schein, Edgar H. *Organizational Culture and Leadership.* San Francisco: Jossey-Bass, 1996.
42. Adapted from Coddington, Dean C., and Keith D. Moore. *Market-Driven Strategies in Health Care,* 204. San Francisco: Jossey-Bass, 1987.
43. Robbins and Coulter, *Management.*
44. This discussion of the work of managers in HSs is adapted from Longest, Beaufort B., Jr. "Managerial Competence at Senior Levels of Integrated Delivery Systems." *Journal of Healthcare Management* 43 (March/April 1998): 117–118.
45. Griffith, John R. "Managing the Transition to Integrated Health Care Organizations." *Frontiers of Health Services Management* 12 (Summer 1996): 4–50.
46. Conrad, Douglas A., and Stephen M. Shortell. "Integrated Health Systems: Promise and Performance." *Frontiers of Health Services Management* 13 (Fall 1996): 3–40.
47. Adapted from Vaill, Peter B. *Managing as a Performing Art: New Ideas for a World of Chaotic Change* 8–9. San Francisco: Jossey-Bass, 1989; reprinted by permission.

SELECTED BIBLIOGRAPHY

Aon Consulting. *America@Work.* Chicago: Aon Consulting Worldwide, Inc., 1998.

Aon Consulting. "Managing the Stages of Change." *Forum* (October 1998): 6–7.

Berwick, Donald M. "Blazing the Trail of Quality: The HFHS Quality Management Process." *Frontiers of Health Services Management* 7 (Summer 1991): 47–50.

Berwick, Donald M., A. Blanton Godfrey, and Jane Roessner, Eds. *Curing Health Care: New Strategies for Quality Improvement.* San Francisco: Jossey-Bass, 1990.

Bodenheimer, Thomas S., and Kevin Grumbach. *Understanding Health Policy: A Clinical Approach.* Stamford, CT: Appleton & Lange, 1995.

Conger, Jay A., and Rabindra N. Kanungo. *Charismatic Leadership in Organizations.* Thousand Oaks, CA: Sage Publications, 1998.

Conrad, Douglas A., and Stephen M. Shortell. "Integrated Health Systems: Promise and Performance." *Frontiers of Health Services Management* 13 (Fall 1996): 3–40.

Couger, Daniel J. *Creative Problem Solving and Opportunity Finding.* Danvers, MA: Boyd & Fraser, 1995.

Dunham, Randall B., and Jon L. Pierce. *Management.* Reading, MA: Addison-Wesley, 1989.

French, John R. P., and Bertram H. Raven. "The Basis for Social Power." In *Studies of Social Power,* edited by Dorwin Cartwright, 150–167. Ann Arbor, MI: Institute for Social Research, 1959.

French, Wendell L., and Cecil H. Bell, Jr. *Organization Development,* 6th ed. Upper Saddle River, NJ: Prentice-Hall, 1999.

Ginter, Peter M., Linda M. Swayne, and W. Jack Duncan. *Strategic Management of Health Care Organizations,* 3rd ed. Malden, MA: Blackwell, 1998.

Griffith, John R. "Managing the Transition to Integrated Health Care Organizations." *Frontiers of Health Services Management* 12 (Summer 1996): 4–50.

Hernandez, S. Robert, and Arnold D. Kaluzny. "Organizational Innovation and Change." In *Essentials of Health Care Management,* edited by Stephen M. Shortell and Arnold D. Kaluzny, 355–380. Albany, NY: Delmar Publishers, 1997.

Kaluzny, Arnold D. "Patients, Populations, and Caregivers: Opportunities and Challenges at the Intersection." *Frontiers of Health Services Management* 15 (Fall 1998): 43–46.

Lewin, Kurt. "Group Decision and Social Change." In *Readings in Social Psychology,* 2nd ed., edited by Guy E. Swanson, Theodore M. Newcomb, and Eugene L. Hartley, 459–473. New York: Holt, Rinehart, 1952.

Longest, Beaufort B., Jr. *Seeking Strategic Advantage Through Health Policy Analysis.* Chicago: Health Administration Press, 1997.

Longest, Beaufort B., Jr. *Health Policymaking in the United States,* 2nd ed. Chicago: Health Administration Press, 1998.

Longest, Beaufort B., Jr. "Managerial Competence at Senior Levels of Integrated Delivery Systems." *Journal of Healthcare Management* 43 (March/April 1998): 115–133.

Longest, Beaufort B., Jr. "Organizational Change and Innovation." In *Handbook of Health Care Management,* edited by W. Jack Duncan, Peter M. Ginter, and Linda E. Swayne, 369–398. Malden, MA: Blackwell, 1998.

Mondy, R. Wayne, Robert M. Noe, and Shane R. Premeaux. *Human Resource Management,* 7th ed. Upper Saddle River, NJ: Prentice-Hall, 1998.

Rakich, Jonathon S., Kurt Darr, and Beaufort B. Longest, Jr. "An Integrated Model for Continuous Quality Improvement and Productivity Improvement in Health Services Organizations." *Clinical Laboratory Management Review* 7 (July–August 1993): 292–303.

Robbins, Stephen P., and Mary K. Coulter. *Management,* 6th ed. Englewood Cliffs, NJ: Prentice-Hall, 1998.

Schein, Edgar H. *Organizational Culture and Leadership.* San Francisco: Jossey-Bass, 1996.

Schermerhorn, John R., Jr. *Management for Productivity,* 4th ed. New York: John Wiley & Sons, 1993.

Schermerhorn, John R., Jr., James G. Hunt, and Richard N. Osborn. *Organizational Behavior,* 6th ed. New York: John Wiley & Sons, 1998.

Schneider, Benjamin. *Organizational Climate and Culture.* San Francisco, CA: Jossey-Bass, 1990.

Shortell, Stephen M., Ellen M. Morrison, and Bernard Friedman. *Strategic Choices for America's Hospitals: Managing Change in Turbulent Times.* San Francisco: Jossey-Bass, 1990.

Vaill, Peter B. *Managing as a Performing Art: New Ideas for a World of Chaotic Change.* San Francisco: Jossey-Bass, 1989.

Van de Ven, Andrew H., and Marshall S. Poole. "Explaining Development and Change in Organizations." *Academy of Management Review* 20 (July 1995): 510–540.

Wallace, Robert B. "Public Health and Preventive Medicine: Trends and Guideposts." In *Public Health & Preventive Medicine,* 14th ed., edited by Robert B. Wallace and Bradley N. Doebbeling, chap. 1. Stamford, CT: Appleton & Lange, 1998.

Zuckerman, Howard S., Arnold D. Kaluzny, and Thomas C. Ricketts, III. "Strategic Alliances: A Worldwide Phenomenon Comes to Health Care." In *Partners for the Dance: Forming Strategic Alliances in Health Care,* edited by Arnold D. Kaluzny, Howard S. Zuckerman, and Thomas C. Ricketts, III, 1–18. Chicago: Health Administration Press, 1995.

Managing
Relationships

13 Ethics

A moral twilight zone has developed in the past 10 years, as the power equilibrium has shifted from physicians to administrators. CEOs are ill prepared to make the decisions traditionally made by doctors and nurses about moral dilemmas.[1]

This chapter examines the ethical aspects of health services management. Because the relationships between ethics and law are numerous and varied, this introductory section serves as a background for both this chapter and Chapter 14.

Ethical issues arise in all types of health services organizations and health systems (HSOs/ HSs). Historically, the most significant ethical issues occurred in acute care hospitals where more advanced technology was applied. In the 1990s changes in where care was delivered caused other types of facilities to be confronted with ethical issues as well. Because of the uniqueness and complexity of HSOs/HSs, ethical issues commonly have legal dimensions; legal issues usually have ethical aspects. Capable managers will see both.

SOURCES OF LAW

Because of the dynamic relationship between ethics and law, it is useful to begin by reviewing the development of law. *Law* is a system of principles and rules of human conduct prescribed or recognized by society and enforced by public authority. This definition applies to both criminal and civil law. *Ethics* is the study of standards of conduct and moral judgment. When referring to a profession, ethics is the group's principles or code.

Criminal law has a moral underpinning in that it reflects society's sense of right and wrong— its moral code (ethics). This also is true for civil law, which governs organizational and individual relationships such as contracts and malfeasance, including medical malpractice. Here, however, the underlying moral principles are more obscure.

Historically, some societies regarded the law as a gift from the gods; Plato's Greece is an example. Plato considered written law an oversimplification that could not account for nuances, conditions, and differences among people and situations in a dispute. He believed that the best method of resolving a dispute was one in which a philosopher applied an unwritten law. His own experiences proved this impossible in practice, however, and Plato later accepted a written form of law in which the authorities become servants of the law and administer it without regard to the parties in dispute.[2] This principle of "a rule of law, not of men" is reflected in the Anglo-American legal system.

Beyond the written law, which reflects the most significant concerns of society, are other considerations. There are times when orderliness and continuity must yield to justice or fairness. Aristotle recognized the importance of unwritten law incorporating concepts of justice too elusive or varied in their application to be readily codified:

> *When therefore the law lays down a general rule, and thereafter a case arises which is an exception to the rule, it is then right, where the lawgiver's pronouncement because of its absoluteness is defective and erroneous, to rectify the defect by deciding as the lawgiver would himself decide if he were present on the occasion, and would have enacted if he had been cognizant of the case in question.*[3]

This tradition was established in England and was known as chancery. American legal practice uses the concept of equity, in which courts seek to do justice to parties in a dispute that is unique and unlikely to recur. Such a principle of law permits the right result to occur in a case in which blindly following the law would provide no remedy or one that is unsatisfactory.

Bodenheimer, a scholar of jurisprudence, divides sources of law into two major categories, formal and nonformal.

> *By formal sources, we mean sources which are available in an articulated textual formulation embodied in an authoritative legal document. The chief examples of such formal sources are constitutions and statutes, executive orders, administrative regulations, ordinances, charters and bylaws of autonomous or semiautonomous bodies, treaties and certain other agreements, and judicial precedents. By nonformal sources we mean legally significant materials and considerations which have not received an authoritative or at least articulated formulation and embodiment in a formalized legal document. Without necessarily claiming exhaustive completeness for this enumeration, we have subdivided the nonformal sources into standards of justice, principles of reason and consideration of the nature of things (natura rerum), individual equity, public policies, moral convictions, social trends, and customary law.*[4]

HSOs/HSs use charters and bylaws of autonomous or semiautonomous bodies as formal sources of law. Courts look to these documents to determine the rights and obligations of those who are affected. Chapter 4 describes how states issue charters to establish corporations and other types of legally sanctioned organizations and discusses the importance of professional staff organization bylaws in the HSO.

Bodenheimer's definition of formal sources of law includes the codes of ethics used by professional associations to guide affiliates. Written provisions with interpretations that guide application and decision making have the virtues of consistency and predictability. Professional codes of ethics usually set a higher standard than the law does. They state a profession's minimally acceptable behavior, its goals and strivings, and its philosophy and mission. Formal sources of law supersede nonformal sources, except when the former lack comprehensiveness or require interpretation. All types of formal law, even treaties, may affect HSOs/HSs; it is incumbent on health services managers to have a basic understanding of formal law and its effect.

RELATIONSHIP OF LAW TO ETHICS

Democratically derived laws in general reflect the majority's views of justice and fairness. Nonetheless, some may consider a law unjust or immoral and are willing to risk punishment for breaking it. A classical example in U.S. history is the Volstead Act, which amended the Constitution to prohibit the manufacture and distribution of alcoholic beverages. Violation of the law was rampant until its repeal in 1933. Another dimension that shows the complexity of the relationship between ethics (morality) and law is the issue of abortion. Abortion is legal, but many people consider it immoral.

Some may view the link between law and ethics as one to one—what is lawful is ethical and what is unlawful is unethical. This is not necessarily true. The law is the minimum performance that is expected in society. Professions demand that members comply with the law but simultaneously hold members to a higher standard. Thus a profession's code of ethics may require its group's members to act in ways that are different from members of society in general.

Henderson developed models showing the relationship of law and ethics.[5] Figure 13.1 suggests the succession of events that results in the public scrutiny of corporate decisions and a determination as to whether they are right, ethical or both. This judgment is necessarily after the fact, despite management's efforts to predict the effects of actions. This model suggests the impossibility of knowing whether those who eventually judge the decision will consider it legal (law enforcement officials) or ethical (a profession or the public). This adds uncertainty to HSO/HS decision making. Predicting an action's legality usually is easier than knowing whether it will be judged ethical.

Figure 13.2 shows the combinations of legal, illegal, ethical, and unethical factors that are involved in corporate decision making. Decisions made in Quadrant I are ethical and legal and easily identified: Managers who obey the law are acting ethically and legally. Quadrant II includes decisions that are ethical but illegal. The American College of Healthcare Executives (ACHE) *Code of*

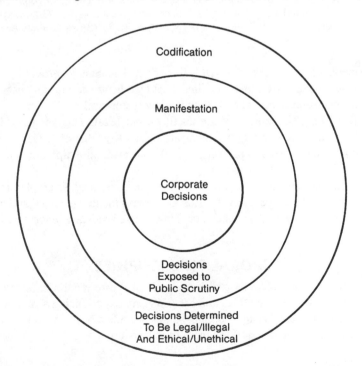

Figure 13.1.   The relationship between law and ethics. (From Henderson, Verne E. "The Ethical Side of Enterprise." *Sloan Management Review* 23 [Spring 1982]: 37–47; reprinted by permission. Copyright © 1982 by the Sloan Management Review Association. All rights reserved.)

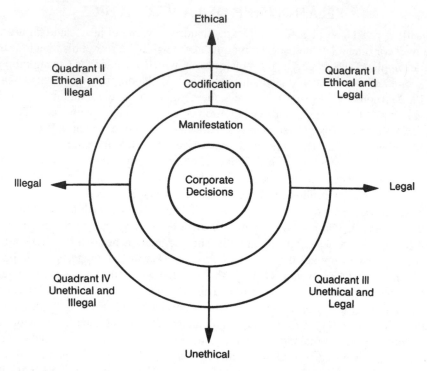

Figure 13.2. A matrix of possible outcomes concerning the ethics and legality of corporate decisions. (From Henderson, Verne E. "The Ethical Side of Enterprise." *Sloan Management Review* 23 [Spring 1982]: 37–47; reprinted by permission. Copyright © 1982 by the Sloan Management Review Association. All rights reserved.)

Ethics requires obeying the law as minimal ethical conduct. This blanket prohibition means that only compelling moral justification exculpates an illegal act by a health services manager; an example is to engage in civil disobedience because obeying the law is immoral.

Quadrant III includes decisions that are unethical but legal. This suggests that ethics, especially in a profession, are likely to require a standard higher than that of the law. Examples include failing to take all reasonable steps to protect patients from medical malpractice or managerial self-aggrandizement to the detriment of patients.

Quadrant IV includes activities that are both illegal and unethical. Examples are easy. Codes of ethics require that the law be obeyed; any decision that breaks the law is illegal and unethical. Failing to meet fire safety regulations, embezzlement, or filing a false Medicare report lie in this quadrant.

MORAL PHILOSOPHIES

Three theories of moral philosophy are used extensively in Western culture: teleology, deontology, and natural law. Two others, virtue ethics and casuistry, are experiencing a revival and are considered here briefly. In sum, these five moral philosophies provide a basis to study morals (ethics) and help determine the moral rightness or wrongness of a decision.

Teleology

The word *teleology* comes from the Greek root *telos,* meaning "end." The most prominent modern theory of morality using this concept is called *utility theory;* a person who follows it is a utilitarian.

The underlying premise is that the moral rightness or wrongness of an act or decision is judged by whether it brings into being more good (utility) or ungood (disutility) than alternative decisions. Classical utilitarianism's most prominent proponent was the English philosopher John Stuart Mill (1806–1873). Utilitarians have no independent right or wrong to guide them. They look at the consequences of an act—the "good" is independent of the "right." Utilitarians are sometimes called consequentialists because they judge actions by their consequences.

Utilitarianism is divided into act utility and rule utility. *Act utility* assesses each decision and determines its consequences when judging moral rightness or wrongness. Act utilitarians judge each action independently, without reference to preestablished guidelines (rules). They measure the amount of good, or (nonmoral) value, brought into being and the amount of evil, or (nonmoral) disvalue, avoided by acting on a particular choice. Each person affected is counted equally. This seems to give a strong sense of objectivity to this moral philosophy. However, because it is episodic, act utilitarianism is incompatible with developing and deriving the ethical principles that are needed for codes of ethics and a personal ethic. Therefore, it receives no further attention.

Rule utility is more formal. It assesses various courses of action (or nonaction) and measures their consequences—the amount of (nonmoral) good or ungood that is produced. The course of action that is morally superior must be taken, even though it may not produce the most good (least ungood) every time it is applied. In modified form, utility theory is the basis for cost–benefit analysis. A crude summary statement describing utilitarianism is "the end justifies the means."

Deontology

Deontology is a theory about morality that is based on the presence of an independent right or wrong. It does not consider consequences as does utilitarianism. The word *deontology* is derived from the Greek *deon,* meaning "duty." The best known proponent of the role of duty was the German philosopher Immanuel Kant (1724–1804). Briefly, his philosophy holds that the end (result) is unimportant because human beings have duties to one another as moral agents, and these duties take precedence over consequences. For Kant, an act is moral if it arises from good will and if one consequently acts from a sense of duty. The Kantian test of morality is whether the act can meet the categorical imperative, which requires that we act in accordance with what we wish to become a universal law. The universal law is that what is right or wrong for one person is right or wrong for everyone, in all places and at all times. According to Kant, an action is right only if it can be universalized without violating the equality of human beings. For example, Kantians see it as logically inconsistent to argue that a terminally ill person should be euthanized (actively causing death) because this is saying that life can be improved by ending it. Deontology may be summarized as never treating humanity simply as a means but rather always as an end.[6] Another summary is to practice the Golden Rule—do unto others as you would have them do unto you.

The work of a contemporary American philosopher, John Rawls, extended Kantian deontology. In *A Theory of Justice,* Rawls developed the elements of a social contract between free, equal, and rational people. To explain this social contract, Rawls used the hypothetical constructs of an original position and a veil of ignorance. The constructs assume that people entering into a social contract are self-interested and rational but know nothing of their individual talents, intelligence, social and economic situation, health, or the like. Rawls argued that such people would agree to certain principles of justice: "First, each person is to have an equal right to the most extensive basic liberty compatible with similar liberty for others. Second, social and economic inequalities are to be arranged so that they are both (a) reasonably expected to be to everyone's advantage, and (b) attached to positions and offices open to all."[7] He reasoned that rational, self-interested people would reject utilitarianism and select instead the concepts of right and justice as necessary to the good. Rawls concluded that rational, self-interested people will protect the least well off because they may be part of that group.

Natural Law

Natural law states that ethics (morality) must be grounded in a concern for human good, and is, therefore, teleological (consequential). Natural law is based on Aristotelian thought as interpreted and synthesized with Christian dogma by St. Thomas Aquinas (1226–1274).[8] It assumes a natural order in relationships and a predisposition among rational people to do, or refrain from doing, certain things. Because human beings are rational, we are able to discover what we should do, and in that attempt we are guided by a partial notion of the eternal law that is linked to our capacity for rational thought. Because natural law guides what rational people do, it is the basis for positive law, some of which is reflected in statutes. Natural law contends that the good cannot be defined only in terms of subjective inclinations; rather, there is a good for human beings that is objectively desirable, although not reducible to desire.[9] A summary statement of the basic precepts of natural law is that one should do good and avoid evil.

Natural law should be contrasted with legal positivism, which became prominent in the late 19th century, and which is based on an aversion to metaphysical speculations and the search for ultimate principles reflected in the work of Aquinas: "The legal positivist holds that only positive law is law; and by positive law he means those judicial norms which have been established by the authority of the state."[10]

Casuistry

Many historical definitions of casuistry are unflattering. Critics argue that it uses sophistry and encourages rationalizations for desired ethical results, uses evasive reasoning, and is quibbling. Nevertheless, contemporary advocates see casuistry as a pragmatic way to understand and solve ethical problems. Casuistry is case-based reasoning in historical context. It avoids excessive reliance on principles and rules, which may provide only partial answers and may not guide decision makers comprehensively. Casuistry allows problem solvers to use

> the concrete circumstances of actual cases, and the specific maxims that people invoke in facing actual moral dilemmas. . . . (C)onsidering similarities and differences between particular types of cases on a practical level open(s) up an alternative approach to ethical theory that is wholly consistent with our moral practice.[11]

At base, casuistry is similar to the law, where court cases and the precedents they establish guide decision makers.

> Cases in ethics are similar: Normative judgments emerge through majoritarian consensus in society and in institutions because careful attention has been paid to the details of particular problem cases. That consensus then becomes authoritative and is extended to relevantly similar cases.[12]

Casuistry happens in organizations, for example, as ethics committees develop a body of experience with various ethical issues.

Both clinical medicine and management education rely on cases. This makes it natural to use a case approach in health services, in which traditional ethics problem solving has applied moral principles to cases—from the general to the specific, or deductive reasoning. Classical casuists, however, used a kind of inductive reasoning—from the specific to the general. They began by stating a paradigm case with a strong maxim (e.g., "thou shalt not kill"), set in its most obvious relevance to circumstances (e.g., a vicious attack on a defenseless person). Subsequent cases added circumstances that made the relevance of the maxim more difficult to understand (e.g., if defense is possible, is it moral?). Classical casuists went from being deontologists to teleologists and back, as suited the case, and adhered to no explicit moral theory.[13] Jonsen argued that modern casuists can profitably copy the classical casuists's reliance on paradigm cases, reference to broad consensus, and acceptance of probable certitude (defined as assent to a proposition, but acknowledging that its opposite might be true.)[14] Casuistry has achieved a prominent place in applied administrative and biomedical ethics. Increasing numbers of cases and a body of experience will lead to consensus and greater certainty in identifying morally right decisions.

Virtue Ethics

Western thought about the importance of virtue can be partially traced to Aristotle. Like natural law, virtue is based on theological ethics but without a primary focus on obligations or duties. Like casuistry, it has received more attention, some of which results from a perception that traditional rule- or principle-based moral philosophies deal inadequately with the realities of ethical decision making. That is to say, rules take us only so far in solving ethical problems. When there are competing ethical rules or difficulties in which to apply, something more than a coin toss is needed. This is where virtue ethicists claim to have a superior moral philosophy.

Contemporary authors argue that ethics has three levels. The first two are observing laws and observing moral rights and fulfilling moral duties that go beyond the law. The third and highest level is the practice of virtue.[15]

> *Virtue implies a character trait, an internal disposition habitually to seek moral perfection, to live one's life in accord with a moral law, and to attain a balance between noble intention and just action. . . . In almost any view the virtuous person is someone we can trust to act habitually in a good way—courageously, honestly, justly, wisely, and temperately.*[16]

In this view, virtuous physicians (or managers) are disposed to the right and good intrinsic to the practice of their profession and will work for the good of the patient. "Virtue ethics expands the notions of benevolence, beneficence, conscientiousness, compassion, and fidelity well beyond what strict duty might require."[17]

Some virtue ethicists argue that, as with any skill or expertise, practice and constant striving to achieve virtuous traits (good works) improve one's ability to be virtuous. Others argue that accepting in one's heart the forgiveness and reconciliation offered by God (faith) "would lead to a new disposition toward God (trust) and the neighbor (love), much as a physician or patient might be judged to be a different (and better) person following changed dispositions toward those persons with whom . . . [they] are involved."[18]

All people should live virtuous lives, but those in the professions have a special obligation to do so. Virtuous managers and physicians are not just virtuous people practicing a profession; they are expected to work for the patient's good even at the expense of personal sacrifice and legitimate self-interest.[19] Virtuous physicians place the good of their patients above their own and seek that good unless pursuing it imposes an injustice on them or their families, or violates their conscience.[20] Similarly, virtuous managers put the good of the patient (through the organization) above their own.

PHILOSOPHICAL BASES FOR ETHICS[21]

Figure 13.3 shows that principles, rules, and specific judgments and actions rely on or are based on ethical theories. Ethical theories do not necessarily conflict; diverse philosophies may reach the

4. **Ethical theories**

3. **Principles**

2. **Rules**

1. **Particular judgments and actions**

Figure 13.3.   Hierarchy of relationships. (From Beauchamp, T.L., and James F. Childress. *Principles of Biomedical Ethics,* 4th ed., 6. New York: Oxford University Press, 1994; reprinted by permission.)

same conclusion about a particular action, albeit through different reasoning or by use of varying constructs.

Ethical theories and derivative principles guide the development of the rules that produce specific judgments and actions. Four principles are important for health services managers: respect for persons, beneficence, nonmaleficence, and justice. Utility is included as an adjunct to beneficence. These principles should be reflected in the organization's philosophy, as well as in the manager's personal ethic.

Respect for Persons

The principle of respect for persons has four elements. The first, *autonomy,* requires that one act toward others in a way that allows them to govern themselves. To choose and pursue a course of action, persons must be rational and uncoerced (unconstrained). Sometimes persons, especially patients, are or become nonautonomous because of physical or mental conditions. They are owed respect, nonetheless, even though special means are needed for them to express their autonomy. Autonomy underlies the need to obtain consent for treatment, as well as the general way in which a HSO views and interacts with patients and staff.

Autonomy is in a state of dynamic tension with paternalism, a concept that suggests that someone else knows what is best for a person. The Hippocratic oath is antecedent to paternalism in the patient–physician relationship. It urges physicians to act in the patient's best interests—as they judge those interests. Giving primacy to autonomy limits paternalism to specific circumstances.

The second element of respect for persons is *truth telling,* which requires managers to be honest in all they do. Depending on how absolute the position, truth telling eliminates "white lies," even if knowing the truth causes harm to the person learning it.

Confidentiality, the third element of respect for persons, requires managers and clinicians to keep secret what they learn about patients and others in the course of their work. This duty applies to managers as well as to staff, organization, and community. Meeting legal requirements may result in morally justified exceptions to confidentiality.

The fourth element is *fidelity*—doing one's duty, keeping one's word. This is sometimes called promise keeping. Like the other three elements, fidelity requires managers to be respectful of persons, whether they are patients, staff, or others.

Beneficence

The second principle, beneficence, is rooted in the Hippocratic tradition and is defined as acting with charity and kindness. Contemporary health services applications of beneficence are broader, including a positive duty. In general, beneficence anchors one end of a continuum; at the other end is the principle of *nonmaleficence,* defined as refraining from actions that aggravate a problem or cause other negative results.

Beneficence is divided into providing benefits and balancing benefits and harms. Conferring benefits is firmly established in medicine, and failing to provide them when one is able to do so violates an ethical obligation of clinicians. Appropriately modified, beneficence applies to managers, too.

The positive duty that is suggested by the principle of beneficence requires HSOs and their managers to do all that they can to aid patients. There is a lesser duty to aid persons who are potential patients rather than actual patients. This distinction and its importance vary with the values, mission, and vision of the HSO/HS and with the population that is being served. Thus a hospital emergency department has no duty under the principle of beneficence to scour neighborhoods for persons in need of assistance. This duty changes, of course, when someone becomes a patient.

The second dimension of beneficence is balancing the benefits and harms of an action. This is the principle of utility, which is the philosophical basis for cost–benefit and risk–benefit analyses. Here, however, utility is but one of several considerations. Its more limited application results from a positive duty to act in the patient's best interests because one cannot act with kindness and charity if risks outweigh benefits. Regardless of its interpretation, utility cannot justify overriding the interests of patients and sacrificing them to the greater good.

Nonmaleficence

The third principle that is applicable to managing HSOs is nonmaleficence. Like beneficence, it has deep historical roots in medicine. In effect, nonmaleficence is *primum non nocere*—first, do no harm. This dictum to guide physicians' actions is equally applicable to health services managers. Nonmaleficence gives rise to specific moral rules, but neither the principle nor derivative rules are absolute; for example, it may be appropriate (with the patient's consent) to inflict harm (e.g., administer cancer chemotherapy) to avoid worse harm (e.g., performing a surgical procedure), and appropriate to compromise truth telling if it would cause significant mental or physical harm.

The principle of nonmaleficence most commonly applies to HSO relationships with patients. It also raises duties that managers have to their staff; there may be circumstances in which duties conflict. Putting staff at unnecessary or extraordinary risk to their health and safety is inconsistent with the manager's duty to them, even when the result meets a duty of patient beneficence. Balancing benefits and harms also suggests application of the concept of utility.

Justice

The fourth principle, justice, is important in managerial decision making such as allocating organizational resources. It also applies to developing and applying human resources policies.

What is justice, and how does one know when it is achieved? Philosophers define justice differently. Often, the definitions require that all people get their just desserts, what they are due. Rawls defined justice as fairness, but how are just desserts and fairness defined? Aristotle defined justice as equals being treated equally, and unequals unequally—a concept that is common in public policy analysis. Equal treatment of equals is reflected in liberty rights such as freedom of speech for all. Unequal treatment of people unequally situated is used to justify progressive income taxes and the redistribution of wealth. Aristotle's concept of justice is expressed in health services when greater resources are expended on those who are more ill and in greater need. For example, organ transplants usually go to the sickest while others wait. These concepts of justice are helpful but do not solve problems of definition and opinion that are so troublesome for managers. Clinicians and managers act justly if they consistently apply clear and prospectively determined criteria in decision making.

Summary

Moral philosophies and derivative principles provide a framework to hone and use a personal ethic to analyze and solve ethical problems. Like philosophers, managers are unlikely to agree fully with only one moral philosophy. Most will be eclectic in developing or reconsidering a personal ethic. In general, however, the principles of respect for persons, beneficence, nonmaleficence, and justice are useful in defining relationships among patients, managers, and organizations. They may carry different weights and take precedence over each other, depending on the issue being considered. Justice requires, however, that they be consistently ordered and weighted when similar problems are considered.

CODES OF ETHICS

A major problem with applied ethics is that many written and unwritten codes influence or guide human behavior. They arise from family, religious training, professional affiliations and allegiances, and an often ill-defined personal code of moral conduct—an amalgam of intellect, reasoning, experience, education, and relationships. Codes may be vague or contradictory. It may seem that there are few answers—only difficult questions and choices. It is hoped that one's professional code of ethics has been internalized and is a major part of one's personal ethic.

Activities that violate a professional code may be subject to disciplinary action. A profession's attribute of service to society tends to minimize one's private life and maximize one's public life. Professions, however, regularly face the dilemma of how much scrutiny to give nonprofessional and private activities. This boundary is especially problematic if, for example, personal conduct scandalizes the profession. Similarly, organizational culture and values (discussed in Chapter 1) have an important interaction with a manager's personal ethic.

Managers must develop a personal ethic despite membership in a professional group and employment in a HSO/HS with an organizational philosophy reflected in values, mission, and vision statements. A personal ethic is a moral framework for decision making and permits the refinement of guidelines, judgments, and actions. It bears repeating that each person is a moral agent whose actions, inactions, and misactions have moral consequences for which that person is responsible. No one's conduct can be excused by a claim that orders were being followed. Orders from lawfully constituted public authorities such as courts pose special problems. Moral agents who believe that such orders are unjust may engage in civil disobedience, for which they must be prepared to bear societally imposed sanctions. Ethical (moral) implications of acts must be considered independently of the act.

On occasion, conflicts arise between the HSO's/HS's ethic, as expressed in its values statement, and a manager's personal ethic. HSOs/HSs are bureaucratic, seemingly with a life of their own. The manager must think carefully about the implications of acquiescing in specific expressions of a HSO's/HS's philosophy. Again, this is the concept of moral agency. It may seem easier to "go along to get along" than to risk one's position and economic association by speaking out. Failing to speak out when we should, however, violates our duty as moral agents. Managers cannot go about their daily tasks without considering the moral context of what they do. Similarities and differences between the ethic of organization and the ethic of self cannot be forgotten.

HEALTH SERVICES CODES OF ETHICS

Institutional Trade Associations

Many of the groups described in Chapter 2 have ethical guidelines. The American Hospital Association (AHA) is the major hospital trade association. Revised guidelines adopted by AHA in 1992 include sections on community role, patient care, and organizational conduct. Members are expected to improve community health status and deliver high-quality, comprehensive services efficiently. Coordinating services with other HSOs is stressed. Specific provisions address informed consent, confidentiality, and ways to resolve value conflicts among patients and families, clinical staff, employees, organization, and community. The AHA code states that patients' religious and social beliefs and customs should be accommodated if possible, but hospital values are not subordinated to them. This reinforces the need to inform patients about organizational values before treatment.

The American Health Care Association (AHCA) is the trade association whose members are for-profit and not-for-profit long-term facilities, including assisted living facilities, nursing facilities, and subacute care providers. AHCA's code of ethics guides the organization and is a model for state affiliates and their members. Provisions include moral responsibility, good business practices, making difficult choices, acting responsibly, obligations to provide quality services, dealing with conflicting values, use of information, responsible advocacy, potential conflicts of interest, respect for others, and fairness in competition. In addition, AHCA publishes a primer on ethics for its members.

The American Association of Health Plans Code of Conduct covering member health plans was revised in 1998. It has three major sections and elements within each: patient information (patient information and patient appeals), patient access (emergency access), and physicians' role in quality improvement (physicians and quality assessment and improvement programs, physicians and practice guidelines, utilization management, physicians and prescription drug formularies, patient confidentiality, patient choice of family and specialty physicians, patient access to specialty care, and transition from one provider to another).

Health Professions

A hallmark of professions is a code of ethics that defines acceptable and unacceptable behavior. Such codes are common in health services, but language usually is general, and vague performance standards make enforcement difficult, if not impossible. Even vigorous enforcement, however, only guides those seeking to do the right thing but who need help determining what that is. Someone at the fringe of a profession is dissuaded neither by principles of ethical conduct nor by legal requirements.

Managers

American College of Healthcare Executives

ACHE adopted its first *Code of Ethics* in 1939, 6 years after its founding. The code has evolved from a general document with vague provisions to one that addresses issues such as conflict of interest, confidential information, honesty in advertising, access to health services, and professional competence. The major revision in 1987 recognized the concept of moral agency and identified a positive duty for affiliates to report violations. In its several iterations the code has become more specific, even though there are many general statements to which applying performance measures would be difficult. ACHE also publishes ethical policy statements to guide affiliates on issues such as medical records confidentiality, decisions near the end of life, and professional impairment.

Information about allegedly unethical behavior is referred to the ACHE Committee on Ethics, which investigates and makes recommendations. Affiliates are entitled to due process, and the code has a grievance (appeals) procedure. The maximum disciplinary action is expulsion. ACHE affiliation is not linked to licensure, but, if it is important to employers and colleagues, expulsion may dampen career potential. The deterrent effects of disciplinary action are speculative; nevertheless, vigorous application enhances a code's importance.

ACHE affiliates hold that a code should be comprehensive and specific in guiding decisions, and that enforcement and disposition of cases should be reported. Affiliates have an interest in learning about ethical problems.[22] A vital, living code prepares affiliates to solve ethical issues. The code, however, focuses on administrative ethics. The biomedical ethical issues that directly or indirectly affect the health services manager receive little attention.

American College of Health Care Administrators

The *Code of Ethics* of the American College of Health Care Administrators (ACHCA), revised in 1994, guides managers of long-term care facilities, usually known as nursing facilities. Members must meet expectations that are divided into prescriptions and proscriptions. The expectations state that the welfare of those receiving care is paramount; managers must remain professionally competent; and other managers must be encouraged to meet their responsibilities to the public, the profession, and other colleagues. The issues that are addressed include quality of services; confidentiality of patient information; continuing education; conflicts of interest; fostering knowledge, supporting research, and sharing expertise; and providing information to the standards and ethics committee of actual or potential code violations. No enforcement or appeals process is described.

Physicians

The American Medical Association (AMA) is the preeminent professional association for allopathic physicians; its *Principles of Medical Ethics* are addressed exclusively. AMA's first code, adopted at its founding in 1847, was based on the code of medical ethics that was developed by the English physician and philosopher Sir Thomas Percival in 1803.[23] Several iterations have appeared since. A major revision of the 1957 code was adopted in 1980. Deleted were prohibitions against voluntarily associating with so-called unscientific practitioners (e.g., chiropractors) and against soliciting patients, which prevented advertising. The paternalism that allowed physicians to break patient confidentiality when it was in the interest of patients or society was replaced by a principle to "safeguard patient confidence within the constraints of the law." Members have a positive duty to "strive to expose those physicians deficient in character or competence, or who engage in fraud or deception."[24] The opinions of AMA's Judicial Council assist in interpreting the principles.

The 1980 principles are noteworthy because they are "the opening to an ethics based on notions of rights and responsibilities rather than benefits and harms. It is the first document in the history of professional medical ethics in which a group of physicians is willing to use the language of responsibilities and rights."[25]

Nurses

The *Code for Nurses,* developed by the American Nurses Association (ANA), was first adopted in 1950 and revised in 1985. The preamble states that clients are the primary decision makers in matters concerning their own health, treatment, and well being, and "the goal of nursing actions is to support and enhance the client's responsibility and self-determination to the greatest extent possible."[26] The introduction states that "justification of behavior as ethical must satisfy not only the individual nurse acting as a moral agent, but also the standards for professional peer review," and notes further that the code "serves to inform both the nurse and society of the profession's expectations and requirements in ethical matters."[27]

The code has 11 provisions; each has an interpretive statement. As in the ACHE and AMA codes, nurses have a positive duty "to safeguard the client and the public when health care and safety are affected by the incompetent, unethical, or illegal practice of any person."[28]

PATIENT BILLS OF RIGHTS

Further guidance about ethical relationships between health services consumers and the HSO/HS and its staff comes from patient bills of rights. Titles vary, but bills of rights or discussions of patient rights have been published by organizations including AHA, the Joint Commission on Accreditation of Healthcare Organizations (Joint Commission), and the Department of Veterans Affairs (DVA). The American Civil Liberties Union (ACLU) presented its position on patient rights in a handbook.[29] AHA's position is more institution oriented, whereas that of ACLU is more strident in patient advocacy; this puts them more or less at polar ends of a continuum. Philosophically, DVA's *Patient Rights* and its companion document *Patient Responsibilities* and the Joint Commission's *Patient Rights and Organization Ethics* lie between AHA's and ACLU's patient rights documents.

All of the documents reflect the law on issues such as confidentiality and consent. AHA's bill recognizes that patient choice may be limited by hospital policies and that health care is a collaborative endeavor between providers and patients. It lists the responsibilities that the patient must fulfill if care is to be effective. The ACLU handbook is more demanding on behalf of patients; it identifies the goals for a patient advocacy program and the authority that advocates should have, outlines the elements of informed consent for treatment of and the process for obtaining it, and details the access that patients should have to their medical records.

Bills of patient rights have no legal effect; rather they set an ethical tone for a HSO's/HS's relationships with those it serves. As defined by Bodenheimer, they are formal sources of law. The effectiveness of a bill of patient rights is limited by the HSO's/HS's willingness to make its contents known and develop processes that encourage and monitor its use. In the late 1990s the U.S. Congress considered but did not pass a bill of rights that would have applied at least to people whose care is paid by federal programs.

ETHICAL ISSUES AFFECTING GOVERNANCE AND MANAGEMENT

Fiduciary Duty

Fiduciary duty, an ethical (and legal) concept that arose from Roman jurisprudence, means that, in certain relationships, a person in a superior position of knowledge and authority and in whom trust is placed has obligations and duties toward others. Ethically, and often legally, many relationships have fiduciary dimensions (e.g., physician–patient, priest–penitent, attorney–client, and professor–student). Fidelity, an element of respect for persons, finds expression in the concept of fiduciary duty. Beneficence and nonmaleficence underpin the ethical aspects of fiduciary duty as well.

Governing body members of corporations organized both for profit and not for profit have a fiduciary duty, the breach of which can lead to personal liability.[30] Fiduciaries have primary duties of loyalty and responsibility:

> *Loyalty means that the individuals must put the interest of the corporation above all self-interest, a principle based on the biblical doctrine that no man can serve two masters. Specifically no trustee is permitted to gain any secret profits personally, to accept bribes, or to compete with the corporation. . . .*[31]

The fiduciary duty of responsibility means that governing body members must exercise reasonable care, skill, and diligence that is in proportion to the circumstances in every activity of governance. In other words, governing body members can be held personally liable for gross negligence, which can be acts of commission or omission.[32]

The law recognizes trustees as a unique kind of fiduciary and holds them to a higher standard of care. Trustees are responsible for assets held in trust for the benefit of another and for whom the law holds to a high standard. Trustees may not use their position for personal gain and must act only in the best interests of the beneficiary of the trust. Historically, governing body members of not-for-profit HSOs/HSs have used the title "trustee," even when there was no trust for which they were fiduciaries (trustees). Unless they are fiduciaries of a trust, however, the technically correct legal term is "director" or "corporate director."

The most significant court case involving the fiduciary duties of HSO governing body members is *Stern et al. v. Lucy Webb Hayes National Training School of Deaconesses and Missionaries et al.*[33] This class action was brought by patients of Sibley Hospital, which was controlled by the Lucy Webb Hayes School, who alleged that they had paid too much for care because several "trustees" had been mismanaging, nonmanaging, self-dealing, and conspiring among themselves and with various financial institutions.[33] The court found no evidence of a conspiracy and determined that the Sibley "trustees" should be held to a lesser standard than a true trustee:

> *The charitable corporation is a relatively new legal entity which does not fit neatly into the established common law categories of corporation and trust. . . . [T]he modern trend is to apply corporate rather than trust principles in determining the liability of the directors of charitable corporations, because their functions are virtually indistinguishable from those of their "pure" corporate counterparts.*[34]

The case is complex. Suffice to say that defendant trustees were found to have violated their fiduciary duties, even when held to the lesser, corporate standard. Mismanagement occurred because certain trustees ignored the investment sections of yearly audits, failed to gather enough information to vote intelligently on opening new bank accounts, and in general failed to exercise even cursory supervision over hospital funds. The nonmanagement that resulted from the same failure to exercise supervision was most starkly shown because trustees repeatedly elected to the investment committee did not object when it did not meet in more than 10 years. Self-dealing was shown because thousands of dollars were kept in non–interest-bearing checking accounts, interest-bearing accounts paid less than market conditions would have permitted, and a trustee advised the approval of and voted to approve a contract for investment services with the corporation of which he was president. The court found, however, that no defendant trustees had gained personally, even though they were associated with organizations that benefited from the transactions. The absence of a conspiracy seemed important to the court's ruling.

The court ordered the named trustees removed but found no personal liability. To prevent future problems, the court ordered the governing body to adopt a written investment policy, conduct a review to determine that all hospital assets conformed to the policy, and devise a regular process for disclosing business affiliations. In the meantime the governing body had adopted AHA–recommended guidelines on conflicts of interest. Although done long after the fact, this evidenced its good faith. The AHA guidelines in Figure 13.4 are the 1990 iteration, which are identical to those adopted by Sibley in 1975 and reflect the corporate director rather than the true trustee standard.

Conflict of Interest

The potential for conflicts of interest exists in any organization. It occurs in HSOs/HSs in several ways. The examples of self-dealing in the Sibley Hospital case are one type. A conflict of interest occurs, too, when someone has multiple obligations that demand loyalty, and decisions based on these loyalties are different or in conflict. It is the problem of serving two masters that was noted earlier. This section addresses conflicts of interest and how to avoid them. The element of fidelity (promise keeping) assists in ethical analysis of conflicts of interest. The principles of beneficence and nonmaleficence also provide an ethical framework to analyze conflicts of interest.

Disclosure of certain interests of governing board members

Whereas, The proper governance of the nation's health care institutions depends on governing board members who give of their time for the benefit of their health communities; and,

Whereas, The giving of this service, because of the varied interests and backgrounds of the governing board members, may result in situations involving a dual interest that might be interpreted as conflict of interest; and, whereas, this service should not be rendered impossible solely by reason of duality of interest or possible conflict of interest; and,

Whereas, This service nevertheless carries with it a requirement of loyalty and fidelity to the institution served, it being the responsibility of the members of the board to govern the institution's affairs honestly and economically, exercising their best care, skill, and judgment for the benefit of the institution; and,

Whereas, The matter of any duality of interest or possible conflict of interest can best be handled through full disclosure of any such interest, together with noninvolvement in any vote wherein the interest is involved;

Now, therefore, be it resolved; That the following policy on duality and conflict of interest is hereby adopted:

- Any duality of interest or possible conflict of interest on the part of any governing board member should be disclosed to the other members of the board and made a matter of record, either through an annual procedure or when the interest becomes a matter of board action.

- Any governing board member having a duality of interest or possible conflict of interest on any matter should not vote or use his personal influence on the matter, and he should not be counted in determining the quorum for the meeting, even where permitted by law. The minutes of the meeting should reflect that a disclosure was made, the abstention from voting, and the quorum situation.

- The foregoing requirements should not be construed as preventing the governing board member from briefly stating his position in the matter, nor from answering pertinent questions of other board members since his knowledge may be of great assistance.

Be it further resolved: That this policy be reviewed annually for the information and guidance of governing board members, and that any new member be advised of the policy upon entering on the duties of his office.

Figure 13.4.   Conflict of interest statement of the American Hospital Association. (From American Hospital Association. *Management Advisory on Functions of Hospital Executive Management,* 2. Chicago: American Hospital Association, 1990; reprinted by permission of the American Hospital Association, copyright 2000.)

The ACHE *Code of Ethics* states that

> A conflict of interest may be only a matter of degree, but exists when the healthcare executive:
> —is in a position to benefit directly or indirectly by using authority or inside information, or
>   allows a friend, relative or associate to benefit from such authority or information. (or)
> —uses authority or information to make a decision to intentionally affect the organization in
>   an adverse manner.[35]

This definition should guide managers in avoiding conflicts of interest. The phrase "a matter of degree" correctly suggests that limited behavior of some types is unlikely to cause or even imply a conflict of interest, whereas exaggerated behavior of the same type does. Arguably, no conflict of interest arises if a vendor buys an inexpensive lunch for a manager. An all-expenses-paid, 2-week vacation suggests a conflict of interest. Large gifts are presumed to encourage or reward certain behavior. The additional code provision that the executive shall "Accept no gifts or benefits offered with the expectation of influencing a management decision"[36] is stringent but appropriate.

Examples of extravagant gifts and kickbacks occurred at the Cedars of Lebanon Hospital, where the chief executive officer (CEO) engaged in unethical and illegal activities.[37] Self-dealing occurred because the CEO was part-owner of a firm that contracted with his hospital for architectural consulting services that were never done. The CEO falsified governing body minutes to cover up the fraudulent contract. In another transaction, the CEO received more than 2,500 shares of stock with a market value of $75,000 in a computer company from which the hospital had purchased a $1.8 million diagnostic computer to be used for multiphasic screening. Underutilization of the machine caused losses of more than $2,000 per day. The CEO also bribed public officials to get approval for construction permits and loans to build an unneeded addition. Finally, to ease a desperate cash flow problem, the CEO broke the law by not paying federal withholding taxes on employees' salaries. The Cedars of Lebanon case contains several examples of law breaking, which makes the activities unethical in themselves. The conflicts of interest are obvious. The important lesson is, however, that the problems occurred because the governing body was inattentive to what its CEO was doing. As a result the hospital was forced into receivership and the CEO went to prison.

Conflicts of interest can be subtle, however. Is it ethical for a manager to use a position of influence and power to gain personal aggrandizement of titles and position at the expense of patient care or other HSO/HS activities? Is it ethical for a manager to be lax in developing and implementing an effective patient consent policy and process? Is it ethical for a manager to screen information provided to the governing body and present it to convey the appearance of competence? Is it ethical for a manager who believes there are quality-of-care problems in a clinical department to fail to investigate? Is it ethical for managers who have concerns about their personal ability to meet the demands of their position to remain in it? Such examples raise ethical questions.

Many conflicts of interest can be identified only through continued questioning and self-analysis. Intensified competition will increase the number of conflicts of interest, but attention to fidelity and the principles of beneficence and nonmaleficence, as well as the ACHE code and the AHA statement, can reduce or eliminate them.

Confidential Information

HSOs/HSs are rife with confidential information about patients, staff, and the organization. Managers have an ethical and a legal obligation to use this information properly. Problems occur if confidential information is used to benefit a manager or other people with whom the manager is associated or related, or to harass or injure. The ACHE code views this problem broadly and asks affiliates to "respect professional confidences" and "to assure [sic] the existence of procedures that will safeguard the confidentiality and privacy of patients, clients and others served."[38]

Misuse of confidential information includes disclosing governing body decisions so that advantageous sales or purchases can be made by the insider's associates; selling or giving patient medical information to the media or attorneys; and providing the HSO's/HS's marketing strategies to competitors. An example that raises potential conflicts of interest and confidential information problems occurs when a manager serves on the governing body of a planning agency or potentially competing HSO/HS. Fidelity to one's own HSO/HS conflicts with the duty to objectively consider another HSO's/HS's certificate of need, for example. In addition, and more subtly, the manager becomes privy to information that is important to that manager's own HSO/HS. One cannot ignore such information. A competitive marketplace makes cooperation with other HSOs/HSs difficult because of potential conflicts of interest and the consequences of antitrust law.

Ethics and Marketing

All HSOs/HSs market and did so even before marketing became an accepted practice in health services. Marketing occurs in the physicians' lounge, at community health fairs, in new employee orientation, and in press releases. Applying the four Ps of marketing—product, price, place, and promotion—to health services is not difficult; health services marketers have adapted them with a newer vocabulary—service, consideration, access, and promotion (SCAP). Although the new milieu of the competitive marketplace makes marketing problematic for many HSOs/HSs, it is generally agreed that competition is desirable. This necessitates marketing.

HSOs/HSs are unique as compared with the typical business enterprise. They differ in historical development, purpose, type of activity, public service orientation, charitable motives, religious affiliation, profit orientation (many are not-for-profit), links to the healing professions, highly educated and trained staff, labor intensity, and the emotional and psychological aspects of services. HSOs/HSs are social enterprises with economic dimensions, not economic enterprises with social dimensions.

The HSO/HS can carry out its mission only if it remains solvent. "No margin, no mission" has become a cliché, but it accurately states the dilemma. The economic survival of HSOs/HSs depends on balancing compensated care with uncompensated care to the under- and uninsured. Even a limited general duty of beneficence obliges HSOs/HSs to provide services that assist all groups and to be a community resource. Some services generate surpluses that subsidize uncompensated care and fund programs for the underserved. Although laudable, such efforts raise other ethical questions.

Need Versus Demand

Discussing health services marketing often causes disagreement about whether it creates or meets demand. This disagreement is complicated by implicit value judgments about which health services merit the creation of demand and which do not. Except for questions about cost–benefit, there is little dispute about the desirability of screening for hypertension or colorectal cancer. Conversely, cosmetic surgery is an oft-cited example of so-called unnecessary demand. Its opponents argue that face lifts, tummy tucks, or liposuction wastes health resources (regardless of payment source) that should be available for better uses. This is a subjective definition of need. Reasonable people could reach different conclusions based on scientific fact as to what people need and whether demand arising from that need should be met. Perhaps cosmetic surgery should be defined as a consumer service, like haircutting or bodybuilding, that happens to use elements of the health system.

Epidemiological studies develop health data about populations, including incidence and prevalence rates of disease, as well as psychological and physical problems outside traditional definitions of disease. Objectivity is lessened when personal values determine what is studied, how data are evaluated, or what to do with results.

All efforts to improve health are beneficial if the World Health Organization definition that "health is a state of complete physical, mental, and social well-being and not merely the absence of disease or infirmity" is applied.[39] In this regard it is instructive to consider wellness activities. The possibilities seem limitless because all facets of life could be affected to improve health status and prevent medical problems. Beyond wellness activities are questions of how to treat demand from those who want to use disposable income as they wish, regardless of how foolish it may seem. Should they be denied elective procedures such as cosmetic surgery because some judge these procedures to provide only a marginal improvement in the quality of life, or because the condition is not life threatening? Such infringement on autonomy would be a major loss of freedom.

Responsible Marketing

The dilemma of responsible marketing is how HSOs/HSs can meet their ethical obligation to serve those potentially in need but avoid creating unnecessary demand. Guidance is offered by AHA: "Advertising should be used to educate the public, to report to the community, to increase awareness of available services, to increase support for the organization, and to recruit employees. Health care advertising should be truthful, fair, accurate, complete, and sensitive to the needs of the public."[40]

Responsible marketing is an important, if elusive, concept. HSOs/HSs whose focus is return on investment will view marketing and competition very differently from those with other goals. At minimum, responsible marketing means tempering customers' desires and potential demand with efforts to judge value and usefulness. This view has elements of paternalism, but it means that HSO/HS decision makers have determined that certain expenditures and goals are more worthwhile than others, which is consistent with the purpose of the mission statement and their expertise as providers.

Future of Competition

A political science theory suggests that, over time, enemies become more like one another. If this theory is true, then such an evolution greatly concerns not-for-profit HSOs/HSs, who see themselves as historically incorporating a mindset and an attitude that are different from those organized for profit. They fear that aggressively competing for market share maximizes financial considerations and minimizes humanitarian motives. Doing more with less and demands for efficiency are not at variance with operationalizing the principles of respect for persons, beneficence, nonmaleficence, and justice. It remains for everyone involved in organizing, planning, and delivering health services to keep these principles firmly in mind.

CONFLICTS OF INTEREST IN MANAGED CARE[41]

There is an inherent potential for conflicts of interest in managed care because goals, purposes, and objectives—the interests—of managed care organizations (MCOs) are different from interests of their members. The tension among the MCO and its members and potential members occurs as early as the marketing stage, when benefit packages and market segments are identified. The potential for conflicts of interest is unavoidable, but its presence and consequent negative effects can be minimized if clinicians and managers are mindful of it. There are potential conflicts of interest when one duty (allegiance) cannot be met without dereliction of another.

Marketing and Operations

Can potential conflicts of interest lead to actual conflicts when no relationship has been established between a MCO and those to whom marketing is directed? Arguably, no. Nonetheless, many MCOs have a morally demanding self-image that includes a public service orientation; for them, marketing that ignores or excludes high-risk groups ("cream skimming") is at variance with historic and current mission and purpose. Furthermore, the MCO may be forced to ignore high-risk groups because it has a greater duty to current patients than to potential patients. It must be asked, however, whether marketing that focuses on healthy, low-risk people is ethical.[42]

Although not a conflict of interest, MCO marketing must take into account the possible need to "keep one's light under a bushel (basket)." If a MCO is, or is thought to be, a leader in certain techniques or medical conditions, then the MCO will be overwhelmed with new members needing that treatment. Adverse selection also results when high-risk people disproportionately join a MCO with an excellent reputation for high-quality care and good results. As the MCO strains against adverse selection, quality may diminish, benefits may be restricted, or premiums may be increased. Thus the MCO's interests are to minimize the appearance of providing superb care; instead, it seeks an image of providing good quality but unexceptional services.

Both the MCO and its members want a financially strong, well-functioning organization that meets member needs in a timely and effective manner. There is ample opportunity for divergence beyond this congruence, however.

As a bureaucracy, MCO managers, physicians, and staff seek to maximize position, power, income, and other rewards with the least disruption of homeostasis. Achieving these goals, especially maximizing income, may minimize service whether or not this is consistent with mission or contract provisions. The bureaucratic response may even be at variance with long-term survival. The member has a primary interest in retaining or regaining health and paying the least to do so. Members also want to maximize access to services that are consistent with perceived needs. The goals of the MCO and members are congruent when members stay well with minimal costs and use existing services appropriately. It is rarely that simple, however.

Using services has the greatest potential for conflicts of interest. In this regard, members may be divided into appropriate users and overusers, whether purposefully or not. The MCO's interests and those of appropriate users are congruent; to be competitive, however, overusers must be controlled. Even appropriate users are a potential financial threat to a MCO in a competitive environment. To trim costs, the MCO may seek to make them underusers, which may result in a conflict of interest.

How do the potential conflicts of interest evidenced by incongruent MCO and member goals become true conflicts? Marketing information describes the available primary care and specialty services. Limitations, especially those on specialty or high-cost services, are downplayed. Beyond marketing, constraints may include reduced hours and services; queues may be allowed, especially for self-limiting medical conditions. The escape valve for queue pressures is treating walk-ins during office hours or, as a last resort, emergency services. The public reacted negatively to the CEO of a major MCO who stated publicly that queues were important in reducing demand related to self-limiting conditions. Such policies are effective in the short term. In the long term, however, they will have an antimarketing effect and cause disenrollment.

Physician Incentives and Other Constraints

Of great concern to members will be subtle and potentially serious constraints affecting MCO–affiliated physicians. Potential conflicts of interest arise between MCO and member and, in terms of professional ethics, between physician and patient. The Hippocratic oath requires that physicians act in the patients' best interests, a paternalistic ethic that suggests safeguards. AMA's *Principles of Medical Ethics* require that patients' interests be foremost as physicians choose the level and content of care. The law reflects both concepts.

Physician treatment decisions are important, but the MCO facilitates or inhibits these decisions. Employment is the clearest example of self-selection bias—the physicians who are unable to accept the MCO's rules will work elsewhere. Nonemployed physicians who are part of a MCO network or MCO–sponsored independent practice association are less directly controlled but are subject to similar constraints. It is theoretically possible for independent physicians to disaffiliate from a MCO they find inhospitable, but the growing number of people in managed care may give them no choice but to participate, even if it is distasteful.

MCO–affiliated physicians face a range of behavior-modifying guidelines: limits on referrals (especially out-of-plan) and hospitalization, financial disincentives (and incentives), quotas on numbers of patients seen (used in staff-model health maintenance organizations [HMOs]), and peer review. Based on a physician's practice pattern, the MCO can take several actions. In order of increasing severity, they are peer pressure, letter of warning/admonition, economic incentives or disincentives, nonrenewal, and dismissal. Constraints are positive when they encourage judicious but appropriate use of medical resources—this explains in part why MCOs use fewer ancillary services and hospital days. When are constraints excessive and members deprived of needed service? When do constraints infringe on the principles of nonmaleficence and beneficence? There are no simple answers because constraints are a function of a MCO's willingness, prompted by the manager as a conscience and moral agent, to institute safeguards that balance competitiveness and financial viability with serving members' needs.

Other examples of constraints can be found in organizational and managerial functioning. A complicated decision-making process (e.g., significant committee involvement and several levels of review) may slow approval of new procedures or types of equipment that deliver technically better care but at greater cost. Such complexities may be more prevalent in not-for-profit than investor-owned MCOs. Complex processes in not-for-profit MCOs may result from a greater degree of democracy, however, and not a deliberate attempt to diminish access. The effect may be the same, nonetheless. For-profit MCOs tend to have a narrower management pyramid and give the CEO more authority. A complex management structure in an investor-owned MCO is less likely to diminish its ability to conserve resources to the potential detriment of members.

The MCO may forgo purchase of high-technology diagnostic and treatment equipment, or it may contract with physicians or hospitals without such technology. These strategies lower costs. Lower costs that enhance financial integrity and support availability of services make organizational and member interests congruent. This strategy has no advantage for those who might have benefited from a technology; for them it is a conflict of interest.

Minimizing Conflicts of Interest in Managed Care

How are conflicts of interest prevented or at least minimized? An indispensable first step is acknowledging that potential conflicts of interest are inherent in the relationship between MCOs and members, as well as between the MCO and patients and between physicians and patients. Awareness permits avoidance. Beyond that, checks and balances are needed. One solution is employing an ombudsman or consumer relations specialist. In addition, there should be due process procedures for members who wish to have a matter reviewed. The success of such programs depends on enlightened management and on the personal characteristics of the people who are involved. MCOs may use the managing physician or gatekeeper concept to determine whether patients receive needed services. This role may conflict with financial and other incentives that constrain affiliated physicians, however. Federally qualified HMOs, for example, must have an effective grievance procedure for members. This requirement offers some protection, but its usefulness requires that members suspect that care was inadequate, a determination they may be incapable of making.

Audits of utilization data and comparisons with other MCOs allow management to determine whether use was appropriate. Awareness of how and where conflicts of interest arise will help prevent them or minimize their effect.[43] Such activities are essential if managers are to meet their ethical obligations to patients.

BIOMEDICAL ETHICAL ISSUES

Resource Allocation

The ethical implications of allocating resources are receiving greater attention. Whether at the macro or micro level, resource allocation is an important application of the principle of justice and necessitates making decisions—who gets what, when, and how. Value-laden criteria such as worth, usefulness, merit, or need are common. Government involvement often brings political motives. Like governments, HSOs/HSs use macroallocation to determine what equipment to buy and whether to begin a new program. Microallocation includes a physician's willingness to refer, a patient's geographic access to services and technologies, and economic considerations. Often, micro-level decisions are guided (in a sense, are predetermined) by the policies and procedures of governments or HSOs/HSs.

A common solution is to use the "greatest good" (utility) principle of utilitarianism for allocation decisions, as is done by economists and policy analysts. It is at best a partial answer because applying only principles of utility may allow us to ignore considerations of human need, fairness, and justice.

Numerous macroallocation theories have been proposed. At one end of a continuum is egalitarianism, which stems from the concept that all human beings are entitled to equal health services. Hyperegalitarianism is extreme egalitarianism, which holds that a technology that is not available to all should not be available to any. At the other end of that continuum is a theory that health services are not a right that is guaranteed by society; rather they are a privilege to be earned. This hyperindividualistic position holds that caregivers such as physicians have no obligation to render services to people who cannot afford them, but they may freely choose to provide them. Between these extremes is a view that society is obliged to encourage, develop, and perhaps even provide health services in limited situations. Fried suggested that a "decent minimum" (routine services) should be available to all, but that high-technology services are limited in several ways and should be available on a different basis.[44]

Helpful theories of microallocation—allocation to individuals—of exotic lifesaving services have been developed by Childress and Rescher. They consider the problem of how (by what criteria) decisions are to be made about who gets what. Both start by applying medical criteria to determine need and appropriateness for treatment. Then they diverge.

Childress rejected subjective criteria (utilitarianism) because these comparisons demean people and run counter to the inherent dignity of human beings. He argued that the only ethical system of allocation is one that views all people needing a specific treatment as equals. To properly recognize human beings, treatment should be provided on a first-come, first-served basis or, alternatively, through random selection, as by a lottery.[45]

Rescher used a two-tiered approach. The first tier consists of basic screening for factors such as constituency served (service area), progress of science (benefit of advancing science), and prospect of success by type of treatment or recipient, such as denying dialysis to the very young or very old. The second tier considers individual patients and judges biomedical factors, including relative likelihood of success for the patient and life expectancy, and social aspects including family role, potential future contributions, and past services rendered. When all factors were equal for two people, Rescher used random selection to make a final choice.[46] Because they result from value judgments, the social aspects are the most difficult. Rescher considered it irrational, however, to choose based on chance (after meeting medical criteria), as Childress advocated.

Each microallocation theory has advantages and disadvantages; the resulting decisions will not satisfy everyone. However, the decision frameworks address issues and problems in an organized fashion. The choice of which people will receive extraordinary lifesaving treatment may be unpredictable, in the case of random allocations (Childress), or rational and almost totally predictable (Rescher). It may be left to chance, and in that sense fair to all needing treatment (Childress), or a matter of primarily subjective criteria (Rescher). Awareness of how choices are made allows the public to know that the system is fair. Kantian principles of respect for persons and not using people as means to ends are reflected in Childress's theory. Rescher's criteria are predominantly utilitarian. Few HSOs/HSs address the ethical issues of resource allocation in an organized, prospective manner.

Consent

Ethical and legal aspects of consent are similar, but ethical expectations are higher. The concept began in the law as protecting a person's right to be free from nonconsensual touching. This right at law and in ethics has expanded and includes autonomy (part of the principle of respect for persons) and self-determination, as well as a reflection of the special relationship of trust and confidence (fiduciary relationship) between physician and patient. This reflects Kant's concept of the equality of human beings. The law recognizes that failing to obtain consent can lead to legal action for battery, an intentional tort. In addition, an action for negligence can be brought if physicians breach a duty to communicate information that is needed by the patient to make a decision.[47]

Both general codes of medical ethics, such as the AMA principles, and specialized codes, such as the 1975 Declaration of Helsinki (relating to biomedical research), recognize the importance of consent. Emphasizing patients' rights or sovereignty is an idealized view. It challenges a tradition of medical paternalism that makes the physician a dominant authoritarian figure who decides what is in the patient's best interest.[48]

Questions of consent arise initially when a patient seeks treatment. Consent usually is implied because the patient has sought treatment. Consent also is implied in life-threatening emergencies. Elective, routine treatment requires only general consent, as compared with special consent obtained for invasive, surgical, or experimental or unusual types of procedures. All consent must be voluntary, competent, and informed.

Voluntary means that consent is given without duress that substantially influenced the decision. Prisoners are a group whose incarceration greatly diminishes their independence; thus it is impossible for them to give voluntary consent to be part of an experiment, for example. Voluntariness also is reduced when inducements to participate are so great that one becomes imprudent and incautious. Similarly, there are circumstances when even small inducements reduce voluntariness; for example, starving people offered food may agree to take part in a risky experiment.

Beyond such obvious problems, voluntariness is an elusive concept. Patients may be under duress to accept physician recommendations because they fear being seen as difficult and losing the physician's goodwill and cooperation. Patients are influenced by family and friends and may be persuaded (perhaps coerced) by them to accept (or reject) treatment. It has been suggested that one's freedom to accept or reject medical treatment is reduced to only that of the right to veto unwanted procedures.[49] Such arguments amplify the need to understand the complex relationships in medicine and preclude simple answers about voluntary consent.

Competent consent means that patients know the nature and consequences of what is contemplated or the decision to be made. The law presumes that unemancipated minors are incompetent, as are people with mental illness or developmental disability.

The third element of consent is that it be informed. Some discussions incorrectly refer to "informed consent" as if being informed were the only criterion. This assumption ignores the other two elements. Historically, the legal standard for informed consent required disclosure of the condition for which treatment was proposed and all significant facts about it, and an explanation of likely consequences and difficulties related to the proposed treatment. This standard was based on the amount of information that a reasonable physician would give in the same or similar circumstances. By comparison, ethical criteria suggest more active patient participation. Criteria developed by the President's Commission for the Study of Ethical Problems in Medicine and Biomedical and Behavioral Research state that patient sovereignty with complete participation in the process is preferred. The Commission recognized that such participation is a goal not easily achieved, however.[50]

A number of courts have adopted a standard that is based on what a typical (reasonable) patient would want to know. A legal criterion that is oriented to patient sovereignty and used in a few jurisdictions asks, "What would *this* patient want to know?" The latter legal standard is consistent with the President's Commission position and reflects the ethical view that a covenant (contract) between patient and physician should guide their relationship.

The consent procedures that HSOs use are covered in Chapter 14. HSOs are likely to apply a legally oriented consent process whose primary purpose is self-protection. Typically, there is little emphasis on an ethical relationship with a higher standard of participation. This utilitarian approach is legally prudent but ignores the positive ethical obligation to the patient that is suggested by the principle of respect for persons.

Ethical Issues in Research

Medicine has always experimented by attempting new means, methods, and techniques. Medical knowledge would stagnate without research. Health services managers may think that experimenting is exclusive to academic medical centers or specialized facilities, where rigorous standards are applied. Many HSOs conduct research, however, some of which may be unknown by nonclinical managers.

All codes of ethics in research emphasize the subject's voluntary, informed consent. Competence receives less attention. A provision in the Nuremberg Code (1949) states that subjects should be able to stop the experiment if they no longer wish to continue to participate in it. This puts a heavy burden on the subject, who may be incapacitated by the research or a medical problem, or may be intimidated by the setting. Subjects, too, usually lack the technical competence to know when they are at risk. This weakness was partly corrected in the Declaration of Helsinki (1964, revised 1975), which recommends establishing an independent committee to review and approve the research protocol. This type of committee, known as an institutional review board (IRB), is described later. IRBs are required by the Department of Health and Human Services (DHHS) for the research that it funds.

Another issue is whether research is therapeutic or nontherapeutic. Therapeutic research occurs when an experimental treatment might benefit the subject—the subject also is the patient. Nontherapeutic research involves healthy subjects or patients with medical problems other than those that might benefit from the experimental treatment. This lack of potential benefit means that non therapeutic research should receive closer attention, and special emphasis should be placed on the quality of consent. Some commentators have argued that nondiagnostic *and* nontherapeutic research on children and incompetent adults should be prohibited.[51]

All codes and guidelines permit nontherapeutic research. They recognize that volunteers for whom the experimental treatment offers no diagnostic or therapeutic advantage are needed for certain research. All codes are utilitarian (except the paternalism in the AMA guidelines) and suggest comparing and balancing risks to subjects in nontherapeutic research with benefits to society. Emphases on voluntary and informed consent in the codes are Kantian and reflect the principles of respect for persons and nonmaleficence.

The DHHS regulations contain a mix of moral philosophies and values. Beneficence and its subsidiary, cost–benefit analysis, determine the benefits of research compared with the risks. A Kantian perspective and principles of respect for persons and nonmaleficence underlie consent, privacy, and confidentiality requirements.

A major problem with research codes other than federal regulations is that they inadequately separate the physician's roles as healer and researcher. This combination carries a heavy ethical burden because the duality of interests puts physician-researchers in a classical conflict-of-interest situation. What is good for the research subject as a patient may not be good for the experimental design. This problem is exacerbated in nontherapeutic research, in which the risk to the subject is not balanced by potential benefit. AMA research guidelines recognize the dilemma but adopt a paternalistic view of the relationship between physician and patient-subject by asking the physician to exercise professional skill and judgment to act in the best interests of the patient-subject.

The U.S. Food and Drug Administration (FDA) does not regulate surgical experimentation. Thus, for example, it does not determine whether coronary artery bypass surgery or radial keratotomy (ophthalmic surgery) are safe and efficacious. Neither does FDA regulate innovative clinical care, defined as new uses of existing treatments, drugs, and devices. Innovative treatment must be distinguished from standard therapy and should require more demanding review and consent procedures. Absent government regulation, HSO/HS managers, staff, and clinicians must monitor innovative uses of drugs or treatments or new types of surgery. A requirement that results must be submitted to peer review by publishing them in the professional literature is a type of control, but it is far removed from the research and protects prospective rather than current patients. The patient's only recourse may be medical malpractice litigation.

Organizational policies must distinguish unauthorized from authorized experimentation. Obtaining a few extra milliliters of amniotic fluid during amniocentesis causes moderate additional risk. Experimenting on unused urine routinely collected for other purposes or performing analyses on the placenta poses no risk to the patient, but requires consent nonetheless. Minor or nonexistent risks do not justify ignoring patients' rights and the duties that are owed them.

End-of-Life Decisions

The historical definition of death as cessation of blood circulation and of circulation-dependent animal and vital functions such as respiration and pulsation proved inadequate as technology advanced. A 1968 Harvard Medical School committee definition of irreversible coma was an important first step in redefining death.[52] These criteria were useful, but the President's Commission noted several criticisms.[53]

The Harvard criteria's emphasis on the physician's paternalistic role is inconsistent with the changes since 1968 that include patient autonomy expressed in living wills and natural death act declarations, family involvement in decision making, and use of institutional ethics committees. These changes diminish the centrality and primacy of the physician's role.

By 1995, 31 states and the District of Columbia had enacted the Uniform Determination of Death Act, which has alternate definitions of death: irreversible cessation of circulatory and respiratory functions, or irreversible cessation of all functions of the entire brain, including the brain stem (brain death).[54] Table 13.1 shows various definitions of death. The progression from physiologic

TABLE 13.1. DEFINITION OF DEATH

Concept of death (philosophical or theological judgment of the essentially significant change at death)	Locus of death (place to look to determine whether a person has died)	Criteria of death (measurements physicians or other officials use to determine whether a person is dead—to be determined by scientific empirical study)
1. Irreversible loss of flow of vital fluids (i.e., the blood and breath)	Heart and lungs	Visual observation of respiration, perhaps with the use of a mirror Feeling of the pulse, possibly supported by electrocardiogram
2. Irreversible loss of the soul from the body	Pineal body(?) (according to Descartes) Respiratory tract?	Observation of breath (?)
3. Irreversible loss of the capacity for bodily integration	Brain	Unreceptivity and unresponsivity No movements or breathing No reflexes (except spinal reflexes) Flat electroencephalogram (to be used as confirmatory evidence) All tests to be repeated 24 hours later (excluded conditions: hypothermia and central nervous system drug depression)
4. Irreversible loss of consciousness or the capacity for social interaction	Probably the neocortex	Electroencephalogram

Adapted from Veatch, Robert M. *Death, Dying, and the Biological Revolution: Our Last Quest for Responsibility*, 53. New Haven, CT: Yale University Press, 1976. © Yale University Press. This table has been modified using material from the 1989 second edition.

Note: Death is defined as a complete change in the status of a living entity characterized by the irreversible loss of those characteristics that are essentially significant to it. The possible concepts, loci, and criteria of death are much more complex than the ones given here. These are meant to be simplified models of types of positions being taken in the current debate. It is obvious that those who believe that death means the irreversible loss of the capacity for bodily integration (3) or the irreversible loss of consciousness (4) have no reservations about pronouncing death when the heart and lungs have ceased to function. This is because they are willing to use loss of heart and lung activity as shortcut criteria for death, believing that, once heart and lungs have stopped, the brain or neocortex will necessarily stop as well.

measures such as respiration and pulse to sociopsychological factors such as the capacity for social interaction has ominous portent.

Life-Sustaining Treatment

Among HSOs, hospitals and nursing facilities often face ethical issues regarding withholding or withdrawing life-sustaining treatment. Historically, potential legal liability caused a reluctance to withdraw life support absent court intervention. The first case receiving national attention, *In re Quinlan*,[55] occurred in 1976 when the New Jersey Supreme Court permitted 21-year-old Karen Ann Quinlan's father to be appointed her guardian. He was authorized to withdraw all extraordinary life-sustaining procedures if the family and physicians concurred that Quinlan had no reasonable possibility of emerging from a persistent vegetative state (PVS)[56] and if the hospital ethics committee confirmed the prognosis. This was one of the earliest enunciations of a role for ethics committees in hospitals. Quinlan was weaned from the respirator and transferred to a nursing facility, where she died after 10 years in PVS.

In 1990 the U.S. Supreme Court first ruled on a case involving life-sustaining treatment, *Cruzan v. Director, Missouri Department of Health*.[57] Nancy Cruzan had been in PVS since her 1983 automobile accident. She was a patient in a Missouri state hospital, where a gastrostomy tube had been inserted for nutrition and hydration. Cruzan's parents brought suit after the facility refused their request to remove the tube. The case was eventually appealed to the U.S. Supreme Court, which held that the U.S. Constitution does not prevent Missouri from requiring "clear and convincing evidence" that an incompetent person in PVS would not wish to be kept alive artificially. The Court distinguished the rights of competent people, who are assumed to have a constitutionally protected right to refuse life-sustaining hydration and nutrition, from the rights of incompetent people. The opinion noted that, although Missouri recognized that there were circumstances when a surrogate may act for a patient in electing to withdraw hydration and nutrition and thus cause death, the state had established a procedural safeguard to ensure that the surrogate's actions conform with the wishes that are expressed by the patient while competent. Allowing a clear and convincing evidence standard recognized broad state latitude to protect and preserve human life in life continuation decisions. It also noted that the state may guard against potential abuses by surrogates who may not act to protect a patient's interests and that the state may decline to include judgments about the quality of a patient's life. The Court did not, however, outline the limits of action that a state could take.

In late 1990 Cruzan's parents were granted a second hearing in state court, which the state of Missouri did not oppose. New evidence convinced a judge that Cruzan would not have wanted to live in PVS, and he ordered the feeding tube removed. Cruzan died a few days later.

Child Abuse

"Baby Doe" is a name taken from the 1982 Indiana case brought after parents declined to treat a newborn with Down syndrome who had duodenal atresia (no opening between the stomach and intestine) and possible other anomalies. A court agreed that nontreatment was one medically recommended option. As expected, the untreated infant died. Baby Doe was unlike Karen Ann Quinlan or Nancy Cruzan in that he was not in PVS, nor was he terminally ill. A simple surgical procedure would have corrected the atresia but not the underlying mental disability.

That case and another in Illinois prompted DHHS to issue regulations prohibiting hospitals that received federal funds from denying care to infants with disabilities. DHHS claimed authority for the regulations under Section 504 of the Rehabilitation Act of 1973, which prohibits discrimination on the basis of disability. The regulations were legally challenged on procedural grounds because the period for public comment was too short. An attempt to promulgate a modified version of the regulations followed in 1983. Like the first, they proposed telephone hotlines to report alleged cases of withholding life-sustaining care from seriously ill newborns. An important change was that the Rehabilitation Act did not require "impossible or futile acts or therapies that merely prolong the process of dying of an infant born terminally ill."[58]

The original controversy prompted Congress to address the issue of newborns with defects, and the Child Abuse Amendments of 1984 established treatment and reporting guidelines for severely disabled newborns. Withholding "medically indicated treatment" from disabled infants is illegal except when

> *in the treating physician's(s') reasonable medical judgment, (i) the infant is chronically and irreversibly comatose; (ii) the provision of such treatment would merely prolong dying, not be effective in ameliorating or correcting all of the infant's life-threatening conditions, or otherwise be futile in terms of survival of the infant; or (iii) the provision of such treatment would be virtually futile in terms of the survival of the infant and the treatment itself under such circumstances would be inhumane.*[59]

The law requires that all infants receive "appropriate nutrition, hydration, and medication," regardless of their condition or prognosis. The law also requires that health facilities designate people to report suspected medical neglect problems to state child protective services agencies that would coordinate and consult with those people and may initiate legal action. The infant care review committees recommended in the regulations are discussed later in this chapter.

Advance Directives

Patient participation in and control of health care decisions were enhanced when the federal Patient Self Determination Act (PSDA) of 1989 took effect December 1, 1991. PSDA requires that HSOs participating in Medicare and Medicaid give *all* patients written information about their rights under state law to accept or refuse treatment and to formulate advance directives.[60] Medical records must document whether a patient has an advance directive, and the HSO must educate staff and community about them. There is some evidence that PSDA has increased the use of advance directives in nursing facility residents. Despite PSDA and widespread state legislation, most patients do not have advance directives.[61]

Living Wills

The concept of living wills was developed several decades ago as a way for a person's wishes regarding medical treatment to be communicated to caregivers if that individual could not communicate them. In theory, living wills allow a person to control treatment, regardless of potential benefit. Absent legislation or case law, living wills have no legal status; patients must rely on the willingness of caregivers to follow their directives.

Natural Death Act Statutes

Interest in living wills and public reaction to situations in which seemingly excessive treatment was provided led to state laws recognizing the patient's right to control treatment. They may be called living wills laws, natural death acts, or death with dignity laws. In early 1983, 14 states had such laws. By 1985 the District of Columbia and 35 states had such laws; by 1999 only Massachusetts, Michigan, and New York did not have them.[62] The content of an advance directive suggested for Virginia is shown as Figure 13.5.

In general, the laws recognize a patient's right to direct caregivers to withhold or withdraw life-sustaining treatment. If statutory requirements are met, then the directives legally bind caregivers. These laws tend to be drafted narrowly and apply when a physician determines that the patient who signed the declaration is terminally ill and has no prospect of recovery. Some states require the directives to be reaffirmed when patients know they have a terminal illness. Some laws include penal-

An advance directive executed pursuant to this article may, but need not, be in the following form, and may (i) direct a specific procedure or treatment to be provided, such as artificially administered hydration and nutrition; (ii) direct a specific procedure or treatment to be withheld; or (iii) appoint an agent to make health care decisions for the declarant as specified in the advance directive if the declarant is determined to be incapable of making an informed decision, including the decision to make, after the declarant's death, an anatomical gift of all or any part of the declarant's body pursuant to Article 2 (§ 32.1-289 et seq.) of Chapter 8 of Title 32.1 and in compliance with any directions of the declarant. Should any other specific directions be held to be invalid, such invalidity shall not affect the advance directive. If the declarant appoints an agent in an advance directive, that agent shall have the authority to make health care decisions for the declarant as specified in the advance directive if the declarant is determined to be incapable of making an informed decision and shall have decision-making priority over any individuals authorized under § 54.1-2986 to make health care decisions for the declarant.

ADVANCE MEDICAL DIRECTIVE

I, . . . , willfully and voluntarily make known my desire and do hereby declare:

If at any time my attending physician should determine that I have a terminal condition where the application of life-prolonging procedures would serve only to artificially prolong the dying process, I direct that such procedures be withheld or withdrawn, and that I be permitted to die naturally with only the administration of medication or the performance of any medical procedure deemed necessary to provide me with comfort care or to alleviate pain (OPTION: I specifically direct that the following procedures or treatments be provided to me:..........................)

In the absence of my ability to give directions regarding the use of such life-prolonging procedures, it is my intention that this advance directive shall be honored by my family and physician as the final expression of my legal right to refuse medical or surgical treatment and accept the consequences of such refusal.

OPTION: APPOINTMENT OF AGENT (CROSS THROUGH IF YOU DO NOT WANT TO APPOINT AN AGENT TO MAKE HEALTH CARE DECISIONS FOR YOU.)

(This section provides for appointment of primary and successor agents for health care decisions, including a general discussion of powers, roles, and relationships and limits the agent's authority to times when the declarant is incapable of making an informed decision.)

OPTION: POWERS OF MY AGENT (CROSS THROUGH ANY LANGUAGE YOU DO NOT WANT AND ADD ANY LANGUAGE YOU DO WANT.)

(This section allows the declarant to select specific powers of the agent for health care decisions.)

OPTION: APPOINTMENT OF AN AGENT TO MAKE AN ANATOMICAL GIFT (CROSS THROUGH IF YOU DO NOT WANT TO APPOINT AN AGENT TO MAKE AN ANATOMICAL GIFT FOR YOU.)

(This section allows the agent for health care decisions to make anatomical gifts of the declarant.)

This advance directive shall not terminate in the event of my disability.

By signing below, I indicate that I am emotionally and mentally competent to make this advance directive and that I understand the purpose and effect of this document.

_____   _____

(Date)   (Signature of Declarant)

The declarant signed the foregoing advance directive in my presence. I am not the spouse or a blood relative of the declarant.

(Witness) _____

Figure 13.5.   Suggested form of Written Natural Death Act Declaration adopted by the State of Virginia. (From *Code of Virginia 1950, 1990 Cumulative Supplement,* Vol. 7A, Title 54.1, Article 8, Section 2984, 197–198.)

ties against caregivers and the organization if directives are ignored. In addition to statutes, appeals court and state supreme court decisions affect how the laws are interpreted and if life-sustaining treatment is withheld or withdrawn. These laws solve some of the issues of control (autonomy), patient and family roles, and, to an extent, organizational and provider efforts to comply with patient wishes.

Problems with Advance Directives

Three studies of advance directives were not encouraging. The one fifth of patients who actually write down their treatment preferences usually do not tell their physicians, and only about one third of that one fifth have this information entered on their medical chart. Of this small number, most statements were too vague to be helpful in guiding specific decisions about treatment.[63]

Furthermore, an advance directive may be ignored because caregivers are unaware of it or disagree with it or because family members make other demands. Fragmented care complicates patients' use of advance directives and poses a special challenge to managers. For example, an advance directive in a medical record at a nursing facility may be left behind when a patient is hospitalized. A study of elderly patients hospitalized for acute illnesses found that 75% of the time the medical record did not indicate that physicians had consulted the patient's living will or designated proxy before making treatment decisions, including whether to resuscitate. This failure occurred because nursing facilities failed to transfer the information, patients were not asked or did not volunteer the information, and hospital staff failed to ask or to ensure that such documents were part of the record. Once documented in the hospital record, advance directives influenced treatment decisions in 86% of cases involving incompetent patients.[64]

Other problems regarding advance directives include determining mental status and whether the patient comprehends the effect of what is being done and establishing the presence of a terminal illness. Ethical problems are more likely if statutory requirements have not been met.

The HSO's/HS's challenge is to develop processes that promote completion of advance directives. Completion rates for advance directives can be improved by altering the time when they are distributed to patients.[65] Patients were far more likely to complete an advance directive at a hospital that distributed information several days before admission rather than the day of admission. Patients were much more likely to read the information provided when it was available before hospitalization. The most common reason given for not completing an advance directive was that it was not seen or was not read—a problem much more common in the hospital that did not provide information in advance.[66] Providing reminders, education, and feedback to attending physicians and a new documentation form used by physicians for advance directives can greatly increase the percentage of patients who have advance directives. After these changes, 87% of physician-attested directives agreed with the treatment preferences of patients interviewed, and physicians' attitudes and interest in advance directives improved.[67] In part, the care of dying patients may not have kept pace with national recommendations because many physicians and nurses disagreed with them or may have been unaware of key guidelines, such as permissibility of withdrawing treatments.[68] Furthermore, the amount of care that dying patients receive varies greatly in different parts of the United States and seems to be a function of how much care is available, not of how much patients need.[69]

Substituted Judgment

Surrogates make decisions for people who are incompetent to make them because they are too young or have a physical or mental disability. Before advance directives, surrogates were appointed on petition to a court, which then determined that a person was incompetent to make decisions about health care. To ease the use of surrogates, many states enacted laws allowing surrogates to make decisions for people without advance directives. By June 1998, 28 states and the District of Columbia had authorized surrogate decision making in such situations.[70]

Powers of attorney are another type of decision making by a surrogate. These delegations of authority are prepared before the fact, however, and may be general or limited. Powers of attorney are "durable" when the authority continues beyond the time that the grantor becomes incompetent. Different names are used, but their effect is that health care agents and surrogate decision makers are granted durable powers of attorney for health care. These limited powers of attorney enable a surrogate to make legally binding decisions on behalf of the person who granted the power of attorney. By 1998 the District of Columbia and 49 states had statutes specifically recognizing the appointment of health care agents.[71] Figures 13.6 and 13.7 show a durable health care power of attorney and health care treatment instructions form, respectively. State requirements must be met when surrogates make decisions.

Durable Health Care Power of Attorney

I, _____, of _____ County, Pennsylvania, appoint the person named below to be my agent to make health and personal care decisions for me **when and only when I lack sufficient capacity to make or communicate a choice regarding a health or personal care decision as verified by my attending physician.** My agent may not delegate the authority to make decisions.

MY AGENT HAS ALL OF THE FOLLOWING POWERS (SUBJECT TO THE HEALTH CARE TREATMENT INSTRUCTIONS THAT FOLLOW IN PART II).

1.   To authorize, withhold or withdraw medical care and surgical procedures;
2.   **To authorize, withhold or withdraw nutrition (food) or hydration (water) medically supplied by tube through my nose, stomach, intestines, or veins;**
3.   To authorize my admission to or discharge from a medical, nursing, residential or similar facility and to make agreements for my care, including hospice care;
4.   To have full access to my medical and hospital records and all information regarding my physical or mental health;
5.   To hire and fire medical, social service and other support personnel responsible for my care;
6.   To take any legal action necessary to do what I have directed.

APPOINTMENT OF AGENT

I appoint the following agent:

Agent: _____
(Name and relationship)

Address: _____

Telephone: Home _____   Work _____

You are not required to appoint an agent. If you don't wish to appoint an agent, write "None" in the above space. If you don't name an agent, health care providers will ask your family for help in determining your wishes for treatment.

If my agent is not available or if my agent is my spouse and becomes divorced from me <u>after</u> the date of this document, I appoint the person or persons named below in the order named. *(It is helpful, but not required, to name alternative agents.)*

First Alternative Agent: Second Alternative Agent:

_____   _____
(Name and relationship)   (Name and relationship)

Address: _____   Address: _____

Telephone: Home _____ Work _____   Telephone: Home _____ Work _____

Figure 13.6.   A sample durable power of attorney for health care decisions. (From the Allegheny County Bar Association/Allegheny County Medical Society, Pittsburgh, Pennsylvania; reprinted by permission.)

Do-Not-Resuscitate Orders

The do-not-resuscitate (DNR) order is another type of advance directive, albeit much closer to the delivery of services. Most patients neither have drawn up living wills nor have executed advance directives that comply with state requirements. This fact emphasizes the need for HSOs to prospectively address issues about resuscitating terminally ill patients and patients for whom life-continuation decisions must be made (e.g., patients in PVS). Typically, HSOs have a DNR policy affirming the legal right of a patient (or a surrogate) to direct caregivers. The DNR policy should identify chemical and mechanical technologies included and when they will be applied. Patients with a DNR order may require surgery and anesthesia management for palliative care, for relief of pain or distress, or to improve the quality of life. These interventions present unique ethical problems that the organization should address prospectively.[72] More recent are nonhospital DNR orders, which allow resuscitation to be refused in medical emergencies. In 1999 statutes in 37 states recognized nonhospital DNR orders.[73] Often, these are known as emergency medical services (EMS) do-not-resuscitate orders, or EMS-DNRs. They make the patient's wishes legally binding in the home or a similar setting and supersede state laws that require EMS technicians to undertake cardiopulmonary resuscitation (CPR).

PART II - HEALTHCARE TREATMENT INSTRUCTIONS
(LIVING WILL)

The following healthcare treatment instructions exercise my right to make decisions concerning my health care. These instructions are intended to provide clear and convincing evidence of my wishes to be followed when I lack the capacity to make or communicate my treatment decisions:

TERMINAL ILLNESS OR PERMANENT UNCONSCIOUSNESS

If I suffer from a terminal condition or a state of permanent unconsciousness such as a permanent coma or persistent vegetative state and there is no realistic hope of significant recovery, all of the following apply:

1. I direct that I be given health care treatment to relieve pain or provide comfort even if such treatment might shorten my life, suppress my appetite or my breathing, or be habit forming;
2. I direct that all life prolonging procedures be withheld or withdrawn;
3. I specifically do not want any of the following as life prolonging procedures: heart-lung resuscitation (CPR), mechanical ventilator (breathing machine), dialysis (kidney machine), surgery, chemotherapy, radiation treatment, antibiotics.

Please indicate whether you want nutrition (food) or hydration (water) medically supplied by a tube into your nose, stomach, intestine or veins if you suffer from a terminal condition or a state of permanent unconsciousness and there is no realistic hope of significant recovery. (Initial only one statement.)

TUBE FEEDINGS

_____ I want tube feedings to be given.

OR

NO TUBE FEEDINGS

_____ I do not want tube feedings to be given.

OTHER EXTREME CONDITIONS

If I should suffer from irreversible brain damage or brain disease with no realistic hope of significant recovery, I would consider such a condition intolerable and I want my health care providers and agent to treat any intervening life-threatening conditions just as they would a terminal condition or state of permanent unconsciousness as I have indicated above.

Initials _____ I agree

Initials _____ I disagree

GOALS (OPTIONAL)

My goals in making medical decisions if I suffer from a terminal illness or other extreme irreversible medical condition are as follows *(insert your personal priorities such as comfort care, preservation of mental functions, etc.)*:_____

_____

_____

AGENT'S USE OF INSTRUCTIONS *(Initial one option only.)*

_____ My agent must follow these instructions.

OR

_____ These instructions are only guidance. My agent shall have final say, and may override any of my instructions.

If I did not appoint an agent, these instructions shall be followed.

LEGAL PROTECTION

On behalf of myself, my executors and heirs I hold my agents and my health care providers harmless, and release and indemnify them against any claim for recognizing my agents' authority or for following my treatment instructions in good faith.

SIGNATURE

Having carefully read this document, I have signed it this _____ day of _____, 19____, revoking all previous health care powers of attorney and medical treatment instructions.

_____

(SIGN FULL NAME HERE FOR HEALTHCARE POWER OF ATTORNEY AND HEALTHCARE TREATMENT INSTRUCTIONS)

WITNESS:_____   WITNESS:_____

Two witnesses at least 18 years of age are required in Pennsylvania and should witness your signature in each other's presence. (It is preferable if the witnesses are not your heirs nor your creditors, nor employed by any of your health care providers.)

NOTARIZATION (OPTIONAL)

(Notarization of document is not required in Pennsylvania, but if the document is both witnessed and notarized, it is more likely to be honored in some other states.)

On this _____ day of _____, 19____, before me personally appeared the aforesaid declarant, to me known to be the person described in and who executed the foregoing instrument and acknowledged that he/she executed the same as his/her free act and deed. IN WITNESS WHEREOF, I have hereunto set my hand and affixed my official seal in the County of _____, State of _____, the day and year first above written.

_____   _____
Notary Public   My commission expires

Figure 13.7.   A sample living will. (From the Allegheny County Bar Association/Allegheny County Medical Society, Pittsburgh, Pennsylvania; reprinted by permission.)

Resulting inconsistencies in applying DNR orders because of lack of DNR policies were shown at three Houston teaching hospitals.[74] Some DNR patients underwent chemotherapy and surgery and were admitted to the intensive care unit (ICU). At the other extreme, some DNR patients received inadequate hydration and nutrition. Staff were confused about what care DNR patients were to receive, perhaps because they disagreed with decisions. In 10% of the cases no decisions had been made about keeping the patient alive. In most no-decision cases the subject of DNR had not been broached with the patient or family. This lack suggests that efforts to decide about resuscitation before a crisis commonly fail. Other studies of DNR orders report similar findings.[75] A key aspect of DNR is whether patient wishes about CPR are clear to physicians. One study found that, in nearly one of three cases, the patient's preference not to receive CPR was at odds with the doctor's perception of what the patient wanted.[76]

Another dimension of DNR orders is whether they are written equitably for patients with different diseases but similar prognoses. A study reported in 1995 that DNR orders were written more often for older patients, women, and patients with dementia or incontinence and less often for patients who are African American, had Medicaid insurance, or were in rural hospitals.[77] An earlier study found similar disparities: DNR orders were much more likely to be written for patients with acquired immunodeficiency syndrome (AIDS) or inoperable lung cancer than for patients with other diseases with equally poor prognoses, such as cirrhosis or heart failure.[78] Neither study assigned causes for the differences.

A more important problem may be forgoing treatment because the physician assumes that it is not in a patient's interests or because the physician believes that the patient would not want it.[79] Such actions do not consider the patient's autonomy as either an independent decision maker or involved participant. In sum, findings such as these suggest major ethical problems involving DNR orders for hospitalized patients.

Summary

It has been suggested that widespread use of advance directives might encourage systematic rationing of health care, especially to older adults. If a right to die becomes a duty to die, then the living will and its progeny, the natural death act declaration, will have become Frankenstein's monster. Indeed, statements made in the 1980s by a state governor and DHHS officials that older people should be required to have living wills raised a storm of protest. Regardless of true motives, such suggestions are perceived as motivated by economics.

The HSO/HS must be alert to the ethical issues of advance directives. Health services managers must consider them prospectively and develop policies that respect patients' wishes, consistent with organizational values.

Euthanasia

It is important to distinguish *euthanasia* from *natural death* or *death with dignity,* the latter of which mean that the patient or a surrogate has directed that life-sustaining treatment be withheld or withdrawn so life is not artificially extended. The Hippocratic tradition prohibited physicians from giving a deadly drug, and euthanasia (Greek for "good death" [*eu* and *thanatos*]) described care that made an inevitable death pain-free. In contemporary use, however, euthanasia often is synonymous with mercy killing—active steps that cause death. It is important to understand the ethical distinctions between providing comfort care and pain control to allow a pain-free, dignified death and hastening death through active intervention.

Ordinary versus Extraordinary Care

Hastening or bringing about death by increasing the dosage of a painkiller beyond that which is needed to control pain would be euthanasia, an action that is illegal in almost all states. As defined here, comfort care and pain relief are ordinary care. Care that offered no hope of benefit would be extraordinary. Historically, hydration and nutrition were considered ordinary, a distinction that is contemporarily hotly contested. The principle of nonmaleficence provides a distinction:

> *Ordinary means are all medicines, treatments, and operations which offer reasonable hope of benefit and which can be obtained and used without excessive expense, pain, or other inconvenience. Extraordinary means are all medicines, treatments, and operations which cannot be obtained or used without excessive expense, pain, or inconvenience, or which, if used, would not offer a reasonable hope of benefit.*[80]

Ordinary and extraordinary do not mean usual and unusual, respectively. This would be confusing because there is variation even among similar hospitals as to which treatments are usual or unusual. Instead, the measure is hope of benefit compared with excessiveness of expense, pain, or other inconvenience. Absent hope of benefit, any medicine, treatment, or operation is extraordinary. If there is hope of benefit, then using the same medicine, treatment, or operation is not excessive, and is ordinary treatment.

The concepts of benefits and burdens of treatment were suggested in the late 1990s. Expressed as proportionality, *proportionate* and *disproportionate* are thought to be more descriptive than *ordinary* and *extraordinary*. Proportionate and disproportionate care are measured like ordinary and extraordinary care. The type of treatment and its complexity or risk, cost, and appropriateness are studied and compared with results to be expected, taking into account the state of sick people and their physical and moral resources.[81] If the benefit justifies the burden using this calculus, then treatment is ethical. Like ordinary and extraordinary, proportionate and disproportionate are primarily qualitative measures of treatment and can be summarized as "Does the benefit justify the burden?"

Types of Euthanasia

There are four permutations of euthanasia: voluntary active, voluntary passive, involuntary active, and involuntary passive. *Voluntary* means that the person has freely consented. *Involuntary* means that the person either has not freely consented or cannot freely consent but is presumed to want to die. *Active* means that there are positive steps to bring about death, an action that could be called killing. *Passive* means that nothing is done to hasten death—the natural course of the disease causes death. All types of euthanasia include comfort care and pain control.

Rule of Double Effect

Like ordinary and extraordinary care, double effect is a subset of nonmaleficence. Classical formulations of the rule of double effect (RDE) require that four conditions or elements be satisfied to justify an act with double effect. Each is a necessary condition; together they form sufficient conditions of morally permissible action.

1. The nature of the act. *The act must be good, or at least morally neutral (independent of its consequences).*
2. The agent's intention. *The agent intends only the good effect. The bad effect can be foreseen, tolerated, and permitted, but it must not be intended.*
3. The distinction between means and effects. *The bad effect must not be a means to the good effect. If the good effect were the direct causal result of the bad effect, the agent would intend the bad effect in pursuit of the good effect.*
4. Proportionality between the good effect and the bad effect. *The good effect must outweigh the bad effect. The bad effect is permissible only if a proportionate reason is present that compensates for permitting the foreseen bad effect.*[82]

As an example, it is ethical under the RDE to use increasing quantities of morphine to ease the pain of a dying patient.

Physician-Assisted Suicide

Physician-assisted suicide, often called aid in dying, is not euthanasia. Despite having characteristics of voluntary, active euthanasia, it differs in a critical aspect. Physician-assisted suicide occurs when a physician provides the means, medical advice, and assurance that death results. The person, not the physician, performs the act that causes death. Broadly defined, it is a good death because it is likely to be pain-free; however, it is not euthanasia, as defined here. Physical disability prevents some people from performing the act needed to commit suicide; they fit in the category of voluntary, active euthanasia. The mental competence of people to be assisted in suicide must be ensured.

In the Hippocratic tradition it is unethical for physicians to deliberately cause death, and, when there is no treatment, physicians are expected to "comfort always." Sometimes pain control caused administration of too much morphine, for example, but such unintended consequences never raised an ethical issue. The ethical prohibition did not consider the patient's wishes and is reflected in laws against homicide as well as in laws making it illegal to commit suicide.

In 1990 the first publicized physician-assisted suicide occurred when a 54-year-old Alzheimer's disease patient, Janet Adkins, was aided in her suicide by Jack Kevorkian, a retired Michigan pathologist. Kevorkian, known to his critics as Dr. Death, gained national prominence with a device that enabled people wishing to commit suicide to administer chemicals to themselves, after initial assistance from a physician. Commentators criticized Kevorkian's actions as flawed procedurally and questioned whether Adkins was competent because she had Alzheimer's disease.[83] The case focused public attention on active, voluntary euthanasia and assisted suicide. Kevorkian's role has varied in the more than 100 suicides he has assisted. In 1999 he was convicted of second-degree murder in a criminal trial in Michigan, where assisted suicide is illegal.[84]

Kevorkian had been criticized on professional and ethical grounds because he did not know his "patients," was unqualified to diagnose or understand illnesses because he is a pathologist, had a conflict of interest because he desired publicity for himself and (initially) his death machine, assisted people who were not terminally ill, and did not assess the mental competence of those who were assisted. Kevorkian hoped to establish a clinic for terminally ill people—an *obitorium*—to assist in suicides. In mid-1995 the U.S. Supreme Court declined to review Kevorkian's activities.[85]

Legal Aspects of Physician-Assisted Suicide

Ballot initiatives in Washington (1991) and California (1992) to legalize physician-assisted suicide were rejected, a result that is inconsistent with polls showing that a large majority of Americans favor physician help in dying for terminally ill patients. A substantial proportion of physicians receive such requests, and about 6% have complied at least once.[86] After narrowly approving physician-assisted suicide in the so-called Death with Dignity Act in 1994 (52% to 48%), Oregon voters were asked by the legislature to repeal the law, which they overwhelmingly rejected in November 1997 (60% to 40%). The law permits physicians to prescribe, but not administer, fatal doses of oral drugs to competent adults with less than 6 months to live. Other requirements are oral and written requests from the patient, consultations by other physicians, a 15-day waiting period, and notification by the physician of pharmacists and state health authorities.[87] Physicians who act in good faith are protected from professional discipline and legal liability.[88] The first suicide under the Oregon law was reported in March 1998.[89] In late 1998 Oregon Medicaid added physician-assisted suicide to end-of-life comfort care services such as pain medication and hospice.[90]

At this writing no nationwide trend to adopt laws similar to Oregon's has developed. In fact, statutes in 38 states criminalize assisted suicide, the common law criminalizes it in 6 states and the District of Columbia, and the legality of assisted suicide is unclear in 5 states.[91] In 1997 a unanimous U.S. Supreme Court ruled that states may ban physician-assisted suicide without violating either the due process or equal protection clauses of the 14th Amendment to the Constitution. The Court did not decide whether states could pass laws, such as in Oregon, giving people the choice of assisted suicide.[92]

Dutch Practice

The vanguard of aid in dying is the Netherlands, where euthanasia and assisted suicide have been practiced since the 1980s and where euthanasia is supported by 92% of the population.[93] In late 1999 the Dutch parliament considered the legalization of euthanasia and physician-assisted suicide. Passage was expected, which would make the Netherlands the first country to legalize these practices.[94] This step was a natural progression from a 1993 law that codified and clarified judicial guidelines permitting physicians to euthanize and assist in suicides if certain rules were followed.[95] The old rules included *voluntary* (patient's voluntary request to die), *competent* (patient must be mentally capable), *terminal* (no hope of recovery), *second opinion* (provided by an independent colleague), and *report* (physician informed coroner when death was not the result of natural causes; public prosecutor used this report to determine the appropriateness of the physician's action).[96]

As evidence that euthanasia and physician-assisted suicides occurred in the Netherlands before the 1993 change in the law, a 1990 government study found that 2% of deaths were caused by those means.[97] Other findings showed that no consent had been obtained from the majority of patients from whom treatment had been withdrawn or withheld or who died from the administration of pain-killing drugs.[98]

Under the proposed law, physicians do not report euthanasia deaths to the coroner. Instead, cases go directly to a three-person committee, consisting of a physician, a lawyer, and an ethicist, for review. If the committee determines that hastening death was appropriate, then the prosecutor does not become involved. It is hoped that the proposed law will bring into the open hidden euthanasia that has occurred historically; effectively, the state will "be issuing retrospective licenses for consensual killing."[99]

As recently as 1993, only 11% of Dutch physicians said that they would not participate in euthanasia or assisted suicide.[100] Oregon physicians were far less willing than Dutch physicians to assist in suicide; 31% stated that they could not do so on moral grounds.[101] Legally sanctioning involuntary active euthanasia is a significant change and moves euthanasia from the exceptional to an accepted way of dealing with serious or terminal illness. Palliative care is one casualty of the Netherlands' history of aid in dying, and hospice care there lags behind other countries.[102]

The proposed Dutch law recognizes existing practice; de facto has become de jure but raises troubling ethical issues nevertheless. Although the practice was undertaken to enhance individual self-determination, data from the Netherlands show that euthanasia has not been limited to those who request it; this highlights the slippery slope, defined as one exception leading to other, more easily accepted exceptions. Others argue, however that data from the late 1990s are contrary and that the slippery slope has not been proved by the Dutch experience.[103]

Issues for Physicians

For many physicians, to assist in dying turns medicine on its head—those who traditionally guarded life are asked to end it. Organized medicine in the United States has condemned proposals that physicians provide aid in dying. Given that few Dutch physicians morally oppose aid in dying, and based on domestic survey findings, this reaction seems overstated. Nonetheless, aid in dying raises basic moral questions that necessitate reexamining the physician–patient relationship. To this point, at least, physicians cannot be required to perform a procedure to which they are morally opposed.

Surveys have found that a majority of physicians in Michigan (Kevorkian's home state) and Oregon favored legalizing assisted suicide, although a sizable minority in Oregon objected on moral grounds.[104] A national survey found 6% of physicians responding who regularly care for the dying had either given at least one lethal injection or written a prescription so patients could kill themselves—at a time when physician assistance in suicide was illegal. The survey also found that one third of doctors would write prescriptions for deadly doses and one fourth would give lethal injections *if* they were legal. Opiates such as morphine were the drugs that were given most often to help patients die.[105] Notably, in 1998 Oregon led the nation in the medical use of morphine, an increase of more than 70% since 1994, when voters approved the first assisted-suicide referendum.[106] By the end of 1999, approximately 30 people had been assisted in their suicides in Oregon.[107]

Demedicalizing aid in dying reduces some ethical problems for physicians but raises others. German law, for example, effectively makes it illegal for physicians to assist in suicides. Because neither suicide nor assisting the suicide of people who are capable of exercising control over their actions *and* who have freely made a responsible choice to commit suicide are illegal, however, unique societal views about suicide and aid in dying have developed in Germany.[108]

Issues for HSOs/HSs

Notably, none of Kevorkian's "work" occurred in a HSO. People came to him. HSOs/HSs will face the ethical issues of aid in dying. Nursing facilities, for example, will have PVS residents or bedridden residents with a terminal illness who are too ill for transfer. Managed care organizations must decide whether they will include aid in dying as a benefit. How will the person's rights compare with those of the HSO/HS? The importance of an organizational philosophy addressing aid in dying is clear. As with physicians, the HSO cannot be forced to participate in activities that compromise its ethic.

The physician's and organization's interests in voluntary or involuntary passive euthanasia are limited to questions of the futility of or hope of benefit from continued treatment. New forms of payment and new organizational arrangements will change HSO/HS economic incentives, even as they become less able to meet the costs of services. Hospitals already have experienced a form of capitation in diagnosis-related groups, which have the incentive to limit services. The increasing difficulty of cost shifting means HSOs/HSs must reduce costs through greater productivity or by changing the content of care (i.e., earlier death reduces costs).

When physicians were less affected by cost reduction, they counterbalanced organizational efforts to limit services. Traditional relationships are changing rapidly, however, and the economic oneness of physician and organization raises myriad ethical issues.

Any fixed-sum payment scheme (e.g., capitation) provides an incentive to minimize services, especially those that are costly. Such incentives cause an inherent conflict of interest between providing services that might be in the patient's best interests and holding to a fixed monetary limit. The result is that certain services, especially those that are high cost, are likely to be withheld and that services will be withdrawn from those deemed to have a poor quality of life or prognosis—the concept of futility care.

Futile Treatment

Futility theory has quantitative and qualitative aspects that focus on the absence of possible benefit from continued treatment. The quantitative determination is made by caregivers and addresses the probability of success if a treatment were attempted or continued. The patient or someone speaking on the patient's behalf makes the qualitative determination and assumes successful treatment, but asks whether the resulting quality of life is such that treatment ought to be undertaken.

In many ways futility theory is old wine in new bottles. Its origins lie in the distinction between ordinary and extraordinary care, which are distinguished by "hope of benefit" and "excessive expense, pain, or other inconvenience." These distinctions make it ethical to withhold any medicine, treatment, or operation that offers no reasonable hope of benefit or that cannot be obtained or used without excessive expense, pain, or inconvenience.

The issue of care arises when patients, surrogates, or both demand care that clinicians consider futile. Two cases involving surrogates are those of Helga Wanglie, a Minneapolis woman in PVS whose husband demanded that all efforts be made to keep her alive, despite a prognosis that doing so offered no hope of benefit; and that of Baby K, an anencephalic (major part of the brain missing) infant whose mother refused to authorize a DNR order and insisted that all treatment continue. HSOs themselves often insist on futile care, as exemplified by *Quinlan* and *Cruzan,* even if surrogates decide that care is futile and should not be provided. Thus futility policies may be important to HSOs/HSs, as well as patients and families.

Applying the futility concept has been described as a unilateral DNR order—a decision made by the physician using a physiological definition of what is futile.[109] The futility policy of Santa Monica Hospital Medical Center defines futile care as

> *Any clinical circumstance in which the doctor and his consultants, consistent with the available medical literature, conclude that further treatment (except comfort care) cannot, within a reasonable possibility, cure, ameliorate, improve or restore a quality of life that would be satisfactory to the patient.*[110]

The first two thirds of this policy is clinical and seeks to quantify the futility of continued care. The last third is patient focused and adds a subjective criterion—a value judgment: "a quality of life that *would be satisfactory to the patient*" (emphasis added). The two portions conflict. If the quality of life is satisfactory to the patient, regardless of how poor others might consider it to be, then clinical judgments about futility are irrelevant. These parts of the policy can be reconciled only if physicians act paternalistically and decide that a certain quality of life would be unsatisfactory to the patient.

Implementation of the policy includes several steps: informing the competent patient and family about the illness, options, and prognosis; emphasizing that the patient will be given all other support; providing names of consultants to give an independent opinion; providing the assistance of nurses, clergy, and others; involving the ethics committee, as appropriate; and giving sufficient time for the patient and family to consider the information. If, after these steps, the family is unconvinced, then "neither the doctor nor the hospital is required to provide care that is not medically indicated, and the family may be offered a substitute physician . . . and another hospital."[111] Most significant is the final step: "If it is determined that the patient can no longer benefit from an acute hospital stay and the patient insists on staying, or the family insists that the patient should remain, the mechanism for personal payment can be invoked."[112] The policy concludes with examples of futile care: irreversible coma or PVS, a terminally ill patient in whom applying life-sustaining procedures would only artificially delay the moment of death, and permanent dependence on ICU care.

The final step in the policy focuses on economics by stating that the hospital can bill the patient for care that was not medically indicated. This harsh result will be used infrequently because third parties pay for most hospital services, especially Medicare for older people and people with disabilities, among whom cases of futile care are likely to occur. In addition to unresolved and complex legal implications, such a policy raises public relations and political issues.

Implications

Futility theory goes well beyond the contemporary concept of autonomy. Patient autonomy is a negative right—the right to be free from unwanted treatment; to be able to say no, thank you. Futility theory limits what is perceived as a positive right, a right to demand care when it is claimed that there is no medical benefit to receiving it. From an ethical standpoint it is arguable no such right exists.

Futility theory is an aggressive approach to issues of extraordinary, disproportionate, and burdensome care. The decision maker is the physician. The sample policy states that there is a need to educate and inform the patient. The patient, the family, or both need not concur with the decision. This is very different from the shared decision making in what is considered the ideal: a nonpaternalistic physician–patient relationship. In fact, the problem that futility theory purports to address may be only partly attributable to patient demands. Research documents many shortcomings in the care of seriously ill, dying patients, especially the effectiveness of patient–physician communication.

The findings of the Study to Understand Prognoses and Preferences for Outcomes and Risks of Treatments (SUPPORT) research are compelling:

> [The] Study to Understand Prognoses and Preferences for Outcomes and Risks of Treatments patients were seriously ill, and their dying proved to be predictable, yet discussion and decisions substantially in advance of death were uncommon. Nearly half of all DNR orders were written in the last 2 days of life. The final hospitalization for half of patients included more than 8 days in generally undesirable states: in an ICU, receiving mechanical ventilation, or comatose. Families reported that half of the patients who were able to communicate in their last few days spent most of the time in moderate or severe pain.[113]

These results occurred in the intervention phase of the SUPPORT study despite the presence of nurses whose tasks were to improve communication and encourage the patient and family to engage in an informed and collaborative decision-making process with a well-informed physician. The authors concluded that more proactive and forceful measures may be needed. It was estimated that patients meeting SUPPORT criteria account for approximately 400,000 admissions per year in the United States. Such findings bolster the rather harsh approach that was taken in the futility policy noted earlier, but there is reason for caution.

In a corollary to the first phase of SUPPORT, investigators examined the impact of prognosis-based futility guidelines on survival and hospital length of stay in a cohort of seriously ill adults. They calculated the hospital days that would not be used if, on the third day, life-sustaining treatment had been stopped or not initiated for patients with an estimated 2-month survival of 1% or less. They found that only 10.8% of hospital days would have been forgone and concluded only modest savings would have resulted.[114]

If large numbers of patients demand futile care, then such guidelines will have several important effects. First, voluntary (patient, surrogates, or both have consented) passive euthanasia will exist in theory but will be rarely needed. Second, involuntary (patient, surrogates, or both have not consented) passive euthanasia will increase dramatically. Third, futile care policies and guidelines may become a means by which physicians feel that they are relieved of the obligation to talk to their patients, the patients' surrogates, or both. Finally, the current system that requires physicians to obtain consent before withdrawing life-sustaining treatment would be reconsidered.

The contradiction between medical science and quality of life in the definition of futile care suggests that a paternalistic quality-of-life decision is masquerading as scientific, objective decision making. If so, then futile care policies are more than a step back for patient autonomy; they are a return to the physician paternalism of Hippocrates.

The most compelling ethical issue raised is that the right to die may become a duty to die. Do futile care policies put HSOs and providers on a slippery slope? Will the policies become broader and more focused on the quality of life that clinicians determine would be acceptable to the patient? These questions can be answered only in retrospect, in itself not a cheery prospect.

Alternatives to Futile Care Policies

Absent data showing that patients, surrogates, or both commonly demand care that caregivers consider futile, futility policies may be solving a nonproblem. This is especially true given the published cases of patients who are forced to accept care. In addition, the SUPPORT investigators' findings as to economic impact should be explored further.

When a problem exists, one solution is the status quo; patients, surrogates, or both must agree to discontinue care after physicians have diagnosed it as futile. Complementing this alternative is enhancing the communication skills of caregivers so that patients and surrogates understand the prognosis. Objective predictions of survival or probability of good result, such as the Acute Physiology and Chronic Health Evaluation (APACHE) system, can assist decision makers (patients, surrogates, or both) to understand the best course of action. APACHE predicts probable outcomes of treatment using several variables; the data assist everyone in the process.

A second, more long-range solution is changing the presumption about care in cases of PVS, terminal illness, and brain death. It is presumed that care must be provided absent directives to the contrary. This presumption, reflecting Baconian theory about science conquering nature, has been reinforced by the law. Recognizing that medicine has limits requires a return to the Hippocratic tradition.[115] The presumption should be that care will be provided if there is a probability it will benefit the patient (i.e., the care contemplated is not futile).

A third solution is to apply a community standard, something each HSO is able to develop. This idea is that of protecting the "commons," the contemporary manifestation of which is communitarianism, a concept championed by Amitai Etzioni. Communitarianism means recognizing resource limits and cooperatively working within them.

HSOs/HSs should address several issues when developing a futile care policy. The first is determining the extent of the problem. Other solutions, such as making education on advance directives more effective and increasing the likelihood that such directives will be on the medical record, may be more appropriate. Most important, a futile care policy may provide guidelines and support for physicians, who will benefit from defining futile care. In turn, the policy may convince patients, surrogates, or both that treatment without hope of benefit should be stopped.

Acquired Immunodeficiency Syndrome[116]

The human immunodeficiency virus (HIV), which leads to AIDS, has proved an elusive foe. Much has been learned about HIV disease since it was identified in the early 1980s. For the United States, both the pessimistic prediction of a major outbreak in the general population and the optimistic prediction that it would be confined to and then eliminated from the homosexual population have proved wrong. There have been scientific breakthroughs in understanding HIV[117] and in treating AIDS, but there is neither a vaccine to prevent infection nor a cure once infected. New strains of HIV continue to be isolated.[118] Rapid mutation of HIV makes developing a vaccine with long-term effectiveness difficult, if not impossible. Even if a vaccine met specific effectiveness criteria, it would take several years of testing and clinical trials to determine whether the vaccine was effective enough to be made available.[119] Meanwhile, prevention and education have received attention that is unprecedented in modern public health.

Incidence and Prevalence

By mid-1999 a cumulative total of 711,344 AIDS cases had been reported to the Centers for Disease Control and Prevention (CDC); of this number, 59% have died.[120] Drugs and improved treatment regimens have increased the life expectancy of people with AIDS, but the outlook for long-term survival of those infected remains grim.

In 1986 it was estimated that 1–1.5 million Americans were infected with HIV.[121] In 1999 CDC estimated that 650,000–900,000 Americans were infected, of which about 300,000 had frank AIDS.[122] These numbers suggest that the HIV epidemic in the United States has plateaued and is waning. There was a 2% decline in the incidence rate (number of new cases) of HIV between 1996 and 1997. In 1997 the death rate from AIDS fell almost 50%, the largest single-year decline for a major cause of death ever recorded. The drop, which is attributed to the use of powerful new drugs, resulted in AIDS falling from 8th to 14th place as a cause of death among Americans. Some segments of the population, notably African American women and Hispanics, have an increasing incidence of HIV infection, however.[123] Increasingly, heterosexual contact is a major source of infection in women; the presence of sexually transmitted diseases (STDs) seems to be an important comorbidity.[174] It has been estimated that AIDS cases among African Americans will surpass those among Caucasians.[125] The first national survey of young homosexual and bisexual men found that the prevalence (existing infections) of HIV among those in their teens and early 20s who have homosexual encounters is 7%; more than one third reported unprotected anal sex in the past 6 months.[126]

Data about the spread of HIV among college students are troubling. In the late 1980s the average seroprevalence rate was 0.20%; the rate on one campus was greater than 0.60%.[127] This meant that, on average, 1 in 500 college students was HIV positive; at the higher level, 2 in 500 were. Seroprevalence was much higher for men (0.5%) than for women (0.02%). This study has not been replicated, however. Because there have been no changes in other indicators or surrogate markers that would suggest a significant change in results, the rates of HIV infection among college students in the 1980s were thought to be correct in 2000.[128] This evidence that college students are not taking the risk of AIDS seriously should be of great concern.

At the end of 1999 it was estimated that almost 40 million people worldwide are infected with HIV—33.6 million adults and children living with HIV/AIDS and another 5.6 million newly infected. Sub-Saharan Africa, where the adult prevalence rate of HIV is 8% (of which 55% are women), accounts for two thirds of the world total. HIV is increasing rapidly in Caribbean nations, where the adult prevalence rate is almost 2%. By comparison, North America has an adult prevalence rate of .56%.[129] HIV and its progression to AIDS is a modern pandemic that threatens to destroy the economic and social fabric of whole regions of the developing world.

Research and Treatment

Disproportionate amounts of federal research monies are spent on AIDS research. In 1997 the leading causes of death in the United States were diseases of the heart (935,350); malignant neoplasms, including neoplasms of lymphatic and hematopoietic tissues (535,480); and cerebrovascular diseases (159,160). Far down the list was HIV infection, with 22,040 deaths.[130] Despite these great differences, federal research on HIV disease is funded at $31,381 per death; heart disease research receives $1,129 per death.[131] Such policy making seems less than rational.

In addition, a great deal of AIDS research is occurring in the private sector, where pharmaceutical companies are developing drugs and vaccines to prevent HIV infection and to treat AIDS. New drugs are proving effective in unique ways: blocking the virus's ability to reproduce its genes, blocking the virus from multiplying in the cells, hindering a virus enzyme needed to process key viral proteins, and stimulating the immune system.[132]

People with AIDS are living longer as a result of more effective medical management and healthier lifestyles, including better nutrition and preventive measures that reduce the risk of reinfection. A significant part of medical management is using combinations of drugs known as highly active antiretroviral therapy.[133] Drugs slow the progression of HIV to AIDS, but this approach is expensive and will become less effective as drug-resistant strains of HIV develop. In addition to antiretroviral therapy, drugs such as aerosolized pentamidine are used to treat the serious pulmonary infections that afflict patients with frank AIDS. All of these efforts are making AIDS a chronic rather than an acute disease. Researchers have concluded, however, that learning to manipulate the human immune system in new ways offers the best hope for progress against HIV.[134]

Political and social pressures from AIDS activists have radically changed how FDA approves drugs to treat HIV and AIDS. Primarily, clinical trials are less rigorous and safety concerns receive less attention if preliminary results show that a drug is effective. In addition, FDA has approved "community testing" rather than limiting clinical trials to hospitals.

A countervailing theory, supported by a prominent virologist and a Nobel laureate, asserts that HIV neither causes AIDS nor is it contagious. Instead, this minority view purports that AIDS is caused by malnutrition, recreational drug use and abuse, and medicines, including zidovudine (AZT). This view notes that 1) if AIDS were caused by a virus or bacterium it would not strike men more frequently than women; 2) millions of people are infected with HIV but do not have AIDS, and there is no convincing proof that HIV is present in everyone who has AIDS; and 3) infectious diseases typically occur soon after infection, not years later as is true with AIDS, and not after the immune system has made large amounts of antibodies to fight the microbe.[135]

Implications for HSOs/HSs

Financial Implications

In its early phase the AIDS epidemic primarily affected middle-class, Caucasian homosexuals, who usually had ample health insurance, although coverage was often lost once they were unable to work. As the epidemic's demographics changed, however, the number of uninsured patients increased dramatically. People with frank AIDS are or almost always become uninsured; Medicare, and perhaps Medicaid, are available if criteria are met. The financial and insurance statuses of people with AIDS have major implications for the economic survival of hospitals and other HSOs, especially nursing facilities and hospice.

Early in the epidemic, the economic and social burdens of treating AIDS were inequitably distributed because people with AIDS were concentrated in inner-city hospitals in major metropolitan areas.[136] The proportion of people with AIDS in nonurban areas appears to be increasing. This wider dispersion will spread the social and economic burdens and bring some relief to urban hospitals. Increasingly, nursing facilities, hospice, and home care have been effective in treating AIDS, which may result in less costly treatment in more appropriate settings. Policies that promote dying at home may improve quality of life (death) but actually increase costs, however.[137]

AIDS has implications for medical education. Decline in medical school applications in the late 1980s and early 1990s may have resulted because of the risks of treating people with HIV. The presence of large numbers of people with AIDS under treatment may cause medical training programs to lose their approval because residents cannot treat a range of illnesses. Concentrations of people with AIDS may cause problems for other types of education, as well as staffing HSOs.

Legal Implications

The legal implications of HIV and AIDS are addressed in Chapter 14. Suffice to say that, to meet their ethical obligations, HSO/HS managers must, at minimum, comply with the law. Ethical obligations are usually more demanding, however.

Ethical and Administrative Implications

Clinical developments have allowed HSOs to treat AIDS patients more effectively. In general, staff are better prepared and have specialized clinical skills. New drugs have increased the longevity of people with AIDS, and this will result in more episodes of hospitalization as well as treatment at other types of HSOs, especially nursing facilities and home health agencies.

The AIDS epidemic raises significant ethical issues for the organization and its managers, including 1) protecting staff who are providing care to infected patients; 2) protecting patients and staff from infected staff; and 3) maintaining the confidentiality of staff and patients with AIDS. Some of these issues are more easily solved than others. A critical context for analysis is that, for unknown reasons, the probability that caregivers will become infected when exposed to blood and body substances from HIV–positive patients is several orders of magnitude greater than the probability that patients will become infected from HIV–positive caregivers. In fact, with two possible exceptions (see p. 664), there are no documented cases in which a HIV–positive caregiver, even with frank AIDS, has infected a patient.

Protecting Staff from Exposure to HIV

The beginning premise is that HSOs must respond to significant infectious diseases by doing everything possible to protect staff. This is supported by fidelity, part of the principle of respect for persons: Through its managers, the HSO has a duty to provide a safe workplace. Rawls's difference principle supports this duty, as does the theory of utility—the greatest good for the greatest number. An effective workforce is achievable only with safe working conditions. Legal obligations reinforce this ethical duty to employees. Having identified the ethical priority to protect staff, the HSO must create and maintain an environment that is compatible with the obligation to provide services to the community, as well as to treat people with AIDS.

In 1987 CDC confirmed that three hospital staff members had become HIV positive after occupational exposure to contaminated blood. The risk to health care workers who work with patients with HIV is well documented, and there have been hundreds of confirmed cases of transmission of HIV, almost all the result of needle sticks or other direct exposure to contaminated blood.[138] Three large studies in the 1980s estimated the risk of contracting HIV after being stuck accidentally with a contaminated needle at about 1 in 250.[139] Estimates from the 1990s are even lower, with the average risk of transmission after percutaneous exposure to HIV–infected blood estimated at approximately 0.3% and after mucous membrane exposure at 0.09%.[140] In the early 1990s it was estimated that 70,000 health care workers nationwide had tested positive for HIV[141] and that HIV among health care workers is significantly underreported.[142] Despite this, a CDC study of 22,000 patients found that no patients who became HIV positive were infected by health care workers.[143]

Although the virus is present in all body substances of people who are HIV positive, it can apparently be spread only by sexual intercourse or intimate contact with body substances, especially blood. The risk for health care workers is low, but the consequences of AIDS make infection a major concern for them and the HSO. CDC and Occupational Safety and Health Administration guidelines for universal precautions should be used in all HSOs.

Some physicians and staff are reluctant or unwilling to treat people with AIDS. There have been reports of surgeons who demand preoperative HIV testing of patients and refuse to operate on patients who test positive. In 1987 the AMA Council on Ethical and Judicial Affairs issued a statement that physicians behave unethically if they refuse to treat people with AIDS whose medical conditions are within their competence.[144] Nurses and other staff have been disciplined for refusing to treat people with AIDS; some have been fired. Given the consequences of contracting HIV, it is unlikely that statements such as AMA's or even disciplinary action by the HSO will cause all caregivers to agree to treat people with AIDS.

In mid-1987 AHA issued recommendations reflecting the growing concern about the clinical management of AIDS patients.[145] These recommendations are consistent with CDC guidelines that universal blood and body substance precautions are the best protection for caregivers. Under the guidelines, all patients' blood and body substances are considered hazardous and all patients are subject to the infection-control guidelines originally established for hepatitis and HIV. This means that isolation and biohazard precautions should be used for all patients, regardless of HIV status, and that health care workers should protect themselves against blood and body substances and patient contact. Under CDC guidelines in effect since 1987, hospitals should judge whether their patients' characteristics are such that all admissions should be tested. In late 1987 AHA spoke out against routine testing of patients or staff and continues to hold that position. Regardless, some hospitals test all admissions for HIV. Patients who refuse to be tested are admitted but are treated using "extra precautions." Using extra precautions is at variance with universal precautions. All HSOs should address and readdress, as necessary, the question of routine HIV testing.

In 1991 CDC guidelines required people performing exposure-prone procedures to know their HIV status, and those who are HIV positive should inform their patients of that fact before engaging in such procedures. CDC has been criticized for not defining exposure-prone activities from which HIV–infected health care workers can be excluded.[146] Subsequent federal legislation required that states adopt these guidelines by regulation or legislation.

The risk of HIV infection for caregivers is low, but the consequences of infection are great. Research at The Johns Hopkins Hospital emergency department found that physicians complied with universal precautions only 38% of the time. Residents and nurses were more compliant, at 58% and 44%, respectively. At 91%, housekeeping staff complied most often. Staff blamed noncompliance on time pressures and interference of precautions with procedural skills. Low levels of compliance occurred despite ready availability of gloves, gowns, and other protective gear, and despite efforts to educate staff about the risks of contracting HIV. The rate of infected patients in The Johns Hopkins Hospital emergency department increased from 5.2% to 6.0% in 1 year.[147] Other research generally confirms compliance problems regarding universal precautions.[148]

Achieving compliance is a challenge for health services managers; further research is needed on how to meet this goal. Enhanced education can be only a small part of the answer. It is very unlikely that caregivers are ignorant of the risk of contracting HIV and the importance of universal precautions. Management must identify and correct structure and process inhibitors that reduce staff willingness or ability to comply with universal precautions. HSOs that follow CDC and AHA guidelines, the ethically and clinically correct and legally prudent course, treat all patients as if they are HIV positive.

Protecting Patients from Staff

HIV–positive caregivers pose an extremely small risk of infecting patients and staff. This risk comes from both HIV and the opportunistic diseases that afflict people with AIDS, including tuberculosis and *Pneumocystis carinii* pneumonia (PCP). Elderly people and people whose immune systems are suppressed are at special risk.

Significant, too, is that HIV induces neuropsychiatric problems such as impaired coordination and cognitive difficulties that may occur before physical symptoms are apparent. In normal clinical practice such deficits in performance may be attributed to random error rather than a medical condition. If so, then serious problems may occur before a pattern is detected; diminished competence may be apparent only in retrospect, probably after a patient has been harmed. Subtle diminutions in competence would greatly complicate the use of HIV–positive staff. The ethical (and legal) duty of employers to monitor staff and prevent harm to patients is well established.

CDC has confirmed that Dr. David Acer, a Florida dentist, infected six patients with HIV. It is still unknown how he transmitted the virus to them. Acer was confirmed as the source after investigators found that the patients' strains of HIV contained genetic material matching his and that he did not follow infection-control procedures.[149] CDC maintains that its investigation was competent and thorough in all respects. There is, however, evidence suggesting that the infected patients had unreported and undetected risk factors for HIV and that the molecular analyses used to determine that Acer and his patients had the same strains of HIV had potentially serious flaws.[150] Since the Acer case in 1990, CDC has evaluated almost 23,000 patients of HIV–infected health care workers in the United States and has found no other cases in which patients were infected by health care workers.[151]

In early 1999 a French study provided strong evidence that an infected orthopedic surgeon accidentally transmitted HIV to a patient during surgery. Of the almost 1,000 patients on whom the orthopedist had performed surgery who were tested, only 1 had contracted HIV. "The evidence . . .

is not entirely conclusive, but provider-to-patient transmission during orthopedic surgery is the most plausible explanation for the . . . infection."[152] That there have been only two cases of HIV transmission from caregiver to patient, one of which is "confirmed" but challenged and the other of which is "not entirely conclusive," suggests that the risk of being infected with HIV by an infected health care worker is infinitesimal.

The ethical (and legal) problems for HSOs are complicated further by the fact that some caregivers are HIV positive but do not yet have frank AIDS and wish to continue treating patients. AMA and the American Dental Association (ADA) have taken the position that ethics require HIV–infected practitioners to either inform their patients of their HIV status or refrain from performing exposure-prone invasive procedures.[153] This is true, despite CDC's estimates that the risk that an infected surgeon will transmit HIV during an invasive procedure is between 1 in 40,000 and 1 in 400,000 and that the risk of transmission from an infected dentist is between 1 in 200,000 and 1 in 2 million.[154]

Despite the uncertainty of statutory and case law, HSOs should know the HIV status of all staff who engage in exposure-prone invasive procedures. It is ethically appropriate and legally prudent to prohibit those who are HIV positive from performing such procedures. This is consistent with positions taken by CDC, AMA, and ADA. Such a rule meets the principle of nonmaleficence. Implementation is difficult because, except for the two cases noted, there are no documented cases of transmission from HIV–positive caregivers to patients. This is true even when caregivers have frank AIDS. Prominent examples include public reports of surgeons and other physicians with frank AIDS performing exposure-prone invasive procedures, but with no confirmed cases of HIV transmission to their patients. This suggests the unique aspects of HIV and the likelihood of cofactors in transmissibility as well as infectivity and progression to frank AIDS, cofactors not present in the general population.

By way of context, hepatitis B virus (HBV) is a greater threat to patients than is HIV. In 1996 a thoracic surgeon was found to have transmitted HBV to 19 patients during surgery despite evidence that he used adequate infection control procedures.[155] This case, plus that of a Spanish cardiac surgeon who infected five of his patients with hepatitis C (HCV), confirms the importance of mandatory testing for HBV, HCV, and HIV in caregivers who perform exposure-prone invasive procedures.[156]

In meeting their ethical duties, staff should want to know whether they pose a risk to patients and other staff. The opportunistic diseases contracted as HIV progresses to frank AIDS may cause infected staff to pose a risk to patients, many of whom are immunosuppressed or physically weakened. Staff with AIDS also may pose risks to other employees and to visitors. These risks should cause managers to err in favor of caution in assigning staff, at least until legal parameters are established. Furthermore, as HIV–positive staff progress toward frank AIDS and become increasingly immunocompromised, infectious diseases common in HSOs will pose risks to them. If the organization is to discharge its ethical obligations to staff, then it must be able to consider such information in job assignment. Given how much is not known about transmissibility of the virus, HIV–positive staff should be placed in non–patient care positions, whether or not they perform exposure-prone invasive procedures. HIV–positive physicians, whether or not employed by the HSO, should be prohibited from performing exposure-prone invasive procedures, even though they may continue treating patients. Protecting staff confidentiality to the greatest extent possible is crucial to the success of any such effort.

Patient Confidentiality and Specialized Treatment Facilities
Consistent with the principle of respect for persons, HSOs must be alert to the special problems of confidentiality when treating AIDS patients. Within legal constraints, however, the HSO's first obligation is to safeguard staff and other patients.

It has been suggested that identifying patients as HIV positive will cause them to receive poor-quality health services. The potential for giving second-class care has existed since HIV was first identified and patient charts and rooms were marked with biohazard notices, as well as other, more subtle codes. There is little evidence that people with AIDS receive care that is different from that provided to other patients. Identifying HIV–positive patients may be an additional stimulus to encourage staff compliance with universal precautions.

Opponents of AIDS units or regionalization of AIDS treatment argue that patient confidentiality will be lost. This risk is overstated because staff know (as they should) which patients have AIDS. Dedicated AIDS units permit greater use of special training and equipment to protect staff and enhance treatment. Moreover, staff who wish to treat AIDS patients may do so. A dedicated unit minimizes a drift toward second-class care because the availability of staff and other resources would be readily apparent, whereas such lapses could be more easily overlooked or hidden on a general medical-surgical floor.

Few HSOs treat enough AIDS patients to justify a dedicated unit, however. Typically, hospitals admit AIDS patients to general medical-surgical floors rather than to dedicated units, even for acute phases of the disease. Managers argue that privacy is better protected; the extra workload is spread among caregivers, especially nurses; and problems with staffing and work assignments are eased. As the AIDS epidemic recedes, dedicated AIDS units become less likely.

Startling differences in mortality in low- versus high-experience hospitals strongly support arguments to regionalize AIDS treatment, however. Patients in dedicated AIDS units and scattered-bed units of hospitals with dedicated AIDS units had a lower odds of dying by factors of 0.61 and 0.56, respectively.[157] All things being equal, it stands to reason that organizations doing more of something will do it better.

Conclusion

HIV has ethical, legal, financial, and management dimensions and implications that make it as complex an issue as managers will ever encounter. Caring for people with AIDS while protecting staff is a major ethical and legal challenge for managers. Hospitals must find ways to provide effective episodic treatment and to assist HSOs, especially nursing facilities and hospice, with the delivery of care. Financing care will remain problematic for all providers.

There were predictions in the late 1980s that HIV would soon break out in the general population; the most dire of these stated that HIV would sweep through society with consequences like those of the Black Death. This has not happened, nor is it likely to occur because it has been almost 20 years since HIV was identified as the cause of AIDS. HIV continues to be confined to specific, relatively small populations.

Improved testing has virtually eliminated the transmission of HIV through contaminated blood and blood products. Work on a vaccine against HIV continues. Dozens of experimental vaccines are in development and more than 20 are in human testing. With an estimated 650,000–900,000 Americans infected with HIV and more than 400,000 deaths from AIDS, HIV merits attention, but with neither the emotion nor in the amount being accorded it. Despite its limited threat, government policy is based on the questionable assumption that HIV is a broad threat to public health. Politicization of HIV and AIDS has caused resource allocation decisions that would be unconscionable in other circumstances.

Encouraging in the effort to solve the health problems associated with AIDS is the fact that the debate has become less shrill. There is an increasing willingness to treat AIDS as primarily a public health problem with political and civil rights dimensions rather than as primarily a political and civil rights problem with public health dimensions.

ORGANIZATIONAL RESPONSES TO ETHICAL PROBLEMS

Thus far, little has been said about how HSOs/HSs can organize to solve administrative and biomedical ethical problems. The starting point in such efforts is the organizational philosophy, which reflects the values of the HSO/HS and establishes moral direction and a framework for the vision and mission. The organization's philosophy is subject to external constraints such as criminal and civil laws and derivative regulations that set a minimum standard. Some external constraints, such as the "conscience clause," support the values of the HSOs and their staffs[158]; others, such as the federal guidelines that protect human research subjects, are a starting point for the HSO's/HS's relationship with patients participating in federally funded research.

As an employee and a leader, the manager's personal ethic influences the organizational philosophy and is influenced by it. In addition, the manager organizes the organization to solve ethical problems. Ethical problem solving occurs in the context of the organizational philosophy, but is affected by the manager's personal ethic, which may be more specific and comprehensive. This dynamic reinforces the importance of the personal ethic.

MEANS TO RESOLVE ETHICS ISSUES

Since the 1970s, HSOs/HSs have established various groups to solve ethical problems; most prominent are institutional ethics committees (IECs), institutional review boards (IRBs), and infant care review committees (ICRCs). IECs provide a broad range of assistance on administrative and biomedical ethical issues. IRBs are specialized IECs that focus on preventing and solving ethical issues in research. ICRCs, too, are specialized IECs that prevent and solve ethical issues that arise in caring for infants with profound impairments.

Institutional Ethics Committees

Progenitors to IECs were abortion selection committees that determined, prior to *Roe v. Wade,* whether a woman's health or life was at sufficient risk to justify an abortion and medical morals committees in Catholic hospitals that assessed certain treatment decisions in light of church teachings.[159] Later, in the 1960s, committees selected recipients of renal dialysis at a time when medically suitable patients greatly exceeded the number of dialysis machines.

The Karen Ann Quinlan decision in 1976 directed the establishment of an ethics committee to review her prognosis. Such committees confirmed prognoses and helped determine whether to continue life support. In some hospitals prognosis committees were called "God squads" because they determined when treatment should be withdrawn. Contemporary IECs have a much broader role. An early source of information about them was a national survey done for the President's Commission for the Study of Ethical Problems in Medicine and Biomedical and Behavioral Research and published in 1983.[160] No hospital with fewer than 200 beds had an IEC. IECs were not ubiquitous in large hospitals, but those with teaching programs likely had one. The study estimated that there were fewer than 100 IECs in U.S. hospitals. The *Quinlan* decision encouraged hospitals to establish IECs; in New Jersey, where they were most common, 71% were formed because of *Quinlan.*

Surveys in 1983 and 1985 by the National Society of Patient Representatives showed rapid growth of IECs—from 26% of hospitals responding to 59%, respectively. The findings are somewhat skewed because the methodology of the survey caused disproportionate numbers of large hospitals to respond. The Babies Doe controversies in the early 1980s caused many hospitals to establish specialized IECs to solve the ethical problems of treating newborns with profound disabilities. The findings of rapid growth were consistent with research by the American Academy of Pediatrics reported later in this chapter. The growth of new IECs slowed in the late 1980s, however.[161] Lack of growth is confirmed by more recent estimates that nationally about 60% of hospitals have IECs; state and regional ethics networks suggest 65%–85%.[162] A 1993 survey by the Catholic Health Association found that 92% of its members who responded have an IEC.[163] Hospital IECs may be mature and may need to determine whether to participate in new ways and in other aspects of the organization.[164] IECs are more likely to be involved in issues of appropriateness of technology, a renewed interest in patients' rights, changing relationships among health care providers, and conflicting social values than in case consultation, which seems to have declined.[165]

The delivery of nonacute health services is moving rapidly from hospitals to other types of HSOs. The growth in need and use of IECs will be greatest in sites such as nursing facilities, HMOs, and HSs. The American Association of Homes and Services for the Aging found that IECs among its members had increased from 29% in 1990 to 45% in 1995; many others were being planned. IECs perform case consultation, make and review policy recommendations, and educate and advise staff and administration. Of those association members with committees, 86% found them useful.[166] IECs in nonacute types of HSOs are likely to develop differently, consistent with their unique activities and roles. It has been suggested that, unlike hospitals, physicians on IECs in nursing facilities will play a minor role and that administrative staff will be much more important. In addition, because nursing facilities are heavily regulated, legal rather than ethical issues are likely to be emphasized.[167]

Organizing IECs

This section recommends that complex HSOs/HSs have an ethics committee with subcommittees for administrative and biomedical ethical issues. An alternative is two ethics committees, one for administrative ethical issues and one for biomedical ethical issues. Specialization is necessary because a committee that is prepared to address biomedical ethics problems may not be prepared for administrative ethics problems. Greater specialization may be needed within the broad categories of administrative and biomedical ethics (e.g., an ICRC). Committee proliferation or overlap must be avoided, but addressing various types of ethical problems separately will improve results. Because of the need to solve general, organizationwide issues and specific, sometimes technical problems, the committee/subcommittees model should be considered.

Veatch suggests three models for organizing IECs: 1) an autonomy model that implements decisions of competent patients whose wishes are known; 2) a social justice model to address broad issues such as HSO/HS health care policies, resource allocation, cost-effectiveness, and the like; and 3) a patient benefit model to make decisions for patients who are unable to make decisions for themselves.[168] He argues that in many respects these roles are mutually exclusive because different tasks emphasize different ethical principles. Ethics committees that use an autonomy model are accountable to the patient, whereas ethics committees concerned with social justice must be accountable to the organization (or the community). The first and third models emphasize biomedical ethical issues. The second could address administrative as well as biomedical issues if it were determined that it is desirable to mix the two in one committee.

Regardless of the model that is used, IEC members will benefit from training on resolving disputes more effectively. Disputes must be resolved because staff have different views about issues and cases. Improved dispute resolution should weld the multidisciplinary group into a cohesive and mutually supportive team that can resolve its differences and focus on the ethical issue.

Purpose and Role of IECs

Since their early, focused beginnings, the purposes of IECs have evolved into two roles of general importance. One is assisting to develop or reconsider the organizational philosophy and derivative vision and mission statements. Here, the experience and range of interdisciplinary membership is likely to produce more reasoned and thorough results. Education is a second role in which members' experience make the IEC a reservoir of expertise. Utilizing the resources of a sophisticated IEC will improve clinical and administrative decision making in a HSO/HS.

Before considering ethical problems, the IEC must develop a statement of its ethic, the framework for which is the organizational philosophy. This exercise facilitates effectiveness by identifying and minimizing differences in members' personal ethics. Only by understanding and enunciating its own ethic can an IEC appreciate how its values differ from a patient's, for example, an understanding that is essential if patient autonomy is to be respected. The IEC's ethic does not determine how ethical problems are solved. Rather, this statement of general principles guides deliberations and recommendations.

Both administrative and biomedical IECs undertake generic activities such as policy development, education, case consultation, and guidance for staff or patients on request. Sample activities for administrative IECs include developing consent procedures, considering the ethics of macro-allocation of resources, and whistle blowing. Biomedical IECs could develop DNR and patient consent policies and advise on withholding or withdrawing life-sustaining treatment.

In terms of biomedical ethics, the major, continuing benefits of IECs that were first reported by the President's Commission include facilitating decision making by clarifying important issues, shaping consistent policies about life-sustaining treatment, and providing a way for professionals to air disagreements. The IECs that focused on solving biomedical clinical problems were not effective at increasing the ability of patients' families to influence decisions or at educating professionals about issues that are relevant to life support decisions. General observations of the President's Commission are still true:

1. *Committees . . . are not involved in large numbers of cases. Existing committees reviewed an average of only one case per year.*

2. *The composition and function of committees identified in the survey would not allay many of the concerns of patients' rights advocates about patient representation and control. Committees were clearly dominated by physicians and other health professionals. The majority of committees did not allow patients to attend or request meetings, although family members were more often permitted to do so. Yet, chairmen generally regarded their committees as effective.*[169]

The latter finding suggests that health services managers must be alert to patient autonomy, a matter that affects several aspects of the organization, but especially microallocation (e.g., at the bedside) and consent. Important for HSOs with culturally diverse patients and their families and staff is that IEC members are sensitive to differing views about significant events such as death and the process of dying.

Membership of IECs

In general, baseline data on IEC membership reported by the President's Commission remain correct. Biomedical IECs are interdisciplinary. Physicians are the most common type of member. Most IECs include a member of the clergy; some include attorneys, laypeople, social workers, and physicians in graduate education programs (residents). Administrators are less likely to be included than physicians, which may reflect their limited interest in clinical matters, a problem that must be rectified. Because of their numbers in HSOs and the biomedical ethical problems they encounter, nurses also may be underrepresented.[170] The President's Commission found no strong community link—an important perspective that could be provided by governing body members and consumers from the service area.[171]

Administrative IECs should be interdisciplinary, although they have fewer clinical staff and more members of governance and management. Clinical staff must be included because it is reasonable to conclude that research showing that organizations are most effective when they involve clinicians in management decision making also applies to solving administrative ethics problems.

Relationships of IECs

IECs should be proactive in developing and revising the organizational philosophy and considering the ethical implications of macroallocation decisions. Similarly, they should be proactive in reviewing and revising consent processes. However, they are likely to be passive and wait to be consulted about conflicts of interest and misuse of confidential information, as with an administrative IEC, or about specific clinical matters, as with a biomedical IEC.

The President's Commission suggested that biomedical IECs will be more effective if they wait to be consulted rather than interpose themselves. Consultation means committees make recommendations, not final decisions.[172] IEC participation in biomedical and administrative decision making may be optional or mandatory. Whether the IEC's advice must be followed could be optional or mandatory as well. Table 13.2 shows the combinations.

Physicians are unlikely to accept mandatory-mandatory involvement by a biomedical IEC. Furthermore, this may be undesirable when the physician has communicated alternatives to the patient and others concerned. Even if the physician refuses to share decision making with an ethics committee, there are benefits to having its analysis and recommendation.

The administrative location of IECs is important. Options include being a standing committee of the governing body, professional staff organization, or administration. Fears that an IEC will be dominated by physicians cause some experts to suggest that it be a governing body or administration committee. Similarly, no committee member should represent a specific interest or group.[173]

Summary

IECs are not without potential problems. Organizational interests, especially legal aspects and avoiding public embarrassment, may overwhelm patient goals.[174] At the extreme, it is suggested that IECs cannot be objective because they are part of an organization; this may cause IECs to fail as patient advocates because, when a dispute arises, they will take management's side to avoid risk.[175] Management must ensure that IECs are not subverted in this manner.

Overall, effectively using IECs is likely to improve clinical and administrative decisions. It should not be assumed that the mere presence of an IEC means that it is successful or useful. It is important that IECs be evaluated to improve their performance.[176]

Infant Care Review Committees

The Child Abuse Act Amendments of 1984 directed DHHS to encourage establishment of ICRCs in hospitals with tertiary-level neonatal care units.[177] ICRCs are specialized IECs that focus on the biomedical ethical problems of infants with life-threatening conditions. In the DHHS guidelines ICRCs are ethics committees that provide information and education, recommend institutional policies and guidelines, and offer counsel and review of issues that are related to infant care. DHHS considers it prudent to establish an ICRC, but the HSO makes the final decision.

DHHS recommends that an ICRC's membership include people from varied disciplines and perspectives because a multidisciplinary approach provides expertise to supply and evaluate perti-

TABLE 13.2.   OPTIONAL VERSUS MANDATORY USE OF AN
IEC

Involvement of committee in decision making	Acceptance and use of advice given by IEC
Optional	Optional
Optional	Mandatory
Mandatory	Optional
Mandatory	Mandatory

nent information. The committee should be large enough to present diverse viewpoints, but not so large that its effectiveness is hindered. The members recommended include a practicing nurse, a senior hospital manager, a social worker, a representative of a disability group, a lay community member, and one of the facility's medical staff, who chairs ICRC.[178] The recommendation to include a representative of a disability group violates the IEC principle that no specific group should be represented.

DHHS suggested that ICRC have adequate staff support, including legal counsel; recommend procedures to ensure that hospital staff and patient or families are informed of its existence, functions, and 24-hour availability; self-educate about pertinent legal requirements and procedures, including state law requiring reports of known or suspected medical neglect; and maintain records of deliberations and summary descriptions of cases considered and their disposition.[179]

The form and activities recommended by DHHS for ICRCs are like those reported in a 1984 study of 710 hospitals with special care pediatric units. The American Academy of Pediatrics found that, of the 426 respondents, 56.5% had ICRCs or IECs. Of hospitals without such a committee, 75% were considering establishing one. The remaining 25% handled ethical problems by other means, including waiting for clarification of legal issues and acting on that information and using a university committee or state board. The committee activity mentioned most often was consulting on difficult ethical decisions, followed by advising parents, advising physicians (when consulted), and educating staff. Developing hospital policies was rated as the third most important ICRC function. Committee composition was similar to that found by the President's Commission study of IECs.[180]

Institutional Review Boards

To protect human subjects, HSOs conducting research should establish IRBs, which are required by many federal agencies that fund or regulate research. DHHS and FDA are the most important in health services. Federal agencies that require IRBs include the Environmental Protection Agency, the National Science Foundation, and the Consumer Product Safety Commission.

Research involving human subjects that is wholly or partly funded by DHHS must be reviewed by an IRB with a process that meets DHHS criteria. FDA regulates the interstate sale of drugs, biologicals, and medical devices and has requirements like those of DHHS. Unlike DHHS, however, compliance with FDA guidelines, including use of IRBs, is necessary regardless of funding source. A few states, notably New York, regulate medical research, but in general there is little regulation beyond that of DHHS and FDA.

Membership and Purpose of IRBs

Both DHHS and FDA require that an IRB be qualified to review research proposals for conformance with the law, standards of professional conduct and practice, and institutional commitment and regulations. IRBs that are acceptable to DHHS have at least five members with varying backgrounds (one must have nonscientific professional interests), who are capable of reviewing research proposals and activities of the type that are commonly performed by the organization.

In addition to provisions needed for consent, an IRB that is acceptable to DHHS must apply several requirements in reviewing research:

- Minimize risk to subjects
- Determine that risks are reasonable relative to anticipated benefits
- Select research subjects equitably
- Obtain and document appropriate consent from research subjects or legally authorized representatives

- Monitor data to ensure safety
- Protect privacy and confidentiality
- Develop special protections when consent is obtained from people who are likely to be vulnerable to coercion or undue influence, such as people with acute or severe physical or mental illness, or people who are economically or educationally disadvantaged

FDA uses the same basic elements of consent as DHHS, but it applies special provisions when the subject has a life-threatening situation that necessitates the use of the test article and the subject cannot give legally effective consent, when time is insufficient to obtain consent from the subject's legal representative, and when no alternative method of generally recognized therapy that provides an equal or greater likelihood of saving the subject's life is available.

IRB Requirements

Regulations issued in 1981 made it clear that only research funded wholly or partly by DHHS had to comply with DHHS requirements for IRBs.[181] This change enlarges the responsibilities of HSO/HS managers and researchers and places greater reliance on their personal ethic and organizational policies and procedures as well. As a practical matter, HSOs/HSs with multiple research funding sources, one of which is DHHS, are likely to use the same DHHS–qualified IRB for all formal research. It is easy to slip, however, and managers must be alert to potential ethical problems in formal research programs, as well as in isolated innovative therapy or surgical experimentation.

Exempt Research and Expedited Review

The 1981 DHHS regulations identified exempt research and research warranting expedited review as new categories to be regulated differently. Exempt research is primarily in the behavioral sciences, including certain educational practices and testing, interview procedures and observation, and use of precollected data. Expedited review applies special procedures for research with minimal risk and in which human subjects have limited involvement. Examples include the collection of hair and nail clippings in a nondisfiguring manner; the collection of deciduous teeth; the use of voice recordings; the study of existing data, documents, records, and pathological or diagnostic specimens; and moderate exercise by volunteers.

Summary

Irrespective of regulations and legal requirements, HSO/HS managers have independent duties under the principles of respect for persons, beneficence, nonmaleficence, and even justice (e.g., equitable selection of research subjects) to protect patients. Managers must establish and maintain systems and procedures to prevent unauthorized research and to provide the necessary protection when innovative treatment is proposed or undertaken.

Specialized Assistance

Ethics Consultation Services

An ethics consultation service (ECS) is a way in which HSOs/HSs can provide specialized staff to advise and assist in solving biomedical ethics problems. Doing so is like establishing a clinical service. The ECS is staffed by ethicists with graduate degrees in philosophy, often at the doctoral level, and clinical staff such as physicians or other caregivers. The clinicians have a special interest or preparation in ethics and provide a bridge between the ethicists and the clinical staff attending the patient. They also serve as a resource for nonclinician ethicists. In this model an ethicist is on call and the clinical member of the ECS participates as needed. The ECS reports to the IEC, and the IEC develops and recommends policy to the governing body. The IEC also is a sounding board for problems that arise in ethics consultation. A variant of this model has a primary consultant who is assisted by other ECS members. Both the primary consultants and those assisting have various backgrounds, but all of them have specialized training in ethics and participate in case reviews, ethics instruction, and ECS staff meetings.[182]

Ethicists

An approach that is less formal but with wider application than the ECS is found in larger hospitals. As with ECSs, full- or part-time ethicists (who may be university or medical school faculty) consult on biomedical ethical issues. Organizations seeking the assistance of an ethicist should consider anyone with specialized preparation in ethics and its application in the health field. Here, as with an ECS, the ethicist is the clinically oriented, problem-solving extension of an IEC, whose role includes facilitation and consensus building.[183]

Ethics Officer

Appointing an ethics officer is a way for a HSO/HS to focus on internal ethics activities. An ethics officer could manage internal reporting systems, assess ethics risk areas, develop and distribute ethics policies and publications, investigate alleged violations, and design training programs. This senior-level executive also could manage corporate compliance programs.[184]

SUMMARY

This chapter identifies administrative and biomedical ethical issues and describes how HSOs/HSs and their administrative and clinical staffs work to solve them. The essential link between the organizational philosophy and the personal ethic of managers is stressed. The ethical aspects of marketing, managed care, and AIDS are discussed.

After being identified in the 1970s, ethics committees have become important parts of HSOs. By the 1990s they were commonplace; many have become specialized, with broad and varied missions. Ethics committees are interdisciplinary to grapple better with problems that often have both ethical and legal dimensions.

HSOs are becoming more adept at solving ethical problems. The HSO/HS, through its managers, has an ethical responsibility to protect patients and further their interests. This duty incorporates principles of respect for persons, beneficence, nonmaleficence, and justice, and is more demanding than the law. It stresses the independent relationship between managers and patients. The manager's duty to protect patients and further their interests transcends other obligations and is one that HSOs/HSs must formalize and aggressively implement.

DISCUSSION QUESTIONS

1. Describe the relationship between law and ethics. Which is the more demanding standard? Why? Identify and be prepared to explain examples other than those described in the chapter.
2. Identify health services laws or regulations based on 1) a utilitarian philosophy, 2) a deontological philosophy, and 3) elements of both. How compatible are these philosophies when included in the same law or regulation?
3. What does a professional code of ethics reflect? How can enforcement be made meaningful? Must a profession police its standards? Why or why not?
4. Describe the uses and limitations of codes of ethics that apply to HSOs/HSs. Should they be communicated to individuals who are served by the organization? If so, how?

5. What is the HSO's/HS's role regarding patients' rights? Are some duties or obligations surpassed by the organization's duty to patients? If so, give examples of where this occurs.

6. Define fiduciary. Give some examples in and out of health services. Are HSOs/HSs and their services unique in terms of this concept? If so, how?

7. Define conflict of interest. Give examples in HSOs or HSs. How can they be minimized? What is the manager's role?

8. What should be the role of managers in allocating resources at the micro and macro levels? What can be done to reduce the likelihood that ethical problems will arise?

9. What types of experimentation might occur in HSOs/HSs? Distinguish surgical experimentation from that involving drugs and devices, in terms of safeguards. How can patients be protected?

10. Identify the types of advance directives. What is their effect on HSOs? How do managers ensure that HSOs interact effectively with patients in terms of such directives?

11. What is euthanasia? What are the types of euthanasia? Distinguish euthanasia from physician-assisted suicide. Develop brief scenarios that highlight the differences between the various types of euthanasia and physician-assisted suicide.

12. Is futility theory compatible with physician-assisted suicide? Given the preliminary findings of the SUPPORT study, why should caregivers and HSOs wish to implement a futile care policy?

CASE STUDY 1: "WHAT'S A MANAGER TO DO?"[185]

S.L. Rine joined the managerial staff of a large health services provider after gaining several years of experience. Rine is an affiliate of the American College of Healthcare Executives (ACHE) and wants to build the best set of credentials in the shortest possible time. Rine wants to become a CEO.

Rine is responsible for several support departments as well as some clinical areas. Rine realized quickly that the HSO is very political. Much of what happens at the senior level is the result of personal relationships.

One of Rine's departments, maintenance, is responsible for all groundskeeping. Rine found that grounds crews were being sent to the homes of senior members of the governing body to maintain their lawns, shrubs, and trees. Rine asked the maintenance director to explain and was told that the practice had a long history; he suggested that it would be best not to make any changes. When Rine asked the director for a cost estimate of the grounds work being done at the private homes, the director refused to give it. He said he did not want to incur the wrath of the governing body members who were benefiting. Rine pondered what to do.

Shortly after talking to the maintenance director, Rine had lunch with the laboratory director. Without discussing specifics Rine described the problem in maintenance. The laboratory director exclaimed, "That's nothing!" and described how two governing body members were selling reagents, supplies, and equipment to the laboratory at what she thought were higher-than-market prices. Rine asked if she had done anything about it; she replied that her predecessor had tried to stop the practice and had been fired. Rine pondered what to do.

QUESTIONS

1. Identify the ethical problem(s) that face the governing body members and the managers. Do similar problems face those who are not directly involved?

2. Are the grounds maintenance and the sale of reagents, supplies, and equipment to the laboratory ethically different? State your reasons. Are the two likely to be distinguished in the real world?

3. What steps should managers like Rine take if they have the moral courage to risk their jobs to try to solve the problems? Short of risking their jobs, what steps could they take?

4. What sources of assistance are there for Rine outside the organization? How should they be involved?

CASE STUDY 2: BITS AND PIECES[186]

John Henry Williams was pleased with his new job in the radiology department of Affiliated Nursing Homes and Rehabilitation Center. He was appointed acting department head because his predecessor, Mary Beth Jacobson, was granted 6 months' maternity leave. John Henry would be responsible for the equivalent of 2½ full-time technicians, an appointment clerk, and $250,000 in equipment. He would have the authority to purchase supplies, including certain types of X-ray film. The annual value of these purchases was around $90,000. Most were obtained from three vendors, companies from which the Center had bought for years.

During her orientation for John Henry, Mary Beth emphasized how much she liked the meetings with sales representatives from the three vendors. Over the years, one had become a personal friend. Most meetings were held at the nice restaurant near the Center. Some were held in her office and, if so, the sales representative always brought along a "little something." When John Henry asked what she meant, Mary Beth gave some examples: perfume, a bottle of French brandy, and a pen set in a leather case. John Henry remembered thinking that his wife would like the perfume, but he was more interested in the lunches. It would be a chance to get away from the dreary cafeteria and his boring brown-bag lunches. Mary Beth described the lunches as nothing fancy. She estimated the cost to the sales representatives as the same as the small gifts—in the $40–$50 range.

John Henry asked Mary Beth whether there was a policy about accepting gifts from vendors. Mary Beth was angered by the question because it implied that something was wrong with what she was doing. She responded curtly that the Center trusted its managers and allowed them discretion in such matters.

John Henry asked if her behavior might suggest to other staff that her decisions were influenced by the gratuities she received from the sales representatives. Mary Beth's anger flashed: "I know you think that this doesn't look right. That isn't fair! I work long hours as a manager and get paid very little extra. It takes more effort and time to order and maintain proper inventory. If things go wrong, I get the blame. These gifts make me feel better about my efforts. My work has been exemplary. I'd be happy to talk to anyone who thinks otherwise!"

QUESTIONS

1. Develop arguments that support Mary Beth's position on the gratuities that she is receiving. List the arguments in order of importance.
2. Describe the importance of business custom in the relationship that Mary Beth has with the sales representatives. Should this influence the ethics of the situation?
3. Develop a policy regarding gratuities that Affiliated Nursing Homes and Rehabilitation Center could use. Identify the underlying ethical principles, and be prepared to defend the policy.
4. Describe incidents from your own experience that are similar to the issues in the case. Did they have detrimental effects on the organization? Were they resolved? If so, how?

CASE STUDY 3: DEMARKETING TO AVOID BANKRUPTCY[187]

Chris Hines had finally gotten far enough into the stack of papers on her desk to see last month's emergency department activity report. She had already digested the grim news about the continued financial losses at Community Hospital. The total deficit was $500,000 and it was only the fourth month of the fiscal year. Because Community Hospital served a largely inner-city population, many of whom were uninsured or whose care was paid by a chronically underfunded Medicaid program, there seemed little hope that the financial situation would improve.

As CEO, Hines knew that over 40% of Community Hospital admissions came through the emergency department and that about one half of these arrived by taxi, by private automobile, or on foot. The other half were brought in by the city-run ambulance service. A few years earlier Hines had tried to implement a plan to increase the number of elective admissions (and thus improve the payer mix) by encouraging physicians to bring their private patients to Community Hospital. It failed, however, largely because the physicians had difficulty getting their patients admitted—emergency department admissions were taking too many beds. Next, Hines tried to work with city officials to implement a new ambulance routing system that would send more patients to other hospitals and give Community Hospital a chance to improve its financial condition. They were unsympathetic.

Hines knew that Community Hospital's endowment would carry the hospital approximately 3 years, but, if it was not breaking even by then, the hospital would close. Because there was nothing that could be done through the city, the key to survival, she concluded, lay with reducing the number of uninsured and Medicaid admissions through the emergency department.

Hines spoke with several marketing consultants, one of whom offered to work without a fee. The consultant recommended a plan to demarket the emergency department. He argued that it was the emergency department's fine reputation in the community that was responsible for the 50% of patients who came to the emergency department other than by city ambulance. He listed ways to make the emergency department less desirable: reducing emergency department staffing to a minimum; closing the parking lot near the emergency department; reducing housekeeping coverage so that the physical plant would be dirty and unkempt; deferring non–safety-related maintenance; changing triage policies and procedures and staffing to increase waiting time for nonemergency patients; using staff who were most likely to be rude and inconsiderate; and encouraging rumors that the closure of the emergency department was imminent.

Demarketing would cause repercussions beyond the emergency department, but the hospital was in desperate straits. Extreme actions seemed justified.

QUESTIONS

1. Identify the ethical issues in the case. Who bears the major responsibility for their presence? Their solution?
2. Outline a strategy that would save Community Hospital without using the plan that was developed by the marketing consultant. How is it superior? How is it inferior?
3. Develop arguments that support the suggested plan from a utilitarian perspective and from a Kantian perspective.
4. Describe the likely effects of the plan on patients, staff, physicians, and managers.

CASE STUDY 4: CHOICES

Randy Glenn had just fallen asleep when the telephone rang. It was the night supervisor at the comprehensive care center and hospital of which Glenn was the CEO. The supervisor was very agitated and had trouble getting her words out. It took a few minutes for the message to become clear. One of Glenn's nightmares had come true. The four-bed intensive care unit (ICU) was full and an emergency case had just been admitted after a car accident. She had been stabilized in the emergency department, but her injuries were severe and transferring her to another facility would likely cause death. She had to get into the ICU in 1–2 hours.

The night supervisor recovered somewhat and described the patients who were currently occupying ICU beds and the new patient:

Patient A: 60-year-old comatose female, with stroke, has been in the ICU for 27 days; prognosis uncertain; retired, no family

Patient B: 1-week-old premature male with Down syndrome; has been in the ICU since birth; hospital repaired a duodenal atresia (no opening between stomach and small intestine), parents opposed the procedure; child's social future uncertain

Patient C: 36-year-old male who had emergency appendectomy, developed severe wound infection and probable septicemia, source of infection unknown; previous anaphylactic shock in reaction to antibiotics necessitates ICU; bachelor; elderly mother lives in city

Patient D: 12-year-old female undergoing chemotherapy for leukemia with experimental drug; has been in remission three times; close monitoring of protocol and potential reaction to drug requires ICU care; family lives in city

New Patient: 24-year-old female; college honor student in physics, scholarship winner; pregnant; engaged; no family known

The supervisor ended by asking, "What should I do? How do I treat five patients with only four beds?" Indeed, what to do? thought Glenn. He wished he had paid more attention in his college ethics course. Glenn pondered alternatives to the supervisor's questions as the garage door opened and the 10-minute trip to the facility began.

QUESTIONS

1. What should Glenn do? Why is it ethically best?
2. Identify the steps involved in reaching a decision.
3. Describe ways to minimize these problems in the future and to deal with them when they occur. (The organization has no money to build additional ICU beds.)
4. What sources of assistance might be available to Glenn at this point? Which should Glenn develop for the future?

CASE STUDY 5: BENEFITING OLDER ADULTS BY INFECTING THEM WITH INFLUENZA

New Horizons is a state-owned institution for the care of indigent older people. As in many nursing facilities, influenza is a major problem among the residents. Influenza usually is not fatal in younger populations, but it has a significant mortality for older people, often because of complications such as pneumonia. A major drug company has been conducting animal studies on a vaccine to protect against influenza. The vaccine is ready for clinical trials.

The administrator of New Horizons, Gregg Greeley, was contacted by the drug company about the feasibility of establishing a research unit. The unit would hold about 20 residents at a time. The presence of drug company employees, including physicians, nurses, and ancillary staff, would provide better care for residents of the unit than is usually available at New Horizons. In addition, funds would be available for better meals and other amenities. However, once the vaccine had been administered, the residents would be deliberately exposed to influenza to determine whether the vaccine protected them.

Many residents at New Horizons have children or relatives who are their guardians. Greeley called some of the guardians and found that they had no problem consenting to the experiment. Several noted that residents in the unit would receive better quality care and, if they contracted influenza, would receive the advantages of that care.

QUESTIONS

1. Which moral philosophy supports the action contemplated by Greeley? Which does not?
2. Should residents have a voice in the decision? If so, how can their wishes be known and implemented?
3. Which interests are being balanced? How and by whom should the interests be weighed?
4. If the experiment proceeds, how should residents be protected? What is Greeley's role?

CASE STUDY 6: KNOWING WHETHER OR WHEN TO STOP

An 18-year-old woman suffered severe head injuries in a car accident in early 1995. After a few weeks in a coma, she opened her eyes but was totally unresponsive for 15 months. Then, nurses noticed a hopeful sign when she twice seemed to obey their orders to move her leg or close her eyes. These responses were rare, but 2 months later her physicians administered drugs to improve alertness and she improved slowly. Over time, she learned to answer multiple-choice questions and do simple math using eye blinks. At one point, she wrote, "Mom, I love you."

Three years after the accident, she was communicating regularly with eye blinks and could move her arms somewhat. After 5 years, she could mouth words and short phrases. Although her attention span was limited to 15 minutes, she liked pampering and took pleasure in teasing her nurses. Her favorite joke was pretending not to know who they were.

Her mother was overjoyed. She reveled in each small bit of progress. Five years and 2 months after the injury, the young woman was sent home, totally dependent on others. Her rehabilitation had cost more than $1 million.[188]

QUESTIONS

1. Should treatment have been withdrawn when the prognosis was certain? Is this a case of futile care? If so, who has the legal right to speak for the patient? Who has the moral right?
2. Identify the issues/questions that arise in terms of macroallocation of resources. Who should be financially responsible for the care? Distinguish situations in which insurance is available and unavailable.
3. What is the role of the health services executive in solving the ethical issues posed by this case?
4. What is the role of the clinicians, such as physicians and nurses, in solving the ethical issues posed by this case? How do they differ from the role of the health services executive?

CASE STUDY 7: SOMETHING MUST BE DONE, BUT WHAT?[189]

Stunned, Carolyn Aubrey, the CEO of Metropolitan Hospital, sank into her chair and stared out the window for a very long time. She realized when Dr. Midmore's wife had angrily insisted on seeing the CEO that something was afoot. But even in her worst nightmares, Aubrey had never imagined that Mrs. Midmore would tell Aubrey that she was suing her husband, an orthopedic surgeon, for divorce because he had given her AIDS. As Mrs. Midmore left

Aubrey's office, she turned back and said, "I was sure you'd want to know—surely you'll have to do something."

Fleetingly, Aubrey thought Mrs. Midmore's statements might be nothing more than the ravings of an angry, vindictive wife, but that was not likely. As she considered what she had just learned, she recalled an incident several years ago involving Dr. Midmore and a male orderly. In retrospect, it suggested that Dr. Midmore might be bisexual. Aubrey thought, too, about the department of surgery meeting last year during which there had been a long discussion about the desirability of knowing the HIV status of all surgical patients. The special risks to surgeons of torn gloves and cuts during orthopedic surgery had been described in detail.

Now it seemed that Dr. Midmore's patients might be at risk. Aubrey called operating room scheduling and learned that Dr. Midmore was maintaining a full surgical load. Aubrey asked her secretary to call the hospital attorney and the medical director and set up an emergency meeting for 7:00 the following morning. Mrs. Midmore had been right, thought Aubrey. We'll have to do something, but what?

QUESTIONS

1. Bearing in mind that HIV-infected caregivers seem to pose a very small risk of infecting patients, even when they engage in exposure-prone procedures, should Aubrey refrain from any action? What are the ethical and legal implications of your response?

2. What steps, if any, should Aubrey take in terms of previous patients who have been treated by Dr. Midmore at Metropolitan Hospital? Why? Is there any obligation in terms of the patients whom Midmore has treated in his office or at other HSOs?

3. Discuss this case using Henderson's models (Figures 13.1 and 13.2).

4. Assume that you are a recent patient on whom Dr. Midmore has performed surgery. What would you want Metropolitan Hospital to do? Why?

NOTES

1. Fleck, Leonard. Speech to the American Hospital Association. *Catholic Health World* 5 (October 15, 1989): 3.
2. Bodenheimer, Edgar. *Jurisprudence: The Philosophy and Method of the Law,* 6. Cambridge, MA: Harvard University Press, 1974.
3. Bodenheimer, *Jurisprudence,* 6.
4. Bodenheimer, *Jurisprudence,* 325.
5. Henderson, Verne E. "The Ethical Side of Enterprise." *Sloan Management Review* 23 (Spring 1982): 41–42. Can a corporation know the difference between right and wrong? In *State v. Christy-Pontiac, GMC, Inc.* (354 N.W.2d 17), the Minnesota Supreme Court held that a corporation could form the specific intent necessary to commit theft and forgery and thus be subject to criminal fines. The irony of the case lies in the fact that corporate officers were found not guilty when tried separately on the same charges (Simonett, John E. "A Corporation's Soul." *Minnesota Bench & Bar* September (1997): 34–35.
6. Kant, Immanuel. "Fundamental Principles of the Metaphysics of Morals." Translated by Thomas K. Abbott. In *Knowledge and Value,* edited by Elmer Sprague and Paul W. Taylor, 535–558. New York: Harcourt, Brace, 1959.
7. Rawls, John. *A Theory of Justice,* 60. Cambridge, MA: Belknap Press, 1971.
8. Bodenheimer, *Jurisprudence,* 23.
9. Arras, John, and Nancy Rhoden. *Ethical Issues in Modern Medicine,* 3rd ed. Mountain View, CA: Mayfield Publishing, 1989.
10. Bodenheimer, *Jurisprudence,* 94.
11. Jonsen, Albert R., and Stephen Toulmin. *The Abuse of Casuistry: A History of Moral Reasoning,* 13. Berkeley: University of California Press, 1988.

12. Beauchamp, Tom L., and LeRoy Walters. *Contemporary Issues in Bioethics,* 4th ed., 21. Belmont, CA: Wadsworth, 1994.

13. Jonsen, Albert R. "Casuistry and Clinical Ethics." *Theoretical Medicine* 7 (1986): 70.

14. Jonsen, "Casuistry," 71.

15. Pellegrino, Edmund D., and David C. Thomasma. *For the Patient's Good: The Restoration of Beneficence in Health Care,* 121. New York: Oxford University Press, 1988.

16. Pellegrino and Thomasma, *For the Patient's Good,* 116.

17. Pellegrino, Edmund D. "The Virtuous Physician and the Ethics of Medicine." In *Contemporary Issues in Bioethics,* 4th ed., edited by Tom L. Beauchamp and LeRoy Walters, 55. Belmont, CA: Wadsworth, 1994.

18. Carney, Frederick S. "Theological Ethics." In *Encyclopedia of Bioethics,* vol. 1, edited by Warren T. Reich, 435–436. New York: The Free Press, 1978.

19. Pellegrino and Thomasma, *For the Patient's Good,* 121.

20. Pellegrino, "The Virtuous Physician," 53.

21. This section is adapted from Darr, Kurt. "Moral Philosophies and Principles." In *Ethics in Health Services Management,* 3rd ed., 23–26. Baltimore: Health Professions Press, 1997; reprinted by permission.

22. Darr, Kurt. "Administrative Ethics and the Health Services Manager." *Hospital & Health Services Administration* 29 (March–April 1984): 120–136.

23. American Medical Association. *Current Opinions of the Judicial Council,* vii. Chicago: American Medical Association, 1982.

24. American Medical Association. *Principles of Medical Ethics.* Chicago: American Medical Association, 1980.

25. Veatch, Robert M. "Professional Ethics: New Principles for Physicians?" *Hastings Center Report* June (1980): 17.

26. American Nurses Association. *Code for Nurses with Interpretive Statements,* i. Kansas City, MO: American Nurses Association, 1985.

27. American Nurses Association, *Code for Nurses,* iii.

28. American Nurses Association, *Code for Nurses,* 1.

29. Annas, George J. *The Rights of Patients: The Basic ACLU Guide to Patient Rights,* 2nd ed. Totowa, NJ: Humana Press, 1992.

30. Southwick, Arthur F. *The Law of Hospital and Health Care Administration,* 2nd ed., 122–123. Ann Arbor, MI: Health Administration Press, 1988.

31. Southwick, *The Law of Hospital,* 123–124.

32. Southwick, *The Law of Hospital,* 126.

33. Stern et al. v. Lucy Webb Hayes. The governing body was called a board of trustees and its members were known as trustees even though no trust was involved and they functioned like corporate directors.

34. Stern v. Hayes, 381 Federal Supplement 1003 (1974).

35. American College of Healthcare Executives. *Code of Ethics.* Chicago: American College of Healthcare Executives, 1999.

36. American College of Healthcare Executives, *Code of Ethics.*

37. Devolites, Milton C. "The Cedars of Lebanon Hospital." Unpublished case study, The George Washington University Department of Health Services Administration, Washington, DC, 1974.

38. American College of Healthcare Executives, *Code of Ethics.*

39. Hanlon, John J., and George E. Pickett. *Public Health: Administration and Practice,* 5. St. Louis: Times Mirror/Mosby, 1984.

40. "Ethical Conduct for Health Care Organizations." Management Advisory, American Hospital Association. [On-line] http://www.aha.org/resource/hethics.html, April 12, 2000.

41. This section is adapted from Darr, Kurt. "Ethics in Marketing and Managed Care." In *Ethics in Health Services Management,* 3rd ed., 213–221. Baltimore: Health Professions Press, 1997; reprinted by permission.

42. A furor resulted from a report that some Medicare HMOs' advertising targeted healthy seniors (Hilzenrath, David S. "Study: HMOs Target Healthiest Seniors." *The Washington Post,* July 14, 1998, C3).

43. Some physicians are "gaming" MCO constraints—sometimes through fraud and deception—so that their patients can get medical treatment that is needed, but that the MCO will not authorize. These actions go well beyond the physician as advocate and raise another set of ethical issues. (Hilzenrath, David S. "Healing vs. Honesty? For Doctors, Managed Care's Cost Controls Pose Moral Dilemma." *The Washington Post,* March 15, 1998, H1.)

44. Harron, Frank, John Burnside, and Tom Beauchamp. *Health and Human Values: A Guide to Making Your Own Decisions,* 148. New Haven, CT: Yale University Press, 1983.

45. Childress, James F. "Who Shall Live When Not All Can Live?" *Soundings, An Interdisciplinary Journal* 53 (Winter 1970): 339–355.

46. Rescher, Nicholas. "The Allocation of Exotic Medical Lifesaving Therapy." In *Unpopular Essays on Technological Progress,* 30–44. Pittsburgh: University of Pittsburgh Press, 1980.

47. Contrast this view with a case in Japan in which a physician told a patient she had gallstones rather than frightening her by telling her she actually had gallbladder cancer. She delayed surgery. The cancer spread and she died. Her family brought suit. The court said the patient herself was to blame because she had not followed the physician's advice to have the surgery and that the physician had no obligation to inform her of the true condition. (Hiatt, Fred. "Japan Court Ruling Backs Doctors." *The Washington Post,* May 30, 1989, A9.)

48. President's Commission for the Study of Ethical Problems in Medicine and Biomedical and Behavioral Research. *Making Health Care Decisions,* Vol. 1. Washington, DC: President's Commission, 1982.

49. Katz, Jay. "Informed Consent—A Fairy Tale." *University of Pittsburgh Law Review* 39 (Winter 1977): 137–174.

50. President's Commission, *Making Health Care Decisions,* vol. 1.

51. Ramsey, Paul. "Research Involving Children or Incompetents." In *The Patient as Person,* 252. New Haven, CT: Yale University Press, 1970. In late 1997 FDA proposed that manufacturers of new drugs study their effects on children when the products are expected to be widely used in pediatrics. Eighty percent of all drugs on the market have not been labeled for use by infants. Only 42% of drugs that are widely prescribed to children have been tested on pediatric populations. ("FDA Wants Pediatric Medicines Tested on Children." *Health Lawyers News* October [1997]: 21.)

52. Harvard Medical School. "A Definition of Irreversible Coma." *Journal of the American Medical Association* 205 (August 5, 1968): 337–338.

53. President's Commission for the Study of Ethical Problems in Medicine and Biomedical and Behavioral Research. *Defining Death: Medical, Legal, and Ethical Issues in the Determination of Death,* 25. Washington, DC: President's Commission, 1981.

54. Personal communication, Uniform Law Commissioners, Chicago, July 26, 1990.

55. In re Quinlan, 70 N.J. 10 (1976).

56. "Permanent" is used instead of "persistent" after a vegetative state has continued longer than a year.

57. Cruzan v. Director, Missouri Department of Health, 110 S. Ct. 2841 (1990).

58. Rehabilitation Act of 1973, PL 93-112, 29 U.S.C. § 701 *et seq.*

59. Child Abuse Act Amendments of 1984, PL 98-457, 98 Stat. 1749 (1984).; "Appendix to Part 1340—Interpretative Guidelines Regarding 45 CFR Section 1340.15—Services and Treatment for Disabled Infants." *Federal Register* (January 13, 1999): 355–356.

60. Patient Self Determination Act of 1989, PL 101-508, 104 Stat. 1388-27 (November 5, 1990).

61. Bradley, Elizabeth H., and John A. Rizzo. "Public Information and Private Search: Evaluating the Patient Self-Determination Act." *Journal of Health Politics, Policy and Law* 24 (April 1999): 239–273.

62. Personal communication, Carol E. Sieger, Choice in Dying, Inc., November 1, 1999.

63. Colburn, Don. "Patients' Directives on Dying Have Little Effect on Care." *The Washington Post,* Health Section, April 15, 1997, 5.

64. Morrison, R. Sean, Ellen Olson, Kristan R. Mertz, and Diane E. Meier. "The Inaccessibility of Advance Directives on Transfer from Ambulatory to Acute Care Settings." *Journal of the American Medical Association* 274 (August 9, 1995): 478–482.

65. Brown, Jonathan Betz, Arne Beck, Myde Boles, and Paul Barrett. "Practical Methods to Increase Use of Advance Medical Directives." *Journal of General Internal Medicine* 14 (1999): 21–26. Mailing written materials to older adults with a substantial baseline placement rate increased the placement of advance directives in the medical record.

66. Cugliari, Anna Maria, Tracy Miller, and Jeffery Sobal. "Factors Promoting Completion of Advance Directives in the Hospital." *Archives of Internal Medicine* 155 (September 25, 1995): 1893–1898.

67. Reilly, Brendan M., Michael Wagner, C. Richard Magnussen, James Ross, Louis Papa, and Jeffrey Ash. "Promoting Inpatient Directives About Life-Sustaining Treatments in a Community Hospital." *Archives of Internal Medicine* 155 (November 27, 1995): 2317–2323.

68. Solomon, Mildred Z., Lydia O'Donnell, Bruce Jennings, Vivian Guilfoy, Susan M. Wolf, Kathleen Nolan, Rebecca Jackson, Dieter Koch-Weser, and Strachan Donnelley. "Decisions Near the End of Life: Professional Views on Life-Sustaining Treatments." *American Journal of Public Health* 83 (January 1993): 14–21.

69. Goldstein, Amy. "Dying Patients' Care Varies Widely by Place, Study Says." *The Washington Post,* October 15, 1997, A1.

70. Choice in Dying, Inc. *State Statutes Governing Surrogate Decisionmaking.* New York: Choice in Dying, Inc., 1998.

71. Choice in Dying, Inc., *State Statutes Governing.*

72. Jacobson, Bonnie S. "Ethical Dilemmas of Do-Not-Resuscitate Orders in Surgery." *AORN Journal* 60 (September 1994): 449–452; "Proposed AORN Position Statement on Perioperative Care of Patients with Do-Not-Resuscitate (DNR) Orders." *AORN Journal* 60 (October 1994): 648, 650; "Statement of the American College of Surgeons on Advance Directives by Patients: 'Do Not Resuscitate' in the Operating Room." *ACS Bulletin* September (1994): 29; Margolis, Judith O., Brian J. McGrath, Peter S. Kussin, and Debra A. Schwinn. "Do Not Resuscitate (DNR) Orders During Surgery: Ethical Foundations for Institutional Policies in the United States." *Anesthesia and Analgesia* 80 (1995): 806–809.

73. Personal communication, Carol E. Sieger, Choice in Dying, Inc., November 1, 1999.

74. Evans, Andrew L., and Baruch A. Brody. "The Do-Not-Resuscitate Order in Teaching Hospitals." *Journal of the American Medical Association* 253 (April 1985): 2236–2239.

75. Bedell, Susanna E., and Thomas L. Delbanco. "Choices About Cardiopulmonary Resuscitation in the Hospital: When Do Physicians Talk with Patients?" *New England Journal of Medicine* 320 (April 1984): 1089–1093.

76. Teno, Joan M., Rosemarie B. Hakim, William A. Knaus, Neil S. Wenger, Russell S. Phillips, Albert W. Wu, Peter Layde, Alfred F. Connors, Neal V. Dawson, and Joanne Lynn, for the SUPPORT Investigators. "Preferences for Cardiopulmonary Resuscitation: Physician-Patient Agreement and Hospital Resource Use." *Journal of General Internal Medicine* 10 (April 1995): 179–186.

77. Wenger, Neil S., Marjorie L. Pearson, Katherine A. Desmond, Ellen R. Harrison, Lisa V. Rubenstein, William H. Rogers, and Katherine L. Kahn. "Epidemiology of Do-Not-Resuscitate Orders: Disparity by Age, Diagnosis, Gender, Race, and Functional Impairment." *Archives of Internal Medicine* 155 (October 23, 1995): 2056–2062.

78. Wachter, Robert M., John M. Luce, Norman Hearst, and Bernard Lo. "Decisions About Resuscitation: Inequities Among Patients with Different Diseases but Similar Prognoses." *Annals of Internal Medicine* 111 (September 1989): 525–532.

79. Morse, Susan. "Final Requests: Preparing for Death." *The Washington Post,* July 15, 1985.

80. Kelly, Gerald. "The Duty to Preserve Life." *Theological Studies* 12 (December 1951): 550.

81. "Declaration on Euthanasia." Rome: Vatican Congregation for the Doctrine of the Faith, June 26, 1980.

82. Beauchamp, Tom L., and James F. Childress. *Principles of Biomedical Ethics,* 4th ed., 207. New York: Oxford University Press, 1994.

83. Gibbs, Nancy. "Dr. Death's Suicide Machine." *Time,* June 18, 1990, 69–70.

84. Walsh, Edward. "Kevorkian Sentenced to Prison." *The Washington Post,* April 14, 1999, A2.

85. Murray, Frank J. "High Court Won't Touch Michigan Suicide-Aid Ban." *The Washington Times,* April 25, 1995, A-1.

86. Meier, Diane E., Carol-Ann Emmons, Sylvan Wallenstein, Timothy Quill, R. Sean Morrison, and Christine K. Cassel. "A National Survey of Physician-Assisted Suicide and Euthanasia in the United States." *New England Journal of Medicine* 338 (April 23, 1998): 1193–1201.

87. Claiborne, William. "An Oregon Statute Is Blunting Death's Sting." *The Washington Post,* April 29, 1998, A1.

88. Lee, Melinda A., and Susan W. Tolle. "Oregon's Assisted Suicide Vote: The Silver Lining." *Annals of Internal Medicine* 124 (January 15, 1996): 267–269. After various court reviews and appeals, Oregon in 1997 became the first state to legalize physician-assisted suicide.

89. Booth, William. "Woman Commits Doctor-Assisted Suicide." *The Washington Post,* March 26, 1998, A7. The Oregon Health Plan, which covers Medicaid patients, and the Blue Cross and Blue Shield plans of Oregon began covering physician-assisted suicide in early 1998 ("Oregon Health Plans Proceed with Caution on Suicide Coverage." *AHA News* 34 [March 16, 1998]: 5).

90. "Assisted-Suicide Coverage Could be Expanded." *AHA News* 34 (November 2, 1998): 6.

91. Personal communication, Choice in Dying, Inc. January 3, 2000.

92. Washington v. Glucksberg, 521 U.S. 702; Vacco v. Quill, 521 U.S. 793. In *Lee v. Harcleroad,* 118 S. Ct. 328, *cert. den.,* the Court declined to review a lower court ruling that a group of terminally ill people and their physicians had no standing to challenge the constitutionality of Oregon's physician-assisted suicide law because it posed no personal danger to them. (Biskupic, Joan. "Oregon's Assisted-Suicide Law Lives On." *The Washington Post,* October 15, 1997, A3.)

93. Truehard, Charles. "Holland Prepares Bill Legalizing Euthanasia." *The Washington Post,* August 15, 1999, A19.

94. Meek, James. "Dutch Wrestle with Morality of Mercy Killings: Parliament is Expected to Legalize Euthanasia, Doctor-Assisted Suicide." *The Washington Times,* November 21, 1999, C12.

95. Simons, Marlise. "Dutch Parliament Approves Law Permitting Euthanasia." *The New York Times,* February 10, 1993, A10.

96. Meek, "Dutch Wrestle."

97. Simons, "Dutch Parliament Approves."

98. Keown, John. "Dutch Slide Down Euthanasia's Slippery Slope." *The Wall Street Journal,* November 5, 1991, A18.

99. Meek, "Dutch Wrestle."

100. Simons, "Dutch Parliament Approves."

101. Lee, Melinda A., Heidi D. Nelson, Virginia P. Tilden, Linda Ganzini, Terri A. Schmidt, and Susan W. Tolle. "Legalizing Assisted Suicide—Views of Physicians in Oregon." *New England Journal of Medicine* 334 (February 1, 1996): 310–315.

102. Hendin, Herbert, Chris Rutenfrans, and Zbigniew Zylicz. "Physician-Assisted Suicide and Euthanasia in the Netherlands." *Journal of the American Medical Association* 277 (June 4, 1997): 1720–1722.

103. Ryan, Christopher James. "Pulling Up the Runaway: The Effect of New Evidence on Euthanasia's Slippery Slope." *Journal of Medical Ethics* 24 (October 1998): 341–344.

104. Bachman, Jerald G., Kirsten H. Alcser, David J. Doukas, Richard L. Lichtenstein, Amy D. Corning, and Howard Brody. "Attitudes of Michigan Physicians and the Public Toward Legalizing Physician-Assisted Suicide and Voluntary Euthanasia." *New England Journal of Medicine* 334 (February 1, 1996): 303–309; Lee, Nelson, Tilden, Ganzini, Schmidt, and Tolle, "Legalizing Assisted Suicide," 310–315.

105. Haney, Daniel Q. "6 Pct. of Physicians in Survey Say They Have Assisted Patient Suicides." *The Washington Post,* April 23, 1998, A9.

106. Claiborne, "An Oregon Statute," A1.

107. McMahon, Patrick, and Wendy Koch. "Assisted Suicide: A Right or a Surrender?" *USA Today,* November 22, 1999, 21A.

108. Battin, Margaret P. "Assisted Suicide: Can We Learn from Germany?" *Hastings Center Report* 22 (March–April 1992): 44–51.

109. Waisel, David B., and Robert D. Truog. "The Cardiopulmonary Resuscitation-Not-Indicated Order: Futility Revisited." *Annals of Internal Medicine* 122 (February 15, 1995): 304–308.

110. Hudson, Terese. "Are Futile-Care Policies the Answer?" *Hospitals & Health Services Networks* February 20 (1994): 26–32.

111. Hudson, "Are Futile-Care Policies," 28.

112. Hudson, "Are Futile-Care Policies," 28.

113. The SUPPORT Principal Investigators. "A Controlled Trial to Improve Care for Seriously-Ill Hospitalized Patients: The Study to Understand Prognoses and Preferences for Outcomes and Risks of Treatments (SUPPORT)." *Journal of the American Medical Association* 274 (November 22/29, 1995): 1595.

114. Teno, Joan M., Donald Murphy, Joanne Lynn, Anna Tosteson, Norman Desbiens, Alfred F. Connors, Jr., Mary Beth Hamel, Albert Wu, Russell Phillips, Neil Wenger, Frank Harrell, Jr., and William A. Knaus for the SUPPORT Investigators. "Prognosis-Based Guidelines: Does Anyone Win?" *Journal of the American Gerontological Society* 42 (November 1994): 1202–1207.

115. Jecker, Nancy S. "Knowing When to Stop: The Limits of Medicine." *Hastings Center Report* 21 (May 1991): 5–8.

116. Adapted from Darr, Kurt. "Dealing with HIV and AIDS." In *Ethics in Health Services Management,* 3rd ed., 223–240. Baltimore: Health Professions Press, 1997; updated and reprinted by permission.

117. "HIV Attacks Specific Defense Cells, Researchers Say." *The Washington Times,* September 11, 1998, A6.

118. Weiss, Rick. "New Strain of AIDS Virus Discovered in Africa." *The Washington Post,* September 1, 1998, A2.

119. Novitt-Moreno, Anne. "AIDS: Will the Future Bring a Cure?" *Current Health 2* 25 (December 1998): 6–13.

120. "HIV/AIDS Statistics," fact sheet, National Institute of Allergy and Infectious Diseases. [On-line] http://www.niaid.nih.gov/factsheets/aidsstat.htm, December 12, 1999.

121. Price, Joyce. "Deaths from AIDS in U.S. Outpace New HIV Infections." *The Washington Times,* February 1, 1996, A3.

122. "HIV/AIDS Statistics," fact sheet.

123. Brown, David. "AIDS Death Rate in '97 Down 47%." *The Washington Post,* October 8, 1998, A1.

124. "STD Control Plays Important Role in Reducing the Spread of HIV." [On-line] http://www.cdc.gov/nchstp/hiv_aids/media/pr_148.htm, January 3, 2000.

125. Brown, David. "Demographic Shift Noted in New Cases of AIDS: Black, Hispanic Gay Men Now Form a Majority." *The Washington Post,* January 14, 2000, A3; "STD Control Plays Important Role in Reducing the Spread of HIV." [On-line] http://www.cdc.gov/nchstp/hiv_aids/media/pr_148.htm.

126. "HIV Found in 7% of Gay Young Men: Education Fails to Halt Spread." *The Washington Times,* February 11, 1996, A3. This article reported results from the first national survey of young homosexual and bisexual men.

127. Gayle, Helene D., Richard P. Keeling, Miguel Garcia-Tunon, Barbara W. Kilbourne, John P. Narkunas, Fred R. Ingram, Martha F. Rogers, and James W. Curran. "Prevalence of the Human Immunodeficiency Virus Among University Students." *The New England Journal of Medicine* 323 (November 29, 1990): 1538–1541.

128. Personal communication, Richard P. Keeling, M.D., January 4, 2000.

129. Brown, David. "AIDS Toll Will Be a Record 2.6 Million." *The Washington Post,* November 24, 1999, A3.

130. National Vital Statistics System. "Provisional Data from the Centers for Disease Control and Prevention/National Center for Health Statistics." *Vital and Health Statistics* 46 (March 17, 1998): Table 6. Provisional Number of Deaths and Death Rates for 72 Leading Causes, Human Immunodeficiency Virus, and Alzheimer's Disease: United States, June 1996 and 1997. (Data are provisional; they were estimated from a 10% sample of deaths.)

131. Istook, Ernest. "Should NIH Weigh Disease Prevalence in Allocating Funds?" *The Washington Post, Health Section,* August 11, 1998, 15.

132. Paul, William E. "A Turning Point in AIDS Research: Building on Firmer Foundations." *Vital Speeches of the Day* 60 (September 15, 1994): 709.

133. Henkel, John. "Attacking AIDS with a 'Cocktail' Therapy." *FDA Consumer* 33 (July/August 1999): 12–17.

134. Brown, David. "At AIDS Conference, a Shift in Direction." *The Washington Post,* July 4, 1998, A8.

135. Weiss, Rick. "And Now for Something Completely Different." *The Washington Post, Health Section,* November 1, 1994, 7.

136. Boodman, Sandra G. "Up Against It: In Newark, a Public Hospital Fights the Twin Plagues of AIDS and Drugs." *The Washington Post, Health Section,* September 5, 1989; "AIDS Update: An Executive Report." *Hospitals* 64 (May 5, 1990): 26–34.

137. "Home Care for Terminally-Ill AIDS Patients May Not Lower Costs." *Research Activities* 186 (July/August 1995): 11.

138. CDC estimated that approximately 800,000 health care workers in the United States would be injured by needles used on patients in 1998. Combined estimates from CDC and EPINet, a computer-based standardized injury tracking system used by approximately 1,500 U.S. hospitals, suggest that more than 2,000 of those workers will test positive for new infections of hepatitis C, another 400 will get hepatitis B, and 35 will contract HIV. HIV is the most feared; but hepatitis B, for which there is a vaccine, and hepatitis C, for which there is no vaccine, are life threatening because they can lead to liver

damage, cirrhosis, and cancer. (Phalen, Kathleen F. "Needle Stick Risk." *The Washington Post, Health Section,* August 11, 1998, 11.)

139. Okie, Susan. "HIV-Infected Workers Undercounted." *The Washington Post,* January 16, 1990, A5.

140. "PHS Guidelines for Management of Health-Care Worker Exposure to HIV." [On-line] http://www.cdc.gov/epo/mmwr/preview/mmwrhtml/00052722.htm, January 3, 2000.

141. Wojcik, Joanne. "Health Care Workers with HIV." *Business Insurance* 26 (August 24, 1992): A11.

142. Okie, "HIV-Infected Workers," A5.

143. Japsen, Bruce. "Study Casts Doubt on Need to Test Healthcare Workers for HIV." *Modern Healthcare* 25 (May 8, 1995): 26.

144. American Medical Association. *Ethical Issues Involved in the Growing AIDS Crisis* (Reports of the Council on Ethical and Judicial Affairs). Chicago: American Medical Association, 1987. The report states that "A physician who knows that he or she has an infectious disease should not engage in any activity that creates a risk of transmission of the disease to others. . . . disclosure of that risk to patients is not enough; patients are entitled to expect that their physicians will not increase their exposure to the risk of contracting an infectious disease, even minimally" (p. 169).

145. American Hospital Association. *AIDS/HIV Infection: Recommendations for Health Care Practices and Public Policy, Report and Recommendations of the Special Committee on AIDS/HIV Infection Policy.* Chicago: American Hospital Association, 1987–1988.

146. Hermann, Donald H. "A Call for Authoritative CDC Guidelines for HIV-Infected Health Care Workers." *Journal of Law, Medicine, and Ethics* 22 (1994): 176.

147. Koska, Mary. "AIDS Precautions: Compliance Difficult to Enforce." *Hospitals* 63 (September 5, 1989): 58.

148. Haddock, Cynthia Carter, Gail W. McGee, Hala Fawal, and Michael S. Saag. "Knowledge and Self-Reported Use of Universal Precautions in a University Teaching Hospital." *Hospital & Health Services Administration* 39 (Fall 1994): 295–307.

149. Price, Joyce. "2 of 6 Who Got HIV from Dentist Are Alive." *The Washington Times,* February 9, 1996, A7.

150. Barr, Stephen. "The 1990 Florida Dental Investigation: Is the Case Really Closed?" *Annals of Internal Medicine* 124 (January 15, 1996): 250–254.

151. Okie, Susan. "French Surgeon Gave a Patient AIDS Virus." *The Washington Post, Health Section,* January 12, 1999, 9.

152. Okie, "French Surgeon Gave," 9.

153. Bayer, Ronald. "The HIV-Infected Clinician: To Exclude or Not Exclude?" *Trustee* 44 (May 1991): 16.

154. Bayer, "The HIV-Infected Clinician," 17.

155. Harpaz, Rafael, Lorenz von Seidlein, Francisco M. Averhoff, Michael P. Tormey, Saswati D. Sinha, Konstantina Kotsopoulou, Stephen B. Lambert, Betty H. Robertson, James D. Cherry, and Craig N. Shapiro. "Transmission of Hepatitis B Virus to Multiple Patients from a Surgeon Without Evidence of Inadequate Infection Control." *New England Journal of Medicine* 334 (February 29, 1996): 549–554.

156. Esteban, Juan I., Jordi Gomez, Maria Martell, Beatriz Cabot, Josep Quer, Joan Camps, Antonio Gonzalez, Teresa Otero, Andres Moya, Rafael Esteban, and Jaime Guardia. "Transmission of Hepatitis C Virus by a Cardiac Surgeon." *New England Journal of Medicine* 334 (February 29, 1996): 555–559.

157. "AIDS Patients Fare Much Better in Dedicated AIDS Units and Magnet Hospitals Compared with General Hospital Units." *Research Activities* 231 (November 1999): 9.

158. Also known as the Church Amendment, the conscience clause was enacted by Congress in 1973. It relieves HSOs whose religious beliefs or moral convictions prohibit performing sterilizations or abortions from adverse consequences and similarly protects staff who refuse to participate in these activities even if organizational values permit them.

159. Ross, Judith Wilson, John W. Glaser, Dorothy Rasinski-Gregory, Joan McIver Gibson, and Corrine Bayley. *Health Care Ethics Committees: The Next Generation,* 1. Chicago: American Hospital Publishing, 1993.

160. President's Commission for the Study of Ethical Problems in Medicine and Biomedical and Behavioral Research. *Deciding to Forego Life-Sustaining Treatment: Ethical, Medical, and Legal Issues in Treatment Decisions,* 443. Washington, DC: President's Commission, 1983.

161. "Right-to-Die: An Executive Report." *Hospitals* 63 (November 20, 1989): 34.

162. Ross, Glaser, Gregory, Gibson, and Bayley, *Health Care Ethics Committees,* ix.

163. Lappetito, Joanne, and Paula Thompson. "Today's Ethics Committees Face Varied Issues." *Health Progress* (November 1993): 34–39, 52.
164. Cohen, Cynthia B., Ed. "Ethics Committees," *Hastings Center Report* 20 (March/April 1990): 29–34.
165. Lappetito and Thompson, "Today's Ethics Committees," 34.
166. American Association of Homes and Services for the Aging. *Summary Report: Survey on Ethics Involvement in Aging Services.* Washington, DC: American Association of Homes and Services for the Aging, 1995.
167. Ross, Glaser, Gregory, Gibson, and Bayley, *Health Care Ethics Committees,* 8.
168. Veatch, Robert M. "Ethics Committees Proliferation in Hospitals Predicted." *Hospitals* 57 (July 1983): 48–49.
169. President's Commission for the Study of Ethical Problems in Medicine and Biomedical and Behavioral Research. *Protecting Human Subjects,* 443. Washington, DC: President's Commission, 1982.
170. Ross, Glaser, Gregory, Gibson, and Bayley, *Health Care Ethics Committees,* 5.
171. Mannisto, Marilyn M. "Orchestrating an Ethics Committee: Who Should Be on It, Where Does It Best Fit?" *Trustee* 38 (April 1985): 18–19.
172. Freedman, Benjamin. "One Philosopher's Experience on an Ethics Committee." *Hastings Center Report* 11 (April 1981): 20–22.
173. Mannisto, "Orchestrating an Ethics Committee," 18–19.
174. Mannisto, "Orchestrating an Ethics Committee," 17–20.
175. Annas, George, and Amy Haddad. "Do Ethics Committees Work?" *Trustee* 47 (July 1994): 17.
176. Scheirton, Linda S. "Measuring Hospital Ethics Committee Success." *Cambridge Quarterly of Healthcare Ethics* 2 (1993): 495–504.
177. Information about DHHS guidelines on ICRCs and the principles of treatment of disabled infants can be found on-line at *http://frwebgate4.access.gpo.gov/cgi-bin/...cID.*
178. Department of Health and Human Services, Office of Human Development Services. "Services and Treatment for Disabled Infants; Model Guidelines for Health Care Providers to Establish Infant Care Review Committees." *Federal Register* 50 (April 15, 1985): 14893.
179. Department of Health and Human Services, "Services and Treatment," 14893.
180. "Summary: Survey of Infant Care Review Committees." Paper delivered at the Annual Meeting of the American Academy of Pediatrics, Chicago, September 18, 1984.
181. Veatch, Robert M. "Protecting Human Subjects: The Federal Government Steps Back." *Hastings Center Report* 11 (June 1981): 9–12.
182. Fletcher, John C., Margo L. White, and Philip J. Foubert. "Biomedical Ethics and an Ethics Consultation Service at the University of Virginia." *HEC Forum* 2 (1990): 89–99.
183. Casarett, David J., Frona Daskal, and John Lantos. "Experts in Ethics? The Authority of the Clinical Ethicist." *Hastings Center Review* 28 (November–December 1998): 6–11.
184. Petry, Edward. "Appointing an Ethics Officer." *Healthcare Executive* 13 (November/December 1998): 35.
185. Adapted from Darr, Kurt. *Ethics in Health Services Management,* 3rd ed., 118–119. Baltimore: Health Professions Press, 1997; reprinted by permission.
186. Adapted from Darr, Kurt. *Ethics in Health Services Management,* 3rd ed., 107. Baltimore: Health Professions Press, 1997; reprinted by permission.
187. Adapted from Darr, Kurt. *Ethics in Health Services Management,* 3rd ed., 210–211. Baltimore: Health Professions Press, 1997; reprinted by permission.
188. Childs, Nancy L., and Walt N. Mercer. "Brief Report: Late Improvement in Consciousness After Post-Traumatic Vegetative State." *New England Journal of Medicine* 334 (January 4, 1996): 24–25; "'Permanent' Coma Can be Misnomer, Texas Case Shows." *The Washington Post,* January 4, 1996, A16.
189. Adapted from Darr, Kurt. *Ethics in Health Services Management,* 3rd ed., 233. Baltimore: Health Professions Press, 1997; reprinted by permission

SELECTED BIBLIOGRAPHY

American College of Health Care Administrators. *Code of Ethics.* Alexandria, VA: American College of Health Care Administrators, 1989.

American College of Healthcare Executives. *Code of Ethics.* Chicago: American College of Healthcare Executives, 1999.

American Medical Association. *Policy Compendium. Current Opinions of the Council on Ethical and Judicial Affairs of the American Medical Association: E-2.07—Clinical Investigation.* Chicago: American Medical Association, 1998.

American Medical Association. *Principles of Medical Ethics.* Chicago: American Medical Association, 1980.

American Nurses Association. *Code for Nurses with Interpretive Statements.* Kansas City, MO: American Nurses Association, 1985.

Angell, Marcia. "A Dual Approach to the AIDS Epidemic." *New England Journal of Medicine* 324 (May 23, 1991): 1498–1500.

Arras, John D., and Bonnie Steinbock. *Ethical Issues in Modern Medicine,* 4th ed. Mountain View, CA: Mayfield Publishing Company, 1995.

Bayer, Ronald. "Public Health Policy and the AIDS Epidemic: An End to HIV Exceptionalism?" *New England Journal of Medicine* 324 (May 23, 1991): 1500–1504.

Beauchamp, Tom L., and James F. Childress. *Principles of Biomedical Ethics,* 4th ed. New York: Oxford University Press, 1994.

Beauchamp, Tom L., and LeRoy Walters. *Contemporary Issues in Bioethics,* 5th ed. Belmont, CA: Wadsworth, 1999.

Bernat, James L. "A Defense of the Whole-Brain Concept of Death." *Hastings Center Report* 28 (March/April 1998): 4–23.

Bodenheimer, Edgar. *Jurisprudence: The Philosophy and Method of the Law.* Cambridge, MA: Harvard University Press, 1974.

Bradley, Elizabeth H., and John A. Rizzo. "Public Information and Private Search: Evaluating the Patient Self-Determination Act." *Journal of Health Politics, Policy and Law* 24 (April 1999): 239–273.

Callahan, Daniel. *False Hopes: Why America's Quest for Perfect Health Is a Recipe for Failure.* New York: Simon & Schuster, 1998.

Centers for Disease Control. "Recommendations for Preventing Transmission of Human Immunodeficiency Virus and Hepatitis B Virus to Patients During Exposure-Prone Invasive Procedures." *MMWR. Morbidity and Mortality Weekly Report* 40 (July 12, 1991): 1–8.

Childress, James F. "Who Shall Live When Not All Can Live?" *Soundings, An Interdisciplinary Journal* 53 (Winter 1970): 339–355.

Childress, James F. "Ethical Criteria for Procuring and Distributing Organs for Transplantation." *Journal of Health Politics, Policy and Law* 14 (Spring 1989): 87–113.

Childress, James F. "Policies for Allocating Organs for Transplantation: Some Reflections." *BioLaw* 2:3 & 4, Special Section (March–April 1995): S:29–S:39.

Cohen, Cynthia B., Ed. "Ethics Committees." *Hastings Center Report* 18 (August/September 1988): 19–34.

Cohen, Cynthia B., Ed. "Ethics Committees." *Hastings Center Report* 19 (January/February 1989): 19–24.

Cohen, Cynthia B., Ed. "Ethics Committees." *Hastings Center Report* 19 (September/October 1989): 21–26.

Cohen, Cynthia B., Ed. "Ethics Committees." *Hastings Center Report* 20 (March/April 1990): 29–34.

Danis, Marion, Leslie I. Southerland, Joanne M. Garrett, Janet L. Smith, Frank Hielema, C. Glenn Pickard, David M. Egner, and Donald L. Patrick. "A Prospective Study of Advance Directives for Life-Sustaining Care." *New England Journal of Medicine* 324 (March 28, 1991): 882–888.

Darr, Kurt. *Ethics in Health Services Management,* 3rd ed. Baltimore: Health Professions Press, 1997.

DeGeorge, Richard T. *Business Ethics,* 5th ed. New York: Macmillan, 1999.

"Dying Well in the Hospital: The Lessons of SUPPORT." *Hastings Center Report* Special Supplement (November/December 1995).

Engelhardt, H. Tristam, Jr. *The Foundations of Bioethics,* 2nd ed. New York: Oxford University Press, 1996.

Fletcher, John C., Margo L. White, and Philip J. Foubert. "Biomedical Ethics and an Ethics Consultation Service at the University of Virginia." *HEC Forum* 2 (1990): 89–99.

Frankena, William K. *Ethics,* 2nd ed. Englewood Cliffs, NJ: Prentice-Hall, 1973.

Harvard Medical School. "A Definition of Irreversible Coma." *Journal of the American Medical Association* 205 (August 5, 1968): 337–338.

Heitman, Elizabeth. "Institutional Ethics Committees: Local Perspectives on Ethical Issues in Medicine." In *Society's Choices: Social and Ethical Decision Making in Biomedicine,* edited by Ruth Ellen Bulger, Elizabeth Meyer Bobby, and Harvey V. Fineberg, 409–431. Washington, DC: National Academy Press, 1995.

Henderson, Verne E. "The Ethical Side of Enterprise." *Sloan Management Review* 23 (Spring 1982): 37–47.

Kant, Immanuel. "Fundamental Principles of the Metaphysics of Morals." Translated by Thomas K. Abbott. In *Knowledge and Value,* edited by Elmer Sprague and Paul W. Taylor, 535–558. New York: Harcourt, Brace, 1959.

Katz, Jay. "Informed Consent—a Fairy Tale." *University of Pittsburgh Law Review* 39 (Winter 1977): 137–174.

Lappetito, Joanne, and Paula Thompson. "Today's Ethics Committees Face Varied Issues." *Health Progress* 74 (November 1993): 34–39, 52.

"Office of Human Development Services, U.S. Department of Health and Human Services, Child Abuse and Neglect Prevention and Treatment Program (Final Rule); and Model Guidelines for Health Care Providers to Establish Infant Care Review Committees (Notice)." *Code of Federal Regulations,* pt. 45, 1340. Washington, DC: Office of the Federal Register, April 1985. (See also "Subchapter E—The Administration for Children and Youth and Families, Child Abuse and Neglect Prevention and Treatment Program." *Code of Federal Regulations,* pt. 45, ch. XIII. Washington, DC: Office of the Federal Register, October 1997.)

Pellegrino, Edmund D., and David C. Thomasma. *For the Patient's Good: The Restoration of Beneficence in Health Care.* New York: Oxford University Press, 1988.

President's Commission for the Study of Ethical Problems in Medicine and Biomedical and Behavioral Research. *Compensating for Research Injuries* (2 vols.). Washington, DC: President's Commission, 1982.

President's Commission for the Study of Ethical Problems in Medicine and Biomedical and Behavioral Research. *Deciding to Forego Life-Sustaining Treatment: Ethical, Medical, and Legal Issues in Treatment Decisions.* Washington, DC: President's Commission, 1983.

President's Commission for the Study of Ethical Problems in Medicine and Biomedical and Behavioral Research. *Defining Death: Medical, Legal, and Ethical Issues in the Determination of Death.* Washington, DC: President's Commission, 1981.

President's Commission for the Study of Ethical Problems in Medicine and Biomedical and Behavioral Research. *Implementing Human Research Regulations.* Washington, DC: President's Commission, 1983.

President's Commission for the Study of Ethical Problems in Medicine and Biomedical and Behavioral Research. *Making Health Care Decisions* (2 vols.). Washington, DC: President's Commission, 1982.

President's Commission for the Study of Ethical Problems in Medicine and Biomedical and Behavioral Research. *Protecting Human Subjects.* Washington, DC: President's Commission, 1982.

President's Commission for the Study of Ethical Problems in Medicine and Biomedical and Behavioral Research. *Screening and Counseling for Genetic Conditions.* Washington, DC: President's Commission, 1983.

President's Commission for the Study of Ethical Problems in Medicine and Biomedical and Behavioral Research. *Securing Access to Health Care* (3 vols.). Washington, DC: President's Commission, 1983.

President's Commission for the Study of Ethical Problems in Medicine and Biomedical and Behavioral Research. *Splicing Life.* Washington, DC: President's Commission, 1982.

President's Commission for the Study of Ethical Problems in Medicine and Biomedical and Behavioral Research. *Whistleblowing in Biomedical Research.* Washington, DC: President's Commission, 1981.

Ramsey, Paul. *The Patient as Person.* New Haven, CT: Yale University Press, 1970.

Rawls, John. *A Theory of Justice.* Cambridge, MA: Belknap Press, 1971.

Rescher, Nicholas. "The Allocation of Exotic Medical Lifesaving Therapy." *Ethics* 79 (April 1969): 173–186.

Rescher, Nicholas. *Unpopular Essays on Technological Progress.* Pittsburgh: University of Pennsylvania Press, 1980.

Ross, Judith Wilson, John W. Glaser, Dorothy Rasinski-Gregory, Joan McIver Gibson, and Corrine Bayley. *Health Care Ethics Committees: The Next Generation.* Chicago: American Hospital Publishing, 1993.

Veterans Affairs Medical Center. *Patient Responsibilities.* Washington, DC: Veterans Affairs Medical Center, 1999.

Veterans Affairs Medical Center. *Patient Rights.* Washington, DC: Veterans Affairs Medical Center, 1999.

Williams, Kenneth J., and Paul R. Donnelly. *Medical Care Quality and the Public Trust.* Chicago: Pluribus Press, 1982.

World Medical Assembly. "Declaration of Helsinki: Recommendations Guiding Medical Doctors in Biomedical Research Involving Human Subjects." Adopted by the 18th World Medical Assembly, Helsinki, Finland, 1964, and revised by the 29th World Medical Assembly, Tokyo, Japan, 1975.

14 Legal Considerations

For law is order, and good law is good order.[1]

Law and ethics are distinguished in Chapter 13. Suffice it to say that organized societies have a code delineating unacceptable behavior and prescribing penalties for those who act in a contrary manner. Law is a system of principles and rules of human conduct that are prescribed or recognized by society and enforced by a public authority, a definition that is broad enough to include criminal and civil law. This chapter focuses on civil law, which relates to private rights and remedies; contracts and commercial relations among individuals are governed by civil law.

PROCESSES THAT PRODUCE THE LAW

The Constitution is the basic law of the United States, and the federal system that it reflects was established after the American Revolution when sovereign states relinquished specific authority to a central government. These enumerated powers are interpreted by the U.S. Supreme Court. Powers that are not delegated to the federal government are reserved to the states. This is important because of the states' police powers, which are noted in Chapter 3. Each state's constitution establishes its form of government and identifies the rights of its residents.

Official or Public Processes

Legislative Process

Statutes are enacted by state legislatures and the U.S. Congress. Comparable legislative activities are performed by local government when ordinances are passed. These laws are binding but may be challenged in court if they violate constitutionally protected rights or were improperly enacted because of procedural irregularity. The legislative branch relies on the executive branch to implement and enforce the laws.

Paradigmatic of these processes is the process that occurs in the U.S. Senate and House of Representatives. The basic legislative process in both houses of Congress is the same. The political party with a majority controls committee and subcommittee membership and determines legislative priorities. Bills related to health care that are introduced in either house are referred to committees or subcommittees and may be amended at various points, including in committee or subcommittee, on the floor, or in conference between the houses. During the legislative process, or to learn more about problems before drafting bills, committees or subcommittees may hold hearings in which people from the health field testify. Hearings are held consistent with the committee chair's interests, however, and there usually is a political dimension. Managers or governing body members of health services organizations/health systems (HSOs/HSs) rarely participate in the legislative process. Testimony, drafts of bills, and other input are provided by professional or trade associations, either by their staffs or through hired lobbyists. A bill that is approved by the Senate and the House and signed by the president becomes law.

Regulatory Process

Once enacted, laws must be implemented and enforced. This is accomplished by executive branch departments and agencies and by independent regulatory bodies. All of these were established by Congress. Rule-making and regulatory activities give them quasi-legislative authority, which is a contemporary development; as recently as the 1930s, the U.S. Supreme Court held that the delegation of legislative authority by Congress was unconstitutional.[2] In addition, executive departments and agencies and independent regulatory bodies have quasi-executive and quasi-judicial powers because they enforce regulations and judge compliance.

Implementing Law—Regulations

Laws are implemented through regulations that are issued by executive departments and agencies and independent regulatory bodies such as the Federal Trade Commission (FTC). The implementation process is governed by the Administrative Procedures Act of 1946, as amended.[3] Requirements include notice of proposed rule making, proposed regulations, and final regulations. The steps before final regulations are issued permit interested parties to comment on provisions. Interim regulations testing the effect of proposed regulations may be issued until final regulations are drafted and approved.

During the period of public comment, HSOs/HSs through their trade associations and lobbyists are able to influence the content of final regulations. It is most cost-effective to influence the process at this point. Primarily, attention is given to the staff who write the regulations. Efforts are sometimes directed at the president or Congress to cause them to intervene. The record of HSOs/HSs and their professional associations has been mixed. Lobbying by provider groups resulted in moderation of Medicare fraud and abuse regulations. Conversely, the National Labor Relations Board (NLRB) did not accept the position of hospitals when its rule-making authority was used to define their labor union bargaining units. Details about NLRB are provided in Chapter 11.

Results of the implementation process appear in the *Federal Register,* which is published each working day. Final regulations are compiled in the *Code of Federal Regulations.*

Multiple Functions of the Regulatory Process

As suggested earlier, the regulatory process melds executive, legislative, and judicial functions. It is legislative because regulations are issued pursuant to laws. The regulations reflect the law and congressional intent and have general (prospective) application. The law's specificity determines the latitude for interpretation in the rule-making process. Regulators have executive authority through their enforcement powers. Compliance is achieved by bringing complaints, issuing directives such as cease-and-desist orders, and levying fines, all of which can occur pending a decision in the agency's hearing and review process or prior to a hearing in an emergency. Finally, the regulatory process is judicial or quasi-judicial when a dispute about compliance arises. Hearings and reviews are held before hearing officers or administrative law judges who are part of that agency. Such officials have a degree of independence because they are appointed for a specific term by the president and can be removed only for cause.

For the HSO/HS, challenging a regulatory decision by engaging in the administrative hearing and review process is time consuming and expensive. Outside legal counsel who are expert in administrative law are needed to work with retainer or in-house corporate counsel. As a practical matter, small HSOs/HSs have little choice but to comply with a regulation or to simply accept an adverse administrative ruling without appeal to the courts. Legal challenges are costly and usually can be undertaken only by a large HSO/HS or association. This may change, however, because some recent federal laws permit successful challengers to recover costs.

An important development of the past several decades is the increasing complexity and significance of administrative law and the rule-making processes. Some political scientists argue that the bureaucracies have become a de facto fourth branch of the federal government. An atypical example is the Baby Doe regulations discussed in Chapter 13, in which federal courts were brought into the rule-making process when procedures were ignored. In general, the parties must exhaust the administrative review process before appeal to the federal courts is allowed.

Judicial Process

Space does not permit a full discussion of the various courts and their jurisdiction and authority. Suffice it to say that state and federal court systems have many similarities. Both have trial courts (county and district courts, respectively), intermediate courts (appeals courts), and supreme courts. Some states reverse the terms *supreme* and *appeals* and make the appeals court the highest court. "Judge" is the title of jurists in courts other than the highest state and federal courts; "justice" is the title of members of state supreme courts and the Supreme Court of the United States. Typically, state governors nominate judges and justices, who are ratified by the state senate. Some states elect judges and justices, although the election of judges is more common. If elected, terms of 10 or 15 years are typical. Federal court judges and justices are nominated by the president with confirmation by the Senate. They serve for life.

Appointment insulates the judiciary somewhat from politics, and this results in more predictable and consistent court-made law. Judges and justices who are appointed by a governor or president are likely to have compatible political philosophies, although the history of the U.S. Supreme Court shows notable exceptions. The need for legislative confirmation and the almost-universal review of nominees by bar committees usually results in the appointment of competent and ethical people.

Stare Decisis and Res Judicata

Two central doctrines make courts a source of formal law. *Stare decisis* is a Latin phrase meaning that courts will stand by precedent and not disturb a settled point.[4] The doctrine of *stare decisis* is based on the principle that the law should be fixed, definite, and known. Courts and litigants are guided by previous cases with similar facts. Predictability and consistency are important attributes of the law. Whimsical changes and uncertainty are to be avoided with judge-made law and legislative enactments. Nevertheless, precedents are sometimes overturned.

The second doctrine is reflected in the Latin phrase *res judicata,* which means a matter has been judged or a thing has been judicially acted on or decided.[5] Thus rehearing will occur only if there is a substantial problem in the original judgment because of factual error, misrepresentation, or fraud, or if significant new information becomes available. *Res judicata* adds stability and predictability to the law because, after appeals are exhausted, the case is settled and usually will not be reopened.

Courts and Health Services

HSOs/HSs often are involved in state and federal courts, as *plaintiffs* (those bringing civil legal action) or *defendants* (those against whom civil legal action is taken). In addition, associations may submit legal briefs as a friend of the court, or *amicus curiae*. Such briefs bring to the court's attention legal precedents and other information from that group's perspective.

Executive Orders

Formal law results from executive orders. Authority for some executive orders, such as the president's role as commander-in-chief of the armed forces, is derived from the U.S. Constitution. Decisions arising from treaties result in executive orders. Other examples occur when Congress delegates authority to the president to act in specific circumstances, such as emergencies. The executive order declaring a region a disaster area, thus qualifying it for federal assistance, is likely to affect HSOs/HSs.

Unofficial or Private Processes

Influence of HSOs/HSs

Health care became highly politicized after massive federal financing of health services began in the mid-1960s with the enactment of Medicare and Medicaid. The legislative and regulatory processes affecting health services were increasingly subject to the influences of lobbyists, political action committees (PACs), and other interest groups, all seeking to ensure that their concerns became known. For HSOs/HSs and their trade associations, participating in federal and state government processes affecting them was a matter of survival.

The change loop [6] in the management model in Figure 1.7 suggests that HSOs/HSs affect their external environment. This occurs when their positions are advocated by them or by a trade association or PAC. Another is by bringing a lawsuit, which is described later in this chapter.

Trade Associations and Interested Parties

Washington, D.C., and its environs are home to thousands of trade associations; among them are many from the health care field. Physical proximity to policy makers and the bureaucrats who develop and enforce federal laws and regulations is considered an advantage. The associations from health care include the American Hospital Association (AHA), the Federation of American Health Systems (FAHS), the American Association of Health Plans (AAHP), the American Medical Association (AMA), and American Nurses Association (ANA). In addition to the major associations, there are hundreds of other special interests, including HSOs and HSs, which may be called interested parties. At best, trade associations and interested parties provide information that enhances the outcomes of the legislative and regulatory processes. Both seek to further their own interests first, but the quasi-public role of member HSOs means that these interests have much in common with those of the public.

Associations and interested parties make their positions known at various points in the legislative and regulatory processes. The myriad bills and their often-complex subject matter makes personal, in-depth knowledge by members of Congress difficult to achieve. This enhances the importance of staff; most interaction occurs between lobbyists and congressional staffers. These interactions are outside public scrutiny, which is not to suggest illegal or immoral acts. It is common for trade associations and interested parties to have access to data that are not available to Congress and regulators. Staffers know that lobbyists will present information most advantageously for the party that they represent. A cardinal rule among lobbyists is that truthfulness is essential. Lobbyists caught lying or purposefully misleading the member or staff irretrievably lose credibility, which is their greatest asset. This description of lobbying and lobbyists does not state the obvious. There are dishonest legislators and special interests who seek to do more than express a viewpoint and make a convincing argument. These are the exception, despite the occasional bad publicity.

Political Action Committees

Since the 1960s, many health care trade associations have organized PACs, which make campaign contributions. PACs permit the aggregation and targeting of contributions and protect contributors who may be charitable organizations, as defined in the Internal Revenue Code, from losing their tax-exempt status. AMA established one of the first health care PACs; AHA soon followed.[6] Defenders of PACs argue that federal election laws prohibit gifts of a size that is likely to influence elected officials. Their position is that PAC contributions only assure access to lawmakers, a subtle but important distinction. This view is reinforced by the fact that many PACs contribute to both parties in a political campaign.

CONTRACTS

A contract is an agreement between two or more parties that identifies rights and obligations. The parties agree to do or not do certain things. Understandings between private people or between private people and government is another source of formal law. Bodenheimer notes:

> There would seem to be no reason, for example, why a collective bargaining agreement, constituting an accord which governs the hiring, discharge, wage rates, working hours, and disciplining of employee groups, should not be deemed a source of law just as much as a labor code enacted by a legislature which deals with exactly the same subjects. It must be kept in mind that a valid collective bargaining agreement may serve in court suits as well as arbitration proceedings as the sole legal foundation for the recognition and adjudication of substantial rights and the obligations on the part of employers and employees.[7]

Decision makers in contract disputes first look to the generally applicable law and then interpret the private agreement in light of it. Thus the contract's provisions become important.

Elements of a Contract

A valid contract has several elements. It is 1) an agreement that is reached after an offer and an acceptance, 2) for which there is consideration (something of value), that is 3) reached by parties who have the legal capacity to contract, and 4) the objective of which is lawful. These requirements seem simple enough, but applying them has resulted in a vast body of statutes, regulations, and case law.

HSOs/HSs contract for goods and services with numerous businesses and people. Examples include contracts to buy supplies, equipment, and services; sell maintenance or laundry services; employ staff; and make collective bargaining agreements. Many transactions are not and need not be in writing (e.g., a dietitian calls a greengrocer to bring vegetables with payment on delivery). However, states treat oral contracts differently from written contracts, and oral contracts may not be legally binding if they exceed a certain dollar amount or if their duration exceeds a certain length of time. Managerial control of contracts is maintained by using purchase orders that, when sent to the seller, constitute an offer to buy or, if sent in response to a previous offer to sell, constitute the acceptance. Increasingly, HSOs/HSs sell services. Hospitals sell laboratory services to physicians or contract with health maintenance organizations (HMOs) to provide hospital care. Visiting nurse agencies sell therapists' services to nursing facilities. HSs contract with consultants. Such services usually are offered at predetermined prices, although cost-plus contracts may be used.

Breach of Contract

When compared to the total number of contracts that HSOs/HSs execute annually, breaches of contract are rare. Defenses are available when a breach of contract occurs. One defense is that the contract is impossible to complete; examples include destruction or unavailability of the subject matter, death or illness, and legal prohibition. When impossibility is not an issue, however, and the contract is simply breached, three types of remedies are available: rescission for a material breach, specific performance, and damages. *Rescission* means that the contract is null and void, and the parties are put into their original positions relative to each other, as far as possible. Specific performance requires the party who is in breach to do what was agreed to in the contract. If neither rescission nor specific performance is the appropriate remedy, then the aggrieved party may seek money damages.

Breaches of contract usually involve lawyers and legal fees and often a trial, even if one party is clearly right and the other is clearly wrong. As a consequence, breaches should be avoided. One of the best ways to avoid them is to involve competent legal counsel in drafting and negotiating contracts. Binding arbitration is a commonly used, low-cost means of resolving disputes. It is standard in commercial contracts and should be included in other types as well.

TORTS

Breach of Contract and Tort Distinguished

A principle of Anglo-American legal tradition is that people are responsible for the harm they cause, whether they have acted intentionally or unintentionally (negligently). Such responsibility falls into the domains of both contract and tort obligations. Tort is derived from the Latin *tortus,* or twisted. As its use in standard English faded, *tortus* acquired a technical meaning in the law.[8]

A tort is a civil wrong, other than a breach of contract, for which courts provide a remedy in the form of an action for damages.[9] To be successful, the action must include certain elements: there must be a duty, a breach of that duty, and resulting harm that is causally linked to the defendant. Defendants may be liable for punitive damages in addition to actual damages, depending on their intent and the circumstances.

Contract liability is distinguished from tort liability primarily by the nature of what is protected:

> *The distinction between tort and contract liability, as between parties to a contract, has become an increasingly difficult distinction to make. It would not be possible to reconcile the results of all cases. The availability of both kinds of liability for precisely the same kind of harm has brought about confusion and unnecessary complexity. . . . Tort obligations are in general obligations that are imposed by law—apart from and independent of promises made and therefore apart from the manifested intention of the parties—to avoid injury to others. By injury here is meant simply the interference with the individual's interest or an interest of some other legal entity that is deemed worthy of legal protection. . . . Contract obligations are created to enforce promises which are manifestations not only of a present intention to do or not to do something, but also a commitment to the future. They are, therefore, obligations based on the manifested intention of the parties to a bargaining transaction.[10]*

This statement suggests that breach of contract and tort are more easily distinguished in theory than in application. This is especially true in the breach of an implied warranty, which is a hybrid of contract and tort. In general, there is an implied warranty that goods are fit (merchantable) for their usual and customarily intended purposes.

> *The doctrine of (strict) liability imposes liability on those responsible for defective goods which pose an unreasonable risk of injury and which do in fact result in injury, regardless of how much care was taken to prevent the dangerous defect. An important distinction has been made between products and services, and the doctrine does not normally apply to the latter. For example, in attempts to hold hospitals strictly liable for injuries caused by blood transfusions, courts generally have held that hospitals are providing a service and not in the business of selling blood; therefore strict liability does not apply.*[11]

The legal concept of implied warranty has been applied extensively to medical products and devices. The legal and financial implications of the distinction between products and services are important for health care providers.

Intentional Torts

Some torts arise from intentional rather than negligent conduct. The actor's intent is not necessarily hostile nor is it based on a desire to harm; rather, there is an intent to "bring about a result which will invade the interests of another in a way that the law will not sanction."[12] Types of intentional torts most likely to affect HSOs/HSs include battery, defamation, false imprisonment, invasion of privacy, tortious interference in contractual obligations, wrongful discharge of an employee, and wrongful disclosure of confidential information. Assault often is linked to battery in criminal proceedings but rarely in civil law. Assault must raise a reasonable apprehension of harmful or offensive contact and can occur with the physical touching necessary for battery. Chapter 13 noted that, to be ethical, consent must be informed, voluntary, and competent. Legal requirements are similar. Although consent is discussed here in the context of intentional torts, a legal action regarding consent can arise in negligence as well.

Written consent is not obtained for routine outpatient visits in which no invasive or potentially dangerous medical treatment is rendered. Consent is presumed when people present themselves for treatment, and this is sufficient for routine care. Because of the likelihood of more significant activities, however, hospitals obtain general consent for the routine treatment of inpatients. Hospital staff obtain the general consent for treatment when patients are admitted. Figure 14.1 is a sample acute care hospital general consent form.

Nonroutine diagnostic, surgical, or other invasive procedures require special consent. Figure 14.2 is a sample acute care hospital special consent form. The HSO's role in obtaining special consent is secondary and usually means obtaining the patient's signature on a form that authorizes the hospital to participate in treatment ordered or rendered by physicians. At some point prior to hospital admission, as in the case of surgery, the attending physician has provided the information that is needed by the patient to give informed consent. This consent is recorded on forms in the physician's office. When the patient is admitted, the HSO determines that the medical record contains a special consent signed by the patient, which reflects the consent process that occurred previously between the physician and patient. HSOs concerned with the ethical aspects of consent make an independent effort to determine that patients whose treatment requires a special consent are really informed. This may be a more legally prudent course of action, but doing so exceeds the legal standard of care.

A major aspect of informed consent is how much to tell the patient, and the physician must judge the extent of the patient's knowledge. States apply one of three legal standards to determine

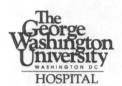

PATIENT AUTHORIZATION FORM

PATIENT IDENTIFICATION

GENERAL POLICY: All patients shall be treated, admitted and assigned accommodations without distinction to race, religion, color, national origin, sexual orientation, age or handicapping condition.

CONSENT TO TREATMENT: I have come to The George Washington University Hospital for medical treatment. I ask the health care professionals at the Hospital to provide care and treatment for me that they feel is necessary. The undersigned consents to the procedures, which may be performed during this hospitalization, or on an outpatient basis including emergency treatment or services. I consent to undergo routine tests and treatment as part of this care. These may include but are not limited to laboratory, radiology, medical or surgical tests, treatments, anesthesia or procedures as directed under the general and special instructions of the physician or surgeon. I understand that I am free to ask a member of my health care team questions about any care, treatment or medicine I am to receive. Because The George Washington University Hospital is a teaching hospital, I understand that my health care team will be made up of hospital personnel and medical students under the direction of my attending physician and his/her assistants and designees. Hospital personnel include, but are not limited to nurses, technicians, interns, residents and fellows. I am aware that the practice of medicine is not an exact science and admit that no one has given me any promises or guarantees about the result of any care or treatment I am to receive or examinations I am to undergo.
_____ (Initial here) I consent to laboratory studies (HIV, HBV, HCV) in the event a health care worker is exposed to my blood or body fluids.
_____ (Initial here) I agree to the disposal or use of any tissue or part removed from my body and/or to the taking of photographs during my treatment for research, teaching or scientific purposes as long as my identity is not disclosed.

PHYSICIANS NOT AS EMPLOYEES: I acknowledge that all physicians furnishing services including, but not limited to radiologists, pathologists, anesthesiologists, emergency department physicians, consultants and assistants to the physician are not employees of the Hospital. I understand that I may receive separate billing from each of these providers for services rendered.

RELEASE OF INFORMATION: The George Washington University Hospital is authorized to release any information necessary, including copies of my hospital and medical records to process payment claims for health care services which have been provided, and to duly authorized local and federal regulatory agencies and accrediting bodies as required or permitted by law. Such records may include information of a psychological or psychiatric nature, pertaining to my mental condition or treatment for conditions relating to the use of alcohol or drugs. In addition, I authorize my insurance carrier, employer or person otherwise responsible for payment to provide The George Washington University Hospital information necessary to determine benefits or process a claim. This release will be valid for the period of time to process the claim or until consent is revoked by myself. I release and forever discharge The George Washington University Hospital, its employees and agents, and my attending physician from any liability resulting from the release of my medical records or information from them for payment purposes. I understand that my name will be displayed in the signage system outside my hospital room.

_____ (Initial here) **PERSONAL VALUABLES: THE GEORGE WASHINGTON UNIVERSITY HOSPITAL WILL NOT BE RESPONSIBLE FOR LOSS OR DAMAGE TO CLOTHES, PERSONAL PROPERTY OR VALUABLES. MONEY AND OR VALUABLES MAY BE SECURED IN THE CASHIER'S OFFICE.**

NON-SMOKING POLICY: In accordance with regulatory agency standards, the Hospital is a non-smoking facility.

FINANCIAL AGREEMENT/ASSIGNMENT OF BENEFITS: I assign any and all insurance benefits payable to me to The George Washington University Hospital. I understand that I am responsible for payment for services rendered at the Hospital including excluded services from my insurance either because the plan deems such services not medically necessary, or for any other reason including pre-certification requirements, second opinions or preexisting conditions. Should the account be referred to any attorney or collection agency for collection, I understand that I will be responsible for attorney or collection expenses. I give permission to my insurance provider(s), including Medicare and Medicaid, to directly pay The George Washington University Hospital for my care instead of paying me. I understand that I am responsible for any health insurance deductibles and co-insurance and non-covered services.

EMERGENCY DEPARTMENT ONLY
PPO PHYSICIAN NOTIFICATION: It is the responsibility of the patient to inform the Hospital of their Primary Care Physician. If the Hospital is unable to contact or utilize the services of your physician, a non-PPO physician may be assigned to you. This could result in an increase in cost to you, the patient. My Primary Care Pyysician is:
_____.

_____ (Initial here) USE OF THE EMERGENCY DEPARTMENT: I understand that my insurance carrier/third party payer has the right to review my record for use of the emergency department. I understand that if the reason for my visit is determined by my insurance/third party payer to be a non-emergency, I will be responsible for the bill.

ADVANCE DIRECTIVE
Do you have an Advance Directive
(Living Will/Health Care Power of Attorney)?   __ Yes __ No
If no, do you want assistance completing one during this admission? __ Yes __ No
If yes, did you bring it with you?   __ Yes __ No
Give name and phone # of person to contact to obtain
   a copy for your medical record.
   Person name: _____ Phone #: _____
A copy must be on your chart within 24 hours of each admission.

I, the undersigned, state that the information that I have provided The George Washington University Hospital is correct to the best of my knowledge. I acknowledge by my signature that I have read and received a copy of this statement. I understand that by signing it, I am agreeing to it.

Unable to sign
( ) Serious Condition
X _____   ( ) _____
   Signature of patient or responsible party

_____ _____   _____ _____
Date   Witness   Hospital Representative   Date
80-010 (7/98)

Figure 14.1.   Sample general consent form. (Reprinted by permission of The George Washington University Medical Center.)

PATIENT'S REQUEST FOR PROCEDURE OPERATION AND TREATMENT

76519

(PATIENT IDENTIFICATION)

1. I, PATIENT _____ (, or

_____ as ☐ Parent ☐ Representative

☐ Guardian (Check One)

acting on his/her behalf,) request the procedure/operation/treatment set out below.

2. I have requested Dr(s). _____ perform

and supervise my procedure/operation/treatment which has been explained to me to be:

_____

_____

My doctor's explanation informed me about my medical condition as well as the common foreseeable benefits and risks of the procedure/operation/treatment as well as of its reasonable alternatives, if any.

3. I know, too, that during my procedure/operation/treatment it may become apparent to my doctor that in his/her professional judgement further procedures, operations, or treatments may be necessary. I therefore authorize modification or extension of this consent to include those additional procedures which in my doctor's professional judgement are medically necessary under these special circumstances and for my .... ☐ no exceptions

4. I understand that if a member of the Department of Anesthesiology is to participate in my care, for general, regional, or monitored anesthesia care, a separate consent will be obtained for these services.

5. If my doctor has indicated to me that I will require a local anesthetic as part of my procedure/operation/treatment, I authorize its administration. I acknowledge that my doctor has explained the benefits and risks of my receiving a local anesthetic as well as a reasonable alternative, if any. Potential risks may include but are not limited to pain at the injection site, or very rarely allergic reaction to the anesthetic. Further, I understand that during my procedure/operation/treatment, unforeseen circumstances may require alternative methods of anesthesia, such as general, and I therefore authorize modification of anesthesia administration which my doctor's professional judgment indicates to be necessary under the circumstances.

6. If it is anticipated that I may require transfusion of blood or blood products during my procedure, I will be required to sign a separate INFORMED CONSENT TO BLOOD TRANSFUSION AND/OR BLOOD COMPONENT ADMINISTRATION form. If in the event of an unanticipated emergency during my operative care and based on the medical judgement of my physician, I require the transfusion of blood or blood products, I understand they will be administered and agree to such action being taken.

7. Knowing that the George Washington University Hospital is a teaching institution, I understand that along with my doctor and his/her assistants and designees, other Hospital personnel such as residents, trainees, nurses, and technicians will be involved in my procedure/operation/ treatment and care. I understand and agree to the presence of appropriate observers for the advancement of medical education and care.

8. I consent to appropriate routine tests and treatment as part of my medical care associated with this procedure/operation/treatment.

9. I agree to the appropriate disposal of any tissue or part removed from my body, to the taking of photographs during the procedure/operation/ treatment for research, teaching, or scientific purposes as long as my identity is not disclosed, and to participate in the

_____ research protocol/program.

PATIENT AFFIRMATION By signing this request form, I am indicating that I understand the contents of this document and agree to its provisions. I know that if I have concerns or would like more detailed information, I can ask more questions and get more information from my attending physician. I am also acknowledging that I know that the practice of anesthesiology, medicine and surgery is not an exact science and that no one has given me any promises or guarantees about the designated procedure/operation/treatment or its results. I fully understand what I am now signing of my own free will.

WITNESS TO AFFIRMATION AND SIGNATURE | DATE | TIME | PATIENT SIGNATURE (or Parent, Guardian or Representative) | DATE/TIME

SIGNATURE OF PHYSICIAN OBTAINING INFORMED CONSENT _____ DATE _____ TIME _____

PHYSICIAN ATTESTATION I, Dr. _____ , attest that this patient or the representative named above has been informed about the common foreseeable risks and benefits of undergoing the procedure/operation/treatment as well as its reasonable alternative(s),if any. Further questions with regard to this procedure have been answered to his/her apparent satisfaction. | PHYSICIAN SIGNATURE | DATE/TIME

76-519 (11/97)

Figure 14.2. Sample special consent form. (Reprinted by permission of The George Washington University Medical Center.)

how much information the patient should be given: 1) that given by a reasonable physician, 2) that given to a reasonable patient, and, as a minority view, 3) what this patient wants. *Therapeutic privilege* is a legal concept that allows information to be withheld if the physician judges that the patient might be harmed or engage in harmful behavior by having it.

The consent process may one day oblige physicians to divulge their mental and physical health status, clinical experience and competence, outcomes for the procedure being contemplated, and whether they have been sued for malpractice or disciplined for poor clinical work. Such information undoubtedly is important to an informed decision, and the law is evolving in that direction. At the forefront of the duty to disclose are *Behringer v. The Medical Center at Princeton* and *Doe v. Noe,*[13] which found that HIV–positive physicians have a duty to disclose that fact to their patients.

As suggested when the ethical aspects of consent were discussed in Chapter 13, myriad factors, including education, intellect, emotional status, and general physical and psychological conditions, make it difficult for patients to give truly informed consent. Informed consent may be an impossible goal. It has been suggested that informed consent can occur only if the patient is as well qualified as the physician. Commonly, however, patients put themselves in their physicians' hands and accept their recommendations, thus minimizing, for those patients, the burden of giving consent.

Negligence

Negligence can be defined as not doing something that a reasonable person who is guided by reasonable considerations that ordinarily regulate human affairs would do, or doing something that a reasonable and prudent person would not do.[14] The test in health services is the actions or non-actions of a reasonable and prudent physician, nurse, or manager. As with the law of contracts, this seems straightforward enough, but volumes have been written to define and apply the concept of "reasonable person." What the reasonable person would do is called the *standard of care.* The standard of care is used to measure the performance of the acts (actions) in question—the alleged negligence. If the plaintiff—the party who brought the lawsuit and must prove the allegations (burden of proof)—convinces the finder of fact (a jury or a judge) by a preponderance of the evidence that the acts (actions) deviated from the standard of care, then the finder of fact will find for the plaintiff. "Preponderance of the evidence" refers to evidence that produces the stronger effect or impression, has a greater weight, and is more convincing as to its truth. Consequently, its effect is greater. If the party having the burden of proof does not meet that burden by a preponderance of the evidence, then the finder of fact must find for the defendant.

The person who engages in tortious conduct is always liable for damages. Commonly, however, HSOs/HSs are named as a defendant because of legal theories discussed subsequently. A successful lawsuit for negligent medical conduct has four elements:

1. The caregiver (physician or other care provider) must have had a duty to provide care of a certain quality (standard of care).
2. There must have been a breach of that duty—the care provided must be less than the established standard of a reasonable provider of that type of care.
3. The breach of duty must have been a substantial factor in causing the harm (*proximate cause*).
4. The patient must have been injured.

Absent any of these elements, the plaintiff patient cannot recover damages on a theory of negligence.

With few exceptions, state law in the United States places no positive legal duty on one person to aid another. This also is true for physicians and other caregivers, unless a duty has been established. Once a duty is established, care may be discontinued only if alternate provisions have been made and the patient is protected from harm. Abandonment is an intentional tort that could support a lawsuit.

Standard of Care

If providers have a duty to provide services of a certain quality, how is that standard determined? The standard of care has evolved from a locality rule that used the provider's geographic location, to a broader standard using the practice in communities of similar size and medical resources, to the current form that expects providers to meet a national standard. In general, providers are held to the standard of care that is appropriate under similar circumstances for that type of practitioner, delivered with the same reasonable and ordinary care, skill, and diligence as those in good standing would ordinarily exercise in like cases. This is the "average standard of the profession test,"[15] which is a national standard. Because providers are of different types, using various theories about disease causation and cure, practitioners must meet the standard for their type of practice.

The breach of the standard of care must be proven by testimony from people who are able to state what is normally expected of that type of practitioner delivering care with ordinary and reasonable care, skill, and diligence. This is done through expert witnesses. Historically, there was a "conspiracy of silence" because physicians refused to testify as expert witnesses against one another. Those who did often were treated badly and faced discrimination, disciplinary actions by their professional society, and ostracism by colleagues. This problem has somewhat but has not disappeared.

There are other ways to establish a breach of the standard of care: citing the treating physician's own statements; calling that physician as a hostile or adverse witness; using standard medical textbooks or similar sources; or invoking a doctrine known as *res ipsa loquitur* (the thing speaks for itself), which is a legal theory that is limited to specific circumstances. On occasion, the negligence is a matter of common knowledge and expert testimony is not needed.

Proof of Negligence and Recovery of Damages

The final elements that are needed to prove negligence are causation and injury. Causation has several aspects:

> *In addition to proving that a physician was negligent, that is, failed to meet the standard of care, and that the patient was injured, a malpractice plaintiff must also prove that the injury resulted from the negligence. Although this element of proof is called "causation," the term has a different sense from that used in medical circles. The law considers an injury to be caused by a negligent act if the injury would not have occurred but for the defendant's act, or if the injury was a foreseeable result of the negligent conduct. The legal cause of an injury is often termed the proximate cause. Note that the plaintiff need not prove that the negligent act caused the result, but only the strong likelihood that it did. Also, the negligence need not be the sole cause, but only a significant factor in the injury. It must be remembered that the purpose of a malpractice trial is not to convict the defendants of malpractice, but to decide whether the loss caused by the injury should be allocated to the defendants. The standards of proof are thus lower than for a criminal trial, for example.*[16]

To assist in solving problems of liability when two causes act together to bring about an event and either one of them alone would have brought the same result, some courts have adopted the concept of substantial factor. Was the defendant's conduct a substantial factor in bringing about the injury? An example of substantial factor occurs when two physicians treat a patient essentially simultaneously in an emergency situation and both are negligent, so that either could have caused the injury. This concept was applied by the California Supreme Court in *Landeros v. Flood,* a medical malpractice case in which the defendant negligently failed to diagnose and report battered child syndrome to authorities and the plaintiff child was returned to the same environment, where battering continued and further injuries occurred. The court found that actors may be liable if their negligence is a substantial factor in causing injury, and they are not relieved of liability because of the intervening act of a third person if such act was reasonably foreseeable at the time of their negligent conduct.[17]

Damages awarded to the plaintiff can be nominal, actual, and/or punitive. Nominal damages are paid when the plaintiff proves the case but cannot prove the extent of damages. Actual damages are awarded for past and future medical expenses and loss of income, as well as for physical pain and mental suffering. The plaintiff is awarded punitive damages when there is a desire to punish the defendant. These also are called exemplary damages and are like a fine levied against a defendant in a criminal case. Punitive damages are appropriate when conduct has been reckless, willful, malicious, or grossly negligent.

Torts and HSOs/HSs

The previous discussion about torts focused on the role of the person who committed the civil wrong, intentionally or unintentionally (negligently). This section identifies and analyzes legal theories that are used to find liability against the HSOs/HSs where there is an employment relationship or where physicians or other licensed independent practitioners (LIPs) are independent contractors. Two legal theories result in legal liability for HSOs/HSs: one is agency; the other is a general legal concept that organizations owe a duty to patients and others. Legal theories holding HSOs/HSs accountable have expanded significantly since the 1960s.

In the past HSOs, notably hospitals, often avoided liability for employees' negligent acts because of the legal theories of governmental immunity and charitable immunity. Governmental immunity derived from the king's sovereign power to be free from civil actions, a concept that has been reduced by statutes such as the Federal Tort Claims Act[18] or court decisions and is rarely available today. Also virtually extinct is the doctrine of charitable immunity, which was based on the concept that assets of a charitable HSO were unacceptably threatened if actions for medical malpractice could be brought against them.

Agency and Corporate Liability

Agency

The master's responsibility for a servant's negligence was established in English common law and is embodied in the Latin phrase *respondeat superior* (let the master answer). Similarly, principals are responsible for their agents' acts. The negligence of a servant or agent is imputed (vicarious liability) to the person who is best able to exercise control—the master or principal—which is known as the law of agency. An important pragmatic consideration underlying *respondeat superior* is that courts sometimes search for a deep pocket, and employers usually have one. This doctrine applies to HSO/HS employees' acting within the scope of their employment. It has limited applicability to caregivers who are independent contractors because they exercise control over the means and methods of performing their tasks, rather than being controlled by the HSO/HS. Therefore, the legal theory of agency cannot be used to hold the HSO/HS liable for their negligent acts. Physicians are the most common type of independent contractor in HSOs. The legal doctrine of apparent or ostensible agency is applied when a patient is wittingly or unwittingly led to believe that the HSO is an employer of a caregiver who would otherwise be defined as an independent contractor. A reasonable person standard is used.

Corporate Liability

The other legal theory used to hold HSOs/HSs liable is based on a general concept that the HSO/HS owes a duty to patients (as well as to others, such as visitors) to protect them from harm. This is known as corporate liability, an area of tort law that expanded rapidly in the last decades of the 20th century. In the past this legal doctrine allowed recovery by visitors and patients injured because the HSO did not maintain buildings, grounds, and equipment in safe condition. In addition, the HSO/HS has a duty to take reasonable steps in selecting and retaining those who provide services as independent contractors. HMOs, for example, may be liable for the negligence of their independent contractor physicians using legal theories such as nondelegable duties by contract or by statute, joint venture, agency, or apparent or ostensible agency.[19] Managed care organizations face similar risks.

Implications for HSOs/HSs

Southwick concludes that these two concepts of organization liability for malpractice have virtually merged into one:

> It should . . . be acknowledged that in the hospital setting there is no longer a viable distinction between the rules of respondeat superior, on one hand, and corporate or independent negligence, on the other. Essentially, the two theories have become one. . . . In the delivery of health care services in an institutional setting it is increasingly difficult to determine factually who is in control of whom. As allied health care professionals proliferate and are accorded a greater degree of independence from the direct supervision and control of the attending physician, the matter of the right to control another's actions becomes a very difficult question both as a matter of fact and of law. It therefore becomes necessary to place either sole or joint liability upon the institution which, in the final analysis, is ultimately responsible for arranging, providing, and coordinating the activities of a host of professional persons, all of whom must work together in the care of patients.[20]

This evolution of law has major consequences for HSOs/HSs. They are not yet guarantors of the results of medical treatment, but the field is moving toward unequivocal accountability for all HSO/HS activities that fall below the standard of care. HSOs use quality assessment, continuous quality improvement, and risk management to establish and maintain high levels of quality. These concepts are considered in Chapters 9 and 10.

ENTERPRISE LIABILITY

The concept of enterprise liability includes elements of strict liability and corporate liability, which were discussed previously, and no-fault, which is discussed later. The 1993 Clinton health reform plan included tort reform, a prominent part of which was enterprise liability. Opposition caused the original proposal that "qualified health plans" bear all liability for medical malpractice to be diminished to a demonstration project. Enterprise liability, also known as organizational liability, continues to be a favorite of tort reformers, however. It changes the locus of liability for patient injuries without other significant alterations to the rules of proof and damages.[21] Channeling liability to hospitals (or other types of HSOs) is justified on several grounds:

> First, insurers would have an improved ability to price insurance, since difficulties in pricing for individual physicians in high-risk specialties would be eliminated; in most other areas of tort law, from environmental to products risk, business enterprises bear the cost of insuring against liability. Second, by eliminating the insurance problems inherent in the fragmented malpractice market, specialties such as obstetrics would no longer face onerous burdens, nor will physicians have to face premiums that fluctuate excessively from year to year. Third, physicians would be freed from the psychological stress inflicted by being named defendants in malpractice suits. Fourth, administrative and litigation costs would be reduced by having only one defendant,

rather than the multiplicity of providers named in the typical malpractice suit. Fifth, and most
important, patterns of poor medical practice would be deterred by placing liability on institutions
rather than individuals, since organizations have superior data collection abilities and manage-
ment tools for managing risks.[22]

Proponents argue that a compensation system that rewards more claimants, especially small ones, in a more evenhanded and rapid fashion than does the current tort system will be an improvement, even if it is not cheaper.[23] Opponents argue that individuals rather than organizations should be accountable for medical care, excessive power will accrue to organizations, and physicians will be pitted against organizations.[24] Enterprise liability is but a logical extension of the evolution of vicarious liability and corporate negligence, which have moved the locus of much medical liability from independent contractor physicians to HSOs, especially hospitals.

MALPRACTICE "CRISES"

The medical malpractice "crises" in the late 1960s/early 1970s and mid-1980s resulted from unexpected substantial increases in physician and hospital tort liability insurance premiums. It is thought that these increases resulted from adverse court decisions in medical negligence cases and insurance carriers' fears that they had underestimated their potential liability. In both crises the premium increases caused physicians in some states to "go on strike" by declining to admit patients or provide certain types of care. Other physicians threatened similar action.

The general concern caused by the first malpractice crisis prompted the establishment in 1971 of a Secretary's Commission on Medical Malpractice in the U.S. Department of Health, Education, and Welfare, now the Department of Health and Human Services (DHHS). Its 1973 report put the first crisis into perspective. It found that a claim was asserted for only 1 of every 226,000 patient visits to doctors; most doctors had never had a medical malpractice suit filed against them; and, regardless of size, most hospitals went through an entire year without a claim filed against them.[25] At that time, medical malpractice insurance premiums were less than 1% of national health care expenditures. Analysis of claims files showed that insurance carriers judged 46% of claims meritorious, a finding contradicting assertions that malpractice claims were largely baseless.

The 1980s malpractice problem was more regionalized; *crisis* was a word that was used rarely. Claims per physician rose nearly by half from 1980 to 1986, and the average claim more than doubled in real terms. Premiums increased by 81% from 1982 to 1985.[26] The problem diminished by the late 1980s as premiums declined with claims.[27] The claims rate increased steadily from 1988 to 1993 but then leveled off into the mid-1990s.[28] By the late 1990s, however, claim costs had begun to rise, a development likely to lead to increased malpractice insurance rates.[29]

Sources describing the second malpractice "crisis" are more diverse. A 1991 New York State report using mid-1980s data supported the 1973 Secretary's Commission finding that malpractice is a real rather than imagined problem. It estimated that the fraction of medical negligence leading to claims is probably under 2% and that "(p)erhaps half the claimants will eventually receive compensation."[30]

Additional evidence of the malpractice problem is found in a report that was released in late 1999 by the Institute of Medicine (IoM) of the National Academy of Sciences. The report estimated that medical mistakes result in between 44,000 and 98,000 deaths annually in the U.S. health services system, making them the eighth leading cause of death. The IoM report focused on hospitals because they have the best data sets. Because few data were available from other types of HSOs, even this high number may understate the problem.[31] Mistakes occurred largely because of the cumulative opportunities for human error that arise in complex medical systems, not because of flagrant recklessness. Most mistakes resulted from medication errors—wrong drug, wrong dosage, wrong time, or wrong patient. In commenting on the report, one of its authors, Donald M. Berwick, stated, "You can't use fear or blaming of individuals as a foundation for safety improvement. We want to set up an environment where more errors will be revealed."[32] Establishing such a quality environment is discussed in Chapter 9.

State boards of medicine (licensing bodies) appear to lack aggressiveness in disciplining physicians, an issue that is raised repeatedly by public interest groups. By 1998, approximately 25% of the physicians who had ever been disciplined by the Drug Enforcement Administration (restriction or revocation of federal narcotics license) or by Medicare (exclusion from Medicare) had received no state sanctions. Also by 1998, 16,638 physicians were listed as having been disciplined by either state medical boards or federal agencies, an increase of 4,652 since 1996.[33] In 1996 the Federation of State Medical Boards reported that 3,880 physicians were disciplined, including 1,607 who lost their licenses or privileges and 1,261 whose practice was restricted.[34] This was a rate of serious disciplinary actions of 3.96/1,000 physicians. It is argued that the rate should be closer to 10/1,000, a rate exceeded by only a few states, including Mississippi.[35]

Effects of Malpractice Suits

There has been an important change in the public perception of malpractice suits. A 1982 survey by AMA found that nearly 50% of those queried thought that malpractice suits were justified. In early 1989, however, the same survey found that view held by only 27%.[36] Business executives are taking a hard line about the effect of medical malpractice claims on health care costs. A 1991 poll found that 79% believed that liability awards and malpractice insurance were the most important factors in driving up health insurance costs, a number far exceeding those who believed technology, inefficient hospitals, and unnecessary care were responsible.[37] Later findings suggested that the number of claims and level of awards by juries would decline, despite data showing significant amounts of medical malpractice.

Defendants win more than two thirds of medical malpractice claims, and, if cases go to trial, defendants prevail more than 80% of the time. Defending a malpractice case consumes 40% of the costs; the average cost of defending a malpractice claim was almost $20,000 in 1995. The expert witnesses who are needed to defend a case account for almost 12% of defense costs.[38]

Fear of malpractice lawsuits affects medical practice and results in distrust and antagonism between physicians and patients (some physicians screen patients for attributes of litigiousness), defensive medicine, and higher fees to recoup higher insurance premiums. Defensive medicine is defined as physicians ordering tests, procedures, or visits, or avoiding high-risk patients or procedures, primarily to reduce their exposure to malpractice liability.[39] Defensive medicine is thought to forestall lawsuits and provide a defense if they are instituted.[40] Although expensive in absolute terms, defensive medicine is insignificant as compared with all health services expenditures. In 1991 defensive medicine costs were estimated at $15 billion, which it was asserted overstated them.[41] A report by the Office of Technology Assessment (OTA) estimated that less than 8% of diagnostic procedures were consciously defensive in nature, even though it concluded that the costs of defensive medicine could not be measured accurately.[42] Alleged diagnostic omissions were considered important in less than 9% of claims and of central importance in 4%, but, compared with other claim types, were more likely to be paid, had a higher median payment, and were more often associated with significant patient injury or death.[43] Although relatively uncommon, these types of claims are difficult to defend. There is evidence that physician concern about iatrogenesis (physician-caused medical problems) from overtesting is counterbalancing the use of ancillary services.

Medical malpractice insurance premiums are another dimension of malpractice. In 1993 medical malpractice insurance costs were estimated by OTA as substantially less than 1% of the nation's overall health care costs,[44] a number that is identical to that cited 20 years earlier. AMA data show that, from 1982 to 1988, liability insurance premiums were only 5.6% of a physician's total budget for professional expenses. Applying this percentage nationally means premiums and damage payments totaled $5.7 billion of the $102.7 billion spent on physicians' services. The physicians surveyed estimated that the costs of defensive medicine and the time that they spent away from the office because of malpractice litigation cost them $19.3 billion. Professional liability costs of $25 billion were only 5% of total health services expenditures of almost $500 billion in 1987.[45]

Another way to understand the impact of medical malpractice is by the amount of premiums that are paid. In 1995 the average annual professional liability insurance premium for a self-employed physician was $15,000, with a low of $5,500 for psychiatry ($7,900 for pediatrics and $9,000 for general/family practice) and a high of $38,600 for obstetrics-gynecology.[46]

Malpractice premium cost changes seem linked in part to the insurance industry's business cycles. Good profits because of high premium income cause new companies to enter the medical malpractice insurance market. Increased competition forces premiums down, and reduced profits force some insurers out of the market. The remaining insurers can then dramatically increase premiums. The cycles are worsened because most carriers rely on nonpremium income from investments as a supplement; thus poor investment policies exacerbate the effects of increased competition.

Reforms of the Malpractice System

Early state efforts at tort reform included limiting noneconomic damages, primarily recovery for pain and suffering; capping plaintiffs' legal fees; and allowing juries to learn how much money plaintiffs received from other sources (modifying the collateral source rule). Some state supreme courts have found such limitations constitutional.[47] In addition, legislative proposals include modifying the joint liability doctrine, allowing defendants to pay in installments, establishing malpractice screening panels, establishing patient compensation funds, granting immunity, and implementing a no-fault scheme.[48] It is argued that such reforms do not address the root of malpractice because the basic system is unchanged. Caps on damages and attorneys' fees lower insurance premiums, but "patients with the most serious injuries are the ones who pay the price for the strategy."[49] Indiana's 1975 tort reforms decreased premiums but resulted in more injured patients getting more money than was paid before. More than 50% of closed claims nationwide were settled without payment, compared with only 33% in Indiana.[50] Mid-1990s data show that tort reforms in California and Indiana produced no savings in health care costs.[51] A further complication is that many such laws have been ruled unconstitutional.[52] There appears to be a trend toward state supreme courts rulings that tort reform caps are unconstitutional.[53]

It is argued that reforms such as no-fault, which compensates injured people without litigation or assigning liability, are key to reducing medical malpractice costs. Workers' compensation, which pays medical expenses and lost income to workers injured on the job, is an example of no-fault. No-fault malpractice systems in Virginia and Florida apply to newborns who suffer neurological damage caused by medical treatment during delivery. Both states allow recovery for medical and rehabilitation expenses as well as compensation to replace lost future wages and noneconomic losses. The compensation for future wages and noneconomic damages is less than successful plaintiffs could obtain under a tort system, and it is argued that these no-fault systems have not performed as expected. Families of newborns who suffered neurological injuries during birth have had difficulty proving that the injuries were iatrogenic (physician caused), especially when the babies were born with cerebral palsy or other birth defects.[54]

No-fault may dramatically increase rather than decrease costs, however. A Maine study found that time, financial costs, and, most significantly, contact with attorneys appear to discourage many patients from seeking redress for medical malpractice injuries. The data suggest that few people who believe that they have experienced iatrogenic illness or injury go to attorneys; those who do so follow long and circuitous routes. More discuss their problems with health services professionals, including those whom they think caused the injuries, and at a much earlier stage.[55] Evidence is mounting that (primary care) physicians who communicate effectively with their patients are sued less often and that physicians who admit errors and apologize for them are less likely to be sued.[56]

The 1993 Clinton health proposal included tort reform, but interest in federal preemption of state medical malpractice law has waned. Future federal regulation is likely to be incremental and tied to excess testing, defensive medicine, and Medicare reimbursement.

NONJUDICIAL MEANS OF RESOLVING DISPUTES

Most lawsuits are settled before trial; some are settled after trial begins. Settlement occurs at the behest of counsel, or the parties perceive the advantages of avoiding a trial: uncertainty of outcome, desire to control the result, and avoiding a trial's negative publicity. State law may require settlement efforts; many courts have mandatory procedures to settle cases.

Resolving disputes in court is expensive and time consuming. Since the mid-1980s much attention has been given to alternative dispute resolution (ADR). ADR includes binding and non binding arbitration (which may be voluntary or nonvoluntary), mediation, mini trials, neutral fact finding, and variations of these techniques; each has attributes that may make it best to resolve a dispute. ADR is private, inexpensive, and efficient—attributes that are especially useful for HSOs/ HSs. Each type of ADR has attributes that make it a better means of resolving a dispute than going to trial. For example, mediation is especially useful when the parties want to maintain a continuing relationship. Professional staff, in particular, should be aware of the advantages of ADR, and their bylaws should reflect its use. A number of private organizations provide mediators, arbitrators, and other experts in ADR.

Several states use screening panels to determine whether medical malpractice claims should proceed to trial. The panels identify nonmeritorious claims, reduce the burden on the courts, promote early disposition or settlement of meritorious claims, and reduce the cost of medical care by decreasing malpractice claims. In 1980 some type of screening panel was used in 26 states.[57] By 1994 only 16 states had screening panels, usually comprising an attorney, a physician, and a consumer or health services manager.[58] Use of the screening panel was mandatory in most of the states that had them, but the panel's decision regarding the health care provider's liability was nonbinding and the plaintiffs could, and often did, file suit following an unfavorable finding. Since 1990, legislatures and supreme courts in 11 states have eliminated screening panels because they were found to be inefficient or infringed on the constitutional right to a speedy trial.[59]

In future, more HSOs/HSs are likely to use mediation or voluntary binding arbitration to settle medical malpractice claims. *Voluntary* means that if the parties choose to have the claim arbitrated, the arbitrator's award is binding and judicial remedies are unavailable. Despite its potential, Michigan's 18-year-old program was eliminated in 1993.[60] By contrast, the presuit voluntary binding arbitration program that was adopted by Florida in 1988 as part of tort reform offers significant potential benefit to plaintiffs and defendants.[61]

Kaiser-Permanente (a large HMO) contracts require enrollees in several states to use binding arbitration for alleged medical malpractice claims and other disputes. Parties retain their own attorneys and share the costs of a three-member arbitration panel. The program has resulted in compensation for a greater number of patients, even though the amounts that are paid are more modest.[62] However, contracts of adhesion, such as Kaiser-Permanente's, are scrutinized closely and may be unenforceable.[63] In addition, given the strong constitutional safeguards of a right to trial by jury, mandatory arbitration is not generally viewed favorably by courts.[64]

Mediation is common in court-annexed programs. For example, the Superior Court of the District of Columbia requires mediation of all cases in its small claims division (claims up to $5,000).

For cases in its civil division, judges may order mediation, evaluation (similar to neutral fact finding), or nonbinding arbitration, which becomes binding arbitration if the parties agree or fail to file a timely request for a trial de novo. A number of cases in the civil division involve medical malpractice. In both divisions, cases that do not settle are scheduled for trial.

This discussion of ADR has focused on medical malpractice, but many other types of problems occur in HSOs/HSs: professional staff appointment and credentialing issues; disputes regarding sales agreements and employment and construction contracts; debt collection; and zoning appeals. ADR is common outside health services and it has significant potential for expanded application in HSOs/HSs.

DEVELOPING LEGAL AREAS

HIV and AIDS Legal Issues and Litigation

In the legal arena human immunodeficiency virus (HIV) and acquired immunodeficiency syndrome (AIDS) are daunting to HSOs/HSs. By 1990 the number of AIDS–related lawsuits was already the largest number that are attributable to any disease in U.S. legal history, and it was predicted that HSOs would become the most important focus of AIDS–related litigation in the near future.[65] By mid-1995, 50% of the lawsuits that were filed under the Americans with Disabilities Act (ADA) of 1990 involved AIDS.[66] (Chapter 13 provides background information on HIV and AIDS.)

One area of litigation results from special risks that are present when staff members work with AIDS patients. Under the Occupational Safety and Health Act of 1970, administered by the Occupational Safety and Health Administration (OSHA), employers must provide employment and a place of employment that is free from recognized hazards that cause or are likely to cause death or serious physical harm.[67] OSHA requires universal blood and body substance precautions, which are likely to be the focus of targeted enforcement and responses to employee complaints. OSHA offers educational programs about AIDS hazards and precautions and requires them of employers.

The second legal dimension concerns the risk to patients and staff from patients infected with HIV and the opportunistic diseases that invariably develop as HIV progresses to frank AIDS. As they protect patients and staff, HSOs/HSs must avoid discriminating against people with AIDS, whom the law defines as having a disability. The rights of people with disabilities to full and equal enjoyment of public accommodations were strengthened in 1990 by ADA, which combined protections for such individuals found in the Civil Rights Act of 1964, the Rehabilitation Act of 1973, and the Civil Rights Restoration Act of 1988.[68] ADA protects people who are HIV positive or have AIDS from discrimination in places of public accommodation, which include professional offices. Physicians or dentists can refuse to treat an HIV–positive or AIDS patient only under limited circumstances, such as cases in which the needed care is outside the provider's expertise.[69] Prudence suggests that the patient must be referred to an appropriate provider, however.

A third legal dimension concerns risk to patients and staff from staff who are infected with HIV. HSOs are subject to Section 504 of the federal Rehabilitation Act of 1973, which prohibits discrimination against otherwise qualified people with disabilities. Protections in the Rehabilitation Act of 1973 for such applicants or employees were strengthened by ADA, which requires that employers make reasonable accommodations for employees with disabilities and provides other protections to them.

> In order to establish a violation of either of these statutes [Section 504 of the Rehabilitation Act and Title II of the ADA], a plaintiff must prove: (1) that he has a disability; (2) that he is otherwise qualified for the employment or benefit in question; and (3) that he was excluded from the employment or benefit due to discrimination solely on the basis of the disability. Regarding the

second requirement, an individual is not otherwise qualified if he poses a significant risk to the health or safety of others by virtue of the disability that cannot be eliminated by reasonable accommodation.[70]

ADA protects HIV–positive applicants and employees. Whether such an employee is "otherwise qualified" in a health services setting is considered later in this section.

In 1987 the U.S. Supreme Court considered a case that is analogous to that of an HIV–positive employee. In *School Board of Nassau County, Florida v. Arline,*[71] a teacher who had three recurrences of tuberculosis was discharged because the school board considered her to be a health risk to students. The Court determined that tuberculosis was contagious and was a "handicapping condition" protected by Section 504 of the Rehabilitation Act of 1973. The Court developed a four-part test: nature of the risk (how the disease is transmitted); duration of the risk (how long the carrier is infectious); severity of the risk (potential harm to third parties); and probability that the disease will be transmitted. The case was remanded to the trial court to determine whether Arline was otherwise qualified and whether she could have been accommodated in alternate employment. A footnote in *Arline* stated that the Court was not deciding whether people with a contagious disease have a physical impairment or whether they have a disability solely because of contagiousness.

Additional federal protection for HIV–positive people is found in the Civil Rights Restoration Action of 1987, which amended the Rehabilitation Act so that people with a contagious disease or infection are protected if they do not "constitute a direct threat to health or safety" and are able to "perform the duties of the job."[72] Federal legislation is buttressed by disability statutes in the 50 states and the District of Columbia.[73] *Arline* may be distinguished from situations in which HSO staff have AIDS: chronic (tuberculosis) versus acute (the opportunistic diseases that eventually afflict people who are HIV positive); type of setting; the risk to students (who are likely to be healthy) versus the risk to ill, possibly immunosuppressed non–AIDS patients; and the well-established legal duties that HSOs have to protect patients. An analysis of cases involving HIV–positive applicants or staff should distinguish those who are HIV positive from those with frank AIDS, who may have other infectious diseases. Such considerations will affect application of ADA in HSOs/HSs as well.

Cases litigating whether HIV–positive health services staff are "otherwise qualified" under ADA seem to turn on the potential risk of harm to patients, even when that harm is remote. A state appeals court in Illinois found that by constructively discharging James Davis, a cook with HIV who prepared and distributed food and cleaned the kitchen and storeroom, a nursing facility had violated ADA by discriminating against him on the basis of his disability. Davis's doctor had written to the nursing facility stating that HIV is not transmitted through preparing and serving food and beverages and that his HIV status did not restrict him from performing his job.[74] Conversely, a federal court case involving William Mauro, a surgical technician with HIV who assisted in exposure-prone invasive procedures, held that ADA and the Rehabilitation Act of 1973 did not apply because Mauro's HIV status disqualified him from working as a surgical technician and that he was not "otherwise qualified" to perform his job. Mauro acknowledged that his duties occasionally required him to place his hands on and into surgical incisions and that this put him at risk for needle sticks and minor lacerations. Mauro's expert witness testified that the risk of transmitting HIV to a patient is very small. However, the trial court applied the four-part test that was enunciated by the Supreme Court in *Arline* and agreed with the defendant hospital that there was a real possibility of transmitting HIV and that, because the consequence of infection is death, the nature, duration, and severity of the risk outweighed the fact that the chance of transmission was slight.[75]

Other legal aspects of AIDS are confidentiality, including reporting HIV infection, and the duty to warn third parties. Legal protections against breaching medical confidentiality are well established. The AIDS epidemic caused most states to pass laws safeguarding the confidentiality and privacy of people who are infected or who are thought to be infected with HIV.[76] All states require physicians to report AIDS cases to the health department. Extending reporting to the results of HIV antibody testing has proved more difficult, however; only about half of the states require it.[77] Contact tracing, a historically important role for health departments, is belatedly being applied to HIV infection.

The concept of duty to warn defines the extent to which caregivers are legally obligated to protect third parties in immediate danger. In *Tarasoff v. Regents of the State of California*[78] the California Supreme Court held that a psychotherapist who reasonably believes that a patient poses a direct threat to a third party must warn the person who is in danger. Many state supreme courts have adopted *Tarasoff*; most limit the duty to warn identifiable third parties at risk of real and probable harm.[79] This legal doctrine may well be applied to HIV infection.

Antitrust

The federal government's interest in prohibiting private business activity that impedes marketplace competition dates from the Sherman Antitrust Act of 1890, which was passed "against a background of rampant cartelization and monopolization of the American economy."[80] In 1914 Congress enacted additional antitrust legislation in the Federal Trade Commission Act and the Clayton Act. The Department of Justice (DOJ) and FTC share responsibility for enforcement. State antitrust laws are patterned after the federal statutes.

Professions

The application of federal antitrust law in the health services field dates from the 1940s. In *AMA v. United States*[81] AMA and its Washington, D.C., affiliate society were convicted of a criminal violation of Section 3 of the Sherman Act because they had conspired to prevent Group Health Association (a HMO) from hiring and retaining physicians. A doctrine that the professions were immune from civil suit under antitrust laws had developed through court decisions (common law), but in 1975 the U.S. Supreme Court held that the learned professions, including physicians, were subject to the antitrust laws.[82] Federal antitrust law is especially powerful and frightening for defendants because successful plaintiffs are entitled to treble damages, that is, three times the damages that can be established. Prevailing plaintiffs in a private antitrust action may petition the court to have their attorneys' fees paid by a losing defendant.[83] The Equal Access to Justice Act of 1985 mandates the award of reasonable attorney's fees unless the "position of the United States was substantially justified or that special circumstances would make the award unjust," and thus offers some protection from an onerous financial burden to defendants in federal cases.[84]

Facilities Planning

The first significant Supreme Court decision to apply antitrust principles in health services delivery was *Hospital Building Co. v. Trustees of Rex Hospital* in 1976.[85] The case involved two defendant hospitals that had cooperated with the local health planning council to develop a long-term community plan. Subsequently, they used the plan to oppose the plaintiff hospital's application for a certificate of need to expand its facility, arguing that this would duplicate facilities that the planning council had recommended for the defendant hospitals. After 14 years of litigation, the final decision applied a modified rule of reason.[86] This means that, absent per se violations of antitrust law (horizontal price fixing, allocation or division of a market, group boycotts and joint refusals to deal, and tie-in sales), the Court compares favorable and unfavorable effects of a restraint of trade on competition.[87]

Mergers

Because of their great potential to reduce competition, mergers have been of special interest to both DOJ and FTC. *United States v. Rockford Memorial Corporation*[88] involved a merger of two not-for-profit hospitals that was challenged by the federal government under the Sherman Act. The court of appeals stated that Clayton Act restrictions on mergers applied to not-for-profit hospitals, despite the government's failure to make this argument. *Rockford* conflicts with *United States v. Carilion Health Systems, Community Hospital of Roanoke Valley,*[89] wherein a federal district court held that Clayton Act merger restrictions did not apply to not-for-profit hospitals. The Supreme Court's refusal to hear an appeal of *Rockford* caused considerable confusion about application of federal antitrust law in not-for-profit hospital mergers. Such uncertainty is especially problematic when hospitals and other types of HSOs face financial difficulties because of the inefficiencies of excess capacity and duplicative services. It has been argued that *Rockford* does not prohibit mergers:

> *Of the five . . . mergers that were cleared to go forward, all were scrutinized by the FTC or Justice Department using the same standards that were applied in the* Rockford *case.*
>
> *It is difficult to deduce from that empirical evidence that the antitrust standards applied by the federal enforcement agencies—as is articulated in* Rockford—*compel a cessation of hospital merger activity.*
>
> *The[se] examples show that antitrust analysis is fact-specific. There are so many different combinations and fact patterns that high-profile cases don't always produce the same antitrust results. This phenomenon is particularly true in health care because of the wide variety of types of facilities and ownership and because of the multiple legal structures that are used in mergers and affiliations.*[90]

In 1996 a joint DOJ/FTC policy statement declared that, absent extraordinary circumstances, the agencies will not challenge a merger between two acute care hospitals in which one of the hospitals 1) averaged less than 100 licensed beds in the last 3 years, 2) averaged a daily census of fewer than 40 inpatients in the last 3 years, and 3) is more than 5 years old. The agencies assume that such a hospital cannot achieve the economies of scale of a larger facility and that anticompetitive effects of merging with a larger competitor would be inconsequential. This suggests that the agencies are willing to recognize that efficiency may be served by allowing acquisition of a weak facility by a stronger company and that this goal may override the usual concern about increases in concentration of the market.[91]

Peer Review

Historically, antitrust actions against physicians and HSOs arose in hospitals in which the professional staff organization (PSO) routinely conducts peer review of its members' performance. When peer decisions cause PSO members to lose or be denied privileges, it is alleged that the actions are anticompetitive because they are based on economics, not on efforts to improve quality. In *Patrick v. Burget* a physician alleged federal antitrust violations when peer review brought an end to his clinic practice and a suspension of his hospital privileges.[92]

The potential chilling effect of such legal actions on peer review and other efforts to improve the quality of care resulted in passage of the Health Care Quality Improvement Act of 1986 (HCQIA).[93] HCQIA provides limited immunity from paying damages in private lawsuits under federal or state law (except civil rights laws) for any "professional review action" (which includes peer review) if that professional review action follows standards that are established in the law. Standards include a reasonable belief that the action was justified in furthering the quality of health care, there was a reasonable effort to obtain the facts, and the physician (or dentist) was given adequate notice and a fair hearing or such other procedures fair under the circumstances. Cases such as *Austin v. McNamara* and *Egan v. Athol Memorial Hospital* show that the peer review protections in HCQIA are achieving their purpose.[94]

HCQIA includes reporting requirements for several types of entities for a variety of professional review actions and establishes a national practitioner data bank to receive reports and provide information to certain people and organizations. Sanctions by boards of medical examiners (state licensing boards) must be reported. In addition, HCQIA requires hospitals and other health care entities that provide health care services and engage in formal peer review to report

1. Professional review actions that adversely affect the clinical privileges of a physician for longer than 30 days
2. Surrender of clinical privileges by a physician
   • While the physician is under investigation by the entity relating to possible incompetence or improper professional conduct
   • In return for not conducting an investigation or proceeding
3. If a professional society takes a professional review action that adversely affects the physician's membership

Reports are sent to the state board of medical examiners, which sends them to the National Practitioner Data Bank (NPDB). In addition, entities (including insurance companies) that make a payment under a policy of insurance, self-insurance, or otherwise to settle (or partially settle) or to satisfy a judgment in a medical malpractice action or claim must report certain information to NPDB. This part of the statute is broader because information about payments for the benefit of LIPs, as well as physicians, must be reported. HSOs must query NPDB when granting privileges and are presumed to know what information is there.

NPDB became operational in late 1990. Whether HCQIA actually will encourage or discourage peer review is unclear. It has been argued that the requirement to report any payment discourages settlement; a straightforward business decision to settle a malpractice case could be interpreted as an admission of culpability by the physician. HCQIA has some loopholes. In a practice known as "corporate shielding," physicians need not be reported to NPDB if the plaintiff agrees to drop them from the lawsuit before settlement; in such instances the HSO pays the settlement.[95] NPDB reporting also is avoided if disciplinary actions against physicians are handled earlier and informally. For example, physicians with quality-of-care problems can be told informally that it would be better if they did not admit any more patients to the hospital and that at the next reappointment cycle they do not seek renewal of privileges. Thus, because there is neither a formal investigation nor a peer review action, no report to NPDB is required.

A 1995 report showed that 75% of all hospitals never reported an adverse action against practitioners in their facilities, and the rate of reporting varied from a low of 0.7 to a high of 8.5/1,000 hospital beds. The wide variation is troubling and suggests differences in the quality of care or in the willingness of hospitals to submit reports.[96] It may be, however, that finding adverse occurrences is a function of data sources, and this makes comparisons among hospitals appropriate only when systems for detection have similar validity.[97]

Summary

It is certain that DOJ and FTC will continue to be attentive to the health services field, even though their focus is likely to change to managed care arrangements, physician joint ventures, networks, and vertical integration.[98] In the early 1990s "sham independent practice associations" (IPAs) that were nothing more than blatant price-fixing arrangements were of special interest.[99] In the mid- to late 1990s, DOJ and FTC applied a "rule of reason" to allow clinical integration (e.g., utilization review, quality assurance, profiling network members) alone to justify price setting by IPAs, even if physicians do not take monetary risk or financially integrate their practices.[100]

It is noteworthy that, although most attention in antitrust litigation has focused on DOJ and FTC, a 1990 study found that state attorneys general have filed or investigated at least 70 health services antitrust cases since 1985. Allegations have included illegal group boycotts or concerted efforts by competitors against a third party, price fixing, anticompetitive mergers, and other suspected antitrust violations. Likely to receive future attention are nursing facilities, third-party payers, hospital mergers, mergers of large HMOs, and "sham" physician unions.[101]

Emergency Medical Treatment and Active Labor Act

The federal Emergency Medical Treatment and Active Labor Act (EMTALA) was passed in 1985.[102] It requires that hospitals participating in Medicare provide a screening examination to people who present at their emergency department. If an emergency condition is determined, then the hospital must treat and stabilize the patient unless the patient requests a transfer in writing with knowledge of the hospital's obligation under EMTALA, or a physician certifies that the benefits to the patient of an unstabilized transfer outweigh the risks. The means of transportation that are used to transfer must meet statutory requirements as to adequacy of equipment and personnel, the receiving facility must agree to accept the transfer, and medical records must be provided to the receiving facility. In 1989 EMTALA was amended to apply to women in any stage of labor, rather than merely active labor.[103] Women in labor are in an emergency condition if transfer cannot occur before delivery or if transfer presents a health threat to the woman or unborn child.[104]

People who are injured because of a failure to meet EMTALA have a cause of action against the hospital, as do facilities that suffer a financial loss because of the transfer. In addition, hospitals and "responsible" physicians are liable for civil money penalties for violating EMTALA.[105] In mid-1998 the work of a joint AHA-Health Care Financing Administration (HCFA) task force caused HCFA to issue revised instructions, investigative procedures, and interpretive guidelines that should clarify health care providers' EMTALA obligations.[106]

Employee Retirement Income Security Act

In 1974 Congress enacted the Employee Retirement Income Security Act (ERISA) to exempt employee benefit plans from state law to allow uniform administration and protect the rights of employees in the plans.[107] ERISA does not comprehensively regulate the content of employer-provided health care plans, including the benefits that are provided through managed care organizations. Instead, it relies on disclosure, administrative requirements, and fiduciary obligations to prevent abusive practices by employer-provided health plans.[108] ERISA has created a legislative void—an area in which the states may not regulate and Congress has not addressed the content of employee health plans. This void is being filled by judge-made federal common law and fragmented legislation at the state and federal levels.[109]

The legal status of fiduciaries and the high standard to which they are held is discussed in Chapter 13. Fiduciaries are important in ERISA. They include the plan itself, the plan administrator and sponsor, the employer, and others acquiring this status because of relationships to the plan or its assets. ERISA states that fiduciaries breach their fiduciary duties by failing to pay a valid claim or by causing losses to the plan, and ERISA holds them personally liable.[110]

The application of ERISA, however, is a case study in what political scientists call the law of unintended consequences. Its preemption of state law is being used successfully by some insurers, health plans, and managed care organizations to deny employees' claims, prominent among which are tort claims under state law. Employees can be denied a right to sue if ERISA preempts state law, which depends on whether the claim has a connection with or reference to a benefit plan.[111] Preemption was found in some cases[112] but not in others.[113] Federal courts seem to agree that a denial of benefits falls under ERISA because the law regulates them specifically. It is less clear whether ERISA applies when a patient's claim involves vicarious liability for the alleged negligence of a contracting physician.[114]

ERISA limits damages to the costs of the denied treatment, which usually are only a fraction of damages. In late 1997 Texas became the first state to allow patient suits for managed care treatment decisions or delays that cause injury,[115] a law that will have no effect if a court determines that state law is preempted because ERISA applies to the employer-sponsored plan that is the defendant in the lawsuit.

Jurisdictional issues underlie suits against employer-sponsored health plans, primarily because of the need to interpret federal preemption of state laws. Plaintiffs prefer to have the case heard in state court because that court is less likely to find that state law is preempted and is likely to be a more sympathetic venue for medical malpractice claims. Conversely, defendants prefer federal court, where there are more likely to be judges who are willing to find a federal preemption of state law.

Problems regarding ERISA's preemption of state medical malpractice law will be exacerbated by continued growth of managed care and HMOs. Only Congress can eliminate the unintended consequences of ERISA and remove a needless level of uncertainty.

Medicare and Medicaid Fraud and Abuse

Since Medicare and Medicaid were enacted in 1965, a great body of law has been built on the amendments, regulations, and court decisions that followed. A special focus of Congress has been what is generically called fraud and abuse, defined broadly to include lying, stealing, providing too few or too many services, improperly coding services, bribes and kickbacks, and self-referrals.[116] Congress has been of some assistance to providers by identifying exceptions and by authorizing DHHS "to issue 'safe harbor' regulations delineating conduct that DHHS determined would not be subject to prosecution or exclusion under the anti-kickback statute."[117] Of the numerous actions defined by Medicare and Medicaid as fraud and abuse, only fraudulent billing and self-referral are considered in detail here.

Fraudulent Billing

In addition to the *qui tam* actions described later, there are civil and criminal penalties for false claims made to Medicare and Medicaid. Fraudulent billing is a common type of false claim. Some infractions are easily determined to be fraudulent: a psychiatrist who billed Medicaid for 4,800 hours in 1 year (40 hours/week = 2,080 hours/year); a physician who, in 48 separate instances, billed Medicaid for performing two abortions on the same patient within a month; and a physician who billed Medicaid for treating a 22-year-old college football player for diaper rash. Other cases are much less clear: A court upheld a $258,000 fine against anesthesiologists whose defense was that, at most, they were guilty of "unartfully" describing services rendered. The court found that the standard of care to be applied was exacting and "unartful descriptions" were a description of services not rendered as claimed.[118] It is suggested that complex Medicare reimbursement, particularly physician reimbursement under resource-based relative value scales, make "unartful" coding and claims difficult to avoid.[119]

Physician Self-Referral

A second example of fraud and abuse is physician self-referral. Amendments to Medicare in 1989 and 1993 to restrict self-referral are known as Stark I and Stark II, respectively, after the congressman who was instrumental in their passage. (Proposed regulations to Stark II were not issued until early 1998.) Stark I restricted referrals for clinical laboratory services by physicians (or their immediate families) who had a financial relationship in the laboratory, for the purpose of furnishing clinical laboratory services for which Medicare paid. Neither could the laboratory bill another payer for service pursuant to the prohibited service.[120] Stark II expanded restrictions on self-referral to 10 additional services: physical therapy; occupational therapy; radiology services, including magnetic resonance imaging, computerized tomography scans, and ultrasound; radiation therapy services and supplies; durable medical equipment and supplies; parenteral and enteral nutrients, equipment, and supplies; prosthetics, orthotics, and prosthetic devices and supplies; home health services; outpatient prescription drugs; and inpatient and outpatient hospital services.[121] Stark II modified some exceptions and added others; clarified the meaning of key terms such as "direct supervision," "fair market value," "entity," and "referral"; and made the self-referral provisions applicable to Medicaid. Among the health care providers affected are group practices and physician independent contractors, integrated delivery systems, drug manufacturers, nursing facilities, physician practice management companies, dialysis providers, and lithotripsy providers.[122]

Penalties for violating self-referral restrictions can be substantial. Civil penalties of thousands of dollars per item or service, plus assessments equaling twice or three times the amount claimed, can be imposed. Some infractions can result in criminal sanctions. In addition, providers can be excluded from participating in Medicare and Medicaid, a penalty that might be the harshest of all.[123]

> *This body of law has had a profound impact on the healthcare industry and on relationships among providers. The bribe and kickback prohibition and accompanying legislation limiting self-referrals discourage doctors from acquiring interests in other health care providers while en-couraging them to form group practices or to become employees of health care entities, thus supporting greater concentration in the health care industry. This may have the ultimate effect of creating a better organized, more competitive health care industry. . . . Fraud and abuse law has, in any event, proved a gold-mine for health lawyers, who must be at the side of their health care clients continually to steer them through the treacherous narrows of these federal and state prohibitions, violation of which can result in imprisonment or impoverishment.[124]*

Healthcare Integrity and Protection Data Bank

Section 221 of the Health Insurance Portability and Accountability Act of 1996[125] created the Healthcare Integrity and Protection Data Bank (HIPDB), the purpose of which is to record adverse actions against health care providers, suppliers, or practitioners. Included are

- Civil judgments against a provider, supplier, or practitioner related to the delivery of healthcare
- Criminal convictions related to the delivery of a healthcare item or service
- (Adverse) actions by federal or state agencies responsible for licensing and certification
- Exclusion of a provider, supplier, or practitioner from federal or state healthcare programs
- Any other adjudicated actions or decisions that the secretary of DHHS establishes by regulations[126]

The Office of the Inspector General of DHHS has proposed expansive regulations that it believes are consistent with congressional intent to interpret health care fraud and abuse broadly. The proposed regulations include reporting all actions that

> *are inconsistent with accepted sound fiscal, business, or medical practices, directly or indirectly resulting in: (1) unnecessary costs to the program; (2) improper payment; (3) services that fail to meet professionally recognized standards of care or that are medically unnecessary; or (4) adverse patient outcomes, failure to provide covered or needed care in violation of contractual arrangements, or delays in diagnosis or treatment.[127]*

Settlements in which no findings or admissions of liability have been made are excluded, as are medical malpractice civil judgments. Reporting is retroactive to August 21, 1996, and heavy penalties can be levied against organizations that fail to report. As with NPDB, the subject of the entry may submit corrections, and a charge will be made for all requests for information to HIPDB.[128] This well-intentioned legislation adds greatly to the necessity that HSOs/HSs have continual access to legal advice to avoid running afoul of the law. As with NPDB, HIPDB is likely to achieve far less than its intended results, and at considerable cost to providers.

Qui Tam Actions

The vast amounts of money that are spent by the federal government result in significant potential for fraud, abuse, and waste. In 1986 Congress enacted the False Claims Act Amendments to strengthen Civil War–era legislation protecting whistleblowers who report fraud, abuse, and waste in federally funded programs.[129] One provision allows such people, known in the law as relators, to sue in the name of the federal government, with the incentive that they will receive 15%–30% of the triple damages and fines that may be imposed. Such suits are known as *qui tam* actions, from the Latin for "who as well for the king for himself sues in the matter." In the late 1990s the majority of *qui tam* actions arose from health care fraud.[130] Examples are instructive.

An apparent *qui tam* action alleged that 132 research center hospitals conspired to miscode procedures and manipulate patient records to obtain $1 billion in federal reimbursement for the use of investigational devices that are not covered under Medicare and Medicaid guidelines. The hospitals argued that diagnosis-related groups pay by diagnosis rather than products used; thus payment was due regardless of treatment.[131]

A clear example of a *qui tam* action occurred at Pineville (Kentucky) Community Hospital, where a new physician found that some physician colleagues were not conducting histories for some patients, physical examinations, and other services that were listed in patient records. Medical records clerks were writing histories and physicals based on information in the medical records or, occasionally, interviews with patients. The document created by the clerk became the basis for the physician's bill to Medicare for a comprehensive history and physical. Similarly, on discharge, the records clerk used information from the medical record to prepare a discharge summary, which was stamped with the physician's signature. The physician's office used this document to bill Medicare for a discharge examination and treatment plan. After repeated efforts to change the practice, the new physician brought a *qui tam* suit. In settlement, the hospital agreed to pay $2.3 million; each of the two physicians involved in the fraudulent practices paid $100,000. Had the case gone to trial and maximum damages and penalties been awarded, the total recovered from defendants could have been $31 million. It was alleged that hospital administration hindered efforts to end the fraudulent practices. Regrettable, but not unexpected, the whistleblower was viewed as the problem by many at the hospital and in the community.[132]

Tax-Exempt Status of HSOs/HSs

Federal tax law has long recognized the special role of organizations performing charitable work. HSOs/HSs organized as not-for-profit corporations may apply to the Internal Revenue Service (IRS) to become a tax-exempt organization under Section 501(c)(3) of the Internal Revenue Code, which exempts them from federal income and excise taxes and permits donors to deduct gifts in calculating federal income taxes. States may accept the IRS determination, which provides other tax advantages. In addition, tax-exempt HSOs/HSs usually avoid local property and other taxes.

From 1956 to 1969 IRS required that a tax-exempt hospital "be operated to the extent of its financial ability for those not able to pay for the services rendered and not exclusively for those who are able and expected to pay."[133] A 1969 IRS Revenue Ruling removed the requirement to render service to those unable to pay and stated that promoting health was a sufficient charitable purpose benefiting the community as a whole. By operating an emergency room that was open to all and providing hospital care for the community members who were able to pay the costs of it, a hospital was promoting the health of a class of people that was broad enough to benefit the community. The IRS position was supported in the legal challenge that followed.[134] The net effect was that there could be less emphasis on treating those unable to pay without losing tax-exempt status. The 1969 Revenue Ruling criteria are reflected in the IRS manual that guides auditors who are instructed to investigate how well the exempt organization meets what is called the "community benefit" standard of Section 501(c)(3) status. The most important question when reviewing community benefit is whether the benefits that are received by the community are at least equal to the value of the tax exemption. Other dimensions of gauging community benefit include the community's perception of the organization and whether charitable gifts are received from people in the community.[135]

Despite a consistent approach by IRS, the issue is far from resolved at all levels of government. The stakes are high. Estimates of the benefits to hospitals of tax-exempt status have ranged from $4.5 to $8.5 billion.[136] One estimate for the benefit to *all* tax-exempt health care organizations was $15 billion.[137] Congress seems to be tying continued charitable status to minimum levels of charity care, which are likely to be a percentage of the benefit of being tax exempt.

Texas, Utah, and Pennsylvania challenged or redefined hospitals' property tax exemption.[138] Local governments in Pennsylvania successfully challenged the tax-exempt status of hospitals.[139] The basic rationale is that tax-exempt hospitals perform too little public service and charity care to justify their special status. Some tax-exempt hospitals paid voluntarily, Hospitals in Vermont, Pennsylvania, Missouri, and Tennessee fought and won.[140]

A significant part of the problem, especially for hospitals, is that many are involved in activities such as integration, diversification, reorganization, mergers, and joint ventures, all of which have a distinct flavor of entrepreneurial business, not charity. In addition, the media have alerted politicians to the high levels of compensation earned by many HSO/HS executives. These developments blur and diminish the actual and perceived community benefit that distinguished not-for-profit HSOs in the past. A public that perceives "not-for-profit" HSOs to be businesses will be disinclined to continue their tax-exempt status.

Another problem for the tax-exempt status of not-for-profit HSOs/HSs, especially hospitals, stems from making core activities available to people other than patients. Filling prescriptions for people who have not been hospitalized or selling hearing aids to the public through an audiology service are the activities of for-profit business. The IRS test is whether the activity furthers the organization's exempt purpose. For example, revenue that is produced by a hospital cafeteria from serving patients and on-call staff is tax exempt because that activity furthers the exempt purpose; revenue from selling prepared food to the public is treated differently.[141] The problem of unrelated business activities has two dimensions: 1) whether unrelated business income jeopardizes tax-exempt status, and 2) the political implications of lobbying by for-profit businesses that believe they are experiencing unfair competition from tax-exempt HSOs/HSs whose tax status gives them an economic advantage and whose referrals allow them to channel patients to their own services.

A tax-exempt organization may participate in a limited amount of activity that is not related to its exempt purpose, provided that the activity is an insubstantial part of its operations. Beyond that proviso, Congress has imposed an unrelated business income tax (UBIT) to eliminate a potential source of unfair competition from tax-exempt entities.[142] The primary test that is applied by IRS is whether the activities benefit patients or nonpatients. For example, providing laboratory services to nonhospital patients is ordinarily taxable, as are pharmacy sales to nonpatients.[143] It is unlikely that a not-for-profit HSO/HS will lose its federal tax-exempt status because of excessive unrelated activity.[144] Nevertheless, the consequences of losing tax exemption are so serious that caution is advisable. The issue of business activity unrelated to the exempt purpose of HSOs/HSs and how it should be taxed is a continuing source of discontent and complaint by investor-owned companies performing similar activities.

IRS looks closely at income that is earned from partnerships and joint ventures between tax-exempt HSOs/HSs and taxable entities such as physicians.[145] An exempt organization in a joint venture that does not further its exempt purpose risks having income from the joint venture classified as unrelated taxable business income and perhaps losing its tax exemption.[146] Such arrangements raise questions of inurement as well. The concept of *inurement* (or "private benefit" if an individual and not an organization is involved) stems from a requirement in Section 501(c)(3) that individuals (including organizations) receive no benefit from an exempt organization's activities. Arm's-length transactions such as reasonable salaries for services performed and lease of space to physicians at fair market value, for instance, are not considered inurement. IRS is especially vigilant about arrangements that return substantial profits or capital gains to physicians who invest little in a joint venture with an exempt HSO. State courts are upholding local government challenges to property tax exemption because of private profit motive.[147] IRS also has defined inurement in terms of "excess benefit transactions," which are defined as economic benefit to an insider that has greater value than what the organization receives in return. This reinforces the importance of arm's-length transactions in tax-exempt organizations.[148]

The results of efforts to qualify various alternative delivery organizations and systems as Section 501(c)(3) charitable organizations have been varied and highly fact dependent. HMOs (even when they are part of an integrated delivery system [IDS]), independent practice associations, and preferred provider organizations have been, in general, unsuccessful. Tax-exempt status has been granted to several IDSs, however.[149] Primary IRS concerns have been meeting the community benefit test; inurement; the efficiencies that are achieved by integrating patient records; and the commitment to charitable care.[150] The trend seems to be that of narrowing tax-exempt status, and it is likely that new legislation will be required to adequately address the plethora of emerging health services delivery mechanisms.

Telemedicine

Even though it will apply to existing legal principles such as breach of contract, negligence, malpractice, and strict liability, the law of telemedicine, like the technology, is evolving and is unlikely to achieve stability for several decades. Several areas—confidentiality, data compression, artificial intelligence, licensure, and consent—are legally problematic.

Confidentiality

Electronic patient records with multiple users and distributed computer systems render information security hard to achieve. This suggests several confidentiality issues: improper disclosure (e.g., leaving visible or easily retrievable data on a screen), unauthorized access (the hacker problem), aggregating data to identify individual patients, and data integrity and authenticity.[151] Providers' liability for failing to maintain the confidentiality of patient information is well established; undetermined is the duty of companies providing telemedical support.[152]

Data Compression

The great amount of data in health services requires special handling so the system is not overwhelmed. Compressing files makes the data stream more manageable, but greater compression ratios increase the risk of image degradation. This means, for example, that teleradiology may be unable to achieve the reliability of in-person reading of X-rays.[153] Resulting faulty diagnoses or treatments will raise liability issues.

Artificial Intelligence

Telemedicine includes aids to decision making, one of which is artificial intelligence (AI). Expert systems are a type of AI that can help practitioners solve medical problems by asking questions, discarding irrelevant information, and producing an explained, reasoned conclusion.[154] An example of expert systems applications is the Acute Physiology and Chronic Health Evaluation (APACHE), which helps manage intensive care unit patients by monitoring various measures and calculating the probability of death.[155] Studies comparing the conclusions of expert physicians with those of AI diagnostic systems found that the systems provided useful but potentially misleading information. In addition, AI could lead to claims of information overload that is distracting to the physician, or it could be used to unfairly call into question a physician's treatment when, in fact, it is the technology that is limited.[156] Such findings suggest that AI's contribution to health services may increase in the future, but there are potential legal problems.

Licensure

States regulate physicians and other LIPs. A LIP who is unlicensed in the state that is the source of a consultation has engaged in unauthorized practice in that state. Conversely, if the LIP was not practicing in the state (e.g., because no physician–patient relationship had been established), reimbursement may be denied. Some states have attempted to address this multidimensional legal issue, but it is far from resolved.[157] AMA recommends that physicians be licensed wherever their patients are; the American College of Radiology recommends that physicians who interpret teleradiology images be licensed at both the transmitting and receiving sites.[158]

Although not necessarily affecting HSOs/HSs directly, at least in the near term, the availability of prescription drugs at websites on the Internet raises complex legal and ethical issues and potentially disastrous health risks for "patients" who self-diagnose and self-prescribe. These websites undergo little or no review by physicians, and remote prescribing raises issues of unlicensed practice.[159] In addition, there are few, if any, controls or prospect of control by state or federal government.

Consent

The use of telemedicine makes the legal aspects of patient consent more complex. Disclosing the involvement of a LIP via telemedicine becomes legally more important as "direct" participation increases, as, for example, in robotic surgery. Prudence suggests that patients be informed when the course of their treatment is directed by someone other than their attending physician.[160]

Summary

Managers will encounter numerous pitfalls as this area of law develops. It has been suggested that the legal concepts originating in the law of computers are likely to provide a reference point for many of the issues that arise in telemedicine.[161]

LEGAL PROCESS OF A CIVIL LAWSUIT

This discussion of the legal process of a civil lawsuit presumes a case involving a tort, not a breach of contract. A civil lawsuit begins when a plaintiff files a complaint in a court with jurisdiction to hear the case. This filing makes the complaint an official document and a matter of public record. It is served on (delivered to) a defendant, usually by a marshal or a sheriff's deputy. The defendant's response to the complaint is known as an answer and must be filed in a limited period of time. The answer may deny the allegations in the complaint in whole or in part, or it may assert specific affirmative defenses, such as that the complaint is barred by the statute of limitations and the suit may not be brought, the plaintiff assumed the risk, or the plaintiff was partly to blame for the injury (contributory negligence). The defendant also may make certain motions before the court— for example, a motion to dismiss because the complaint fails to state a cause of action, or a motion to dismiss because the complaint was filed in a court that lacks jurisdiction. Few cases are dismissed at this stage. The next phase is discovery, which allows the parties to learn about their opponent's case. The plaintiff seeks information to support the allegations of tortious conduct; the defendant seeks to determine the strength of the plaintiff's case, and vice versa.

During discovery, the plaintiff's side is likely to make motions in court for the production of documents that are needed to prepare its case. The defendant may ask the court to deny the motions for reasons such as statutory privilege, relevance, and reasonableness of demands. In addition, the parties obtain information through written interrogatories (questions) and by taking sworn depositions (statements) of the parties, other people with knowledge of the alleged injuries, or those who will testify as expert witnesses. With rare exceptions, all states protect the results of peer review by health services providers from discovery. The discovery phase may take months or years; statutes determine the time. Procedural maneuvering to prevent a party (usually the plaintiff) from obtaining documents and information adds time and expense.

Many cases are settled during the discovery phase or when it is complete, primarily because the parties have learned enough about the accuracy of the allegations and the strength of the opposition's case to make an informed decision. Some ways that states determine the merit of a medical malpractice claim were discussed earlier, along with the alternative means of settling cases.

If the case has merit but there is no settlement, then a trial date is set. The trial begins with opening statements by counsel in which they outline their cases and suggest what they will attempt to prove. The plaintiff's case is presented first, and it must be proven by a preponderance of the evidence that the elements of a tort are present. This is done by introducing evidence consisting of documents and testimony by people who may have observed the event or can offer other information and by expert witnesses. Often, there is no direct evidence about the event but the circumstances that lead to an inference of tortious conduct. Both parties will object to introduction of evidence that damages their case. The judge rules on the admissibility of evidence and any motions that are made by counsel during the trial. If present, a jury hears and sees the evidence and makes findings of fact.

Witnesses are questioned in several steps. The party calling the witness asks questions first; this is called direct examination. After direct examination, opposing counsel asks questions to cross-examine the witness. Cross-examination permits counsel to "impeach" the witness by raising questions about the accuracy of the witness's memory, veracity, reputation, and the like. This tests the witness's testimony and allows the finder of fact (the jury or judge sitting without a jury) to weigh it. After cross-examination, redirect examination allows counsel to "rehabilitate" the witness—to correct undesirable impressions left by cross-examination. The last round of questions is called re-cross-examination. A major theory of the law is that truth will emerge from this adversarial process and that the finder of fact can determine the witnesses' reliability.

The defendant's case is presented following the plaintiff's and involves the same steps. When the evidence has been heard and seen, the jury is charged—given instructions—by the judge. This means that the judge instructs the jury in writing that, if it determines that certain facts are present, then the law requires it to find in certain ways. Jury instructions are crucial, and both sides submit proposed instructions that the judge may use. Proposed instructions are cast by each party in the light that is most favorable to its case. If there is no jury, then the judge will consider the evidence and render a decision. In some jurisdictions the decision to find for the plaintiff or defendant is separate from a decision on damages, if the finding is for the plaintiff.

At various times during the trial, the parties make motions for the judge to consider and make rulings. For example, the defendant usually moves for a directed verdict after the plaintiff's case has been presented. This motion asks the judge to rule that plaintiff has not presented enough evidence to support the claim (a *prima facie* case) and, as a matter of law, the plaintiff is not entitled to damages. If granted, which is rare, the trial ends because the judge has found for the defendant. Both parties may move for a directed verdict after all of the evidence has been presented. When the jury finds for one of the parties, the other may ask for a judgment notwithstanding the verdict or, alternatively, for a new trial. If the judge grants the former, which is rare, then the jury verdict is overturned and judgment is entered for the other party. If the latter is granted, then a new trial is set in the future. Motions are supported or opposed by briefs from the parties that cite legal precedents and arguments as to why that motion should be granted or denied.

If the defendant loses and the jury awards damages that the defendant believes are excessive as a matter of law, then the defendant can petition the court for *remittitur,* which allows the judge to decrease the award, if granted. Again, the defendant's brief argues that the evidence and the law do not support the verdict. The plaintiff submits a brief in opposition. Similarly, the doctrine of *additur* allows a court to increase an inadequate jury award.

The losing party may appeal the verdict. Appeals are based on alleged errors made by the trial court and that represent misapplication of the law by the judge. These appeals are entered in the appeals court (the intermediate level) or, on further appeal, in the supreme court of a state. Typical errors alleged by the losing party are permitting (or failing to allow) the admission of evidence, failing to grant a motion, the content of jury instructions, and the judge's decision to qualify or refuse to qualify expert witnesses.

Trial and appeals court proceedings are very expensive. Discovery before trial requires paying for the reproduction of documents at a high rate per page, deposing the parties and witnesses, and paying the costs of expert witnesses. Usually, such costs must be paid as they are incurred. There are major costs to defendants who must answer interrogatories, produce documents, and cope with the disruption and other aspects of defending the suit. Trial appearances by attorneys command higher fees than those charged for other work. In addition, court costs must be paid. Appeals require that the stenographic record of the trial be transcribed. This record is several thousand pages long even for a short trial and costs thousands of dollars to prepare. High stakes, however, warrant such costs. Contingency fees for attorneys are suggested as a cause of the large number of medical malpractice suits. However, such financial arrangements permit injured patients to seek redress even though they cannot pay the costs for an attorney to prepare and try the case.

SPECIAL CONSIDERATIONS FOR THE MANAGER

This section provides information about preventing medical malpractice and identifies special considerations once a complaint is served. HSOs/HSs should be perceived as having an independent ethical obligation to the patient and community that is separate from and more demanding than that arising from their legal obligations.

Managers face a range of problems in effectively handling the legal and quasi-legal matters that arise regularly. These matters run the gamut from dealing with patients who have a grievance with the HSO and are potential litigants to providing instruction for staff members on the maintenance and confidentiality of medical records.

Record Keeping

Without adequate medical records, health care providers have great difficulty proving that what they did met the standard of care. Medical records hold no special legal magic. The information that is contained in medical records is admissible only under an exception to the hearsay rule of evidence. They are used to refresh the recollection of caregivers who participated in treatment and made entries in the record. In addition, the record is the basis for opinions by medical experts. The complexity and extent of events and treatment, the mobility of caregivers, and fading memories necessitate that medical records be complete, accurate, and legible.

It is not unknown for people who fear the ramifications of poor-quality care or a lawsuit to alter medical records. Such acts violate a basic ethical duty and break the law. In a malpractice claim, however, alterations are likely to be discovered, and they not only make juries more willing to award damages but also could persuade a judge to punish the defendant by allowing an award of punitive damages. Effective risk management requires that a responsible person obtain custody of the medical record at the first indication of a potentially compensable event. This control should be exercised continuously until the dispute has been resolved, including any appeal.

A common problem with paper medical records is that handwritten entries are difficult to read or are illegible. Many physicians have poor handwriting. The medical records committee or its equivalent must make special, continuing efforts to monitor and improve the legibility of medical record entries. It also must work to ensure that records are properly organized, authenticated, completed properly and in a timely fashion, and readily available when they are needed. The advantages and disadvantages of electronic medical records are discussed in Chapter 6.

Effective Use of House and Retainer Counsel

HSOs/HSs obtain legal advice in two basic ways. Most common, smaller organizations pay an attorney a retainer to be available for consultation. The retainer guarantees consultation as needed. Considering the law's importance in managing HSOs/HSs and the need for ongoing advice and counsel, however, this may not be the most desirable option. Larger HSOs/HSs employ full-time in-house counsel. In this arrangement, the attorney is a staff assistant to management and the governing body. One of these methods is essential because HSOs/HSs can no longer rely on free advice from an attorney member of the governing body. Health services law is so specialized and frequently applied that casual or informal relationships are insufficient.

The effective use of legal counsel poses the same problems for management as does interacting with other technical staff. Specifics vary depending on whether there is in-house or retainer counsel. A major advantage of in-house counsel is that they are likely to be integrated into systems that alert management to legal problems or prevent them from occurring, such as heading the risk management program. Furthermore, frequent contact with in-house counsel enhances managers' knowledge of the law and potential legal problems, and they are likely to seek guidance in a timely manner. In-house counsel is committed to one organization and not distracted by other clients. Finally, the attorney will become expert in the HSO's/HS's unique characteristics and special problems. In sum, these considerations offer enhanced effectiveness. Legal expertise can be obtained in other ways, too. Increasing numbers of law school graduates with dual degrees and clinical backgrounds enable HSOs/HSs to hire managers and program directors with legal training, thus enhancing their ability to comply with the law.

Having in-house counsel does not, however, eliminate the need to retain outside counsel. Specialized areas of the law and litigation are referred to outside attorneys. Like medicine, the practice of law has become highly segmented. The appropriate skills optimize the outcome.

Testifying

During their professional careers, health services managers are likely to testify in a legal proceeding. Common testimony is that used to provide information about how the HSO/HS is organized or how it functioned in a specific circumstance. Less common is providing information about an incident about which the manager has firsthand knowledge.

Written interrogatories ask managers and staff to answer questions about the organization, staffing, functions, and similar topics and are prepared with the assistance of counsel. Interrogatories assist counsel in requesting specific documents and information and often are the first step in the discovery process. Managers may be deposed by counsel for the opposing party. The deponent (manager) swears (or affirms) to answer questions truthfully. The HSO's/HS's attorney is present and may object to the questions, but they usually are answered. A verbatim record is made. If the deposition is used in court, then the judge rules on the objections that counsel made during the deposition.

Expert witnesses are ubiquitous in legal proceedings involving HSOs/HSs. The experience and education of health services managers qualifies them to be expert witnesses regarding the organization and management of HSOs/HSs about which they are knowledgeable. Once qualified by the court, the expert renders an opinion as to whether the organization, management, and performance of a HSO/HS met the standard of care. Hypothetical questions may be used to establish the standard of care, but they are less common than in the past. Questions are as likely to be formulated in terms of whether performance conformed with the standard of care.

Being an expert witness requires no special skills beyond a knowledge of one's field and a clear understanding of how it applies to the case. The finder of fact weighs the testimony of witnesses, and it is incumbent on the expert to testify in an honest and forthright manner.

SUMMARY

This chapter provides a basic overview of the legal aspects of health services management and develops a general framework for managers to understand the legal dimensions of problems. Greater understanding and appreciation of the law and its processes necessitate additional education, especially in health services law. It should be clear, however, that the legal implications of HSO/HS management have increased and are likely to continue to do so. This trend requires that managers have a basic understanding of the law as it affects the HSO/HS and of how to interact effectively with legal counsel. As with the practice of medicine, prevention is more efficient than solving legal problems after they occur.

Managers know all too well that legal problems often have ethical dimensions and vice versa. A basic aspect of this dynamic is that areas of the law are inadequately developed, and, in many instances, ethics and the law do not agree. This tension complicates the manager's decision making. The pragmatic reality, however, is that decisions must be made and actions taken. Regardless of the administrative and clinical aspects, the HSO/HS, through its managers, has an ethical responsibility to protect patients and to act in their best interests. This standard is more demanding than that defined in the law.

DISCUSSION QUESTIONS

1. Identify formal sources of law that can be found in HSOs/HSs. How are they used? Is the emphasis on self-government and independence for groups such as the PSO consistent with external forces acting on HSOs/HSs, especially hospitals?

2. Describe three sources of law that are external to HSOs/HSs. Distinguish the development of law in each branch of the federal government. What factors play a role in forming the law, and how do they interact? Is there a role for HSO/HS managers? If so, what?

3. How are standard of care and its breach determined? What are the roles of courts? Legislatures? Clinicians? Managers?

4. Is the HSO's/HS's role to act in the best interests of patients (described in Chapter 13) compatible with its defense of lawsuits for alleged malpractice? Explain.

5. State and federal regulatory processes are increasingly important to all HSOs/HSs. Identify examples of regulations that affect HSOs/HSs. Discuss the pros and cons of the regulatory processes identified from the standpoint of society and of the HSO/HS.

6. Contracts enable HSOs/HSs to conduct business. Identify the types of clinical and nonclinical contracts. How are HSO/HS managers involved in 1) negotiating contracts, 2) monitoring compliance, and 3) resolving disputes?

7. The law distinguishes intentional from unintentional (negligence) torts. What intentional torts affect HSOs/HSs? What should be the HSO's/HS's manager's role in consent processes?

8. Meticulous record keeping is important to good medical treatment; it is crucial to defending a malpractice action successfully. Describe the manager's role in the process of record keeping.

9. With greater frequency attorneys are on the full-time staff of larger HSOs/HSs. What should managers seek in selecting an attorney? Identify the pitfalls of using in-house and retainer counsel.

10. All organizations benefit from using alternative dispute resolution (ADR). Describe ADR. Identify how various types of ADR could be used to settle disputes in HSOs/HSs.

CASE STUDY 1: REPORTING SUSPECTED CHILD ABUSE OR NEGLECT

Monkota state law requires health services professionals to report suspected child abuse or neglect to welfare authorities or the police. Roosevelt Hospital is a major teaching institution in the state's only metropolitan area. It has large emergency and outpatient departments. All attending physicians, house officers (residents), and clinical employees are told about the state law during new employee orientation. This information is reiterated during hospital-sponsored continuing education programs. Roosevelt Hospital has written standard operating procedures that describe how to comply with the law. Forms to report suspected child abuse and neglect are provided.

You are the chief operating officer (COO) at Roosevelt. Last week, your assistant told you that far fewer suspected child abuse and neglect cases are being reported this year, which suggested to him that staff may not be reporting cases as aggressively. The matter must wait a few days, however, because you are going to the American College of Healthcare Executives convocation, where you will be advanced to Fellow.

You attend to the problem the following week. Because most emergency and outpatient care is provided by house officers, you ask to meet with the chief resident. She seems reluctant to discuss the matter, but with prompting she confirms your assistant's assessment of the data. She tells you that pediatric residents are the most unwilling to report suspected abuse and neglect when doing so is not in the child's best interests. She tells you that most residents and the attending staff agree about selective reporting.

To your horror, the chief resident recounts two cases in which reports were made, but the parents retained custody of the children. Both children suffered major trauma when the parents vented their frustration and anger about being reported. One child became paraplegic because of a spinal cord injury; the other had to have the fingers on one hand amputated because of burns sustained when his hand was held in a deep-fat fryer.

The chief resident points out that the Hippocratic oath requires physicians to do what they believe is in the patient's best interests. Somewhat sharply, she reminds you that the child is the patient and the physician's moral duty lies in treating the child, not in intimidating the parents. In addition, effective medical care requires mutual trust. Trust will disappear if parents perceive the hospital and physician as agents of the government informing on them, and parents will not bring children in for treatment. She also notes that investigation may not substantiate the suspected abuse or neglect. The fact of being investigated by welfare authorities and police, however, stigmatizes the parents and violates the privacy of the family.

It is clear that the topic is both important and sensitive. You are obliged to identify for the chief resident the opposing arguments from your perspective and that of the hospital.

QUESTIONS

1. What arguments can the COO make based on the law? Are these arguments based in morals or codes of ethics?

2. Instead of addressing the issue with the chief resident, should the COO use formal managerial control over nursing and other employees to solve the problem? Why or why not?

3. Should the hospital try to modify state law by becoming involved in the political process? If so, what should it do and who should do it?

4. How much informal pressure should the COO put on the residents? What are the acceptable means of doing so?

CASE STUDY 2: EFFECTIVE CONSENT

Alex Burkowski finished reading the incident report written by the supervisor of the cardiac catheterization laboratory and rescanned the letter from the former patient, Mr. Walter. As Burkowski read, he could not help thinking that this was the silly kind of thing that consumed too much of his time. He wondered whether he or "Smokey Bear" fought more fires.

As the director of risk management, Burkowski cochaired the ad hoc interdisciplinary committee that had been established to review the consent policies at the large multispecialty group practice at which he was employed. Now, he would have to try to get that committee restarted. At best, it would move at glacial speed; at worst, it would be an exercise in futility.

Burkowski summarized the problem:

Patient Walter admitted for catheterization. Patient alert during procedure; his cardiologist came to head of table to speak to him. Patient became alarmed and wanted to know who was performing procedure (catheter visible to patient on television monitor). Cardiologist told him a qualified cardiology resident was doing procedure. Procedure completed uneventfully. Patient very angry; told lab supervisor no one told him someone other than "his doctor" would do procedure, especially a "learner." Cardiologist can't remember if he informed patient about resident. No consent form in file.

Walter had threatened to sue, but Burkowski knew the law and understood that, absent an injury, it would be very difficult for Walter to win damages. Burkowski started to write the memorandum to the committee, but he was not sure what to say.

QUESTIONS

1. What are the legal issues here? Whose concern are they? Do HSOs with medical education programs have a special legal obligation to patients in cases like this? If so, how is it met?

2. Outline the memorandum that Burkowski should write to the committee.

3. Is Burkowski a part of the problem? If you were Burkowski's boss, what would you do? Why?

4. What is the ethical obligation here? What should the organization do regardless of the legal implications?

CASE STUDY 3: THE MISSING NEEDLE PROTECTOR

E.L. Straight is director of clinical services at Hopewell Hospital. As in most hospitals, there are a few physicians who deliver acceptable, but marginal-quality care. They tend to make more mistakes than the others and have more patients who go "sour." After Straight took the position 2 years ago, new programs were developed and things seemed to be getting better.

Dr. Cutrite has practiced at Hopewell longer than anyone can remember. He was once a brilliant general surgeon, but he has slipped physically and mentally, and Straight is considering how to reduce his surgical privileges. The process is incomplete, however, and Cutrite continues to perform surgery.

The operating room supervisor came to Straight's office one Monday afternoon. "We've got a problem," she said, somewhat nonchalantly, but with a hint of disgust. "I'm almost sure we left a plastic needle protector from a disposable syringe in a patient's belly—a Mrs. Jameson. You know what I mean, the protectors that are reddish-pink. They're impossible to see in a wound."

"Where did it come from?" asked Straight.

"I'm not sure," answered the supervisor. "All I know is that the syringe was in a used surgical pack when we did the count." She went on to describe the safeguards of counts and records. The discrepancy was noted when the records were reconciled at the end of the week. A surgical pack was shown as having a syringe that was not supposed to be there. When the scrub nurse working with Cutrite was questioned, she remembered that he had used the syringe, but, when it was included in the count at the conclusion of surgery, she did not think about the protective sheath, which must have been on it.

"Let's get Mrs. Jameson back into surgery," said Straight. "We'll tell her we have to check her incision and deep sutures. She'll never know we're really looking for the needle cover."

"Too late," responded the supervisor. "She went home the day before yesterday."

Damn, thought Straight. "Have you talked to Cutrite?"

The supervisor nodded affirmatively. "He won't consider telling Mrs. Jameson that there might be a problem and readmitting her," she said. "He warned us not to do anything, either," she added. "Cutrite claims it cannot possibly hurt her. Except for some discomfort, she'll never know it's there."

Straight called the chief of surgery and asked hypothetically about the consequences of leaving a small plastic cap in a patient's belly. The chief knew something was up, but did not pursue it. He simply replied that it was likely there would be occasional discomfort, but probably no life-threatening consequences. "Although," he added, somewhat darkly, "one is never sure."

Straight liked working at Hopewell Hospital and wanted to avoid a confrontation with Cutrite, who had declined professionally but was still powerful politically. Straight had resisted fingernail biting for years, but that old habit was suddenly overwhelming.

QUESTIONS

1. What should Straight do? Why?
2. What sources of guidance can Straight use?
3. What steps should be taken to avoid similar problems in the future?
4. Is there anything disturbing about the attitudes of the operating room supervisor and chief of surgery? Explain.

CASE STUDY 4: IS THIS THE MOST EFFICIENT WAY?

Joan Vinson, the hospital COO, hated giving depositions. Plaintiffs' lawyers probed and pushed and leapt at any word that might give them an advantage. When a deposition was over she always felt wrung out, and there was a lingering feeling, a subtle implication, that somehow she was dishonest.

The latest case involved a claim that an emergency department (ED) triage nurse had misjudged the severity of a patient's arm injury. Delayed treatment allegedly exacerbated the injury, and the plaintiff had a slight, permanent movement deficit. Usually this would not result in a lawsuit, but he was a semiprofessional stock car driver and the complaint alleged that the injury would make him less likely to win. The complaint demanded $50,000 in damages.

The hospital attorney told Vinson that the plaintiff would have difficulty proving damages and that the case would likely settle for less than half the requested amount. He recommended, however, moving as slowly as possible because it was a contingency fee case. Moving slowly would increase the plaintiff's attorney's expenses and would make him more willing to settle.

Vinson was certain that the triage nurse had erred. It had been a very busy night in the ED. The triage nurse was working a double shift because her replacement had called in sick. When the plaintiff came to the ED, the nurse had been working for 14 hours and was exhausted.

Vinson wanted to settle the suit, but she felt compelled to follow the attorney's advice. It just seemed to her that there had to be a better way to handle such problems, especially when liability was not really an issue.

QUESTIONS

1. What policy issue is present here? Describe the roles of in-house and retainer counsel in a case such as this. Might either have a conflict of interest in terms of settling the case? Why?

2. Distinguish cases in which HSO staff are clearly negligent from those in which reasonable people could disagree. Identify the negative and positive aspects of contesting all cases, regardless of merit.

3. What recommendations would you make to prevent the untoward event described in this case? Be prepared to support them.

4. Based on personal experience or facts that are known to you, describe an untoward event resulting from interacting with a HSO. What was the result? Did the HSO act ethically?

CASE STUDY 5: STAKEHOLDERS

A small-town attorney named Franklin Jones was first elected to the Virginia state senate in 1978. Jones served his constituents well, performed his committee assignments diligently, and enjoyed a good reputation among members of his party as well as his political opponents. Jones was reelected to each 2-year term by substantial margins. Health care issues were an area of special interest for Jones, and by 1988 he had sufficient seniority to be appointed chairman of the powerful subcommittee on health.

In the late 1990s the president of the senate, who was a member of Jones's political party, was told by reliable, unnamed sources that Jones was enjoying a lifestyle beyond his means. He owned several upscale automobiles and a large pleasure boat, lived in a very affluent neighborhood by the ocean, and often was seen dining at expensive restaurants. Reluctantly, the senate president asked for a confidential investigation of the matter. Several months later the report showed the following about Jones:

1. Jones was asked to join the boards of several not-for-profit health groups that subsequently received tens of thousands of dollars in grants and gifts from organizations that are subject to the purview of the subcommittee on health.

2. Jones owned small amounts of stock in several publicly traded for-profit health services companies, which had received advance information on new regulations that were being developed by the state Medicaid office.

3. A letter from a constituent, who was the president of a large Medicaid managed care company, had prompted Jones to hold hearings on reimbursement rates in that program. The subcommittee on health concluded that reimbursement was too low and issued a report that recommended a new payment schedule.

The president of the senate was very distressed. There seemed to be enough questions raised to warrant a criminal investigation, but he was not sure what to do.

QUESTIONS

1. Describe the role of health services managers in the political process. Identify the limits in their professional and personal activities.
2. Distinguish the investigation's three findings in terms of ethics and the law.
3. Apply the American College of Healthcare Executives *Code of Ethics* (see Chapter 13) in analyzing the investigation's findings.
4. Propose ways in which the problems suggested by the findings could (or should) be prevented.

NOTES

1. Aristotle. *Politics,* 287. Translated by Benjamin Jowett. New York: The Modern Library, 1943.
2. United States v. Shreveport Grain and Elevator Company, 287 U.S. 77 (1932).
3. Administrative Procedures Act of 1946, 60 Stat. 993 (1946).
4. *Black's Law Dictionary,* 6th ed., 1406. St. Paul, MN: West Publishing, 1990.
5. *Black's Law Dictionary,* 1305.
6. Federal Election Commission data for 1994 and 1996, respectively, show disbursements from PACs for ANA as $1,084,508 and $784,891; the American Academy of Ophthalmology as $877,155 and $606,975; AHA as $1,041,177 and $881,176; AMA as $2,386,947 and $2,319,197; and FAHS as $126,121 and $121,487. By comparison, the largest PAC disbursement in 1995–1996 was made by Emily's List, a pro-choice group, which disbursed $12,494,230.
7. Bodenheimer, Edgar. *Jurisprudence: The Philosophy and Method of the Law,* rev. ed., 340. Cambridge, MA: Harvard University Press, 1974.
8. Keeton, W. Page, Ed. *Prosser and Keeton on the Law of Torts,* 5th ed., 2. St. Paul, MN: West Publishing, 1984.
9. Keeton, *Prosser and Keeton,* 2.
10. Keeton, *Prosser and Keeton,* 655–656.
11. Southwick, Arthur F. *The Law of Hospital and Health Care Administration,* 2nd ed., 67–68. Ann Arbor, MI: Health Administration Press, 1988.
12. Prosser, William L. *Handbook of the Law of Torts,* 4th ed., 31. St. Paul, MN: West Publishing, 1971.
13. Behringer v. The Medical Center at Princeton, 249 N.J. Super. 597, 592 A.2d 1251 (1991); Doe v. Noe, Ill. App. Ct. Dec. 26, 1997.
14. *Black's Law Dictionary,* 1032.
15. *American Jurisprudence,* 2nd ed., Cumulative Supplement, Section 205, Vol. 61, St. Paul, MN: West Publishing, 1997.
16. Southwick, *The Law of Hospital,* 69.
17. Landeros v. Flood, 17 Cal. 3d 399 (1976).
18. Federal Tort Claims Act of 1946, 60 Stat. 842 (August 2, 1946).
19. Baumberger, Charles H. "Vicarious Liability Claims Against HMOs." *Trial* 34 (May 1998): 30–33, 35.
20. Southwick, *The Law of Hospital,* 580.
21. Furrow, Barry R., Thomas L. Greaney, Sandra H. Johnson, Timothy S. Jost, and Robert L. Schwartz. *Health Law: Cases Materials and Problems,* 3rd ed., 353. St. Paul, MN: West Publishing, 1997.
22. Furrow, Greaney, Johnson, Jost, and Schwartz, *Health Law,* 353.
23. Furrow, Greaney, Johnson, Jost, and Schwartz, *Health Law,* 354.
24. Thornhill, Michael C., and William H. Ginsburg. "Enterprise Liability: Cure or Curse." *Whittier Law Review* 16 (Spring 1995): 143–156.
25. U.S. Department of Health, Education, and Welfare. *Report of the Secretary's Commission on Medical Malpractice,* 14. Washington, DC: U.S. Department of Health, Education and Welfare, 1973.
26. Kosterlitz, Julie. "Malpractice Morass." *National Journal* 23 (July 6, 1991): 1683.

27. "Malpractice: Calm Before the Storm?" *Medicine & Health Perspectives* 43 (September 18, 1989): 37.
28. Gonzalez, Martin L. "Medical Professional Liability Claims and Premiums." In *Socioeconomic Characteristics of Medical Practice, 1997,* 39. Chicago: American Medical Association, 1998.
29. Moskowitz, Daniel B. "Will Medical Liability Outlays Boost Total Health Care Costs?" *Medicine & Health* 35 (September 8, 1997): 1–2.
30. Localio, A. Russell, Ann G. Lawthers, Troyen A. Brennan, Nan M. Laird, Liesi E. Hebert, Lynn M. Peterson, Joseph P. Newhouse, Paul C. Weiler, and Howard H. Hiatt. "Relation Between Malpractice Claims and Adverse Events Due to Negligence: Results of the Harvard Medical Practice Study III." *New England Journal of Medicine* 325 (July 25, 1991): 249.
31. "Medical-Errors Toll May Be Understated: Doctor Testifies to Senate Health Panel." *The Washington Times,* December 14, 1999, A6.
32. Weiss, Rick. "Medical Errors Blamed for Many Deaths." *The Washington Post,* November 30, 1999, A1.
33. "16,638 Questionable Doctors." Health Letter 14 (March 1998): 1–2. (Published by Public Citizen, Health Research Group, 1600 20th Street NW, Washington, DC 20009)
34. *National Health Lawyers Association News* 1 (May 1997): 28–29.
35. "16,638 Questionable Doctors," 2–3.
36. "Malpractice: Calm Before the Storm?", 37.
37. Smith, Lee. "A Cure for What Ails Medical Care." *Fortune* (July 1, 1991). 59.
38. Moskowitz, "Will Medical Liability Outlays," 2.
39. Office of Technology Assessment. *Defensive Medicine and Medical Malpractice.* Washington, DC: Congress of the United States, 1994. The OTA defines positive defensive medicine as physicians ordering extra tests or procedures; avoiding certain procedures or patients is negative defensive medicine.
40. U.S. Department of Health, Education, and Welfare, *Report of the Secretary's Commission,* 14.
41. Rubin, Robert J., and Daniel N. Mendelson. "How Much Does Defensive Medicine Cost?" *Journal of American Health Policy* 4 (July/August 1994): 7–15.
42. Office of Technology Assessment, *Defensive Medicine and Medical Malpractice.*
43. Kravitz, Richard L., John E. Rolph, and Laura Petersen. "Omission-Related Malpractice Claims and the Limits of Defensive Medicine." *Medical Care Research and Review* 54 (December 1997): 456–471.
44. Gabin, Jan H. "Health Care Reformation and the Need for Tort Reform." *New Jersey Medicine* 92 (May 1995): 329.
45. Hudson, Terese. "Experts Disagree Over the Cost of Defensive Medicine." *Hospitals* 64 (August 5, 1990): 74.
46. Gonzalez, "Medical Professional Liability," 44.
47. Goldstein, Avram. "Va. High Court Upholds Malpractice Cap." *The Washington Post,* January 9, 1999, B3. The unanimous opinion upheld the constitutionality of Virginia's $1 million cap on medical malpractice damage awards, including punitive damages, lost wages, future medical costs, and interest on unpaid judgments against doctors and hospitals. Supporters argue that the cap has stabilized the physicians' malpractice insurance market and eased their ability to get malpractice insurance.
48. Wencl, Annette, and Margaret Brizzolara. "Medical Negligence: Survey of the States." *Trial* 32 (May 1996): 21.
49. Grant, Ruth Ann. "Tinkering on Tort Reform Not Enough to Solve Problem: Experts." *AHA News* 27 (March 18, 1991): 2.
50. Grant, "Tinkering on Tort Reform," 5.
51. Citizen Action. *Health Care Statistics and the Effect of Caps on Noneconomic Damages,* 17–18. Washington, DC: Citizen Action, 1996.
52. Best v. Taylor Machine Works 179 Ill.2d 367, 689 N.E.2d 1057 (1997).
53. Smith, William C. "Prying Off Tort Reform Caps: States Striking Down Limits on Liability and Damages, and Statutes of Limitations." *ABA Journal* 85 (October 1999): 28–29.
54. Wencl, Annette, and David Strickland. "No-Fault Med Mal: No Gain for the Injured." *Trial* 33 (May 1997): 20.
55. Meyers, Allan R. " 'Lumping It': The Hidden Denominator of the Medical Malpractice Crisis." *American Journal of Public Health* 77 (December 1987): 1544–1548.

56. Darr, Kurt. "Communication: The Key to Reducing Malpractice Claims." *Hospital Topics* 75 (Spring 1997): 4–6.
57. Carlin, Peter E. "Medical Malpractice Pre-trial Screening Panels: A Review of the Evidence." *Intergovernmental Health Policy Project* (newsletter), October 30, 1980, 13, 15.
58. Lowes, Robert L. "Can Malpractice Really Be Kept Out of Court?" *Medical Economics* 71 (August 22, 1994): 111.
59. Lowes, "Can Malpractice," 111.
60. Lowes, "Can Malpractice," 112–114.
61. Parenti, Gail Leverett. "Voluntary Binding Arbitration of Medical Malpractice Claims: Meaningful Tort Reform at Last." *Trial Advocate Quarterly* 15 (Winter 1996): 16–20.
62. Felsenthal, Edward. "What Happens When Patients Arbitrate Rather than Litigate?" *The Wall Street Journal,* February 4, 1994, B-1.
63. "Arbitration Accepted as a Means for Resolution of Medical Malpractice Disputes." *American Journal of Orthodontics and Dentofacial Orthopedics* 3 (March 1997): 349–351. This reference includes a form to contract for arbitration of medical malpractice disputes. In *Engalla v. The Permanente Medical Group, Inc.* (43 Cal. Rptr.2nd 621, 1995), a California court of appeals reversed the trial court and upheld an arbitration clause, despite the fact that it resulted from a contract of adhesion and there were numerous problems in commencing arbitration.
64. White, Jeffrey Robert. "Mandatory Arbitration: A Growing Threat." *Trial* 35 (July 1999): 32–34, 36.
65. "AIDS-Related Lawsuits Will Continue to Rise, Report Shows." *AHA News* 26 (April 16, 1990): 3.
66. Pranschke, Sybil C., and Barbara M. Wright. "HIV and AIDS—Employers Grapple with Difficult Issues." *Benefits Quarterly* 11 (Third Quarter, 1995): 41.
67. Occupational Safety and Health Act of 1970, PL 93-237, 42 U.S.C. § 3142-1.
68. Americans with Disabilities Act of 1990, PL 101-336, 42 U.S.C. § 12101 *et seq*; Civil Rights Act of 1964, PL 105-220, 112 Stat. 1092; Rehabilitation Act of 1973, PL 93-112, 29 U.S.C. § 701 *et seq*; Civil Rights Restoration Act of 1988, PL 100-259, 102 Stat. 28 (March 22, 1988); Stein, Robert E. "The Americans with Disabilities Act of 1990." *Arbitration Journal* 46 (June 1991): 6–7.
69. Labowitz, Kenneth E. "Refusal to Treat HIV-AIDS Patients: What Are the Legal Obligations?" *Trial* 28 (March 1992): 58.
70. Furrow, Greaney, Johnson, Jost, and Schwartz, *Health Law,* 487–488.
71. School Board of Nassau County, Florida v. Arline 480 U.S. 273 (1987).
72. Bayer, Ronald, and Larry Gostin. "Legal and Ethical Issues Relating to AIDS." *Bulletin of the Pan American Health Organization* 24 (1990): 456.
73. Bayer and Gostin, "Legal and Ethical," 456.
74. Raintree Health Care Center v. Human Rights Commission, 655 N.E.2d 944 (1995).
75. Mauro v. Borgess Medical Center, 886 F.Supp. 1349 (1995). The trial court decision was affirmed on appeal at 137 F.3d 398 (6th Cir. Feb. 25, 1998). A federal court held that, despite the virtually nonexistent risk of infection (see Chapter 13), an HIV–positive surgeon was not "otherwise qualified" under Section 504 and ADA and could be prohibited from performing exposure-prone procedures in *Scoles v. Mercy Health Corporation of Southeastern Pennsylvania* (887 F.Supp.765 [1994]); a federal court upheld the suspension of a neurosurgical resident from his residency in *Doe v. University of Maryland Medical System Corporation* (50 F.3d 1261 [1995]) because he posed a significant risk to his patients' health and safety that could not be eliminated by reasonable accommodation.
76. Bayer and Gostin, "Legal and Ethical," 457.
77. Okie, Susan. "AIDS: Health Officials Launch New Campaign to Determine How Widespread the Virus Is." *The Washington Post, Health Section,* September 2, 1997, 13.
78. Tarasoff v. Regents of the State of California, 17 Cal. 3d 425 (1976).
79. Bayer and Gostin, "Legal and Ethical," 461–462.
80. Posner, Richard A. *Antitrust Law: An Economic Perspective,* 23. Chicago: University of Chicago Press, 1976.
81. AMA v. United States, 130 F. 2d 233, (D.C. Cir. 1942); affirmed, 317 U.S. 519 (1943).
82. Goldfarb v. Virginia State Bar, 421 U.S. 773 (1975).
83. Bierig, Jack R. "Antitrust for Physicians." In *Physician's Survival Guide: Legal Pitfalls and Solutions* 63–84. Chicago: American Medical Association and National Health Lawyers Association, 1991.

84. Equal Access to Justice Act of 1988, PL 99-80, 99 Stat. 186 (August 5, 1985); Sisk, Gregory C. "The Essentials of the Equal Access to Justice Act: Court Awards of Attorney's Fees for Unreasonable Government Conduct (Part Two)." *Louisiana Law Review* 56 (Fall 1995): 18.

85. Hospital Building Co. v. Trustees of Rex Hospital, 425 U.S. 738 (1976); reversed and remanded, 691 F.2d 678 (4th Cir. 1982); certiorari denied 464 U.S. 890 (1982) and 464 U.S. 904; rehearing denied 464 U.S. 1003 (1983).

86. Southwick, *Law of Hospital,* 227–229.

87. Southwick, *Law of Hospital,* 250.

88. United States v. Rockford Memorial Corp., 898 F.2d 1278 (7th Cir. 1990); certiorari denied, 498 U.S. 920 (1990).

89. United States v. Carilion Health Systems, Community Hospital of Roanoke Valley, 707 F.Supp. 840 (W.D. Va, 1989); affirmed without opinion, 892 F.2d 1042 (4th Cir. 1989).

90. Higgins, Daniel B. "Rockford Will Not End Hospital Mergers." *Hospitals* 65 (April 5, 1991): 76.

91. Brock, Thomas H. "Antitrust and the Healthcare Field," 2–3. Photocopy handout at the American College of Healthcare Executives, Congress on Healthcare Management, Chicago, March 1998.

92. Patrick v. Burget, 800 F.2d 1498 (9th Cir. 1986); reversed, 486 U.S. 94 (1988); rehearing denied 487 U.S. 1243 (1988). Dr. Patrick prevailed in the antitrust claims in the trial court. The court of appeals reversed the decision because the peer review activity that was established by Oregon and that conduct by state activities is exempt from federal law. The Supreme Court reversed the appeals court on a finding that the state judiciary did not supply active supervision and raised the question of whether state court review could constitute state action.

93. Health Care Quality Improvement Act of 1986, PL 99-660, 100 Stat. 3784.

94. Austin v. McNamara, 731 F.Supp. 934 (C.D. Cal. 1990); affirmed 979 (F.2d) 726 (9th Cir. 1992). Egan v. Athol Memorial Hospital, 971 F.Supp. 37 (D. Mass. 1997), affirmed per curiam 134 F.3d 361 (1st Cir. 1998), certiorari denied, 119 S.Ct. 409 (1998).

95. This problem was reported soon after the Data Bank became operational (Rushford, Greg. "Data Bank Has a Deficit." *Legal Times* 13 [April 22, 1991]: 1). The problem continues (Editorial. "The National Practitioner's Data Bank." *Trauma* 3 [April 1996]: 1–5).

96. "About 75% of Hospitals Not Reporting to Data Bank." *Hospital Peer Review* 20 (June 1995): 91–92.

97. Nettleman, Mary D., and Ann Pettinger Nelson. "Adverse Occurrences During Hospitalization on a General Medicine Service." *Clinical Performance and Quality Health Care* 2 (April/May/June 1994): 67–72.

98. Berg, Robert N. "Vertical Integration: The Next Antitrust Regulatory Frontier." *Journal of the Medical Association of Georgia* 84 (May 1995): 228–229. Physician networks or mergers in three states were the focus of DOJ business review letters, with special concern as to the control exerted over a market. (Busey, Roxane C. "DOJ Raises Concerns About Mergers and Large Physician Networks." *Healthcare Financial Management* 50 [August 1996]: 65, 67, 69, 71–72.)

99. McGinn, Paul R. "Next Antitrust Target—IPAs." *American Medical News* 33 (October 26, 1990): 30.

100. Pretzer, Michael. "Will the Big, Bad Antitrust Wolf Blow Your IPA Down?" *Medical Economics* 74 (April 7, 1997): 40–44, 47.

101. Burda, David. "Study by State Attorneys General Finds at Least 70 Antitrust Cases in Healthcare Since 1985." *Modern Healthcare* 20 (December 17, 1990): 41.

102. Emergency Medical Treatment and Active Labor Act of 1985, PL 99-272, 100 Stat. 174.

103. Furrow, Greaney, Johnson, Jost, and Schwartz, *Health Law,* 547.

104. Furrow, Greaney, Johnson, Jost, and Schwartz, *Health Law,* 539.

105. Furrow, Greancy, Johnson, Jost, and Schwartz, *Health Law,* 540.

106. Baker, Constance H., and Therese M. Goldsmith. "From Triage to Transfer: HCFA's Update on EMTALA." *Health Law Digest* 26 (October 1998): 3–14.

107. Employee Retirement Income Security Act of 1974, PL 93-406, 88 Stat. 829 (September 2, 1974). To fall within ERISA, an employee benefit plan must be a plan, fund, or program that is established or maintained by an employer or an employee organization for the purpose of providing for its participants or beneficiaries medical, surgical, or hospital care; or benefits in the event of sickness, accident disability, death, or unemployment; or vacation benefits, apprenticeship, or other training programs; or day care centers, scholarship funds, or prepaid legal services. Non–ERISA plans are those in which the

1) employer makes no premium contributions; 2) employees' participation is voluntary; 3) employer does not endorse the plan and its only functions are to allow insurers to undertake marketing to employees and to collect (through payroll deductions) and remit premiums to the insurer; and 4) employer receives no compensation to administer the plan other than reasonable payment for services involving payroll deductions. (Perez, Robert Armand, Sr. "ERISA Preemption: Denying Employees' Rights to Benefits." *Trial* 33 [May 1997]: 72–74.)

108. Farrell, Margaret G. "ERISA Preemption and Regulation of Managed Health Care: The Case for Managed Federalism." *American Journal of Law & Medicine* 23:2&3 (1997): 251.

109. Farrell, "ERISA Preemption and Regulation," 252.

110. Perez, "ERISA Preemption," 72–74.

111. Perez, "ERISA Preemption," 72–74.

112. Metropolitan Life Insurance Company v. Taylor, 481 U.S. 58 (1987); Visconti v. U.S. Health Care, 857 F.Supp.1097 (E.D.Pa. 1994).

113. Dukes v. U.S. Health Care, 57 F.3d 350 (3d Cir. 1995); Pacificare of Oklahoma, Inc. v. Burrage, 59 F.3d 151 (10th Cir. 1995).

114. Farrell, "ERISA Preemption and Regulation," 273–275.

115. Huff, Charlotte. "Chinks in ERISA's Armor." *Hospitals & Health Networks* 71 (November 20, 1997): 39.

116. Furrow, Greaney, Johnson, Jost, and Schwartz, *Health Law,* 638.

117. Furrow, Greaney, Johnson, Jost, and Schwartz, *Health Law,* 648.

118. Furrow, Greaney, Johnson, Jost, and Schwartz, *Health Law,* 641–642.

119. Furrow, Greaney, Johnson, Jost, and Schwartz, *Health Law,* 642.

120. Crane, Thomas S., Richard G. Cowart, Robert G. Homchick, Ellen P. Pesch, Sanford V. Teplitzky, and Harvey Yampolsky. "Stark II Proposed Regulations." *Health Law Digest* 26 (February 1998): 3–4.

121. "Spotlight on the Stark II Regulations." *Health Lawyers News* 2 (February 1998): 6.

122. Crane, Cowart, Homchick, Pesch, Teplitzky, and Yampolsky, "Stark II Proposed Regulations," 4–5.

123. Furrow, Greaney, Johnson, Jost, and Schwartz, *Health Law,* 643.

124. Furrow, Greaney, Johnson, Jost, and Schwartz, *Health Law,* 639.

125. Health Insurance Portability and Accountability Act of 1996, PL 104-191, 110 Stat. 1936 (August 2, 1996).

126. "New Healthcare Integrity and Protection Data Bank Casts Wide Net." *Health Lawyers News* 2 (December 1998): 7.

127. "New Healthcare Integrity," 7.

128. "New Healthcare Integrity," 7–8.

129. False Claims Act Amendments of 1986, PL 99-562, 100 Stat. 3153 (October 27, 1986).

130. "Qui Tam Statistics." *False Claims Act and Qui Tam Quarterly Review* 12 (January 1998): 41.

131. Scott, Lisa. "Whistleblower Suit Alleges Patient Records Doctored." *Modern Healthcare* 25 (August 21, 1995): 34. Another example of a *qui tam* suit occurred in *United States ex rel. Brandimarte v. Wurtzel,* Civ. Action No. 94-2398 (E.D. PA. Nov. 3, 1995), in which defendants settled allegations of making false and fraudulent claims for psychotherapy services under the Medicare and Medicaid programs by paying $500,000 to the United States and $50,000 toward the whistleblower's legal fees and costs.

132. Rice, Berkeley. "When A Doctor Accuses Colleagues of Health Fraud." *Medical Economics* 72 (August 7, 1995): 172–174, 177–179, 183–184, and 189–190.

133. Havighurst, Clark C. *Health Care Law and Policy: Readings, Notes, and Questions,* 204. Westbury, NY: Foundation Press, 1988.

134. Havighurst, *Health Care Law,* 204–205.

135. Wolfson, Jay. "Overcoming Challenges to Tax-Exempt Status." *Healthcare Financial Management* 50 (April 1996): 60.

136. The General Accounting Office estimated that the benefit of tax-exempt status to not-for-profit hospitals was worth $4.5 billion in saved income, use, sales, and property taxes, reduced costs through tax-exempt bond financing, and receipt of charitable donations. (Hudson, Terese. "Not-for-Profit Hospitals Fight Tax-Exempt Challenges." *Hospitals* 64 [October 20, 1990]: 36.) At $8.5 billion, a private estimate was much higher (Copeland, John, and Gabriel Rudney. "Federal Tax Subsidies for Not-for-Profit Hospitals." *Tax Notes* [46 March 26, 1990]: 1559–1576).

137. Pound, Edward T., Gary Cohen, and Penny Loeb. "Tax Exempt!" *U.S. News & World Report* (October 2, 1995): 37.

138. Fischer, Kevin B. "Tax Exemption and the Health Care Industry: Are the Challenges to Tax-Exempt Status Justified?" *Vanderbilt Law Review* 49 (January 1996): 163.

139. Hudson, Terese. "Not-for-Profit Hospitals Fight Tax-Exempt Challenges." *Hospitals* 64 (October 20, 1990): 36. As a result of the successful challenges, some hospitals agreed to make payments in lieu of taxes.

140. Fischer, "Tax Exemption," 163.

141. Henry, Wayne. "Tax-Exempt Challenges Warrant Hospitals' Attention." *Healthcare Financial Management* 45 (January 1991): 32.

142. Stanley, J. Mark, and David R. Ward. "UBIT May Hit Common Transactions." *Tax Advisor* 25 (September 1994): 557.

143. Furrow, Greaney, Johnson, Jost, and Schwartz, *Health Law,* 49.

144. Henry, "Tax-Exempt Challenges," 32.

145. Furrow, Greaney, Johnson, Jost, and Schwartz, *Health Law,* 47.

146. Korman, Rochelle, and William F. Gaske. "Joint Ventures Between Tax-Exempt and Commercial Health Care Providers." *Tax Notes* 74 (March 24, 1997): 1582.

147. In Pinnacle Health Hospitals v. Dauphin County Board of Assessment Appeals (PA CCP 1998), a Pennsylvania appellate court upheld revocation of a not-for-profit hospital's local property tax exemption because certain activities (e.g., excessive chief executive officer compensation and executive bonus plan), combined with ownership of a for-profit subsidiary, showed a private profit motive.

148. Proskauer Rose, LLP. *Client Alert* (newsletter), November 1998, 1.

149. Fischer, "Tax Exemption," 185. *Geisinger Health Plan v. Commissioner,* 30 F.3d 494 (3d Cir. 1994), narrowly defined community benefit with regard to HMOs. The basic requirements granting IDSs tax-exempt status are found in IRS determination letters, which are not legally binding.

150. Fischer, "Tax Exemption," 185–186.

151. McMenamin, Joseph P. "Telemedicine: Technology and the Law." *For the Defense* 39 (July 1997): 11.

152. McMenamin, "Telemedicine," 11.

153. McMenamin, "Telemedicine," 13.

154. McMenamin, "Telemedicine," 13.

155. McMenamin, "Telemedicine," 13.

156. McMenamin, "Telemedicine," 14.

157. Daar, Judith F., and Spencer Koerner. "Telemedicine: Legal and Practice Implications." *Whittier Law Review* 19 (Winter 1997): 16–18.

158. Cepelewicz, Barry B. "Telemedicine and Provider Liability: New Technology Creates New Risks." *Health Law Report* 7 (December 1997): 12.

159. Neergaard, Lauran. "Patients Bypass Doctors' Visits with On-Line Prescription Sales." *The Washington Times,* December 25, 1998, B11.

160. Daar and Koerner, "Telemedicine: Legal," 25.

161. McMenamin, "Telemedicine," 14.

SELECTED BIBLIOGRAPHY

American Medical Association and National Health Lawyers Association. *Physician's Survival Guide: Legal Pitfalls and Solutions.* Chicago: American Medical Association and National Health Lawyers Association, 1991.

Baumberger, Charles H. "Vicarious Liability Claims Against HMOs." *Trial* 34 (May 1998): 30–33, 35.

Bodenheimer, Edgar. *Jurisprudence: The Philosophy and Method of the Law,* rev. ed. Cambridge, MA: Harvard University Press, 1974.

Blum, John D., Ed. *Achieving Quality in Managed Care: The Role of Law.* Chicago: American Bar Association, 1997.

Centers for Disease Control and Prevention. "Recommendations for Preventing Transmission of Human Immunodeficiency Virus and Hepatitis B Virus to Patients During Exposure-Prone Invasive Procedures. *MMWR. Morbidity and Mortality Weekly Report* 40 (July 12, 1991): 1–8.

Corbin, Arthur L. *Corbin on Contracts.* St. Paul, MN: West Publishing, 1952.

Fischer, Kevin. "Tax Exemption and the Health Care Industry: Are the Challenges to Tax-Exempt Status Justified?" *Vanderbilt Law Review* 49 (January 1996): 161–195.

Flynn, Ruth E. "Demand for Public Access to the National Practitioner Data Bank: Consumers Sound Their Own Death Cry." *Hamline Journal of Public Law & Policy* 18 (Fall 1996): 251–279.

Havighurst, Clark C. *Health Care Law and Policy: Readings, Notes, and Questions.* Westbury, NY: Foundation Press, 1990. (Supplement, 1992)

Henry, Wayne. "Tax-Exempt Challenges Warrant Hospitals' Attention." *Healthcare Financial Management* 45 (January 1991): 30, 32, 34–38.

"HIV-infected Physicians and the Practice of Seriously Invasive Procedures." *Hastings Center Report* 19 (January–February 1989): 32–39.

Keeton, W. Page, Ed. *Prosser and Keeton on the Law of Torts,* 5th ed. St. Paul, MN: West Publishing, 1984.

Nolan, Virginia E., and Edmund Ursin. "Enterprise Liability Reexamined." *Oregon Law Review* 75 (Summer 1996): 467–492.

Richardson, Eric N., and Salvatore J. Russo, Eds. "Calming AIDS Phobia: Legal Implications of the Low Risk of Transmitting HIV in the Health Care Setting." *University of Michigan Journal of Law Reform* 28 (Summer 1995): 733–798.

Southwick, Arthur F. *The Law of Hospital and Health Care Administration,* 2nd ed. Ann Arbor, MI: Health Administration Press, 1988.

Stein, Robert E. "The Americans with Disabilities Act of 1990." *Arbitration Journal* 46 (June 1991): 6–15.

Wing, Kenneth R. *The Law and the Public's Health,* 4th ed. Ann Arbor, MI: Health Administration Press, 1995.

15 Leadership

*Leadership is not domination, but the art of persuading people
to work toward a common goal.*[1]

The quality of leadership in a health services organization/health system (HSO/HS) affects how work is done, how well the organization or system performs, and whether its objectives are achieved.[2] Burns, in a classical work, established that leadership in organizations is of two distinct types: transactional and transformational.[3] Both types are considered in this chapter.

Transactional leadership occurs throughout a HSO/HS because managers directly supervise people, which establishes "supervisor–subordinate" relationships. Leadership in these relationships is a transactional process in which the needs of followers are met if they perform to the leader's expectations; leaders and followers undertake transactions through which each receives something of value. Good leadership skills and techniques facilitate the transactions that are essential if these pervasive relationships are to function properly.

In the second type of leadership—more likely to be practiced in HSOs/HSs by senior managers—the purpose is significant change in the status quo. In practicing transformational leadership, managers are more focused on creating change than on exchanges.[4] In their transformational leadership roles, managers may focus on changes that are organizationwide or systemwide in scope and relate to such things as

- The HSO's/HS's mission and values
- Attaining or modifying the level of support for the mission among internal and external stakeholders
- Allocating responsibility for the HSO's/HS's operation and performance
- Developing new strategies or implementing existing ones differently
- Altering the balance among the economic, professional, and social interests of the HSO/HS and those who work in it
- Establishing new or discarding existing relationships with other organizations or systems with which interdependencies are shared

735

In contrast to the transactional leadership process that occurs in direct supervisor–subordinate relationships, a transformational leader must have a vision for the entire HSO/HS, and lead followers both inside and outside it if the vision is to be realized.[5] Often, when people speak of leadership, they mean transformational leadership. When a HSO/HS is perceived as successful because of strong and effective leadership, this means generally that leadership has made good decisions regarding mission, objectives, structure, service mix, quality, and new technologies, not that its leaders (managers) have summoned extra motivation and performance from people, or helped plan their tasks, coordinated their work, or taught them new skills. These latter activities, which characterize transactional leadership, are important, but they are not the only determinants of senior-level managers' success in their transformational leader roles.[6]

Senior managers lead by managing organizational culture.[7] They focus on decisions and activities that affect the entire organization or system, including those that are intended to ensure its survival and overall good health.[8] They also lead by providing strategic direction and vision to the HSO/HS and ensuring that its mission and objectives are achieved.[9] Effective organization- or system-level leaders also lead by inculcating certain values; building intra- and interorganizational coalitions; and interpreting and responding to various challenges and opportunities from the external environment, which includes taking steps to alter the environmental constraints placed on the HSO/HS.

Because of their relationship to the success of leaders in HSOs/HSs in both transactional and transformational leadership roles, the extensive research and theories about leadership and leaders are discussed in this chapter. However, it is necessary to first define leadership precisely and to model it as a process.

LEADERSHIP DEFINED AND MODELED

Leadership is defined in different ways, although most definitions have common elements. Cartwright and Zander define leadership as the acts and activities of one person that contribute to performance by others.[10] Fiedler and Chemers define it as an "unequal influence and power relationship"[11] in which followers accept the leader's right to make certain decisions for them. Holt's definition of leadership is "the process of influencing others to behave in preferred ways to accomplish organizational objectives."[12] Blake and Mouton define leadership as the managerial activity through which managers maximize productivity, stimulate creative problem solving, and promote morale and satisfaction among those who are led.[13] In Jago's view leadership is a process that uses noncoercive influence as a means of directing and coordinating the activities of the members of a group toward attaining the group's objectives.[14] Bass notes that "leadership occurs when one group member modifies the motivation or competencies of others in the group."[15] In one of the most comprehensive definitions of leadership, Yukl defines it as

> *the process wherein an individual member of a group or organization influences the interpretation of events, the choice of objectives and strategies, the organization of work activities, the motivation of people to achieve the objectives, the maintenance of cooperative relationships, the development of skills and confidence by members, and the enlistment of support and cooperation from people outside the group or organization.*[16]

These definitions include individuals, groups, organizations, goals/objectives, influence, and acceptance. In sum, they suggest that the leader's role is to determine what is to be accomplished by others, whether individuals or entire HSOs/HSs, and to influence others to contribute to achieving objectives. At the level of supervisor–subordinate relationships, leadership focuses on what a specific individual or group is to accomplish. At the level of organization or system leadership, the focus is on what the HSO/HS is to accomplish. These definitions further imply that those being led must accept the leader's role and influence over them. As Bass stated, "Leaders are agents of change, persons whose acts affect other people more than other people's acts affect them."[17]

Taking these definitions into account, a comprehensive definition of this complex, multidimensional activity is to view leadership *as a process of one individual influencing another individual or group to achieve particular objectives.* A leader can be defined as one who practices leadership, that is, as an individual who influences another individual or group to achieve particular objectives. These definitions of leadership and leader apply to organizational or system-level leadership (transformational leadership) as well as leadership at the level of supervisor–subordinate relationships (transactional leadership). In both situations leadership means determining what is to be accomplished and influencing others to contribute to its accomplishment. Figure 15.1 shows a simplified model of this process.

The processes of transactional and transformational leadership differ. For example, managers at the supervisor–subordinate level lead individuals and small groups whose members tend to be relatively homogeneous in the work that they do and in their preparation for doing it. This stands in contrast to the transformational leadership of an entire organization or system, in which there is likely to be great diversity and heterogeneity among those who must be led. Another very important difference in the leader roles of managers at different organizational levels is the amount and sources of power available to them. As is discussed in the next section, power is crucial to the ability to exert influence, and the ability to influence is essential to the ability to lead.

POWER AND INFLUENCE

Influence is important to the leadership process and to success in the leader role because influence is the means by which "people successfully persuade others to follow their advice, suggestion, or order."[18] The essence of leadership is the ability to influence followers. To have influence, however, one also must have power. Power is the potential to exert influence. More power means more potential to influence others. Therefore, to understand influence, one must first understand power.

Sources of Power

Those who wish to exert influence must first acquire power by utilizing the various sources of power that are available to them. The classical scheme for categorizing the bases of interpersonal power includes legitimate, reward, coercive, expert, and referent power.[19]

Legitimate power is power that is derived from a person's position in an organization. It also is called formal power or authority and exists because organizations find it advantageous to assign certain powers to individuals so that they can do their jobs. Based on their position, all managers have some degree of legitimate power or authority. Of course, managers at different levels of HSOs/HSs have different amounts of legitimate power or authority.

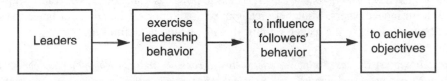

Figure 15.1. The process of leadership.

Reward power is based on the leader's ability to reward desirable behavior. Reward power stems partly from the legitimate power that is granted to the leader by the organization. In other words, managers by virtue of their positions are given control over certain rewards to buttress their legitimate or positional power. Rewards include pay increases, promotions, work schedules, recognition of accomplishments, and status symbols such as office size and location.

Coercive power is the opposite of reward power and is based on the leader's ability to punish people or prevent them from obtaining desired rewards. As described in Chapter 16, rewards and punishments are powerful motivational tools, although managers playing their leader roles are, in general, better served by reward power than coercive power.

Expert power derives from having knowledge valued by the HSO/HS, such as expertise in problem solving or critical tasks. Expert power is personal to the individual who possesses the expertise. Thus it is different from legitimate, reward, and coercive power, which are prescribed by the organization or system, even though people may be granted these forms of power because they possess expert power. For example, certain health professionals enter management positions because of their superior levels of expertise. When they make this shift, they acquire legitimate, reward, and coercive power in addition to their expert power. It also is noteworthy that, in organizations in which work is highly technical or professional, such as a typical HSO/HS, expert power alone makes some people very powerful. For example, the power of the professional staff is based on clinical knowledge and skills. Physicians with scarce expertise, such as transplant surgery, gain more power than physicians whose expertise is more readily replaceable. Expert power is not reserved for those with clinical or technical skills, however. The ability to effectively manage increasingly complex HSOs/HSs is a source of power for those with the expertise.

Referent power results when individuals engender admiration, loyalty, and emulation to the extent that they gain the power to influence others. This is sometimes called charismatic power. Charismatic leaders typically have a vision for the groups or organizations that they lead, strong convictions about the correctness of the vision, and great self-confidence about their ability to realize the vision, and they are perceived by their followers as agents of change.[20] It is rare for a leader, whether transactional or transformational, to gain sufficient power to heavily influence followers simply from referent or charismatic power. As with expert power, referent power cannot be given by the HSO/HS as can legitimate, reward, and coercive power.

The five bases of power are not necessarily independent and, in fact, can be complementary. Leaders who use reward power wisely strengthen their referent power. Conversely, leaders who abuse their coercive power will quickly weaken or lose referent power. Effective leaders are those who can translate power into influence, who understand the sources of their power and act accordingly. For example, if a person's power derives from expertise, it may be dangerous to try to lead in areas that lie outside that expertise. Effective leaders "understand—at least intuitively—the costs, risks, and benefits of using each kind of power and are able to recognize which to draw on in different situations and with different people."[21]

Effective Use of Power

Interpersonal and political skills distinguish individuals who effectively use power and translate it into influence as they lead others. However, access to power is not enough. One must know how to use power to influence others. Mintzberg recognized this important fact and attributes the successful use of power largely to the leader's political skills, which he defines as

> *the ability to use the bases of power effectively—to convince those to whom one has access, to use one's resources, information, and technical skills to their fullest in bargaining, to exercise formal power with a sensitivity to the feelings of others, to know where to concentrate one's energies, to sense what is possible, and to organize the necessary alliances.*[22]

TABLE 15.1.   SOURCES OF POWER IN ORGANIZATIONS

Position power
- Formal authority
- Control over rewards
- Control over punishments
- Control over information
- Ecological control

Personal power
- Expertise
- Friendship/loyalty
- Charisma

Political power
- Control over decision processes
- Coalitions
- Co-optation
- Institutionalization

From Yukl, Gary A. *Leadership in Organizations*, 4th ed., 179. Upper Saddle River, NI: Prentice-Hall 1998; reprinted by permission

Yukl's comprehensive model of the sources of power in organizations, shown in Table 15.1, includes the importance of political skills in the effective exercise of power. He argues that people in organizations derive power, in part, from their positions in the organizational design. Position power includes the authority that is granted to managers by the organization and its inherent control over certain resources, processes, and information. However, power in organizational settings also depends on attributes of the interpersonal relationship between leaders and followers. Personal power includes relative task expertise, friendship and the loyalty that some people engender in others, and sometimes the leader's charismatic qualities. Finally, power also depends on certain political processes and skills. Political power derives from the leader's control over key decisions, ability to form coalitions, ability to co-opt or diffuse and weaken the influence of rivals in the organization, and ability to institutionalize the leader's power by exploiting ambiguity to interpret events in a manner that is favorable to the leader.[23]

Depending on circumstances, power from the sources shown in Table 15.1 is available in different degrees to leaders in HSOs/HSs. For example, at the level of departments, where leadership comes primarily through the transactions that occur in supervisor–subordinate relationships, first-level managers have the power to influence or lead because they have formal authority over the department and the people in it. First-level managers also have some control over resources, rewards, punishments, and information (position power), and may have more expertise in the work than others in the department (personal power derived from expertise). Such managers may have little political power, but this is not a problem if position and personal power sources are sufficient to lead the department.

In contrast, senior-level managers, who lead at the organization or system level, derive power from the same menu of sources but in a different mix. For example, the chief executive officer (CEO) of a HSO/HS possesses political power by virtue of the authority to control decision processes, form coalitions of key decision makers, or co-opt opponents. The CEO may have considerable charisma, extremely loyal assistants, and deep friendships with key physicians and governing body members, all of which provide the CEO with personal power. The CEO's position power can be great in terms of control over resources and information available in the HSO/HS. Finally, the CEO may be in a strong position to control access to the sources of power in the organization or system.[24] This is an important source of power in itself.

Much of what is known about power and influence is pertinent to an understanding of leadership. By definition, leadership involves one person influencing others, and power is the ability to

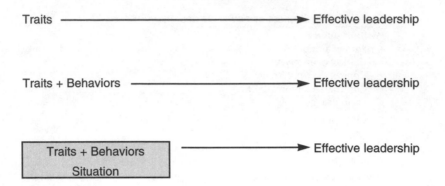

Figure 15.2.   Comparing three approaches to leadership.

influence others. Power and influence alone, however, do not fully explain leadership effectiveness or the success or failure of leaders.

APPROACHES TO UNDERSTANDING LEADERSHIP

The study of leadership has followed several paths, none of which has produced a definitive theory of effective leadership. Much of the theorizing about leadership and many of the studies of the subject can be classified into one of three basic approaches. One approach has been based on the proposition that traits, skills, abilities, or characteristics that are inherent in some people explain why they are better leaders than others. Theories and studies developed around this assumption belong to the trait approach to understanding leadership and leaders. Another approach, which grew directly out of the inability of traits to explain leadership effectiveness fully, was based on the assumption that particular behaviors might be associated with successful leaders. A third approach, an integrative approach to understanding leadership, focuses on how leaders, followers, and the situations in which they find themselves interact and work.

These approaches to an explanation of how leadership is practiced successfully (traits and skills, leader behavior, and situational) contribute to understanding leadership, and the key theories, findings, and conceptualizations that are developed in each approach are examined in this chapter. Figure 15.2 illustrates the evolutionary relationships these approaches bear to one another.

One can best understand the leadership phenomenon by integrating all three conceptual approaches or perspectives, rather than by thinking of them as competing approaches. Each approach is discussed, and the chapter concludes with an integrative model of the leadership process that incorporates elements of trait, behavior, and situational perspectives.

LEADER TRAITS AND SKILLS

The link between interpersonal and political skills, and the fact that some personal characteristics such as expertise and personal charisma are important bases of power, suggest that certain traits and skills are associated with effective leaders. As has been noted,

> *Leaders do not have to be great men or women by being intellectual geniuses or omniscient prophets to succeed, but they do need to have the "right stuff" and this stuff is not equally present in all people. Leadership is a demanding, unrelenting job with enormous pressures and grave*

responsibilities. It would be a disservice to leaders to suggest that they are ordinary people who happened to be in the right place at the right time. Maybe the place matters, but it takes a special kind of person to master the challenges of opportunity.[25]

Most studies of leadership in the first half of the 20th century sought to find leader traits in physical characteristics, personality, and ability. Researchers theorized that it was possible to identify traits that distinguished leaders and followers, or successful and unsuccessful leaders. These studies focused on the traits that are associated with effective leaders in business, but they also looked at leaders in government, the military, and religious organizations. Of course, to prove that traits explained leadership, it was necessary to find traits that all leaders had in common. This proved very difficult. The many different traits studied included physical characteristics such as height, weight, and appearance and personality traits such as alertness, originality, integrity, and self-confidence, as well as intelligence or cleverness.

None of the hundreds of studies that were conducted in search of universal leader traits was successful. A landmark review of the subject by Stogdill in 1948 analyzed all the major studies of leader traits and concluded that "a person does not become a leader by virtue of the possession of some combination of traits . . . the pattern of personal characteristics of the leader must bear some relevant relationship to the characteristics, activities, and goals of the followers."[26] This conclusion was useful in later research that studied leadership in the context of specific situations.

Stogdill's conclusion discouraged additional research to identify universal leader traits. However, people interested in the selection of effective managers through the identification of people with leadership potential continued to search for traits that might at least be associated with successful leaders. They used improved methodologies and added administrative and technical abilities to the traits of intelligence and personality studied earlier. Many of these studies, in fact, showed associations between certain traits and leader effectiveness. In a later review of these newer, more sophisticated studies, Stogdill confirmed his original negative assessment of efforts to identify universal leader traits. He concluded, however, that it is possible to develop a trait profile that characterizes successful leaders:

> *The leader is characterized by a strong drive for responsibility and task completion, vigor and persistence in pursuit of goals, venturesomeness and originality in problem solving, drive to exercise initiative in social situations, self-confidence and sense of personal identity, willingness to accept consequences of decision and action, readiness to absorb interpersonal stress, willingness to tolerate frustration and delay, ability to influence other persons' behavior, and capacity to structure social interaction systems to the purpose at hand.*[27]

The idea that traits, whether of intelligence, personality, or ability, are associated with leader effectiveness continues to be assessed. Although there is no longer a search for universal leader traits, the traits that are associated with leader effectiveness continue to be refined. Table 15.2 lists traits and skills that frequently characterize successful leaders. Kirkpatrick and Locke summarize contemporary thought about the role of traits in determining leadership effectiveness as follows:

> *Although research shows that the possession of certain traits alone does not guarantee leadership success, there is evidence that effective leaders are different from other people in certain key respects. Key leader traits include drive (a broad term that includes achievement, motivation, ambition, energy, tenacity, and initiative), leadership motivation (the desire to lead but not to seek power as an end in itself), honesty and integrity, self-confidence (which is associated with emotional stability), cognitive ability, and [expert] knowledge. There is less clear evidence for traits such as charisma, creativity, and flexibility. We believe that the key leader traits help the*

TABLE 15.2.   TRAITS AND SKILLS FOUND IN SUCCESSFUL LEADERS

Traits	Skills
Adaptable to situations	Clever (intelligent)
Alert to social environment	Conceptually skilled
Ambitious, achievement oriented	Creative
Assertive	Diplomatic and tactful
Cooperative	Fluent in speaking
Decisive	Knowledgeable about the work
Dependable	Organized (administrative ability)
Dominant (power motivation)	Persuasive
Energetic (high activity level)	Socially skilled
Persistent	
Self-confident	
Tolerant of stress	
Willing to assume responsibility	

From Yukl. Gary A. *Leadership in Organizations*, 4th ed., 237. Upper Saddle River, NJ: Prentice-Hall, 1998; reprinted by permission.

leader acquire necessary skills; formulate an organizational vision and an effective plan for pursuing it; and take the necessary steps to implement the vision in reality.[28]

Goleman has made an important contribution to understanding the role of "emotional intelligence" in leadership success.[29] He identifies five components of emotional intelligence: self-awareness, self-regulation, motivation, empathy, and social skill. These components are defined in Table 15.3, and the hallmarks of their presence in leaders are given. Goleman concludes that successful leaders vary in many ways, but notes

I have found, however, that the most effective leaders are alike in one crucial way: they all have a high degree of what has come to be known as emotional intelligence. It's not that IQ and technical skills are irrelevant. They do matter, but mainly as "threshold capabilities"; that is, they are the entry-level requirements for executive positions. But my research, along with other current studies, clearly shows that emotional intelligence is the sine qua non *of leadership. Without it, a person can have the best training in the world, an incisive, analytical mind, and an endless supply of smart ideas, but still won't make a great leader.*[30]

Because the search for universal leader traits was unsuccessful, researchers began to expand their views on the role of leader traits in leadership effectiveness. They came to view traits as predispositions to behaviors, adopting the view that "a particular trait, or set of them, tends to predispose (although do not cause) an individual to engage in certain behaviors that may or may not result in leadership effectiveness."[31] They began to appreciate that traits had an impact, but not in the way imagined in the earlier search for the universal traits of leaders. These researchers came to understand that "what seems to be most important is not traits but rather how they are expressed in the behavior of the leader."[32]

LEADER BEHAVIOR AND LEADERSHIP STYLE

Research into behavioral aspects of leadership was premised on the exciting possibility that, if leader behaviors that explained leadership effectiveness could be identified, then people could be taught how to be leaders. Education may not increase intelligence levels or change personality profiles, but it can be used to teach behaviors. The trait theories maintained that leaders are effective

TABLE 15.3. THE FIVE COMPONENTS OF EMOTIONAL INTELLIGENCE AT WORK

Component	Definition	Hallmarks
Self-awareness	The ability to recognize and understand your moods, emotions, and drives, as well as their effect on others	Self-confidence Realistic self-assessment Self-deprecating sense of humor
Self-regulation	The ability to control or redirect disruptive impulses and moods The propensity to suspend judgment—to think before acting	Trustworthiness and integrity Comfort with ambiguity Openness to change
Motivation	A passion to work for reasons that go beyond money or status A propensity to pursue goals with energy and persistence	Strong drive to achieve Optimism, even in the face of failure Organizational commitment
Empathy	The ability to understand the emotional makeup of other people Skill in treating people according to their emotional reactions	Expertise in building and retaining talent Cross-cultural sensitivity Service to clients and customers
Social skill	Proficiency in managing relationships and building networks An ability to find common ground and build rapport	Effectiveness in leading change Persuasiveness Expertise in building and leading teams

From Goleman, Daniel. "What Makes a Leader?" *Harvard Business Review* 76 (November–December 1998): 95; reprinted by permission.

because of characteristics they were born with. People either have them or they do not. However, if specific behaviors were associated with leadership success, then programs could be designed to train people to practice the behaviors. The studies in leader behavior focused on describing leadership behaviors, developing concepts and models of leadership styles (styles being thought of as combinations of behaviors), and examining the relationships between leadership styles and leadership effectiveness. These studies added a new and important dimension to the understanding of leadership.

Early Leader Behavior Studies

The most important early research into leader behavior took place in the late 1940s at Ohio State University and the University of Michigan, where researchers conducted studies designed to better understand behavior that contributes to effective leadership. Most behavioral studies of leadership are based on the pioneering work done in the leadership studies that were conducted at these two universities.

The studies conducted at Ohio State University identified two aspects of leader behavior that are thought to explain effective leadership at the supervisor–subordinate level. The researchers sought to answer the basic questions of how a leader's behavior has an impact on the performance of a workgroup and their satisfaction with work. Two aspects of leader behavior, labeled "consideration" and "initiating structure,"[33] were the focus of these studies. Consideration was defined as the degree to which a leader acts in a friendly and supportive manner, shows concern for subordinates, and looks out for their welfare. Initiating structure was defined as the degree to which a leader defines and structures the work to be done by the workgroup and the extent to which attention was focused on achieving objectives that were established by the leader. These dimensions were not viewed as ends of a spectrum of behavior but as two distinct and separate dimensions. Researchers hypothesized that leaders who scored high on both dimensions of leader behavior would be most effective, that is, would achieve high subordinate or workgroup performance and satisfaction. However, follow-up studies failed to support this hypothesis in all situations.[34] Reinterpretation of some of these study results eventually led to the conclusion that the combination of initiating structure behavior and consideration behavior that produces leadership effectiveness is dependent on the situation in which leadership is exercised.[35]

The studies at Ohio State University were paralleled by researchers at the University of Michigan. Based on extensive interviews of leaders and followers in a variety of organizations, Likert and his colleagues identified two distinct styles of leader behavior, "job centered" and "employee centered."[36] The leader behaviors identified are similar at both universities: job-centered behaviors at Michigan correspond to the initiating structure category that was identified at Ohio State, and employee-centered behaviors at Michigan correspond to the consideration category that was identified at Ohio State.

In the University of Michigan studies, leaders who were employee centered emphasized interpersonal relations, took a personal interest in the needs of their subordinates, and readily accepted differences among workgroup members. These leaders were considerate, supportive, and helpful with subordinates. In contrast, job-centered leaders emphasized technical or task aspects of the job, were more concerned with accomplishing the workgroup's tasks than anything else, and regarded group members as a means to this end. These leaders spent their time planning, scheduling, coordinating, and closely supervising the work of the group's members.

Initially, researchers believed that job-centered and employee-centered leader behaviors were mutually exclusive and at opposite ends of a continuum. Later, they found leaders could exhibit either set of behaviors or a combination of them. Studies that were conducted in a variety of organizations found that effective leaders, at the level of supervisor–subordinate relationships, were employee centered and focused on the needs of the workgroups they led. These studies also demonstrated that, in addition to being employee centered, effective workgroup leaders established high performance objectives for the group, but permitted the group members to participate in establishing the objectives.[37]

Fundamentally, mutual reinforcement of the results of the leader behavior studies by University of Michigan and Ohio State University researchers enhanced the credibility of the results. This research was the intellectual foundation for later theories and studies that explained effective leadership styles by identifying the optimal mix of leader behaviors to achieve effectiveness (remember that leadership style was defined as a particular combination of behaviors). Some of the most important of these later studies and associated models of leadership style are presented here.

Likert's System 4 Management Model

One important theory that seeks to explain the relative effectiveness of various leadership styles was developed by Likert.[38] As a participant in the University of Michigan leadership research program, he was influenced by findings about the relationship of job-centered and employee-centered leader behaviors to leader effectiveness. He concentrated on employee-centered behaviors because he believed that the degree to which leaders allow followers to influence their decisions is a key element in effective leadership at the level of supervisor–subordinate relationships.

Figure 15.3 is a schematic of Likert's model showing the ways in which leaders relate to followers on the dimension of follower participation in decisions about their work. He called this model System 4 management because it contains four distinct systems (or styles) of interpersonal relationships.

Likert considers participative or democratic leadership styles to be superior to autocratic styles in terms of their contribution to productivity and follower satisfaction. In his model, System 1 lead-

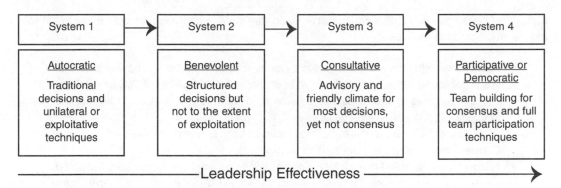

Figure 15.3.   Likert's System 4 management model. (Adapted from Likert, Rensis. *Past and Future Perspectives on System 4*, 3–5, 9. Ann Arbor, MI: Rensis Likert Associates.)

are are autocratic and rely on authority granted by the organization as the basis for their leadership. Such leaders show little confidence or trust in their followers. System 2 leaders are more benevolent toward followers, although they use authoritarian approaches. System 3 leaders consult with followers about decisions but stop short of permitting full participation in decisions.

System 4 leaders give followers full participation in decision making. They endorse open channels of communication and other behaviors that ensure a high level of reciprocal influence between leader and followers. They also use group methods of supervision rather than close, one-to-one supervision. System 4 leaders show high levels of confidence and trust in followers in most matters. The main benefit of System 4 leadership, according to Likert, is that it encourages the acceptance of decisions and commitment to them, both of which contribute directly to productivity and to follower satisfaction.[39]

Likert's views on the benefits of participatory leadership stimulated substantial research on its effects. Miller and Monge provide a good meta-analytical review of this research for readers who want more detail.[40] It is sufficient to say that the participative leader style provides a number of benefits and advantages to HSOs/HSs, including the following:

- Participation encourages followers to identify with the HSO/HS more closely. This enhances motivation, especially in such citizenship behaviors as cooperation, protecting fellow employees and organizational property, avoiding waste, and, in general, going beyond the call of duty. If people have some voice in their jobs, they tend to be more enthusiastic in performing them.
- Participation can be a means to overcome resistance to change. Those who participate in decisions that cause change will understand the changes and will be less likely to resist.
- Participation enhances personal growth and development of those who work in a HSO/HS. By participating in decisions, followers gain experience and become more proficient in decision making.
- Participation enables a wider range of ideas and experiences to be brought to bear on a problem. Often, followers are familiar with a situation and can solve related problems better than can the leaders.
- Participation increases organizational flexibility because followers gain a wider range of experience about the job situation.

In general, HSO/HS managers rely heavily on participative decision making.[41] For example, the participative leadership style is critical to the success of continuous quality improvement (CQI) activities. A HSO's/HS's professional employees will not tolerate being left out of CQI decisions that are related to patient care. A participative leadership style is facilitated by adherence to the following managerial guidelines:

- People who are permitted to participate in decisions should have expertise and skill in the matters under consideration, or expertise must be developed before they can participate effectively.
- The consequences of error should be considered. When others participate, do they raise or lower the risk that mistakes will be made?
- Avoid abrupt shifts in leadership style. Steps should be taken to prepare followers for any change in style to reduce skepticism and build confidence.
- Followers must be willing to participate. Some people do not want the responsibility that participation entails. Furthermore, the climate of respect between manager/leader and subordinates/followers should be such that followers are not afraid to voice opinions.
- A participative style of leadership must be used with sincerity and integrity. Specifically, the manager/leader who frequently asks subordinates/followers to participate but who has no intention of following their recommendations will soon lose support and acceptance. Once mistrust arises, followers may cease viewing the participative style as legitimate. This does not mean that leaders can never reject followers' recommendations; however, if recommendations are rejected, then the manager must explain the decision.

Blake and McCanse's Leadership Grid

Another model depicting the variety of leadership styles was developed by Blake and Mouton[42] and revised by Blake and McCanse.[43] This model uses two variables of leadership orientation: "concern for people" and "concern for production." The people orientation focuses on enhancing the leader's relationships with followers or on the relationships among followers. The production orientation focuses on tasks and objectives in relation to work. These two orientations are used to create the leadership grid shown in Figure 15.4, a significant tool to help people understand variation in leadership styles.

By plotting various locations on the grid created by the concern for people and concern for production axes, Blake and McCanse identified five distinct leadership styles. Table 15.4 contains the typical characteristics of these five styles. Blake and McCanse took the position that the 9,9, or team management, leadership style universally is the most effective leader orientation, just as Likert had done regarding System 4 management.

The position that there is "one best way" to lead workgroups troubled other researchers to whom it seemed that what worked best in one situation did not necessarily work best in another. It should be noted that the importance of situational variation is clear cut only in hindsight. Researchers pursuing both trait theories and behavioral theories began with the premise that it was important to discover the set of traits that was characteristic of successful leaders or the behavioral style of leadership that explained leadership effectiveness. It was only after much work that researchers realized that there was neither one set of traits that invariably explained leader success nor a specific behavioral style that always worked best. Only then could it be understood that situational variables were needed to more fully explain leadership effectiveness. One model of leadership that bridges the pure behavioral theories and the emerging situational theories deserves special recognition for this important role and is considered next.

Tannenbaum and Schmidt's Continuum of Leader Behavior

Tannenbaum and Schmidt[44] developed a model of leader behavior in which styles of leadership were arrayed as a continuum ranging from autocratic to laissez-faire, as depicted in Figure 15.5.

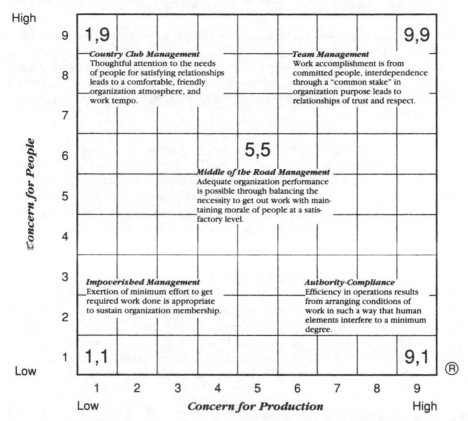

High

9 **1,9**   **9,9**

Country Club Management   *Team Management*
Thoughtful attention to the needs   Work accomplishment is from
8 of people for satisfying relationships   committed people, interdependence
leads to a comfortable, friendly   through a "common stake" in
organization atmosphere, and   organization purpose leads to
work tempo.   relationships of trust and respect.

7

6   **5,5**

Middle of the Road Management
Adequate organization performance
5   is possible through balancing the
necessity to get out work with main-
taining morale of people at a satis-
4   factory level.

3 *Impoverished Management*   *Authority-Compliance*
Exertion of minimum effort to get   Efficiency in operations results
required work done is appropriate   from arranging conditions of
to sustain organization membership.   work in such a way that human
2   elements interfere to a minimum
degree.

1 **1,1**   **9,1**   ®
Low

    1   2   3   4   5   6   7   8   9
  Low   *Concern for Production*   **High**

(left axis, vertical) *Concern for People*

Figure 15.4.   The leadership grid. (Blake, Robert R., and Anne Adams McCanse. *Leadership Dilemmas—Grid Solutions,* 29. Houston: Gulf Publishing Company, 1991. Copyright 1991 by Scientific Methods, Inc. Reproduced by permission of the owners.)

Their model has polar ends with varying decision-making authority shared by managers/leaders and subordinates/followers and shows alternative ways for managers/leaders to approach decision making, depending on how much participation they want from subordinates/followers. Styles on the left are more authoritarian, and those on the right are more participative.

Tannenbaum and Schmidt provide descriptions of the various styles presented in Figure 15.5, indicating the degree of decision-making authority that is held by the manager. Below these descriptions are commonly used labels that describe the basic leader behavior being exhibited along the continuum, from autocratic to laissez-faire.

- Autocratic leaders (Style 1 in the model) are those who make and announce decisions. The role of subordinates is to carry out orders without an opportunity to materially alter decisions already made by the manager/leader.
- Consultative leaders "sell" decisions to their followers by carefully explaining the rationale for the decision and its effect on followers—Style 2 in the model. Style 3 leaders permit slightly more subordinate involvement—the leader presents decisions to followers but invites questions so that understanding and acceptance are enhanced.
- Participative leaders may present tentative decisions that will be changed if subordinates can make a convincing case for a different decision—Style 4 in the model. Style 5 leaders present a problem to subordinates, seek their advice and suggestions, and then make the decision. This

leadership style makes greater use of participation and less use of authority than autocratic and consultative styles.

- Democratic leaders (Style 6) define the limits of the situation and problem to be solved and permit followers to make the decision.
- Laissez-faire leaders (Style 7) permit followers to function within limits set by the leader's superior. The manager/leader does not interfere and participates in decision making with no more influence than other members of the group. Leader and follower roles are indistinguishable in this style.

Tannenbaum and Schmidt describe possible leadership styles much as do Likert, Blake and McCanse, and others who searched for the best style. Here the similarity ends, however, and the importance of their contribution to understanding leadership effectiveness results from their conclusion that the best style depends on the particular situation. In their view the choice of a style should be based on forces that are internal to the manager/leader (e.g., value system, confidence in subordinates/followers, tolerance for ambiguity and uncertainty), forces within subordinates/ followers (e.g., expectations, need for independence, ability, knowledge, experience), and forces in the situation (e.g., type of organization, nature of the problem to be solved or the work to be done, time pressure). No single leadership style is correct all of the time. Leaders/managers must adapt and change to fit the situation.[45]

An autocratic style might be appropriate in an operating room because work activity must be performed precisely and immediately, perhaps under crisis conditions. However, if physicians who are autocratic in the operating room become HSO/HS managers, a very different style may be necessary, especially when other professionals are supervised. Subordinates' characteristics—training, education, motivation, and experience—influence the leader's authority style. If subordinates are

TABLE 15.4.   THE MAJOR LEADERSHIP GRID STYLES

Style	Description
1,1 Impoverished Management	This type of leadership is often referred to as laissez-faire leadership. Leaders in this position have little concern for people or productivity, avoid taking sides, and stay out of conflicts. They do just enough to get by.
1,9 Country Club Management	Managers in this position have great concern for people and little concern for production. They try to avoid conflicts and concentrate on being well liked. To them the task is less important than good interpersonal relations. Their goal is to keep people happy. (This is a soft Theory X approach and not a sound human relations approach.)
9,1 Authority–Compliance	Managers in this position have great concern for production and little concern for people. They desire tight control in order to get tasks done efficiently. They consider creativity and human relations to be unnecessary.
5,5 Middle of the Road Management	Leaders in this position have medium concern for people and production. They attempt to balance their concern for both people and production but are not committed to either.
9,9 Team Management	This style of leadership is considered to be ideal. Such managers have great concern for both people and production. They work to motivate employees to reach their highest levels of accomplishment. They are flexible and responsive to change, and they understand the need to change.

Adapted from Blake, Robert R., and Anne Adams McCanse. *Leadership Dilemmas—Grid Solutions*, 29. Houston: Gulf Publishing Company, 1991; reprinted by permission.

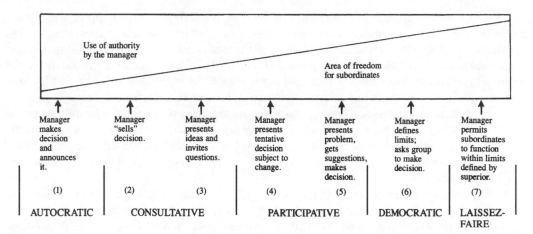

Figure 15.5. Continuum of leader decision-making authority. (Tannenbaum, Robert, and Warren H. Schmidt. "How To Choose a Leadership Pattern." HARVARD BUSINESS REVIEW 51 (May-June 1973), 162-168, reprinted by permission. Copyright 1973 by the President and Fellows of Harvard College; all rights reserved.)

skilled professionals, the manager may readily seek their opinions and use a consultative or participative style. Similarly, the work being performed can determine which style is appropriate. If it is routine, clerical, and must have a specific sequence flow, then the manager may be more consultative than democratic in determining what, how, and when work will be performed. However, if work is creative and flexible and other departments do not rely on timely completion, the manager may use a participative or democratic style. Certainly, the business office manager will use a different leader authority style than would the manager of a medical research department.

The Tannenbaum and Schmidt model identifies a set of leadership styles, but it couples this with the concept that certain factors dictate choosing one style over the others. In this way the model provides a bridge between early trait and behavioral theories of leadership and more sophisticated situational or contingency theories of leadership, described in the next section.

SITUATIONAL OR CONTINGENCY THEORIES OF LEADERSHIP

By the early 1960s it had been determined that traits or particular behaviors could not fully explain leader success or leadership effectiveness, and it was found that behavior that was appropriate in one circumstance produced failure in others. Researchers then turned to incorporating situational factors, or contingencies, into leadership models. From among the many resulting models or theories that seek to explain how situational variables help determine the relative effectiveness of leadership styles, four of the most important are described: the Fiedler model, Hershey and Blanchard's situational model, the Vroom-Yetton participation model, and path–goal theory.

Fiedler's Contingency Theory

Fiedler's research focused on specifying situations in which certain leader styles would be particularly effective.[46] The phrase *contingency theory* refers to Fiedler's hypothesis that effective leadership is contingent on whether the elements in a particular leadership situation fit the style of the leader. He sought to identify leader styles that fit particular situations and that could be used to improve leader effectiveness by: 1) changing leader styles to fit situations, 2) selecting leaders whose styles fit particular situations, 3) moving leaders in organizations to situations that fit their styles, or 4) changing situations to better fit leader styles.

Fiedler's leadership model is complex, but the underlying theory can be appreciated by understanding the leader styles that he examined and the way in which he assessed situations. He was interested in whether a leader was more task or relations motivated or oriented. The task-motivated leader is more concerned about task success and task-related problems. Such leaders are motivated primarily by achieving task objectives and are not motivated to establish good relationships with followers unless the work is going well and there are no serious task-related problems.

In contrast, the relations-motivated leader is more concerned with good leader–follower relations, is motivated to have close interpersonal relationships, and will act in a considerate, supportive manner when relationships need to be improved. For such leaders, the achievement of task objectives is important only if the primary affiliation motive is adequately satisfied by good personal relationships with followers.

Fiedler considered the two orientations to be polar. He measured these two orientations in leaders by using the least preferred co-worker (LPC) score. The LPC questionnaire asked leaders to think of the present or past co-worker with whom they least liked to work. The LPC questionnaire has a number of attribute sets, such as pleasant–unpleasant, with an 8-point rating scale. The LPC score is the sum of the ratings for the attribute sets. A high score reflects a leader who is primarily relations motivated; a low score reflects a leader who is primarily task motivated. In effect, the score reflects the degree of regard leaders hold for their least preferred co-worker. Leaders with low LPC scores, interpreted as reflecting disregard for the least preferred co-worker, are considered to have a task-motivated leadership style. Leaders with high LPC scores, interpreted as reflecting favorable assessments of the co-worker they least prefer, are considered to have a relations-motivated leadership style.

According to Fiedler's theory, the relationship between a leader's LPC score and leadership effectiveness depends on a complex situational variable that he called situational favorability. Favorability is determined by three aspects of a situation:

1. Leader–follower relations, which can be good or poor (good leader–follower relations imply that the leader is able to obtain compliance with minimum effort, whereas poor relations imply compliance with reservation and reluctance, if at all)
2. Task structure, which can be structured (specific instructions and standard procedures provide for task completion) or unstructured (the task has only vague and inexplicit procedures without step-by-step guidelines)
3. Leader position power, which can be strong or weak, and refers to the extent to which the leader has authority (including reward, coercive, and legitimate power) to evaluate the performance of followers (workgroup members) and reward or punish them

Figure 15.6 shows how the style of effective leadership varies with the situation and illustrates information relevant to the Fiedler contingency theory of leadership. The bottom portion shows combinations of the three situational favorability aspects: leader–follower relations (good–poor), the task structure (structured–unstructured), and the leader's position power (strong–weak). The result is eight unique combinations that Fiedler calls octants.

Octant 1 shows good leader–follower relations, a structured task, and a leader with strong position power. Octant 8 shows poor leader–follower relations, an unstructured task, and a leader with weak position power. An intermediate octant, Octant 4, shows good leader–follower relations, an unstructured task, and a leader with weak position power. Octant 1 is most favorable and Octant 8 least favorable in Fiedler's schema to measure the favorability of particular situations for leaders.

With a way to measure certain leader traits and to scale the favorability of the situations faced by leaders, Fiedler tested the relationships. His results, in the upper portion of Figure 15.6, show that relationship-motivated leaders (high LPC scores) do well (relative to task-motivated leaders)

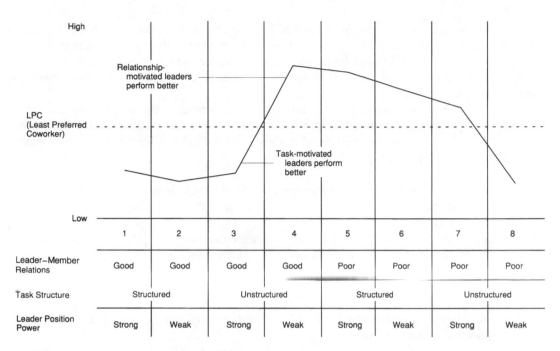

Figure 15.6. How the style of effective leadership varies with the situation. (From Fiedler, Fred E., and Martin E. Chemers. *Leadership and Effective Management,* 80. Glenview, IL: Scott, Foresman, 1974; reprinted by permission.)

in moderately favorable situations. Conversely, task-motivated leaders (low LPC scores) do relatively well in situations that are either very favorable or very unfavorable.

Fiedler[47] attributes success of relationship-motivated leaders in situations with intermediate favorability to the leader's nondirective, permissive approach; a more directive approach could cause anxiety in followers, conflict in the workgroup, and lack of cooperation. He attributes success of the task-motivated leader in very favorable situations to the fact that, because the leader has power, formal backing, and a well-structured task, followers are ready to be directed in their tasks. He attributes success of the task-motivated leader in very unfavorable situations to the fact that, without the leader's active and aggressive intervention and control, the group might fall apart.

Complex theories typically have ample room for criticism, and Fiedler's is no exception.[48] Most research, however, supports the model.[49] Fiedler's research is especially important because it represents the first comprehensive attempt to incorporate situational variables directly into a leadership theory. This new dimension was refined in many subsequent studies. Furthermore, his model has considerable utility in management practice, especially in suggesting to managers the importance of systematically assessing their position power, leader–follower relations, and task structures in relationship to their leadership styles and, in turn, how this affects their effectiveness as leaders.

Hershey and Blanchard's Situational Leadership Model

Hershey and Blanchard[50] developed a leadership model that attempts to explain effective leadership as interplay among 1) the leader's relationship behavior, defined as the extent to which leaders maintain personal relationships with followers through open communication and by exhibiting supportive behaviors and actions toward them; 2) the leader's task behavior, which is the extent to which leaders organize and define roles of followers and guide and direct them; and 3) the followers' readiness level, which Hershey and Blanchard define as readiness to perform a task or function or to pursue an objective. This model focuses on followers as the key situational variable, specifically their readiness to perform. The central premise is that the most effective leadership style is determined by the readiness level of the people whom the leader is attempting to influence.[51] Even though their model focuses on only one situational variable, Hershey and Blanchard call it the situational leadership model.

Appreciation of the situational leadership model requires an understanding of how it incorporates leadership styles, as well as a concept called "follower readiness." Hershey and Blanchard assume that the relative presence (high–low) of task and relationship behaviors can be used to identify four distinct leadership styles (S1–S4) as follows:

- S1, or Telling (high task–low relationship)—the leader makes the decision. The leader defines roles and tells followers what, how, when, and where to do various tasks, emphasizing directive behavior.
- S2, or Selling (high task–high relationship)—the leader makes the decision and then explains it to followers. The leader provides both directive behavior and supportive behavior.
- S3, or Participating (low task–high relationship)—the leader and followers share decision making. The main role of the leader is to encourage and assist followers in contributing to sound decisions.
- S4, or Delegating (low task–low relationship)—the followers make the decision. The leader provides little direction or support.

Follower readiness in the situational leadership model refers to a person's readiness to perform a particular task. Readiness is assessed by two factors, ability and willingness. Ability refers to knowledge, experience, and skill that an individual or group possesses. Willingness is the extent to which an individual or group has the motivation, confidence, and commitment that is needed to accomplish a specific task.[52]

Hershey and Blanchard use the ability of followers and their willingness (divided into commitment/motivation and confidence) to develop a four-stage continuum of follower readiness, from low (R1) to high (R4):

- R1—Followers are unable and unwilling to take responsibility for performing a task (i.e., they do not possess the necessary ability and they feel insecure about taking responsibility).
- R2—Followers are unable but willing to do job tasks (i.e., they do not possess the necessary ability, but they are motivated and feel confident if the leader provides guidance).
- R3—Followers are able but unwilling to do what the leader wants (i.e., they possess the necessary ability, but they feel insecure about doing what the leader wants).
- R4—Followers are able and willing to do what is asked of them (i.e., they possess the necessary ability, and they feel confident about their ability to do what is asked of them).

In the Hershey and Blanchard model of situational leadership the four leadership styles (Telling, Selling, Participating, and Delegating) are best used with specific levels of follower readiness (see Figure 15.7). Leadership effectiveness results when the leader's style matches followers' readiness. The model suggests that, as followers reach high levels of readiness (R4), the leader responds by decreasing task *and* relationship behaviors. At R4, the leader need do very little because followers are willing and able to take responsibility. At the lowest level of follower readiness (R1), followers need explicit direction because they are unable and unwilling to take responsibility. At moderate or intermediate levels (R2 and R3), different leadership styles are needed. At R2, at which the followers are unable but willing, the leader must exhibit high levels of task and relationship behaviors. High-level task behavior compensates for followers' lack of ability, and high-level rela-

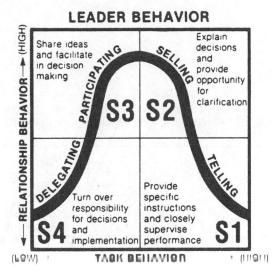

Figure 15.7. The situational leadership model. (Adapted from Hershey, Paul, and Kenneth H. Blanchard. *Management of Organizational Behavior,* 7th ed., 186. Upper Saddle River, NJ: Prentice-Hall, 1996; reprinted by permission.)

tionship behavior may help them to psychologically "buy into" the leader's wishes. At R3, at which followers are able but unwilling or insecure, a leadership style that incorporates high levels of relationship behaviors may help overcome unwillingness or insecurity among followers.

Although there has been almost no research confirming the relationships theorized in the situational leadership model, it is widely used by managers because it is intuitively appealing.[53] The model clearly illustrates certain aspects of leader behavior that are quite important. Leaders must be concerned about the readiness of their followers to be led, and they must recognize that the level of readiness can be affected by leaders' actions. This model also provides a useful reminder to leaders that it is important to treat followers as individuals, with real differences among them. Moreover, the model reminds leaders to treat the same follower differently over time, as the follower changes in terms of readiness.[54]

Vroom and Yetton's Model

Vroom and Yetton[55] developed a model based on how leader behavior affects the quality of decision making in problem-solving situations. This model was presented in Figure 7.8 with a focus on problem-solving styles. It is presented in Figure 15.8 with a focus on leadership styles. As originally developed, the model features a decision tree and questions to guide users. A revised version developed by Vroom and Jago[56] replaces decision rules with mathematical functions and is so complex that microcomputer software is needed to fully understand it. The earlier version is presented here to explain the model's logic and use.

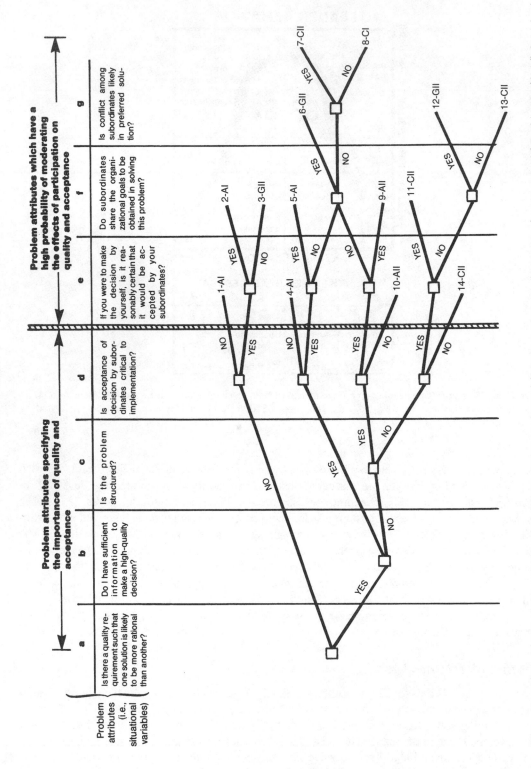

Figure 15.8.   The Vroom-Yetton problem-solving and decision-making style model. (Vroom, Victor H. "A New Look at Managerial Decision Making." *Organizational Dynamics* 1 (Spring 1973): 70; reprinted by permission. Copyright 1973. American Management Association, New York. All rights reserved.)

The Vroom-Yetton model assumes that five leader behaviors can be used: two types of autocratic decision making (AI and AII), two types of consultation (CI and CII), and one behavior that represents joint decision making by leader and followers as a group (GII). These leader behaviors are defined as follows:

AI. You (the leader) solve the problem or make the decision yourself, using information available to you at the time.

AII. You obtain the necessary information from your subordinates, then decide the solution to the problem yourself. You may or may not tell your subordinates what the problem is in getting the information from them. The role that is played by your subordinates in making the decision is clearly one of providing necessary information to you rather than generating or evaluating alternative solutions.

CI. You share the problem with the relevant subordinates individually, getting their ideas and suggestions, without bringing them together as a group. Then you make the decision, which may or may not reflect your subordinates' influence.

CII. You share the problem with your subordinates as a group, obtaining their collective ideas and suggestions. Then you make the decision, which may or may not reflect your subordinates' influence.

GII. You share the problem with your subordinates as a group. Together you generate and evaluate alternatives and attempt to reach agreement (consensus) on a solution. Your role is much like that of a chairperson. You do not try to influence the group to adopt "your" solution, and you are willing to accept and implement any solution that has the support of the entire group.[57]

Figure 15.8 illustrates the model's seven contingency questions (*a–g* across the top of the figure) and a decision tree to direct a leader to situation-dependent prescribed leader behavior. The leader chooses from among five behaviors (AI, AII, CI, CII, or GII) and is guided by answering questions in the *a*-through-*g* sequence.

The Vroom-Yetton model is in general supported by the work of several researchers.[58] Beyond its wide acceptance, the model has great practical value to managers. It demonstrates that managers can effectively vary their leadership styles to fit particular situations, a point that is critical to accepting the situational approach to leadership.[59]

House and Mitchell's Path–Goal Model

Like the other situational or contingency approaches described previously, the path–goal model of leadership predicts the leadership behaviors that will be most effective in particular situations. This model is the most generally useful situational model of leadership effectiveness. The path–goal model is named for its focus on how leaders influence followers' perceptions of their work goals and the paths that they follow to attain these goals. House, in the original conception of this model, posited that the leader's function is to increase the personal payoffs to followers for attaining their work-related goals, and to make the path to these payoffs smoother.[60] As House and Mitchell, who helped develop the theory further, note

According to this theory, leaders are effective because of their impact on subordinates' motivation, ability to perform effectively, and satisfaction. The theory is called path-goal because its major concern is how the leader influences the subordinates' perceptions of their work goals, personal goals and paths to goal attainment. The theory suggests that a leader's behavior is mo-

tivating or satisfying to the degree that the behavior increases subordinate goal attainment and clarifies the paths to these goals.[61]

This leadership theory relies on the Ohio State University and University of Michigan leadership studies previously discussed and on the expectancy theory of motivation described more fully in Chapter 16. In the expectancy theory, expectancy is the perceived probability that effort will affect performance, instrumentality is the perceived probability that performance will lead to outcomes, and the value attached to an outcome by a person is its valence. The expectancy model of motivation focuses on describing the relationships among expectancy, instrumentality, and valence. The path–goal model of leadership focuses on factors that affect expectancy, instrumentality, and valence. Leaders can increase the valences that are associated with work-goal attainment, the instrumentalities of work-goal attainment, and the expectancy that effort will result in work-goal attainment.

Path–goal theory is a situational theory because its basic premise is that the effect of leader behavior on follower performance and satisfaction depends on the situation, specifically including follower characteristics and task characteristics. Restated, different leader behaviors are best for different situations. According to House and Mitchell,[62] there are four categories of leader behavior; each is best suited to a particular situation:

> *Directive leadership:* The leader tells followers what to do and how to do it, requires that they follow rules and procedures, and schedules and coordinates the work. This leader behavior is similar to initiating structure in the Ohio State University studies.
>
> *Supportive leadership:* The leader is friendly and approachable and exhibits consideration for the status, well-being, and needs of followers. This leader behavior is similar to consideration in the Ohio State University studies.
>
> *Participative leadership:* The leader consults with followers, asks for opinions and suggestions, and considers them.
>
> *Achievement-oriented leadership:* The leader establishes challenging goals for followers, expects excellent performance, and exhibits confidence that they will meet expectations.

House believes that effective leaders use all four styles of leader behavior as the situation dictates, and match styles to situations, which can vary along two dimensions. One dimension is the nature of the people who are being led. Followers may or may not have the ability to do the job. They differ, too, as to the perceived degree of control that they have over their work. They may feel controlling or controlled. The second dimension is the nature of the task, which may be routine or new and ambiguous.

Figure 15.9 illustrates how the four leader behavior styles are matched to subordinate characteristics and the nature of the task to produce leader effectiveness. Leaders face different situations, and the path–goal model suggests that effective leaders diagnose the situation and match behavior to it. For example, directive leadership could be used when followers are not well trained and the work that they are doing is partly routine and partly ambiguous. Supportive or participative leadership might be most appropriate if followers are doing routine work and have experience doing it. Achievement-oriented leadership is most effective if followers are doing innovative and ambiguous work and have a high level of knowledge and skill that are related to the work.

The path–goal model of leadership suggests that the functions of effective leaders include 1) making the path to achieving work goals easier by providing coaching and direction when needed, 2) removing or minimizing frustrating barriers that interfere with followers' abilities to achieve work goals, and 3) increasing payoffs for followers when they achieve work-related goals.

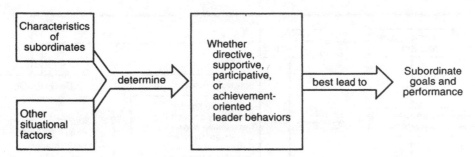

Figure 15.9. Path–goal model of leadership. (From Longest, Beaufort B., Jr. *Health Professionals in Management,* 236. Stamford, CT: Appleton & Lange, 1996; reprinted by permission.)

House and Mitchell intend the path–goal theory to be a partial explanation of the motivational effects of leader behavior, and they do not include all relevant variables. Despite limited validation of much of the path–goal theory, it is a useful construct because it merges leadership and motivation theories. It also provides a pragmatic framework that is valuable to managers who are trying to match their leader behavior to subordinate/follower characteristics and task characteristics.

Furthermore, path–goal theory is useful because it illustrates substitutes for leadership. For example, if being an effective leader means clarifying the path to a follower's goal, then the existence of clear organizational rules and plans that may also clarify the path is a partial substitute for leadership. Substitutes for leader behaviors are anything that clarifies role expectations, motivates employees, or satisfies employees. This phenomenon is significant for HSOs/HSs because much of their workforce is highly professional and possesses a body of knowledge with standard practices to guide their work. To the extent that these factors reduce the need for leaders to guide the work, they are a substitute for leadership.

TOWARD AN INTEGRATIVE FRAMEWORK FOR LEADERSHIP

This chapter describes three approaches to understanding leadership: traits and skills, leadership behavior, and situational or contingency theories of leadership. These different approaches to leadership effectiveness and success have yielded numerous models, each seeking to explain the phenomenon of leadership effectiveness. Individually, however, none of the theories or models does so fully. Levey suggested, "We will probably never be able to achieve a truly elegant and rigorous general theory of leadership."[63] This pessimistic view reflects the complexity and the tremendous variety of variables that are involved in the leadership process. It is possible, however, to integrate the different theories to more fully illustrate the processes and interactions involved in leadership effectiveness, whether in transactional or transformational leadership.

One of the most comprehensive leadership models or frameworks was developed by Yukl.[64] Figure 15.10, an adaptation of his integrative model, illustrates that leadership contributes to the end results of individual, workgroup, and organizational performance. It shows that these results are partly determined by complex interactions among leader traits and skills, personal power of the leader, leader behavior, and situational variables. These variables are mediated or influenced by intervening variables, the presence of which reminds us that leadership is not the only determinant of individual, group, or organizational performance. Indeed, outcomes in HSOs/HSs are influenced by many factors.

The model oversimplifies very complex relationships, but it does illustrate the most important interactions among key variables in effective leadership. For example, it shows that leader behavior is influenced by leader traits and skills, power, and situational variables and characteristics or cir-

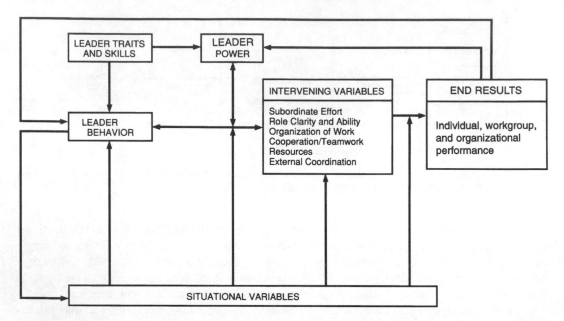

Figure 15.10. Integrating conceptual framework of leadership. (Adapted from Yukl, Gary A. *Leadership in Organizations,* 3rd ed., 269. Englewood Cliffs, NJ: Prentice-Hall, 1989. Copyright 1989, Prentice-Hall, Inc.)

cumstances, as well as by information about intervening variables and results of previous leadership behaviors. In this sense, leader behaviors are simultaneously dependent and independent variables that influence and are influenced by intervening variables and results. The model also shows how a leader's personal power is determined by results, the leader's traits and skills, and situational variables such as the type and extent of authority that is possessed by the leader as a result of organizational position.

This integrative model is useful for understanding both transactional and transformational leadership. In supervisor–subordinate interfaces that characterize so much of the work of middle- and first-level managers in HSOs/HSs, the model suggests that transactional leadership effectiveness results from interactions among multiple variables. These variables include leader traits and skills, leader power, and leader behavior selected to fit situational variables, all of which are mediated or influenced by intervening variables such as follower efforts and abilities, the HSO's/HS's design features, and the availability of resources.

The exercise of leadership is even more complex at the senior level of management.[65] However, everything the model suggests about the complexity of leadership at the leader–follower interface holds true for transformational leadership that is exerted at the top levels of HSOs/HSs. Effective leadership here also requires blending traits, skills, power, and behaviors to meet the situation. However, as noted earlier, senior-level managers who attempt to be transformational leaders face several additional and unique issues. They must establish shared values and principles as a common part of the HSO's/HS's culture. They must affirm the mission of the organization or system, and resolve conflicts among competing but legitimate organizational objectives. They must take steps to legitimize the HSO's/HS's claims for support from internal and external stakeholders and develop and pursue strategies that ensure organizational autonomy, stability, and self-control in an increasingly turbulent environment.[66]

Successful leaders at the HSO/HS level must not only develop a clear vision for the HSO/HS but also must use their legitimate, expert, and referent power to ensure that important stakeholders understand this vision. Leaders who effectively articulate and communicate their visions will have a distinct advantage in having them considered. Conger observed that

> *While we have learned a great deal about the necessity of strategic vision and effective leadership, we have overlooked the critical link between vision and the leader's ability to powerfully communicate its essence. In the future, leaders will not only have to be effective strategists, but rhetoricians who can energize through the words they choose. The era of managing by dictate is ending and is being replaced by an era of managing [leading] by inspiration. Foremost among the new leadership skills demanded of this era will be the ability to craft and articulate a message that is highly motivational.*[67]

Effective leadership is highly dependent on effective motivation and communication. These management topics are the focus in Chapters 16 and 17, respectively. These two chapters are crucial to a complete understanding of effective leadership.

SUMMARY

Leadership is a process of one individual influencing another individual or group to achieve particular objectives. Leaders help determine what is to be accomplished by workgroups, organizations, or systems and influence others to contribute to accomplishing these purposes. Power and influence in relation to leadership, including the sources of a leader's power, are covered. Transactional and transformational leadership are described in this chapter.

Various approaches to the study of leadership are described. Theories of leadership that are based on leader traits and skills, including intelligence, personality, and ability, are reviewed. The important research into leader behavior conducted at Ohio State University and the University of Michigan is presented as a prelude to reviewing the main behavioral models of leadership: Likert's System 4 model, Blake and McCanse's managerial grid, and Tannenbaum and Schmidt's continuum of leader behavior. Four key situational theories of leadership are reviewed: Fiedler's contingency theory, Hershey and Blanchard's situational leadership model, the Vroom-Yetton model, and the House-Mitchell path–goal theory of leadership.

How these theories of leadership build on one another, differ, and are complementary is described. Particular emphasis is given to situational theories of leadership, and an integrative model of leadership is used to link current information about leadership at the level of supervisor–subordinate relationships and at the level of HSO/HS leadership, at which senior-level managers are increasingly expected to be transformational leaders.

DISCUSSION QUESTIONS

1. Distinguish between the roles of leaders at the level of supervisor–subordinate relationships and those at the level of HSO/HS leadership (discuss transactional and transformational leadership in your response).
2. Define and model leadership.
3. Describe the relationship between influence and leadership and between power and influence.
4. Compare the three basic conceptual approaches to the study of leadership (traits and skills, leader behavior, and situational or contingency approaches) and explain why different approaches to the study of leadership have been taken.

5. Outline key contributions to the understanding of leadership made by the leadership studies at Ohio State University and the University of Michigan.
6. Some have argued that leaders are born, not made, and that all great leaders have certain common traits. Discuss this viewpoint about leadership.
7. Briefly describe three models of leader behavior presented in this chapter.
8. Briefly describe four situational models of leadership presented in this chapter.
9. Sketch and discuss the model used in the chapter to integrate the various theories of leadership.
10. Assume that you have been invited to give a lecture on leadership effectiveness. What three key points would you emphasize?

CASE STUDY 1: CHARLOTTE COOK'S PROBLEM

Charlotte Cook is a registered nurse (RN) who has three certified nursing assistants (CNAs) (Sally, John, and Betty) reporting to her at Longview Nursing Facility. Cook is 48 years old and has worked for Stanley George, the CEO, for 10 years.

Cook is confronted with a leadership problem. Sally, who has worked for Cook for 5 years, is 40 years old, cooperative, dependable, skilled, and an excellent performer. John, who is 28, transferred from another nursing unit 2 months ago after working there for 1 year. The CEO told Cook that he was transferring John because John could not get along with his RN supervisor on that unit. The RN supervisor is 2 years younger than John and they had a personality clash. In fact, rumors circulated that John disliked his RN supervisor because she was not satisfied with either his performance or his attitude. Furthermore, the RN supervisor's predecessor and John had been very close socially, she was not demanding of John, and she often made exceptions for him. This had made the other CNAs on that unit resent John, and they had nothing to do with him. Betty is 30 years old and has worked for Cook for the year she has been at Longview. Her performance is acceptable, although she requires some direct supervision. She and Cook have a good relationship.

Four weeks ago John began complaining to Sally and Betty. He criticized Mr. George and Ms. Cook and was generally "anti-everything" about Longview and its staff, particularly the RN supervisor on his previous unit and Cook. He was uncooperative, often did his job poorly, and gossiped constantly with the patients. Cook has noticed that John always seems to be with Betty during their free time and that Betty tends to agree with him about things on the unit. Cook feels that, if the situation is ignored, matters could get worse.

Presume that CNAs are difficult to recruit and retain and that Cook does not want to discharge John, at least for the present.

QUESTIONS

1. What leadership style should Cook use with Sally? With John?
2. How should Cook approach and interact with Betty?
3. What should Cook do if John does not change?
4. Did Mr. George do the correct thing in transferring John?
5. What could Mr. George have done to remedy the situation at the time he transferred John?

CASE STUDY 2: THE PRESIDENTIAL SEARCH

Memorial Hospital is a 500-bed teaching hospital located in a thriving city. In recent years other hospitals in the area have reduced Memorial's market share. The outgoing president had been preoccupied with issues of a deteriorating physical plant and loss of professional staff to other area hospitals and systems.

The governing body formed an ad hoc search committee to find a new hospital president. The committee plans to use a national executive search firm but wants to develop a clear picture of the person who will lead the HSO back to preeminence in the city before talking with the search firm.

Mr. Adams, a hospital trustee and president of a large financial services company, is chair of the ad hoc committee. He has convened the committee to develop a list of capabilities the president should possess so that this information can be provided to the search firm.

Assume that you are a member of this committee.

QUESTIONS

1. What capabilities should the new president possess? Rank them in order.
2. Should this person be more skilled at the supervisor–subordinate interface or at organization-level leadership? How will the committee distinguish between skill at the two types of leadership?
3. Some committee members point out that the situation at Memorial is unique, therefore, finding a person who was successful at another hospital will not guarantee success at Memorial. What would be your position on this issue?

CASE STUDY 3: IS LEADERSHIP THE ISSUE?

There are 22 hospitals in a large eastern city. Each is independent of the others, except that three of the largest are affiliated with the local medical school for purposes of teaching medical students. The others range in size from 180 beds to 600 beds; about half are sponsored by religious organizations. There is one large public hospital, and three hospitals are investor owned. The others are not-for-profit community hospitals.

The state planning commission has argued for years that there are excess beds and overuse of services in the community and that this could be relieved through merger and consolidation of some of the hospitals. All of the hospitals have resisted this strategy and continue to be autonomous.

QUESTIONS

1. What role should the hospital CEOs play in addressing the question of merger or consolidation to solve the excess bed problem? Who else should play a role? Is this a "leadership" problem?
2. Assume that you are one of the hospital CEOs and that you want your institution to merge with one or more of the other hospitals. What problems do you face? How could these problems be overcome?
3. A local newspaper ran a series of articles on the issue, culminating with a harsh editorial that challenged hospital leaders to meet to discuss merger or consolidation as a way to solve the excess bed problem and reduce costs. Assume that you are one of the CEOs and that you want to convene such a meeting. How would you approach other CEOs to arrange this meeting? How might they respond? Why?

CASE STUDY 4: LEADERSHIP QUESTIONNAIRE [68]

For each of the following 10 pairs of statements, divide five points between the two according to your beliefs, perceptions of yourself, or according to which of the two statements characterizes you better. The five points may be divided between the A and B statements in any way you wish with the constraint that only whole positive integers may be used (i.e., you may not split evenly, giving 2.5 points to each). Weigh your choices between the two according to the one that better characterizes you or your beliefs.

___ 1. A. As a leader, I have a primary mission of maintaining stability.
___   B. As a leader, I have a primary mission of change.
___ 2. A. As a leader, I must cause events.
___   B. As a leader, I must facilitate events.
___ 3. A. I am concerned that my followers are rewarded equitably for their work.
___   B. I am concerned about what my followers want in life.
___ 4. A. My preference is to think long range; what might be.
___   B. My preference is to think short range; what is realistic.
___ 5. A. As a leader, I spend considerable energy in managing separate but related goals.
___   B. As a leader, I spend considerable energy in arousing hopes, expectations, and aspirations among my followers.
___ 6. A. Although not in a formal classroom sense, I believe that a significant part of my leadership is that of teacher.
___   B. I believe that a significant part of my leadership is that of facilitator.
___ 7. A. As leader, I must engage with followers at an equal level of morality.
___   B. As a leader, I must represent a higher morality.
___ 8. A. I enjoy stimulating followers to want to do more.
___   B. I enjoy rewarding followers for a job well done.
___ 9. A. Leadership should be practical.
___   B. Leadership should be inspirational.
___10. A. What power I have to influence others comes primarily from my ability to get people to identify with me and my ideas.
___   B. What power I have to influence others comes primarily from my status and position.

Scoring Key

Transformational	Transactional
Your point(s)	Your point(s)
1. B _____	1. A _____
2. A _____	2. B _____
3. B _____	3. A _____
4. A _____	4. B _____
5. B _____	5. A _____
6. A _____	6. B _____
7. B _____	7. A _____
8. A _____	8. B _____
9. B _____	9. A _____
10. A _____	10. B _____
Column totals: _____	_____

Note: The higher column total indicates that you agree more with, and see yourself as more like, either a transformational leader or a transactional leader.

CASE STUDY 5: LESSONS WHERE YOU FIND THEM[69]

A management consultant asked the group of mid-level executives he was working with to consider several facts about how geese fly and suggested an associated lesson from each fact as follows:

Fact 1: As each bird flaps its wings, it creates an uplift draft for the bird following. By flying in a "V" formation, the whole flock adds a greater flying range than if one bird flew alone.

Lesson 1: People who share a common direction and sense of community can get where they're going quicker and more easily because they are traveling on the strength of one another.

Fact 2: Whenever a goose falls out of formation, it suddenly feels the drag and resistance of trying to fly alone and quickly gets back into formation to take advantage of the lifting power of the bird immediately in front.

Lesson 2: If we have as much sense as geese, we will stay in formation and be willing to accept help when we need it and give help when it is needed.

Fact 3: When the lead goose gets tired, it rotates back into the formation, and another goose flies in the point position.

Lesson 3: Geese instinctively share the task of leadership and do not resent the leader.

Fact 4: The geese in formation honk from behind to encourage those up front to keep up their speed.

Lesson 4: We need to make sure our honking from behind is encouraging and not something else.

Fact 5: When a goose gets sick, is wounded or is shot down, two geese drop out of formation and follow it down to earth to help and protect it. They stay with their disabled companion until it is able to fly again or dies. They then launch out on their own or with another formation or catch up with the flock.

Lesson 5: If we have as much sense as geese, we, too, will stand by one another in difficult times and help the one who has dropped out regain his place in the formation.

QUESTIONS

1. Do you think the lessons suggested by the consultant have any relevance to leadership in HSOs/HSs? If so, what is it?
2. How does the leadership behavior of geese differ from managers' leadership roles?

CASE STUDY 6: SUPERVISORY BEHAVIOR QUESTIONNAIRE[70]

Instructions: This questionnaire is part of an activity that is designed to explore supervisory behaviors. It is not a test; there are no right or wrong answers.

Think about supervisors (managers) you have known or know now, and then select the *most-effective* supervisor and the *least-effective* supervisor (*effective* is defined as being able to substantially influence the effort and performance of subordinates).

Read each of the following statements carefully. For the *most-effective* supervisor, place an X over the number that indicates how true or untrue you believe the statement to be. For the *least-effective* supervisor, place a circle around the number that indicates how true you believe the statement to be.

Most effective X
Least effective . . . . . O

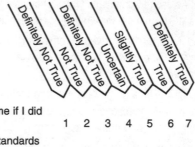

1. My supervisor would compliment me if I did outstanding work.   1   2   3   4   5   6   7

2. My supervisor maintains definite standards of performance.   1   2   3   4   5   6   7

3. My supervisor would reprimand me if my work were consistently below standards.   1   2   3   4   5   6   7

4. My supervisor defines clear goals and objectives for my job.   1   2   3   4   5   6   7

5. My supervisor would give me special recognition if my work performance were especially good.   1   2   3   4   5   6   7

6. My supervisor would "get on me" if my work were not as good as he or she thinks it should be.   1   2   3   4   5   6   7

7. My supervisor would tell me if my work were outstanding.   1   2   3   4   5   6   7

8. My supervisor establishes clear performance guidelines.   1   2   3   4   5   6   7

9. My supervisor would reprimand me if I were not making progress in my work.   1   2   3   4   5   6   7

SUPERVISORY BEHAVIOR QUESTIONNAIRE SCORING SHEET

Instructions: For each of the three scales (A, B, and C), compute a *total score* by summing the answers to the appropriate questions and then subtracting the number 12. Compute a score for both the most-effective and the least-effective supervisors.

Question Number	Most Effective	Least Effective	Question Number	Most Effective	Least Effective	Question Number	Most Effective	Least Effective
2.	+ ( )	+ ( )	1.	+ ( )	+ ( )	3.	+ ( )	+ ( )
4.	+ ( )	+ ( )	5.	+ ( )	+ ( )	6.	+ ( )	+ ( )
8.	+ ( )	+ ( )	7.	+ ( )	+ ( )	9.	+ ( )	+ ( )
Subtotal	( )	( )	Subtotal	( )	( )	Subtotal	( )	( )
	− 12	− 12		− 12	− 12		− 12	− 12
Total Score	___	___	Total Score	___	___	Total Score	___	___
	A	A		B	B		C	C

Next, on the following graph, write in a large "X" to indicate the total score for scales A, B, and C for the most effective supervisor. Use a large "O" to indicate the scores for the least-effective supervisor.

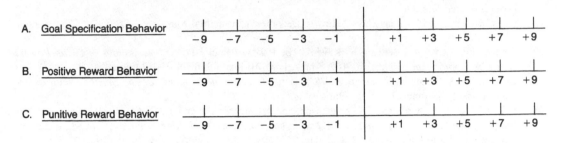

QUESTIONS

1. Describe the profile of attributes or characteristics of the most-effective supervisor reflected in the A, B, and C scales above.
2. Describe the profile of attributes or characteristics of the least-effective supervisor reflected in the A, B, and C scales above.

NOTES

1. Goleman, Daniel. *Emotional Intelligence,* 149. New York: Bantam Books, 1995.
2. Connors, Edward J. "Reflections on Leadership in Health Care." *Hospital & Health Services Administration* 35 (Fall 1990): 309–320; also see the readings in Part III, "Leadership and Competitive Advantage." In *Contemporary Issues in Leadership,* edited by William E. Rosenbach and Robert L. Taylor, 121–194. Boulder, CO: Westview Press, 1998.
3. Burns, James M. *Leadership.* New York: Harper & Row, 1978.
4. Pointer, Dennis D., and Julianne P. Sanchez. "Leadership: A Framework for Thinking and Acting." In *Essentials of Health Care Management,* edited by Stephen M. Shortell and Arnold D. Kaluzny, 99–132. Albany, NY: Delmar Publishers, 1997.
5. Bass, Bernard M. *Leadership and Performance Beyond Expectations.* New York: Academic Press, 1985; Longest, Beaufort B., Jr., Kurt Darr, and Jonathon S. Rakich. "Organizational Leadership in Hospitals." *Hospital Topics* 71 (1993): 11–15.
6. Tichy, Noel M., and Mary A. Devanna. *The Transformational Leader.* New York: John Wiley & Sons, 1990.
7. McLaughlin, Charles P., and Arnold D. Kaluzny. "Total Quality Management in Health: Making It Work." *Health Care Management Review* 15 (Summer 1990): 7–14.
8. Deal, Terrence E. "Healthcare Executives as Symbolic Leaders." *Healthcare Executive* 5 (March/April 1990): 24–27; Nutt, Paul C. "How Top Managers in Health Organizations Set Directions That Guide Decision Making." *Hospital & Health Services Administration* 36 (Spring 1991): 57–75.
9. Zuckerman, Howard S. "Redefining the Role of the CEO: Challenges and Conflicts." *Hospital & Health Services Administration* 34 (Spring 1989): 25–38.
10. Cartwright, Dorwin, and Alvin Zander. *Group Dynamics: Research and Theory.* New York: Harper & Row, 1968.
11. Fiedler, Fred E., and Martin E. Chemers. *Leadership and Effective Management,* 4. Glenview, IL: Scott, Foresman, 1974.
12. Holt, David H. *Management: Principles and Practices,* 2nd ed., 450. Englewood Cliffs, NJ: Prentice-Hall, 1990.
13. Blake, Robert R., and Jane S. Mouton. *The Versatile Manager: A Grid Profile.* Homewood, IL: Irwin, 1981.

14. Jago, Arthur G. "Leadership: Perspectives in Theory and Research." *Management Science* 28 (March 1982): 315–336.

15. Bass, Bernard M. *Bass and Stogdill's Handbook of Leadership,* 20. New York: The Free Press, 1990.

16. Yukl, Gary A. *Leadership in Organizations,* 4th ed., 5. Upper Saddle River, NJ: Prentice-Hall, 1998.

17. Bass, *Bass and Stogdill's,* 19–20.

18. Keys, Bernard, and Thomas Case. "How to Become an Influential Manager." *Executive* 4 (November 1990): 38.

19. French, John R.P., and Bertram H. Raven. "The Bases of Social Power." In *Studies of Social Power,* edited by Dorwin Cartwright, 150–167. Ann Arbor, MI: Institute for Social Research, 1959.

20. Conger, Jay A., Rabindra Kanungo, and Associates. *Charismatic Leadership: The Elusive Factor in Organizations.* San Francisco: Jossey-Bass, 1988.

21. Morlock, Laura L., Constance A. Nathanson, and Jeffrey A. Alexander. "Authority, Power, and Influence." In *Health Care Management: A Text in Organization Theory and Behavior,* 2nd ed., edited by Stephen M. Shortell and Arnold D. Kaluzny, 268. New York: John Wiley & Sons, 1988.

22. Mintzberg, Henry. *Power in and Around Organizations,* 26. Englewood Cliffs, NJ: Prentice-Hall, 1983.

23. Yukl, *Leadership in Organizations,* 178–179.

24. Mintzberg, *Power in and Around Organizations.*

25. Kirkpatrick, Shelly A., and Edwin A. Locke. "Leadership: Do Traits Matter?" *Executive* 5 (May 1991): 59.

26. Stogdill, Ralph M. "Personal Factors Associated with Leadership." *Journal of Psychology* 25 (January 1948): 64.

27. Stogdill, Ralph M. *Handbook of Leadership: A Survey of the Literature,* 81. New York: The Free Press, 1974.

28. Kirkpatrick and Locke, "Leadership," 48.

29. Goleman, *Emotional Intelligence;* Goleman, Daniel. "What Makes a Leader?" *Harvard Business Review* 76 (November–December 1998): 93–102.

30. Goleman, "What Makes," 94.

31. Pointer and Sanchez, "Leadership," 109.

32. Van Fleet, David D., and Gary A. Yukl. "A Century of Leadership Research." In *Contemporary Issues in Leadership,* 2nd ed., edited by William E. Rosenbach and Robert L. Taylor, 67. Boulder, CO: Westview Press, 1989.

33. Stogdill, Ralph M., and Alvin E. Coons, Eds. *Leadership Behavior: Its Description and Measurement* (Research Monograph No. 88). Columbus: Bureau of Business Research, Ohio State University, 1957.

34. Fleishman, Edwin A. "Twenty Years of Consideration and Structure." In *Current Developments in the Study of Leadership,* edited by Edwin A. Fleishman and James G. Hunt, 1–37. Carbondale: Southern Illinois University Press, 1973.

35. Gibson, James L., John M. Ivancevich, and James H. Donnelly, Jr. *Organizations: Behavior, Structure, Processes,* 7th ed. Homewood, IL: Irwin, 1991.

36. Likert, Rensis. *New Patterns of Management.* New York: McGraw-Hill, 1961.

37. Katz, Daniel, and Robert L. Kahn. "Some Recent Findings in Human Relations Research in Industry." In *Readings in Social Psychology,* edited by Guy E. Swanson, Theodore M. Newcomb, and Eugene L. Hartley, 650–665. New York: Holt, Rinehart & Winston, 1952; Katz, Daniel, and Robert L. Kahn. *The Social Psychology of Organizations.* New York: Wiley, 1966, 1978.

38. Likert, Rensis. *Past and Future Perspectives on System 4.* Ann Arbor, MI: Rensis Likert Associates, 1977; Likert, Rensis. "An Integrating Principle and an Overview." In *The Great Writings in Management and Organizational Behavior,* edited by Louis E. Boone and Donald D. Bowen, 216–238. New York: Random House, 1987.

39. Likert, *Past and Future Perspectives.*

40. Miller, Katherine I., and Peter R. Monge. "Participation, Satisfaction, and Productivity: A Meta-analytic Review." *Academy of Management Journal* 29 (December 1986): 727–753.

41. Nutt, Paul C. "How Top Managers in Health Organizations Set Directions That Guide Decision Making." *Hospital & Health Services Administration* 36 (Spring 1991): 57–75.

42. Blake, Robert R., and Jane S. Mouton. *The Managerial Grid III: The Key to Leadership Excellence.* Houston: Gulf Publishing, 1985.

43. Blake, Robert R., and Anne Adams McCanse. *Leadership Dilemmas—Grid Solutions.* Houston: Gulf Publishing Company, 1991.

44. Tannenbaum, Robert, and Warren H. Schmidt. "How to Choose a Leadership Pattern." *Harvard Business Review* 51 (May–June 1973): 162–180.

45. Tannenbaum and Schmidt, "How to Choose."

46. Fiedler, Fred E. "A Contingency Model of Leadership Effectiveness." In *Advances in Experimental Social Psychology,* edited by Leonard Berkowitz, 149–190. New York: Academic Press, 1964; Fiedler, Fred E. *A Theory of Leadership Effectiveness.* New York: McGraw-Hill, 1967.

47. Fiedler, *A Theory of Leadership Effectiveness.*

48. Schriesheim, C.A., and Steven Kerr. "Theories and Measures of Leadership: A Critical Appraisal of Current and Future Directions." In *Leadership: The Cutting Edge,* edited by James G. Hunt and Lars L. Larson, 9–45. Carbondale: Southern Illinois University Press, 1977.

49. Peters, Lawrence H., Darnell D. Hartke, and John T. Pohlman. "Fiedler's Contingency Theory of Leadership: An Application of the Meta-analysis Procedures of Schmidt and Hunter." *Psychological Bulletin* 97 (March 1985): 274–285.

50. Hershey, Paul, and Kenneth H. Blanchard. *Management of Organizational Behavior,* 7th ed. Upper Saddle River, NJ: Prentice-Hall, 1996.

51. Hershey and Blanchard, *Management of Organizational Behavior.*

52. Hershey and Blanchard, *Management of Organizational Behavior.*

53. Yukl, *Leadership in Organizations.*

54. Bateman, Thomas S., and Carl P. Zeithaml. *Management: Function and Strategy,* 2nd ed. Homewood, IL: Irwin, 1992.

55. Vroom, Victor H., and Phillip W. Yetton. *Leadership and Decision Making.* Pittsburgh: University of Pittsburgh Press, 1976.

56. Vroom, Victor H., and Arthur G. Jago. *The New Leadership.* Englewood Cliffs, NJ: Prentice-Hall, 1988.

57. Vroom and Yetton, *Leadership and Decision Making,* 13.

58. Yukl, *Leadership in Organizations.*

59. Hershey and Blanchard, *Management of Organizational Behavior.*

60. House, Robert J. "A Path-Goal Theory of Leader Effectiveness." *Administrative Science Quarterly* 16 (September 1971): 321–339.

61. House, Robert J., and Terence R. Mitchell. "Path-Goal Theory of Leadership." *Journal of Contemporary Business* 3 (Autumn 1974): 84.

62. House and Mitchell, "Path-Goal Theory of Leadership."

63. Levey, Samuel. "The Leadership Mystique." *Hospital & Health Services Administration* 35 (Winter 1990): 479.

64. Yukl, *Leadership in Organizations.*

65. Avolio, Brice J., and Bernard M. Bass. "Transformational Leadership, Charisma and Beyond." In *Emerging Leadership Vistas,* edited by James G. Hunt, B. Rajaram Baliga, H. Peter Dachler, and Chester A. Schriesheim, 29–49. Lexington, MA: Lexington Books, 1988.

66. Burns, Lawton R., and Selwyn W. Becker. "Leadership and Managership." In *Health Care Management: A Text in Organization Theory and Behavior,* edited by Stephen M. Shortell and Arnold D. Kaluzny, 2nd ed., 142–186. New York: John Wiley & Sons, 1988.

67. Conger, Jay A. "Inspiring Others: The Language of Leadership." *Executive* 5 (February 1991): 31.

68. Adapted from Wall, Jim. *Bosses,* 129–133, 142–150, 256–260. New York: The Free Press, 1988; reprinted by permission.

69. Adapted from an anonymous letter to Ann Landers appearing in *The Washington Post,* August 1, 1998, E9; reprinted by permission.

70. From Sims, Henry P., Jr. "Patterns of Effective Supervisory Behavior." In *The 1981 Annual Handbook for Group Facilitators,* edited by John E. Jones and J. William Pfeiffer, 10th ed., 95–99. San Diego, CA: University Associates, 1981; reprinted by permission.

SELECTED BIBLIOGRAPHY

Bass, Bernard M. *Bass and Stogdill's Handbook of Leadership.* New York: The Free Press, 1990.

Bateman, Thomas S., and Carl P. Zeithaml. *Management: Function and Strategy,* 2nd ed. Homewood, IL: Irwin, 1992.

Conger, Jay A. "Inspiring Others: The Language of Leadership." *Executive* 5 (February 1991): 31–45.

Connors, Edward J. "Reflections on Leadership in Health Care." *Hospital & Health Services Administration* 35 (Fall 1990): 309–320.

Deal, Terrence E. "Healthcare Executives as Symbolic Leaders." *Healthcare Executive* 5 (March/April 1990): 24–27.

Fiedler, Fred E. "A Contingency Model of Leadership Effectiveness." In *Advances in Experimental Social Psychology*, edited by Leonard Berkowitz, 149–190. New York: Academic Press, 1964.

Fiedler, Fred E. *A Theory of Leadership Effectiveness*. New York: McGraw-Hill, 1967.

Fiedler, Fred E., and Martin E. Chemers. *Leadership and Effective Management*. Glenview, IL: Scott, Foresman, 1974.

Goleman, Daniel. *Emotional Intelligence*. New York: Bantam Books, 1995.

Goleman, Daniel. "What Makes a Leader?" *Harvard Business Review* 76 (November–December 1998): 93–102.

Hershey, Paul, and Kenneth H. Blanchard. *Management of Organizational Behavior,* 7th ed. Upper Saddle River, NJ: Prentice-Hall, 1996.

House, Robert J. "A Path-Goal Theory of Leader Effectiveness." *Administrative Science Quarterly* 16 (September 1971): 321–339.

House, Robert J., and Terence R. Mitchell. "Path-Goal Theory of Leadership." *Journal of Contemporary Business* 3 (Autumn 1974): 81–97.

Keys, Bernard, and Thomas Case. "How to Become an Influential Manager." *Executive* 4 (November 1990): 38–51.

Kirkpatrick, Shelly A., and Edwin A. Locke. "Leadership: Do Traits Matter?" *Executive* 5 (May 1991): 48–60.

Levey, Samuel. "The Leadership Mystique." *Hospital & Health Services Administration* 35 (Winter 1990): 479–480.

Likert, Rensis. *Past and Future Perspectives on System 4*. Ann Arbor, MI: Rensis Likert Associates, 1977.

Longest, Beaufort B., Jr. *Health Professionals in Management*. Stamford, CT: Appleton & Lange, 1996.

Longest, Beaufort B., Jr., Kurt Darr, and Jonathon S. Rakich. "Organizational Leadership in Hospitals." *Hospital Topics* 71 (1993): 11–15.

McLaughlin, Charles P., and Arnold D. Kaluzny. "Total Quality Management in Health: Making It Work." *Health Care Management Review* 15 (Summer 1990): 7–14.

Mintzberg, Henry. *Power In and Around Organizations*. Englewood Cliffs, NJ: Prentice-Hall, 1983.

Nutt, Paul C. "How Top Managers in Health Organizations Set Directions That Guide Decision Making." *Hospital & Health Services Administration* 36 (Spring 1991): 57–75.

Pointer, Dennis D., and Julianne P. Sanchez. "Leadership: A Framework for Thinking and Acting." In *Essentials of Health Care Management,* edited by Stephen M. Shortell and Arnold D. Kaluzny, 99–132. Albany, NY: Delmar Publishers, 1997.

Rosenbach, William E., and Robert L. Taylor, Eds. *Contemporary Issues in Leadership*. Boulder, CO: Westview Press, 1998.

Stogdill, Ralph M. "Personal Factors Associated with Leadership." *Journal of Psychology* 25 (January 1948): 35–71.

Stogdill, Ralph M. *Handbook of Leadership: A Survey of the Literature*. New York: The Free Press, 1974.

Stogdill, Ralph M., and Alvin E. Coons, Eds. *Leadership Behavior: Its Description and Measurement* (Research Monograph No. 88). Columbus: Bureau of Business Research, Ohio State University, 1957.

Tichy, Noel M., and Mary A. Devanna. *The Transformational Leader*. New York: John Wiley & Sons, 1990.

Van Fleet, David D., and Gary A. Yukl. "A Century of Leadership Research." In *Contemporary Issues in Leadership,* 2nd ed., edited by William E. Rosenbach and Robert L. Taylor, 65–90. Boulder, CO: Westview Press, 1989.

Vroom, Victor H., and Arthur G. Jago. *The New Leadership.* Englewood Cliffs, NJ: Prentice-Hall, 1988.

Vroom, Victor H., and Phillip W. Yetton. *Leadership and Decision Making.* Pittsburgh: University of Pittsburgh Press, 1976.

Yukl, Gary A. *Leadership in Organizations,* 4th ed. Upper Saddle River, NJ: Prentice-Hall, 1998.

16 Motivation

The good news is that the area of motivation has garnered more attention than any other topic in the study of individual behavior. Thus, there is an extraordinarily large body of work on which to draw. The bad news is that even with this abundance of theorizing, empirical studies, and practical experience, we are still somewhat unclear and tentative as to how best to go about motivating our health care work force.[1]

Managers in health services organizations and health systems (HSOs/HSs) may be adept at planning and organizing human and physical resources, but, unless they can motivate people to work toward achieving organizational objectives, acceptable levels of organizational performance will not be attained. This chapter and the others in Part III deal with the important managerial function of directing. To be effective in directing, managers must get other people to do what needs to be done.[2] Critical to the manager's ability to inspire others to make significant contributions to the HSO's/HS's objectives are answers to questions such as: Why do people act as they do? How does one person obtain the cooperation of others? The answers to such questions involve many variables, but a key element is motivation. As the opening quotation for this chapter suggests, much is known about motivation from studies in many settings, a great deal of which is generalizable.

To fully appreciate motivation as a crucial concept in effectively managing HSOs/HSs is to view motivation as a means to understanding the ways in which people behave in these organizations and systems.[3] The behaviors of people employed in HSOs/HSs are important because these organizations and systems benefit from several specific types of behaviors from their workers. First, however, people must be motivated to enter the HSO/HS workforce. Then they must be motivated to continue their employment or contractual relationship with the HSO/HS, and they must be motivated to attend work regularly, punctually, and predictably. These behaviors are motivated behaviors. People also must be motivated to perform their work at acceptable levels, in terms of both the quantity and quality of work. Finally, the HSO/HS needs certain good citizenship behaviors from its workforce.[4] People can be motivated to exhibit such behaviors as cooperation, altruism, protecting fellow workers and the HSO's/HS's property, and generally going above and beyond the call of duty. The presence of good citizenship behaviors invariably makes the manager's job easier and contributes directly to organizational performance.[5]

Managers in HSOs/HSs must motivate all of these behaviors. The list suggests the extensive and pervasive part that motivation plays in management success. In concept, motivation is at once simple and complex. Motivation is simple because it is now known that behavior is goal directed and is induced by increasingly well-understood forces, some of which are internal to the individual, others external. Motivation is complex because mechanisms that induce behavior include very complicated and individualized needs, wants, and desires that are shaped, affected, and satisfied in different ways for different people. This chapter explores the concept of motivation by examining the major theories and models that have been developed to explain human motivation in the workplace. However, it is first necessary to define motivation.

MOTIVATION DEFINED AND MODELED

Why does one person work harder than another? Why is one more cooperative than another? In part, these differences occur because people have varying needs and act differently to satisfy them. People's needs are, in effect, deficiencies that cause them to undertake a pattern of behavior intended to fill the deficiency. For example, at a very simple level human needs are physiological. A hungry person needs food, is driven by hunger, and is motivated to satisfy the need or, stated another way, to overcome the deficiency. Other needs are more complex; some are psychological (e.g., the need for self-esteem) and some are sociological (e.g., the need for social interaction). In short, unmet needs trigger and energize human behaviors. This fact is the basis for a model of the motivation process.

As shown in Figure 16.1, the motivation process is cyclical. It begins with an unmet need and cycles through the individual's assessment of the results of efforts to satisfy the need, which may confirm the continuation of an unmet need or permit identification of a new need. In between, the

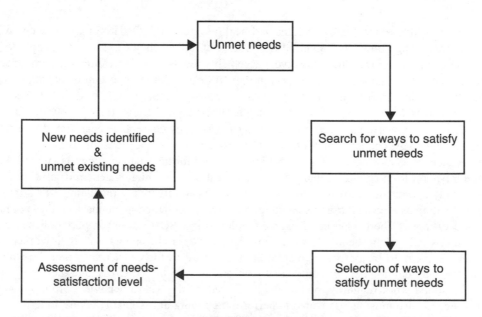

Figure 16.1.   The motivation process. (From Longest, Beaufort B., Jr. *Health Professionals in Management,* 247. Stamford, CT: Appleton & Lange, 1996; reprinted by permission.)

person searches for ways to satisfy the unmet need and chooses a course of action, which means exhibiting goal-directed behavior intended to satisfy the unmet need.

The model is oversimplified, but it contains the essential elements of the process by which human motivation occurs. Motivation is driven by unsatisfied needs and results in goal-directed behaviors in the person experiencing it, although it also can be influenced by factors that are external to the individual. This model also suggests a definition of motivation: an internal drive that stimulates behavior that is intended to satisfy an unmet need. Most contemporary definitions include these terms or express the same concept. For example, motivation has been defined as "a goal-directed, internal drive which is always aimed at satisfying needs"[6] or as "a state of feeling or thinking in which one is energized or aroused to perform a task or engage in a particular behavior."[7] It is important to note that the direction, intensity, and duration of this state can be influenced by factors outside the individual experiencing the state, including the ability of managers and HSOs/HSs to contribute to or impede the satisfaction of the individual's needs. Thus it may be concluded that motivation 1) is driven by unsatisfied or unmet needs, 2) results in goal-directed behaviors, and 3) is influenced by factors that may be internal or external to the individual experiencing motivation.

Motivation is a key determinant of individual performance in work situations and is of obvious importance in achieving a HSO's/HS's organizational objectives. However, motivation alone does not fully explain performance. It is only one of many variables affecting performance. Intelligence, physical and mental abilities, previous experiences, and the nature of the work environment also determine performance. Good equipment and pleasant surroundings facilitate high levels of performance. The variables affecting performance can be conceptualized as follows:

$$\text{Performance} = f(\text{ability/talent/experience} \times \text{environment} \times \text{motivation})$$

This equation shows that performance is a function of or results from an interaction of variables, an interaction that goes beyond being merely additive.[8] Without motivation, no amount of ability or talent, and no environmental conditions, can produce acceptable performance. However, motivation alone will not result in a satisfactory level of performance.

Unfortunately, managers vary widely in their effective use of knowledge about human motivation, in part because of the different views they hold about the basic nature of people in work situations. In the 1960s Douglas McGregor postulated two opposing views held by managers on human nature in workplaces: Theory X, the negative view, and the positive view, Theory Y.[9] The central tenet of McGregor's argument is that managers' views of human beings are based on assumptions that they make about human nature, and their behaviors toward people, including efforts to motivate them, are largely influenced by these assumptions.

In McGregor's Theory X conceptualization, some managers view people in the workplace in such essentially negative ways as assuming that they

- Inherently dislike work and try to avoid it when possible
- Must be coerced and controlled to get them to put forth adequate effort toward achieving organizational objectives
- Prefer being closely directed, leaving responsibility to others

In contrast, he argues in Theory Y that other managers view people in the workplace in much more positive ways, assuming

- Work is as natural for people as play or rest, and people do not inherently dislike work.
- People will exercise self-direction and self-control in pursuing objectives to which they are committed.

- Commitment to objectives is a function of the rewards associated with their achievement.
- People, under proper conditions, learn not only to accept but to seek responsibility.
- The capacity to exercise a relatively high degree of imagination, ingenuity, and creativity in the solution of organizational problems is widely, not narrowly, distributed in the workforce.

Managers' attitudes about people and the assumptions that they make about human nature and people's approach to work shapes how managers motivate employees. In fact, all contemporary motivation theories integrate in one way or another McGregor's observation of the importance of managers' attitudes about people in determining their approach to motivation.

The wide variation in the ability of managers to apply effectively what is known about human motivation also results, in part, from the fact that there is neither an undisputed theory about motivation nor a comprehensive perspective on how managers effect it in the workplace.[10] Instead, as the opening quote for this chapter points out, many competing theories have been posited to explain motivation. These theories are examined in the following sections.

MOTIVATION THEORIES

Because human motivation is complex and not fully understood, a confusing diversity of theories has been developed to explain it. There is disagreement as to how motivation occurs in people, as well as about its causes. Meanwhile, knowledge about motivation remains piecemeal and many theorists vie to explain it. One implication is that students of management must integrate many theories to gain understanding of what is known about motivation. The remaining sections of this chapter are organized around the theories of motivation, with the final section integrating what is known from these theories. The most important motivation theories can be divided into two broad categories: content theories and process theories.

Content theories focus on the internal needs and desires that initiate, sustain, and eventually terminate behavior. They focus on *what* motivates people. In contrast, process theories seek to explain *how* behavior is initiated, sustained, and terminated. Combined, these theories define variables that explain motivated behavior and show how these variables interact and influence each other to produce certain behavior patterns. Table 16.1 summarizes examples from a managerial perspective of the most important theoretical developments in both categories. It serves as an outline for the discussion of content and process theories of motivation that follow.

CONTENT THEORIES

The process of motivation shown in Figure 16.1 begins with a need deficiency—an unfulfilled need. Content theorists seek to determine how managers motivate people by studying their needs (e.g., what motivates them, what energizes their behavior). These theories of motivation focus on identifying human needs and helping people understand the things and behaviors that can satisfy them. Perhaps the most widely recognized content theory of motivation—and certainly one of the most important and enduring—was developed by Abraham Maslow.

Maslow's Hierarchy of Needs

Maslow, a psychologist, formulated a theory of motivation that stressed two fundamental premises.[11] First, human beings are wanting beings whose needs depend on what they already have. In Maslow's view, only needs not yet satisfied influence behavior; an adequately fulfilled need is not a motivator. Second, people's needs are arranged in a hierarchy. Once a need is fulfilled, another emerges and demands fulfillment. Maslow's needs theory stressed the idea that, within the hierar-

TABLE **16.1.** MANAGERIAL PERSPECTIVE OF CONTENT AND PROCESS THEORIES OF MOTIVATION

Theoretical base	Theoretical explanation	Founders of the theories	Managerial application
Content	Focuses on factors within person that energize, direct, sustain, and stop behavior; factors can only be inferred	Maslow—five-level needs hierarchy Alderfer—three-level hierarchy (ERG) Herzberg—two major factors called hygiene, motivators McClelland—three learned needs acquired from society: achievement, affiliation, and power	Managers need to be aware of differences in needs, desires, and goals because each individual is unique in many ways
Process	Describes, explains, and analyzes how behavior is energized, directed, sustained, and stopped	Vroom—an expectancy theory of choices Adams—equity theory based on comparisons individuals make Locke—goal-setting theory that conscious goals and intentions are determinants of behavior Skinner—reinforcement theory concerned with learning that occurs as consequence of behavior	Managers need to understand process of motivation and how individuals make choices based on preferences, rewards, and accomplishments

Adapted from Gibson, James L., John M. Ivancevich, and James H. Donnelly, Jr. *Organizations: Behavior, Structure, Processes*, 8th ed., 149. Homewood, IL: Irwin, 1994.

chy, "higher" needs become dominant only after "lower" needs are satisfied. Figure 16.2 illustrates Maslow's needs hierarchy, with examples of each category of need that could be fulfilled in a HSO/HS.

From lowest to highest order, the five categories of needs identified by Maslow begin with basic physiological needs, such as air, water, food, shelter, and sex, which are necessary for survival. People can satisfy many of these needs through the resources that their paychecks purchase. Once survival needs are met, attention is turned to ensuring continued survival by protecting oneself against physical harm and deprivation. People seek to meet their safety and security needs. They concern themselves about job security. Health insurance and other benefits that are provided by employers also help people meet these needs. The third level of needs is for social activity, which relates to people's social and gregarious nature, and includes such things as the need for belonging, friendship, affection, and love. The ability to have friendships at work and to engage in social activity in the workplace helps satisfy these needs. It is important to note that these third-level needs are something of a breaking point in the hierarchy because the needs move away from the physical or quasi-physical needs of the first two levels. This level reflects people's needs for association or companionship, belonging to groups, and giving and receiving friendship and affection.

The fourth level, ego needs, includes two different types of needs: the need for a positive self-image and for self-respect, and the need for recognition and respect from others. Examples of ego needs are the need for independence, achievement, recognition from others, self-esteem, and status. Opportunities for advancement within HSOs/HSs can help people fulfill these needs. The fifth level and top of the hierarchy of needs developed by Maslow is self-actualization needs. These needs include realizing one's potential for continued growth and development; in effect, they represent the need to become everything a person is capable of being. Self-actualization needs are evidenced in

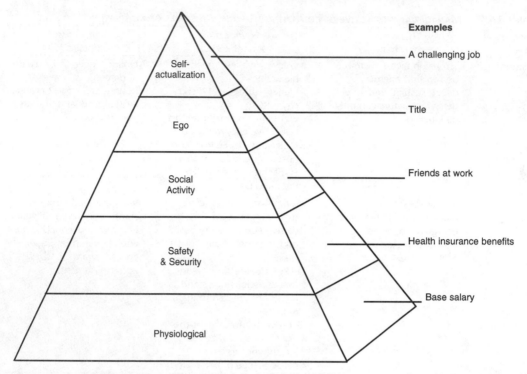

Figure 16.2.   Maslow's needs hierarchy. (From Longest, Beaufort B., Jr. *Health Professionals in Management*, 251. Stamford, CT: Appleton & Lange, 1996; reprinted by permission.)

people by their need to be creative and to have opportunities for self-expression and self-fulfillment. A challenging job is a primary means for satisfying such needs in contemporary society.

Probably because of its great intuitive appeal, as well as the ease with which most people can understand it, Maslow's theory has been widely adopted. However, it is only a theory. Maslow offered no significant empirical substantiation. In a remarkable bit of candor he once wrote of his concern that his theory was "being swallowed whole by all sorts of enthusiastic people, who really should be a little more tentative. . . ."[12]

Numerous studies have failed to validate the theory exactly as Maslow specified it, although these studies have found that, in general, people do have numerous needs and that they seek to fulfill them.[13] In this sense, Maslow's work contributes important insight into the nature of motivation and especially how need deficiencies influence actions to fill these needs. This is consistent with the motivation process model in Figure 16.1. Most important, Maslow's theory provided a conceptual framework that was used to build and test more sophisticated theories about needs and how they affect human behavior.

Alderfer's ERG Theory

Building on Maslow's theoretical base, an improved theory was developed by Clayton Alderfer, who agreed with Maslow that each individual's needs are arranged in a hierarchy.[14] However, in Alderfer's view the hierarchy of needs is more accurately conceptualized as having only three distinct categories, not five as Maslow had hypothesized. The name of this theory, ERG, is derived from the first letter of the three types of needs that Alderfer posited. Existence needs include material and physical needs—needs that can be satisfied by such things as air, water, money, and working conditions. Relatedness needs include all needs that involve other people—needs that are satisfied by meaningful social and interpersonal relationships. Growth needs, the third type of needs in Alderfer's scheme, include all needs satisfied by an individual through creative or productive contributions.

Alderfer's ERG theory is obviously similar to Maslow's hierarchy of needs. Alderfer's existence needs are similar to Maslow's physiological and safety needs, his relatedness needs are similar to Maslow's affection and social activity category, and his growth needs are similar to the esteem and self-realization needs that were identified by Maslow. The theories differ, however, in an important aspect: the manner in which needs predominate in influencing behavior.

Maslow theorized that unfulfilled lower-level needs are predominant and that the next-higher level of need is not activated until the predominant (unmet lower level) need is satisfied. He called this the satisfaction-progression process. In contrast, Alderfer argued that his three categories of needs form a hierarchy only in the sense of increasing abstractness or of decreasing concreteness: As an individual moves from existence to relatedness to growth needs, the means to satisfy the needs become less and less concrete. In Alderfer's theory, people focus first on needs that are satisfied in relatively concrete ways; then they focus on needs that are satisfied more abstractly. This is similar to Maslow's idea of satisfaction-progression. However, Alderfer proposed that a frustration regression process also is present in determining which category of needs predominates at any time. By this he meant that people who are frustrated in their efforts to satisfy their growth needs may regress and focus on satisfying more concrete relatedness or even more concrete existence needs. In Alderfer's view, the coexistence of the satisfaction-progression and the frustration-regression processes leads to a cycling among categories of needs.

To clarify Alderfer's concept of cycling, consider the following case:

Jennifer Smith, a young registered nurse, is a single parent of two children. Although she finds the social interactions with co-workers rewarding, she is concerned about the security of her position and her pay. She is an excellent nurse who enjoys her work. When a vacancy occurred for the nurse manager position on her unit, she considered the opportunities this presented for professional growth and development, as well as for a higher salary, and applied for the position. Smith looked forward to the challenges she would face when promoted.

However, a more experienced nurse was promoted. Smith's disappointment showed and she became concerned about her future. Several co-workers noticed her reaction and made special efforts to ease her disappointment. They told her that other opportunities would come and that, with a little more experience, she would be promoted. The newly promoted nurse manager was sensitive to this situation and made a point of telling Smith what a valuable contribution she was making. After a few weeks, Smith returned to the level of enjoyment she obtained from her work before this episode. In terms of needs, Smith cycled from having existence and relatedness needs predominate, to the growth needs represented by the promotion, and then back to relatedness needs, all in a few weeks. In other words, she experienced a satisfaction-progression process *and* a frustration-regression process.

Another way in which Alderfer's ERG theory differs from Maslow's theory is his view that, when individuals satisfy their existence and relatedness needs, these needs become less important. The opposite is true for growth needs, however; as growth needs are satisfied, they become increasingly important. People who become more creative and productive raise their growth goals and are dissatisfied until the new goals are reached. In the case of "Jennifer Smith," this means that, when she becomes a nurse manager, she will then want to become a nursing director, and then a vice president for nursing.

An important implication of the ERG theory for managers in HSOs/HSs is that they should assume that all employees have the potential for continued growth and development. Recognition of this fact leads naturally to their assurance of "ongoing opportunities for training and development, transfer, promotion, and career planning for all employees."[15]

Herzberg's Two-Factor Theory

Frederick Herzberg, in developing another well-known content theory of motivation, took a different approach to the study of what factors motivate human behavior in the workplace.[16] He started with questions of what satisfies or dissatisfies people about their work, assuming that the answers would contribute to understanding what motivates people.

The research that led to Herzberg's model of motivation was based on interviews with 200 engineers and accountants in Pittsburgh who were asked to recall a time when they felt exceptionally good about their jobs. Other questions were intended to determine why they felt satisfied and whether these feelings affected performance, personal relationships, and well-being. Finally, the events that returned their attitudes to "normal" were identified. A second set of interviews asked the same people to describe incidents that were related to some event on the job that made them feel exceptionally negative about their jobs.

Herzberg and associates concluded that job satisfaction consisted of two separate and independent dimensions, and they postulated a "two-factor" theory of motivation. They argued that one set of factors, called satisfiers or motivators, resulted in satisfaction when they were adequate. The other factors, labeled dissatisfiers or hygiene factors, caused dissatisfaction when they were deficient. Herzberg argued that the absence of some job conditions can dissatisfy employees. However, the presence of the same conditions does not necessarily lead to a high degree of motivation. Herzberg called these conditions hygiene (or maintenance) factors because they are necessary to maintain a reasonable level of satisfaction. Managers who eliminate factors that create job dissatisfaction do not necessarily increase motivation. Many of Herzberg's hygiene factors had been thought by managers to be motivators, but actually they are more potent dissatisfiers when absent. Herzberg identified 10 hygiene or maintenance factors: organizational policy and administration, technical supervision, interpersonal relations with supervisor, interpersonal relations with peers, interpersonal relations with subordinates, salary, job security, personal life, work conditions, and status.

In Herzberg's theory, the presence of job conditions other than motivational factors (satisfiers) tends to build high levels of motivation and job satisfaction. However, the absence of these conditions does not prove to be highly dissatisfying. Herzberg identified six motivational factors or satisfiers: achievement, recognition, advancement, the work itself, the possibility of growth, and responsibility.

In the two-factor model of motivation, hygiene factors affect job dissatisfaction, and motivators affect job satisfaction. According to Herzberg, managers must improve or control hygiene factors to minimize dissatisfaction, but achieving satisfaction depends on other factors. This insight, which is the central element in the two-factor theory, made a major contribution to understanding the dynamics of job satisfaction. Earlier theories viewed job satisfaction (people's attitude toward their jobs) as unidimensional. Job satisfaction was at one end of a continuum, and job dissatisfaction was at the other. Herzberg posited that two distinct continua affect job satisfaction. One affects dissatisfaction and the other affects satisfaction. The opposite of satisfaction is not dissatisfaction—it is no satisfaction. The opposite of dissatisfaction is not satisfaction—it is no dissatisfaction. If managers are to effectively motivate people, then they must be concerned with one set of factors to minimize dissatisfaction and another to help people achieve satisfaction.

Although Herzberg's two-factor theory extended the understanding of motivation, like other theories of motivation examined in this chapter, it has limitations.[17] The most valuable contribution of the two-factor theory of motivation is that it has caused managers to think about the factors that contribute to motivation and what managers can do to enhance opportunities to achieve intrinsic satisfaction from work. Herzberg's research, in fact, provided the conceptual framework for the job enrichment movement in the United States. Job enrichment makes a job more satisfying by adding variety and responsibility.[18] In Herzberg's view, job enrichment "seeks to improve both task efficiency and human satisfaction by means of building into people's jobs, quite specifically, greater scope for personal achievement and recognition, more challenging and responsible work, and more opportunity for individual advancement and growth."[19]

Herzberg's identification of motivation factors can be very useful to managers in HSOs/HSs as they enrich jobs along five important dimensions that incorporate motivators:

1. Skill variety—By adding to the skill base needed to perform a job, the work becomes more interesting and challenging.
2. Task identity—By permitting people to complete whole, identifiable pieces of work, the work becomes more important and satisfying to people.
3. Task significance—By making clear to them that their work has relevance to organizational objectives, people gain a greater sense of achievement through its accomplishment.
4. Autonomy—By increasing their participation in decision making and permitting the exercise of independent judgment, people feel a greater sense of responsibility in their work.
5. Feedback—By increasing the amount of information that people receive about their job performance, especially when it recognizes good performance, they gain a sense of achievement, recognition, and growth when good performance is tied to advancement in the job.

McClelland's Learned Needs Theory

Another important contribution to content theory was made by David McClelland.[20] McClelland's theory, called the learned or acquired needs theory, posits that people learn their needs through life experiences; they were not born with this knowledge. This theory builds on the much earlier work of Henry Murray,[21] who theorized that people acquire an individual profile of needs by interacting with their environment. McClelland also was influenced by the work of John Atkinson.[22] Both McClelland and Atkinson suggested that people have three sets of needs: 1) the need for achievement, including the need to excel, to achieve in relation to standards, to accomplish complex tasks, and to resolve problems; 2) the need for power, including the need to control or influence how others behave and to exercise authority over others; and 3) the need for affiliation, including the need to associate with others, to form and sustain friendly and close interpersonal relationships, and to avoid conflict.

McClelland theorized that people are not born with these needs. Instead, he believed that they are learned or acquired through unique experiences as people grow and develop. For example, children learn the need to achieve because of encouragement and reinforcement of autonomy and self-reliance by adults who influence their early years. McClelland also suggested that everyone has these three sets of needs that operate simultaneously in individuals, and the intensity of these needs differs from person to person. One set of these needs predominates and affects an individual's decisions and behaviors, and that determines how people "fit" particular work situations.

For example, it has been noted that "achievers do not always make the best managers because organizations are based on diffused authority and group activities, and achievers are often uncomfortable in situations of group responsibility and control."[23] In contrast, people who are predominantly influenced by a need for power are generally better suited to be managers because they are comfortable with executive decision making and are likely to aggressively control work activities in their areas of responsibility.

People who are most heavily influenced by a need for affiliation might not make good managers because they have difficulty making decisions and taking actions that interfere with social compatibility, even when such decisions are vital to organizational effectiveness. Holt correctly observed that "few affiliators are happy or successful in line management and executive positions, where emotionally difficult decisions must often be made, such as disciplining employees, enforcing policies, and retrenching outdated technologies."[24] Nonetheless, such people are vital to HSOs/HSs because affiliators are adept at bringing together groups or individuals with diverse interests and viewpoints, coordinating interdependent tasks, and helping solve conflicts. Therefore, people with strong affiliation needs are valuable in HSOs/HSs.

People with high achievement needs might fit well in many positions in HSOs/HSs, especially those with extensive and rigorous demands for excellence. In McClelland's view certain characteristics identify people with high needs for achievement:[25] 1) clear desire for personal responsibility; 2) strong preference for quick and concrete feedback on their performance; 3) ability to derive intrinsic satisfaction from doing a job well or solving problems; and 4) tendency to set moderately difficult (in contrast to easy or difficult) performance goals. This last characteristic of high achievers surprises many managers who assume that people with high levels of need for achievement would set high goals for themselves or relish having their superiors do so. Instead, people with high achievement needs prefer goals that lie within their capabilities.

Perhaps the most important contribution of McClelland's theory of motivation in the workplace is the importance of matching particular dominant needs of people with the work situation. If this is done carefully, then people will be motivated and their individual performance, as well as overall organizational performance, will reflect this.

Managerial Implications of the Content Theories of Motivation

It is well established that human motivation originates from the needs of people and their search to satisfy them. The common thread running through each of the four content theories of motivation is their focus on needs that motivate human behavior. Figure 16.3 compares the needs identified in each of the content theories that have been examined. Each theory defines human needs differently, but all of them agree that managers help motivate people, at least in part, by helping them identify and meet their needs in the workplace.

The synopsis of each content theory that is contained in Table 16.2 compares key points of the theories. None is a complete model of human motivation, and in fact together they do not fully explain human motivation. It is not sufficient to understand what motivates people; managers must also understand the processes by which behavior is initiated, directed, sustained, and terminated. A discussion of several process motivation theories developed by other researchers follows in the next section, but first it is important to understand some of the implications of the content theories of motivation for HSO/HS practicing managers.

The most important value of the content theories is their contributions to managers' abilities to help people understand their needs and to find ways to satisfy them within the workplace. These are extraordinarily complex tasks in view of the fact that each person has a unique and constantly changing set of needs. Managers can help the people whom they manage to identify and meet their needs by empathizing with them. Combining empathy with effective two-way communication about needs and the potential to satisfy them within the context of the workplace results in progress toward identifying and fulfilling needs. Effective managers use many approaches in their efforts to enhance motivation by helping people fulfill their needs. Among the more common approaches are adjustments in leadership and communication styles, modification of economic and noneconomic

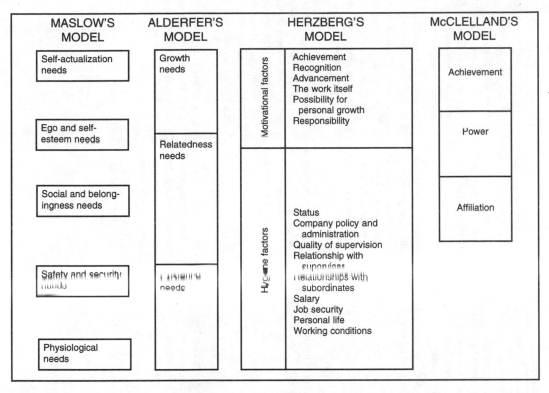

Figure 16.3. A comparison of the needs identified in the content theories of motivation. (From D'Aunno, Thomas A., and Myron D. Fottler. "Motivating People." In *Essentials of Health Care Management,* edited by Stephen M. Shortell and Arnold D. Kaluzny, 80. Albany, NY: Delmar Publishers, Inc., 1997; reprinted by permission.)

rewards in the workplace, reassignment of people to situations in which their needs can be better fulfilled by the nature of the work, and providing different levels of participation in work-related decisions to reflect different levels of need for such participation among people.

The content theories of motivation, with their singular focus on motivational factors—on *what* motivates behavior—provide many useful insights for managers. Other models are needed to provide insight into the process of motivation, to explain the mechanisms through which motivation occurs.

PROCESS THEORIES

Process theorists focus on how individuals' expectations and preferences for outcomes that are associated with or resulting from their performance actually influence performance. An important element in the process theories of motivation examined here is that of people as decision makers who weigh the personal advantages and disadvantages of their behavior. Table 16.1 summarizes the major models of processes by which motivation occurs. Vroom's expectancy theory, Adams's equity theory, Locke's goal-setting theory, and Skinner's reinforcement theory describe *how* motivation occurs in human beings.

Vroom's Expectancy Theory

In the early 1960s, Vroom, like the content theorists who preceded him, theorized that not only are people driven by their needs but they also make choices about what they will and will not do to ful-

Content motivation theories	Assumptions made	How motivation is measured	Practical application value	Problems and limitations
Maslow's needs hierarchy	Individuals attempt to satisfy basic needs before directing behavior toward higher-order needs.	Maslow, as a clinical psychologist, used his patients in asking questions and listening to answers. Organizational researchers have relied on self-report scales.	Makes sense to managers and gives many a feeling of knowing how motivation works for their employees	Does not address issue of individual differences, has received limited research support, and fails to caution about dynamic nature of needs—needs change.
Alderfer's ERG theory	Individuals who fail to satisfy growth needs become frustrated, regress, and refocus attention on lower-order needs.	Self-report scales are used to assess 3 needs categories.	Calls attention to what happens when and if needs satisfaction does not occur; frustrations can be a major reason performance levels are not attained or sustained.	Not enough research conducted; available research is self-report in nature, which raises the issue of measurement's quality; another issue is whether individuals really have only 3 needs areas.
Herzberg's two-factor theory	Only some job features and characteristics can result in motivation; some of the characteristics that managers have focused on may result in a comfortable work setting but do not motivate employees.	Asks employees in interviews to describe critical job incidents	Talks in terms that managers understand; identifies motivators that managers can develop, fine-tune, and use	Assumes that every worker is similar in needs and preferences; fails to meet scientific measurement standards; has not been updated to reflect changes in society with regard to job security and pay needs
McClelland's learned needs	Needs of a person are learned from society; training and education can enhance and influence a person's needs strength.	Thematic Apperception Test (TAT), a projective technique that encourages respondents to reveal their needs	If a person's needs can be assessed, then management can intervene through training to develop needs that are compatible with organizational goals.	Interpreting TAT is difficult; effect that training has on changing needs has not been tested sufficiently

From Gibson, James L., John M. Ivancevich, and James H. Donnelly, Jr. *Organizations: Behavior, Structure, Processes,* 8th ed., 163. Homewood, IL: Irwin, 1994; reprinted by permission.

fill their needs based on three conditions: 1) the person must believe that effort to perform at a particular level will make the desired performance or behavior more likely, 2) the desired performance or behavior must lead to some concrete outcome or reward, and 3) the person must value the outcome.[26] Figure 16.4 shows the three central components and the relationships in the expectancy theory model.

Expectancy is the probability that individuals perceive that their efforts will lead to a desired level of performance. The person must believe that effort will cause something to happen; if it is believed that more effort will lead to improved performance, expectancy will be high. If, in a different situation, the same person believes that more effort will not improve performance, the expectancy that effort will lead to performance will be low. An example is a person with low job-related aptitude or skills; no matter how much effort this person exerts, it is unlikely that performance will improve. Thus expectancy will be low.

Instrumentality is the probability perceived by individuals that their performance will lead to desired outcomes or rewards. If a person believes that better performance will be rewarded, then the instrumentality of performance to reward will be high. Conversely, if the person believes that improved performance will not be rewarded, then the instrumentality of improved performance will be low.

Outcomes are listed only once in Figure 16.4, but they play two important roles in the expectancy theory. "Level of performance" (in the center of Figure 16.4) actually represents an outcome of the "individual effort to perform." Vroom calls this a first-order outcome. Examples of first-order outcomes include productivity, creativity, absenteeism, quality of production, or other behaviors that result from the individual's effort to perform. The "outcomes" component listed on the right side of Figure 16.4 is a second-order outcome that results from the attainment of first-order outcomes. That is, these outcomes are the reward (or punishment) that is associated with performance. Examples include merit pay increases, esteem of co-workers, supervisory approval, promotion, and flexible work schedules.

Crucial to Vroom's expectancy theory is the concept that people have preferences for outcomes. Vroom terms the value an individual attaches to a particular outcome its valence. When people have a strong preference for a particular outcome, it receives a high valence; similarly, a lower preference for an outcome yields a lower valence. People have valences for both first- and second-order outcomes. For example, someone might prefer a merit pay increase over a more flexible work schedule (second-order outcomes). This individual might prefer to produce quality work (a first-order outcome) because it is believed this will lead to a merit pay increase (a second-order out-

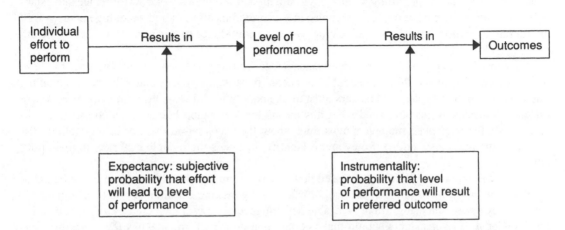

Figure 16.4.   Simplified model of expectancy theory.

come), which might be high on the person's list of preferences (which, in Vroom's terminology, would be assigned a high valence).

These three components of the expectancy theory (expectancy, instrumentality, and valence for outcomes) can be combined into an equation to express the motivation to work:

$$\text{Motivation} = \text{Expectancy} \times \text{Instrumentality} \times \text{Valence}$$

or

$$M = E \times I \times V$$

It is important to note that, because the equation is multiplicative, a low value assigned to any variable will yield a low result. For example, if a person is certain that effort will lead to performance (an E value of 1.0 is assigned) and that performance will lead to reward (an I value of 1.0 is assigned) but does not have a very high valence or preference for the reward involved (a V value such as 0.5 is assigned), the result ($1.0 \times 1.0 \times 0.5 = 0.5$) is low, indicating that motivation is low. For motivation to be high, expectancy, instrumentality, and valence values all must be high.

Managerial Implications of Expectancy Theory

For the manager, expectancy theory explains a great deal about motivated behavior. It can help managers focus on leverage points that help them influence the motivation of those they manage. For motivated behavior to occur, three conditions must be met: 1) the person must have a high expectancy that effort and performance actually are linked; 2) the person must have a high expectancy that performance will lead to outcomes or rewards; and 3) the person must have a preference for (assign a high valence value to) the outcomes that result from effort, including first- and second-order outcomes.

Managers who know their workers' preferences in terms of second-order outcomes have an advantage in developing effective approaches to motivation. It is important to remember that implicit in Vroom's model is the fact that individuals have different preferences about outcomes. The design of motivation approaches must be flexible enough to address differences in individual preferences regarding the rewards of work.

Bateman and Zeithaml identified three crucial implications for management work that are inherent in expectancy theory.[27] First, they argued that managers should take steps to increase expectancies. This means providing a work environment that facilitates work performance and establishes realistic performance objectives. It also means providing support and encouragement, as well as training at appropriate levels to give employees the confidence to perform their work at the expected levels.

Second, Bateman and Zeithaml urged managers to identify positively valent outcomes for those they manage. This means thinking about what needs are satisfied by jobs and what needs could be, but are not, satisfied by them. Managers must think about how and why different employees assign different valences to outcomes and what this means for motivating behavior. In considering outcomes with high valences, managers must think about the needs-based theories of motivation (discussed in the previous section) if they are to identify the needs that people can meet in their work situations.

Third, Bateman and Zeithaml stressed that managers must make performance instrumental to positive outcomes. Managers can do this, for example, by making certain that good performance is followed by praise and recognition, favorable performance reviews, pay increases, or other positive results. Conversely, managers should make certain that poor performance has fewer positive outcomes and more negative outcomes. Instrumentality, in the context of equity theory, means that there is a perceived relationship between performance and outcome, positive or negative.

Adams's Equity Theory

An important extension of expectancy theory comes from the realization that, in addition to preferences as to the rewards associated with performance, individuals also assess whether rewards are equitably distributed within organizations. Equity theory posits that people calculate the ratios of their efforts to the rewards they receive and compare them to the ratios they believe exist for others in similar situations. They do this because they have a strong desire to be treated fairly.

Adams developed and tested his equity theory of motivation in the early 1960s.[28] He theorized that people judge equity with the following equation:

$$\frac{O_P}{I_P} = \frac{O_o}{I_o}$$

where

O_P is the person's perception of the outcomes received.

I_P is the person's perception of personal inputs.

O_O is the person's perception of the outcomes that a comparison person (or comparison other) is receiving.

I_O is the person's perception of the inputs of the comparison person (or comparison other).

This formula suggests that equity exists when an individual's perception of the ratio of inputs (efforts) made to outcomes (rewards) received is equivalent to that of a "comparison other" or referent. Conversely, inequity exists when the ratios are not equivalent.

It is noteworthy that perception, not reality, is considered in this equation. Furthermore, there are options as to the comparison others or referents in the equation. These options include people in similar circumstances (co-workers or someone whose circumstances are thought to be similar); a group in similar circumstances (e.g., all registered nurses in the HSO/HS); or the perceiving person under different circumstances (e.g., earlier in the present position or circumstances when the person worked in another HSO/HS). Choice of referent is a function of the information that is available as well as perceived relevance. Finally, it is important to note that there may be many different inputs and outcomes. Inputs are what people believe they contribute to their jobs, such as experience, time, effort, dedication, and intelligence. Outcomes are what they believe they get from their jobs, such as pay, promotion, status, esteem, monotony, fatigue, and danger.

Equity theory recognizes that people are concerned both with the absolute rewards that they receive for their efforts and the equity of these rewards compared with what others receive. People routinely make judgments about the relationship between their inputs and outcomes and the inputs and outcomes of others. In effect, equity theory recognizes that people are interested in distributive fairness—getting what they believe they deserve for their work. Extensive research supports the fact that, even with all the variables involved in making comparisons, people consider equity regularly.[29]

When faced with situations that they perceive to be inequitable, people seek to restore equity in a number of different ways. Their alternatives are contained in the equity equation shown previously. They might use some or all of these alternatives simultaneously or in sequence before a feeling of equity is restored or attained. Using pay as an example of something about which equity is important, people who feel an inequity (i.e., feel that their pay is too low) can decrease their input by reducing effort or performance to compensate for this perceived inequity. Alternatively, they could seek to modify their comparisons or referents. For example, they might try to persuade low performers who are receiving equal pay to increase their efforts, or they might try to discourage high performers from exerting so much effort. Others who are feeling an inequity in their pay, perhaps in desperation, may distort reality and rationalize that the perceived inequities are somehow justified. Finally, as a last resort to perceived inequities, people can leave an inequitable situation if they conclude that the inequities will not be resolved.[30] Thus people can attempt to restore equity by changing the reality or the perception of the inputs and outcomes in the equity equation. However, each mechanism they use can present serious problems for managers and for HSOs/HSs.

Managerial Implications of Equity Theory

Equity theory makes an important contribution to understanding human motivation because it shows that motivation is significantly influenced by both absolute and relative rewards. It also shows that, when people perceive inequity, they act to reduce it. Thus it is important for managers to minimize inequities—real and perceived—in the workplace. This means helping people to understand the differences among jobs and rewards and making certain that reward differences actually reflect different performance requirements among jobs.

The bottom-line implication of equity theory for managers is that people who feel equitably treated in their workplaces are more satisfied than are those who feel inequitably treated. Whereas satisfaction alone does not ensure high levels of performance, dissatisfaction in the workplace has negative consequences such as higher absenteeism and turnover rates, lower citizenship behaviors, more grievances and lawsuits, stealing, sabotage, vandalism, more job stress, and other costly negative consequences for HSOs/HSs and the people who work in them.

The equity theory emphasizes the importance of managers' treating subordinates fairly. However, motivation is complex, and treating people fairly often means treating them differently; treating people differently suggests inequity.

Locke's Goal-Setting Theory

An increasingly popular process theory builds on the pervasiveness of the "goal-directedness" of human behavior.[31] In proposing his theory to explain motivation, Locke viewed goal setting as a cognitive process through which conscious goals, as well as intentions about pursuing them, are developed. Goals and intentions developed in this way become primary determinants of behavior.[32] Thus, in Locke's theory of motivation, the intent to work toward goals that they have established is an important part of people's motivation.[33] The central premise in this process theory is that people focus their attention on the concrete tasks that are related to attaining their goals and persist in the tasks until the goals are achieved.[34]

In general, research affirms the importance of goals in motivation.[35] Other studies confirm Locke's original theory that goal specificity (the degree of quantitative precision of the goal) and goal difficulty (the level of performance required to reach the goal) are important to motivation.[36] It also is well established that goals that are both specific and challenging lead to an increase in performance because they make it clearer to the individual what is to be done.[37] Finally, understanding the role of goals in motivation has been enhanced by research that shows the relationship of goal acceptance to performance. One line of research shows that acceptance of goals significantly increases performance.[38] Other studies show that people are more likely to accept goals (other than those that they set for themselves), especially difficult goals, when they participate in establishing them.[39]

Managerial Implications of Goal-Setting Theory

Goals that can effectively motivate desirable behaviors in the workplace have certain characteristics. Managers should keep these characteristics in mind as they set goals for staff or encourage them to set goals for themselves. The most important characteristic of goals, in terms of their ability to motivate, is that they must be acceptable to the people whom managers wish to motivate. Acceptability increases when work-related goals do not conflict with personal values and when people have clear reasons to pursue the goals. Goals must be challenging but attainable, specific, quantifiable, and measurable.[40]

It also is important for managers to provide timely and specific feedback on progress toward achieving established goals. The most widely adopted method of using goal-setting theory to enhance the contributions of people in organizations is management by objectives (MBO). MBO is a process through which people participate in developing specific, attainable, and measurable personal objectives (goals). MBO works when individual objectives mesh with and support the attainment of organizational objectives.[41]

Figure 16.5 shows MBO applied in HSOs/HSs and illustrates how manager–subordinate pairs jointly establish objectives (goals). Jointly developed goals can have the desired degrees of speci-

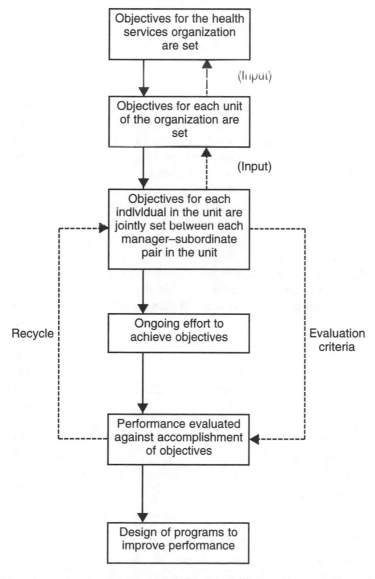

Figure 16.5.　The MBO process in HSOs/HSs. (From Longest, Beaufort B., Jr. *Health Professionals in Management,* 226. Stamford, CT: Appleton & Lange, 1996; reprinted by permission.)

ficity and difficulty that are needed to maximize their usefulness in motivating behavior. Participating in development increases acceptability to those trying to achieve the objectives. It also is important that managers make certain that subordinates have the ability and the support that are necessary to achieve their goals. Finally, consistent with reinforcement theory, which is examined next, it is important that goal achievement serve as a basis for rewards in the workplace.

Skinner's Reinforcement Theory

Reinforcement theory is a counterpoint to the goal-setting theory of motivation, which holds that behavior is driven by the establishment of goals and intentions. Behavior is a cognitive activity that is largely internal, although a process like MBO subjects individual goals and intentions to negotiation. By contrast, reinforcement theory holds that behavior is associated with externally imposed consequences that are learned from experience.

Reinforcement theory suggests that consequences of behavior are reinforcers, and, when positive consequences immediately follow an act, the act likely will be repeated. The converse is true for negative consequences. At the heart of reinforcement theory is operant conditioning, the concept that people learn through experience what to do or not do to ensure positive consequences or avoid negative ones. The most widely read and quoted operant-conditioning theorist is B.F. Skinner, who theorized that reinforcement concepts explain all human behavior.[42] Figure 16.6 illustrates his conceptualization of how reinforcement theory motivates human behavior.

In this model, a person responds to a stimulus. The response (behavior) triggers consequences, positive or negative, that will affect future responses. People learn from the consequences of previous experiences. When faced with the same or a similar stimulus, they follow one of two paths. If previous consequences were positive or desirable, then the person is likely to respond in the same manner (shown as Path 4 in Figure 16.6). If the consequences were negative or undesirable, then the person will likely follow Path 5 in Figure 16.6, which represents a new response.

Managerial Implications of Reinforcement Theory

Reinforcement theory has been useful in explaining some aspects of the way in which people work. For example, studies have shown it to partially explain absenteeism, tardiness, work effort, and the amount and quality of work performed, although it explains little of the level of job satisfaction that people feel.[43]

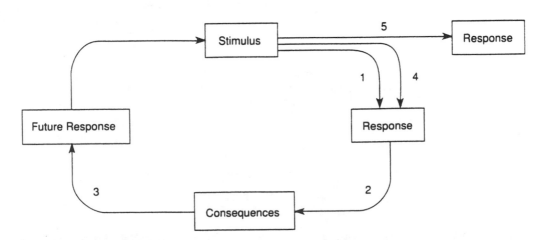

Figure 16.6.　The reinforcement theory of motivation.

For managers, the most important concepts in reinforcement theory are that people repeat behavior that is rewarded and avoid behavior that is punished, and that managers encourage preferred behaviors by reinforcing them. Positive reinforcement is achieved by doing something positive after preferred behavior is exhibited. Merit pay or expressions of approval that are linked to desired behavior, especially when visible to co-workers, are positive reinforcers. Conversely, managers must be careful not to reward undesired behavior. Workers learn to make demands when managers repeatedly agree to them. Managers can gradually end this behavior by refusing to agree to such demands. Workers will learn that unwarranted demands will not be met and will stop making them. Nonreinforcement, or withholding positive reinforcement for a previously learned response, can be used to eliminate undesired behavior.

Punishment differs from nonreinforcement. Punishment is an undesirable consequence of a behavioral response; it also can be removal of a desirable consequence. In the case of workers making unreasonable demands, for example, managers may be able to change this behavior by punishing it with an undesirable consequence such as a letter of reprimand. Alternatively, managers may punish behavior by withholding or removing a desirable consequence, such as ending social interactions. As a general rule, managers do not like to punish those they manage. Punishment typically angers and embitters people, leading to dissatisfaction and perhaps to turnover. Beyond this, punishment only stops undesirable behavior; managers are still left with the task of increasing desired behavior. Even so, punishment is widely used to alter behavior inside and outside the workplace. Sometimes punishment is the only means available to change human behavior, but most often reinforcement theory works best when it focuses on positive reinforcement of desired behavior or nonreinforcement of undesired behavior and not on punishment.

TOWARD AN INTEGRATIVE FRAMEWORK FOR MOTIVATION

A set of content theories and another set of process theories of motivation have been described thus far. Each of the theories contributes to an understanding of the phenomenon of human motivation, although none fully explains motivation. Each of the theories must be viewed as part of a larger, incomplete mosaic. One of the best efforts to integrate the theories into a meaningful whole is that of Porter and Lawler.[44] Figure 16.7 adapts and extends their integrative model, which illustrates the relationships among effort, performance, rewards, and satisfaction. It also shows that effort alone does not explain performance. As noted earlier in the chapter, an individual's performance also is determined by the person's abilities and by constraints in the work situation, such as uncoordinated workflow or inadequate budgets for technology or training. The model emphasizes that people are motivated differently. People have their own intrinsic and extrinsic reward preferences and expectancies regarding the linkages between their efforts and performance levels. Although this model does not capture all of the intricacies of the theories examined, it does integrate many aspects of motivation into a meaningful whole.

The integrative model of motivation is useful in identifying where some of the typical problems of motivation arise in the workplace. As D'Aunno and Fottler have suggested, some of the most significant problems arise because managers do not clearly define what they want in terms of performance.[45] This can be seen in problems such as unclear objectives, inappropriate or unrealistic objectives, inadequate job descriptions, and inadequate or imprecise performance standards.

Another area in which motivation problems typically arise is in the linkage between performance and rewards.[46] These problems can take the form of inappropriate rewards, inadequate rewards, poor timing of rewards, low probability of receiving rewards, and inequity in the distribution of rewards. A third area of motivational problems identified from Figure 16.7 reflects the fact that ability and situational constraints also affect performance. It is important for managers to remove or minimize these barriers to performance as part of their overall motivation efforts. Inability to per-

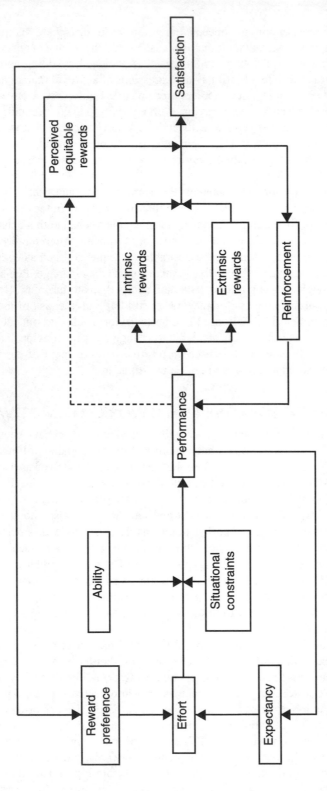

Figure 16.7.   A model of motivation integrating content and process theories. (Adapted from Porter, Lyman W., and Edward E. Lawler, III. *Managerial Attitudes and Performance*, 165. Homewood, IL: Irwin, 1968.)

form can be addressed through increased education and training and in some cases matching people with jobs more carefully. Situational constraints, such as inadequate resources or organization designs that impede performance, can be addressed once they are identified.

Finding solutions to these and other motivational problems is a significant managerial challenge in HSOs/HSs. However, managers can find concrete ideas for solutions in the motivation theories that are integrated into the model in Figure 16.7. The simplest, and perhaps best, advice is to recruit and select motivated staff. People who have demonstrated appropriate levels of performance in the past are motivated to perform and will quite likely continue to perform well. However, there are other things that managers can do to help motivate the people whom they manage.

A critical step in motivating people is choosing appropriate ways to reward desired performance, remembering that rewards can be intrinsic (e.g., derived from the work itself) or extrinsically provided by managers or the HSO/HS to the person being rewarded. Reward selection is made more difficult because people have different valences or preferences about rewards. Some people would rather have more challenging assignments, or more vacation time, than more money. For others, the reverse may be true. The point for managers to remember is that rewards must be important to the person receiving them if they are to be effective motivators. Often, valences can be determined simply by discussing their preferences with employees. Viewed broadly, their responsibilities to provide suitable rewards can lead managers into such areas as process improvement, job redesign and job enrichment, changes in leadership styles, and increasing the degree of participative decision making, in addition to the more typical focus on pay levels and benefits.

Selection of suitable rewards is only a part of using rewards as effective motivators. Managers must link rewards to job performance; that is, rewards must be made contingent on performance and the linkage must be explicit. The more that a person is told about the relationship between performance (with clearly established expectations about performance) and rewards, the more likely the rewards will help motivate desired performance. The performance–reward linkage is strengthened if the rewards follow desirable performance as soon as possible and by providing extensive feedback to individuals. Finally, it is important to remember that people have a strong preference for being treated fairly and equitably. Their perceptions about the linkage between performance and rewards at work is fundamental to their sense of fairness. Managers must pay careful attention to the equity implications of their use of rewards.

Managers' efforts to help motivate people are greatly enhanced if the organization or system is concerned about the quality of work life (QWL). Organizations that institute QWL programs foster environments in which staff well-being and satisfaction are enhanced. Full-fledged QWL programs have several dimensions or foci of attention: 1) adequate and fair compensation; 2) a safe and healthful work environment; 3) a commitment to the full development of employees; 4) a social environment that fosters personal identity, freedom from prejudice, and a sense of community; 5) careful attention to personal privacy, dissent, and due process; 6) a work role that minimizes infringement on personal leisure and family needs; and 7) commitment to socially responsible organizational actions.[47]

HSOs/HSs differ in their commitment to the quality of work life, although most have strong commitments to providing good work environments. Indeed, for many this commitment is a key feature of the organizational culture. There is evidence that organizations that pay attention to QWL dimensions reap the benefits of improved organizational performance as a result of reduced turnover, absenteeism, accidents, theft, and sabotage and increased levels of creativity, innovation, and quality of work. They also facilitate the efforts of their managers to help increase the motivation of staff to contribute to organizational performance by improved individual performance.[48]

SUMMARY

Motivation is an internal drive in individuals and a stimulus to behavior that is intended to satisfy an unsatisfied need felt by the individual. Thus motivation stimulates goal-directed behavior. Managers have a responsibility to motivate people so that their behavior contributes to achieving organizational objectives. The chapter contains overviews of major content and process theories of motivation.

Content theories focus on the internal needs and desires that initiate, sustain, and eventually terminate behavior. They focus on *what* motivates people. Four content theories of motivation are presented: Maslow's hierarchy of needs theory, Alderfer's ERG theory, Herzberg's two-factor theory, and McClelland's learned needs theory.

Process theories seek to explain *how* behavior is initiated, sustained, and terminated. Four process theories of motivation are also presented: Vroom's expectancy theory, Adams's equity theory, Locke's goal-setting theory, and Skinner's reinforcement theory. Table 16.1 summarizes examples of the most important theoretical developments in both categories from a managerial perspective and serves as an outline for the discussion of content and process theories of motivation in the chapter.

Combined, the content and process theories of motivation define variables that explain motivated behavior and show how these theories interact to produce certain behavior patterns. An integrative model ties the content and process theories together. The chapter describes how these theories build on one another, differ, and are complementary.

DISCUSSION QUESTIONS

1. Describe five types of behavior a HSO/HS needs from its members.
2. Use the motivation process model in Figure 16.1 to identify an example of a need deficiency you have experienced. Review the goal you established and pursued to fulfill this need deficiency. Was the goal attained? Was the need fulfilled? If it was not fulfilled, what was your response or reaction?
3. What is the relationship between a manager's view of human nature and the approach the manager might take to motivate staff?
4. Compare and contrast McGregor's Theory X and Theory Y.
5. How does Herzberg's two-factor theory of motivation relate to Maslow's hierarchy of needs model of motivation?
6. Discuss McClelland's approach to motivation. What categories of needs do people have according to McClelland?
7. How do process theories of motivation differ from content theories?
8. Draw a general model of expectancy theory. Use this model to discuss how expectations relate to performance.
9. Define equity theory. How are people in the workplace likely to react to perceived inequities?
10. Discuss the relationship of MBO to Locke's goal-setting theory of human motivation.
11. Identify several typical problems that managers face in motivation and suggest steps that might be taken to address each problem.

CASE STUDY 1: A POTENTIAL CONFLICT

Brad Smith is director of the laboratory at Memorial Hospital. With a professional staff of 67, the laboratory is large, complex, and very busy. Smith does an excellent job, but just keeping up with the demands of the job requires considerable evening and weekend work. He intends to obtain a master's degree (part time in the evening) and use it as a stepping stone to a higher-level management position in the health field. With an outstanding undergraduate record and excellent scores on the Graduate Management Admission Test (GMAT), he was readily admitted into the program, but on two occasions the demands of his job prevented him from beginning graduate studies.

Smith earns a good salary, as does his wife, but they have already started their family and need both incomes to maintain their standard of living. Smith has no choice but to continue to work and attend school only part time.

QUESTIONS

1. Why does Brad Smith want to attend graduate school? What needs could it help him fulfill?
2. Is there another way these needs could be satisfied?
3. Does Memorial Hospital have any responsibility to Brad Smith in this situation? How could the hospital help him?

CASE STUDY 2: THE YOUNG ASSOCIATE'S DILEMMA

Jane O'Hara faced a serious choice. Five years after receiving her master's degree in health administration from a prestigious midwestern university, she was advancing quickly in a large accounting firm. She was receiving assignments with some of the firm's most important clients, and her salary had increased steadily. She was certain that she made at least $15,000 more per year than classmates working in hospitals. The only thing that bothered her about her position, besides the travel, was a nagging feeling that she wanted to become the chief executive officer of a large hospital.

One of O'Hara's clients is a large eastern teaching hospital that has a vice president for finance who is about 5 years from retiring. He is set in his ways; O'Hara judges him to be about a decade behind the sophisticated financial management techniques in her "bag of tools." She was surprised when he offered her a position as his assistant—with a strong hint that he wanted to groom a replacement. The salary is about what she makes with the accounting firm, and the hospital position has slightly better fringe benefits.

When she discussed the offer with her managing partner, he showed a resigned interest in learning what it would take to retain her. Over the next several weeks the firm developed a counteroffer that included a $7,000 salary increase and a clear indication that she was "pegged" for a partnership position in a few years.

O'Hara took a long weekend to consider her choice.

QUESTIONS

1. Identify and describe the motivation variables present in this case.
2. Would these two positions permit O'Hara to fulfill different needs? If so, what are they?
3. What would you do if you were O'Hara? Why?

CASE STUDY 3: CLOCKWORK

At present, Eastern Regional Psychiatric Hospital requires all employees except department heads and above to use a time clock. Categories below this level are paid only for hours recorded on their time cards. Certain professional employees, including registered dietitians, social workers with master's degrees, and medical technologists, have asked to be removed from the rigorous controls of the time clock.

QUESTIONS

1. What factors prompted these employees to make their request?
2. What might happen if the request were not granted?
3. If the request were granted, then how would other employees react?

CASE STUDY 4: BILL'S PROMOTION

Community Hospital had an opening for a dietary supervisor. Kathy Harris applied, and her background was judged to be suitable by the human resources department and the director of dietary services.

A few days after Harris started she encountered problems. The previous dietary supervisor had been discharged, and most of the dietary aides assumed that Bill Warner would be promoted to the position. The director of dietary services told Harris that Warner had been considered but was thought to be too young for that much responsibility.

It soon became evident that, although Warner was cooperative, many employees were not. Dietary services employees who were unhappy with an assignment would tell Harris that, if Warner had been appointed, such problems would not occur. Many comments were made as Harris continued her duties. Some were very embarrassing. One person suggested that she had friends in senior management who gave her the job out of friendship rather than because she was competent.

Then Harris got an idea. Because Warner was close to the employees, she delegated authority to him to coordinate daily job assignments. Warner was delighted and did an excellent job. As a result, Harris had less contact with individual dietary services employees, and she began to depend on Warner in these relationships. Warner was apparently happy, and the employees were satisfied. One day, Warner suggested to Harris that he be given a raise to reflect his new responsibilities. Because he was doing an effective job she requested that his job description be reviewed by human resources and that he be given a promotion and pay raise. However, the vice president for human resources denied the request because "Harris had no approval for the action she had taken in the first place."

QUESTIONS

1. If you were Kathy Harris, what would you do?
2. In dealing with Warner, was Harris using Theory X or Y? Discuss.
3. How does a promotion policy affect employee motivation?
4. What problems now exist in motivating Warner?
5. What should the director of the dietary services department do?

CASE STUDY 5: WHAT NEEDS ARE MOST IMPORTANT TO YOU?[49]

This exercise will give you an opportunity to assess the most important needs that are fulfilled by your work.

Instructions: For each of the following questions, rank your responses from 5 to 1, using 5 as most important or true for you, and 1 to designate the least important.

Example

The work I like best involves:

A 4 Working alone.
B 3 A mixture of time spent with people and time spent alone.
C 1 Giving speeches.
D 2 Discussion with others.
E 5 Working outdoors.

1. Overall, the most important thing to me about a job is whether or not:
A __ The pay is sufficient to meet my needs.
B __ It provides the opportunity for fellowship and good human relationships.
C __ It is a secure job with good employee benefits.

D __ It gives me freedom and the chance to express myself.

E __ There is opportunity for advancement based on my achievements.

2.   If I were to quit a job, it would probably be because:

A __ It was a dangerous job, such as working with inadequate equipment or poor safety procedures.

B __ Continued employment was questionable because of uncertainties in business conditions or funding sources.

C __ It was a job people looked down on.

D __ It was a one-person job, allowing little opportunity for discussion and interaction with others.

E __ The work lacked personal meaning to me.

3.   For me, the most important rewards in working are those that:

A __ Come from the work itself—important and challenging assignments.

B __ Satisfy the basic reasons why people work—good pay, a good home, and other economic needs.

C __ Are provided by fringe benefits—such as hospitalization insurance, time off for vacations, security for retirement, and so on.

D __ Reflect my ability—such as being recognized for the work I do and knowing that I am one of the best in my organization or profession.

E __ Come from the human aspects of working—that is, the opportunity to make friends and to be a valued member of a team.

4.   My morale would suffer most in a job in which:

A __ The future was unpredictable.

B __ Other employees received recognition, when I didn't, for doing the same quality of work.

C __ My co-workers were unfriendly or held grudges.

D __ I felt stifled and unable to grow.

E __ The job environment was poor—no air conditioning, inconvenient parking, insufficient space and lighting, primitive toilet facilities.

5.   In deciding whether to accept a promotion, I would be most concerned with whether:

A __ The job was a source of pride and would be viewed with respect by others.

B __ Taking the job would constitute a gamble on my part, and I could lose more than I gained.

C __ The economic rewards would be favorable.

D __ I would like the new people I would be working with, and whether we would get along well.

E __ I would be able to explore new areas and do more creative work.

6.   The kind of job that brings out my best is one in which:

A __ There is a family spirit among employees and we all share good times.

B __ The working conditions—equipment, materials, and basic surroundings—are physically safe.

C __ Management is understanding and there is little chance of losing my job.

D __ I can see the returns on my work from the standpoint of personal values.

E __ There is recognition for achievement.

7.   I would consider changing jobs if my present position:

A __ Did not offer security and fringe benefits.

B __ Did not provide a chance to learn and grow.

C __ Did not provide recognition for my performance.

D __ Did not allow close personal contacts.

E __ Did not provide economic rewards.

8. The job situation that would cause the most stress for me is:
   A __ Having a serious disagreement with my co-workers.
   B __ Working in an unsafe environment.
   C __ Having an unpredictable supervisor.
   D __ Not being able to express myself.
   E __ Not being appreciated for the quality of my work.
9. I would accept a new position if:
   A __ The position would be a test of my potential.
   B __ The new job would offer better pay and physical surrounding.
   C __ The new job would be secure and offer long-term fringe benefits.
   D __ The position would be respected by others in my organization.
   E __ Good relationships with co-workers and business associates were probable.
10. I would work overtime if:
   A __ The work was challenging.
   B __ I needed the extra income.
   C __ My co-workers also were working overtime.
   D __ I must do it to keep my job.
   E __ The organization recognized my contribution.

Scoring Directions: Place the values you gave to A, B, C, D, and E for each question in the spaces provided in the scoring key. Notice that the letters are not always in the same place for each question. Then add each column and obtain a total score for each of the motivational levels.

Scoring Key						
Question 1	A	C	B	E	D
Question 2	A	B	D	C	E
Question 3	B	C	E	D	A
Question 4	E	A	C	B	D
Question 5	C	B	D	A	E
Question 6	B	C	A	E	D
Question 7	E	A	D	C	B
Question 8	B	C	A	E	D
Question 9	B	C	E	D	A
Question 10	B	D	C	E	A
TOTAL SCORE					
	I	II	III	IV	V
	MOTIVATION LEVELS				

The five motivational levels are as follows:

Level I   Physical needs
Level II   Safety needs
Level III Social needs
Level IV Esteem needs
Level V   Self-realization needs

Those levels that received the highest scores are the most important needs identified by you in your work. The lowest levels show the needs that have been relatively well satisfied or deemphasized by you at this time.

CASE STUDY 6: THE HOLDBACK POOL

Dr. Lloyd Brooks is involved in a new disease management program for his patients with diabetes. As a means to improve patient care and possibly to contain costs, the health maintenance organization (HMO) Dr. Brooks works with has instituted this disease management program. The program includes detailed guidelines for managing diabetes. The guidelines are intended to keep the disease under control, give patients a better quality of life, and minimize costs that are associated with treating complications of diabetes.

The HMO uses financial incentives, almost exclusively, to motivate physician behavior. Specifically, it uses a holdback, bonus pool of money that physicians in the HMO can share at the end of the fiscal year. This means that the more money the physicians save the HMO during the course of a year, the larger the pool of money to be shared, and the larger the bonus check for each physician.

QUESTION:

1. Discuss this case in terms of the expectancy theory of motivation.
2. What are the implications of the holdback pool for motivating the physicians? For patient care?
3. What are the implications for motivation in this case, considering the fact that managing diabetes cases effectively may require higher short-term costs to achieve the objectives of longer, healthier lives for patients and cost savings in the long run?
4. What changes in the HMO's efforts to motivate physician behavior do you recommend?

NOTES

1. O'Connor, Stephen J. "Motivating Effective Performance." In *Handbook of Health Care Management,* edited by W. Jack Duncan, Peter M. Ginter, and Linda E. Swayne, 431. Malden, MA: Blackwell, 1998.
2. Baron, Robert A. "Motivation in Work Settings: Reflections on the Core of Motivation." *Motivation and Emotion* 15 (March 1991): 1–8; Keys, Bernard, and Thomas Case. "How To Become an Influential Manager." *Executive* 4 (November 1990): 38–51; Turnipseed, David L. "Evaluation of Health Care Work Environments via a Social Climate Scale: Results of a Field Study." *Hospital & Health Services Administration* 35 (Summer 1990): 245–262.
3. Ulrich, Dave, and Dale Lake. *Organizational Capability.* New York: John Wiley & Sons, 1990; Ulrich, Dave, and Dale Lake. "Organizational Capability: Creating Competitive Advantage." *Executive* 5 (February 1991): 77–92; Kongstvedt, Peter R. "Changing Provider Behavior in Managed Care Plans." In *The Managed Care Handbook,* 3rd ed., edited by Peter R. Kongstvedt, 427–439. Gaithersburg, MD: Aspen Publishers, 1996.
4. Greenberger, David, Stephen Strasser, Roy J. Lewicki, and Thomas S. Bateman. "Perception, Motivation, and Negotiation." In *Health Care Management: A Text in Organization Theory and Behavior,* 2nd

ed., edited by Stephen M. Shortell, Arnold D. Kaluzny, and associates, 101–102. New York: John Wiley & Sons, 1988.

5. Bateman, Thomas S., and Dennis W. Organ. "Job Satisfaction and the Good Soldier: The Relationship Between Affect and Employee Citizenship." *Academy of Management Journal* 26 (December 1983): 587–595.

6. O'Connor, "Motivating Effective Performance," 438.

7. D'Aunno, Thomas A., and Myron D. Fottler. "Motivating People." In *Essentials of Health Care Management,* edited by Stephen M. Shortell and Arnold D. Kaluzny, 68. Albany, NY: Delmar Publishers, 1997.

8. O'Connor, "Motivating Effective Performance," 438.

9. McGregor, Douglas T. *The Human Side of Enterprise.* New York: McGraw-Hill, 1960.

10. Vroom, Victor H., and Arthur G. Jago. *The New Leadership: Managing Participation in Organizations.* Paramus, NJ: Prentice-Hall, 1988.

11. Maslow, Abraham H. "A Theory of Human Motivation." *Psychological Review* 50 (July 1943): 370–396; Maslow, Abraham H. *Motivation and Personality,* 2nd ed. New York: Harper & Row, 1970.

12. Maslow, Abraham H. *Eupsychian Management,* 56. Homewood, IL: Dorsey-Irwin, 1965.

13. Hall, Douglas T., and Khalil E. Nongaim. "An Examination of Maslow's Needs Hierarchy in an Organizational Setting." *Organizational Behavior and Human Performance* 3 (February 1968): 12–35; Lawler, Edward E., III, and J. Lloyd Suttle. "A Causal Correlational Test of the Need Hierarchy Concept." *Organizational Behavior and Human Performance* 7 (April 1972): 265–287; Wahba, Mahmoud A., and Lawrence G. Bridwell. "Maslow Reconsidered: A Review of Research on the Needs Hierarchy Theory." In *Motivation and Work Behavior,* 4th ed., edited by Richard M. Steers and Lyman W. Porter, 51–67. New York: McGraw-Hill, 1987.

14. Alderfer, Clayton P. "A New Theory of Human Needs." *Organizational Behavior and Human Performance* 4 (May 1969): 142–175; Alderfer, Clayton P. *Existence, Relatedness, and Growth: Human Needs in Organizational Settings.* New York: The Free Press, 1972.

15. D'Aunno and Fottler, "Motivating People," 76.

16. Herzberg, Frederick, Bernard Mausner, and Barbara Snyderman. *The Motivation to Work.* New York: John Wiley & Sons, 1959; Herzberg, Frederick. "One More Time: How Do You Motivate Employees?" *Harvard Business Review* 65 (September–October 1987): 109–117.

17. House, Robert J., and Lawrence A. Wigdor. "Herzberg's Dual-Factor Theory of Job Satisfaction and Motivation: A Review of the Evidence and a Criticism." *Personnel Psychology* 20 (Winter 1967): 369–389; Whitset, David A., and Eric K. Winslow. "An Analysis of Studies Critical of the Motivator-Hygiene Theory." *Personnel Psychology* 20 (Winter 1967): 391–416.

18. Hackman, J. Richard, Greg R. Oldham, Robert Janson, and Kenneth Purdy. "A New Strategy for Job Enrichment." *California Management Review* 16 (Fall 1975): 57–71.

19. Paul, William J., Jr., Keith B. Robertson, and Frederick Herzberg. "Job Enrichment Pays Off." *Harvard Business Review* 47 (March–April 1969): 61.

20. McClelland, David C. *The Achieving Society.* Princeton, NJ: Van Nostrand, 1961; McClelland, David C. *Power: The Inner Experience.* New York: Irvington Publishers, 1975; McClelland, David C. *Human Motivation.* Glenview, IL: Scott, Foresman, 1985.

21. Murray, Henry A. *Explorations in Personality.* New York: Oxford University Press, 1938.

22. Atkinson, John W. *An Introduction to Motivation.* New York: Van Nostrand, 1961; Atkinson, John W., and Joel O. Raynor. *Motivation and Achievement.* Washington, DC: Winston, 1974.

23. Holt, David H. *Management: Principles and Practices,* 2nd ed., 422. Englewood Cliffs, NJ: Prentice-Hall, 1990.

24. Holt, *Management,* 430.

25. McClelland, *Human Motivation.*

26. Vroom, Victor H. *Work and Motivation.* New York: John Wiley & Sons, 1964.

27. Bateman, Thomas S., and Carl P. Zeithaml. *Management: Function and Strategy,* 2nd ed. New York: McGraw-Hill, 1993.

28. Adams, J. Stacy. "Toward an Understanding of Inequity." *Journal of Abnormal and Social Psychology* 67 (November 1963): 422–436; Adams, J. Stacy. "Inequity in Social Exchanges." In *Advances in Experimental Social Psychology,* Vol. 2, edited by Leonard Berkowitz, 267–299. New York: Academic Press, 1965.

29. Walster, Elaine H., G. William Walster, and Ellen Berscheid. *Equity: Theory and Research.* Boston: Allyn & Bacon, 1978; Mowday, Richard T. "Equity Theory Predictions of Behavior in Organizations." In *Motivation and Work Behavior,* 4th ed., edited by Richard M. Steers and Lyman W. Porter, 89–110. New York: McGraw-Hill, 1987.

30. Holt, David H. *Management,* 433–434.

31. Locke, Edwin A. "Toward a Theory of Task Motivation and Incentives." *Organizational Behavior and Performance* 3 (May 1968): 157–189; Locke, Edwin A. "The Ubiquity of the Technique of Goal Setting in Theories of and Approaches to Employee Motivation." In *Motivation and Work Behavior,* 4th ed., edited by Richard M. Steers and Lyman W. Porter, 111–120. New York: McGraw-Hill, 1987.

32. Wood, Robert E., and Edwin A. Locke. "Goal Setting and Strategy Effects on Complex Tasks." In *A Theory of Goal Setting and Task Performance,* edited by Edwin A. Locke and Gary P. Latham, 293–319. Englewood Cliffs, NJ: Prentice-Hall, 1990.

33. Tubbs, Mark E., and Steven E. Ekeberg. "The Role of Intentions in Work Motivation: Implications for Goal-Setting Theory and Research." *Academy of Management Review* 16 (January 1991): 180–199.

34. Latham, Gary P., and Edwin A. Locke. "Goal-Setting—A Motivational Technique That Works." In *Motivation and Work Behavior,* 4th ed., edited by Richard M. Steers and Lyman W. Porter, 120–134. New York: McGraw-Hill, 1987; Locke, Edwin A., and Gary P. Latham. *A Theory of Goal Setting and Task Performance.* Englewood Cliffs, NJ: Prentice-Hall, 1990; Muchinsky, Paul M. *Psychology Applied to Work: An Introduction to Industrial and Organizational Psychology,* 5th ed. Pacific Grove, CA: Brooks/Cole, 1996; Muchinsky, Paul M. *People at Work: The New Millennium.* Pacific Grove, CA: Brooks/Cole, 2000.

35. Mento, Anthony J., Robert P. Steel, and Ronald J. Karren. "A Meta-analytic Study of the Effects of Goal Setting on Task Performance: 1966–1984." *Organizational Behavior and Human Decision Processes* 39 (February 1987): 52–83.

36. Naylor, James C., and Daniel R. Ilgen. "Goal Setting: A Theoretical Analysis of a Motivational Technique." In *Research in Organizational Behavior,* edited by Barry M. Staw and Larry L. Cummings, Vol. 6, 95–140. Greenwich, CT: JAI Press, 1984.

37. Latham, Gary P., and J.J. Baldes. "The Practical Significance of Locke's Theory of Goal Setting." *Journal of Applied Psychology* 60 (February 1975): 120–134.

38. Erez, Miriam, and Frederick H. Kanfer. "The Role of Goal Acceptance in Goal Setting and Task Performance." *Academy of Management Review* 8 (July 1983): 454–463.

39. Erez, Miriam, P. Christopher Earley, and Charles L. Hulin. "The Impact of Participation on Goal Acceptance and Performance: A Two-Step Model." *Academy of Management Journal* 28 (March 1985): 50–66; Schwartz, Robert H. "Coping with Unbalanced Information About Decision-Making Influence for Nurses." *Hospital & Health Services Administration* 35 (Winter 1990): 547–559.

40. Bateman, Thomas S., and Carl P. Zeithaml. *Management.*

41. Drucker, Peter F. *The Practice of Management.* New York: Harper & Brothers, 1954; Duncan, W. Jack. *Great Ideas in Management.* San Francisco: Jossey-Bass, 1989.

42. Skinner, B.F. *Science and Human Behavior.* New York: The Free Press, 1953; Skinner, B.F. *Contingencies of Reinforcement.* New York: Appleton-Century-Crofts, 1969; Skinner, B.F. *Beyond Freedom and Dignity.* New York: Alfred A. Knopf, 1971.

43. O'Connor, Stephen J. "Motivating Effective Performance," 458–459.

44. Porter, Lyman W., and Edward E. Lawler, III. *Managerial Attitudes and Performance.* Homewood, IL: Irwin, 1968.

45. D'Aunno, Thomas A., and Myron D. Fottler. "Motivating People," 87.

46. D'Aunno and Fottler, "Motivating People," 87.

47. Bateman and Zeithaml, *Management*; Muchinsky, *People at Work.*

48. Hackman, J. Richard, and J. Lloyd Suttle. *Improving Life at Work: Behavioral Science Approaches to Organizational Change.* Glenview, IL: Scott, Foresman, 1977; Lawler, Edward E., III. "Strategies for Improving the Quality of Work Life." *American Psychologist* 37 (1982): 486–493.

49. From Manning, George, and Kent Curtis. *Human Behavior: Why People Do What They Do,* 17–20. Cincinnati, OH: Vista Systems/South-Western, 1988; reprinted by permission. Copyright 1988 by South-Western Publishing Co. All rights reserved.

SELECTED BIBLIOGRAPHY

Adams, J. Stacy. "Toward an Understanding of Inequity." *Journal of Abnormal and Social Psychology* 67 (November 1963): 422–436.

Adams, J. Stacy. "Inequity in Social Exchanges." In *Advances in Experimental Social Psychology,* Vol. 2, edited by Leonard Berkowitz, 267–299. New York: Academic Press, 1965.

Alderfer, Clayton P. "A New Theory of Human Needs." *Organizational Behavior and Human Performance* 4 (May 1969): 142–175.

Alderfer, Clayton P. *Existence, Relatedness, and Growth: Human Needs in Organizational Settings.* New York: The Free Press, 1972.

Atkinson, John W. *An Introduction to Motivation.* New York: Van Nostrand, 1961.

Atkinson, John W., and Joel O. Raynor. *Motivation and Achievement.* Washington, DC: Winston, 1974.

Baron, Robert A. "Motivation in Work Settings: Reflections on the Core of Motivation." *Motivation and Emotion* 15 (March 1991): 1–8.

Bateman, Thomas S., and Carl P. Zeithaml. *Management: Function and Strategy,* 2nd ed. New York: McGraw-Hill, 1993.

D'Aunno, Thomas A., and Myron D. Fottler. "Motivating People." In *Essentials of Health Care Management,* edited by Stephen M. Shortell and Arnold D. Kaluzny, 67–98. Albany, NY: Delmar Publishers, 1997.

Drucker, Peter F. *The Practice of Management.* New York: Harper & Brothers, 1954.

Gibson, James L., John M. Ivancevich, and James H. Donnelly, Jr. *Organizations: Behavior, Structure, Processes,* 8th ed. Homewood, IL: Irwin, 1994.

Greenberger, David, Stephen Strasser, Roy J. Lewicki, and Thomas S. Bateman. "Perception, Motivation, and Negotiation." In *Health Care Management: A Text in Organization Theory and Behavior,* 2nd ed., edited by Stephen M. Shortell, Arnold D. Kaluzny, and associates, 81–141. New York: John Wiley & Sons, 1988.

Hall, Douglas T., and Khalil E. Nongaim. "An Examination of Maslow's Need Hierarchy in an Organizational Setting." *Organizational Behavior and Human Performance* 3 (February 1968): 12–35.

Herzberg, Frederick. "One More Time: How Do You Motivate Employees?" *Harvard Business Review* 65 (September–October 1987): 109–117.

Herzberg, Frederick, Bernard Mausner, and Barbara Snyderman. *The Motivation to Work.* New York: John Wiley & Sons, 1959.

Holt, David H. *Management: Principles and Practices,* 2nd ed. Englewood Cliffs, NJ: Prentice-Hall, 1990.

House, Robert J., and Lawrence A. Wigdor. "Herzberg's Dual-Factor Theory of Job Satisfaction and Motivation: A Review of the Evidence and a Criticism." *Personnel Psychology* 20 (Winter 1967): 369–389.

Keys, Bernard, and Thomas Case. "How To Become an Influential Manager." *Executive* 4 (November 1990): 38–51.

Kongstvedt, Peter R. "Changing Provider Behavior in Managed Care Plans." In *The Managed Care Handbook,* 3rd ed., edited by Peter R. Kongstvedt, 427–439. Gaithersburg, MD: Aspen Publishers, 1996.

Latham, Gary P., and J. James Baldes. "The Practical Significance of Locke's Theory of Goal Setting." *Journal of Applied Psychology* 60 (February 1975): 122–124.

Latham, Gary P., and Edwin A. Locke. "Goal-Setting–A Motivational Technique that Works." In *Motivation and Work Behavior,* 4th ed., edited by Richard M. Steers and Lyman W. Porter, 120–134. New York: McGraw-Hill, 1987.

Lawler, Edward E., III. "Strategies for Improving the Quality of Work Life." *American Psychologist* 37 (1982): 486–493.

Lawler, Edward E., III, and J. Lloyd Suttle. "A Causal Correlational Test of the Need Hierarchy Concept." *Organizational Behavior and Human Performance* 7 (April 1972): 265–287.

Locke, Edwin A. "Toward a Theory of Task Motivation and Incentives." *Organizational Behavior and Performance* 3 (May 1968): 157–189.

Locke, Edwin A. "Purpose Without Consciousness: A Contradiction." *Psychological Reports* 24 (June 1969): 991–1009.

Locke, Edwin A. "The Ubiquity of the Technique of Goal Setting in Theories of and Approaches to Employee Motivation." In *Motivation and Work Behavior,* 4th ed., edited by Richard M. Steers and Lyman W. Porter, 111–120. New York: McGraw-Hill, 1987.

Locke, Edwin A., and Gary P. Latham. *A Theory of Goal Setting and Task Performance.* Englewood Cliffs, NJ: Prentice-Hall, 1990.

Longest, Beaufort B., Jr. *Health Professionals in Management.* Stamford, CT: Appleton & Lange, 1996.

Maslow, Abraham H. "A Theory of Human Motivation." *Psychological Review* 50 (July 1943): 370–396.

Maslow, Abraham H. *Motivation and Personality,* 2nd ed. New York: Harper & Row, 1970.

McClelland, David C. *Human Motivation.* Glenview, IL: Scott, Foresman, 1985.

McGregor, Douglas T. *The Human Side of Enterprise.* New York: McGraw-Hill, 1960.

Mowday, Richard T. "Equity Theory Predictions of Behavior in Organizations." In *Motivation and Work Behavior,* 4th ed., edited by Richard M. Steers and Lyman W. Porter, 89–110. New York: McGraw-Hill, 1987.

Muchinsky, Paul M. *Psychology Applied to Work: An Introduction to Industrial and Organizational Psychology,* 5th ed. Pacific Grove, CA: Brooks/Cole, 1996.

Muchinsky, Paul M. *People at Work: The New Millennium.* Pacific Grove, CA: Brooks/Cole, 2000.

Naylor, James C., and Daniel R. Ilgen. "Goal Setting: A Theoretical Analysis of a Motivational Technique." In *Research in Organizational Behavior,* edited by Barry M. Staw and Larry L. Cummings, Vol. 6, 95–140. Greenwich, CT: JAI Press, 1984.

O'Connor, Stephen J. "Motivating Effective Performance." In *Handbook of Health Care Management,* edited by W. Jack Duncan, Peter M. Ginter, and Linda E. Swayne, 431–470. Malden, MA: Blackwell, 1998.

Porter, Lyman W., and Edward E. Lawler, III. *Managerial Attitudes and Performance.* Homewood, IL: Irwin, 1968.

Skinner, B.F. *Beyond Freedom and Dignity.* New York: Alfred Knopf, 1971.

Tubbs, Mark E., and Steven E. Ekeberg. "The Role of Intentions in Work Motivation: Implications for Goal-Setting Theory and Research." *Academy of Management Review* 16 (January 1991): 180–199.

Turnipseed, David L. "Evaluation of Health Care Work Environments via a Social Climate Scale: Results of a Field Study." *Hospital & Health Services Administration* 35 (Summer 1990): 245–262.

Ulrich, Dave, and Dale Lake. *Organizational Capability.* New York: John Wiley & Sons, 1990.

Ulrich, Dave, and Dale Lake. "Organizational Capability: Creating Competitive Advantage." *Executive* 5 (February 1991): 77–92.

Vroom, Victor H. *Work and Motivation.* New York: John Wiley & Sons, 1964.

Vroom, Victor H., and Arthur G. Jago. *The New Leadership: Managing Participation in Organizations.* Paramus, NJ: Prentice-Hall, 1988.

Wahba, Mahmoud A., and Lawrence G. Bridwell. "Maslow Reconsidered: A Review of Research on the Needs Hierarchy Theory." In *Motivation and Work Behavior,* 4th ed., edited by Richard M. Steers and Lyman W. Porter, 51–67. New York: McGraw-Hill, 1987.

Wood, Robert E., and Edwin A. Locke. "Goal Setting and Strategy Effects on Complex Tasks." In *A Theory of Goal Setting and Task Performance,* edited by Edwin A. Locke and Gary P. Latham, 293–319. Englewood Cliffs, NJ: Prentice-Hall, 1990.

17 Communication

Someone once said that if we could solve the problems inherent in communications, we would indeed solve most of the problems not only of the organization but of the world.[1]

Successfully carrying out the management functions of planning, organizing, staffing, directing, and controlling, as well as sound decision making by managers, depends on effective communication. Without it, decision making would take place in an information vacuum; objectives and the strategies and plans to achieve them would go no further than the person who originated them; the health services organization or system (HSO/HS) would be organized and staffed only as a conglomeration of isolated people and departments or organizations; directing people as to what, when, how, or why to do their work would be impossible; and control would be impossible without performance information and a meaningless exercise without the communication of results to influence future performance. Similarly, all of the managerial roles (whether thought of as interpersonal, informational, and decisional roles or strategist, designer, and leader roles, as discussed in Chapter 1) depend on effective communication. Managers cannot effectively lead, plan, design their organizations, develop relationships, disseminate information, or negotiate without communicating.

Typically, the relationships and interactions in which managers in HSOs/HSs are involved are highly information dependent. This is true in relationships and interactions that occur within the HSO/HS, such as those among managers and between managers and other professionals or members of the governing body, as well as in relationships and interactions with the HSO's/HS's external stakeholders. External stakeholders include individuals, groups, or organizations outside the HSO/HS that have a stake in its decisions and actions and attempt to influence those decisions and actions.[2] Examples of external stakeholders are patients, health plans, and government.

In short, the degree to which understanding is transmitted and received effectively through communication plays a critical part in accomplishing work results, whether the work is direct, support, or management. People communicate facts, ideas, feelings, and attitudes while working. If communication is adequate, then work is done more effectively. In any organized activity, communication is essential because it permits people to influence and react to one another.

When managers communicate, four things may be accomplished: information is transmitted, someone is motivated, something is controlled, or emotions and feelings are expressed.[3] Some communication provides the information that people need to understand what to do. Information about a HSO's/HS's mission and objectives, operating plans and activities, resources, and alternatives are necessary for people to make their best contribution to organizational performance. Managers also must provide a great deal of information to external constituencies, especially potential customers, third-party payers, and regulators, if their HSOs/HSs are to function effectively within their environments.

Although motivation is a process that is internal to the person experiencing it (see Chapter 16), managers can affect motivation by informing others about rewards based on performance, by providing information that builds commitment to the HSO/HS and its objectives, and by helping employees understand and fulfill their personal needs. Managers also communicate with interface and external stakeholders to motivate or influence them to act in ways that benefit the HSO/HS. Examples include motivating consumers to select the HSO/HS as a provider of medical services, motivating health plans to pay adequate rates for services, or influencing public policy makers to establish fair regulations (see Chapter 8). To the extent that communication provides a path by which managers can influence behavior, it serves a motivation function.

Many kinds of communications facilitate the control of performance in HSOs/HSs. Activity reports, policies to establish standard operating procedures, budgets, and face-to-face directives are examples. Such communications enhance control when they clarify duties, authorities, and responsibilities.

Finally, by permitting people to express their emotions and feelings, such as satisfaction, dissatisfaction, happiness, or anger, emotive communication permits necessary venting to occur among people in the HSO/HS. Emotive communication helps managers increase acceptance of the HSO/HS and its actions both internally and with external stakeholders and constituencies.

COMMUNICATION DEFINED AND MODELED

Communication is the creation or exchange of understanding between sender(s) and receiver(s). This definition does not restrict communication to words alone; it includes all methods (verbal and nonverbal) by which meaning is conveyed. Even silence conveys meaning and is part of communication.

Managers in HSOs/HSs must be concerned with two types of communication: that which is internal to the organization or system and that which is external and occurs between the HSO/HS and its external stakeholders. Intraorganizational communication occurs within HSOs/HSs and depends on the effectiveness of formal channels and networks to transmit information and understanding throughout the organization or system. These channels and networks carry communications multidirectionally—downward, upward, horizontally, and diagonally.

In addition to vital communication within HSOs/HSs, managers—especially senior-level managers—must be concerned with communication between their HSO/HS and external stakeholders. Examples of communication with external stakeholders include marketing the HSO's/HS's services, maintaining good community relations, influencing (lobbying) political constituencies, or building alliances. An important aspect of communication with external stakeholders, discussed more fully later in this chapter, is receiving information from them. No HSO/HS can be well managed unless its managers know a great deal about its external environment. The best way to acquire such information is by systematically communicating with the relevant actors in that environment.

Both intraorganizational communication and communication with external stakeholders involve the creation or exchange of understanding between sender(s) and receiver(s). Both types use the mechanism discussed in the next section. Understanding is the objective in communication, unless, of course, the objective in a communication is obfuscation. Unfortunately, complete understanding seldom results because of the many environmental and personal barriers to effective communication. These barriers and how to overcome them are discussed later in this chapter.

A Model of the Communication Process

Figure 17.1 is a model of the basic mechanism of the communication process. In this model the sender—which can be one or more individuals, departments, or units of a HSO; the HSO itself; or a HS—has ideas, intentions, and information it wishes to convey. A sender uses words and symbols to encode ideas and information into a message for its intended receiver.

Words alone may be insufficient to ensure that the message is understood. Because words may have different meanings for people, or people may not understand certain words, it is often useful to augment the message with symbols. In HSOs/HSs symbols such as things, pictures, or actions play a role in communication. For example, uniforms frequently permit the quick identification of staff. Pictures or visual representations are another type of symbol, and are efficient and helpful in communication. Consider how many words would be needed to explain a HSO's/HS's organization structure in lieu of the information in an organization chart. Or, imagine the difficulty of communicating the information in a magnetic resonance image using only words. Finally, action or inaction communicates. A smile or a hearty handshake has meaning. A promotion or pay increase conveys a great deal to the recipient and to others. Lack of action also has symbolic meaning. As has been noted,

> *Failure to act is an important way of communicating. A manager who fails to praise an employee for a job well done or fails to provide promised resources is sending a message to that person. Since we send messages both by action and inaction, we communicate almost all the time at work, regardless of our intentions.*[4]

Actions or inactions that are inconsistent with words or other symbols transmit contradictory messages. The manager who tells an employee, "I have confidence in your ability, your performance is excellent, and I want to expand your duties by delegating more to you," acts inconsistently by becoming angry if a small error occurs. The receiver who says, "I am listening," to the sender

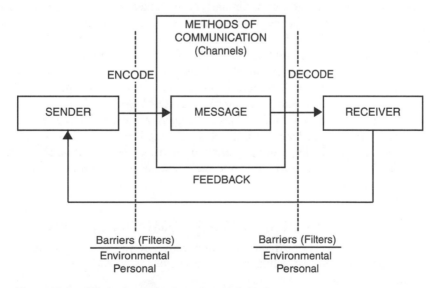

Figure 17.1. The basic mechanism of communication.

and then looks at the clock impatiently or starts to walk away during the conversation sends a mixed message.

The channels or methods of communication are the means by which messages are transmitted. Channels include face-to-face or telephone conversations, email, facsimile messages, letters, memoranda, policy statements, operating room schedules, reports, electronic message boards, video teleconferences, newspapers, television and radio commercials, and newsletters for internal or external distribution.

The selection of channels is important in the communication process. Effective communication often involves multiple channels to transmit a message. For example, a major change in a HSO's/HS's human resources policy, such as modifying the benefits package, may be announced in a letter from the vice president of human resources to all employees, graphically illustrated by posters in key locations, and then reinforced in group meetings in which managers explain the policy and answer questions. A decision to lobby the state legislature for more generous Medicaid reimbursement might result in messages that are transmitted through channels such as letters to legislators, direct contact between HSO/HS managers and trustees and legislators, and newspaper advertisements stating the HSO's/HS's position. Other HSOs/HSs might participate through an association to produce and distribute television commercials or use other channels to increase support for their position.

Messages transmitted over any channel must be decoded by the receiver. Decoding means interpreting the words and symbols in the message. The decoding that is done by receivers is affected by their prior experiences and frames of reference. Decoding involves the receiver's perceptual assessment both of the content of the message and the sender and of the context in which the message is transmitted. The fact that messages must be decoded (interpreted) by the receiver raises the possibility that the message that the sender intends is not the message the receiver gets. The closer the decoded message is to that intended by the sender, the more effective the communication.

The most effective way to determine whether messages are received as intended is through feedback. "Without feedback, you have a one-way communication process. Feedback makes possible a two-way process, reversing the sender and receiver roles so that information can be shared, recycled, and fine-tuned to achieve an unambiguous mutual understanding."[5] In intraorganizational communication, in which interdependencies among individuals and units of a HSO/HS are significant, the feedback loop is very important in ensuring that enough information is exchanged to effectively manage these interdependencies. Similarly, communication with external stakeholders is improved greatly by feedback to senders, who can adjust the message if it is not received as intended. When a sender encodes and transmits a message to a receiver, who decodes the message and indicates understanding by giving feedback, effective two-way communication occurs.

Feedback can be direct or indirect. Direct feedback is the receiver's response to the sender regarding a message. Indirect feedback is more subtle and involves the consequences of a message. Internally, indirect feedback on a policy to change the HSO's/HS's benefit package might include higher levels of employee satisfaction if the change is liked or increased turnover if the change is disliked. Externally, indirect feedback on attempts to change Medicaid reimbursement might include an increase in rates if the legislature agrees with the HSO/HS, no action if they disagree, or even hostile action if they disagree with the message or are upset by the methods used to communicate it.

ELEMENTS OF EFFECTIVE COMMUNICATION

Shortell identifies key elements of effective communication in a model developed for physicians and hospitals.[6] The following list summarizes these elements, and Figure 17.2 illustrates their interrelationships.

- An effective communicator must have a desire to communicate that is influenced by both personal values and the expectation that the communication will be received in a meaningful way.
- An effective communicator must have an understanding of how others learn, including how others perceive and process information. For example, is the receiver analytical or intuitive? Does the receiver prefer abstract or concrete information? Is the receiver better able to interpret information received verbally or in writing?
- The receiver of the message should be cued as to the purpose of the message, that is, whether the message is to provide information, elicit a response or reaction, or arrive at a decision.
- The content, importance, and complexity of the message should be considered in determining the channels through which the message is communicated.
- The achieved or ascribed credibility of the sender affects how the message will be received; "trust" (an achieved credibility) is most significant.
- The time frame that is associated with the content of the message (long versus short) must be considered in choosing the channels through which and the manner in which the message is communicated. That is, faster channels and more precise cues are needed with shorter time frames.

Applying these elements can improve a manager's communication, especially if it is considered in conjunction with the process model that is described in Figure 17.1. No matter how skillfully one communicates, however, there are almost always barriers that must be overcome for

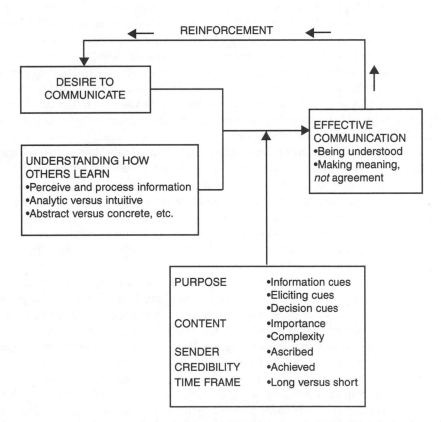

Figure 17.2.   Elements of effective communication: a guiding framework. (From Shortell, Stephen M. *Effective Hospital-Physician Relationships,* 87. Chicago: Health Administration Press, 1991; reprinted by permission.)

communication to be effective. These barriers apply whether communication is within a HSO/HS or between it and external stakeholders.

BARRIERS TO EFFECTIVE COMMUNICATION

The environmental and personal barriers illustrated in Figure 17.1 are ubiquitous in the communication process within HSOs/IISs and between them and external stakeholders. These barriers can block, filter, or distort messages as they are encoded, sent, decoded, and received.

Environmental Barriers

Environmental barriers are created by certain characteristics of a HSO/HS and its environmental context. Two of the most common of these barriers to effective communication are competition for attention and competition for time on the part of senders and receivers. Multiple and simultaneous demands requiring the attention of the sender may cause a message to be packaged inappropriately, or may cause the message to be incorrectly decoded by the receiver. A receiver may hear the message without comprehending it because it is not getting complete attention—the receiver is not really listening. Similarly, time constraints may be a barrier to effective communication by prohibiting the sender from thinking through and properly structuring the message to be conveyed, or by giving the receiver too little time to determine its meaning.

Other environmental barriers that can filter, distort, or block a message include the HSO's/ HS's managerial philosophy, multiplicity of hierarchical levels, and power/status relationships between senders and receivers. Managerial philosophy can inhibit or promote effective communication. Managers disinterested in promoting intraorganizational communication upward or disseminating information downward will establish procedural and organizational blockages. Requirements that all communication "flow through channels"; inaccessibility; lack of interest in employees' frustrations, complaints, or feelings; and insufficient time allotted to receiving information are symptoms of a philosophy that retards communication. Furthermore, managers who fail to act on complaints, ideas, and problems signal to those wishing to communicate upward that the effort is unlikely to have much effect. This discourages information flow.

Managerial philosophy also has a significant impact on a HSO's/HS's communications with external stakeholders. This topic is addressed more fully in a later section, but suffice it to say here that philosophy leads managers to react in particular ways in communicating with external stakeholders in a crisis. For example, if there is a chance that patients could have been exposed to a dangerous infection while hospitalized because of improper handling of contaminated material, then managers could react by covering up the incident or by contacting all who may have been exposed so that they could be tested. Varying reactions to events reflect different managerial philosophies and ethical values about communicating.

Multiple levels in a HSO's/HS's hierarchy, and other organizational complexities such as size or scope of activity, present barriers that tend to cause message distortion. As messages are transmitted up or down, people will interpret them according to their personal frames of reference and vantage points. When the communication chain has multiple links, information can be filtered, dropped, or added, and emphasis can be rearranged as the message is retransmitted. As a result, the message may be distorted or even totally blocked. For example, a message sent from the chief executive officer (CEO) to employees through several layers of an organization is received in a different form than that originally sent. Or, a report prepared for the CEO that passes through the hierarchy may not reach its destination because it is lying on a desk and is, in essence, blocked.

Power/status relationships also can present barriers to effective communication by distorting or inhibiting the transmission of messages. A discordant superior–subordinate relationship can dampen the flow and content of information. Furthermore, an employee's past experiences may inhibit communication because of fear of reprisal, negative sanctions, or ridicule. For example, a subordinate may not inform a superior that something is wrong or that a plan will not work as a result of poor superior–subordinate rapport. Power/status communication barriers are prevalent in HSOs/HSs in which many professionals interact and status relationships create a complex situation. Does the nurse with 20 years of experience tell a new medical resident that a procedure or treatment about to be ordered is not efficacious? How is the nurse's message encoded—bluntly or obliquely?

A final environmental barrier occurs when messages require the use of specific terminology that is unfamiliar to the receiver or when messages are especially complex. Each profession has its own jargon. HSO/HS managers may use terminology in a different way from those responsible for direct care. Both may use terminology that is unfamiliar to external stakeholders. Communications between people who use different terminology can be ineffective simply because people attribute different meanings to the same words. When a message is both complex and contains terminology that is unfamiliar to the receiver, misunderstanding is likely. This barrier is widespread in communication within HSOs/HSs as well as between them and many of their external stakeholders.

Personal Barriers

Another set of potential barriers—personal barriers—always are present when people communicate. They arise from people's nature, especially in their interaction with others, and apply equally to communication within HSOs/HSs and between them and external stakeholders. When people encode and send messages or decode and receive them, they do so according to their frames of reference or beliefs. They may consciously or unconsciously engage in selective perception, and communications may be influenced by emotions such as fear or jealousy.

Socioeconomic background and previous experiences that are an individual's frame of reference shape how messages are encoded and decoded, or even whether communication is attempted. For example, someone whose cultural background is "don't speak unless spoken to" or "never question elders" may be inhibited in communicating. Naïve people tend to accept communication at face value without filtering out erroneous information or observing gaps in information that they receive. Self-aggrandizing people may disseminate information in which messages are distorted for personal gain. Furthermore, unless one has had the same experiences as others, it is difficult to completely understand their messages. People who have health insurance may have difficulty understanding the concerns of people without health insurance. Those who have never experienced pain or childbirth or witnessed death may be unable to fully understand messages about these experiences.

Closely related to one's frame of reference are beliefs, values, and prejudices. They can cause messages to be distorted or blocked in either transmission or reception. This occurs because people and their personalities and backgrounds differ; they have preconceived opinions and prejudices in areas such as politics, ethics, religion, equity in the workplace, and lifestyle. These biases, beliefs, and values filter and distort communication.

Selective perception is one of the most difficult personal barriers to overcome for both the sender and the receiver. People tend to screen derogatory information and amplify words, actions, and meanings that flatter them—there is a tendency to filter out the "bad" of a message and retain the "good." Selective perception can be conscious or unconscious. When it is conscious, often because one fears the consequences of the truth, intentional distortion results. This happens frequently when patients receive bad news about their condition, but it also occurs in management situations. For example, supervisors whose units have high turnover may fear the consequences of this fact if their superiors notice it. They might amplify the argument that turnover is the result of low wages over which they have no control (or responsibility), or delete, alter, or minimize the importance of this information in reports to their superiors.

Sometimes jealousy, especially when coupled with selective perception, may result in conscious efforts to filter and distort incoming information, transmit misinformation, or both. For example, the manager with an able assistant who routinely makes that manager look good may block or distort information that would reveal the truth to superiors. Sometimes petty personality differences, the feeling of professional incompetence or inferiority, or greed can lead to jealousy, resulting in communication distortion.

Two other personal barriers to communication arise because people receiving messages tend to evaluate the source (the sender) and because people often prefer the status quo. Both of these personal barriers to effective communication are common in HSOs/HSs. Receivers often evaluate the source to decide whether to filter out or discount some of the message. However, this can bias communicators. For example, a hostile union–management atmosphere or one in which employees do not trust management may cause employees to ignore messages from management; or managers may ignore messages from physicians with whom they frequently disagree. Source evaluation may be necessary to cope with the barrage of communication received by people in HSOs/HSs, but one must recognize the risk that legitimate messages may be misunderstood.

The preference for the status quo can be a barrier when it results in a conscious effort by the sender or receiver to filter out information in sending, receiving, or retransmitting that would upset the present situation. Internally, conditions that promote fear of sending bad news or a lack of candor among participants can lead to the erection of this barrier. Externally, communicators in a HSO/HS do not want to upset important stakeholders and may react by transmitting messages designed to protect the status quo.

A final personal barrier to effective communication is a lack of empathy, which means being insensitive to the frames of reference or emotional states of other people in the communication relationship. Sensitivity promotes understanding. Empathy helps the sender encode a message for maximum understanding and helps the receiver correctly interpret it. For example, subordinates who empathize with superiors may discount an angry message because they are aware that extreme pressure and frustration can cause such messages to be sent even when they are not warranted.

Similarly, a sender who is sensitive to the receiver's circumstance may decide how best to encode a message or that it is better left unsent. For example, if the receiver is having a "bad day," a reprimand may be interpreted as stronger than it is intended. Or, if a receiver has just had a traumatic experience, such as a family illness or financial setback, the empathetic sender could delay bad news until later. Managers concerned about a HSO's/HS's community image might delay announcing a generous across-the-board wage increase or a large price increase just after a major local employer announces a plant closing because of adverse economic conditions.

Managing Barriers to Effective Communication

Awareness that environmental and personal barriers to effective communication exist is the first step in minimizing their impact, but positive actions are needed to overcome them. Although the steps to overcome the barriers depend on circumstances, several general guidelines can be suggested.

Environmental barriers are reduced if receivers and senders ensure that attention is given to their messages and that adequate time is devoted to listening to what is being communicated. In addition, a management philosophy that encourages the free flow of communications is constructive. Reducing the number of links (levels in the organizational hierarchy or steps between the HSO/HS as a sender and external stakeholders as receivers) reduces opportunities for distortion. The power/status barrier is more difficult to eliminate because it is affected by interpersonal and interprofessional relationships. However, consciously tailoring words and symbols so that messages are understandable and reinforcing words with actions significantly improves communication among different power/status levels. Finally, using multiple channels to reinforce complex messages decreases the likelihood of misunderstanding.

Personal barriers to effective communication are reduced by the conscious efforts of sender and receiver to understand each other's frame of reference and beliefs. Recognizing that people engage in selective perception and are prone to jealousy and fear is a first step toward eliminating or at least diminishing these barriers. Empathy with those to whom messages are directed may be the surest way to increase the likelihood that the messages will be received and understood as intended.

Effectively communicating among component organizations in a HS can be especially demanding. Barriers resulting from organizational complexity in HSs can be formidable. Adapting Porter's approach to achieving effective linkages among business units in a diversified corporation suggests ways in which managers can overcome some of these barriers.[7]

- Use devices or techniques that cross organizational lines, such as partial centralization and interorganization task forces or committees to actively facilitate communication. At the governance level, HSs can enhance communication through interlocking boards, defined as boards with overlapping membership. Interlocking boards can enhance communication among components in a HS.
- Use management processes that are cross-organizational in areas such as planning, control, incentives, capital budgeting, and management information systems to enhance communication.
- Use human resource practices that facilitate cooperation among the HSOs in a HS, such as cross-organizational job rotation, management forums, and training, because these increase the likelihood that managers in one part of the HS will understand their counterparts elsewhere in the system and that they will communicate more effectively.
- Use management processes that effectively and fairly resolve conflicts among HSOs in a HS to enhance communication. The key to such processes is that corporate management installs and operates a process that fairly settles disputes among component organizations in the system. Equitable settlement of disputes facilitates effective communication.

FLOWS OF INTRAORGANIZATIONAL COMMUNICATION

Intraorganizational communication flows downward, upward, horizontally, and diagonally. Each direction has its appropriate uses and unique characteristics. Typically, downward flow is communication between superiors and subordinates in organizations; upward flow uses the same channels but in the opposite direction. Horizontal flow is manager to manager or worker to worker. Diagonal flow cuts across functions and levels. Although this violates an organization's chain of command, it may be permitted in situations in which speed and efficiency of communication are particularly important.

Downward Flow

Downward communication primarily involves passing on information from superiors to subordinates in HSOs/HSs. It commonly consists of information, verbal orders, or instructions from an organizational superior to subordinate on a one-to-one basis. It also may include speeches to employee groups or in meetings. Myriad written methods such as handbooks, procedure manuals, newsletters, bulletin boards, and the ubiquitous memorandum also are channels of downward communication. Computerized information systems contribute greatly to downward flow in many HSOs/HSs.

Upward Flow

Objectives of upward communication include providing managers with decision-making information, revealing problem areas, providing data for performance evaluation, indicating the status of morale, and in general, underscoring the thinking of subordinates. Upward flow becomes more important with increased organizational complexity and scale in HSOs and with their participation in HSs. Managers rely on effective upward communication; they encourage it by creating a climate of trust and respect as integral to the organizational culture.[8]

In addition to being directly useful to managers, upward communication flow helps employees satisfy personal needs. It permits those in positions of lesser authority to express opinions and perceptions to those with greater authority; as a result, they feel a heightened sense of participation. The hierarchical chain of command is the main channel for upward communication in HSOs/HSs, but this may be supplemented by grievance procedures, open-door policies, counseling, employee questionnaires, exit interviews, participative decision-making techniques, and ombudsmen.[9]

Horizontal and Diagonal Flows

In complex HSOs/HSs, which are frequently subject to abrupt demands for action and reaction, horizontal flow also must occur. For example, the work of interdependent patient care units must be coordinated. HSOs/HSs using matrix designs, as described in Chapter 3, illustrate the value of horizontal communication and coordination in these organizations and systems. Committees, task forces, and cross-functional project teams are all useful mechanisms of horizontal communication.

The least common communication in HSOs/HSs are diagonal flows. Diagonal flows, however, are growing in importance. For example, diagonal communication occurs when the director of a hospital pharmacy alerts a nurse in medical intensive care about a potential adverse reaction between two medications. Diagonal flows violate the usual pattern of upward and downward communication flows by cutting across departments, and they violate the usual pattern of horizontal communication because the communicators are at different levels in the organization. Yet, such communication is essential in HSOs/HSs.

Committees, task forces, quality improvement teams, and cross-functional project teams made up of members from different levels or component areas of the organization or system each can serve as mechanisms of diagonal communication. The prevalence of committees in HSOs/HSs can be attributed to a need for horizontal and diagonal communication. They permit representatives of different organizational units to discuss common concerns and potential problems face to face and to coordinate activities. Committees are useful boundary-spanning devices. However, they tend to be time consuming and expensive, and their decisions often are compromises that may be ineffectual solutions to problems.

Communication Networks

Downward, upward, horizontal, and diagonal communication flows can be combined into patterns called communication networks, which are communicators that are interconnected by communication channels.[10] Figure 17.3 illustrates the five common networks: chain, Y, wheel, circle, and all-channel. The chain network is the standard format for communicating upward and downward and follows line authority relationships. An example is a staff nurse who reports to a nurse manager, who reports to a nursing supervisor, who reports to the vice president for nursing, who reports to a HSO's CEO.

The Y pattern (if inverted) shows two people reporting to a superior who reports to another. An example is two staff pharmacists who report to the pharmacy director, who reports to the vice president for professional affairs, who reports to the president. The wheel pattern shows four subordinates reporting to one superior. Subordinates do not interact, and all communications are channeled through the manager at the center of the wheel. This pattern is rare in HSOs/HSs, although elements of it can be found where four vice presidents report to a president if the vice presidents have little interaction. Even though this network pattern is not routinely used, it may be used when

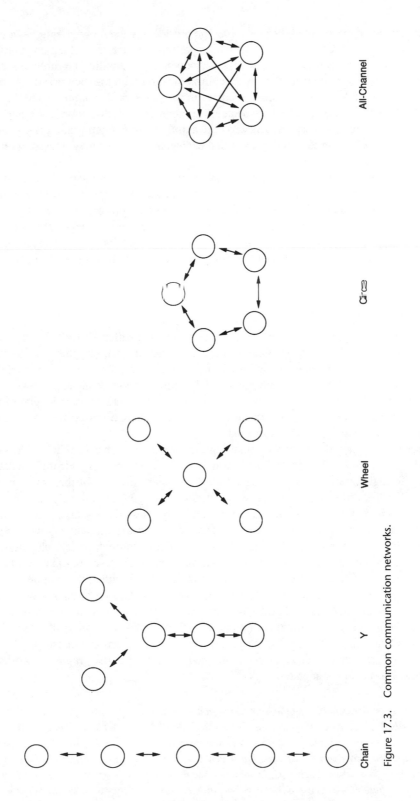

Chain   Y   Wheel   Circle   All-Channel

Figure 17.3.   Common communication networks.

urgency or secrecy is required. For example, the president with an organizational emergency might communicate with vice presidents in a wheel pattern because time does not permit using other modes. Similarly, if secrecy is important, such as when investigating possible embezzlement, then the president may require that all relevant communication with the vice presidents be confidential.

The circle pattern allows communicators in the network to communicate directly only with two others, but because each communicates with another communicator in the network, the effect is that everyone communicates with everyone, and there is no central authority or leader. The all-channel network is a circle pattern except that each communicator may interact with all other communicators in the network.

Communication networks vary along several dimensions, and none is best in all situations. The wheel and all-channel networks tend to be fast and accurate compared with the chain or Y-pattern networks, but the chain or Y-patterns promote clear lines of authority and responsibility. The circle and all-channel networks enhance morale among those in the networks better than other patterns because everyone is equal in the communication activity, but these patterns result in relatively slow communication. Managers in HSOs/HSs must choose communication networks to fit various communication situations.

Informal Communication

Coexisting with formal communication flows and networks within HSOs/HSs are informal communication flows, which have their own networks. Like the informal organization structures discussed in Chapter 3, informal communication flows and networks result from interpersonal relationships in organizations and systems. The common name for informal communication flows is the *grapevine,* a term that arose during the Civil War, when telegraph lines were strung between trees, much like a grapevine.[11] Messages transmitted over those flimsy lines were often garbled. As a result, any rumor was said to have come from the grapevine.

Informal communication flows in an organization are as natural as the patterns of social interaction that develop in all organizational settings. Like the informal organization structure (see Chapter 3), informal communication coexists with the formal flows established by management. There is no doubt that informal communication channels can be and routinely are misused in HSOs/HSs, especially in transmitting rumors. For example, in times of crisis, organizations and systems are rife with rumors; frequently they are wrong. However, informal communication can be useful. Downward flows move through the grapevine much faster than through formal channels. In a HSO/HS much of the coordination among units occurs through informal give-and-take in informal horizontal and diagonal flows. In the case of upward flow, informal communication can be a rich source of information about performance, ideas, feelings, and attitudes. Because of their potential usefulness and pervasiveness, managers should understand informal communication and use it to advantage.

Similar in concept to formal communication flows, informal flows follow predictable patterns and form identifiable networks. Figure 17.4 illustrates four common patterns that the grapevine can take. The single strand pattern is how many people think that the grapevine works. Instead, it is more likely to be a cluster pattern.

> *Managers occasionally get the impression that the grapevine operates like a long chain in which A tells B, who tells C, who then tells D, and so on, until 20 persons later, Y gets the information— very late and very incorrect. [See the single-strand network in Figure 17.4.] Sometimes the grapevine may operate this way, but it generally follows a different pattern. Employee A tells three or four others (such as C, D, and F). [See the cluster network in Figure 17.4.] Only one or two of these receivers will pass the information forward, and they usually will tell more than one person. Then as the information becomes older and the proportion of those knowing it gets*

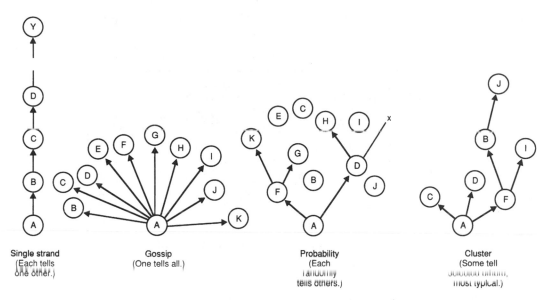

Figure 17.4.   Grapevine networks. (From Newstrom, John W., and Keith Davis. *Organizational Behavior: Human Behavior at Work,* 9th ed., 445. New York: McGraw-Hill, 1993. Reproduced with permission of McGraw-Hill, Inc.)

larger, it gradually dies out because not all those who receive it repeat it. This network is a cluster chain, because each link in the chain tends to inform a cluster of other people instead of only one person.[12]

Informal communication is present in every HSO/HS and can either aid or inhibit effectiveness. Managers can use this to achieve organization objectives. This is done by paying attention to informal communication (even inaccurate rumors reflect some aspects of employees' feelings and views) and by occasionally and selectively using informal communication, especially when speed is critical.

Summary of Intraorganizational Communication Flows

Both the multidirectional communication flows and the networks they form within HSOs/HSs have a purpose, and each is an important tool for managers. To the extent that these flows are planned and designed into the HSO/HS, they are part of its formal organization design and they represent formal communication channels and networks. To the extent that they are natural communication between and among people arising outside the formal design, they are informal communication channels and networks.

Understandable messages, whether they flow through formal channels or informal ones that exist "up and down hallways, in and out of offices, around water coolers, over transoms, and between friends and colleagues,"[13] are as crucial to the life of a HSO/HS as the circulation of blood is to human life. Figure 17.5 summarizes the key uses of downward, upward, horizontal, and diagonal communication in HSOs/HSs.

COMMUNICATING WITH EXTERNAL STAKEHOLDERS

HSOs/HSs typically maintain relationships with a large number of external stakeholders.[14] As defined earlier, stakeholders include individuals, groups, or organizations that are interested in the

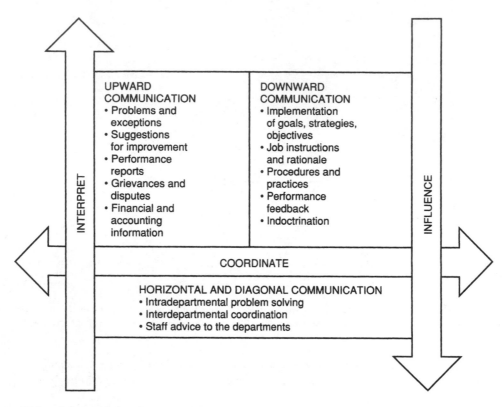

Figure 17.5.   Communication flows in HSOs/HSs. (From Daft, Richard L., and Richard M. Steers. *Organizations: A Micro/Macro Approach,* 538. Reading, MA: Addison-Wesley, 1986; reprinted by permission.)

HSO's/HS's decisions and actions and attempt to influence them. A stakeholder map like that for the Indiana State Department of Health in Figure 17.6 illustrates the diversity of a HSO's/HS's external stakeholders.

Effective communication between a HSO/HS and each external stakeholder is necessary because HSOs/HSs are affected, sometimes quite dramatically, by what external stakeholders think or do. The relationships and communication between HSOs/HSs and their external stakeholders can be complex because these organizations and systems are dynamic, open systems in the context of complex and turbulent external environments, as discussed in Chapter 8. For most HSOs/HSs, the sheer number and variety of external stakeholders complicate communication with them.

Communication between HSOs/HSs and their stakeholders also is complicated by the nature of the relationships. Positive relationships with external stakeholders usually make it easier to manage the relationships, and communication tends to be more effective than when relationships are negative. Figure 17.7 uses a large hospital to illustrate the extraordinary diversity of stakeholders with which relationships must be maintained. The figure also shows that these relationships are not the same. Some are positive (shown by the plus [+] symbol in Figure 17.7), some are negative (shown by the minus [−] symbol), and some are neutral (shown by the zero [0] symbol). It is important to note that the arrows connecting the hospital with its stakeholders go in both directions. Managers must be concerned about communication to *and* from external stakeholders.

Boundary spanning is another name for the process through which HSOs/HSs communicate with external stakeholders, and boundary spanners carry out this process. On the one hand, boundary spanners obtain information from external stakeholders that can be useful to the HSO/HS.

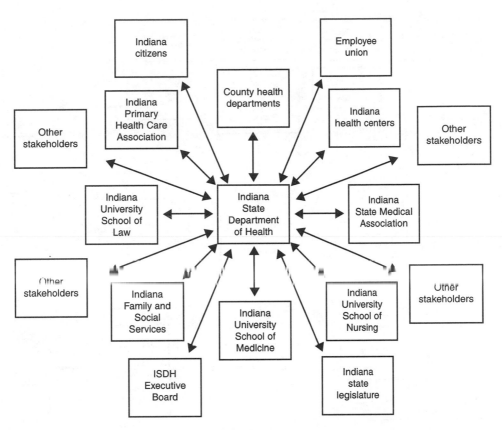

Figure 17.6.   Indiana State Department of Health stakeholder map. (From Ginter, Peter M., Linda M. Swayne, and W. Jack Duncan. *Strategic Management of Health Care Organizations,* 3rd ed., 458. Malden, MA: Blackwell, 1998; reprinted by permission.)

Strategic planning and marketing in HSOs/HSs are examples of boundary spanning. On the other hand, boundary spanners also represent the HSO/HS to external stakeholders. This activity includes marketing, public relations, guest or patient relations, government relations, or community relations. Because information is the object of boundary-spanning activities, communication is critical to success. A HSO's/HS's ability to glean useful information from external stakeholders or to be effectively represented to them depends on effective communication.

Although the communication process with all external stakeholders essentially is the creation of understanding between sender and receiver, each stakeholder must be considered in terms of its unique dimensions if effective communication is to occur. This is especially true of two important sets of external stakeholders in the typical HSO/HS: the public sector with which the organization or system interacts and the geographical community in which the organization or system is located. Communicating with these important external stakeholders is examined in the following sections.

Communicating with the Public Sector

HSOs/HSs are affected by public policies—the formal decisions made in the public sector. The fact that HSOs/HSs are the targets of so much public policy stems from their fundamental contributions to the physical and psychological well-being of people, as well as their role in the nation's economy. In view of these important contributions, government at all levels is keenly interested in their performance. This interest is reflected vividly in the numerous public policies that directly affect

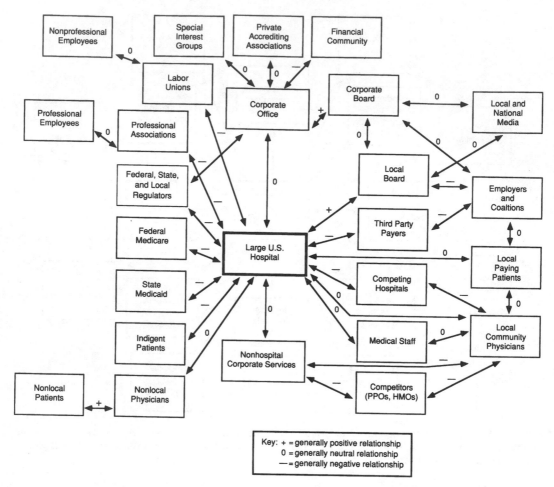

Figure 17.7.   Stakeholders in a large hospital. (From Fottler, Myron D., John D. Blair, Carlton J. Whitehead, Michael D. Laus, and Grant T. Savage. "Assessing Key Stakeholders: Who Matters to Hospitals and Why?" *Hospital & Health Services Administration* 34 [Winter 1989]: 530; reprinted by permission. Copyright 1989, Foundation of the American College of Healthcare Executives.)

HSOs/HSs, including policies affecting the provision and financing of health care services as well as the production of inputs (e.g., the education of health professionals, the development of health technology) to those services.[15] The importance of public policy to HSOs/HSs makes effective communication with the public sector very important. A public policy issues life cycle model and suggested ways for HSOs/HSs to affect such issues are discussed in Chapter 8.

Managers have two important categories of communication responsibilities regarding the public sector environment of a HSO/HS.[16] First, they must analyze this environment to acquire sufficient information and data to understand the strategic consequences of events and forces in the public policy environment. Such analysis yields an assessment of the impacts, in terms of both opportunities and threats, of public policies on the HSO/HS, and permits managers to make strategic adjustments that reflect planned responses to them.

Second, HSO/HS managers are responsible for influencing the formulation and implementation of public policies. They do so through their strategist and leader roles using their political competency. This responsibility derives from the fact that effective managers seek to make the external environment, including the public policy component, favorable to the HSO/HS. Inherent in this responsibility are requirements to identify public policy objectives that are consistent with their organization's or system's values, mission, and objectives and to seek through appropriate and ethical means, such as lobbying individually or through associations, to help shape public policies accordingly.

Communicating with the Community

HSOs/HSs usually consider their communities to be external stakeholders requiring intensive communication. As with all effective communication, those between HSOs/HSs and their communities involve the creation of understanding between senders and receivers. However, this communication involves several special considerations, such as the fact that HSOs/HSs identify their communities in different ways. Effective communication depends on the sender identifying the receiver in the exchange. Thus the first step in a HSO's/HS's effective communication with its community is to identify the community carefully.

The meaning of community usually implies physical location, although for some organizations or systems it is not this straightforward. For example, community may be a function of specialized services provided (such as pediatrics or psychiatric services) or of cohorts of patients served (patients needing rehabilitation services). The impact of some HSOs/HSs extends far beyond their immediate geographical locations, as they attract international patients, draw students widely and return graduates to serve those areas, or conduct research that influences diagnosis and treatment without respect to physical boundaries. HSs may have numerous and broadly dispersed physical locations. However, physical location is not the only way a HSO/HS identifies its community. All HSOs/HSs are concerned to some extent with their relationships with the people and other organizations in their immediate geographic location. For most HSOs/HSs, physical location is their "community of first loyalty."[17] Although not equally relevant to all HSOs/HSs, relationships between them and their geographical communities are important and require a great deal of communication.

In addition to identifying the community, another important aspect of how HSOs/HSs communicate with their communities is the nature of the relationships between them. Perhaps more than with other external stakeholders, the basis for effective communications between HSOs/HSs and their communities is clear understanding and acceptance of the expectations each has of the other and of the responsibilities each bears for the other. Communities wonder what contributions to community life to anticipate from HSOs/HSs, while managers ponder their organization's or system's role in the community as well as what the community provides in the way of customers or patients, employees, infrastructure, or resources. Until such questions are answered, effective communication flows may be hampered by misunderstanding relationships, responsibilities, and expectations.

Managers in HSOs/HSs need to consider carefully the nature of the relationship that their organization or system bears to its community as a foundation on which to build effective communication. As Figure 17.8 suggests, these organizations and systems can do much more for their communities than simply provide health care services. In building the foundational relationship with its community, a HSO's/HS's managers can be guided by the answers to several questions:[18]

- Does our HSO/HS enhance health in our community across a broad front of efforts reflecting the variety of determinants of health?
- Do we provide benefits that we are uniquely positioned to provide to our community through how and for whom we choose to pursue our core, health-enhancing mission?
- Are our economic contributions to our community broadly defined and fully met?
- Are our philanthropic activities in our community established broadly and generously and collaboratively pursued?
- Are we in full compliance with legal requirements and obligations?
- Are our fiduciary and ethical obligations fully met?

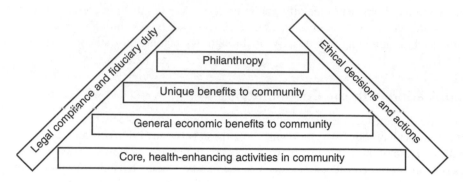

Figure 17.8.   The benefits HSOs/HSs can provide to their communities.

Listening to External Stakeholders

When HSOs/HSs listen to external stakeholders, they want to be good receivers in the communication process, and they approach the task in a systematic, analytical way called stakeholder analysis.[19] This increases the chances of acquiring useful or necessary information.

Although approaches for systematically listening to external stakeholders vary, in general, these efforts include a set of interrelated activities that are akin to the environmental assessments that HSOs/HSs make in the context of strategic management (see Chapter 8). In conducting environmental assessments, HSOs/HSs scan their environments to identify strategically important issues, monitor the issues, forecast trends in the issues, assess the importance of the issues, and diffuse information obtained to those in the organization or system who need it.[20] In stakeholder analyses HSOs/HSs also scan to identify important stakeholders, forecast or project the trends in stakeholders' views or positions, assess the implications of the stakeholders' views and positions for the HSO/HS, and diffuse the information about stakeholder views and positions developed in the first three steps to those who need it.

Scanning activities involve acquiring and organizing important information about a HSO's/HS's external stakeholders. In most instances, this is a straightforward task that readily leads to the development of a stakeholder map, such as shown in Figure 17.6 for the Indiana State Department of Health.

Determination of whom a HSO's/HS's external stakeholders are is frequently a matter of judgment. To ensure quality in these judgments, it is useful to have multiple people make them. This can be accomplished through use of ad hoc task forces, committees, or outside consultants. Several expert-based techniques may help determine whom the stakeholders are. Most useful are the delphi technique, the nominal group technique, brainstorming, focus groups, and dialectic inquiry.[21]

Scanning is followed by monitoring that tracks the stakeholders' views and positions on matters that are important to the HSO/HS. Monitoring is critical when views and positions are dynamic, not well structured, or ambiguous as to strategic importance. Monitoring stakeholder views and positions clarifies the degree to which they are, or the rate at which they are becoming, strategically important. Like their use in scanning, expert opinions can help managers determine which stakeholders to monitor; consultants may do the actual monitoring.

Effective scanning and monitoring cannot provide managers with all the information they need about the views and positions of external stakeholders. Because these views, positions, and perspectives are frequently dynamic, managers will benefit from forecasts as to likely changes in stakeholders' views and perceptions. Such forecasts give managers time to factor these views and preferences into their decisions.

Scanning and monitoring the views and positions of a HSO's/HS's external stakeholders, and even accurately forecasting trends in their views and positions, do not ensure good stakeholder analysis. Managers also must be concerned about the importance of the information. That is, they must assess and interpret the strategic importance and implications of this information. At a minimum, this means characterizing stakeholders as positive, negative, or neutral, as shown in Figure 17.7. Although the determination of positive, negative, or neutral positions is relatively easy to make, assessments of stakeholders' importance is not an exact science. Intuition, common sense, and best guesses all play a role. Beyond the difficulties of collecting and analyzing enough information to make an informed assessment, other problems arise from the personal prejudices and biases of those judging a HSO's/HS's external stakeholders and their relative importance. This can result in assessments that fit preconceived notions about which stakeholders are strategically important rather than the realities of a situation.[22]

The final step in conducting stakeholder analyses involves diffusing the results to those in the HSO/HS who need the information. This step frequently is undervalued in the process and sometimes overlooked. Unless diffusing the results is done effectively, however, it does not matter how well the other steps are performed.

There are two basic ways that information about the external stakeholders of a HSO/HS can be diffused into the organization or system. One is to rely on the power of senior-level managers to dictate diffusion and use of the information. Alternatively, reason can be used to persuade or educate those involved in the HSO's/HS's decision making to use the information. Combinations of power- and reason-based approaches work best.

Diffusion of strategically important information obtained from or about the HSO's/HS's external stakeholders completes the process of stakeholder analysis. Given the vital linkage between HSOs/HSs and external stakeholders such as customers, payers, and regulators, it is unlikely that any organization or system can succeed without an effective process through which its managers listen to the stakeholders and respond to their communication.

Communicating When Things Go Badly

Occasionally, things go badly even in a well-managed HSO/HS. A HSO may lose its accreditation by the Joint Commission on Accreditation of Healthcare Organizations or its state licensure because of fire code violations. A HS may encounter serious financial difficulties, perhaps threatening its continued operation or raising the specter of major layoffs or closure of some of its component HSOs. Serious clinical errors may occur, perhaps causing a patient's death. For example, suppose a diabetic patient being treated in the hospital for complications of that disease dies unexpectedly, and the results of blood tests on a sample taken several hours before the patient's death show insulin levels that are 200 times too high. There are several possible explanations, but few are good. The possibilities include a fatal overdose of insulin given by accident or on purpose in a criminal act committed by any of several people. How should the hospital handle this situation? Whose interests are to be protected? What information is to be communicated? To whom? By whom? There are few hard-and-fast rules to guide managers in communicating under circumstances such as these, either with those within the hospital or with its external stakeholders, although the ethical guidelines described in Chapter 13 are relevant.

When things go wrong, internal and external communications take on greater importance. How managers communicate in such circumstances affects resolution of the problem and the internal and external perception of the HSO/HS after the problem is resolved. Actions taken by HSOs/HSs in response to serious problems and communications about the actions can be characterized along a continuum of reactive to proactive.[23] At one end of the continuum depicted in Figure 17.9, reactive responses include concealing a problem—doing and saying nothing. Less extreme, but

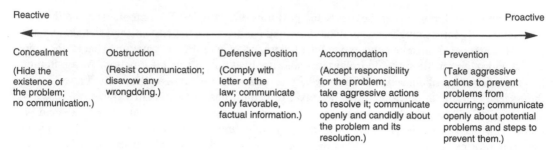

Reactive   Proactive

Concealment	Obstruction	Defensive Position	Accommodation	Prevention
(Hide the existence of the problem; no communication.)	(Resist communication; disavow any wrongdoing.)	(Comply with letter of the law; communicate only favorable, factual information.)	(Accept responsibility for the problem; take aggressive actions to resolve it; communicate openly and candidly about the problem and its resolution.)	(Take aggressive actions to prevent problems from occurring; communicate openly about potential problems and steps to prevent them.)

Figure 17.9.   Continuum of actions and communications to stakeholders in difficult times.

highly reactive, is to admit that a problem may exist, but deny any wrongdoing and take no action to find the cause of the problem or resolve it. Such an obstructionist position could be taken by the HSO/HS regarding further communication about a problem.

A similar reaction is one that is best labeled defensive. The HSO's/HS's managers and spokes-people act and communicate about a problem in a way that complies with the letter of the law. Such actions and communications are intended to minimize legal liability, reflecting in part how expensive liability for serious problems involving human health and life can be. However, some HSOs/HSs take defensive positions with internal and external communications whenever problems arise. They may communicate defensively even when the problems are layoffs, mergers, or closures, problems in which many inside and outside the affected HSO/HS have a legitimate interest.

Figure 17.9 illustrates these reactive responses and two that are more proactive: accommodation and prevention. Accommodation involves accepting responsibility for a problem and aggressively resolving it. Communications are characterized by openness and candor about the problem, its causes, and the actions being taken to resolve it. Prevention is further along the continuum and focuses on taking concerted actions to prevent problems. Continuous quality improvement (see Chapter 9) is an important approach in prevention, as are risk management and performance improvement (see Chapter 10). Communications, as in the case of accommodation, are open and candid, but they focus on the existence and probabilities of potential problems and the steps that have been taken to prevent them.

HSOs/HSs are better served in managing difficult situations by actions and communications that are proactive rather than reactive. Reactive responses (concealment, obstruction, and defensive positions) imply crisis management and invite the scrutiny of those affected by the problem. Technically, managers who choose accommodation are reacting to a problem, too, but their response is positive and proactive in that they take responsibility, actively seek to resolve the problem, and communicate openly and candidly about the problem and their actions regarding it. Prevention involves focused action to avoid problems. Here, managers communicate to interested parties that problems might occur but that actions have been taken to prevent them or minimize their impact. Problems in HSOs/HSs are inevitable, but many can be prevented. Furthermore, the consequences of problems can be managed far more effectively if managers have established a foundation of understanding and trust with those within the HSO/HS as well as with its external stakeholders by communicating about potential problems and about their actions to prevent problems or prepare for them.

SUMMARY

Communication is defined as the creation or exchange of understanding between sender(s) and receiver(s). Communication is not restricted to words; it includes all methods (verbal and nonverbal) through which meaning is conveyed. The communication process is described in Figure 17.1. Particular attention is given to the means of overcoming environmental and personal barriers to effective communication.

Managers in HSOs/HSs must be concerned with two basic types of communication: within the HSO/HS and with external stakeholders. Intraorganizational communication within complex HSOs/HSs depends on formal channels and networks to transmit information and understanding in all directions and on widespread acknowledgment of the existence and effective use of these channels. The channels carry communication multidirectionally—downward, upward, horizontally, and diagonally—and have characteristics that make them useful for the purposes that are illustrated in Figure 17.5. Coexisting with formal intraorganizational communication is an informal flow (the grapevine) that consists of channels and networks that arise from the interpersonal relationships of HSO/HS staff.

Increasingly, senior-level managers in HSOs/HSs are concerned with communication between their organizations and systems and their external stakeholders. HSOs/HSs are interdependent with external stakeholders, and relationships with them must be carefully managed. Effective formal and informal communication that flows to and from these stakeholders is important in successfully managing those relationships. Examples include marketing the HSO's/HS's services, monitoring regulatory changes in government agencies, or lobbying for more favorable reimbursement rates.

DISCUSSION QUESTIONS

1. Draw a model of the communication process. Describe the interrelationships of its parts.
2. Discuss the importance of feedback in communicating.
3. Discuss the various types of communication networks and describe the advantages and disadvantages of each.
4. Discuss the purpose of the downward communication flow in a HSO/HS.
5. Discuss the purpose of the upward communication flow in a HSO/HS.
6. Discuss the role of committees in relation to communication in a HSO/HS.
7. What are barriers to communication? How can they be overcome?
8. Discuss the role of symbols in communication.
9. Think of a situation in which a HSO/HS receives bad press. How might the HSO/HS respond along the reactive–proactive continuum? How should it respond to stakeholders?
10. What are the basic differences between formal and informal communication channels?

CASE STUDY 1: ABC NURSING FACILITY

As the manager in charge of several important projects at the ABC Nursing Facility, Janelle Wilkins has been confronted by some behavior and leadership problems with the project team leader, Emilio Jones, whom she assigned to develop a new staffing plan for the nursing service. Jones has been on the job approximately 3 months, and Wilkins has had several meetings with him. He is leading a team of six people drawn from the nursing facility staff.

In a recent memorandum to Jones, Wilkins said:

Mr. Jones:

You mentioned to me that you have had a difficult time getting the people working on the staffing project I assigned to you to work as a team. You also mentioned that you feel frustrated because I haven't given you enough direction or backed you up in trying to replace two of the team's members.

The purpose of this memorandum is to strongly suggest that you look to yourself as a source of these problems, rather than elsewhere. It is important that you avoid complaining about things that aren't being done for you, and start doing things on your own. Don't always look to others as the source of your problems. Working with people is a difficult challenge.

You have to stand or fall on your own. You cannot expect me to settle all of the problems that arise. You have to develop confidence in yourself and learn to work with the people on the team you are leading. If your problems persist, it will be necessary to replace you.

QUESTIONS

1. What was communicated in the memorandum?
2. What effect will the memorandum have?
3. How else might Wilkins have communicated with Jones?

CASE STUDY 2: THE BUSINESS OFFICE

At 4:45 P.M. on Friday, Mary Hite, an employee in the business office, walked into the office of Henry Staffs, business office manager, and asked to talk with him privately. Hite told Staffs that she had been elected by the other employees of the business office to speak on their behalf about practices that they wished would be modified or eliminated. One practice concerned employee evaluations, which they thought were unfair, poorly executed, and used as an excuse for not paying higher salaries. A second practice not accepted well was the arbitrary way in which management determined employee vacation schedules. Hite said that one employee was given 2 days' notice before he had to take his first week of vacation and 5 days' notice before his second week. Staffs listened attentively and told Hite that, because it was so late in the day, he would consider these requests the first part of next week. During the following week, Hite noticed that Staffs was out of town and that no action was taken concerning her remarks. Her fellow employees tended to treat her like a heroine for representing them before Staffs.

When she picked up her check the next Friday afternoon, Hite was shocked to find a discharge notice and 2 weeks' severance pay in the envelope.

QUESTIONS

1. What should Staffs have done when Hite came to see him?
2. What messages did Staffs communicate to Hite and the other employees?
3. What will be the outcome of the action he took?
4. Is there any way that Staffs can improve communication in the business office?

CASE STUDY 3: GOOD WORK IS EXPECTED[24]

A 600-bed general acute hospital, located in a large city in the eastern United States, brought in an outside management consulting firm to analyze its operations. After 5 weeks, the consultants reported to management. One area that they investigated was communication between superiors and subordinates. To its dismay, management learned that there were numerous discrepancies between what superiors said and did and what their subordinates said their superiors said and did. For example, when the consultants conducted a confidential questionnaire survey with 20% of managers and workers, they received the following responses to the question, "Do you tell your subordinates when they do a good job?"

	Top management says of itself	Middle management says of top management	Middle management says of itself	Lower-level management says of middle management	Lower-level management says of itself	Workers say of lower-level management
Always	93%	82%	95%	63%	98%	39%
Often	7	14	5	15	2	23
Sometimes		4		12		18
Seldom				6		11
Never				4		9

Management was quite upset by the findings. As a result, at the next meeting of the governing body, the president proposed that the hospital bring back the consultants to advise them about how to deal with this problem. The proposal was accepted unanimously.

When middle- and lower-level managers learned of this action, they expressed surprise. One noted, "Just because the data indicate poor communication, there is no need to get excited. After all, workers say lots of things that aren't accurate." Another explained, "Look, I expect subordinates to do a good job. I only tell them when they are doing a poor one. If I praised them every time they did something right, they'd all have swelled heads. My approach is to say nothing."

QUESTIONS

1. What do the responses to the question, "Do you tell your subordinates when they do a good job?" indicate?
2. What do you think of the comments from the two managers? Are they valid?
3. What types of recommendations would you expect from the consultants? Explain.

CASE STUDY 4: GROUP HEALTH COOPERATIVE OF PUGET SOUND'S HARD ROCK SELL[25]

The Puget Sound Group Health Cooperative in Seattle, Washington, one of the oldest and most respected HMOs, wanted to increase enrollment of young, low-risk subscribers. It was only logical when the newly recruited marketing staff chose the local hard rock music station as their medium and shaped the message accordingly.

"Hey, are you TIRED OF SICK CARE? How about joining THE HEALTH CARE plan?" rasped the announcer.

Within hours after the advertising spot was first aired, an eruption equivalent to that of Mount St. Helens began in the Seattle medical community. The local medical society was enraged by the implication that doctors not in the HMO made people sick. The cooperative's medical staff was enraged by the degradation of having their services offered on a hard rock station (although one wonders why so many of them were listening to it). There was concern that the spots would upset the cooperative's efforts to recruit private physicians in outlying communities into a partnership with it and thus seriously hamper efforts to open these new markets. The spot was never used again.

QUESTIONS

1. Who were Group Health's stakeholders in this situation?
2. What message was being transmitted to these stakeholders?

3. How should senior management try to communicate with young, low-risk potential subscribers?

CASE STUDY 5: HOW MUCH SHOULD WE SAY?

The executive committee of the governing body and the senior management team of a large eastern HS were meeting to decide how much information to release to the media about the system's financial condition. Following an extensive period of growth and aggressive acquisition of hospitals and physician practices, the HS experienced serious financial difficulties, leading to a Chapter 11 filing (bankruptcy protection).

A key decision linked to the bankruptcy filing had been to separate the HSOs in the system into geographic clusters and include only some in the filing. Other HSOs in the system were not included. The stakeholders of the HS itself and of its various component HSOs were very concerned about the financial condition of the system and its future prospects. Many were interested in exactly how this disastrous situation had come about.

QUESTIONS

1. Draw a stakeholder map of this HS.
2. Discuss the options available for how communication with external stakeholders could be undertaken. Which option would be best?
3. Discuss the effect the relationships that this HS had previously established with its community would have on the HS's communication with this important external stakeholder in this crisis situation.

NOTES

1. Schulz, Rockwell, and Alton C. Johnson. *Management of Hospitals and Health Services: Strategic Issues and Performance,* 3rd ed., 66. St. Louis: Mosby–Year Book, 1990.
2. Blair, John D., and Myron D. Fottler. "Effective Stakeholder Management: Challenges, Opportunities and Strategies." In *Handbook of Health Care Management,* edited by W. Jack Duncan, Peter M. Ginter, and Linda E. Swayne, 20. Malden, MA: Blackwell, 1998.
3. Scott, William G., Terence R. Mitchell, and Philip H. Birnbaum. *Organization Theory: A Structural and Behavioral Analysis,* 4th ed., 3. Homewood, IL: Irwin, 1981.
4. Newstrom, John W., and Keith Davis. *Organizational Behavior: Human Behavior at Work,* 9th ed., 102. New York: McGraw-Hill, 1993.
5. Holt, David H. *Management: Principles and Practices,* 3rd ed., 483. Englewood Cliffs, NJ: Prentice-Hall, 1992.
6. Shortell, Stephen M. *Effective Hospital-Physician Relationships,* 70–92. Chicago: Health Administration Press, 1991.
7. Porter, Michael E. *Competitive Advantage: Creating and Sustaining Superior Performance.* New York: The Free Press, 1985.
8. Robbins, Stephen P., and Mary K. Coulter. *Management,* 6th ed. Englewood Cliffs, NJ: Prentice-Hall, 1998.
9. Luthans, Fred. *Organizational Behavior,* 8th ed. New York: McGraw-Hill, 1997.
10. Scott, William G., Terence R. Mitchell, and Philip H. Birnbaum. *Organization Theory: A Structural and Behavioral Analysis,* 4th ed., 165. Homewood, IL: Irwin, 1981.
11. Newstrom and Davis, *Organizational Behavior,* 441.
12. Newstrom and Davis, *Organizational Behavior,* 444–445.
13. Holt, *Management,* 487.

14. Longest, Beaufort B., Jr. "Interorganizational Linkages in the Health Sector." *Health Care Management Review* 15 (Winter 1990): 17–28.
15. Longest, Beaufort B., Jr. *Health Policymaking in the United States,* 2nd ed., Chapter 1. Chicago: Health Administration Press, 1998.
16. Longest, Beaufort B., Jr. *Seeking Strategic Advantage Through Health Policy Analysis.* Chicago: Health Administration Press, 1997.
17. Friedman, Emily. *The Right Thing,* 228. San Francisco: Jossey-Bass, 1996.
18. Longest, Beaufort B. Jr. "The Civic Roles of Healthcare Organizations." *Health Forum Journal* 41 (September/October 1998): 40–42.
19. Fottler, Myron D., John D. Blair, Carlton J. Whitehead, Michael D. Laus, and Grant T. Savage. "Assessing Key Stakeholders: Who Matters to Hospitals and Why?" *Hospital & Health Services Administration* 34 (Winter 1989): 525–546.
20. Fahey, Liam, and V.K. Narayaman. *Macroenvironmental Analysis for Strategic Management.* St. Paul, MN: West Publishing, 1986; Ginter, Peter M., Linda M. Swayne, and W. Jack Duncan. *Strategic Management of Health Care Organizations,* 3rd ed., 53–58. Malden, MA: Blackwell, 1998; Longest, *Seeking Strategic Advantage,* 63–79.
21. Ginter, Swayne, and Duncan, *Strategic Management,* 60–64.
22. Thomas, James D., and Reuben R. McDaniel, Jr. "Interpreting Strategic Issues. Effects of Strategy and the Information-Processing Structure of Top Management Teams." *Academy of Management Journal* 33 (1990): 288–298.
23. Carroll, Archie B. "A Three-Dimensional Conceptual Model of Corporate Performance." *Academy of Management Review* 4 (1979): 497–505; Holt, *Management.*
24. Adapted from Hodgetts, Richard M. *Management: Theory, Process and Practice,* 5th ed., 452. Fort Worth, TX: Dryden Press, 1990; reprinted by permission.
25. From Smith, David Barton, and Arnold D. Kaluzny. *The White Labyrinth: A Guide to the Health Care System,* 2nd ed., 115. Ann Arbor, MI: Health Administration Press, 1986; reprinted by permission.

SELECTED BIBLIOGRAPHY

Blair, John D., and Myron D. Fottler. "Effective Stakeholder Management: Challenges, Opportunities and Strategies." In *Handbook of Health Care Management,* edited by W. Jack Duncan, Peter M. Ginter, and Linda E. Swayne, 19–48. Malden, MA: Blackwell, 1998.

Carroll, Archie B. "A Three-dimensional Conceptual Model of Corporate Performance." *Academy of Management Review* 4 (1979): 497–505.

Fottler, Myron D., John D. Blair, Carlton J. Whitehead, Michael D. Laus, and Grant T. Savage. "Assessing Key Stakeholders: Who Matters to Hospitals and Why?" *Hospital & Health Services Administration* 34 (Winter 1989): 525–546.

Ginter, Peter M., Linda M. Swayne, and W. Jack Duncan. *Strategic Management of Health Care Organizations,* 3rd ed. Malden, MA: Blackwell, 1998.

Longest, Beaufort B., Jr. "Interorganizational Linkages in the Health Sector." *Health Care Management Review* 15 (Winter 1990): 17–28.

Longest, Beaufort B., Jr. *Seeking Strategic Advantage Through Health Policy Analysis.* Chicago: Health Administration Press, 1997.

Longest, Beaufort B., Jr. "The Civic Roles of Healthcare Organizations." *Health Forum Journal* 41 (September/October 1998): 40–42.

Longest, Beaufort B., Jr. *Health Policymaking in the United States,* 2nd ed. Chicago: Health Administration Press, 1998.

Luthans, Fred. *Organizational Behavior,* 8th ed. New York: McGraw-Hill, 1997.

Newstrom, John W., and Keith Davis. *Organizational Behavior: Human Behavior at Work,* 9th ed. New York: McGraw-Hill, 1993.

Porter, Michael E. *Competitive Advantage: Creating and Sustaining Superior Performance.* New York: The Free Press, 1985.

Robbins, Stephen P., and Mary K. Coulter. *Management,* 6th ed. Englewood Cliffs, NJ: Prentice-Hall, 1998.

Schulz, Rockwell, and Alton C. Johnson. *Management of Hospitals and Health Services: Strategic Issues and Performance,* 3rd ed. St. Louis: C.V. Mosby, 1990.

Shortell, Stephen M. *Effective Hospital-Physician Relationships.* Chicago: Health Administration Press, 1991.

Smith, David Barton, and Arnold D. Kaluzny. *The White Labyrinth: A Guide to the Health Care System,* 2nd ed. Ann Arbor, MI: Health Administration Press, 1986.

Thomas, James B., and Reuben R. McDaniel, Jr. "Interpreting Strategic Issues: Effects of Strategy and the Information-Processing Structure of Top Management Teams." *Academy of Management Journal* 33 (1990): 288–298.

Author Index

Page references followed by *f* and *t* indicate figures and tables, respectively. References followed by *n* indicate notes.

Subject Index

Page references followed by *f* and *t* indicate figures and tables, respectively. References followed by *n* indicate notes.